FORDNEY'S Medical Insurance

15TH EDITION

FORDNEY'S
Medical Insurance

LINDA M. SMITH, CPC, CPC-I, CEMC, CMBS

Training and Consulting
MedOffice Resources
Greene, New York

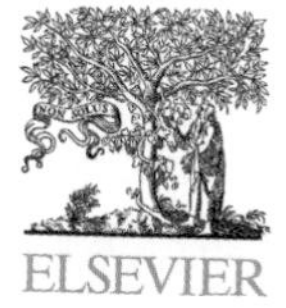

ELSEVIER

ISBN: 978-0-323-59440-0

FORDNEY'S MEDICAL INSURANCE,
FIFTEENTH EDITION

Notices

Practitioners and researchers must always rely on their own experience and knowledge in evaluating and using any information, methods, compounds or experiments described herein. Because of rapid advances in the medical sciences, in particular, independent verifi cation of diagnoses and drug dosages should be made. To the fullest extent of the law, no responsibility is assumed by Elsevier, authors, editors or contributors for any injury and/or damage to persons or property as a matter of products liability, negligence or otherwise, or from any use or operation of any methods, products, instructions, or ideas contained in the material herein.

ISBN: 978-0-323-59440-0

Publishing Director: Kristin Wilhelm
Senior Content Strategist: Linda Woodard
Senior Content Development Manager: Ellen Wurm-Cutter
Senior Content Development Specialist: Maria Broeker
Publishing Services Manager: Deepthi Unni
Senior Project Manager: Kamatchi Madhavan
Project Manager: Haritha Dharmarajan
Designer: Renee Duenow

Printed in Canada

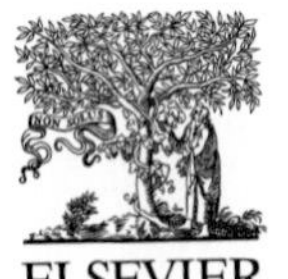

3251 Riverport Lane
St. Louis, Missouri 63043

ABOUT THE AUTHOR

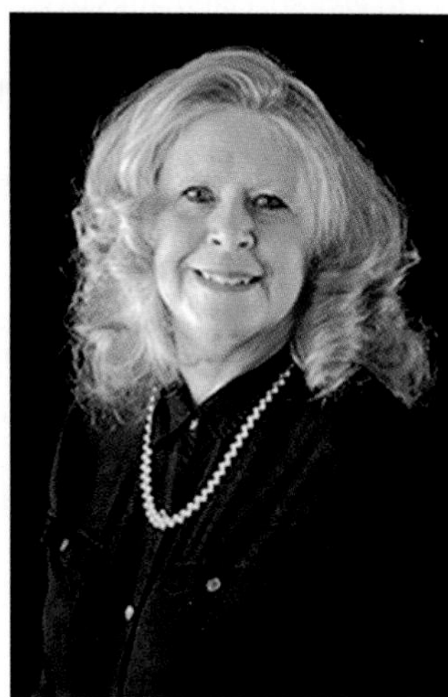

Linda M. Smith has worked in the health care industry for more than 40 years. She started her career as a medical assistant and progressed through health care, spending time in various positions. Throughout that time, the health care industry went through dramatic changes. Health care providers experienced a multitude of billing and reimbursement changes, while also facing the challenges of an ever-increasing focus on regulatory guidelines and compliance. Simultaneously, the need for trained staff and resources to assist with billing, reimbursement, and compliance issues increased, which led her to found her own company, MedOffice Resources, in 2000. MedOffice Resources provides training to health care organizations and to various business and technical schools. She and her associates provide training in the areas of medical ethics, medical terminology, anatomy and physiology, medical coding and billing, and value-based incentive programs. Billing, coding, and auditing services are also offered to health care organizations. Health care facilities, practices, providers and their office staff have been using the services of MedOffice Resources for the past 18 years to strengthen their staff's skills and strengthen their organizations.

Ms. Smith is a certified professional coder (CPC). She has also earned the credentials E/M coding specialist (CEMC) and is an approved professional medical coding curriculum instructor (CPC-I) through the American Academy of Professional Coders (AAPC). She is a frequent presenter at AAPC chapter events in New York State. Additionally, Ms. Smith holds the credential of certified medical billing specialist (CMBS) through the Medical Association of Billers.

Ms. Smith was given the opportunity to work with Marilyn Fordney, the original author of the *Insurance Handbook for the Medical Office.* She worked with Fordney as a contributor to the textbook. After Ms. Fordney's retirement, Smith took on the editor position for the fifteenth edition.

ACKNOWLEDGMENTS

I would like to acknowledge and dedicate this fifteenth edition of the *Insurance Handbook* to Marilyn Fordney, the original author of this textbook. Marilyn published the first edition of the *Insurance Handbook* in 1977 and has followed it through the many changes in our health care industry. It has served as the training tool and building block for so many of us in the field. The publication's longevity speaks for itself.

It was a privilege to have been asked to be a contributor in the thirteenth and fourteenth editions of the *Handbook*, but truly an honor to be asked to follow in Marilyn's footsteps as the primary editor of this fifteenth edition. Marilyn is a remarkable woman with a beautiful heart. Thank you, Marilyn, for all you have contributed to our field.

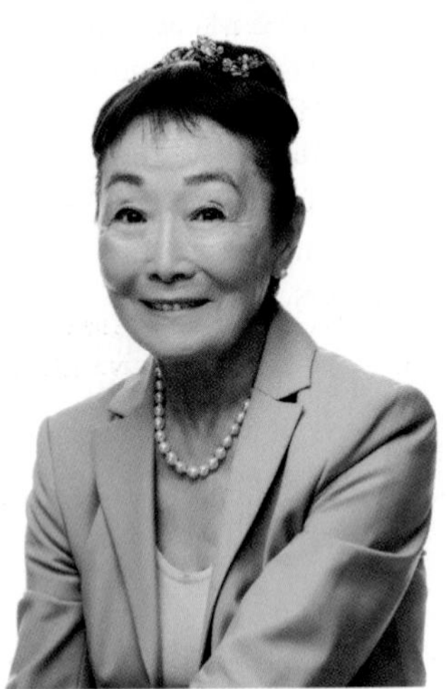

I would also like to give special thanks to Cheryl Fassett, who has been an outstanding contributor in eight chapters of this fifteenth edition. Cheryl's expertise in our field coupled with her outstanding talent and love for writing has made this experience even more enjoyable. Cheryl's work is both remarkable and exemplary.

Thank you to contributors Nanette Sayles and Rachael D'Andrea, who have brought their experience and expertise in facility billing to update the *Insurance Handbook*. Their diligence in meeting deadlines and doing an excellent job is greatly appreciated.

And to the former owner of Practicare Medical Management, Hal Harkavy, a sincere thank you for asking me to join you in your journey into the world of outsourced medical billing. There is so much that you taught me for which I will always be thankful.

Thank you to the many students who have given me the opportunity to share my knowledge of the medical billing and coding field. I can only hope that you will find the passion for it that will provide you with all the opportunities I have had the pleasure of. You have been my motivation and my reward.

I am indebted to many individuals on the staff at Elsevier for encouragement and guidance. I express special appreciation to Maria Broeker, senior content development specialist, and Linda Woodard, senior content strategist, at Elsevier.

And lastly, thank you to my husband, John Wells, and my family who always support and encourage me. You are my reason for everything.

Linda M. Smith, CPC, CPC-I, CEMC, CMBS

CONTRIBUTORS AND REVIEWERS

CONTRIBUTORS

Rachael D'Andrea, MS, RHIA, CPHQ, CDIP, CHTS-TR
Professor, Health Information Management
Lake Sumter State College, Leesburg, Florida
Professor, Health Information Management and Health Care Administration
Charter Oak State College
New Britain, Connecticut

Cheryl Fassett, CPC, CPB, CPPM, CPC-I
Practice Manager
Riverside Associates in Anesthesia, PC
Binghamton, New York

Nanette Sayles, EdD, RHIA, CCS, CHPS, CHDA, CPHI, CPHIMS, FAHIMA
Associate Professor, Health Information Management
East Central College
Union, Missouri

14TH EDITION EDITORIAL REVIEW BOARD

Sandra Alexander, MPA, BAS, CMA (AAMA)
Program Director/Coordinator, El Centro College, Dallas, Texas

Deborah A. Balentine, MEd, RHIA, CCS-P, CHTS-TR
Adjunct Instructor, Truman College, City College of Chicago, Chicago, Illinois

Kimberly, Head, DC
Director of Healthcare Programs, Continuing Education Health Sciences, Collin College, Plano, Texas

Geri Kale-Smith, MS, CMA
Coordinator, Medical Office Programs, Associate Professor, Health Careers Division, Harper College, Palatine, Illinois

Colleen O. Kim, BS
Certified SHIP Counselor, Senior Management Fraud Counselor, Adjunct Professor, Manchester Community College, Manchester, Connecticut

Jennifer K. Lester, RBA, CMAA, CBCS
Certified Allied Health Instructor, Adjunct Instructor, Charleston Jobs Corps Center, Kanawha Valley Community & Technical College, Charleston, West Virginia

Michelle C. Maus, MBA
Program Chair/Assistant Professor of Healthcare Administration, Tiffin University, Tiffin, Ohio

PREVIOUS EDITION REVIEWERS

Pamela Audette, MBA, MT(ASCP), RMA
Assistant Professor and Program Director, Finlandia University, Hancock, Michigan

Megan Baez, CPC, CMA (AAMA)
Medical Coding & Billing Instructor, Everest University, Lakeland, Florida

Kelly Berge, MSHA, CPC, CBCS
Assistant Dean, Online, Berkeley College, Clifton, New Jersey

Ruth Berger, MS, RHIA
Instructor, Health Information Technology, Chippewa Valley Technical College, Eau Claire, Wisconsin

Peggy Black, RN, CCS, AHIMA-Approved ICD-10-CM/PCS Trainer
Medical Coding and Billing Instructor, Winter Park Tech, Winter Park, Florida

Carrie Cosson, CMA (NCCT), RMA (AMT)
Medical Assisting Instructor, Everest University, Lakeland, Florida

Gerard Cronin, DC, CCA
Assistant Professor, Salem Community College, Carneys Point, New Jersey

Brian Edward Dickens, MBA, RMA, CHI
Program Director–MA, Southeastern College, Greenacres, Florida

Jennifer Flippin, CPC
Medical Billing and Coding Program Coordinator, Pinnacle Career Institute, Kansas City, Missouri

Carol Hendrickson, MS Ed, CCS-P
Medical Coding & Health Information Management Instructor, Pasco Hernanado Community College, New Port Richey, Florida

Mary A. Johnson, BA, CPC
Program Manager, Medical Record Coding, Central Carolina Technical College, Sumter, South Carolina

Judith Leonhart, MBA
Instructor, Adult Education, OCM BOCES, Liverpool, New York

Angela MacLeod, MS, RHIA
Medical Coding & Billing Instructor, Certified Medical Assistant Program Director, Gogebic Community College, Ironwood, Michigan

Cassondra Major, MBA
Academic Program Director, Medical, Everest College, Henderson, Nevada

JanMarie C. Malik, MBA, RHIA, CCS-P
Coding, Billing, Reimbursement, and Office Procedures Instructor, Shasta Community College; National University, Redding, California

Laura Melendez, BS, RMA, RT BMO
Allied Health Instructor, Medical Assisting, Southeastern College, Greenacres, Florida

Deborah Newton, MA, PhD
Program Director, Medical Billing/Coding, Great Falls College Montana State University, Great Falls, Montana

Bhamini Patel, BSHIM, CPC, CPC-H
Medical Coding and Billing Instructor, Everest University, Lakeland, Florida

Jeanice Porta, BSEd, CPC, CPC-I
Medical Coding/Billing Instructor, Lee County High Tech Center North, Cape Coral, Florida

Susan Shear, MHA, CPC
Assistant Professor, Medical Information Technology, Bluegrass Community and Technical College, Danville, Kentucky

Tara Shepherd, CMA (AAMA)
Allied Health Director, Apollo Career Center, Lima, Ohio

Phaedra Spartan, RMA, CMAS, BS, MSHA
Healthcare Programs, Director, Medical, Vatterott College, Springfield, Missouri

Mia K. Thompson, MIBC, MAA
Program Director, Everest Institute, Marietta, Georgia

Deanne Ulrich, CPC-A
Instructor, Business, Hawkeye Community College, Waterloo, Iowa

Chris Welch, MBA, CPC, CMC, CEC, CMPE
Medical Insurance Billing and Coding, Program Director, Everest University, Orange Park, Florida

Nancy C. Withee, CPC, CPMA
Program Coordinator, Medical Office Administration and Health Information Technology, Great Bay Community College, Portsmouth, New Hampshire

WELCOME TO THE FIFTEENTH EDITION

Marilyn Fordney first published the *Insurance Handbook* in 1977. At that time, few people were aware of how important the subject of health insurance would become. The *Insurance Handbook* now celebrates its fifteenth year. I am confident that Marilyn Fordney had no idea that her textbook would become the basis of knowledge for so many of us in the field. Marilyn Fordney is a dedicated professional and a forward thinker whose work provided a strong foundation to many of us entering the field. The longevity of this publication speaks for itself, and through the years, Fordney's *Insurance Handbook* has become the leader in its field. The *Handbook* is widely accepted across the nation among educators and working insurance billing specialists and coders.

Because of the ever-changing nature of health care, putting the fifteenth edition together has been challenging and exciting. Because changes occur daily in the insurance industry, the *Insurance Handbook* is revised every 2 years to keep the information current.

PURPOSE

The goals of this textbook are to prepare students to excel as insurance billing specialists and to increase efficiency and streamline administrative procedures for one of the most complex tasks of the physician's business: insurance coding and billing.

Why Is This Book Important to the Profession?

In the past two decades, health care professionals and the community have witnessed the emergence of an administrative medical specialty known variously as insurance billing specialist, medical biller, or reimbursement specialist. Thus the *Handbook* has been written to address the specialty of medical billing as another branch of the administrative medical assistant profession.

As the complexity of the health care field increased, the need for both basic and advanced training have become essential. There are national organizations offering certification in the field, which has quickly become the method of attaining higher recognition for advanced skill levels. The *Handbook* will serve as a training tool to establish a strong foundation of knowledge and will help bridge the learning process into the more advanced levels of expertise. Insurance claims are being submitted for patients on the recommendation of management consultants to control cash flow, obtain correct reimbursement amounts, honor insurance contracts, compete with other medical practices, and maintain a good relationship with patients. Even offices that do not routinely complete insurance claims for patients make exceptions for elderly patients or patients with mental incompetence, illiteracy, diminished eyesight, or a poor command of the English language. When the amount of the bill is hundreds or thousands of dollars or when a surgical report is required, the physician's office should submit the bill to obtain maximum reimbursement. Individuals who administer the federal government's Medicare program increasingly promote electronic transmission of insurance claims for medium-sized and large medical practices. Because of these factors, as well as federal mandates to document care electronically, the amount of knowledge and skills that one must have has substantially increased. This textbook addresses all clerical functions of the insurance billing specialist, and illustrations throughout the text feature generic forms created to help simplify billing procedures.

Who Will Benefit From This Book?

Many colleges are now offering associate degree programs in medical billing and coding. At the same time schools and colleges also offer 1-year certificate programs for those interested in a career as an insurance billing specialist. The student may find programs that offer medical insurance as a full-semester, 18-week course on campus or as a hybrid course (mix of online and face-to-face classroom instruction). Some schools include medical billing and coding as part of a medical assisting program's curriculum, so the individual has knowledge in all administrative functions of a physician's office. The *Insurance Handbook* may be used as a learning tool and resource guide in all of those programs as well as in vocational or commercial training institutes and welfare-to-work programs. The *Insurance Handbook* also serves as a text for in-service training in the private medical office. The *Handbook* may be used for independent home study if no formal classes are available in the community. The layperson who is not pursuing a career in the medical field will find the textbook useful when working with a claims assistance professional or for billing his or her insurance plans. Insurance companies and their agents have found the *Handbook* to be a valuable reference tool when answering clients' questions.

Originally the *Handbook* was designed primarily for students who plan to seek employment in an outpatient setting (such as a physician's office or clinic). To keep pace with the ever-changing health care environment, the fifteenth edition has added a section for billing in the ambulatory surgical center setting. Furthermore, the fifteenth edition of the textbook has been expanded to provide a strong foundation of knowledge to students who may seek employment in the hospital inpatient setting.

Because of the strong base of knowledge that the insurance billing specialist will need to understand the federal guidelines associated with our industry, the fifteenth edition has designated two separate chapters to address them in depth. The student will receive a thorough understanding of compliance issues associated with privacy, security, and the Health Insurance Portability and Accountability Act in Chapter 2 of the textbook. Chapter 3 will provide an in-depth training in the essentials of compliance related to health care fraud and abuse.

Many types of insurance coverage are available in the United States. In Unit 2 of the *Handbook* (Introduction to Health

Insurance), the types most commonly encountered in physicians' offices and clinics have been emphasized in simple, nontechnical explanations and tables.

Over the years, medical documentation and the electronic health record have become essential components of the medical billing process. The insurance billing specialist must be knowledgeable of documentation requirements to assist providers and to ensure compliance in billing. In recent years the federal government targeted this issue with the introduction of Medicare compliance policies related to documentation; such issues are therefore covered to help physicians comply with possible reviews or audits of their billing practices. A strong emphasis has also been placed on the diagnostic and procedural chapters of the textbook. Finally, the *Handbook* may be used as a stand-alone reference source or as an educational tool to increase the knowledge of someone currently working as an insurance billing specialist in any health care setting.

CONTENT

General Features

Each chapter has been updated to reflect current policies and procedures.

- All chapters have been completely restructured for better organization and flow of content, with legal information included where applicable to insurance billing and coding. The information presented is not a substitute for legal advice, and the physician and his or her insurance billing specialist should always seek legal counsel about specific questions of law as they relate to medical practice.
- Compliance Alerts are interspersed throughout all chapters for emphasis.

! COMPLIANCE ALERT

- Objectives are provided at the beginning of each chapter, sequenced to match the technical content, and help to guide instructors in preparing lecture material and inform readers about what material is presented.
- By reviewing the key terms that introduce each chapter, students are alerted to important words for the topic. Key abbreviations follow the key terms; spellouts of the abbreviations are provided in a section that follows the Glossary near the back of the textbook.
- Boxed examples are provided throughout each chapter.
- Key points are presented at the end of each chapter, summarizing and emphasizing the most important technical information in the chapter.

Many experts in the field reviewed the chapters in previous editions so that improvements in content, clarity of topics, and deletions could be considered. The unique color-coded icons have been visually updated and are featured throughout the textbook to denote and clarify information specific to each type of payer. This system makes the learning process more effective by helping students to identify each insurance payer with a specific color and graphic. These icons follow:

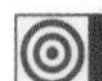
PROPERTY AND CASUALTY CLAIMS

All payer guidelines, including all private insurance companies and all federal and state programs.

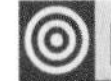
MEDICAID

State Medicaid programs.

MEDICARE

Federal Medicare programs, Medicare/Medicaid, Medicare/Medigap, and Medicare Secondary Payer (MSP).

TRICARE

TRICARE Standard (formerly CHAMPUS), TRICARE Prime, and TRICARE Extra.

CHAMPVA

Civilian Health and Medical Program of the Department of Veterans Affairs.

WORKERS' COMPENSATION

State workers' compensation programs.

MANAGED CARE

All managed care organizations.

MATERNAL AND CHILD HEALTH PROGRAM

State and federal program for children younger than 21 years of age and with special health needs.

Disability Income Insurance

Insurance programs that replace income lost as a result of illness, injury, or disease.

CONSUMER-DIRECTED HEALTH PLANS

Self-directed health plans that often pair a high-deductible preferred provider organization (PPO) plan with a tax-advantaged account.

INDEMNITY HEALTH INSURANCE

Traditional or fee-for-service health plans.

ORGANIZATION

- Chapters 1 through 3 explain the role of the insurance billing specialist and provide them with a thorough understanding of the associated responsibilities. Legislation related to health care and the federal guidelines that affect our industry are laid out for the student. This is coupled with a strong emphasis on the compliance process and their obligation to comply in all situations. Chapters 4 through 10 will provide the student with an introduction into health insurance. These chapters will provide the basics of health care and introduce readers to the various types of insurance carriers they will more than likely need to be familiar with. Thorough, up-to-date information is presented for Medicare, Medicaid, TRICARE, private plans, workers' compensation, managed care plans, disability income insurance, and disability benefit programs.
- Chapters 11 to 13 contain information related to medical documentation and the electronic health record that is critical for the insurance billing specialist to understand. The student will learn and develop diagnostic coding and procedural coding skills. Chapters 14 and 15 will teach students the claims submission process. The textbook offers a unique block by block approach to completion of an insurance claim form.
- A new unit (5) has been added in the fifteenth edition, titled Revenue Cycle Management, and includes Chapters 16 and 17. These chapters focus on the skills necessary to receive payment for health care services. Chapter 16 provides problem solving techniques to use when dealing with insurance carriers. Chapter 17 provides the student with office and insurance collection strategies. Unit 6 of the *Handbook,* which covers facility billing, has been expanded. Chapter 18 is new to the textbook to introduce the student to ambulatory surgical centers (ASCs) and the challenges of billing for this newer type of facility. The chapter outlines the process for billing in the ASC setting. Chapter 19, Hospital Outpatient and Inpatient Billing, is intended especially for those students interested in pursuing a career in the hospital setting. It presents information about the *International Classification of Disease, Tenth Revision, Procedure Classification System* (ICD-10-PCS). Additionally, step-by-step procedures are stated for processing a new patient for admission and to verify insurance benefits. It has been updated to provide the most current issues impacting insurance billing specialists in the hospital setting.
- Chapter 20, "Seeking a Job and Attaining Professional Advancement," provides information pertinent to seeking a position as an insurance billing specialist, a self-employed claims assistance professional, or an electronic claims processor using high-tech procedures. The chapter explains career advancement and certification opportunities for the insurance billing specialist.

ANCILLARIES

Workbook

Users of the *Workbook* that accompanies this edition of the textbook will find the following features:

- Competency-based education is discussed. A point system has been applied to code and claims completion for *Workbook* assignments for instructors who need to document and gather statistics for competency-based education. The worksheets for each assignment are available on the Evolve website. *Textbook* learning objectives, *Workbook* performance objectives for all assignments, use of the tutorial software with reinforcement by *Workbook* assignments, the test section at the end of the *Workbook,* the quizzes of key terms featured on the website, and incorporation of classroom activities and suggestions from the *TEACH Instructor's Resource Manual* (available on the companion Evolve website) provide a complete competency-based educational program.
- Self-assessment quizzes for each chapter are available on the Evolve website for student use.
- Patient records and ledgers have been updated and reworded to correspond with the 2018 procedural codes and ICD-10-CM diagnostic code books.
- All chapters have fill-in-the-blank, multiple-choice, mix-and-match, and true/false review questions. Answers have been put into the *TEACH Instructor's Resource Manual* (available on the companion Evolve website).

General Features

For students, the *Workbook* that accompanies the textbook is a practical approach to learning insurance billing. It progresses from easy to more complex issues within each chapter and advances as new skills are learned and integrated. Chapter outlines serve as a lecture guide. Each chapter has performance objectives for assignments that indicate to students what will be accomplished. Key terms are repeated for quick reference when studying. Key abbreviations followed by blank lines are listed alphabetically so that students can assemble their own reference list for each chapter, thus reinforcing the abbreviations' spellouts. Patients' medical records, financial accounting statements, and encounter forms are presented as they might appear in the physician's files, so that students may learn how to abstract information to complete claim forms properly and accurately. Patient records and ledgers have been completely updated for technical clinical content and reworded to correspond with the 2018 procedural and ICD-10-CM diagnostic code books. Easily removable forms and other sample documents are included in the *Workbook* for completion and to enhance keying skills. Insurance claim forms and letterheads are available on the Evolve website. Some assignments give students hands-on experience in keying insurance claims on the CMS-1500 claim forms using standardized guidelines developed by the National Uniform Claim Committee. Current procedural and diagnostic code exercises are used throughout the *Workbook* to facilitate and enhance coding skills for submitting a claim or posting to a patient's financial account statement. Critical thinking problems are presented in each chapter. Special appendixes are included at the end of the *Workbook.* These include a simulated practice, the College Clinic, with a group of physicians who employ the student. The appendix may be used as reference tools to complete workbook problems. These appendixes include the following:

- Appendix A details information for a simulated practice called *College Clinic.* Information is provided about the group of physicians and a mock fee schedule is included with codes and fees (including Medicare).

Student Software Challenge (Located on Evolve)

The Student Software Challenge ICD-10 located on Evolve is user-friendly software that provides students with another opportunity for hands-on learning. This software simulates a realistic experience by having students gather necessary documents and extract specific information to complete the CMS-1500 insurance claim form. All source documents appear on screen and may be viewed simultaneously in a separate window. The Student Software Challenge also allows users to print the claim form for evaluation and edit it to correct errors.

The main objective is to complete CMS-1500 forms for each case and insert accurate data, including diagnostic and procedural code numbers. Instructors may want their students to work through the first case or basic cases (1 through 4) strictly for learning and to use Case 5 for testing and grading. Cases 6 through 10, which are advanced and insurance specific (for example, Medicare, TRICARE), may be used for practice or testing. This simulated learning methodology makes possible an easier transition from classroom to workplace.

Additional features of the Student Software Challenge for the fifteenth edition of this textbook include the following:

- Blank interactive forms that can be typed into and printed or saved to be turned in to the instructor. This creates clean claims that are easier to read and grade.
- Complete fee schedule to simplify the insertion of fees on the CMS-1500 claim form or financial accounting record.

Other Student Evolve Resources

In addition to the Student Software Challenge, students also have access to an interactive UB-04 form filler and various documents and forms. Also included are insurance cases to accompany SIM Chart for the Medical Office, which is a simulated online EHR.

TEACH Instructor's Resource Manual (Located on Evolve)

The *TEACH Instructor's Resource Manual* is available on the Evolve site; it contains lesson plans, *Workbook* answer keys, a test bank, and PowerPoint slides. This resource allows instructors the flexibility to quickly adapt the textbook for their individual classroom needs and to gauge students' understanding. The *TEACH Instructor's Resource Manual* features the following:

- Guidelines for establishing a medical insurance course
- Answer keys to the *Workbook* and Student Software Challenge assignments and tests with rationales, optional codes, and further explanations for most of the code problems
- Lesson plans for each chapter
- Suggested classroom activities and games
- Ideas on how to use the text as an adjunct to an administrative medical assisting or medical office procedures course
- Pretests for each chapter

Evolve Companion Website

Evolve is an interactive learning environment that works in coordination with the textbook. It provides internet-based course management tools that instructors can use to reinforce and expand on the concepts delivered in class. It can be used for the following:

- To publish the class syllabus, outline, and lecture notes
- To set up "virtual office hours" and e-mail communication
- To share important dates and information through the online class calendar
- To encourage student participation through chat rooms and discussion boards

Evolve also provides online access to free Learning Resources designed specifically to give students the information they need to quickly and successfully learn the topics covered in this textbook. These Learning Resources include the following:

- Self-assessment quizzes to evaluate students' mastery through multiple-choice, true/false, fill-in-the-blank, and matching questions. Instant scoring and feedback are available at the click of a button.
- Technical updates to keep up with changes in government regulations and codes as well as other industry changes.
- SimChart for the Medical Office application cases focused on the Billing and Coding module. SCMO customers can utilize this resource to reinforce practice management and EHR skills.
- Performance Evaluation Checklists.

Elsevier Adaptive Learning (Additional Purchase Required)

Elsevier Adaptive Learning is a uniquely personalized and interactive tool that enables students to learn faster and remember longer. It's fun; it's engaging; and it's constantly tracking student performance and adapting to deliver content precisely when it's needed to ensure information is transformed into lasting knowledge.

- Greater student performance
- Long-term knowledge storage
- Individualized learning
- Cognitive skills training
- Time management Dashboards and reporting
- Mobile app

SUMMARY

The *Handbook* and its ancillaries provide a complete competency-based educational program. *Handbook* learning objectives, *Workbook* performance objectives, assignments, tests, Student Software Challenge, and incorporation of lesson plans and suggested classroom activities from the *TEACH Instructor's Resource Manual* ensure that students know everything they need to succeed in the workforce. Escalating costs of medical care, the effect of technology, and the rapid increase of managed care plans have affected insurance billing procedures and claims processing and have necessitated new legislation for government and state programs. Therefore it is essential that all medical personnel who handle claims continually update their knowledge. This may be accomplished by reading bulletins from state agencies and regional insurance carriers, speaking with insurance representatives, or attending insurance workshops offered at local colleges or local chapters of professional associations, such as those mentioned in Chapters 1 and 20. It is hoped that this textbook will resolve any unclear issues pertaining to current methods and become the framework on which the insurance billing specialist builds new knowledge as understanding and appreciation of the profession are attained.

Linda M. Smith, CPC, CPC-I, CEMC, CMBS
Greene, New York

CONTENTS

FORDNEY'S

Medical Insurance

UNIT 1

Career Role and Responsibilities

1

Role of an Insurance Billing Specialist

Linda M. Smith

OBJECTIVES

After reading this chapter, you should be able to:

1. Identify the background and importance of accurate insurance claims submission, coding, and billing.
2. Assess responsibilities assigned to insurance billing and coding specialists and electronic claims processors.
3. Name and discuss the office procedures performed in a health care organization during a workday that may affect billing.
4. Specify the educational requirements for a job as an insurance billing specialist and a coder.
5. Describe the variety of career advantages open to those trained as insurance billing specialists.
6. List qualifications, attributes, and skills necessary to be an insurance billing specialist.
7. State the personal image to be projected as an insurance billing specialist.
8. Describe professional behavior when working as an insurance billing specialist.
9. Differentiate between professional ethics and medical etiquette.
10. Specify instances when an employer, an employee or an independent contractor can be liable when billing for medical services.
11. Identify common practices and limitations of a claims assistance professional's scope of practice to his or her clients.
12. Explain how insurance knowledge and medical knowledge can be kept current.

KEY TERMS

American Medical Association
cash flow
claims assistance professional
claims examiners
cycle
electronic mail
errors and omissions insurance
ethics
etiquette
facility billing
independent contractor
insurance billing specialist
list service
medical billing representative
professional billing
reimbursement specialist
respondeat superior
revenue
self-pay patient
senior billing representative

KEY ABBREVIATIONS

AMA
ASHD
CAP
e-mail
listserv
MSO
NPP

BACKGROUND OF INSURANCE CLAIMS, CODING, AND BILLING

Welcome to the world of medical billing, an exciting, ever-changing, and fast-growing career field. To help focus on important terms and definitions, some of the basic words in this and subsequent chapters appear in **bold** or *italic* type.

Medical insurance billing specialists' primary goal is to assist in the revenue cycle, both helping the patient to obtain maximum insurance plan benefits and ensuring a cash flow to the health care organization they are employed by. **Revenue** is the total income produced by a medical practice or health care organization, and the **cycle** is the regularly repeating set of events for producing it.

Over the years, medical billing has become very complex. The charge for a baby being born in the late 1960s probably was as little as $250. It was probably a flat fee that covered a 3-day hospital stay and a doctor's fee. The receipt for the birth probably looked like a receipt from a hardware store and contained the name of the patient, the total cost of care, and three options for payment (cash, check, or money order). Today the cost for giving birth can run to more than $37,000 for an uncomplicated delivery and nearly double that for a cesarean delivery. And as the charge for services has increased, so has the complexity of billing for them. There are numerous payers that the billing specialist must be familiar with, each with their own guidelines. The billing is performed using a computer, patient conditions and services must be coded, and there are a variety of methods of reimbursement for the services. It is often difficult for health care organizations to obtain maximum payment for services. The health care industry is one of the most heavily regulated industries in the United States. There are laws that must be followed and many billing and coding guidelines. Physicians and health care organizations rely on professional insurance billing specialists to handle this very complex part of their business. An insurance billing specialist must be knowledgeable of the health care system and all of the components, interrelationships, and interdependencies, such as hospitals, outpatient laboratories, insurance companies, federal government, patients, patient families, other physicians, and co-workers.

Two billing components exist: facility billing and professional billing. **Facility billing** is charging for services done in hospitals, acute care hospitals, skilled nursing or long-term care facilities, rehabilitation centers, or ambulatory surgical centers. **Professional billing** is charging for services performed by physicians or *non-physician practitioners* (**NPPs**). An NPP is a provider of health care services, such as a physician assistant, nurse practitioner, advanced registered nurse practitioner, certified nurse anesthetist, physical therapist, speech therapist, licensed clinical social worker, or certified registered nurse practitioner, who has not obtained a medical degree but is allowed to see patients and prescribe medications. These professionals are sometimes referred to as *physician extenders.* Professional billing is also relevant to other ancillary providers such as ambulance services, radiology and laboratory services, and physical therapists. This textbook will address both facility billing and professional billing. Whether you are employed to perform facility or professional billing functions, the basic setup of a business office encompasses the following units or combined departments: reception of the patient, rendering of medical services, documentation of the services, and financial accounting. You must understand the function of each department in relation to the business office and the health care organization as a whole and how they affect the revenue cycle. The flow of information between departments is one of the most vital components of an organization.

In the health care organization, office procedures performed throughout a workday include the following:

- *Scheduling appointments* involves assigning time slots for patients' visits. Canceling and rescheduling may also be involved. If the time is not properly assigned, there may be an influx or low volume of patients at a given time. Paperwork required for the visit must also be produced. It is important to record why the patient requires a visit.
- *Registering patients* may involve preregistration for visits by using a questionnaire referred to as a *patient registration form.* Financial and personal data are collected and accurately recorded (input) in a timely manner. Incorrect information affects the back-office procedures and submission and payment of claims.
- *Documenting* pertinent clinical notes and assigning a diagnosis and service code to the patient's condition and visit is done by the provider of service. The notes in the patient's health record include the reason for the visit, history, physical examination, diagnostic tests, results, diagnosis, and plan of treatment. The insurance billing specialist may be required to contact the insurance company to obtain authorization for treatment by secondary providers. He or she must also ensure that forms are properly completed, and data are input into the system. Both proper documentation and assignment of the correct code for service affect the revenue cycle.
- Posting (inputting) a *charge entry* for patient care service rendered into the system by the charge entry staff member. The insurance biller must make certain that the insurance is correct in the system and must ensure that the diagnosis coincides with the service rendered. For example, an obstetrics/gynecology visit should not have a diagnosis related to ophthalmology. Many times, individuals have the same names, so billing service dates and the name of the patient seen must be accurate. The charge entry staff member must ensure that the correct charge is assigned to the correct patient. Proper charge entry ensures timely billing and reimbursement.
- *Bookkeeping and accounting* is the posting of payments received (cash, checks, electronic funds transfer, or debit and credit cards) to patients' financial accounts. The bookkeeper or accountant must pay special attention to adjustments, denials, and write-offs. These entries may require investigation for validation. He or she may also receive insurance payer remittance advices and may be assigned to follow up on denials.

ROLE OF THE INSURANCE BILLING SPECIALIST

Several job titles are associated with medical billing personnel. The professional title used may depend on the region within the United States. Some of the most popular titles include insurance billing specialist, electronic claims processor, medical biller, **reimbursement specialist, medical billing representative,** and **senior billing representative.** In large health care organizations it is common to find a billing department made up of many people; within the department, each position is specialized, such as Medicare billing specialist, Medicaid billing specialist, coding specialist, insurance counselor, collection manager, and revenue cycle manager. In this handbook the title *insurance billing specialist* will be used throughout to represent this broad spectrum of titles.

Insurance carriers also employ insurance billing specialists who may serve as **claims examiners.** Claims examiners are also referred to as claims adjustors or claims representatives. Their role is to analyze and process incoming claims, checking them for validity and determining if the services were reasonable and necessary.

Some health care organizations contract with management services organizations (**MSOs**), which perform a variety of business functions, such as accounting, billing, coding, clinical documentation improvement, collections, computer support, compliance oversight, legal advice, marketing, payroll, and management expertise. An insurance billing specialist may find a job working for an MSO as a part of this team.

Individuals called claims assistance professionals (CAPs) work for the consumer. They help patients organize, file, and negotiate health insurance claims of all types; assist the consumer in obtaining maximum benefits; and tell the patient how much to pay the health care organization to make sure there is no overpayment. It is possible for someone who has taken a course on insurance billing to function in this role.

Job Responsibilities

Whether employed by a medical practice, a hospital, or other health care organization as an insurance billing specialist, you should be able to perform any and all duties assigned pertaining to the business office. Front and back office personnel work together to ensure a strong revenue cycle and enhanced reimbursement. Examples of generic job descriptions are shown in Figs. 1.1 and 1.2 to illustrate the job duties, skills, and requirements that might be encountered for various insurance billing and coding positions.

Administrative office duties have gained in importance in the medical billing process. In some health care organizations, an insurance billing specialist may act as an insurance counselor, taking the patient to a private area of the office before being seen by the provider. The insurance counselor will discuss the practice's financial policies and review the patient's insurance coverage. The counselor confirms the deductible or copayment amount and verifies with the insurance company whether any preauthorization, precertification, or second-opinion requirements exist. Insurance counselors help to obtain payment in full when expensive procedures are necessary. Insurance counselors ensure that the health care organization will be paid for services rendered and to develop good communication lines.

Front desk staff are responsible for collecting payment from self-pay patients. Self-pay patients are those who do not have any medical insurance and are liable for the entire bill. Front desk staff are also responsible for collecting any copayments or deductible amounts from the patient at each visit before the patient is treated.

After the patient has been treated, documentation of services should be confirmed as completed. Documentation of services is vital to good patient care and must be done comprehensively for proper reimbursement. A coding specialist may review diagnostic and procedural coding to ensure that the codes are supported in the documentation and that they are correct.

Federal and state insurance programs require the provider of services to submit claims for the patient. Other insurance payers may see claim submission as the patient's obligation; however, most health care organizations submit all claims for patients as a courtesy. The insurance billing specialist must submit insurance claims promptly, ideally within 1 to 5 business days, to ensure continuous cash flow. Cash flow is the amount of actual money generated and available for use by the health care organization within a given period. Without money coming in, overhead expenses cannot be met and an organization will face financial difficulties.

In some organizations the insurance biller may act as a collection manager, who answers routine inquiries related to account balances and insurance submission dates; assists patients in setting up a payment schedule that is within their budget; follows up on delinquent accounts; and traces denied, "adjusted," or unpaid claims (Fig. 1.3).

Having large accounts receivables (total amount of money owed for health care services rendered) in a health care organization is often a direct result of failure to verify insurance plan benefits, obtain authorization or precertification, or collect copayments and deductibles or inadequate claims filing. The rush to get a claim "out the door" cannot be justified when an organization has thousands or millions of dollars in unpaid or denied claims. Accounts receivables will be low and revenue high if the organization takes the extra time to ensure that the claim is 100% accurate, complete, and verified.

Educational and Training Requirements

A high school diploma or equivalent and previous experience in a health care setting may not always be enough for positions as an insurance billing specialist. Typically a postsecondary certificate or an associate's degree is required to enter the field. Postsecondary certificates and associate's degree programs usually include courses in medical terminology, anatomy and physiology, insurance claims completion, procedural and diagnostic coding, health care reimbursement methods, ethics and medicolegal knowledge, computer skills, and general office skills. Completion of an accredited program for coding certification or an accredited health information technology program is necessary for a job as a coder.

The curriculum that might be offered in a 1-year certificate program for a medical insurance specialist is shown in Fig. 1.4. Courses in your locale are labeled with different titles and time frames; the information in Fig. 1.4 is specifically from a community college in Pennsylvania. A 2-year educational course can result in obtaining an associate's degree. Many accredited programs include an externship, which is a training program with private businesses that gives students brief practical experience in their field of study. It is usually short term but allows the student to gain firsthand insight into the field.

Experience and a moderate to high degree of knowledge of the health insurance business are necessary if your goal is to become a self-employed insurance billing specialist or CAP. In addition to insurance terminology, claims procedures, and coding, you must know commercial insurance payers' requirements as well as Medicare and state Medicaid policies and regulations. You also need proficiency in running a business, including marketing and sales expertise.

To reach a professional level of billing or coding expertise, certification is available from many national associations, depending on the type of certification desired. Refer to Chapter 20 for more information on this topic.

Career Advantages

According to the US Bureau of Labor Statistics, employment in the field is expected to grow faster than jobs in other

GENERIC JOB DESCRIPTION FOR ENTRY LEVEL INSURANCE BILLING SPECIALIST

Knowledge, skills, and abilities:
1. Minimum education level consists of certificate from 1-year insurance billing course, associate degree, or equivalent in work experience and continuing education.
2. Knowledge of basic medical terminology, anatomy and physiology, diseases, surgeries, medical specialties, and insurance terminology.
3. Ability to operate computer, printer, photocopy, and calculator equipment.
4. Written and oral communication skills including grammar, punctuation, and style.
5. Ability and knowledge to use procedure code books.
6. Ability and knowledge to use diagnostic code books.
7. Knowledge and skill of data entry.
8. Ability to work independently.
9. Certified Procedural Coder (CPC) or Certified Coding Specialist (CCS) status preferred.

Working conditions:
Medical office setting. Sufficient lighting.

Physical demands:
Prolonged sitting, standing, and walking. Use of word processor or computer equipment. Some stooping, reaching, climbing, and bending. Occasional lifting of ______ lbs to a height of 5 feet. Hearing and speech capabilities necessary to communicate with patients and staff in person and on telephone. Vision capable of viewing computer monitors, calculators, charts, forms, text, and numbers for prolonged periods.

Salary:
Employer would list range of remuneration for the position.

Job responsibilities:	**Performance standards:**
1. Abstracts health information from patient records.	1.1 Uses knowledge of medical terminology, anatomy and physiology, diseases, surgeries, and medical specialties. 1.2 Consults reference materials to clarify meanings of words. 1.3 Meets accuracy and production requirements adopted by employer. 1.4 Verifies with physician any vague information for accuracy.
2. Exhibits an understanding of ethical and medicolegal responsibilities related to insurance billing programs.	2.1 Observes policies and procedures related to federal privacy regulations, health records, release of information, retention of records, and statute of limitations for claim submission. 2.2 Meets standards of professional etiquette and ethical conduct. 2.3 Recognizes and reports problems involving fraud, abuse, embezzlement, and forgery to appropriate individuals.

Fig. 1.1 Generic job description for an insurance billing specialist.

Continued

3. Operates computer to transmit insurance claims.	3.1 Operates equipment skillfully and efficiently. 3.2 Evaluates condition of equipment and reports need for repair or replacement.
4. Follows employer's policies and procedures.	4.1 Punctual work attendance and is dependable. 4.2 Answers routine inquiries related to account balances and dates insurance forms submitted.
5. Transmits insurance claims accurately.	5.1 Updates insurance registration and account information. 5.2 Processes payments and posts to accounts accurately. 5.3 Handles correspondence related to insurance claims. 5.4 Reviews encounter forms for accuracy before submission to data entry. 5.5 Inserts data for generating insurance claims accurately. 5.6 Codes procedures and diagnoses accurately. 5.7 Telephones third-party payers with regard to delinquent claims. 5.8 Traces insurance claims. 5.9 Files appeals for denied claims. 5.10 Documents registration data from patients accurately. 5.11 Maintains separate insurance files.
6. Enhances knowledge and skills to keep up to date.	6.1 Attends continuing education activities. 6.2 Obtains current knowledge applicable to state and federal programs as they relate to insurance claim submission. 6.3 Keeps abreast and maintains files of current changes in coding requirements from Medicare, Medicaid, and other third-party payers. 6.4 Assists with updating fee schedules and encounter forms with current codes. 6.5 Assists in the research of proper coding techniques to maximize reimbursement.
7. Employs interpersonal expertise to provide good working relationships with patients, employer, employees, and third-party payers.	7.1 Works with employer and employees cooperatively as a team. 7.2 Communicates effectively with patients and third-party payers regarding payment policies and financial obligations. 7.3 Executes job assignments with diligence and skill. 7.4 Assists staff with coding and reimbursement problems. 7.5 Assists other employees when needed. 7.6 Assists with giving fee estimates to patients when necessary.

Fig. 1.1, cont'd.

GENERIC JOB DESCRIPTION FOR AN ELECTRONIC CLAIMS PROCESSOR

Knowledge, skills, and abilities:
1. Minimum education level consists of certificate from 1-year insurance billing course, associate degree, or equivalent in work experience and continuing education.
2. Knowledge of basic medical terminology, anatomy and physiology, diseases, surgeries, medical specialties, and insurance terminology.
3. Ability to operate computer and printer, as well as photocopy and calculator equipment.
4. Written and oral communication skills including grammar, punctuation, and style.
5. Ability and knowledge to use procedure code books.
6. Ability and knowledge to use diagnostic code books.
7. Knowledge and skill of data entry.
8. Ability to work independently.
9. Certified Electronic Claims Processor (CECP) status preferred.

Working conditions:
Medical office setting. Sufficient lighting.

Physical demands:
Prolonged sitting, standing, and walking. Use of computer equipment. Some stooping, reaching, climbing, and bending. Occasional lifting of _____ lbs to a height of 5 feet. Hearing and speech capabilities necessary to communicate with patients and staff in person and on telephone. Vision capabilities necessary to view computer monitors, calculators, charts, forms, text, and numbers for prolonged periods.

Salary:
Employer would list range of remuneration for the position.

Job responsibilities:	**Performance standards:**
1. Acts as a link between the medical provider or facility and third-party payers.	1.1 Uses knowledge of medical terminology, anatomy and physiology, diseases, surgeries, and medical specialties. 1.2 Understands computer applications and equipment required to convert and transmit patient billing data electronically. 1.3 Consults reference materials to clarify meanings of words. 1.4 Meets accuracy and production requirements adopted by employer. 1.5 Verifies with physician any vague information for accuracy. 1.6 Reduces volume of paperwork and variety of claim forms providers need to submit claims for payment.
2. Converts patient billing data into electronically readable formats.	2.1 Inputs data and transmits insurance claims accurately, either directly or through a clearinghouse. 2.2 Answers routine inquiries related to account balances and dates insurance data transmitted to third-party payers.

Fig. 1.2 Generic job description for an electronic claims processor.

Continued

	2.3 Updates and maintains software applications with requirements of clearinghouses and third-party payers.
3. Uses software that eliminates common claim filing errors, provides clean claims to third-party payers, expedites payments to providers or facilities, and follows up on delinquent or denied claims.	3.1 Codes procedures and diagnoses accurately. 3.2 Telephones third-party payers about delinquent claims. 3.3 Traces insurance claims. 3.4 Files appeals for denied claims.
4. Exhibits an understanding of ethical and medicolegal responsibilities related to insurance billing programs and plans.	4.1 Observes policies and procedures related to federal privacy regulations, health records, release of information, retention of records, and statute of limitations for claim submission. 4.2 Meets standards of professional etiquette and ethical conduct. 4.3 Recognizes and reports problems involving fraud, abuse, embezzlement, and forgery to appropriate individuals.
5. Operates computer equipment to complete insurance claims.	5.1 Operates equipment skillfully and efficiently. 5.2 Evaluates condition of equipment and reports need for repair or replacement.
6. Follows employer's policies and procedures.	6.1 Must have punctual work attendance and be dependable.
7. Enhances knowledge and skills to keep up to date.	7.1 Attends continuing education skills activities. 7.2 Obtains current knowledge applicable to state and federal programs as they relate to transmission of insurance claims. 7.3 Keeps abreast and maintains files of current changes in coding requirements from Medicare, Medicaid, and other third-party payers. Assists in the research of proper coding techniques to maximum reimbursement.
8. Employs interpersonal expertise to provide good working relationships with patients, employer, employees, and third-party payers.	8.1 Works with employer and employees cooperatively as a team. 8.2 Communicates effectively with patients and third-party payers regarding payment policies and financial obligations. 8.3 Executes job assignments with diligence and skill. 8.4 Assists staff with coding and reimbursement problems. 8.5 Assists other employees when needed. 8.6 Assists with giving fee estimates to patients when necessary.

Fig. 1.2, cont'd.

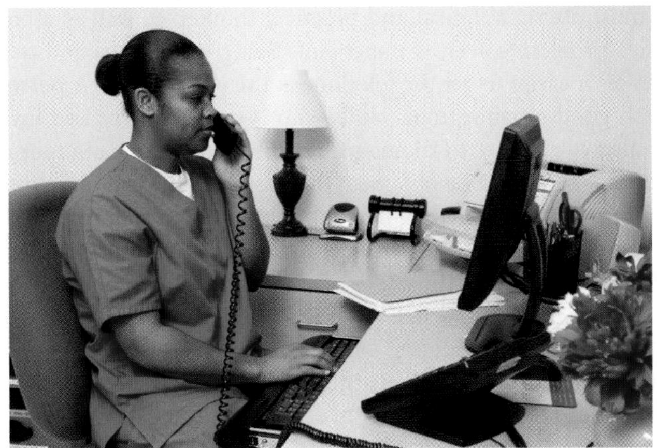

Fig. 1.3 Insurance biller talking to a patient on the telephone about copayment required for an office visit under the patient's insurance plan.

occupations. The demand for health services and related jobs is expected to increase over the next 10 years, as the population ages. Jobs are available in every state, ranging from entry level to management positions. Insurance billing specialists can receive a salary of $8000 part-time to $50,000 full-time or more per year, depending on knowledge, experience, duties, responsibilities, locale, and size of the employing institution. Jobs are available with insurance and managed care companies, medical clearinghouses, ambulatory surgical centers, clinics, hospitals, multispecialty medical groups, and private physicians' practices. Many insurance billing specialists will have the good fortune to advance their careers and move into higher paying positions that come with additional learning, certifications, and experience. These positions may be with consulting firms, instructors at educational facilities, lecturers, or consumer advocates. Other branches of the advanced career field include specialty coding,

MEDICAL INSURANCE SPECIALIST CERTIFICATE PROGRAM

PROGRAM DESCRIPTION: The Medical Insurance program prepares you for employment in the area of medical insurance and health care claims processing. This program also serves the needs of health care personnel interested in upgrading their professional skills. Training in computerized medical billing, CPT-4 and ICD-10-CM coding, and processing medical insurance claims are included in the curriculum. Students may be enrolled on a full-time or part-time basis, and may complete the program by attending either day or evening classes. Accelerated or fast track courses are also available for those wishing to complete this program within a short time period. The program graduates students with marketable skills that are in demand. They are employed in hospitals, insurance companies, private medical laboratories, billing bureaus, and doctors' offices. Graduates may apply credits toward other certificate or associate degree programs.

The following courses are included in this program:

First Semester	
Medical Terminology	3 Credits
Administrative Medical Office Management	4 Credits
Biology	3 Credits
Keyboarding	3 Credits
Computer I	2 Credits
	TOTAL 15 Credits
Second Semester	
Principles and Applications of Medical Insurance	3 Credits
Current Issues of Medical Insurance	3 Credits
Medical Financial Management	3 Credits
Word Processing	3 Credits
Basic Principles of Composition	3 Credits
	TOTAL 15 Credits

Fig. 1.4 Example of a 1-year medical insurance specialist certificate program offered at a community college. Basic coding is taught as a part of the course in Administrative Medical Office Management and advanced coding is covered in Principles and Applications of Medical Insurance. Biology may be titled Anatomy and Physiology in some colleges. (Reprinted with permission from Community College of Allegheny County, Pittsburgh, PA.)

auditing, compliance, and documentation improvement specialists. These advancement opportunities and certifications will be discussed further in Chapter 20.

Self-Employment or Independent Contracting

After gaining experience, many people establish independently owned and self-operated businesses within their communities as medical insurance billing specialists, coders, claim assistance professionals, or collectors. However, the responsibilities are greater in this area because such work demands a full-time commitment, a lot of hard work, long hours to obtain clients, and the need to advertise and market the business. The self-employed insurance billing specialist is responsible for everything: advertising, billing, bookkeeping, and so on. Some billers work from their homes and others rent or lease an office.

Flexible Hours

The nature of medical billing lends itself to flexible hours and flexible job options. The medical insurance billing specialist may want to come in early to transmit electronic claims during off-peak hours or stay late to make collection calls. Many times, medical billing positions have various combinations of work flexibility such as telecommuting, part-time, contract, and work-at-home opportunities. There is an increase in the number of employers who will provide a work-at-home option to highly competent billers and coders who have proven their technical skills and work ethic. In most cases where working from home is allowed, it will be on a hybrid basis, which allows the employees to complete part of their work from home but be required to spend time in the office as well. The availability of work-from-home jobs vary on a case-by-case basis and depends on the employer's policy. Many employers see this type of arrangement as a way to save time, money, and overhead costs, while building productivity and increasing job satisfaction.

Disabled Workers

A career as an insurance billing specialist or a collector of delinquent accounts can be rewarding for persons with disabilities. The financial management responsibilities and other jobs involving telephone communications are an opportunity for someone who is visually impaired because he or she is usually a good listener when properly and specifically trained. Special equipment, such as a Braille keyboard, magnified computer screen, audible scanner, or digital audio recorder, may be necessary to enhance job performance.

Working independently from a home office may appeal to a physically disabled person when there is no need to commute to the health care organization on a daily basis. Accessing information remotely via the computer is a manageable method for success. However, it is important first to gain experience before trying to establish a work-at-home situation.

Inquire at your local vocational rehabilitation center for training disabled individuals.

Qualifications and Attributes

An individual must have a variety of characteristics or qualities to function well as an insurance billing specialist. Strong critical thinking and reading skills with good comprehension are a must. Being a logical and practical thinker, as well as a creative problem solver, is important. Being meticulous and neat makes it easier to get the job done at the workstation. A person with good organizational skills who is conscientious and loyal is always an asset to the employer. Because a large amount of specific data must be obtained, this work requires an individual who is detail oriented. A person with a curious nature will dig deeper into an issue and not be satisfied with an answer unless the "whys" and "whats" are defined. This also helps one to grow while on the job and not become stagnant. Equally important are time management and social skills. This list is by no means complete; perhaps you can think of additional attributes that might lead to a more successful career.

Skills

A person who completes insurance claims must have many skills. One needs the following skills to be proficient:

- Solid foundation and working knowledge of medical terminology, including anatomy, physiology, disease, and treatment terms, as well as the meanings of abbreviations
  Application: Interpretation of patient's chart notes and code manuals.
  Documented Diagnosis: ASHD.
  Locating the diagnostic code using an abbreviation is difficult; therefore, you must be able to translate it. In this case the abbreviation ASHD must be translated to arteriosclerotic heart disease.
- Expert use of procedural and diagnostic code books and other related resources
  Application: Code manuals, official coding guidelines, and other reference books are used to assign accurate codes for each case billed.
- Precise reading skills
  Application: Differentiate between the technical descriptions of two different but similar procedures.
  Procedure (CPT) Code No. 43352 Esophagostomy (fistulization of esophagus, external; cervical approach)
  Procedure (CPT) Code No. 43020 Esophagotomy (cervical approach, with removal of foreign body)
  Note that the addition of the letter *s* to the surgical procedure in the first part of the example changes the entire procedure.
- Basic mathematics
  Application: Calculate fees and adjustments on the insurance claim forms and enter them into the patient accounts. It is essential that these figures be accurate.
- Knowledge of medicolegal rules and regulations of various insurance programs
  Application: Avoid filing of claims considered fraudulent or abusive because of code selection and program policies. Fraud and abuse will be covered in Chapter 3.
- Knowledge of compliance issues
  Application: Federal privacy, security, and transaction rules in addition to fraud, waste, and abuse.
- Basic keyboarding and computer skills
  Application: Good keyboarding and data entry skills and knowledge of computer programs are essential because the industry increasingly involves practice management software and electronic claims submission.

- Proficiency in accessing information through the internet
  Application: Obtain federal, state, and commercial insurance regulations and current information as needed through the internet. Sign on as a member of a list service (listserv), which is a service run from a website where questions may be posted. Find one composed of working coders to obtain answers on how to code complex, rare, or difficult medical cases.
- Knowledge of billing and collection techniques
  Application: Use latest billing and collection ideas to keep cash flow constant and avoid delinquent accounts.
- Expertise in the legalities of collection on accounts.
  Application: Avoid lawsuits by knowing state and federal collection laws as they apply to medical collection of accounts receivable.
- Ability to generate insurance claims with speed and accuracy
  Application: If you develop your own business as a medical claims and billing specialist, you may be paid according to the amount of paid claims the health care practice is reimbursed. Because you will rely on volume for an income, the more expeditious you become, the more money you earn. Therefore accuracy in selecting the correct codes and data entry and motivation in completing claims also become marketable skills.

Personal Image

To project a professional image, be attentive to apparel and grooming (Fig. 1.5). In a work setting, a uniform may be required, or you might be expected to wear business attire that is conservative and stylish but not trendy. For women, this includes a business suit, dress, or skirt of appropriate length; slacks; sweaters; blouses; and dress shoes. For men, a business suit or dress slacks and jacket, shirt, tie (optional), and dress shoes are appropriate.

When hired, it is important to discuss appropriate dress code with the supervisor. Keep in mind that fragrances can be offensive or cause allergies to some clients and patients; therefore use good judgment. Fingernails should be carefully manicured and appropriate to the dress code. For women, subdued eye makeup is appropriate for day use. Consult the employer for the office policy regarding body piercings and tattoos.

Remember that you are in a professional environment and must present yourself in such a way.

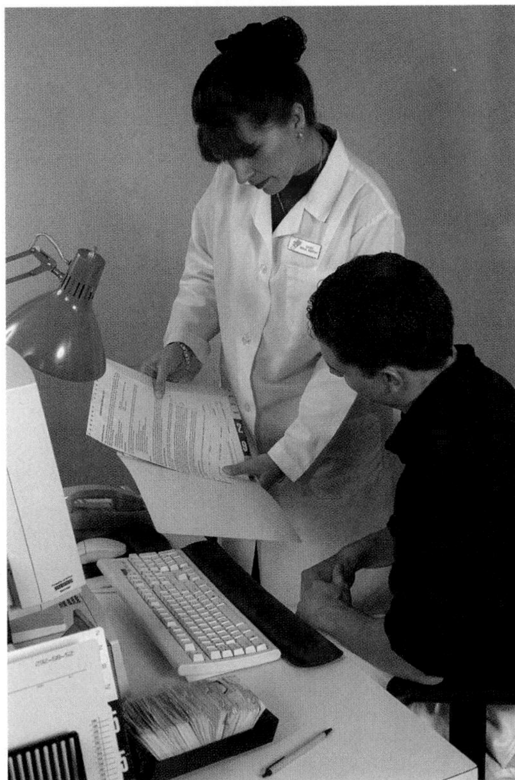

Fig. 1.5 Male and female medical personnel who project a clean, fresh, and professional image.

Behavior

Many aspects make an individual a true professional: getting along with people rates high on the list, as does maintaining confidentiality of patients' health information. An insurance billing specialist depends on many co-workers for information needed to bill claims; therefore it is necessary to be a team player and treat patients and co-workers with courtesy and respect. Consider all co-workers' duties as important because they are part of the team helping you reach the goal of processing the billing and obtaining maximum reimbursement for the patient and physician. Communicate effectively. Be honest, dependable, and on time. Never take part in office gossip or politics. Be willing to do the job and be efficient in how you carry it out.

MEDICAL ETIQUETTE

Before beginning work as an insurance billing specialist, it is wise to have a basic knowledge of medical etiquette as it pertains to the medical profession, the insurance industry, and the medical coder. Medical etiquette has to do with how medical professionals conduct themselves. Customs, courtesy, and manners of the medical profession can be expressed in three simple words: *consideration for others.*

In every business that interacts with customers or clients, the focus begins with good customer service. If you work in an office in which patients go by your desk, acknowledge them with a smile, a nod, or a greeting. Patients may arrive for their appointments ill or injured and suffering from a lot of negativity. If a mistake is made, there is power in an apology given at the first sign of trouble. Attentiveness and a helpful, friendly atmosphere can smooth out the kinks and wrinkles of stressful and negative situations. All people have the need to feel special and they gravitate toward individuals who make them feel that way. All of these personal skills mean good customer service and satisfaction and can lead to professional success for you and the health care organization.

Several points about medical etiquette bear mentioning, as follows:

1. Always connect another health care provider who is calling on the telephone to your provider immediately, asking as few questions as possible.
2. Follow the basic rules of etiquette with co-workers while working in the office, such as acknowledging people who

enter your office or come to your desk by saying, "I'll be with you in a moment."

3. Identify yourself to callers and people you call.
4. Do not use first names until you know it is appropriate to do so.
5. Maintain a professional demeanor and a certain amount of formality when interacting with others. Remember to be courteous and always project a professional image.
6. Observe rules of etiquette when sending e-mail messages and placing or receiving cellphone calls.

Electronic Mail Etiquette

Electronic mail (e-mail) is the transmitting, receiving, storing, and forwarding of text, voice messages, attachments, or images by computer from one person to another. Every computer user subscribing to an online service may establish an e-mail address (Example 1.1).

Because this is a more cost-effective and efficient method of sending a message to someone and obtaining a quicker response, you may be composing, forwarding, and responding via e-mail with staff in other locations, with patients, and with insurance billers (Fig. 1.6). It is important to set some standards to follow when communicating via e-mail. The messages you send are a reflection of your professional image.

EXAMPLE 1.1 Electronic Mail Address

Electronic mail (e-mail) address mason@gmail.com means:
Mason individual user (Mason)

@	at
gmail	site (America Online, an online service provider)
com	type of site (commercial business)

1. Identify yourself and the reason for the message.
2. Compose the message in a clear and concise manner using good grammar and proper spelling. Make sure it cannot be misconstrued.
3. Include a descriptive subject line. If a reply changes the topic, then change the subject line.
4. Do not put confidential information in an e-mail message (e.g., patient-identifiable information).
5. Encrypt (code) all files about patients and e-mail attachments and limit the size of attachments.
6. Recognize that all e-mail is discoverable in legal proceedings, so be careful with content and choice of words.
7. Do not use all capital letters for more than one word.
8. Insert a blank line between paragraphs.
9. Surround URLs (long web addresses) with angle brackets [ ] to avoid problems occurring at the end of a line because of the word wrap feature.
10. Do not use variable text styles (bold or italic) or text colors.
11. Quote sparingly when automatically quoting the original message in replies. Some programs allow you to select some text in the original message by pressing a keyboard shortcut, and only that text will be quoted in the reply. Quotation marks should be inserted to differentiate original and new text.
12. Avoid sending or forwarding junk messages (e.g., welcome messages, congratulation messages, jokes, chain messages).
13. Avoid "emoticons," a short sequence of keyboard letters and symbols used to convey emotion, gestures, or expressions (e.g., "smiley" [(; :–)]).
14. Do not respond immediately if a person's e-mail makes you angry or emotional. Put the message aside until the next day and then answer it diplomatically.

Address →	To: apcmonitor@shore.net
Subject Line →	Subj: **anesthesia modifiers**
Date →	Date: Thursday, April 7, 2016
Sender Address →	From: brownm@aol.com
Salutation →	Dear Madam or Sir:
Left → Justified Brief Message With Proper Grammar	Question: Is conscious sedation considered anesthesia in relationship to modifier -73 and -74? A speaker at a recent conference said "yes" but another said it had not yet been clarified by CMS. Our fiscal intermediary manual has an example that said modifier -52 would be used in conjunction with a colonoscopy with conscious sedation. What is correct?
Complimentary Closing →	Sincerely,
Signature Line →	Mary Brown
Title →	Insurance Billing Specialist
Location →	Smith Medical Center
E-mail address →	brownm@aol.com
Confidentiality Statement →	IMPORTANT WARNING: This e-mail (and any attachments) is only intended for the use of the person or entity to which it is addressed, and may contain information that is privileged and confidential. You, the recipient, are obligated to maintain it in a safe, secure and confidential manner. Unauthorized re-disclosure or failure to maintain confidentiality may subject you to federal and state penalties. If you are not the intended recipient, please immediately notify us by return e-mail, and delete this message from your computer.

Fig. 1.6 Electronic mail message sent to *APC's Weekly Monitor* asking a question about the use of modifiers.

15. Do not write anything that is racially or sexually offensive.
16. Insert a short signature at the end of the message that includes your name, affiliation, and e-mail and/or URL address.

PROFESSIONAL ETHICS

Ethics are not laws but standards of conduct generally accepted as moral guides for behavior by which an insurance billing or coding specialist may determine the propriety of his or her conduct in a relationship with patients, the physician, co-workers, the government, and insurance companies. You are entrusted with holding patients' medical information in confidence, collecting money for your health care organization, and being a reliable resource for your co-workers. To act with ethical behavior means carrying out responsibilities with integrity, decency, honesty, competence, consideration, respect, fairness, trust, and courage.

The earliest written code of ethical principles and conduct for the medical profession originated in Babylonia about 2500 B.C. and is called the *Code of Hammurabi.* Then, about the fifth century B.C., Hippocrates, a Greek physician who is known as the "Father of Medicine," conceived the Oath of Hippocrates.

In 1980 the American Medical Association (AMA) adopted a modern code of ethics, called the *Principles of Medical Ethics,* for the benefit of the health professional and to meet the needs of changing times. The Principles of Medical Ethics of the AMA (Box 1.1) guide physicians' standards of conduct for honorable behavior in the practice of medicine.

BOX 1.1 Principles of Medical Ethics of the American Medical Association

Preamble

The medical profession has long subscribed to a body of ethical statements developed primarily for the benefit of the patient.

As a member of the profession, a physician must recognize responsibility not only to patients, but also to society, to other health professionals, and to self. The following principles adopted by the AMA are not laws but standards of conduct that define the essentials of honorable behavior for the physician.

I. A physician shall be dedicated to providing competent medical service with compassion and respect for human dignity.
II. A physician shall deal honestly with patients and colleagues, and strive to expose those physicians deficient in character or competence, or who engage in fraud or deception.
III. A physician shall respect the law and also recognize a responsibility to seek changes in those requirements that are contrary to the best interests of the patient.
IV. A physician shall respect the rights of patients, of colleagues, and of other health professionals, and shall safeguard patient confidences within the constraints of the law.
V. A physician shall continue to study, apply, and advance scientific knowledge; make relevant information available to patients, colleagues, and the public; obtain consultation; and use the talents of other health professionals when indicated.
VI. A physician shall, in the provision of appropriate patient care, except in emergencies, be free to choose whom to serve, with whom to associate, and the environment in which to provide medical services.
VII. A physician shall recognize a responsibility to participate in activities contributing to an improved community.

It is the insurance billing specialist's responsibility to inform administration or his or her immediate supervisor if unethical or possibly illegal billing or coding practices are taking place. Illegal activities are subject to penalties, fines, and/or imprisonment and can result in loss of morale, reputation, and the goodwill of the community.

The following are principles of ethics for the insurance billing specialist:

- Never make critical remarks about a health care organization or provider to a patient or anyone else. Maintain dignity; never belittle patients.
- Notify your supervisor if you discover that a patient may have questionable issues of care, conduct, or treatment with your health care organization or another provider.
- Maintain a dignified, courteous relationship with all persons in the office—patients, staff, and health care providers—as well as with insurance adjusters, pharmaceutical representatives, and others who come into or telephone the office.

Anyone who uses the internet for health-related reasons has a right to expect that organizations that provide health products, services, or information online will uphold ethical principles. The Internet Healthcare Coalition has developed an eHealth Code of Ethics, which is available at its website (www.ihealthcoalition.org).

It is *illegal* to report incorrect information to government-funded programs, such as Medicare, Medicaid, and TRICARE. Federal legislation has been passed on fraud and abuse issues that relate to federal health care programs. However, private insurance payers operate under different laws and it is *unethical but may not be illegal, depending on state laws,* to report incorrect information to private insurance payers. Incorrect information may damage the individual and the integrity of the database, allow reimbursement for services that should be paid by the patient, or deny payment that should be made by the insurance company.

Most professional organizations for insurance billing specialists or coders have established a code of ethics for their members to follow (Fig. 1.7).

In the final analysis, most ethical issues can be reduced to right and wrong with the focus being the moral dictum to do no harm.

SCOPE OF PRACTICE AND LIABILITY

Most health care professions have a well-defined scope of practice that easily draws a boundary on things that professionals can do and things they are not supposed to do. The field of medical billing and coding does not have such a well-defined scope of practice. Instead, professionals in this field are guided by job descriptions, codes of ethics, coding policies, internal compliance policies, insurance carrier policies, and health care regulations. Regardless of whether they are involved in facility or professional billing, they must be aware of their own liability.

Employer Liability

As mentioned, insurance billing specialists can be either self-employed or employed by physicians, clinics, hospitals, or

STANDARDS OF ETHICAL CODING

Coding professionals should:

1. Apply accurate, complete, and consistent coding practices for the production of high-quality healthcare data.
2. Report all healthcare data elements (e.g. diagnosis and procedure codes, present on admission indicator, discharge status) required for external reporting purposes (e.g. reimbursement and other administrative uses, population health, quality and patient safety measurement, and research) completely and accurately, in accordance with regulatory and documentation standards and requirements and applicable official coding conventions, rules, and guidelines.
3. Assign and report only the codes and data that are clearly and consistently supported by health record documentation in accordance with applicable code set and abstraction conventions, rules, and guidelines.
4. Query provider (physician or other qualified healthcare practitioner) for clarification and additional documentation prior to code assignment when there is conflicting, incomplete, or ambiguous information in the health record regarding a significant reportable condition or procedure or other reportable data element dependent on health record documentation (e.g. present on admission indicator).
5. Refuse to change reported codes or the narratives of codes so that meanings are misrepresented.
6. Refuse to participate in or support coding or documentation practices intended to inappropriately increase payment, qualify for insurance policy coverage, or skew data by means that do not comply with federal and state statutes, regulations and official rules and guidelines.
7. Facilitate interdisciplinary collaboration in situations supporting proper coding practices.
8. Advance coding knowledge and practice through continuing education.
9. Refuse to participate in or conceal unethical coding or abstraction practices or procedures.
10. Protect the confidentiality of the health record at all times and refuse to access protected health information not required for coding-related activities (examples of coding-related activities include completion of code assignment, other health record data abstraction, coding audits, and educational purposes).
11. Demonstrate behavior that reflects integrity, shows a commitment to ethical and legal coding practices, and fosters trust in professional activities.

Fig. 1.7 American Health Information Management Association (AHIMA) Codes of Ethics, revised and adopted by AHIMA House of Delegates, 2008. (Copyright © 2008 American Health Information Management Association. All rights reserved.)

ancillary service providers. The health care organization you are employed by is legally responsible for its own conduct and any actions of its employees performed within the context of their employment. This is referred to as *vicarious liability,* also known as ***respondeat superior,*** which literally means "let the master answer." However, this does not mean that an employee cannot be sued or brought to trial. Actions of the insurance biller may have a definite legal ramification on the employer, depending on the situation. For example, if an employee knowingly submits a fraudulent Medicare or Medicaid claim at the direction of the employer and subsequently the business is audited, both the employer and employee can be brought into litigation by the state or federal government. An insurance biller always should check with his or her employer to determine whether he or she is included in the medical professional liability insurance policy, otherwise known as *malpractice insurance.* If not included, he or she could be sued as an individual. It is the health care organization's responsibility to make certain all staff members are protected.

Employee Liability

Billers and coders can be held personally responsible under the law for billing errors and have been listed as defendants in billing-fraud lawsuits. If you knowingly submit a false claim or allow such a claim to be submitted, you can be liable for a civil violation. If you conceal information or fail to disclose it to obtain payment, you can be held liable. If you are not the person preparing a false claim, but you mail or electronically file it, you can be implicated in mail or wire fraud.

If any staff member within a health care organization, or any provider of services asks you as the insurance biller to do something that is the least bit questionable, such as writing off patient balances for certain patients automatically, contact your supervisor and make sure you have a legal document or signed waiver of liability relieving you of the responsibility for such actions. If you notice a problem, it is your responsibility to correct it and to document your actions in writing.

Independent Contractor Liability

Independent contractors are those who may have decided to establish their own self-operated business as a medical insurance billing specialist or coder. These individuals perform services for health care organizations under contract and are not covered under the organization's professional liability insurance.

Independent contractors should purchase **errors and omissions insurance,** which provides protection against loss of money caused by failure through error or unintentional omission on the part of the individual or service involved in any aspect of preparation or submission of an insurance claim. Independent contractors can often purchase errors and omission insurance though professional organizations they may belong to.

Claims Assistant Professional Liability

An individual who works as a CAP acts as an informal representative of patients, helping them to obtain insurance reimbursement. A CAP reviews and analyzes existing or potential policies, renders advice, and offers counseling, recommendations, and information. A CAP may not interpret insurance policies or act as an attorney. The legal ability of a CAP to represent a policyholder is limited. When a claim cannot be resolved after a denied claim has been appealed to the insurance company, the CAP must be careful in rendering an opinion or advising clients that they have a right to pursue legal action. Always check in your state to see whether there is a scope of practice. In some states, a CAP could be acting outside the scope of the law by giving advice to clients on legal issues, even if licensed as an attorney but not practicing law full time. If the client wishes to take legal action, it is his or her responsibility to find a competent attorney specializing in contract law and insurance. In some states, giving an insured client advice on purchase or discontinuance of insurance policies is construed as being an insurance agent.

A number of states require CAPs to be licensed, depending on the services rendered to clients. CAPs who perform only the clerical function of filing health insurance claims do not have to be licensed. Check with your state's department of insurance and insurance commissioner to determine whether you should be licensed.

FUTURE CHALLENGES

As you begin your study to become an insurance billing specialist, remember that you are expected to profitably manage a health care organization's financial affairs or patient accounts; otherwise, you will not be considered qualified for this position. In subsequent chapters, you will learn the valuable information and skills necessary to help you achieve this goal. You will be expected to do the following:

- Know billing regulations for each insurance program and managed care plan in which the health care organization is a participant.
- Know the aspects of compliance rules and regulations.
- State various insurance rules about treatment and referral of patients.
- Become proficient in computer skills and use of various medical software packages.
- Learn electronic billing software and the variances of each payer.
- Develop diagnostic and procedural coding expertise.
- Know how to interpret insurance carrier's remittance advice summary reports, explanation of benefit documents, or both.
- Attain bookkeeping skills necessary to post, interpret, and manage patient accounts.
- Keep current and stay up to date by reading the latest health care industry association publications, participating in e-mail listserv discussions, joining a professional organization for networking, and attending seminars on billing and coding. Train so that you become familiar with other aspects of the health care organization.
- Discover opportunities to advance your career.
- Strive toward becoming certified as an insurance billing specialist and/or coder and, once certified, seek continuing education credits to become recertified.

Becoming an insurance billing specialist is the first step into an exciting career that has endless opportunities. Chapter 20 will provide information into some of the more advanced roles that the billing specialist can work towards and the professional organizations that offer certification.

KEY POINTS

This is a brief chapter review, or summary, of the key issues presented. To further enhance your knowledge of the technical subject matter, review the key terms and key abbreviations for this chapter by locating the meaning for each in the Glossary at the end of this book, which appears in a section before the index.

1. The person who does facility or professional billing has become a proficient specialist known by a number of job titles, such as insurance billing specialist or reimbursement specialist.
2. Individuals who help patients organize and file claims are called *CAPs*.
3. Insurance claims must be promptly submitted to ensure continuous cash flow for a health care organization. If not, overhead expenses cannot be met and the organization will face financial difficulties.
4. Because of the increased technical knowledge that a biller must have, education and training must be more comprehensive and skills must be developed in coding and claims completion. When proficiency is reached, a person can work for a health care organization or may possibly set up his or her own billing service. In this career, jobs can be rewarding for persons with disabilities.
5. Individuals who do billing and complete insurance claims must have many skills, such as knowledge of medical terminology and abbreviations, expert use of procedural and diagnostic code books, precise reading skills, ability to perform basic mathematic calculations, knowledge of medicolegal rules and regulations of various insurance programs, ability to understand and apply compliance issues, basic computer skills (keyboarding and software applications), proficiency in accessing information via the internet, ability to carry out billing and collection techniques, expertise in the legalities of collection on accounts, and ability to generate insurance claims expediently and accurately.
6. Becoming a professional is a gradual process and one must project an appropriate image and develop as a courteous and respectful team player.
7. Etiquette in a medical setting must be adhered to routinely and one must behave ethically at all times.
8. A health care organization that employs an insurance billing specialist is legally responsible for any actions its employees perform within the context of their employment. This is referred to as vicarious liability, also known as *respondeat superior.*
9. Remember, ignorance of the law is not a protection for anyone working in a health care organization, so one must stay up to date and well informed on state and federal statutes.

STUDENT ASSIGNMENT

Read the Introduction in the *Workbook,* which explains how you will be working as an insurance billing specialist during this course.

- Study Chapter 1.
- Answer the fill-in-the-blank, multiple-choice, and true/false questions in the *Workbook* to reinforce the theory learned in this chapter and help prepare for a future test.
- Complete the assignments in the *Workbook* to help develop critical thinking and writing skills. As you proceed through the assignments in the *Workbook,* you will broaden your knowledge of medical terminology and gain an entry-level skill in diagnostic and procedural coding and insurance claim completion.
- Turn to the Glossary at the end of this book for a further understanding of the key terms and key abbreviations used in this chapter.

2

Privacy, Security, and HIPAA

Cheryl Fassett

OBJECTIVES

After reading this chapter, you should be able to:

1. Name the two provisions of the Health Insurance Portability and Accountability Act (HIPAA) that relate most to health care.
2. Explain the difference between *Title I: Health Insurance Reform* and *Title II: Administrative Simplification.*
3. Define and discuss HIPAA roles, relationships, and key terms, including HIPAA in the practice setting.
4. Describe the Privacy Rule under HIPAA.
5. Define and discuss protected health information (PHI).
6. Identify the difference between disclosure and use of PHI and discuss exceptions to HIPAA.
7. Illustrate the difference between privileged and nonprivileged information.
8. Explain patient rights under HIPAA.
9. Explain responsibilities of the health care organization to protect patient rights under HIPAA.
10. State the guidelines for HIPAA privacy compliance.
11. List the three major categories of security safeguards under HIPAA.
12. Discuss the Security Rule and how it relates to coding and billing.
13. Define the provisions of the Health Information Technology for Economic and Clinical Health Act (HITECH Act).
14. Explain the purpose of the HIPAA Omnibus Rule.
15. List consequences of noncompliance with HIPAA and the HITECH Act.
16. Discuss how HIPAA affects all areas of the health care office, including the organization and staff responsibilities in protecting patient rights.
17. Discuss what to expect from a health care organization when it comes to various HIPAA policies and procedures.

KEY TERMS

American Recovery and Reinvestment Act
authorization
authorization form
breach of confidential communication
business associate
clearinghouse
confidential communication
confidentiality
consent
covered entity
designated record sets
disclosure
electronic media
health care organization
The Health Information Technology for Economic and Clinical Health Act
HIPAA Omnibus Rule
incidental use and disclosure
individually identifiable health information
Minimum Necessary Rule
mitigation
National Provider Identifier
nonprivileged information
Notice of Privacy Practices
Patient Protection and Affordable Care Act of 2010
portability
preexisting condition
privacy
privacy officer, privacy official
privileged information
protected health information
psychotherapy notes
security officer
Security Rule
transaction
use

KEY ABBREVIATIONS

ARRA
CMS
DHHS
EIN
ePHI
FBI
FTP
HIPAA
HITECH
HHS
IIHI
NPI
NPP
OCR
OIG
P&P
PHI
PO
PPACA
TPO

HEALTH INSURANCE PORTABILITY AND ACCOUNTABILITY

One of the most important pieces of legislation to have an impact on health care organizations, health care workers, and patients is the Health Insurance Portability and Accountability Act (HIPAA) of 1996, Public Law 104-191. The Act is made up of five titles. Among these five titles, there are two provisions that relate most to health care: *Title I: Health Insurance Reform* and *Title II: Administrative Simplification.* The HIPAA legislation projected long-term benefits that include the following:

- Lowered administrative costs
- Increased accuracy of data
- Increased patient and customer satisfaction
- Reduced revenue cycle time
- Improved financial management

Title I: Health Insurance Reform

The primary purpose of HIPAA *Title I: Health Insurance Reform* is to provide continuous insurance coverage for workers and their dependents when they change or lose jobs. This aspect of HIPAA affects individuals as consumers. Previously, when an employee left or lost a job and changed insurance coverage, coverage was limited for preexisting conditions. A **preexisting condition** is an illness or injury that began prior to when the insurance went into effect. HIPAA now limits the use of preexisting condition exclusions. It also prohibits discrimination for past or present poor health, and guarantees certain individuals the right to purchase new health insurance coverage after losing a job. HIPAA also allows renewal of health insurance coverage regardless of an individual's health condition. It is important to understand, too, what HIPAA Title I does *not* do. HIPAA does not force employers to offer health insurance. It also does not regulate how much insurance companies can charge for premiums.

Title II: Administrative Simplification

HIPAA *Title II: Administrative Simplification* focuses on the health care practice setting and aims to reduce administrative costs and burdens. Standardizing electronic transmissions of billing and payment information reduces the number of forms and methods used in the claims processing cycle. This reduces the effort needed to process paper or nonstandard electronic claims. Additional provisions are meant to ensure the privacy and security of an individual's health data. Title II also focuses on reducing fraud, waste, and abuse in health care by increasing both the funding to combat fraud and abuse and the penalties associated with fraudulent activities.

There are four main parts of HIPAA Title II (Administrative Simplification) that will directly pertain to your work in a health care organization:

- Standard Transactions and Code Sets
- Unique Identifiers
- Privacy and Confidentiality
- Security of Health Transactions

These main parts will be discussed in detail in this chapter.

Defining HIPAA Roles, Relationships, and Key Terms

Department of Health and Human Services

The Department of Health and Human Services (**DHHS** or **HHS**) is the US government's principal agency for protecting the health of all Americans and providing essential human services. HIPAA legislation required the DHHS to establish national standards and identifiers for electronic transactions as well as to implement privacy and security standards. When speaking about HIPAA, *Secretary* refers to the DHHS Secretary or any officer or employee of DHHS who has the authority to oversee HIPAA issues.

Office of E-Health Standards and Services

The Office of E-Health Standards and Services is an office of the Centers for Medicare and Medicaid Services (**CMS**). It enforces the insurance portability and transaction and code set requirements for Medicare and Medicaid programs. **Portability** is defined as an employee's right to maintain health care benefits under a group health plan when leaving a job. When this occurs, the former employee has the option to continue his or her group health plan benefits; however, he or she is responsible for the *total* cost of the benefit.

The Office for Civil Rights

The Office for Civil Rights (**OCR**) enforces privacy and security rules. It is a part of DHHS. The OCR protects our rights under nondiscrimination laws and HIPAA privacy laws. It investigates violations of these rights as well as patient safety issues.

Key HIPAA Terms

Electronic media refers to the mode of electronic transmission, including the following:

- Internet (online mode—wide open)
- Extranet or private network using internet technology to link business parties
- Leased telephone or dial-up telephone lines, including fax modems (speaking over the telephone is not considered an electronic transmission)
- Transmissions that are physically moved from one location to another using removable or digital memory medium such as magnetic tape or disk, optical disk, or digital memory card

Electronic forms of media can include optical disk (compact disk [CD] or DVD), USB flash drive, or file transfer protocol (**FTP**) over the internet. Voice-over-modem faxes, which use a telephone line, are not considered electronic media, although a fax from a computer (for example, using the WinFax program) is considered an electronic medium.

A ***transaction*** refers to the transmission of information between two parties to carry out financial or administrative activities related to health care. These data transmissions include information that completes the insurance claim process and are discussed later in the text.

Under HIPAA, the term ***covered entity*** applies to any health care provider, health care organization, health plan, or clearinghouse that transmits health information in electronic form for any number of transactions.

HIPAA's definition of a health care organization extends to anyone who provides health care services to a patient. In addition to physicians, this includes hospitals, ambulance service providers, clinics, physician's assistants, nurse practitioners, social workers, chiropractors, dentists, nursing homes, pharmacies, and others. A health care clearinghouse is an organization that acts as a go-between for a health care organization and the entity to which health care information is transmitted. It is an independent organization that receives insurance claims from the health care office, performs software edits, and reformats data as needed into proper format. It then sends the claims electronically to various third-party payers.

HIPAA requires the designation of a privacy officer or privacy official (PO) to develop and implement the covered entities' policies and procedures (P&P). The organization's PO may hold another position within the health care organization or may not be an employee of the organization at all. Sometimes the PO is a contracted professional who is available to the health care organization in an advisory capacity or interim compliance officer. This advisory role may be filled by an attorney or other professional with extensive compliance experience.

A business associate is a person or entity that performs certain functions or activities using health care information on behalf of a covered entity. It is considered an extension of the health care organization and is held to the same standards under HIPAA. Covered entities should have a business associate agreement in place with all entities that work with them. These need to specifically outline how the business associate complies with HIPAA legislation. For example, if the health care organization's medical billing is performed by an outside service, the billing service is a business associate of the covered entity (the health care organization). See Boxes 2.1 and 2.2 for additional information on business associates.

HIPAA's federal privacy regulations apply unless the state laws are more stringent regarding privacy, a situation referred to as state preemption. A state law is considered to be more stringent if it does the following:

- Gives an individual greater access to his or her health information
- Prohibits disclosure that would be allowed under HIPAA
- Narrows the duration of an authorization to release information

For example, under HIPAA, a covered entity is required to provide an individual access to the their health records in a timely manner (30 or 60 days with a possible extension) from the time they are requested. Under New York State law, a provider must permit visual inspection within ten days and furnish a copy within a reasonable time. In this situation, New York State law would preempt HIPAA and a provider will have to provide visual inspection at least within a shorter time frame.

State preemption is a complex technical issue. It refers to instances when state law takes precedence over federal law. The PO determines when the need for preemption arises.

Refer to Box 2.1 for titles of additional HIPAA-related terms.

BOX 2.1 Overseers of HIPAA Functions

A covered entity transmits health information in electronic form in connection with a *transaction* covered by HIPAA. The covered entity may be (1) a health plan carrier, such as Blue Cross/Blue Shield; (2) a health care clearinghouse through which claims are submitted; or (3) a health care organization, such as the primary care physician, hospital, or laboratory.

A business associate is a person who, on behalf of the covered entity, performs or assists in the performance of a function or activity involving the use or disclosure of individually identifiable health information (IIHI). These functions include claims processing or administration, data analysis, processing or administration, utilization review, quality assurance, billing, benefit management, practice management, and repricing. For example, if a provider's practice contracts with an outside billing company to manage its claims and accounts receivable, the billing company would be a business associate of the provider (the covered entity).

A health care provider is a person trained and licensed to provide care to a patient and also a place that is licensed to give health care. A provider may work in a hospital, skilled nursing facility, inpatient/outpatient rehabilitation facility, home health agency, hospice program, physician, diagnostic department, outpatient physical or occupational therapy department, or rural clinic or with a home dialysis supplier.

Privacy and security officers oversee the HIPAA-related functions. These individuals may or may not be employees of a particular health care practice. A privacy officer or privacy official (PO) is designated to help the health care organization remain in compliance by setting policies and procedures (P&P) and by training and managing the staff regarding HIPAA and patient rights. The PO is usually the contact person for questions and complaints.

A **security officer** protects the computer and networking systems within the practice and implements protocols such as password assignment, backup procedures, firewalls, virus protection, and contingency planning for emergencies.

BOX 2.2 HIPAA Help

If a health care provider either transmits directly or uses a business associate, such as a billing company or clearinghouse, to send information electronically for any of the transactions listed, the health care provider is a covered entity and must comply with HIPAA.

TRANSACTION AND CODE SET REGULATIONS

HIPAA has been part of a great shift in processing electronic data. HIPAA requires the use of standard code sets to represent health care concepts and procedures. This reduces the number of forms and standardizes the method used to process claims. It allows providers, facilities, and other health care organizations to code and submit claims in the exact same format for every payer, thereby reducing cost and effort. This was not the case before HIPAA; every health plan could require a different format and additional nonstandard information. It made the billing process time consuming and difficult.

The standard code sets required in HIPAA include the following:

- *International Classification of Disease, Ninth Revision, Clinical Modification* (ICD-9-CM), Volumes I to III (replaced in 2016 by ICD-10-CM for diagnostic coding, and ICD-10-PCS for inpatient procedure coding)

- *Current Procedural Terminology* (CPT) for medical procedure coding
- *Healthcare Common Procedure Coding System* (HCPCS) for medical procedures and supply coding
- *Current Dental Terminology* (CDT) for dental procedure coding

HIPAA electronic transaction standards requires all covered entities to use version 5010 ANSI X12. Not only does this ensure that all claims are submitted in the same format, but all payers are then required to communicate payment, denial, and pended claims in the same format as well. These transaction and code set standards created a common language among providers and other health care organizations and payers that increases the efficiency of the claims process. Types of transactions that transmit sensitive data are as follows:

- Claims and encounter information
- Payment and remittance advice
- Claims status
- Eligibility
- Enrollment and disenrollment
- Referrals and authorizations
- Coordination of benefits
- Premium payments

NATIONAL IDENTIFIERS

HIPPA Title II also mandates the creation of a National Identifier system. This assigns unique identifiers to every health care organization, employer, health plan, and patient. While the first two types of identifiers have already been implemented, the health plan identifiers were not officially mandated until the **Patient Protection and Affordable Care Act of 2010 (PPACA)**. Patient identifiers are still in the discussion phase. Proponents claim the use of unique patient identifiers will increase patient safety and help with the digitizing of health care data. Those against it raise concerns over privacy. The purpose of the identifiers is to further standardize electronic transmissions of claim data.

The Internal Revenue Service assigns employer identifier numbers (**EINs**) to employers. Also known as tax identification numbers (TINs), they identify an employer in all electronic transactions from payroll to health plan enrollment.

National Provider Identifiers (NPIs) are used to submit and process health care claims. NPIs are assigned to every provider, group practice, health care facility, pharmacy, and other health care organization. If you submit a claim for a provider in a group practice, both provider's NPI and the group practice's NPI must appear on the claim.

THE PRIVACY RULE: CONFIDENTIALITY AND PROTECTED HEALTH INFORMATION

> *What I may see or hear in the course of the treatment or even outside of the treatment in regard to the life of men, which on no account one must spread abroad, I will keep to myself holding such things shameful to be spoken about.*
>
> ***Hippocrates, 400 B.C.***

The Hippocratic Oath, federal and state regulations, professional standards, and ethics all address patient privacy. For years, health care organizations locked health records in file cabinets and refused to share patient health information. Patients now have specific rights regarding how their health information is used and disclosed because federal and state laws regulate the protection of an individual's privacy. Knowledge of and attention to the rights of patients are important to being compliant in a health care organization. Health care staff are entrusted with private information that can identify a person such as name, date of birth, and social security number. They also have access to private health information and are expected to recognize when certain health information can be used or disclosed.

Health care organizations and their employees can be held accountable for using or disclosing patient health information inappropriately. Following privacy and security procedures prevents the misuse of health information

Current technology allows easy access to health care information. HIPAA imposes new requirements on health care organizations with regards to this. Since computers are essential to the health care organizations, confidential health data is now sent across networks, e-mailed over the internet, and even accessed by hackers. Sometimes few safeguards are taken to protect data and prevent information from being intercepted or lost. With the implementation of standardized electronic transactions of health care information, the use of technology poses new risks for privacy and security. HIPAA addresses these concerns. Regulations now closely govern how the industry handles its electronic activities. The HIPAA **Privacy Rule** establishes national standards to protect individuals' health records and other personal health information. It applies to all covered entities that conduct certain health care transactions electronically.

Key Terms in the Privacy Rule

Privacy, Confidentiality, and Use

Privacy is the condition of being secluded from the presence or view of others. **Confidentiality** is using discretion in keeping secret information. Integrity plays an important part in the health care setting. Health care workers need a solid understanding of HIPAA's basic requirements. An employee must have strong moral principles and must be committed to protecting the privacy and rights of the practice's patients.

Health care organizations and their staff use and disclose health information on a regular basis. Records are also shared between providers in the course of patient care. Information is released to health plans to process claims. ***Use*** means the sharing, application, utilization, examination, or analysis of health information within the organization. For example, when a patient's billing record is accessed to review the claim submission history, the individual's health information is in use. Records are also shared between providers in the course of patient care; information is released to health plans to process claims.

Protected Health Information

Protected health information (PHI) is any information that identifies an individual and describes his or her health

EXAMPLE 2.1 Protected Health Information in a Health Care Organization

Intake forms	Encounter sheets
Laboratory work requests	Physician notes
Physician–patient conversations	Prescriptions
Conversations that refer to patients by name	Insurance claim forms
Physician dictation tapes	X-ray films
Telephone conversations with patients	E-mail messages

status, age, sex, ethnicity, or other demographic characteristics, whether that information is stored or transmitted electronically. It refers to any part of the patient's health information that is transmitted by electronic media, maintained in electronic form or transmitted, or maintained in any other form or medium. See Example 2.1 for examples of PHI. Traditionally, privacy focused on protecting paper health records that held patient's health information, such as laboratory results and radiology reports. HIPAA Privacy Rule expands these protections to apply to PHI. The individual's health information is protected regardless of the type of medium in which it is maintained. This includes paper, the health care organization's computerized practice management and billing system, spoken words, and x-ray films.

Disclosures, Consent, and Authorizations

HIPAA imposes requirements to protect not only disclosure of PHI outside of the organization but also internal uses of health information. PHI may not be used or disclosed without permission from the patient or someone authorized to act on behalf of the patient. However, the rule does allow the use or disclosure of PHI if it is specifically for the purposes of treatment, payment, or health care operations (**TPO**).

Disclosure means the release, transfer, provision of access to, or divulging information to people or entities outside the health care organization. An example of a disclosure is giving information about a patient you are scheduling for a procedure to the health care facility's outpatient surgery center. See Table 2.1 for examples of uses and disclosures of PHI.

Consent is the verbal or written agreement that gives approval to some action, situation, or statement. In health care, a consent is a document that gives health care organizations permission to use or disclose PHI for TPO. Although many health care organizations obtain signed consents from their patients, the Privacy Rule does not require a covered entity to obtain consent for routine uses and disclosures. See Figs. 2.1 to 2.2 for an example of a consent for release of information form.

Treatment includes coordination or management of health care between providers or referral of a patient to another provider. PHI can also be disclosed to obtain reimbursement or payment for services. Other health care operations include performance reviews, audits, and training programs.

In contrast to a consent, the HIPAA Privacy Rule requires a signed **authorization** for any uses and disclosures that are not routine and are not otherwise allowed by the Rule. Authorization is an individual's formal, written permission to use or disclose his or her personally identifiable health information for purposes other than TPO. For example, if you change primary care providers, you will need to sign an authorization to have your health records sent to your new provider. Health care organizations must be careful when obtaining authorizations for marketing, research, and **psychotherapy notes.** The **authorization form** must state if a health care organization receives remuneration for specific marketing or research activities. See Box 2.3, which details the regulations for disclosing the minimum necessary PHI, de-identification of PHI, marketing related to the patient, and fundraising activities related to patients. See Fig. 2.3 for an example of an authorization for release of information.

Individually Identifiable Health Information

Individually identifiable health information (IIHI) is any part of an individual's health information, including demographic information (for example, address or date of birth), collected from the individual by a covered entity. This information relates to the individual's past, present, or future physical or mental health or condition; the provision of health care to the individual; or the past, present, or future payment for the provision of health care. IIHI data identify the individual or establish a reasonable basis to believe that the information can be used to identify the individual. For example, if you as a health care provider are talking to an insurance representative, you will likely give information such as the patient's date of birth and last name. These pieces of information would make it reasonably easy to identify the patient. If a staff member in a health care organization is talking to a pharmaceutical representative about a drug assistance program that covers a new pill for heartburn and says that the organization has a patient living in your town who is indigent and has stomach problems, the staff member is not divulging information that would identify the patient.

Designated Record Set

HIPAA gives an individual the right to access his or her health information in a designated record set maintained by each covered entity and its business associates. **Designated record sets** include health records, billing and claims records, and health plan enrollment records. A designated record set is one that contains information used to make decisions about a patient. A covered entity is not required to provide explanatory notes or create new information in the record set. A patient is not guaranteed access to information that is not part of a designated record set. Some examples of information that a covered entity is not required to release to a patient are peer reviews, patient safety control records, and business planning records. Other information not included in a designated record set are appointment schedules, requests for diagnostic testing, and birth and death records.

Minimum Necessary Rule

Another way that HIPAA restricts access to PHI within an organization is through the **Minimum Necessary Rule.** This requires that the amount of PHI accessed be limited to the minimum amount necessary for a medical staff member

TABLE 2.1 Title II: Administrative Simplification: Uses and Disclosures of Protected Health Information

Permitted Disclosures (No Authorization Required)	What It Means for Your Health Care Organization
Disclose PHI to patient	A health care provider may discuss the patient's own medical condition with him or her. **Doing so does not require signed authorization from the patient.**
Disclose PHI for treatment	Treatment includes speaking with the patient, ordering tests, writing prescriptions, coordinating his or her care, and consulting with another health care provider about the patient. **"Treatment" does not require signed authorization from the patient.**
Disclose PHI for payment	Payment includes obtaining the patient's eligibility or benefits coverage information from the insurance payer, obtaining preapproval for treatment, and billing and managing the claims process. **"Payment" does not require signed authorization from the patient.**
Disclose PHI for health care operations	Do not confuse this with performing surgery. The term *health care operations* refers to the business activities in which your organization participates. Examples include case management, certification, accreditation, medical reviews, and audits to detect fraud and abuse. **"Operations" do not require signed authorization from the patient.**
Disclose PHI for public purposes	PHI may be disclosed for public health purposes, such as reporting a communicable disease, injury, child abuse, domestic violence, judicial and administrative proceedings, law enforcement, coroner or medical examiner, or research purposes, if PHI is "de-identified." This is not an all-inclusive list but **these examples do not require signed authorization from the patient.**
Disclose PHI for workers' compensation	You may disclose PHI as authorized by the laws relating to workers' compensation. Such disclosures to programs that provide benefits for work-related injuries or illness **do not require signed authorization from the patient.**
Disclosures That Require Patient's Opportunity to Agree or Object	**What It Means for Your Health Care Organization**
Disclose PHI to persons involved with the patient	You must provide patients with an opportunity to object to sharing PHI with family, friends, or others involved with their care. The health care provider can use professional judgment when disclosing PHI to a person involved with the patient's care when the patient is not present. **This requires the patient to have the opportunity to agree or object.**
Disclosures (Authorization Required)	**What It Means for Your Health Care Organization**
Disclose psychotherapy notes	Psychotherapy notes may not be disclosed without authorization except for use by the notes' originator (therapist) for treatment. **Signed authorization *is* required.**
Disclose PHI to a child's school for permission to participate in sports	You may not disclose a child's PHI to a school to permit the student's participation in a sports activity. **Signed authorization *is* required.**
Disclose PHI to employer	You may not disclose PHI to a patient's employer unless the information is necessary to comply with OSHA, MSHA, or other state laws. **With certain exceptions, signed authorization *is* required.**
Disclose PHI to insurer	You may not disclose PHI to an insurer for underwriting or eligibility without authorization from the patient (for example, if the patient is trying to obtain a life insurance policy). **Signed authorization *is* required.**
Disclose PHI for fundraising or marketing	If your health care practice does fundraising or marketing, you may not disclose PHI without prior authorization from the patient. **Signed authorization *is* required.**

MSHA, Mine Safety and Health Administration; *OSHA,* Occupational Safety and Health Administration; *PHI,* protected health information.

to do their job. It should only be shared on a need-to-know basis. For example, a coding specialist will need access to the entire patient's health record to code a visit. However, the receptionist for a medical office will most likely not need to see the entire record to schedule an appointment for a patient. The Minimum Necessary Rule applies to business associates as well. If a physician is referring a patient to a prosthetic manufacturer (business associate), he would be violating the minimum necessary rule if he sent the patient's entire health record. The prosthetic manufacturer does not need to know everything the patient was treated for in the past.

Privileged and Nonprivileged Information

When working with health records, all health care staff members are responsible for maintaining the confidentiality of patients' health information. Example 2.1 lists some of the PHI that is typical in a health care organization and that falls under HIPAA compliance regulations.

The patient record and any photographs obtained are confidential documents and require an authorization form signed by the patient to release information (see Figs. 2.1 to 2.4). If the form is a photocopy, it is necessary to state that the patient approves the photocopy or write to the patient and obtain an original signed document.

RELEASE OF MEDICAL INFORMATION

PATIENT INFORMATION

Patient Name ____________________

Address ____________________ Social Security # ____________________

City ____________ State ______ ZIP ____________ Birth date ____/____/____

Phone (Home) ____________ Work ____________

RELEASE FROM:

Name ____________________

Address ____________________

City ____________ State ______ ZIP ______

RELEASE TO:

Name ____________________

Address ____________________

City ____________ State ______ ZIP ______

INFORMATION TO BE RELEASED:

1. GENERAL RELEASE:

___Entire Medical Record (excluding protected information)
___Hospital Records only (specify)____________
___Lab Results only (specify) ____________
___X-ray Reports only (specify) ____________
___Other Records (specify) ____________

2. INFORMATION PROTECTED BY STATE/FEDERAL LAW:
If indicated below, I hereby authorize the disclosure and release of information regarding:

___Drug Abuse Diagnosis/Treatment
___Alcoholism Diagnosis/Treatment
___Mental Health Diagnosis/Treatment
___Sexually Transmitted Disease

PATIENT AUTHORIZATION TO RELEASE INFORMATION:

Authorization is valid for 60 days only from the date of my signature. I reserve the right to revoke this authorization at any time prior to 60 days (except for action that has already been taken) by notifying the medical office in writing.

I understand that my records are protected under HIPAA (Health Insurance Portability and Accountability Act) Standards for Privacy of Individually Identifiable Information (45 CFR Parts 160 and 164) unless otherwise permitted by federal law. Any information released or received shall not be further relayed to any other facility or person without my written authorization. I also understand that such information will not be given, sold, transferred, or in any way relayed to any other person or party not specified above without my further written authorization.

I hereby grant authorization to release the information listed above. I certify that this request has been made voluntarily and that the information given above is accurate to the best of my knowledge.

____________________ ____________
Signature of Patient/Legally Responsible Party Date

____________________ ____________
Witness Signature Date

Fig. 2.1 Consent for release of information form. (Modified from Bonewit-West, K., Hunt, S., & Applegate, E. (2013). *Today's medical assistant: Clinical & administrative procedures* (2nd ed.). St. Louis: Saunders.)

The purpose of the Privacy Rule is to ensure that patients who receive medical treatment can control the manner in which specific information is used and to whom it is disclosed. Confidential communication is a privileged communication that may be disclosed only with the patient's permission. Everything you see, hear, or read about patients remains confidential and does not leave the office. Never talk about patients or data contained in health records where others may overhear. Some employers require employees to sign a confidentiality agreement (Fig. 2.5). Such agreements should be updated periodically to address issues raised by the use of new technologies.

Privileged Information

Privileged information is related to the treatment and progress of the patient. The patient must sign an authorization to release this information or selected facts from the health record. Some states have passed laws allowing certain test results (for example, disclosure of the presence of the human immunodeficiency virus [HIV] or alcohol or substance abuse) and other information to be placed separate from the patient's health record. Some states require a special authorization form is used to release this information.

Nonprivileged Information

Nonprivileged information consists of ordinary facts unrelated to treatment of the patient, including the patient's name, city of residence, and dates of admission or discharge. This information must be protected from unauthorized disclosure under the privacy section of HIPAA. The patient's authorization is not necessary for the purposes of treatment, payment, or health care operations, unless the record is in a specialty health care facility such as an alcohol treatment center or a special service unit of a general hospital such as a psychiatric unit. Professional judgment is required. The information is disclosed on a legitimate need-to-know basis. An attending physician may require complete access to the health record because the information may have some effect on the treatment of the patient. An x-ray technician would not necessarily need to know everything in the record.

Exceptions to HIPAA

Unauthorized release of information is called breach of confidential communication and is considered a HIPAA violation. Violations may lead to substantial fines.

COLLEGE CLINIC
4567 Broad Avenue
Woodland Hills, XY 12345-0001
Phone: 555/486-9002
Fax: 555/487-8976

CONSENT TO THE USE AND DISCLOSURE OF HEALTH INFORMATION

I understand that this organization originates and maintains health records which describe my health history, symptoms, examination, test results, diagnoses, treatment, and any plans for future care or treatment. I understand that this information is used to:

- plan my care and treatment.
- communicate among health professionals who contribute to my care.
- apply my diagnosis and services, procedures, and surgical information to my bill.
- verify services billed by third-party payers.
- assess quality of care and review the competence of health care professionals in routine health care operations.

I further understand that:

- a complete description of information uses and disclosures is included in a *Notice of Information Practices* which has been provided to me.
- I have a right to review the notice prior to signing this consent.
- the organization reserves the right to change their notice and practices.
- any revised notice will be mailed to the address I have provided prior to implementation.
- I have the right to object to the use of my health information for directory purposes.
- I have the right to request restrictions as to how my health information may be used or disclosed to carry out treatment, payment, or health care operations.
- the organization is not required to agree to the restrictions requested.
- I may revoke this consent in writing, except to the extent that the organization has already taken action in reliance thereon.

☐ I request the following restrictions to the use or disclosure of my health information.

____

Date	Notice Effective Date
Signature of Patient or Legal Representative	Witness
Signature	Title
Date ______________	__ Accepted __ Rejected

Fig. 2.2 An example of a consent form used to disclose and use health information for treatment, payment, or health care operations (TPO). This is not required under HIPAA, but you may find that some health care organizations use it. (From Fordney, M. T., French, L. (2003). *Medical insurance billing and coding: a worktext.* Philadelphia: Elsevier.)

Confidentiality between the physician and patient is automatically waived in the following situations:

1. When the patient is a member of a managed care organization (MCO) and the health care organization has signed a contract with the MCO, the MCO has a right to access the health records of their patients, and, for utilization management purposes, the MCO has a right to audit the patient's financial records. Other managed care providers need to know about the patients if they are involved in the care and treatment of members of the MCO.
2. When patients have certain communicable diseases that are highly contagious, state health agencies require providers to report them. This is true even if the patient does not want the information reported.
3. When a medical device breaks or malfunctions, the Food and Drug Administration (FDA) requires health care organizations to report information that will allow it to be advised of the break or malfunction.
4. When a patient is a suspect in a criminal investigation or to assist in locating a missing person, material witness, or suspect, police have the right to request certain information.

BOX 2.3 HIPAA Help

These key terms are addressed in the Notice of Privacy Practices (NPP) that applies to the patient's right to request restrictions on certain uses and disclosures of protected health information (PHI).

- **Minimum necessary.** Privacy regulations require that use or disclosure of only the minimum amount of information necessary to fulfill the intended purpose be permitted. There are some exceptions to this rule. You do not need to limit PHI for disclosures to health care organizations for treatment, the patient, DHHS for investigations of compliance with HIPAA, or as required by law. Minimum Necessary determinations for *uses of PHI* must be made within each organization and reasonable efforts must be made to limit access to only the minimum amount of information needed by staff members. In smaller offices, employees may have multiple job functions. If a medical assistant helps with the patient examination, documents vital signs, and then collects the patient's copayment at the reception area, the assistant will likely access clinical and billing records. Simple procedure and policy (P&P) about appropriate access to PHI may be sufficient to satisfy the Minimum Necessary requirement. Larger organizations may have specific restrictions regarding who should have access to different types of PHI, because staff members tend to have more targeted job roles. Remain knowledgeable about your office's policy regarding Minimum Necessary. If you are strictly scheduling appointments, you may not need access to the clinical record. An x-ray technician will most likely not need to access the patient billing records. Minimum Necessary determinations for *disclosures of PHI* are distinguished by two categories within the Privacy Rule:
  1. For disclosures made on a routine and recurring basis, you may implement policies and procedures, or standard protocols, for what will be disclosed. These disclosures would be common in your practice. Examples may include disclosures for workers' compensation claims or school physical forms.
  2. For other disclosures that would be considered nonroutine, criteria for determining the Minimum Necessary amount of PHI should be established and each request for disclosure should be reviewed on an individual basis. A staff member such as the privacy officer (PO), will likely be assigned to determine this situation when the need arises.

As a general rule, remember that you must limit your requests to access PHI to the Minimum Necessary to accomplish the task for which you will need the information.

- **De-identification of confidential information.** Other requirements relating to uses and disclosures of PHI include health information that does not identify an individual or leaves no reasonable basis to believe that the information can be used to identify an individual. This "de-identified" information is no longer individually identifiable health information (IIHI). Most health care organizations will never need to de-identify patient information and the requirements for de-identifying PHI are lengthy. The regulations give specific directions on how to ensure that all pieces of necessary information are removed to fit the definition. De-identified information is not subject to the privacy regulations because it does not specifically identify an individual.
- **Marketing.** When communicating about a product or service, the goal is to encourage patients to purchase or use the product or service. For example, a dermatologist may advertise for a discount on facial cream when you schedule a dermabrasion treatment. You will not likely be involved in marketing but keep in mind the general rule that PHI (including names and addresses) cannot be used for marketing purposes without the specific authorization of the patient. Sending appointment reminders and general news updates about your organization and the services you provide is not considered marketing and does not require patient authorization.
- **Fundraising.** Again, you will likely not be involved in fundraising activities but HIPAA allows demographic information and dates of care to be used for fundraising purposes without patient authorization. The disclosure of any additional information requires patient authorization. Your organization's Notice of Privacy Practices will state that patients may receive fundraising materials and are given the opportunity to opt out of receiving future solicitations.

5. When the patient's records are subpoenaed or there is a search warrant, the courts have the right to order health care organizations to release patient information.
6. When there is a suspicious death or suspected crime victim, health care organizations must report cases to proper law enforcement authorities.
7. When the physician examines a patient at the request of a third party who is paying the bill, the payer has the right to request information. An example of this would be a workers' compensation carrier requesting an independent medical examination on a patient.
8. When state law requires the release of information to police that is for the good of society, proper authorities are allowed to access certain information. Examples of this would be cases of child abuse, elder abuse, domestic violence, or gunshot wounds.

Patients' Rights

Right to Privacy

All patients have a right to privacy. It is important never to discuss patient information other than with the physician, an insurance company, or an individual who has been authorized by the patient.

Do's and Don'ts of Confidentiality

Don't: Discuss a patient with acquaintances, yours or the patient's.

Don't: Leave patients' records or appointment books exposed on your desk. If confidential documents are on your desk, patients can easily see them as they walk by. Either turn the documents over or lock them in a secure drawer when you leave your desk, even if you are gone for only a few moments.

Don't: Leave a computer screen with patient information visible, even for a moment, if another patient may see the data. If patient information is on your computer, either turn the screen off or save it on disk, lock the disk in a secure place, and clear the information from the screen.

Do: Make sure the person making a telephone inquiry is who they say they are. Use one of the following methods of verification:

- Ask for one or more of the following items: patient's full name, home address, date of birth, Social Security number, mother's maiden name, dates of service.
- Ask for a callback number and compare it with the number on file.

REQUIRED ELEMENTS OF HIPAA AUTHORIZATION

Identification of person (or class) authorized to request

Identification of person (or class) to whom covered entity is to use/disclose

Description of information to be released with specificity to allow entity to know which information the authorization references

Description of each purpose of the requested use or disclosure

Expiration date, time period, or event

Statement that is revocable by written request

Individual's (patient's) signature and date

Statement of representative's authority

Authorization for Release of Information

PATIENT NAME: Levy (LAST) Chloe (FIRST) E. (MI) ______ (MAIDEN OR OTHER NAME)

DATE OF BIRTH: 02 - 12 - 1950 (MO DAY YR) SS# 320 - 21 - 3408 MEDICAL RECORD #: 3075

ADDRESS: 3298 East Main Street CITY: Woodland Hills STATE: XY ZIP: 12345-0001

DAY PHONE: 013-340-9800 EVENING PHONE: 013-549-8708

I hereby authorize Gerald Practon, MD **(Print Name of Provider) to release information from my medical record as indicated below to:**

NAME: Margaret L. Lee, MD

ADDRESS: 328 Seward Street CITY: Anytown STATE: XY ZIP: 45601-0731

PHONE: 013-219-7698 FAX: 013-290-9877

INFORMATION TO BE RELEASED:

	DATES:
☒ History and physical exam	6-8-20XX
❑ Progress notes	
❑ Lab reports	
❑ X-ray reports	
❑ Other: ______	

I specifically authorize the release of information relating to:
- ❑ Substance abuse (including alcohol/drug abuse)
- ❑ Mental health (including psychotherapy notes)
- ❑ HIV related information (AIDS related testing)

X ______

SIGNATURE OF PATIENT OR LEGAL GUARDIAN DATE

PURPOSE OF DISCLOSURE: ❑ Changing physicians ☒ Consultation/second opinion ❑ Continuing care ❑ Legal ❑ School ❑ Insurance ❑ Workers Compensation ❑ Other (please specify): ______

1. I understand that this authorization will expire on 09/01/20XX (Print the Date this Form Expires) days after I have signed the form.
2. I understand that I may revoke this authorization at any time by notifying the providing organization in writing, and it will be effective on the date notified except to the extent action has already been taken in reliance upon it.
3. I understand that information used or disclosed pursuant to this authorization may be subject to redisclosure by the recipient and no longer be protected by Federal privacy regulations.
4. I understand that if I am being requested to release this information by Gerald Practon, MD (Print Name of Provider) for the purpose of: ______
   a. By authorizing this release of information, my health care and payment for my health care will not be affected if I do not sign this form.
   b. I understand I may see and copy the information described on this form if I ask for it, and that I will get a copy of this form after I sign it.
   c. I have been informed that Gerald Practon, MD (Print Name of Provider) will/will not receive financial or in-kind compensation in exchange for using or disclosing the health information described above.
5. I understand that in compliance with XY (Print the State Whose Laws Govern the Provider) statute, I will pay a fee of $ 5.00 (Print the Fee Charged). There is no charge for medical records if copies are sent to facilities for ongoing care or follow up treatment.

Chloe E. Levy 6/1/XX OR ______

SIGNATURE OF PATIENT DATE PARENT/LEGAL GUARDIAN/AUTHORIZED PERSON DATE

RECORDS RECEIVED BY DATE RELATIONSHIP TO PATIENT

FOR OFFICE USE ONLY

DATE REQUEST FILLED ______ BY: ______

IDENTIFICATION PRESENTED ______ FEE COLLECTED $ ______

Fig. 2.3 Completed authorization for release of information form for a patient who is seeking a consult or second opinion. The required elements for HIPAA authorization are indicated. Note: This form is used on a one-time basis for reasons other than treatment, payment, or health care operations (TPO). When the patient arrives at the new physician's office, a consent for TPO form will need to be signed. (From *Federal Register* 64[212]: Appendix to Subpart E of Part 164: Model Authorization Form, November 3, 1999.)

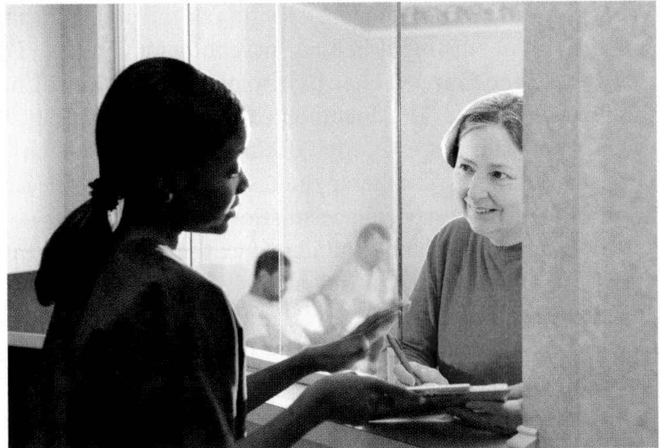

Fig. 2.4 Patient signing a consent form.

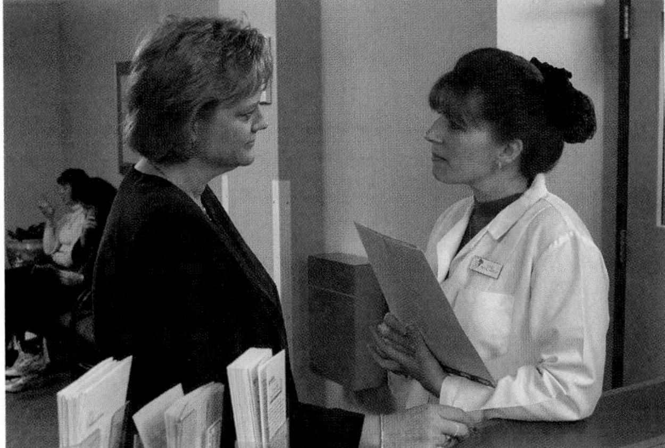

Fig. 2.5 Insurance billing specialist consulting with the supervisor or office manager about office policies regarding release of a patient's health record.

- Ask the patient to fax a sheet with his or her signature on it so that you can compare it with the one on file.
- Some health care facilities may assign a code word or number such as a middle name or date that is easy for patients to remember. If a patient does not know the code word, then ask for personal identifying information as mentioned.

Do: Obtain proper authorization from the patient to release information to another person.

Do: Use care when leaving messages for patients on answering machines or with another person. Leave your name, the office name, and the return telephone number. Never attempt to interpret a report or provide information about the outcome of laboratory or other diagnostic tests to the patient. Let the physician handle it.

Do: Properly dispose of notes, papers, and memos by using a shredding device.

Do: Be careful when using the copying machine, because it is easy to forget to remove the original insurance claim or health record from the document glass.

Do: Use common sense and follow the guidelines mentioned in this chapter to help you maintain your professional credibility and integrity (Fig. 2.5).

Do: Access only the minimum amount of privileged information necessary to complete your job.

Privacy Rules: Patient Rights Under HIPAA

Patients are granted the following six federal rights that allow them to be informed about PHI and to control how their PHI is used and disclosed:

1. *Right to Notice of Privacy Practices (NPP),* a document in plain language that is usually given to the patient at the first visit or at enrollment. The staff must make a reasonable best effort to obtain a signature from the patient acknowledging receipt, and also have it signed by a witness. If the patient cannot or will not sign, this should be documented in the patient's record. The NPP must be posted at every service site and be available in paper form for those who request it. A health care organization's website must have the NPP placed on the site and must deliver a copy electronically on request. A NPP must be in plain language and contain the following information:
   - How the covered entity may use or disclose PHI
   - The patient's rights regarding PHI and how to file a complaint
   - The covered entities legal duties including how it is required by law to maintain the privacy of the PHI
   - Who the patient may contact for further information about the covered entity's privacy policies
2. *Right to request restrictions on certain uses and disclosures of PHI.* Patients have the right to ask for restrictions on how a health care organization uses and discloses PHI for TPO. For example, a patient who had a successfully treated sexually transmitted infection many years ago can request that, whenever possible, this material not be disclosed. A health care organization is not required to agree to these requests but must have a process to review the requests, accept and review any appeal, and give a sound reason for not agreeing to a request. Restrictions must be documented and followed.
3. *Right to request confidential communications* by alternative means or at an alternative location. For example, patients may request a provider call them at work rather than at their home. Patients do not need to explain the reason for the request. The health care office must have a process in place both to evaluate requests and appeals and to respond to the patient. Patients may be required by the office to make their requests in writing. A written document protects the practice's compliance endeavors.
4. *Right to access (inspect and obtain a copy of) PHI.* Privacy regulations allow the health care organization to require that the patient make the request for access in writing. Generally a request must be acted on within 30 days. If the covered entity is unable to respond to the request within 30 days, a one-time 30-day extension may be permitted. If an extension is taken, the health care organization must notify the patient within the initial 30-day period and provide the date that the information will be available. A health care organization may charge a reasonable, cost-based fee for copies of PHI.

BOX 2.4 HIPAA Help

According to the HIPAA Privacy Rule, the term *psychotherapy notes* means notes that are recorded in any medium by a mental health professional. These document or analyze the contents of conversation during a private counseling session or a group, joint, or family counseling session and that are separated from the rest of the individual's health record. Under this rule, a health care professional is not obligated to disclose these notes to third party payers or even to the patient. Some information, such as prescriptions, session start and end times, treatment modalities, and any summary of diagnosis or prognosis, are not considered to be part of the psychotherapy notes. To be safeguarded, psychotherapy notes must be kept separate from the patient's health record.

This may include only the costs for supplies and labor for copying, postage when mailed, and preparing a summary of the PHI if the patient has agreed to this instead of complete access. If a patient requests an electronic copy of his or her information or requests that it be transmitted to another person, the covered entity generally must produce it in the form requested if readily producible. Under HIPAA Privacy Rule, patients do not have the right to access the following:

- Psychotherapy notes (Box 2.4)
- Information compiled in reasonable anticipation of, or for use in, legal proceedings
- Information exempted from disclosure under the Clinical Laboratory Improvements Act (CLIA) (CLIA will be discussed in Chapter 3)

The office may deny patient access for the previously mentioned reasons without giving the patient the right to review the denial. If the health care provider denies access because the patient would be a danger to him- or herself or someone else as a result of accessing the confidential health information, the patient has the right to have the denial reviewed by another licensed professional who did not participate in the initial denial decision.

Psychotherapy notes have special protection under HIPAA. Disclosure of a patient's mental health records requires specific patient permission. This means that when an insurance payer requests the health records to review the claim, a patient authorization is required.

Certain clinical data are excluded from the definition of psychotherapy notes. When an individual is using the services of a mental health professional, not all information gathered and recorded in the health record of the mental health provider is considered part of the psychotherapy notes. The law lists the following specific items that are excluded from such notes:

- Medication prescription and monitoring
- Counseling session start and stop times
- Modalities and frequencies of treatment furnished
- Results of clinical tests
- Any summary of the following items: diagnosis, functional status, treatment plan, symptoms, prognosis, and progress to date

In general, psychotherapy notes are defined as the information that is the recorded (in any manner) documentation and/or analysis of conversation. This information should be kept separate from the medical section of the patient health record to be distinguished as psychotherapy notes. For example, Jane Doe tells her psychologist the details of her childhood trauma. The documented conversation specific to her trauma (for example, what occurred and how she felt) is considered the psychotherapy notes and cannot be released without Jane Doe's specific permission.

It is also important to understand that patients do not have the right to obtain a copy of psychotherapy notes under HIPAA (see Box 2.4). However, the treating mental health provider can decide when a patient may obtain access to this health information.

State law must always be considered. Some states allow patients access to their psychotherapy notes. In these cases, state law would take precedence over HIPAA as a result of the state preemption allowance as described earlier.

5. *Right to request an amendment of PHI.* Patients have the right to request that their PHI be amended. As with other requests, the health care organization may require the request to be in writing. There must be a process to accept and review both the request and any appeal in a timely fashion. The request may be denied for the following circumstances:
   - The provider who is being requested to change the PHI is not the creator of the information. For example, a health care provider cannot amend a record sent by a referring physician.
   - The PHI is believed to be accurate and complete as it stands in the health care organization's health records.
   - The information is not required to be accessible to the patient such as a psychotherapy note.

   Generally, the health care organization must respond to a patient's request for amendment within 60 days. If a request is denied, the patient must be informed in writing of the reason for the denial. The patient must also be given the opportunity to file a statement of disagreement.
6. *Right to receive an accounting of disclosure of PHI.* Health care organizations should maintain a log of all disclosures of PHI, either on paper or within the organization's computer system. The process for providing an accounting should be outlined in the health care organization's policy manual. Patients may request an accounting or tracking of disclosures of their confidential information and are granted the right to receive this accounting once a year without charge. Additional accountings may be assessed a cost-based fee (Boxes 2.5 and 2.6). Items to be documented must include the following:
   - Date of disclosure
   - Name of the entity or person who received the PHI, including their address, if known
   - Brief description of the PHI disclosed
   - Brief statement of the purpose of the disclosure

   Disclosures made for TPO, facility directories, and some national security and law enforcement agencies are not required to be recorded.

   Facility directories are listings of patients within the facility. Under HIPAA, facilities such as hospitals and nursing homes must be careful about releasing information about the patients in their care. Patient directories may list a patient's name,

BOX 2.5 HIPAA Help

In summary, patients have the right to the following:

- Be informed of the organization's privacy practices by receiving a Notice of Privacy Practices (NPP)
- Have their information kept confidential and secure
- Obtain a copy of their health records
- Request to have their health records amended
- Request special considerations in communication
- Restrict unauthorized access to their confidential health information

Patients cannot prevent their confidential health information from being used for treatment, payment, or routine health care operations (TPO), nor may they force amendments to their health record. As you become acclimated to your organization's policies and procedures regarding the handling of protected health information (PHI), you will be better able to recognize that your position plays an important part in HIPAA compliance.

BOX 2.6 HIPAA Help

Health care organizations and staff are not likely to read the *Federal Register* from cover to cover. However, it is important that you are familiar with it. The *Federal Register* is a daily newspaper published by the National Archives and Records Administration. It contains federal regulations, proposed rules, and other important documents. New legislation that affects the health care world will always appear in this publication.

You should be familiar with the general forms used in your practice setting. Be aware of the following:

- **Written acknowledgment.** After providing the patient with the Notice of Privacy Practices (NPP), a "good faith" effort must be made to obtain written acknowledgment from the patient receiving the document. If the patient refuses to sign or is unable to sign, this must be documented in the patient record.
- **Authorization forms.** Use and disclosure of protected health information (PHI) is permissible for treatment, payment, or routine health care operations (TPO) because the NPP describes how PHI is used for these purposes. The health care organization is required to obtain signed authorization to use or disclose health information for situations beyond TPO. This functions as protection for the practice. Health care staff must learn about the particular "authorization" forms used in their office. Psychotherapy notes are handled separately under HIPAA. Such notes have additional protection, specifically that an authorization for any use or disclosure of psychotherapy notes must be obtained.

Your organization will be expected to handle requests made by patients to exercise their rights. You must know your office's process for dealing with each specific request. With your understanding of HIPAA and your organization's policy manual, you will be guided in procedures specific to your health care organization.

general condition, and location in the hospital. A patient must be given the opportunity to opt out of the directory. Information may only be released to visitors who ask for a patient by name. Clergy may be given directory information without having to ask for the patient by name.

Information pertaining to infectious disease outbreaks may be released to public health officials. Law enforcement may be given information pertaining to the whereabouts of a fugitive, as well as in cases of suspected abuse or violence. Media must be directed to the facility spokesperson. Public figures such as elected officials and celebrities must be given the same privacy standards as other patients.

Verification of Identity and Authority

Remember, before any disclosure, you must verify the identity of persons requesting PHI if they are unknown to you. You may request identifying information, such as date of birth, Social Security number, or even a code word stored in your practice management system that is unique to each patient. Public officials may present badges, credentials, official letterheads, and other legal documents of authority for identification purposes. Patients and patient representatives should be prepared to show a valid picture ID such as a driver's license.

You must also verify that the requestor has the right to receive the PHI and identify the need for the PHI. Exercising professional judgment fulfills your verification requirements for most disclosures because you are acting on "good faith" in believing the identity of the individual requesting PHI. It is good practice when making any disclosure to note the authority of the person receiving the PHI and how this was determined. This shows due diligence on your part with respect to HIPAA.

Validating Patient Permission

Before making any uses or disclosures of confidential health information other than for the purposes of TPO, your office must have appropriate patient permission. Always check for conflicts between various permissions your office may have on file for a given patient. This information should be maintained either in your practice management system or in the health record, where it can be easily identified and retrieved.

For example, if a covered entity has agreed to a patient's request to limit how much of the PHI is sent to a consulting physician for treatment but then receives the patient's authorization to disclose the entire health record to that physician, this would be a conflict. In general, the more restrictive permission would take precedence. Privacy regulations allow resolving conflicting permissions either by obtaining new permission from the patient or by communicating orally or in writing with the patient to determine the patient's preference. Be sure to document any form of communication in writing.

Obligations of the Health Care Organization

Training

Under HIPAA regulations, a covered entity must train all members of its staff. This training must include the practice's P&P with respect to PHI as it pertains to their function within the organization. This training will address how each employee's role relates to PHI in his or her office or department. HIPAA training focuses on how to handle confidential information securely in the health care setting. Training should be completed as part of a new hire orientation and then annually. All training must be documented.

Safeguards: Ensuring That Confidential Information Is Secure

Every covered entity must have appropriate safeguards to ensure the protection of an individual's confidential health information. Such safeguards include administrative, technical, and physical measures that will reasonably safeguard PHI from

BOX 2.7 Examples of Safeguards

Administrative	Technical	Physical
Verifying the identity of an individual picking up health records	Create username and password required to access patient records from computer	Locked, fireproof filing cabinets for storing paper records
Apply sanctions against workforce members who fail to comply with security policies and procedures	Establish procedures to obtain necessary ePHI during an emergency	Establish procedures that allow facility access in support of restoration of lost data under the disaster recovery plan
Perform regular records review of information system activity, such as audit logs, access reports, and security incident tracking reports	Implement procedures that terminate an electronic session after a predetermined time of inactivity	Implement physical safeguards for all workstations that access ePHI, to restrict access to authorized users
Identify a security official who will be responsible for the development of policies and procedures	Implement a mechanism to encrypt and decrypt ePHI	Implement policies and procedures to limit physical access to electronic information systems by identifying authorized individuals by title and/or job function

ePHI, Electronic protected health information.

any use or disclosure that violates HIPAA, whether intentional or unintentional (Box 2.7). Examples of security safeguards are discussed later in this chapter.

Complaints to Health Care Practice and Workforce Sanctions

Individuals, both patients and staff, must be provided with a process to make a complaint concerning the P&P of the covered entity. If a violation involves the misuse of PHI, this incident should be reported to the organization's PO. Should there be further cause, the OCR also may be contacted.

Staff members are subject to appropriate sanctions for failure to comply with the P&P regarding PHI set forth in the organization. The types of sanctions applied vary, depending on the violation and its mitigating factors. Sanctions can range from a warning to suspension to termination. This information should be covered in the policy and procedures manual. Written documentation of complaints and sanctions must be kept on file.

Mitigation

Mitigation means to "alleviate the severity" or "make mild." In reference to HIPAA, the covered entity has a duty to take appropriate steps in response to breaches. If a breach is discovered, the health care organization is required to mitigate, to the extent possible, any harmful effects of the breach. For example, if you learn that you have sent health records by fax to an incorrect party, steps should be taken to have the recipient destroy the PHI. Mitigation procedures also apply to activities of the practice's business associates. Being proactive and responsible by mitigating reduces the potential for a more disastrous outcome from the breach or violation.

Refraining from Intimidating or Retaliatory Acts

HIPAA privacy regulations prohibit a covered entity from intimidating, threatening, coercing, discriminating against, or otherwise taking retaliatory action against the following:

- Individuals, for exercising HIPAA privacy rights
- Individuals, for filing a complaint with DHHS; for testifying, assisting, or participating in an investigation about the covered entity's privacy practices; or for reasonably opposing any practice prohibited by the regulation

THE SECURITY RULE: ADMINISTRATIVE, TECHNICAL, AND PHYSICAL SAFEGUARDS

The **Security Rule** comprises regulations related to the security of **electronic protected health information (ePHI)**. This refers to any PHI that is produced, saved, transferred, or received in an electronic form. The Security Rule provides regulations related to electronic transactions and code sets, privacy, and enforcement. Security measures encompass all administrative, physical, and technical safeguards in an information system. The Security Rule addresses only ePHI, but the concept of preserving PHI that will become ePHI makes attention to security for the entire office important. The P&P required by the Security Rule must be maintained for 6 years after they are no longer in use. The Security Rule is divided into three main sections: administrative safeguards, technical safeguards, and physical safeguards.

Administrative safeguards prevent unauthorized use or disclosure of ePHI through administrative actions. Policy and procedures to manage this include the selection, development, implementation, and maintenance of security measures to protect ePHI. These management controls guard data integrity, confidentiality, and availability and include the following:

- Information access controls authorize each employee's physical access to ePHI. This is management of passwords for each individual employee. These restrict access to records in accordance with the employee's responsibility in the health care organization. For example, usually the health information management (HIM) clerk who has authorization to retrieve health records will not have access to billing records located on the computer. Each user should have a unique user name and an unshared, undisclosed password to log in to any computer with access to PHI. Identifying each unique user allows the functions of auditing and access controls to be implemented. Passwords for all users should be changed on a regular basis and should never be common names or words.

- Internal audits review who has had access to PHI to ensure that there is no intentional or accidental inappropriate access. This applies to both the practice management system and the paper records or charges.
- Risk analysis and management is a process that assesses the privacy and security risks of various safeguards and the cost in losses if those safeguards are not in place. Each organization must evaluate its vulnerabilities and the associated risks and decide how to lessen those risks. Reasonable safeguards must be implemented to protect against known risks.
- Termination procedures should be formally documented in the P&P manual and include terminating an employee's access to PHI. Other procedures include changing office security pass codes, deleting user access to computer systems, deleting terminated employees' e-mail accounts, and collecting any access cards or keys.

Technical safeguards are technologic controls that are put in place to protect and control access to information on computers in the health care organization. These include the following:

- Access controls through limitations created for each staff member based on job category. For example, a receptionist, administrative medical assistant, clinical medical assistant, bookkeeper, or insurance billing specialist will have different levels of access depending on their assigned tasks.
- Audit controls keep track of log-ins to the computer system, administrative activity, and changes to data. This includes changing passwords, deleting user accounts, and creating new user accounts.
- Automatic log-offs prevent unauthorized users from accessing a computer when it is left unattended. The computer system or software program should automatically log off after a predetermined period of inactivity.

Physical safeguards also prevent unauthorized access to PHI. These physical measures and P&P protect a covered entity's electronic information systems and related buildings and equipment from natural and environmental hazards as well as unauthorized intrusion by a hacker or employee who should not have access. Appropriate and reasonable physical safeguards should include the following:

- Media and equipment controls are documented in the P&P manual regarding management of the PHI. Typical safeguard policies include how the office handles the retention, removal, and disposal of paper records as well as recycling computers and destroying obsolete data disks or software programs containing PHI.
- Physical access controls limit unauthorized access to areas in which equipment and medical charts are stored. Locks on doors are the most common type of control.
- Secure workstation locations minimize the possibility of unauthorized viewing of PHI. This includes ensuring that password-protected screen savers are in use on computers when unattended and that desk drawers are locked.

! COMPLIANCE ALERT

Computer Confidentiality

Confidentiality Statement

Most information in patients' health records and the health care organization's financial records is considered confidential and sensitive. Employees who have access to such computer data should have integrity and be well chosen because they have a high degree of responsibility and accountability. It is wise to have those handling sensitive computer documents sign an annual confidentiality statement (see Fig. 2.6). This way the statement can be updated when an individual's responsibilities increase or decrease. The statement should contain the following:

- Written or oral disclosure of information pertaining to patients is prohibited.
- Disclosure of information without consent of the patient results in serious penalty or immediate dismissal.

Prevention Measures

Employees can take a number of preventive measures to maintain computer security.

1. Obtain a software program that stores files in coded form.
2. Never leave disks or tapes unguarded on desks or anywhere else in sight.
3. Use a privacy filter over the computer monitor so that data may be read only when the user is directly in front of the computer.
4. Log off the computer terminal before leaving a workstation. Check and double check the credentials of any consultant hired.
5. Read the manuals for the equipment, especially the sections titled "Security Controls," and follow all directions.
6. Store confidential data on disks rather than only on the computer's hard drive. Disks should be stored in a locked, secure location, preferably one that is fireproof and away from magnetic fields.
7. Make sure the computer system has a firewall and proper antivirus/antispyware software installed. Hackers can also access digital copiers, laser printers, fax machines, and other electronic equipment with internal memories. Develop passwords for each user and access codes to protect the data. A password is a combination of letters, numbers, or symbols that an individual is assigned to access the system. Passwords should be changed at regular intervals and never written down. A good password is composed of more than eight characters and is case sensitive. *Case sensitive* means that the password must be entered exactly as stored using upper- or lowercase characters. Delete obsolete passwords from the system. Change any passwords known by an employee who is fired or resigns. Individuals with their own passwords allow the employer to distinguish work done by each employee. If errors or problems occur, focus may then be directed toward correcting the individual user.
8. A strong password:
   - Is at least eight characters long.
   - Does not contain your user name, real name, or company name.
   - Does not contain a complete word.
   - Is significantly different from a previous password.
   - Contains characters from these four categories: uppercase, lowercase, numbers, symbols.
     - Example: Iluv2pla2BA4$
9. Send only an account number when e-mailing a colleague with specific questions. Never send the patient's name or other identifying information over unsecured e-mail.

HEALTH INFORMATION TECHNOLOGY FOR ECONOMIC AND CLINICAL HEALTH ACT

The Health Information Technology for Economic and Clinical Health Act (HITECH Act) was a provision of the

EMPLOYEE CONFIDENTIALITY STATEMENT

As an employee of ABC Clinic, Inc. (employer), having been trained as an insurance billing specialist with employee responsibilities and authorization to access personal medical and health information, and as a condition of my employment, I agree to the following:

A. I recognize that I am responsible for complying with the Health Insurance Portability and Accountability Act (HIPAA) of 1996 policies regarding confidentiality of patients' information, which, if I violate, may lead to immediate dismissal from employment and, depending on state laws, criminal prosecution.

B. I will treat all information received during the course of my employment, which relates to the patients, as confidential and privileged information.

C. I will not access patient information unless I must obtain the information to perform my job duties.

D. I will not disclose information regarding my employer's patients to any person or entity, other than that necessary to perform my job duties, and as permitted under the employer's HIPAA policies.

E. I will not access any of my employer's computer systems that currently exist or may exist in the future using a password other than my own.

F. I will safeguard my computer password and will not show it in public.

G. I will not allow anyone, including other employees, to use my password to access computer files.

H. I will log off of the computer immediately after I finish using it.

I. I will not use e-mail to transmit patient information unless instructed to do so by my employer's HIPAA privacy officer.

J. I will not take patient information from my employer's premises in hard copy or electronic form without permission from my employer's HIPAA privacy officer.

K. Upon termination of my employment, I agree to continue to maintain the confidentiality of any information learned while an employee and agree to relinquish office keys, access cards, or any other device that provides access to the provider or its information.

Mary Doe
Signature

September 14, 20XX
Date

Mary Doe
Print name

Brenda Shield
Witness

Fig. 2.6 An example of an employee confidentiality agreement that may be used by an employer when hiring an insurance billing specialist.

American Recovery and Reinvestment Act (ARRA) of 2009 signed into law by President Obama. ARRA contained incentives for adopting health care information technology that are designed to speed up the adoption of electronic health record systems for many health care organizations. Because this legislation promoted a massive expansion in the exchange of ePHI, the purpose of the HITECH Act was to strengthen the HIPAA privacy protections and rights. The HITECH Act updated and enhanced the privacy and security responsibilities of covered entities that were established under HIPAA. The HITECH Act brought significant compliance changes to three very specific areas:

1. Business associates
2. Notification of breach
3. Civil penalties for noncompliance with the provisions of HIPAA

Business Associates

Under HIPAA, the covered entity is responsible and liable for all activities related to their business associates. If a covered entity becomes aware of a breach involving a business associate, the covered entity is expected to terminate the contract if the breach was not corrected. The HITECH Act brought greater responsibility to the business associate. It requires all business associates to comply with the HIPAA Security Rule by February 17, 2010, in the same manner that a covered entity would. Business associates are expected to implement physical and technical safeguards as outlined in the Security Rule. They are expected to conduct a risk analysis, to develop and implement related policies and procedures, and to comply with written documentation and workforce training requirements. The business associate is now subject to the application of civil and criminal penalties, just as a covered entity is.

Notification of Breach

The HITECH Act defines a breach as the unauthorized acquisition, access, use, or disclosure of PHI, in a manner not permitted by HIPAA, which poses a significant risk of financial, reputational, or other harm to the affected individual.

Under the HITECH Act, if a breach were to occur, the HITECH Act requires a covered entity to notify the affected party directly without delay. In no case should notification be later than 60 calendar days after the discovery of a breach. Enforcement of the notification of breach began on February 22, 2010.

The standard for reporting breaches was modified in 2013 under the HIPAA Omnibus Rule. Any breach is presumed reportable unless the covered entity or business associated can demonstrate that there is a low probability that the information has been compromised. This is based on a risk assessment of certain factors or unless the breach fits within certain exceptions. Health care organizations must develop policies that apply to these standards.

Breach notification is not required when any of the following occur:

1. The breach was unintentional access or use by someone who acquired the PHI in good faith through the normal scope of their job. For example, if a billing specialist receives and opens an e-mail from a nurse, and then notifies the nurse of the misdirected e-mail and deletes it, a breach notification is not required.
2. There is a good faith belief that the unauthorized person could not have retained the PHI. For example, if a laptop is lost and recovered and analysis shows that information on the laptop had not been accessed or altered, a breach notification is not required.
3. A health care organization may be asked by law enforcement to delay breach notification if such notification would impede an investigation.

In health care, all files and electronic data must be encrypted and destroyed when the records no longer need to be retained. If an organization has used an appropriate method to encrypt and destroy files, it is relieved of the breach notification rule as it applies to that PHI.

Breach notification must be sent in writing via first class mail to each individual affected. If the patient is deceased, the next of kin must be notified. If an address is unknown, an effort must be made to reach the individual through other means. If the breach affects 500 or more individuals, the notice must also be provided to local media outlets such as newspaper and television news. DHHS must also be notified within 60 days of the breach for breaches affecting 500 or more people. For smaller breaches, DHHS can be notified annually or within 60 days of the end of the year the breach was discovered. A list of covered entities that have had breaches is maintained by DHHS. Organizations on this list must submit logs of breaches to the DHHS on an ongoing annual basis.

HIPAA Compliance Audits

The HITECH Act further requires DHHS to provide periodic audits to ensure that covered entities and business associates are complying with HIPAA Privacy and Security Rules and Breach Notification standards. The OCR has developed an audit program that is used to assess HIPAA privacy and security programs and compliance efforts. It examines mechanisms for compliance, identifies best practices, and discovers risks and vulnerabilities that may not be identified through other means. All covered entities, including health plans, health care clearinghouses, health care providers, and business associates, are eligible for an audit. Over the past decade, OCR audits have focused on how covered entities have implemented controls and processes to meet HIPAA Privacy and Security and Breach Notification Rules.

Increased Penalties for Noncompliance With the Provisions of HIPAA

There are both civil and criminal penalties for failure to comply with HIPAA regulations. The HITECH Act significantly increased the penalty amounts that may be imposed for violations related to failure to comply with HIPAA rules. These are as follows:

- $100 to $50,000 if the covered entity did not know about the violation
- $1000 to $50,000 if the violation was due to reasonable cause
- $10,000 to $50,000 if the violation was due to willful neglect and was corrected
- $50,000 or more if the violation was due to willful neglect and was not corrected

The HITECH Act set a maximum penalty of $1.5 million for all violations of an identical provision in a calendar year. Penalties may also be applied on a daily basis if the OCR sees fit to do so. An example of when this may occur would be if a health care organization refuses to give patients copies of their records when requested. In this case, OCR may apply the penalty per day that the practice was in violation, or 365 days for an entire year.

Individuals also can be held personally responsible for HIPAA violations, with criminal actions as follows:

- Knowing violations: up to $50,000 and/or 1 year in prison
- Misrepresentation or offenses under false pretenses: up to $100,000 and/or 5 years in prison
- Intent to sell, distribute, etc.: up to $250,000 and/or 10 years in prison

HIPAA Omnibus Rule

The final **HIPAA Omnibus Rule** is an update to the 1996 HIPAA law and 2009 HITECH Act that modified both privacy and security rules for covered entities and their business associates. The new rule was effective March 26, 2013. The rule enhances patients' privacy rights and protections, especially regarding genetic information. It strengthens the OCR's ability to enforce the HIPAA privacy and security protections in the face of the expanded use of electronic health records. The new rule also expands many of the requirements of business associates who receive PHI and their subcontractors, holding them to the same standards of covered entities. As mentioned earlier, the Omnibus Rule also clarifies when breaches of unsecured health information must be reported to DHHS. The rule streamlines the authorization process. It increases the restrictions on use of PHI in research and marketing and raises the penalties for negligent disclosures.

The new rule requires covered entities to update policies applicable to deceased persons. It states that a covered entity may disclose PHI to a coroner or medical examiner for the purpose of identifying a deceased person and determining the cause of death.

The Omnibus Rule strengthens the need for timeliness in response to a patient's request for records. It also adds a provision permitting providers to disclose proof of a child's immunization records to schools if the school is required by law to have such proof. The rule also makes it easier for parents and others to disclose the child's immunization records by giving them the ability to authorize the disclosure through oral consent.

Consequences of Noncompliance With HIPAA and the HITECH Act

Different governing bodies handle the prosecution of HIPAA violations. DHHS handles issues regarding transaction code sets and security. Complaints can be filed against a covered entity for not complying with these rules. The OCR oversees privacy issues and complaints and refers criminal issues to the Office of the Inspector General (OIG). The OIG provides the workup for referral cases, which may involve the Federal Bureau of Investigation (FBI) and other agencies.

Since the 2003 HIPAA Privacy Rule compliance date, the OCR has investigated more than 160,000 complaints. Sometimes the investigation finds that no violation occurred. When a violation has occurred, the OCR attempts to resolve the situation with one of the following:

- Voluntary compliance where the OCR may provide training and technical assistance to bring an entity into compliance;
- Corrective action where the OCR outlines a step-by-step process to correct the violation and ensure it does not happen again; and/or
- Resolution agreement where the covered entity is obligated to perform certain tasks and report to the OCR for 3 years. It often includes a monetary penalty.

DHHS announced its first enforcement action resulting from a violation of the HITECH Act Breach Notification Rule in 2012, which placed a monetary settlement of $1.5 million per breach on the accused. This enforcement action sent a clear message to the health care community that the OCR expects health care organizations to have a carefully designed and active HIPAA compliance plan in place.

More recent settlements have brought millions of dollars in restitution. In May 2017, HHS announced that St. Luke's–Roosevelt Hospital Center, Inc. paid $387,200.00 to settle violations. Allegedly, staff disclosed PHI revealing sensitive information about HIV to a patient's employer. During the investigation, the OCR learned that the same hospital had a similar breach 9 months earlier and had not addressed the weak areas in their P&P to ensure it would not happen again.

In the same month, Memorial Hermann Health System agreed to pay $2.4 million to HHS and to follow a corrective action plan to settle their violations. In 2015 a patient had presented to the facility with a fraudulent identification card. Staff alerted the appropriate law enforcement authorities and the patient was arrested. This was a permissible disclosure. However, the health care organization went on to issue a press release containing the patient's name in the title. The corrective action plan requires Memorial Hermann Health System to update their P&P and to train their staff.

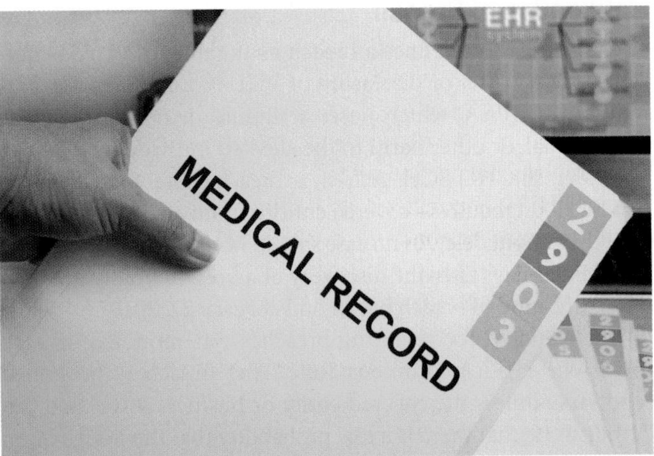

Fig. 2.7 HIPAA, privacy, and security affect every level of the health care organization. (From iStock photo.com)

Again, in 2017, Memorial Healthcare System paid HHS $5.5 million and agreed to a corrective action plan to settle HIPAA violations. They self-reported to HHS a potential breach of PHI for 115,143 individuals where some employees had inappropriately disclosed the information to other office staff. A former employee's login credentials had been used for a year to access more than 80,000 patient records. HHS found that the organization had failed to review activity or terminate the former employee's access despite having identified this risk several years before the breach.

In January 2017, HHS announced the first settlement based on untimely breach notification. Presence Health in Illinois agreed to pay $475,000 and complete a corrective action plan when it failed to notify affected individuals within 60 days of discovering a breach. Though the notification was otherwise handled correctly, the OCR sent a clear message to other organizations. Every aspect of the HIPAA rules and Breach Notification Rules must be followed to the letter.

These and other OCR Resolution Agreements can be reviewed on the DHHS website (https://www.hhs.gov/hipaa/for-professionals/compliance-enforcement/agreements/index.html).

APPLICATION TO THE HEALTH CARE SETTING

HIPAA affects all areas of the health care office, from the reception area to the provider (see Fig. 2.7). In addition to being educated and trained in job responsibilities, every staff member must be educated about HIPAA and trained in the P&P pertinent to the organization.

Reasonable safeguards are measurable solutions based on accepted standards that are implemented and periodically monitored to demonstrate that the office is in compliance. Reasonable efforts must be made to limit the use or disclosure of PHI. If you are the front desk receptionist and you close the privacy glass between your desk and the waiting area when making a call to a patient, this is a reasonable safeguard to prevent others in the waiting room from overhearing.

Incidental uses and disclosures are permissible under HIPAA only when reasonable safeguards or precautions have been implemented to prevent misuse or inappropriate disclosure of PHI. When incidental uses and disclosures result from failure to apply reasonable safeguards or adhere to the minimum necessary standard, the Privacy Rule has been violated. If you are in the reception area and you close the privacy glass before having a confidential conversation but are still overheard by an individual in the waiting room, this would be incidental. You have applied a reasonable safeguard to prevent your conversation from being overheard. The OCR has addressed what is permissible with regard to incidental disclosures. Examples follow.

1. As discussed earlier in this chapter, use caution when handling patient and insurance inquiries over the phone or via e-mail. Ensure that the person you are releasing information to has the right to receive it.
2. Health care professionals may discuss laboratory test results with a patient or other provider in a joint treatment area. A health care professional is an individual who has been trained in a health-related field, whether clinical or administrative. The professional may be licensed, certified, or registered by a state or government agency or professional organization.
3. A physician may discuss a patient's condition or plan of care in the patient's treatment area or hospital room.
4. A pharmacist may discuss a prescription with a patient over the pharmacy counter or with a physician or the patient by telephone.
5. A physician may give instructions to a staff member to bill a patient for a certain procedure even if other individuals in the reception room can overhear the conversation.
6. A patient's name may be called out in the reception room; however, some offices prefer to use first names and not call out last names.

Organization and Staff Responsibilities in Protecting Patient Rights

The covered entity must implement written P&P that comply with HIPAA standards. P&P are tailored guidelines established to inform each employee of their role within the organization. It is important that PHI is addressed in these guidelines. HIPAA requires each organization to implement P&P that comply with privacy and security rules. The organization should have a P&P manual to train providers and staff and to serve as a resource for situations that need clarification. Revisions to P&P must be made as needed and appropriate to comply with laws as they change. Documentation must be maintained in written or electronic form and retained for 6 years after its creation or when it was last in effect, whichever is later.

Health care organizations face challenges in applying the HIPAA requirements; do not let these overwhelm you. Appropriate steps are required to build protections specific to your health care organization. Compliance is an ongoing effort involving teamwork. Understand your office's established P&P. Monitor your own activities to ensure that you are following the required procedures. Do not take shortcuts when your actions involve patient privacy and security.

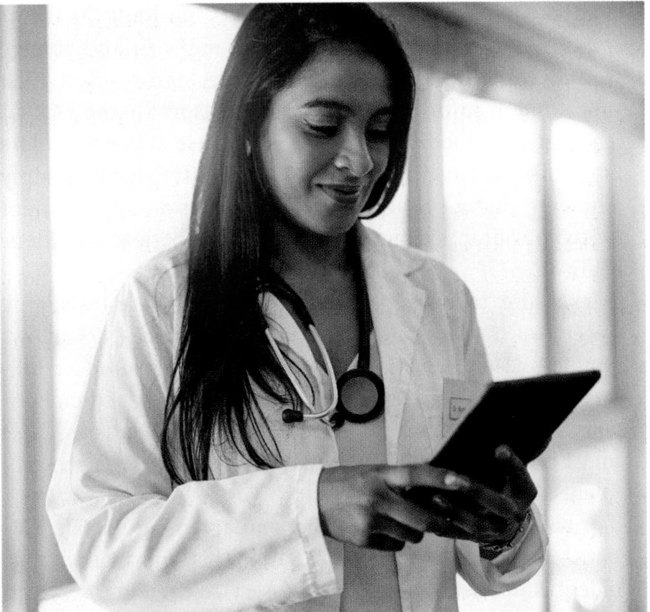

Fig. 2.8 Privacy and security must be considered in every aspect of your job, from phone conversations to computer use to physical surroundings. (From iStock photo.com)

BEST PRACTICES TO AVOID COMMON HIPAA VIOLATIONS

As an insurance billing specialist, you will likely answer the telephone and speak during the course of your business, and there may be uncertainties about what questions you can and cannot answer. Reasonable and appropriate safeguards must be taken to ensure that all confidential health information in your office is protected from unauthorized and inappropriate access, in both verbal and written forms (Fig. 2.8).

- Consider that conversations occurring throughout the office may be overheard. The reception area and waiting room are often linked and it is easy to hear the scheduling of appointments and exchange of confidential information. It is necessary to observe work areas and maximize efforts to avoid unauthorized disclosures. Simple and affordable precautions include using privacy glass at the front desk and having conversations away from settings where other patients or visitors are present. Health care providers can move their dictation stations away from patient areas or wait until no patients are present before dictating. Telephone conversations made by providers in front of patients, even in emergency situations, should be avoided. Providers and staff must use their best professional judgment.
- Be sure to check in both the patient's health record and your computer system to determine whether there are any special instructions for contacting the patient regarding scheduling or reporting test results. Follow these requests as agreed by the office.

- Patient sign-in sheets are permissible, but limit the information you request when a patient signs in and change the sheet periodically during the day. A sign-in sheet must not contain information such as a reason for the visit or the patient's medical condition. Because some providers specialize in treating patients with sensitive issues, simply showing that a particular individual has an appointment with your practice may pose a breach of patient confidentiality.
- Make sure to have patients sign a form acknowledging receipt of the Notice of Privacy Practices. The NPP allows you to release the patient's confidential information for billing and other purposes. If your practice has other confidentiality statements and policies besides HIPAA mandates, these must be reviewed to ensure that they meet HIPAA requirements.
- Formal policies for transferring and accepting outside PHI must address how your office keeps this information confidential. When using courier services, billing services, transcription services, or e-mail, you must ensure that transferring PHI is done in a secure and compliant manner. Data that must be removed from e-mail before being sent are as follows:
  - Name of patient
  - Address information other than city, state, and zip code
  - Telephone and fax numbers
  - E-mail address
  - Social Security number
  - Health record number
  - Health plan beneficiary number
  - Account number
  - Certificate/license numbers
  - Vehicle identifier
  - Device identifiers
  - Device serial number
  - Website address
  - Biometric identifiers
  - Full-face photograph
  - Geographic subdivisions smaller than state
  - Dates (except for years) related to birth, death, admission, and discharge
  - Any other unique identifying number, code, or characteristic, unless otherwise permitted
- Computers are used for a variety of administrative functions, including scheduling, billing, and managing health records. Computers are typically present at the reception area. Keep the computer screen turned so that viewing is restricted to authorized staff. Screen savers should be used to prevent unauthorized viewing or access. The computer should automatically log off the user after a period of being idle, requiring the staff member to reenter his or her password.
- Keep your username and password confidential and change them often. Do not share this information. An authorized staff member, such as the PO, will have administrative access to reset your password if you lose it or if someone discovers it. Also, practice management software can track users and follow their activity. Do not open yourself up to HIPAA violations by giving out your password. Safeguards include password protection for electronic data and storing paper records securely.
- Safeguard your work area; do not place notes with confidential information in areas that are easy to view by nonstaff. Cleaning services will access your building, usually after business hours; ensure that you safeguard PHI.
- Place patient health records face down at reception areas so that the patient's name is not exposed to other patients or visitors. When placing health records on the door of an examination room, turn the chart so that identifying information faces the door. If you keep medical charts on countertops or in receptacles, it is your duty to ensure that nonstaff persons will not access the records.
- Do not post the health care provider's schedule in areas viewable by nonstaff individuals. Schedules are often posted for the convenience of the professional staff but this may be a breach of patient confidentiality.
- Fax machines should not be placed in patient examination rooms or in any reception area where nonstaff persons may view incoming or sent documents. Only staff members should have access to the faxes.
- If you open office mail or take telephone calls pertaining to health record requests, direct these requests to the appropriate staff member.
- Send all privacy-related questions or concerns to the appropriate staff member.
- Immediately report any suspected or known improper behavior to your supervisor or the PO so that the issue may be documented and investigated. If you have questions, contact your supervisor or the PO.
- Never discuss patients casually with co-workers, friends, or family. Be mindful of your surroundings. Avoid sharing any patient information on social media. Even if you do not mention the patient by name, someone may recognize the patient.
- Do not respond to inquiries about a patient no matter how well meaning they may seem. Many people who do not work within the health care system are unaware that this is a HIPAA violation.
- Electronic files can be accessed on stolen or misplaced computers and smartphones. Home computers that do not have appropriate security may be easily hacked. Even texting can be hacked so it is important to only used phones to transmit patient data over secure applications that use encryption.
- Do not access health records for patients out of curiosity or as a favor to a family member or friend. You are only allowed the minimum amount of access necessary to do your job. This is a common HIPAA violation that costs health care organizations every year.
- Be sure to get the proper written consents when disclosing any PHI. If you are not sure if a disclosure is allowed under the Privacy Rule, it is best to get the consent before releasing the information.

Under HIPAA, health care providers and their employees are required to protect PHI and limit the use of it to the minimum amount necessary. Penalties for violating HIPAA are high. As you enter the health care field, it is important to be aware of some common pitfalls and how to avoid them.

Be alert to other activities in your office. Help your co-workers change work habits that do not comply with HIPAA. Do not ignore unauthorized uses and disclosures of PHI and do not allow unauthorized persons to access data. You have an obligation to your employer and to the patients you serve.

KEY POINTS

This is a brief chapter review of the key issues presented. To further enhance your knowledge of the technical subject matter, review the key terms and key abbreviations for this chapter by locating the meaning for each in the Glossary at the end of this text, which appears in a section before the Index.

1. The Health Insurance Portability and Accountability Act (HIPAA) has affected confidentiality and disclosure of protected health information (PHI) and completion and electronic transmission of insurance claims. It has also affected how health care organizations address fraud and abuse in claims submission and implementation of compliance and practice standards.
2. While employed by a health care organization, the insurance billing specialist's duty is to have complete knowledge and understanding of HIPAA mandates. Always carry out policies and procedures that comply with federal regulations, and keep up to date with these statutes. This will assist both the physician and the patients.
3. The primary purpose of HIPAA *Title I: Health Insurance Reform* is to provide continuous insurance coverage for workers and their insured dependents when they change or lose jobs. *Title II: Administrative Simplification* focuses on the health care practice setting and aims to reduce administrative costs and burdens.
4. Serious civil and criminal penalties, such as fines and imprisonment, apply for HIPAA noncompliance.
5. *PHI* refers to data that identify an individual and describe his or her health status, age, sex, ethnicity, or other demographic characteristics, whether that information is or is not stored or transmitted electronically.
6. Under HIPAA, PHI may not be used or disclosed without permission from the patient or someone authorized to act on behalf of the patient. Use or disclosure is permitted if it is specifically required for treatment, payment, or routine health care operations (TPO). The two types of disclosure required by the HIPAA Privacy Rule are to the individual who is the subject of the PHI and to the Secretary of the DHHS to investigate compliance with the rule.
7. When comparing privileged and nonprivileged information, privileged information is related to the treatment and progress of the patient. The patient must sign an authorization to release this information or selected facts from the health record. Nonprivileged information consists of ordinary facts unrelated to treatment of the patient, including the patient's name, city of residence, and dates of admission or discharge.
8. Under HIPAA, a Notice of Privacy Practices (NPP) document must be given to the patient at the first visit or at enrollment. The NPP explains the individual's rights and the health care organization's legal duties regarding PHI. Use and disclosure of PHI is permissible for TPO because the NPP describes how PHI is used for these purposes. Thus a consent form is not required. The health care organization is required to obtain a signed authorization form to use or disclose health information for situations beyond the TPO. This is a protection for the practice. Psychotherapy notes are handled separately under HIPAA. Such notes have additional protection, specifically that an authorization for any disclosure of psychotherapy notes must be obtained.
9. *Disclosure* means the release, transfer, provision of access to, or divulging information to a person or entity outside the health care organization. *Use* means the sharing, employment, application, utilization, examination, or analysis of IIHI within an organization that holds such information. When a patient's billing record is accessed to review the claim submission history, the individual's health information is in use.
10. The three major categories of security safeguards are administrative, technical, and physical measures that will reasonably protect PHI from any use or disclosure that is in violation of HIPAA.
11. DHHS and the OCR perform HIPAA audits and place substantial fines on covered entities that do not follow HIPAA regulations.

You must strongly consider the lessons learned from the privacy, transaction, and security rules in conjunction with OIG compliance recommendations. The most important points are to read your organization's P&P manual and to ask questions about the general operations of your organization. Always use the best practice approach to be an informed and effective employee.

STUDENT ASSIGNMENTS

- Study Chapter 2.
- Answer the fill-in-the-blank, multiple-choice, and true/false questions in the *Workbook* to reinforce the theory learned in this chapter and help prepare for a future test.
- Complete the assignments in the *Workbook* to give you experience in making decisions regarding situations of fraud, abuse, incidental disclosures, compliance violations, consents, or authorizations.
- Turn to the Glossary at the end of this text for a further understanding of the key terms and key abbreviations used in this chapter.

3

Compliance, Fraud, and Abuse

Cheryl Fassett

OBJECTIVES

After reading this chapter, you should be able to:

1. Define compliance.
2. Discuss the difference between fraud and abuse.
3. List examples of fraud and abuse in the health care setting.
4. Identify the federal and state laws that regulate health care fraud and abuse.
5. Understand the penalties for fraud and abuse.
6. Identify the various fraud and abuse audit programs.
7. Discuss the basic components of an effective compliance program.
8. Discuss potential risk areas for physician groups, hospitals and billing companies.

KEY TERMS

abuse
assumption coding
auditing
Civil False Claims Act
Civil Monetary Penalty
Clinical Laboratory Improvement Amendments
clustering
compliance
compliance plan
Comprehensive Error Rate Testing
corrective action plan
cost reports
Criminal False Claims Act
DRG creep
embezzlement
Emergency Medical Treatment and Labor Act
Federal Deposit Insurance Corporation
fraud
Fraud Enforcement and Recovery Act
Health Care Fraud Prevention and Enforcement Action Team
Health Care Fraud and Abuse Control
medical necessity
Medicare Administrative Contractor
Medicare Integrity Program
monitoring
Occupational Safety and Health Administration
Office of Inspector General
Operation Restore Trust
patient dumping
phantom bills
qui tam
Recovery Audit Contractor
Self-Disclosure Protocol
undercoding
upcoding
Zone Program Integrity Contractor

KEY ABBREVIATIONS

CERT
CLIA
CMP
CMS
DHHS
DOJ
EMTALA
FCA
FDIC
FERA
HCFAC
HEAT
MAC
MIP
OIG
ORT
OSHA
P&P
RAC
SDP
ZPIC

COMPLIANCE DEFINED

Compliance in the health care industry is the ongoing process of meeting regulations, recommendations, and expectations of federal and state agencies that pay for health care services and regulate the industry (Fig. 3.1). Health care compliance involves the following:

- The claims reimbursement processes
- Managed care procedures
- Protection of patients' privacy
- Various guidelines and statutes
- Licensure
- Patient safety
- Attention to the law

Health care is one of the most highly regulated industries, holding the health care worker to the highest levels of scrutiny. Any individual working in health care and any business that is involved with the health care industry must conform to the principles and practices identified by state and federal agencies. A compliance strategy provides a standardized process for handling business functions, much like a user's manual. This will enable consistent and effective management and staff performance.

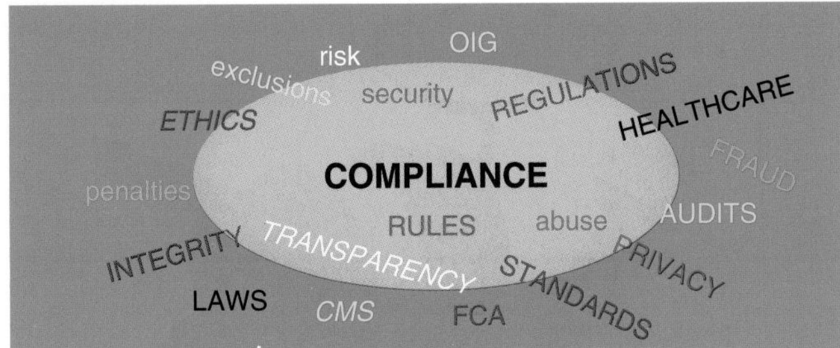

Fig. 3.1 Compliance involves many players, laws, and standards. A compliance plan is a set of policies, procedures, and guidelines to ensure an organization conducts its business in accordance with applicable laws and regulations.

The first step toward achieving compliance is understanding the laws that regulate the industry. Failure to comply with the associated mandates can lead to criminal penalties and/or civil fines.

FRAUD AND ABUSE LAWS

The Center for Medicare and Medicaid Services (CMS) has stated that those who commit health care fraud steal billions of dollars each year from federal and state government programs. This results in higher costs for everyone in the health care system. With many regulations and laws in place, there are very tight controls on medical billing. All individuals involved in the provision of health care services and in billing for those services are held to very high standards. In light of complex government regulations and constant scrutiny, it is important for those involved in the reimbursement process to clearly understand fraud and abuse.

Fraud can occur when deception is used in claim submission to obtain payment from the payer. Individuals who knowingly, willfully, and intentionally submit false information to benefit themselves or others commit fraud. Fraud can also be seen in mistakes that result in excessive reimbursement. No proof of intent is required for fraud to be considered. As you will learn later in this textbook, insurance claims require codes that describe what was wrong with the patient (diagnosis codes) and what service was provided to the patient (procedural codes). Codes must be reported accurately on claim forms. A fraudulent claim may be one that has been coded to maximize payment. It may be a claim that is filed for services that never took place, or for a patient who was never seen. Further examples of health care fraud are listed in Box 3.1.

Abuse means incidents or practices by health care organizations, not usually considered fraudulent, that conflict with accepted sound medical business or fiscal practices. An example of abuse in billing practices may be to submit excessive charges for services or supplies, or bill for noncovered services such as an annual preventative physical for a Medicare patient. Additional examples of health care abuse are listed in Box 3.2.

Defining Fraud and Abuse Roles, Relationships, and Key Terms

Centers for Medicare and Medicaid Services

CMS is the federal agency that administers and oversees the Medicare program and monitors the Medicaid program run by each state. CMS is committed to providing health care services

BOX 3.1 Examples of Fraud

- Bill for services or supplies not provided (**phantom bills** or invoice ghosts)
- Alter fees on a claim form to obtain higher payment
- Forgive the deductible or copayment
- Alter health records to generate fraudulent payments
- Leave relevant information off a claim (for example, failing to reveal whether a spouse has health insurance coverage through an employer)
- Upcode (for example, submit a code for a complex fracture when the patient had a simple fracture)
- Shorten (for example, dispense less medication than billed for)
- Split billing schemes (for example, bill procedures over a period of days when all treatment occurred during one visit)
- Use another person's insurance card to obtain medical care
- Change a date of service
- Post adjustments to generate fraudulent payments
- Solicit, offer, or receive a kickback, bribe, or rebate in return for referring a patient to a physician, physical therapist, or pharmacy or for referring a patient to obtain any item or service that may be paid for in full or in part by Medicare or Medicaid
- Restate the diagnosis to obtain insurance benefits or better payment
- Apply deliberately for duplicate payment (for example, bill Medicare twice, bill Medicare and the beneficiary for the same service, or bill Medicare and another insurer in an attempt to be paid twice)
- Unbundle or explode charges (for example, bill a multichannel laboratory test as if individual tests were performed)
- Collusion between a health care organization and an employee of a third-party payer when the claim is assigned (if the health care organization deliberately overbilled for services, overpayments could be generated with little awareness on the part of the Medicare beneficiary)
- Bill based on gang visits (for example, a physician visits a nursing home and bills for 20 visits without furnishing any specific services to or on behalf of individual patients)
- Knowingly bill for the same item or service more than once or another party bills the federal health care program for an item or service also billed by the health care organization

BOX 3.2 Examples of Medical Billing Abuse

- Refer excessively to other providers for unnecessary services
- Charge excessively for services or supplies
- Perform a battery of diagnostic tests when only a few tests are required for services
- Violate Medicare's physician participating agreement
- Call patients for repeated and unnecessary follow-up visits
- Bill Medicare beneficiaries at a higher rate than other patients
- Submit bills to Medicare and not to third-party payers (for example, claims for injury from an automobile accident, in a store, or at the workplace)
- Breach an assignment agreement
- Fail to make required refunds when services are not reasonable and necessary
- Require patients to contract to pay their health care organization's full charges, in excess of the Medicare charge limits
- Require a patient to waive rights to have the health care organization submit claims to Medicare and obligate a patient to pay privately for Medicare-covered services
- Require patients to pay for services not previously billed, including telephone calls with the physician, prescription refills, and medical conferences with other professionals
- Require patients to sign a global waiver agreeing to pay privately for all services that Medicare will not cover and using these waivers to obligate patients to pay separately for a service that Medicare covers as part of a package or related procedures

to Medicare and Medicaid beneficiaries while also partnering with various entities and law enforcement agencies to prevent and detect health care fraud and abuse.

The Office of the Inspector General

Since its establishment in 1976, the Office of Inspector General's (OIG) mission has been to protect the health and welfare of the beneficiaries of Department of Health and Human Services (DHHS) programs and to safeguard the integrity of the Medicare and Medicaid programs. The OIG was established to find and eliminate fraud, abuse, and waste. The OIG undertakes nationwide audits as well as investigations to review the claim submission processes of health care organizations and reimbursement patterns within the program. The OIG makes recommendations to the DHHS Secretary and the US Congress on correcting problematic areas addressed in the federal programs.

Health Care Fraud and Abuse Control Program

Efforts to combat fraud were consolidated and strengthened under Public Law 104-191, the Health Insurance Portability and Accountability Act (HIPAA) of 1996. The Act established a comprehensive program to combat fraud committed against all health plans, both public and private. The legislation required the creation of a national Health Care Fraud and Abuse Control (HCFAC) Program, under the joint direction of the Attorney General and the Secretary of the DHHS acting through the department's Inspector General (DHHS/OIG). The HCFAC Program coordinates federal, state, and local law enforcement activities to combat health care fraud and abuse.

HIPAA legislation has radically changed the focus and mission within the OIG. HIPAA pushed the OIG into a new era, guaranteeing funds for the OIG programs and mandating initiatives to protect the integrity of all health care programs.

HIPAA requires DHHS and the Department of Justice (DOJ) to detail the amounts deposited to the Medicare Trust Fund as well as the source of such deposits in an annual report. The Affordable Care Act (ACA) provides additional tools and resources to help fight fraud that will help to boost HCFAC Program activities. These resources include the following:

- Enhanced screenings and enrollment requirements
- Increased data sharing across government
- Expanded overpayment recovery efforts
- Greater oversight of private insurance abuses

The text that follows contains very important information from federal fraud and abuse laws that is crucial for anyone in the health care field to become familiar with and to follow to avoid violations that can result in criminal penalties and civil fines.

False Claims Act (1863)

The False Claims Act (FCA) of 1863 is still the US government's main recourse against fraud and abuse. Originally written to protect the government from being sold shoddy equipment in the Civil War, it now extends that protection from military supplies to health care.

A false claim is one for services or supplies that were not provided specifically as presented or for which the health care organization is otherwise not entitled to payment. Presenting a claim for an item or service based on a procedure code known to result in greater payment or to submit a claim for services not medically necessary is also a violation of the FCA. The government uses the FCA in conjunction with other fraud and abuse laws and as a primary enforcement tool.

It is not necessary to prove intent to defraud. Liability can occur when a person knowingly presents or makes a false record that creates a false claim. There are both civil and criminal aspects to the FCA.

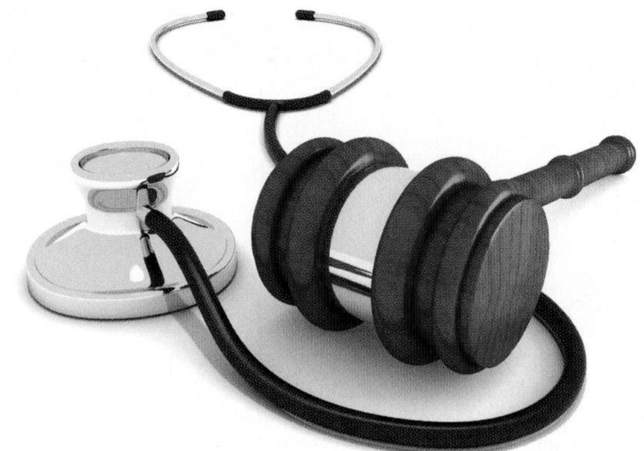

Fig. 3.2 It is crucial that an insurance billing specialist understands fraud and abuse laws. (From iStock photo.com)

Criminal False Claims Act (18 US Code §287)

The Criminal False Claims Act (1863) stated that anyone who knowingly makes or presents a false or fraudulent claim to any department or agency of the United States shall be imprisoned up to 5 years and shall be subject to a fine. Though the law did not apply specifically to the health care industry, HIPAA amendments officially linked the FCA to health care (Fig. 3.2). HIPAA updated the criminal code to include the following:

- *Theft or Embezzlement Statute (18 US Code §669).* This law brings fines and imprisonment against any person who embezzles, steals, or intentionally misapplies any of the moneys, funds, property, or other assets of any public or private health care benefit program. In addition to health care organizations that deal with the Medicare and Medicaid programs, this law applies to financial service industries, bookkeeping and accounting firms, and all business types and industries.

Embezzlement means stealing money that has been entrusted to one's care. The insurance billing specialist has been entrusted to process and manage health care finances in an organization. They should take extreme precautions to protect themselves and the organization who employs them. If an undiscovered embezzler leaves an employer, the person's replacement could be accused some months later of doing something he or she did not do. Be aware of what constitutes fraudulent activity and bring any potential issues to management upon discovery.

- *False Statement Relating to Health Care Matters Statute (19 US Code §1035).* Any person who conceals facts, makes fraudulent statements, or falsifies documentation in

BOX 3.3 Key Components in the AAPC and AHIMA Codes of Ethics

Integrity
Respect
Commitment
Competence
Fairness
Responsibility
Professionalism

Both organizations require their members to adhere to legal and ethical principles in coding, health information management, and every aspect of their jobs. They require members to avoid circumstances that may go against the laws and regulations of the health care industry.

For detailed discussion of each of these components, please refer to the AAPC Code of Ethics page (https://www.aapc.com/aboutus/code-of-ethics.aspx) and the AHIMA Code of Ethics page (http://bok.ahima.org/Profile).

AAPC, American Academy of Professional Coders; *AHIMA*, American Health Information Management Association.

connection with health care services is committing fraud. This holds true for both the delivery of and payment for these services. In doing this, a person is subject to fines and imprisonment.

- *Health Care Fraud Statute (18 US Code §1347).* Any individual who knowingly attempts or carries out a scheme to defraud any health care benefit program is committing fraud and is subject to fines and imprisonment. If serious bodily injury or death occurs, the person may face life imprisonment.
- *Obstruction of Criminal Investigations of Health Care Offenses Statute (18 US Code §1518).* A person is subject to fines and imprisonment when he or she prevents, obstructs, or misleads a federal health care criminal investigator.

Civil False Claims Act (31 US Code §3729-3733)

The Civil False Claims Act authorizes the United States to recover monetary damages from people who file fraudulent claims for payment by the federal government.

A coding or billing specialist who has knowledge of fraud or abuse should take the following measures:

- Notify the provider both personally and in writing.
- Document the false statement.
- Notify the health care organization's manager.
- Maintain a written audit trail with dated memoranda.
- Do not discuss the problem with anyone who is not immediately involved.

The American Academy of Professional Coders (AAPC) and the American Health Information Management Association (AHIMA), as well as most other professional organizations, have established a code of ethics for their certified members. Health care workers who follow these guidelines will be on the right path to avoid fraud and abuse (Box 3.3).

Penalties for Violating the False Claims Act

Civil penalties for violations of the FCA can result in fines of up to three times the programs' loss plus $11,000 per claim filed. Criminal penalties for submitting false claims may include fines, imprisonment, or both (Box 3.4).

BOX 3.4 Penalties for Violating the False Claims Act

Civil penalties:
Up to $20,000 per false claim plus triple the damages (money the government lost because of the claim)
Criminal penalties:
Up to 10 years in jail and $100,000
Administrative sanctions:
Up to $20,000 per line item per false claim and exclusion from participation in government programs

The FCA was amended in 2009 and 2010 under the Fraud Enforcement and Recovery Act of 2009 (FERA) and the Patient Protection and Affordable Care Act (PPACA). One significant change to the FCA under PPACA was clarification that overpayments under Medicare and Medicaid must be reported and returned within 60 days of discovery. Failure to report and return an overpayment exposes a health care organization to liability under the FCA.

The year 2017 saw the largest recovery to date for health care fraud under the FCA. A combined effort by the Medicare Fraud Strike Force, 30 state Medicaid Fraud Control units, the Federal Bureau of Investigation (FBI), and the OIG resulted in a recovery of $1.3 billion. It involved 412 defendants, 115 of whom were physicians, nurses, and other medical professionals. The investigation targeted medically unnecessary prescriptions as well as illegal distribution of opioids and other narcotics. It also involved false claims for treatments that were not provided. Many defendants paid kickbacks for beneficiary information they used to bill Tricare, Medicaid, and Medicare.

For hundreds of real-life examples of health care fraud and abuse, go to the DOJ site (https://www.justice.gov/briefing-room).

Qui Tam Provision

In common law, a writ of qui tam is a writ whereby a private individual who assists a prosecution can receive all or part of any penalty imposed.

The qui tam (pronounced kwee tam) provision in the FCA offers financial incentives to private citizens who act as informants and report suspected fraud on behalf of the federal government. This involves fraud by government contractors and other entities that receive or use government funds. The informant or individual who files a qui tam suit is known as a "relator" or a "whistleblower." A whistleblower can be anyone—an employee, a patient, another physician, or someone who works for a billing company or third-party payer. The whistleblower who assists in the qui tam action shares in any money recovered from penalties imposed.

Qui tam cases for health care fraud and abuse are big business. According to the US DOJ, $2.5 billion was recovered from health care FCA cases in 2016 alone (Fig. 3.3). Some cases from that year include the following:

- Wyeth and Pfizer, Inc. paid $784.6 million for reporting fraudulent prices on two acid reflux drugs.
- Novartis Pharmaceuticals Corp. paid $390 million for giving kickbacks to pharmacies for recommending two of their drugs.

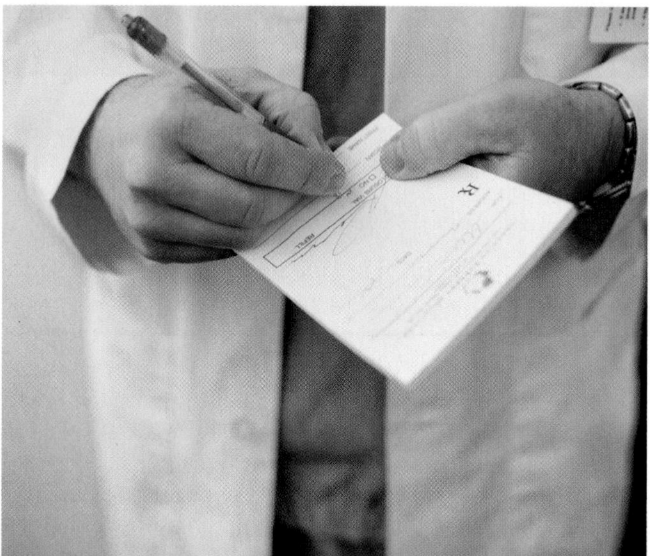

Fig. 3.3 Many fraud cases in 2016 centered around pharmaceuticals and kickbacks. (From iStock photo.com)

- Tenet Healthcare Corp. paid $513 million when four of their hospitals paid kickbacks in return for patient referrals.
- Millennium Health paid $260 million for submitting claims for unnecessary urine drug testing and genetic testing and violating both Anti-Kickback and Stark laws for giving free items to physicians who referred patients for expensive testing.
- RehabCare Group Inc. paid $160 million for inducing nursing homes to submit false claims to Medicare for unnecessary rehabilitation services.

In all of these cases, found on the DOJ website, a whistleblower shared in the recovered monies.

Exclusion Statute (42 US Code §1320a-7)

Under the Exclusion Statute, the OIG is required to exclude individuals, health care providers, and health care organizations who commit criminal offenses from future participation in any federal health care programs. Offenses that can earn exclusion from these programs range from Medicare fraud to patient abuse to financial misconduct.

According to OIG, no payment will be made to an excluded individual for anything he or she furnishes, orders, or prescribes. This payment exclusion extends to anyone who employs or contracts with the excluded individual as well as any hospital or provider where the excluded individual is allowed to provide services.

Health care organizations are required to screen all prospective providers, employees, and contractors against the OIG's List of Excluded Individuals and Entities before hire. Organizations that hire or contract with excluded individuals may be subject to civil monetary penalties. Be sure to check the updated exclusion listings at the OIG website (https://oig.hhs.gov/faqs/exclusions-faq.asp).

Stark Laws (42 US Code §1395nn)

The Stark Law is commonly referred to as the Physician Self-Referral Law. The original Stark Law pertained only to referrals to clinical laboratories. It was later expanded the service list to include the following:

- Clinical laboratory services
- Radiology services
- Physical and occupational therapy services
- Durable medical equipment and supplies, including prosthetics and orthotics
- Radiation therapy services and supplies
- Outpatient speech-language pathology services
- Parenteral and enteral equipment and supplies
- Inpatient and outpatient hospital services
- Home health services
- Outpatient prescription drugs

The Stark Law prohibits the submission of claims for services or referral of patients if the referring physician has a financial relationship with the entity that provides the services. The Stark Law carries exceptions, so it is important to understand the referral processes and in-office ancillary services used by each health care organization. Penalties for violations of the Stark Law include fines and exclusion from participation in the federal health care programs.

Anti-Kickback Statute (42 US Code §1320a-7b[b])

Under the Anti-Kickback Statute (1972), paying for referrals is a crime. A kickback may include any type of gift, reward, or inducement. Accepting discounts, rebates, or other reductions in price may violate this statute if it involves services payable under a federal program such as Medicare or Medicaid. For example, if a hospital provides physicians with free office space or tickets to a golf tournament in exchange for their patient referrals, they would both be guilty of paying and receiving kickbacks. Penalties for paying or accepting kickbacks can include fines, jail terms, and exclusion from participating in federal health care programs. Penalties up to $50,000 per kickback plus three times the amount of the remuneration can be imposed. The Patient Protection and Affordable Care Act (2010) strengthened this statute by clarifying that to prove fraud, the government needs to only prove intent to break the law, not to violate this statute specifically.

Civil Monetary Penalties Law (41 US Code §1320a-7a)

The Social Security Act allows the DHHS to impose monetary penalties and program exclusions for violations of the Anti-Kickback Statute and other various violations. The US Congress enacted this Civil Monetary Penalty (CMP) statute to help combat health care fraud and abuse. CMP imposes civil monetary penalties and assessments against a person or organization for making false or improper claims against any federal health care program. Penalties can range from $2000 to $100,000 per violation and may also include an assessment of up to three times the amount claimed for each item or service. CMP also allows a health care organization or provider to be excluded from government programs. CMP does not require that intent to defraud is proven.

Safe Harbors

A safe harbor is a provision of a statute or a regulation that specifies certain business arrangements that will be deemed not to violate a given rule. There are safe harbors that protect individuals from prosecution under the Anti-Kickback Statue. Certain arrangements are not violations of the Anti-Kickback Statute and are clearly allowed if they fall within a "safe harbor."

In 2013 a safe harbor that allows hospitals to provide physician practices with electronic health record systems and training to operate them was extended by CMS and the OIG through 2021. Before this it could have been viewed as a kickback arrangement for referrals if a hospital provided physician practices with this type of resource. However, this safe harbor was essential in CMS' effort to assist smaller practices in the health care community to adopt electronic health records technology.

Operation Restore Trust

Launched in 1995, Operation Restore Trust (ORT) was a program designed to combine the efforts of federal and state agencies to combat fraud, waste, and abuse in the Medicare and Medicaid programs. It was a joint effort overseen by the OIG and CMS allowing the public to report issues that might indicate fraud, abuse, or waste. ORT identified problems and weaknesses within the federally funded programs, recovering more than $25 million in its first year. It also trained state and local organizations to detect fraud and abuse and implemented statistical methods to identify health care organizations for audits and investigations.

Additional Laws and Compliance

Other laws pertaining to fraud and abuse include the Federal Deposit Insurance Corporation (FDIC) mail and wire fraud provisions, as follows:

- *§1341: Frauds and swindles.* An individual is subject to both fines and imprisonment when devising a scheme to defraud or obtain money or property by means of false pretenses by use of the US Postal Service. When an individual submits false paper claims via mail, he or she is also committing mail fraud.
- *§1343: Fraud by wire, radio, or television.* An individual will be fined and/or imprisoned for devising a scheme to defraud or obtain money or property by means of false pretenses, representations, or promises by wire, radio, or television. A health care organization that is committing billing fraud through electronic claim submission may also be found guilty of wire fraud.

The US government is clearly committed to the investigation and prosecution of health care fraud and abuse. It is imperative that health care entities develop their own compliance program to identify and prevent fraud.

Compliance Audits and Oversight

One of the greatest challenges for health care providers, workers, and organizations is the growing number of government and third-party fraud and abuse audit programs that scrutinize payment of health care services (Fig. 3.4).

Recovery Audit Program

CMS's Recovery Audit Program is tasked with identifying and correcting improper Medicare payments. Recovery Audit Contractors (RACs) are companies that contract with Medicare to recoup money from inappropriately paid claims. An improper payment may be an overpayment where a claim that did not meet Medicare's rules and guidelines was paid by a Medicare Administrative Contractor (MAC), or a provider was paid based on an incorrect fee schedule. It may also be an underpayment where a claims review will show that the procedure should have been coded for a higher level of service.

RACs receive information from Medicare about paid claims and data mine for potential claim payment errors using computer programs. They look for facilities, suppliers, and individual providers whose billings are higher than the majority of other suppliers or providers in an area. If a RAC finds a provider has received an improper payment, the provider is given the opportunity to discuss the determination before having to return the overpayment. This differs from the standard CMS appeal process. They look specifically for underpayments and overpayments. RACs are paid a percentage of the money they recover and are highly motivated to find claim errors.

Medicare and Medicaid Integrity Programs

HIPAA includes a provision establishing the Medicare Integrity Program (MIP). This provision gives the CMS specific authority to enter into contracts with entities to promote the integrity of the Medicare program.

The goals of the MIP are to identify and reduce Medicare overpayments through a series of audits and reviews of health care organizations' claims and cost report data. Objectives of MIP include identifying plan beneficiaries with additional insurance and educating health care organizations. Program integrity contractors help expand the scope of the MIP. This effort has recovered several billions of dollars in the fight against fraud, waste, and abuse in the Medicare program. Similar programs have recently extended into state Medicaid programs and are referred to as Medicaid Integrity Programs. These work to identify and recover inappropriate Medicaid payments.

Zone Program Integrity Contractors

Zone Program Integrity Contractors (ZPICs) replaced the Medicare Program Safeguard Contracts (PSCs) and Medicare Drug Integrity Contractors (MEDICs) that were established in HIPAA. A ZPIC is a fraud-investigating contractor hired by CMS to audit and review on their behalf. ZPICs focus on reviewing claims for health care organizations that have suspicious billing patterns. A ZPIC audit is typically done based on a high frequency of specific services, data analysis, or a call to a tip line. It compares a health care organization's services to those of similar organizations. If fraud and abuse are detected, ZPICs report this to the OIG for further investigation.

Comprehensive Error Rate Testing

The CMS implemented the Comprehensive Error Rate Testing (CERT) program to measure accuracy of payments in the Medicare fee-for-service (FFS) program at both national and regional levels. CERT audits are performed to determine if a MAC is paying claims correctly. Claims are randomly selected for CERT review. The health care organization receives a letter

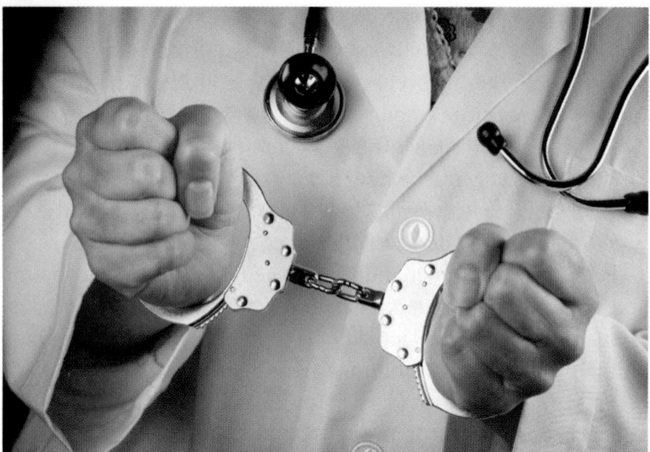

Fig. 3.4 Many types of audits actively search for wrongdoers who commit health care fraud. Fraud and abuse can result in large fines and even jail time. (From iStock photo.com)

from CMS requesting medical documentation to substantiate services that have been paid. Instructions for returning the documentation are provided and all documentation related to the services in question must be sent to the CERT Documentation Contractor within 75 days of the request. Failure to submit documentation will result in a CERT denial and recoupment of Medicare payments. CERT error rates are calculated based on review of records and are then used to form OIG target issues. CERT errors are also used by CMS to measure performance of Medicare contractors.

Health Care Fraud Prevention and Enforcement Action Team

In 2009 the DOJ and DHHS established the Health Care Fraud Prevention and Enforcement Action Team (HEAT) to build and strengthen existing programs to combat Medicare and Medicaid fraud and to crack down on fraud perpetrators. HEAT efforts have included expansion of the DOJ-DHHS Medicare Fraud Strike Force that has been successful in fighting fraud. In 2011, HEAT coordinated the largest-ever federal health care fraud takedown, involving $530 million in fraudulent billing. It continues its efforts, which are outlined in annual reports issued by the DHHS Press Office.

Special Alerts, Bulletins, and Guidance Documents

Health care organizations and their staff should follow all special fraud alerts published by the OIG to alert the industry of specific patterns or trends related to fraudulent or abusive activities regarding the Medicare and Medicaid programs. Special advisory bulletins report industry practices and arrangements that may indicate fraud and abuse. Other guidance documents include updates, response letters, and alerts important to more specifically targeted matters. All notices are available at the OIG website and on their mailing list.

The OIG's Self-Disclosure Protocol (SDP) was originally established in 2006. It has been refined many times over the years, most recently in the ACA (2010). The SDP is a vehicle for providers and health care organizations to voluntarily disclose self-discovered evidence of potential fraud and work together with the OIG in resolving issues efficiently and fairly. The latest revision of this protocol streamlined the disclosure process and made the potential sanctions more proportionate with the disclosed violations.

BOX 3.5 Benefits of a Compliance Program

- Speed the claims processing cycle
- Optimize proper payment on claims
- Minimize billing mistakes
- Reduce the likelihood of a government audit
- Avoid conflict with various federal laws and statutes
- A good faith effort in maintaining compliance
- Create a culture of integrity

COMPLIANCE PROGRAMS

A compliance plan is a comprehensive set of policies, procedures, and guidelines designed to ensure that an organization conducts its business in accordance with applicable laws and regulations. The OIG offers compliance guidelines for various types of health care organizations such as physician groups, hospitals, and billing companies. These guidelines provide acceptable principles for business operations.

The OIG started publishing various compliance program guidelines in 1998. At that time the guidance recommended by the OIG was voluntary. It was provided as a way for health care organizations to effectively reduce the risk of legal action and create a good faith effort in combating fraud, waste, and abuse. Under the PPACA, mandatory compliance program requirements were implemented and became effective January 1, 2011, for Medicare Advantage (MA) and Medicare Part D programs. Under this legislation, the DHHS Secretary has the authority to define providers, suppliers, and health care organizations that must adopt a compliance plan.

The goal of a compliance plan is to prevent and reduce improper conduct. An effective program ensures proper billing practices and decreases the chance for fraud and abuse within a health care organization. The organization's governing authority should be knowledgeable about the contents of the plan and exercise reasonable oversight of its implementation and effectiveness, and high-level management should be assigned overall responsibility for the program (Box 3.5).

A well-designed compliance program can do the following:

- Speed the claims processing cycle
- Optimize proper payment or claims
- Minimize billing mistakes
- Reduce the likelihood of a government audit
- Avoid conflict with Stark laws and the Anti-Kickback Statute
- Show a good faith effort to submit claims appropriately
- Relay to staff that there is a duty to report mistakes and suspected or known misconduct

A health care organization's claims processing supervisor should research industry sector program guidance to help with specific concerns regarding the specialty or facility setting. Check the OIG website (https://oig.hhs.gov/compliance/compliance-guidance/index.asp) to view addenda, comments, and drafts of additional compliance guidance subjects.

Increased Productivity and Decreased Penalties With a Compliance Plan

The presence of an OIG compliance program can significantly lessen imposed penalties in the event of an OIG audit or other discovery of fraudulent billing activities. These policies and procedures can be found in the health care organization's policy and procedure (P&P) manual. Employees at every level of a health care organization can benefit from knowledge of P&P as they pertain to both HIPAA and OIG compliance guidelines.

Because health care organizations rely on the expertise of their billing and coding staff to process claims accurately and promptly, they also look to these staff members for advice and guidance. An insurance billing specialist will be expected to understand the complexities of the various laws and regulations governing the medical claims process.

Compliance plans effectively become a consensus among the players; providers, claims processing staff, and payers all agree to process claims in accordance with shared values. Consider the organization's OIG compliance program as a way to integrate regulatory requirements directly into claims processing procedures. OIG views the experienced billing specialists as the critical screen for the health care organization's claims. The common denominators in the key benefits identified by OIG are efficiency, consistency, and integrity.

Seven Basic Components of a Compliance Plan

OIG outlines the following seven components of an effective program guidance plan specifically for individual and small group physician practices:

- Conducting internal monitoring and auditing
- Implementing compliance and practice standards
- Designating a compliance officer or contact
- Conducting appropriate training and education
- Responding appropriately to detected offenses and developing corrective action
- Developing open lines of communication
- Enforcing disciplinary standards through well-publicized guidelines

Under the PPACA, these elements were adjusted as follows:

- Written policies, procedures and standards of conduct
- Compliance program oversight
- Training and education
- Open lines of communication
- Auditing, monitoring, and disclosure
- Consistent discipline
- Corrective actions

Written Policies, Procedures, and Standards of Conduct

Policies and procedures should be explained to new employees within the first 90 days of employment and then reviewed annually with the entire organization. They should be clearly written and explain expectations. They should detail the organization's commitment to ethical behavior and create an atmosphere of integrity from management down. Policies and procedures should be reviewed and updated at regular intervals.

Written standards and procedures address risk areas that a health care organization needs to monitor and follow. In addition to these risk areas, policies should be developed that address the following:

1. Definition of reasonable and necessary
2. Proper medical documentation
3. Corporate integrity (Stark Laws, Anti-Kickback Statute)
4. Federal sentencing guidelines
5. Record retention

A health care organization's P&P manual should be easily accessible to review the standards and protocol for these issues.

Compliance Program Oversight

The compliance officer is the key individual who oversees the organization's compliance program monitoring with the support of the compliance committee. The number of members on the compliance committee is not important; it is important to have a well-rounded committee drawing on staff members from many departments including human resources, claims auditing, billing, legal, and medicine.

The compliance committee acts as a review board. Committees may consist of provider-client staff and billing company staff or a combination of the provider-client, their practice manager, and the billing company staff. The committee, empowered by management, legitimizes the compliance program within the organization. In addition to possessing professional experience in claims processing and auditing, committee members are expected to use good judgment and high integrity to fulfill committee obligations. The compliance committee is tasked with developing and reviewing policies and procedures, training staff, and auditing and enforcing disciplinary standards.

Training and Education

Significant elements of an effective compliance program involve proper education and training of staff. Every employee and individual who interacts with the health care organization may be accountable for potential misconduct and should be considered in the organization's training sessions.

General compliance training sessions should be required at least annually. For staff members involved in coding and billing, a separate training session should be held to cover internal procedures, federal and state laws regarding fraud and abuse, and specific government and other payer reimbursement policies. Periodic professional courses in continuing education should be available to staff members as well as health care providers. Coding and billing personnel should receive training at least annually to remain updated on diagnostic and procedural codes for each year.

Effective training can reduce potential errors, penalties, and fines. An educated staff makes fewer errors and reduces the organization's risks.

Open Lines of Communication

Effective lines of communication provide a channel for employees to report suspected or known misconduct without immediately reporting to an external agency. In this way, the health care organization can resolve issues internally. Open door policies ensure an environment in which staff members feel secure to ask about the organization's existing P&P and to report questionable activities. Each employee should know the steps to take in reporting any suspicious business activity.

All health care employees should understand the organization's procedure for reporting misconduct. It is important that employees follow these guidelines to protect their reputation and credibility within the workplace. Depending on the size of the practice, the methods for contacting managerial staff may include anonymous telephone calls through a hotline or written report forms.

Auditing, Monitoring, and Disclosure

A comprehensive auditing and monitoring program will not eliminate misconduct within an organization. It will, however, minimize the risk of fraud and abuse by identifying the risk areas. The compliance officer, with the committee's assistance, should identify problem areas and have established auditing priorities and procedures as part of the organization's compliance program.

Auditing provides a systematic and objective review of a transaction. **Monitoring** is not as structured as an audit. It is more of a spot check for quality control. To determine areas that should be audited and monitored, a compliance committee should consider issues that have been reported to them. The OIG *Work Plan* is also a good place to start.

Special attention should be paid to the risk areas associated with claims submission and processing. Also, a thorough review of the organization's standards and written P&P should be conducted to ensure proper guidelines for complying with state and federal laws and insurance payer requirements.

A compliance program should allow an internal reporting of audit results. These are key to continued education within a health care organization. An audit will not necessarily yield errors. Positive feedback is equally important to staff and providers.

If compliance issues are uncovered during an audit, the health care organization should consider self-disclosure. The FCA allows for reduced damages should the violating person or organization furnish information on the violation within 30 days of discovery. To qualify under the self-disclosure guidelines, an organization needs to conduct a thorough investigation and take corrective action to terminate any improper conduct.

Consistent Discipline

Every health care organizations is made up of people, and people make mistakes. For this reason, health care organizations must have established disciplinary guidelines. These must be made well known to employees and other agents who contract with the organization. Employees all want to know what will happen if mistakes are made and what progressive forms of discipline await in situations involving misconduct. Disciplinary standards include the following:

- Verbal warning
- Written warning
- Written reprimand
- Suspension or probation
- Demotion
- Termination of employment
- Restitution of any damages
- Referral to federal agencies for criminal prosecution

Whether the misconduct was intentional or negligent, all levels of employees need to know what is expected of them. The health care organization must publish this information and distribute it to all employees.

When faced with the discovery of an offense or an error, inaction may be interpreted as indifference. This could jeopardize the reputation of the health care organization. The health care organization should have a process for investigating problems and taking necessary corrective action. A **corrective action plan** is a method to address detected offenses. Corrective action plans may include any of the above disciplinary actions as well as appropriate education and training to ensure the errors do not occur again.

Some issues that raise concern include the following:

- Significant changes in claims that are rejected
- Software edits that show a pattern of misuse of codes or fees
- An unusually high volume of charges, payments, or rejections
- Notices from insurance payers regarding claims submitted by the organization

Health care staff members should be encouraged to report concerns for any suspected or known misconduct, with an established chain of command to do so. Some incidences of misconduct may violate criminal, civil, or administrative law. If the situation warrants it, the compliance officer should report the misconduct promptly to the appropriate government authority.

Fraud and abuse should be reported. Contact the DHHS OIG as follows:

- Telephone hotline: 1-800-HHS-TIPS (1-800-447-8477)
- TTY: 1-800-377-4950
- Website: https://oig.hhs.gov/fraud/report-fraud/index.asp

Please note: Suspected fraud and abuse can no longer report fraud to the OIG via e-mail.

OIG COMPLIANCE PROGRAM GUIDELINES

The Office of the Inspector General has issued compliance program guidelines for various types of health care organizations. These are published in the *Federal Register*. Each outlines steps for creating an effective program, as well as addressing specific risk areas that each type of health care organization will want to focus on.

Individual and Small Group Physician Practices

All providers have a responsibility to make sure that claims submitted for their services are accurate. An effective compliance program will assist a physician practice in achieving this goal. A compliance program should complement patient care. The OIG outlines four specific areas of potential risk for physicians and small group practices. The guidelines can be read in their entirety in the *Federal Register*, Vol. 65, No. 194, October 5, 2000.

Coding and Billing

Coding and billing is one of the main areas of fraud investigations for small groups. Attention should be paid to proper health record documentation requirements and using appropriate diagnosis codes to reflect the need for services.

Specific risk areas identified by OIG include the following:

- Billing for items or services not rendered or not provided as claimed
- Submitting claims for equipment, medical supplies, and services that are not reasonable and necessary
- Double billing resulting in duplicate payment
- Billing for noncovered services as though covered
- Known misuse of provider identification numbers, which results in improper billing
- Unbundling, as in billing for each component of the service instead of billing or using an all-inclusive code
- Failure to use coding modifiers properly
- Clustering: reporting one level of service for all patient visits, regardless of the patient's presenting problem or the amount of work or time spent with the patient
- Upcoding the level of service provided: reporting a higher level of service for patient visits, regardless of the patient's presenting problem or the amount of work or time spent with the patient
- Undercoding a service provided: reporting a lower level of service for patient visits or submitting false representation of service provided

Reasonable and Necessary Services

Although the OIG does not want to dictate proper patient care, it does look at medical necessity in determining if treatment is appropriate. *Medical necessity* refers to the activities that are reasonable and appropriate based on the accepted clinical standard of care. Most insurance carriers will deny payment if they feel the service is not reasonable for the given medical condition. Documentation in the health record should support all clinical decisions.

Documentation

The OIG expects every physician to have timely, accurate, and complete documentation for each patient. The health record may be used to validate the appropriateness of treatment among other things. It must be legible and complete. If an encounter or treatment is not documented, it did not happen in the eyes of the insurance carrier.

Improper Inducements, Kickbacks, and Self-Referrals

All physicians should be aware of the federal and state laws that govern ethical practice. It is illegal to give or receive any type of remuneration for a referral. Remuneration can influence medical decision making, cause overuse of services and supplies, and increase the costs billed to government payers like Medicaid and Medicare. Specific attention should be given to the physician or group practice's relationship with hospitals, laboratories, pharmacies, suppliers, and vendors. Physicians should also be careful not to offer any inducements to patients. They should not routinely waive copays or deductibles.

Third-Party Medical Billing Companies

The OIG recognizes that health care organizations are increasingly relying on third-party billing companies. Some billing companies also provide coding services and other practice management services. Billing companies should familiarize themselves with the compliance guidelines for the type of health care entity they service. It is important that they promote a culture of compliance with regard to the prevention, detection, and resolution of any questionable practices. Risk areas include coding and billing, claims submission, credit balances, and integrity of data systems. The guidelines can be read in their entirety in the *Federal Register,* Vol. 63, No. 243, December 18, 1998.

Coding

As discussed earlier in this chapter, insurance claims require reporting of codes to describe what was wrong with the patient (diagnosis codes) and what services were provided to the patient (procedural codes). This will require someone who is involved in the health care organization to assign those codes, based on what the service provider has documented. Assignment of the codes may be done by the service provider, a certified coder, or another individual working for the health care organization. In some cases, coding may be performed by the third-party medical billing company. In addition to the coding and billing items listed in the individual and small group practices risk section, billing companies that offer coding services should also be aware of the following issues:

- Internal coding practices, including software and coding edits, should be reviewed to ensure they follow federal guidelines.
- Assumption coding should be avoided. A service or diagnosis should not be coded if the documentation does not support it.
- Documentation may be the service provider's responsibility, but coders should be aware of what is required for proper documentation and assist in educating the provider when needed. If documentation is not clear, the coder should query the provider.
- Claims should never be submitted for services provided by unqualified or unlicensed clinical personnel.
- All documentation must be available at the time of coding so that codes may be assigned as accurately as possible.
- Billing companies should be sure not to employ sanctioned individuals.
- Billing companies should promote the confidentiality of all medical, financial, and personal information in their possession.

Claims Submission

Policies and procedures should ensure the following:

- Proper and timely documentation is obtained before billing.
- Claims are only submitted when documentation supports the services.
- Diagnosis coding is based solely on documentation.
- Confusing or lacking documentation is verified with the provider.

- Compensation to coding and billing specialists should not provide incentive to upcode.
- Claims will undergo a pre- and postsubmission review.

Credit Balances

Credit balances occur when payments and allowances posted to a claim exceed the amount of the claim. This typically occurs when too much money has been paid by the insurance, the patient, or a combination of the two. It is the responsibility of both the health care organization and the billing company to have a system in place to accurately identify such overpayments in a timely manner. Refunds must be issued on a regular and timely basis.

Integrity of Data Systems

The health care industry relies on computer systems to transmit medical and billing information. Billing companies must have systems in place to not only back up data but also to prevent data corruption by outside sources such as hackers. The system should be checked regularly for viruses and monitored for unauthorized access and disclosures.

Hospitals

Over the last few decades, the ways in which hospitals provide and are reimbursed for services has changed. As a result, the OIG has published multiple guidelines for hospitals. The first publication was in the *Federal Register,* Vol. 63, No. 35, February 23, 1998. A supplemental guidance was published in the *Federal Register,* Vol. 70, No. 19, January 31, 2005. The OIG feels that compliance programs should lead the governing bodies of hospitals. These programs provide guidance to help them adhere to the regulatory laws of health care.

Hospitals have the same risks as those identified for other entities. They must ensure proper documentation, coding, and billing practices. They must adhere to all regulations pertaining to anti-kickbacks and self-referrals. They must be sure to properly refund credit balances. In addition to these, however, they face other risks.

- Hospitals are paid by Medicare for inpatient services through reporting of Medicare Severity Diagnosis-Related Groups (MS-DRGs), which will be discussed later in this textbook. **DRG creep** occurs when an inappropriate diagnosis-related group with a higher payment is attributed to a particular patient for inpatient coding. This is similar to upcoding.
- Outpatient services can be incorrectly billed for an inpatient. This creates a duplicate billing if these services are included in the hospital's inpatient payment through the Prospective Payment System.
- CMS requires institutional health care providers, such as hospitals, to submit annual **cost reports.** These contain information facility utilization data, costs and charges by cost center, and financial settlement data. False cost reports can be submitted to reflect higher operating costs. This also occurs when an institution shifts data from one area to another to show falsely inflated costs related to patient care.
- When a hospital bills for a discharge instead of a transfer, it commits fraud. Under Medicare guidelines, only the discharging hospital may report the full DRG. A transferring hospital must submit per diem charges instead. A per diem charge would be a "per day" charge. When hospitals discharge a patient, the patient's freedom of choice must be considered when referring them for rehabilitation, long-term care, home health care, or durable medical equipment.
- Excessive payments for medical directorships, low rent for office space, interest-free loans, and high payments in health care organization acquisitions can all spell kickback in an OIG investigation.
- Joint ventures and other business arrangements with suppliers, physicians, or health care organizations who are in a position to refer business to the hospital should be entered with care.
- Hospitals must avoid **patient dumping.** The phrase *patient dumping* was coined through the occurrence of private hospitals refusing to examine or treat the poor or uninsured in the emergency department and transferring them to public hospitals. The **Emergency Medical Treatment and Labor Act (EMTALA)** requires that anyone that comes to an emergency room be evaluated and stabilized regardless of their ability to pay. Uninsured patients with emergency medical conditions or in active labor cannot be turned away.

Hospital laboratories must also comply with laboratory guidelines and other legislation such as the **Clinical Laboratory Improvement Amendments (CLIA).** Every diagnostic test is categorized by its level of complexity. Under CLIA every laboratory is certified to be able to run a certain level of test. The goal of CLIA is to ensure quality laboratory tests regardless of the laboratory that runs them. CLIA is overseen by the **Occupational Safety and Health Administration (OSHA).** There are additional OIG compliance guidelines for home health care agencies, Medicare Part C carriers, clinical laboratories, nursing facilities, research programs, ambulance suppliers, and pharmaceutical manufacturers. These can be found on the OIG site at https://oig.hhs.gov/compliance/compliance-guidance/.

COMPLIANCE AS A CAREER

Compliance is a growing specialty in the health care field. Hospitals and large practices have compliance teams. Small groups and billing companies need someone to oversee their compliance programs. Even if a health care worker's job is not specifically focused on compliance, with training he or she can provide support and knowledge to the organization's compliance efforts. There are a few organizations that offer certification and training in compliance.

According to the AAPC's annual salary survey, a compliance credential was one of three credentials that earned significant salary increases in 2016. On average, salaries for those with the health care compliance certification (CPCO) credential earned 5.8% more in 2016 than in 2015, earning an average of approximately $75,000.

The AAPC offers a health care compliance certification as well as a CPCO preparation class. They also offer many compliance resources at https://www.aapc.com/healthcare-compliance/. The Health Care Compliance Association (HCCA) also offers a certification (CHC) as well as resources at https://www.hcca-info.org/default.aspx.

WHAT TO EXPECT FROM THE HEALTH CARE ORGANIZATION

Health care workers must be aware of the potential liabilities when submitting claims for payment that are deemed to be fraudulent or inappropriate by the federal or state government. The government may impose significant financial and administrative penalties when health care claims are not submitted appropriately, including criminal prosecution against the offending party. According to the OIG, fraud can result from deliberate unethical behavior or simply from mistakes and miscues that cause excessive reimbursement.

Billing specialists involved in the claims processing procedures in the health care organization should understand the importance and urgency in following the legal and ethical path when performing their duties. An honest mistake could lead to a situation that puts the health care organization at risk for investigation of fraud, waste, or abuse if it continues and is not corrected.

Although every health care organization or practice has different policies and procedures, each should have the following:

- An expectation that all employees will adhere to all laws and guidelines that regulate and pay for health care services
- Privacy/security/compliance officer (even if one person)
- A P&P manual
- Employee training and education (at least annually and whenever there are changes in business operations that affect staff members directly)

KEY POINTS

This is a brief chapter review of the key issues presented. To further enhance your knowledge of the technical subject matter, review the key terms and key abbreviations for this chapter by locating the meaning for each in the Glossary at the end of this text, which appears in a section before the Index.

1. The difference between fraud and abuse is that fraud can occur when deception is used in a claim submission to obtain payment from the payer. Individuals who knowingly, willfully, and intentionally submit false information to benefit themselves or others commit fraud. *Abuse* means incidents or practices by health care organizations, not usually considered fraudulent, that are inconsistent with accepted sound medical business or fiscal practices.
2. The Centers for Medicare and Medicaid Services, the Office of the Inspector General, and various other regulatory agencies oversee and investigate health care fraud and abuse.
3. The False Claims Act (1863) is the baseline legislation for health care fraud today.
4. Qui tam or whistleblower lawsuits are those in which an individual files a claim on behalf of the federal government. The whistleblower shares in any recovered funds.
5. Stark laws prohibit the submission of claims for services or referral of patients if the referring physician has a financial relationship with the entity who provides the service.
6. The Anti-Kickback Statute prohibits any type of gift, reward, or inducement for referrals.
7. RACs, ZPICs, MIPs, CERT, and HEAT are various types of audits aimed at recovering monies for government payers who have been fraudulently billed.
8. A compliance program is a set of policies, procedures, and guidelines designed to ensure that an organization conducts business in accordance with laws and regulations.
9. An effective compliance program has seven steps: written policies and procedures; program oversight; training and education; open lines of communication; auditing, monitoring and disclosure; consistent discipline; and corrective actions.
10. The OIG has published several compliance program guidelines for various types of health care organizations.

STUDENT ASSIGNMENT

- Study Chapter 3.
- Answer the fill-in-the-blank, multiple-choice, and true/false questions in the *Workbook* to reinforce the theory learned in this chapter and help prepare for a future test.
- Complete the assignments in the *Workbook* to give you experience in making decisions regarding situations of fraud, abuse, incidental disclosures, compliance violations, consents, or authorizations.
- Turn to the Glossary at the end of this text for a further understanding of the key terms and key abbreviations used in this chapter.

UNIT 2

Introduction to Health Insurance

4

Basics of Health Insurance

Cheryl Fassett

OBJECTIVES

After reading this chapter, you should be able to:

1. Describe the history of insurance in the United States.
2. Explain the reasons for the rising cost of health care.
3. Discuss how the Affordable Care Act reforms health care.
4. Discuss the legal principles of insurance and state the four concepts of a valid insurance contract.
5. Explain the difference between an implied and an expressed health care organization–patient contract and discuss different types of patients.
6. Discuss how insurance works and define common insurance terms.
7. List and describe the choices a person has when it comes to choosing and obtaining health insurance.
8. Describe the types of health insurance coverage, including federal, state, and private health insurance plans.
9. Explain the life cycle of an insurance claim from date of service to third-party payer processing and payment.
10. List the types of computerized signatures for documents and insurance claims.
11. Describe the proper information to post to the patient's financial account after claims submission and payment received.

KEY TERMS

accounts receivable management
Affordable Care Act
assignment
birthday rule
blanket contract
cancelable
capitation
claim
coinsurance
competitive medical plan
conditionally renewable
consumer directed health plan
contract
conversion privilege
coordination of benefits
copayment
cost sharing
daysheet
deductible
disability income insurance
electronic signature
emancipated minor
encounter form
Exchanges
exclusions
exclusive provider organization
expressed contract
fee-for-service
flexible spending account
guaranteed renewable
guarantor
Health Care and Education Reconciliation Act
health insurance
health maintenance organization
health reimbursement account
health savings account
implied contract
indemnity health insurance
independent or individual practice association
major medical
mandated benefits
Maternal and Child Health Program
Medicaid
medical savings account
medically necessary
Medicare
Medicare/Medicaid
noncancelable policy
nonparticipating physician or provider
optionally renewable
participating physician or provider
Patient Protection and Affordable Care Act
physician's representative
point-of-service plan
preauthorization
precertification
predetermination
preexisting conditions
preferred provider organization
premium
revenue cycle
State Children's Health Insurance Program
state disability insurance
TRICARE
Unemployment Compensation Disability
Veterans Health Administration (CHAMPVA)
workers' compensation insurance

KEY ABBREVIATIONS

ACA	FSA	MSA	SCHIP
A/R	HCERA	nonpar	SDHP
CDHP	HDHP	NPP	SDI
CHAMPVA	HMO	par	SHOP
CMP	HRA	PMS	SOF
COB	HSA	POS plan	UCD
COBRA copay	IPA	PPACA	VA
DOS	MCHP	PPO	WC
EPO	Medi-Medi	ROA	

HISTORY OF HEALTH INSURANCE IN THE UNITED STATES

Health insurance is a contract between a policyholder and a third-party payer or government program. It reimburses the policyholder for all or a portion of the cost of medical and/or preventive care on the basis of the contract purchased. Its main purpose is to help offset some of the high costs accrued during illness or when an injury has occurred.

To understand the current health care system, a billing specialist needs to understand the history of health care in the United States. The current health care system did not always exist.

Health care insurance originated in the mid-1800s in the United States with the Franklin Health Assurance Company of Massachusetts. It offered coverage for nonfatal injury in railroad and steamboat accidents. About 10 years later, the Travelers Insurance Company of Hartford marketed a plan that is similar to today's health insurance. In 1911 Montgomery Ward and Company offered benefits to its ill or injured employees. These commercial plans paid only for lost wages when an individual was sick or received an injury. This was the first group plan.

Only large employers offered health insurance to their employers before 1920. As doctors learned more about diseases and effective treatments and more people took advantage of new medical technology, the cost for health care increased. To help ease the burden of health care costs, Baylor Hospital in Dallas created a system that eventually became known as Blue Cross to help people pay their hospital bills. Its counterpart, Blue Shield started gaining recognition in the late 1930s as a way for doctors to secure payment for health care services. By the 1960s, the success of the Blue Cross and Blue Shield model encouraged other insurers to enter the health care market.

The shortage of labor during World War II also had an impact on the health care market. Employers began to offer health insurance as an added benefit to the employment package. Soon it was commonplace for employers to provide health insurance. Most private insurance companies sold policies that included hospital care, surgical fees, and health care organizations' services. In addition to those benefits, many plans began offering catastrophic coverage, preventive care, dental insurance, disability income insurance, and long-term or home health care insurance for the chronically ill, disabled, and developmentally disabled.

In 1965 federal legislation was passed to assist the elderly and the poor with their health insurance expenses. This led to the Medicare and Medicaid programs. Although both programs started small, expenditures in Medicare and Medicaid grew dramatically. They currently make up a large percentage of all health care expenses in the United States.

As additional benefits were offered by insurance carriers and the public used more health care services, medical costs and **premium** rates increased. Developing technologies also played a role. An increase in the aging population with more advanced health care needs has pushed health care spending even higher.

To deal with the rising costs of health care, the federal government adopted cost-containment legislation for the **Medicare, Medicaid,** and **TRICARE** programs. The concept of managed care began in the 1930s when Kaiser Industries developed a prepaid, integrated health care insurance model for their employees. In the 1980s, insurance carriers began to see the benefits of managed care. Managed care insurance carriers are more involved in health care decisions such as how much care a patient will receive and who will provide it. This was recognized as a method to help control rising health care expenditures. As a result, many new types of insurance plans arose to control the cost of medical care and help those who could not afford insurance.

HEALTH CARE REFORM

Over the past 75 years, leaders of the United States, from President Roosevelt to President Trump, have announced reforms of the health care system. A major restructuring of the United States health care system was necessary during the 1990s for the following reasons:

- A growing percentage of Americans were not covered by private or government insurance.
- Employers had to pay rising health care premiums and did not want to cut wages to cover these costs.
- Government needed to reduce the deficit by controlling increases in the Medicare and Medicaid programs.
- Physicians and hospital costs soared due to inflation, high-tech equipment, expensive medications, and so on.
- The health care system was riddled with inefficiency and fraud.
- Patients overused health care services.

On March 23, 2010, under President Obama, the Patient Protection and Affordable Care Act (PPACA) was signed into law. The related Health Care and Education Reconciliation Act (HCERA), which modifies certain provisions of PPACA, was signed into law on March 30, 2010. These two laws together are commonly referred to as the Affordable Care Act (ACA) or Obamacare. The ACA brought sweeping health insurance reforms. It holds insurance companies accountable, lowers costs, guarantees choice, and enhances the quality of health care for all Americans. Implementation of the ACA began in 2010 and will continue through 2020 (Table 4.1).

The goal of the ACA was to make health care available and affordable for the 32 million Americans who did not have health insurance. The plan expects to provide coverage to 94% of Americans. The ACA provides tax cuts for the middle class and aims to reduce premiums for families and small business.

Individual Mandate

The ACA includes an individual mandate, which requires most Americans to have health insurance coverage or face a penalty. Because of this, the constitutionality of the Act was challenged in March 2012. On June 28, 2012, the Supreme Court of the United States upheld the PPACA in its entirety.

As a result of this mandate, if an individual does not have health insurance, he or she will pay a tax penalty of $95 per individual or 1% of taxable income, whichever is greater, for 2014. In 2015, the fine rose to $325 per individual or 2% of taxable income, and 2016 saw an increase to $695 per individual or 2.5% of income. For every year after 2016 the government must refigure the fine based on a cost-of-living adjustment.

Health Benefit Exchanges

A primary goal of the ACA was to make health care cheaper and easier to access for the uninsured population. To address this, a key provision of the ACA insurance reform was the creation of Exchanges. An Exchange is an organized marketplace where uninsured individuals and small-business owners can find all the qualified private health plans available in their area. Exchanges were created to lower health care costs by creating a competitive regional private insurance market. Exchanges are administered by the Department of Health and Human Services (DHHS) and Centers for Medicaid and Medicare Services (CMS) along with nonprofit organizations. Small Business Health Options Program (SHOP) Exchanges serve a similar function for small employers and the self-employed. The Exchanges first opened on January 1, 2014.

The Exchanges offer a central site for researching, comparing, and purchasing health insurance coverage. They make the process of finding a health insurance policy easier and more efficient. Exchanges create larger individual and small employer insurance pools. In doing this, they provide individuals and small employers with access to the policies that were written using the ACA's uniform set of national rules.

Individuals and small businesses of up to 100 employees can purchase qualified coverage through exchanges and take advantage of federal subsidies. States are permitted to allow businesses with more than 100 employees to purchase coverage in the SHOP Exchange beginning in 2017. Through establishment of Health Benefit Exchanges, millions of Americans and small businesses have access to more choices of affordable coverage. By holding insurance companies accountable to keep premiums down and prevent insurance industry abuses, the ACA will end discrimination against Americans with preexisting conditions.

The Future of the Affordable Care Act

As discussed, the ACA has affected health care in many positive ways. However, as with any act of legislation, there have been people who opposed the ACA from the start. Some have argued that the government should not be allowed to force people to buy insurance. Some feel that the health plans that are offered on the Exchanges and through employers are not actually "affordable." With the election of President Trump, efforts began to try to repeal or replace the ACA. At this time the future of it is unclear.

LEGAL PRINCIPLES OF INSURANCE

The role of a medical insurance billing specialist is to complete the insurance claim accurately, assist in claims submission, and obtain accurate and timely reimbursement. However, before developing the skill of coding and completing insurance claim forms, it is necessary to understand how insurance works. Legal situations occur daily in the performance of these job duties. They involve confidentiality of health records, accurate insurance claim transmission, fraud and abuse issues, credit and collection laws, and so on. A billing specialist cannot escape liability by pleading ignorance. It cannot be overemphasized that keeping up to date on health care plan policies and procedures is essential. Most legal issues of private health insurance claims fall under civil law. Issues with the Medicare, Medicaid, and TRICARE programs fall under federal laws. The private health care insurance industry is regulated by state law and is not considered a federally regulated industry.

Insurance Contracts

The first concept a billing specialist needs to be familiar with is the insurance contract or policy. A contract is a legal and binding written document that exists between two or more parties. Essentially, any agreement between two or more persons that is enforceable by law is considered a contract. There is no standard health insurance contract. Individuals who take out a policy receive an original document composed by the insuring company.

The following four items are part of a valid insurance contract:

1. The person must be a mentally competent adult and not under the influence of drugs or alcohol when signing the contract.
2. The insurance company must make the offer (the signed application) and the applicant must accept the offer (issuance of the policy), without concealment or misrepresentation of facts on the application.
3. An exchange of value (the first premium payment) submitted with the application, known as a *consideration*, must be present.

TABLE 4.1 Timeline for Implementation of the Affordable Care Act From 2010 to 2020

Year	Timeline
2010	• Implementation of rules to prevent insurance companies from denying coverage to children with preexisting conditions. • Prohibits insurance companies from dropping coverage because of technical errors in insurance contracts when patients get sick. • Prohibits insurance companies from imposing lifetime dollar limits on essential benefits. • Regulates annual limits on insurance coverage. • Provides consumers with an easy way to appeal to their insurance company and to an outside board if the company denies coverage of a claim. • Creates an easy-to-use website where consumers can compare health insurance coverage options. • Tax credits to small businesses that provide insurance benefits to their workers. • Relief for seniors who hit the Medicare prescription drug "doughnut hole." • New insurance plans must cover certain preventive services without cost-sharing (that is, deductibles, copays, or coinsurance). • A prevention and public health fund to invest in proven prevention public health programs. • Further crack down on health care fraud through new resources and screening procedures for health care organizations. • Access to insurance for uninsured Americans with preexisting conditions. • Extends coverage for young adults. • Provided coverage for early retirees. • Rebuilds the primary care workforce. • Holds insurance companies accountable for unreasonable rate hikes. • Allows states to cover more people on Medicaid through additional federal funding. • Provides payments for rural health care organizations.
2011	• Provides prescription drug discounts. • Covers free preventive care for seniors through annual wellness visits and personalized prevention plans. • Improves health care quality and efficiency. • Improves care for seniors after they leave the hospital. • Provides for new innovations to bring down costs. • Increased access to services at home and in the community. • Strengthens community health centers. • Brings down health care premiums. • Addresses overpayments to big insurance companies and strengthens Medicare Advantage.
2012	• Links payment to quality outcomes. • Encourages integrated health systems through Accountable Care Organizations. • Reduces paperwork and administrative costs by implementation of electronic health records. • Helps understand and fight health disparities through collection of racial, ethnic, and language data. • Provides new voluntary options for long-term care insurance.
2013	• Improves preventive health coverage through additional funding to state Medicaid programs. • Expands authority to bundle payments and pay health care organizations at a flat rate for an episode of care. • Increases Medicaid payments for primary care doctors. • Provides additional funding for the State Children's Health Insurance Program.
2014	• Eliminates discrimination as a result of preexisting conditions or gender. • Eliminates annual limits on insurance coverage. • Ensures coverage for individuals participating in clinical trials. • Makes care more affordable. • Establishes Health Insurance Exchanges. • Creates small business tax credits. • Increases access to Medicaid. • Promotes individual responsibility. • Ensures free choice through establishment of health insurance exchanges.
2015	• Pays health care organizations based on value, not volume. Health care organizations receive higher payments based on the quality of care they provide. • Annual health insurance industry fees will be imposed on health insurance companies to fund some of the provisions of the Affordable Care Act. The fees continue to increase yearly until 2018.
2016	• States will be permitted to form health care choice compacts and allow insurers to sell policies in any state participating in the compact. • Reduces Medicare payments to certain hospitals for hospital-acquired conditions by 1%.
2018	• Provides for a 40% excise tax to be imposed on high-cost group health plans.
2020	• Eliminates Medicare Part D (doughnut hole) coverage gap.

Data from https://obamacarefacts.com/health-care-reform-timeline.

4. A legal purpose must exist, which is an insurable interest in the case of a health insurance policy. This means that the policyholder expects to continue in good health but the insurance policy will provide something of value if an accident or illness strikes.

A policy can be challenged and coverage may not be in effect if the purchaser of the insurance policy or subscriber makes a fraudulent statement. After a policy has been in force for 2 years (3 years in some states), it may not be challenged. If a policy is **guaranteed renewable,** the insurer is obligated to continue coverage as long as premiums are paid.

HEALTH CARE ORGANIZATION–PATIENT CONTRACTS AND FINANCIAL OBLIGATION

Implied or Expressed Contracts

A health care organization and its staff must be aware of the health care organization's obligations to each patient and liabilities in regard to service, as well as the patient's responsibilities to the health care organization. The health care organization–patient contract begins when the health care organization accepts the patient and agrees to treat him or her. This action can be either an implied or an expressed contract. An **implied contract** is created by the actions of the parties involved. It is not written or spoken. For example, if Mary Johnson goes to Dr. Doe's office and Dr. Doe provides a medical service to her, this is an implied contract. If the patient is unconscious when treatment is rendered, treatment is based on an implied-in-fact contract. An **expressed contract** can be verbal or written. However, most health care organization–patient contracts are implied.

Self-Pay Patients

For patients who do not have health insurance, the contract for treatment is between the health care organization and the patient. The patient is liable for the entire bill and is considered a self-pay patient.

Guarantor

A **guarantor** is a person who accepts treatment or signs a form agreeing to pay. This creates an expressed contract (Fig. 4.1). Usually a patient of legal age (18 or 21, depending on state law) is his or her own guarantor. If the patient is a child of a divorced parent, the custodial parent bears the responsibility of the child's medical expenses unless the divorce decree states otherwise. An adoptive parent may be the custodial parent or guarantor and therefore solely liable for the child's bill. A father is usually responsible for his children's debts if they are minors and are not emancipated.

Emancipated Minor

An **emancipated minor** is a person younger than 18 years of age who:

- Lives independently,
- Is totally self-supporting,
- Is married or divorced,
- Is a parent even if not married,
- Is in the military and possesses decision-making rights, or
- Is a college student living away from home, even when financially dependent on parents.

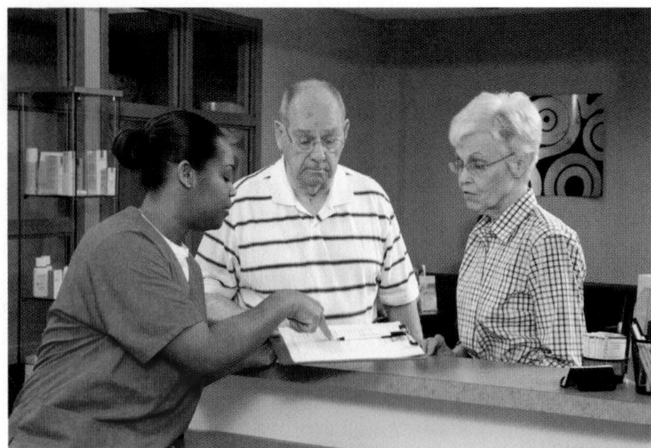

Fig. 4.1 Receptionist explaining where a guarantor's signature goes on a patient registration form for the medical services rendered to a family member.

Parents are not liable for the medical expenses incurred by an emancipated minor. The patient record should contain the minor's signed statement that he or she is emancipated.

Employment and Disability Examinations

When an employer requests an examination for employment or an insurance company requests an examination for a disability claim, the health care organization's contract is with the insurance carrier, not the patient. Because the patient is not seeking the medical service or treatment, the organization does not owe a duty of care to the person being examined.

Workers' Compensation Patients

Workers' compensation (**WC**) cases involve a person being injured on the job. These cases may be referred to as industrial accidents or illnesses. In these types of cases, the contract exists between the health care organization and the insurance company. When there is a dispute as to whether the injured party was hurt at work, a Patient Agreement form must be signed by the patient who agrees to pay the health care organization's fees if the case is declared to be non–work related.

THE INSURANCE POLICY

Insurance policies are complex and contain a great deal of language that is difficult to understand. This can cause misunderstanding by patients or anyone trying to obtain information from the policy. Basic health insurance coverage includes benefits for hospital, surgical, and other medical expenses.

Major medical benefits contracts are designed to offset large medical expenses caused by prolonged illness or serious injury. Some of these policies include coverage for extended care or skilled nursing health care organization benefits.

In a health insurance policy, the insured is known as a subscriber, member, policyholder, or recipient and may not necessarily be the patient seen for the medical service. The subscriber may or may not be the guarantor. The insured is the individual or organization protected in case of loss under the terms of an insurance policy. In group insurance, the employer is considered the insured and the employees are the risks. However, when completing an insurance claim form, the covered employee is listed as the insured.

A policy might also include *dependents* of the insured. Generally, this term refers to the spouse and children of the insured but under some contracts, parents, other family members, and domestic partners may be covered as dependents. Under the ACA, health plans must allow employees to keep their children on their plans until age 26.

Policy Application

Before a policy is issued, the insurance company decides whether it will enter into a contract with the applicant. Information is obtained about the applicant so that the company can decide whether to accept the risk. Generally the application form has two sections: the first part contains basic information about the application, and the second part concerns the health of the individual.

An insurance policy is a legally enforceable agreement. If a policy is issued, the applicant becomes part of the insurance plan. The policy becomes effective only after the company offers the policy and the person accepts it and then pays the initial premium. If a premium is paid at the time the application is submitted, the insurance coverage can be put into force before the policy is delivered. Depending on the laws in some states, the applicant also can have temporary conditional insurance if the agent issues a specific type of receipt.

Policy Renewal Provisions

Health insurance policies may have renewal provisions that state the circumstances under which the company may refuse to renew, may cancel coverage, or may increase the premium. It is important for the insurance billing specialist to understand that a patient's coverage may change from appointment to appointment. It is always a good routine to verify insurance information each time the patient comes for an appointment. A billing specialist may check **eligibility** verification to see if the patient is a member of the insurance plan and that the member identification number is correct. This may seem redundant but it avoids a delay in payment.

In private health insurance, there are five classifications of renewal provisions:

1. A **cancelable** policy grants the insurer the right to cancel the policy at any time and for any reason. The insurance company notifies the insured that the policy is canceled and refunds any advance premium the policyholder has paid. In some states, this type of policy is illegal.
2. In an **optionally renewable** policy, the insurer has the right to terminate coverage on the premium or anniversary date. The insurer may not cancel the policy at any time in between.
3. **Conditionally renewable** policies grant the insurance company a limited right to refuse to renew a health insurance policy at the end of a premium payment period. Reasons stated in the policy may relate to age, employment status, or both but may not relate to the insured's health status.
4. The guaranteed renewable classification is desirable because the insurer is required to renew the policy as long as premium payments are made. However, these policies often have age limits.
5. In a **noncancelable policy,** the insurer cannot increase premium rates and must renew the policy until the insured reaches the age specified in the contract. Some disability income policies have noncancelable terms.

Policy Terms

To keep the insurance in force, a person must pay a monthly, quarterly, or annual fee called a premium. If the premium is not paid, a grace period of 10 to 30 days is usually given before insurance coverage ceases.

Most policies have a **deductible,** which is a specific amount of money that must be paid each year before the policy benefits begin. Generally, the higher the deductible, the lower the cost of the policy. Most policies also have a **cost-sharing** requirement. This means the insured will assume a percentage of the fee called **coinsurance** (for example, 20%) or pay a specific dollar amount called a **copayment or copay** (for example, $5 or $10) for covered services.

Routinely waiving deductibles and copayments is fraudulent because by agreeing to participate with an insurance, the health care organization has agreed to accept a patient portion. The federal government can assess penalties for not collecting coinsurance for patients seen under the Medicare program. Generally, deductibles, coinsurance, and copayments should be collected at the time of service. The Medicare program is an exception to this rule. It does not recommend collecting the deductible in advance from the beneficiary.

A provider may consider writing off a portion of the amount owed by the patient in cases of financial hardship. It is good practice to get a patient's request for this consideration in writing. Additional documentation should be kept on file to prove the patient's financial status.

Health insurance policies define an accident as an unforeseen and unintended event. Some policies cover accidents that occur from the first day the policy is in force. Others may contain an elimination period or a waiting period before benefits for illness or accident become payable.

Generally, it is the patient's responsibility to give a written notice of claim to the insurance company within a certain time limit. However, some insurance carriers and Medicare guidelines require that the provider of service be obligated to submit the claim. Usually as a courtesy, the claim is filed for the patient by the health care organization.

The insurance billing specialist must be able to abstract proper information from the patient record, which is used to code the diagnoses and services rendered, to complete an insurance claim form, to make entries to a patient's financial accounting record, and to follow up on unpaid claims. If any one of these procedures is not done properly, the third-party payer may not pay the claim correctly. Following up on unpaid claims is done by contacting the claims representative, called a claims adjudicator or an adjuster.

EXAMPLE 4.1 Coordination of Benefits for Dual Coverage Case

Mr. Smith has Insurance A and Insurance B. The claim is for $100. The claim is sent to Insurance A. Insurance A allows $80 for the procedure and pays $80. The claim is then sent to Insurance B. Insurance B also allows $80 for the procedure. The claim that was sent to Insurance B was not for $100 but for the remaining $20. The $20 is within the amount allowed by Insurance B; therefore Insurance B pays the $20. Some carriers try to play by their own rules by stating that because Insurance A paid $80 and the $80 equals the amount Insurance B pays, Insurance B will pay no more for the claim. These rules were established by the National Association of Insurance Commissioners and approved by every State Insurance Commissioner. Therefore be observant of insurance claims like this.

Coordination of Benefits

A **coordination of benefits (COB)** statement is included in most policies and contracts with health care organizations. When the patient has more than one insurance policy, insurance companies must coordinate the reimbursement of benefits to determine which carrier is going to be the primary payer and which carrier is the secondary payer. This prevents the duplication or overlapping of payments for the same medical expense. The combination of payments from the primary and secondary carriers cannot be more than the amount of the health care organization's charges (Example 4.1).

Carriers may pend or delay a claim, stating they are attempting to coordinate benefits with the other carrier. This process can be time consuming and may take 90 days or more to resolve. A billing specialist should be diligent in following up on this situation so that the stalled cash flow issue can be resolved. In some situations, the patient ultimately may be responsible for the bill; if the patient understands that, they will pay sooner and resolve the account balance quicker.

Birthday Rule

The **birthday rule** is an informal rule that the health insurance industry has widely adopted for the COBs when children are listed as dependents on two parents' health plans. Under the birthday rule, the health plan of the parent whose birthday comes first in the calendar year is designated as the primary plan. This applies to the month and day only, not the year of birth. If both mother and father have the same birthday, the plan of the person who has had coverage longer is the primary payer. According to the National Association of Insurance Commissioners, the birthday rule is not insurance law. Some insurance plans do not follow these customs and it may be necessary to contact the plan for confirmation.

In cases of divorce, remember it is not the health care organization's responsibility to enforce family court laws. The divorce decree is between the parents of the child. Have the parent accompanying the child pay the bill at the time of service. The responsible party can reimburse him or her. If a copy of the court decision is presented, bill the insurance of the parent deemed responsible.

General Policy Limitations

Health insurance policies may contain **exclusions** or limitations of the policy. Exclusions are services that are never covered by the health insurance policy. These exclusions are outlined in the insurance policy. They may include items such as acupuncture, eyeglasses, contact lenses, dental treatment or surgery, services related to sex transformations, and cosmetic and aesthetic treatments. Most insurance policies also have limitations for covered services that are not deemed medically necessary.

Medically necessary is defined as accepted health care services and supplies that are appropriate for the evaluation and treatment of an injury, illness, or disease and its symptoms. The concept of medical necessity is based on the accepted standards of care. For example, a patient may request to have an electrocardiogram (ECG) performed because he or she has a family history of heart disease. However, the insurance may not pay for the service unless the patient presents with shortness of breath, chest pain, or other signs or symptoms that may indicate medical necessity for the procedure to be performed.

In the past, insurance companies issued policies that did not provide benefits for conditions that existed and were treated before the policy was issued. These are called **preexisting conditions.** The ACA prohibited insurers from denying coverage or charging higher premiums to any person with preexisting conditions.

Mandated benefits are state and/or federal laws that require coverage for treatment of specific health conditions for some categories of dependents, such as children placed for adoption. Health care benefits may be mandated by state law, federal law, or in some cases both. For example, under the Newborns' and Mothers' Health Protection Act of 1996, health plans may not limit benefits for any length of hospital stay related to childbirth for the mother or newborn child. Additionally, there is a federal mandate that requires health plans to provide someone who is receiving benefits related to a mastectomy with coverage for reconstruction of the breast. The Americans with Disabilities Act (ADA) requires insurance companies to provide the same benefits to disabled and nondisabled individuals with regard to premiums, deductibles, and limits on coverage.

Case Management Requirements

Many private third-party payers have certain requirements that must be met before they approve hospital admissions, inpatient or outpatient surgeries, and elective procedures. First, eligibility requirements must be obtained. These are conditions that must be met before the patient receives benefits under a specific insurance plan or government program. The carrier can refuse to pay part of or the entire fee if these requirements are not met.

Precertification refers to discovering whether a treatment such as surgery, hospitalization, or tests is covered under a patient's contract. **Preauthorization** relates not only to whether a service or procedure is covered but also to finding out whether it is medically necessary. **Predetermination** means discovering the maximum dollar amount that the carrier will pay for surgery, consulting services, radiology procedures, and so on.

A health care organization should obtain precertification or predetermination when a procedure is tentatively scheduled.

COLLEGE CLINIC
4567 Broad Avenue
Woodland Hills, XY 12345-0000

Phone: 555/486-9002 **Fax: 555/590-2189**

Insurance Precertification Form

Date: 5/4/XX
To: Insurance Carrier Cal-Net Care From: Janet Office Mgr.
Address 9900 Baker Street
Los Angeles, CA 90067

Check those that apply: Admission certification ✓ Outpatient ___ Inpatient ✓
Surgery certification ✓ Emergency situation ✓

Patient's name Ronald Stranton Date of Birth: 4-14-49
Patient's address 639 Cedar Street Sex: Male ✓ Female ___
Woodland Hills, XY 12345 Social Security No. 527-XX-7250
Insured's Name Same Policy Group ID No. A59
Insured's Address ___ Employer: Aerostar Aviation

Treating physician Clarence Cutler, M.D. NPI #: 430 500 47XX
Primary Care Physician Gerald Practon, M.D. NPI #: 462 7889 7XX

Name of Hospital College Hospital Admission Date: 5/4/XX
Estimated Length of Stay: 3-5 d
Admitting Diagnosis Volvulus Diagnosis Code: 560.2
Complicating conditions to substantiate need for inpatient hospitalization
Complete bowel obstruction
Date current illness or injury began 5/2/XX
Procedure/surgery to be done Reduction of Volvulus Procedure code 44050

Second opinion needed Yes ___ No ✓ Date performed ___

Telephone precertification: Emergency Cert. 5/4/XX
Name of representative certifying McKenzie Kwan
Direct-dial telephone number of representative 1-800-463-9000 ext. 227

Reason(s) for denial ___
Certification approved Yes ✓ No ___ Certification approval No. 69874
Authorization for services Yes ✓ No ___ Authorization No. 69874E

Note: The information contained in this facsimile message is confidential and privileged information intended only for the use of the individual or entity named above. If the reader of this message is not the intended recipient, you are hereby notified that any dissemination, distribution, or copying of this communication is strictly prohibited. If you have received this communication in error, please immediately notify me by telephone and return the original facsimile to me via the U.S. Postal Service. Thank you.

Fig. 4.2 Insurance precertification form. This form can be faxed to the insurance company or used when telephoning to obtain approval for hospitalization under a patient's insurance policy or managed care plan.

The information that may be required to obtain precertification approval by fax or telephone is shown in Fig. 4.2. A form similar to the one shown in Fig. 4.3 can be used to obtain predetermination by mail. Preauthorization forms can also be used to document the information received when verifying the patient's insurance coverage by telephone. It should become part of the patient's record and be used for reference when billing future insurance claims.

After the information is received from the third-party payer, give the patient an estimate of fees for the proposed surgery; state how much the insurance is expected to pay, and make the patient aware of any balance amounts that may be due by him or her. It is further recommended that the patient sign a statement that he or she is aware of his or her responsibility and agrees to pay it on receipt of the bill. An example of suggested wording for a letter is given in Fig. 4.4. This written estimate makes collection quicker and easier.

CHOICE OF HEALTH INSURANCE

A person can obtain health insurance through a group plan or an individual contract. Any insurance plan issued directly to an individual and his or her dependents is called an individual contract. Usually this type of policy has a higher premium and often

COLLEGE CLINIC
4567 Broad Avenue
Woodland Hills, XY 12345-0001

Phone: 555/486-9002 **Fax: 555/487-8976**

INSURANCE PREDETERMINATION FORM

Perry Cardi, MD
Physician

Patient: Leslee Austin
Address: 209 Refugio Road
City Woodland Hills State XY
Social Security # 629-XX-9260
Insurance Company American Insurance
Insurance Co. Address 4040 Broadway Ave
Valley Vista, XY 12345
Policy holder Leslee Austin
Relationship to insured: Self X Spouse ___ Child ___ Other ___
Type of coverage: HMO X PPO ___ 80/20 ___ 70/30 ___ Other ___
Procedure/Service Cardioversion (CPT 92960)
Diagnosis Atrial fibrillation (ICD–9–CM 427.31)

Telephone # (555) 486-8452
Date of Birth 04-07-44
ZIP 12345-0001
Accident Yes ___ No X
Member # Am 45692
Group # 123P
Telephone # (555) 238-5000

BENEFITS:
Coverage effective date: From 02/01/XX To 01/31/XX
Preexisting exclusions: Lupus erythematosus
Major medical Yes X No ___
Deductible Yes ___ No X Amount $___
Per family: Yes ___ No X Amount $___
Deductible paid to date: Amount $___
Out of pocket expense limit: Amount $___
Per: ___

Maximum benefit or benefit limitation: $1,000,000 lifetime
Second opinion requirements: Yes ___ No X
Precertification/Preauthorization Yes X No ___
Reference # 432786
Authorized by: Lucille Vasquez

COVERAGE:

Procedures/Services	YES	NO	COVERAGE DETAILS AND LIMITS
Office visits	X		Physical exam; one per year
Consultations	X		
ER visits	X		
X-ray	X		
Laboratory	X		Need authorization
Office surgery	X		Need authorization
Hospital surgery	X		
Anesthesia	X		Need authorization
DME	X		

Physician payment schedule: RVS ___ RBRVS ___ UCR ___ Other X

Payment sent to: Provider X Patient ___ Time limit after submission? 30 days
Verification by: Karen Reynolds Date: 07-14-XX

Fig. 4.3 Insurance predetermination form. This form can be sent to the insurance company to find out the maximum dollar amount that will be paid for primary surgery, consulting services, postoperative care, and so on.

the benefits are less than those obtainable under a group health insurance plan. Sometimes this is called personal insurance.

A group contract is any insurance plan that covers a group of employees or other group and their eligible dependents. They are insured under a single policy issued to their employer or leader. Individual certificates are given to each insured individual or family unit. A group policy usually provides better benefits and offers lower premiums than individual contracts. The coverage for each person in the group is the same. A new employee must sign a waiver if he or she declines enrollment. Under the PPACA, employers may change the kind of medical benefits they offer their employees. For example, an employer may choose to increase copayments and deductibles or choose a plan that offers fewer benefits.

Some individuals can obtain comprehensive group coverage through plans sponsored by the professional organizations to which they belong. This is called a **blanket contract.**

Conversion Privilege

If the person leaves the employer or organization or the group contract is terminated, the insured may continue coverage under an individual policy if the group contract has a

COLLEGE CLINIC
4567 Broad Avenue
Woodland Hills, XY 12345-0000

Phone: 555/486-9002 **Fax: 555/487-8976**

Current date

Patient's name
Address
City, State, ZIP code

Dear

This letter gives you an estimate of the fees for your proposed surgery. Verification of coverage and benefit information has been obtained from your insurance company. Listed are your benefits for the proposed surgical expenses and the estimated balance after your insurance carrier pays.

Surgical procedure: Craniotomy
Date of surgery: February 21, 20XX
Name of hospital: College Hospital
Hospital address: 4500 Broad Ave., Woodland Hills, XY 12345

		Insurance pays	Estimated balance
Surgeon's fee	2548.09	1344.24	1203.85
Preoperative visit			
Preoperative tests			

You have a policy deductible of $1000 which ___ has ✓ has not been met.

The surgery requires the use of an anesthesiologist, assistant surgeon, and a pathologist. These physicians will bill you separately for their services. The hospital will also bill you separately.

This office will file your insurance claim for the surgical procedure, so the insurance payment should come directly to us. If the insurance carrier sends you the payment, then you are responsible to get the payment to this office within five days. Your balance after surgery should be approximately $1203.85. You are responsible for any remaining balance after our office receives the insurance payment.

This notice gives our estimation of the balance for which you will be responsible. Please sign below to indicate you have received and understand this notification.

Signature Date

Thank you for choosing our medical practice. If you have any questions, please call me.

Sincerely,

Karen Martinez, CMA
Administrative Medical Assistant

Fig. 4.4 Sample letter to a patient supplying an estimate of the fees for proposed surgery.

conversion privilege. Usually, conversion from a group policy to an individual policy increases the premium and could reduce the benefits.

Cobra

The Consolidated Omnibus Budget Reconciliation Act (COBRA) of 1985 requires employers with 20 or more workers to extend group health insurance coverage in light of certain events. Coverage is extended to the employee and his or her dependents at group rates for up to 18 months. Qualifying events include being laid off, reduction in hours, or voluntary or involuntary termination. In the event of the death of a covered employee, a divorce from a covered employee, or an employee becoming entitled to Medicare, the extension of coverage for the spouse or dependents may be extended to 36 months. In all these situations the former employee, the spouse, or the dependent is responsible for paying the premiums for the coverage.

Medical Savings Accounts

A medical savings account (MSA) is a type of tax-free savings account that allows individuals and their employers to set aside money to pay for health care expenses. An employer can set up an MSA for his or her employees and make an annual contribution to the MSA, which is tax deductible for both employer and employee. MSA balances can be carried over from year to year. MSAs are portable, allowing individuals to take their MSA with them when they retire, change jobs, or relocate. When health care services are provided, the patient files a claim with the MSA to receive reimbursement and uses the explanation of benefits (EOB) from the insurance company as documentation. Medicare beneficiaries are eligible to enroll in a similar tax-advantaged savings account, which may be referred to as a Medicare medical savings account.

Health Savings Accounts

The Medicare Reform Act was signed into law in December 2003, giving Americans a tool for defraying medical costs called health savings accounts (HSAs). HSAs are open to anyone younger than 65 years of age who enrolls in a high-deductible health plan. Employers and/or employees may fund an HSA up to a set Internal Revenue Service (IRS)–mandated dollar amount each year. In 2017 this amount was $3400 for a single insured plan and $6750 for a family plan. The IRS also sets annual out-of-pocket expenses, including deductibles and copayments. For 2017, for example, these may not exceed $6550 for single coverage and $13,100 for family coverage. If a high-deductible health plan has a higher out-of-pocket maximum, it may not be an HSA-eligible plan. These accounts are a tax-favored savings plan in which a working person can deposit money in an HSA and deduct the amount of the deposits from taxable income. Withdrawals from HSAs are tax-free when used for qualifying medical expenses. Money left unspent in an HSA may be rolled over year after year.

Health Reimbursement Arrangements

An alternative plan is a health reimbursement account (HRA). HRAs are typically offered in tandem with high-deductible plans. The employer owns the account and only the employer is eligible to make contributions. The employer is allowed to determine contribution limits and define covered expense. Employers can determine whether the balance can be rolled over from one year to the next. If the employee leaves, the money remains with the employer.

Flexible Spending Accounts

Another option is a health care flexible spending account (FSA). FSAs are employer sponsored. They allow a specific amount of wages to be put aside for qualified medical expenses and dependent care. In 2017 an individual could put up to $2600 in an FSA each year, with the cap increasing by the annual inflation rate in subsequent years. Money deducted from an employee's paycheck and deposited into an FSA is not subject to payroll taxes, resulting in substantial payroll tax savings. Before the Affordable Care Act, one disadvantage of using an FSA was that funds not used by the end of the plan year were lost to the employee, known as the "use it or lose it" rule. Under the terms of the ACA and effective in 2013 plan years, the employee is allowed to carry over up to $500 per year to the following year without losing the funds.

High-Deductible Health Plans

High-deductible health plans (HDHPs) give tax advantages that assist in saving for future medical expenses. They have annual out-of-pocket limits and higher annual deductibles than traditional health insurance plans. They are typically combined with an HSA or HRA.

TYPES OF HEALTH INSURANCE COVERAGE

Many forms of health insurance coverage are currently in effect in the United States. These are referred to as third-party payers. Types of third-party payers include private insurance, government plans, managed care contracts, and workers' compensation. A brief explanation of the programs discussed in this text is given here, but for an in-depth study, refer to the appropriate chapters that follow.

COMPETITIVE MEDICAL PLAN

A **competitive medical plan (CMP)** is a type of managed care organization created by the Tax Equity and Fiscal Responsibility Act of 1982 (TEFRA). This federal legislation allows for enrollment of Medicare beneficiaries in managed care plans.

CONSUMER DIRECTED HEALTH PLANS

These plans are a rapidly emerging approach to health care services that are also referred to as self-directed health plans (**SDHPs**). **Consumer directed health plans (CDHPs)** allow the consumer to design and customize his or her own health plan, based on his or her specific needs and circumstances. Typically, the CDHP involves the pairing of a high-deductible preferred provider organization plan with a tax-advantaged account, such as an HSA.

DISABILITY INCOME INSURANCE

Disability income insurance is a form of insurance that replaces income when the insured is unable to work as a result of illness, injury, or disease. This type of insurance should not be confused with workers' compensation, because those injuries must be work related. Some states require employers to have this type of coverage for their employees.

EXCLUSIVE PROVIDER ORGANIZATION

An **exclusive provider organization (EPO)** is a type of managed health care plan in which subscriber members are eligible for benefits only when they use the services of a limited network of health care organizations. EPOs combine features of both health maintenance organizations and preferred provider organizations. Employers agree not to enter into an agreement with any other plan for coverage of eligible employees. EPOs are regulated under state health insurance laws.

HEALTH MAINTENANCE ORGANIZATION

A **health maintenance organization (HMO)** is an organization that provides a wide range of comprehensive health care services for a specified group at a fixed periodic payment. The emphasis is on preventive care. Health care organizations are prepaid by **capitation.** Capitation is a payment system based on a flat rate per patient in the plan. Health care organizations are prepaid based on the number of HMO members. An HMO can be sponsored by the government, medical schools, hospitals, employers, labor unions, consumer groups, insurance companies, or hospital medical plans.

INDEMNITY HEALTH INSURANCE

Indemnity health insurance plans are referred to as traditional or **fee-for-service** health plans. They are designed to allow patients maximum flexibility and choice when it comes to health care organizations. Subscribers pay a fixed monthly premium and services are paid at a percentage of covered benefits after an annual deductible is met. Health care organizations are paid each time a service is rendered on a fee-for-service basis.

INDEPENDENT OR INDIVIDUAL PRACTICE ASSOCIATION

An **independent or individual practice association (IPA)** is a type of managed care plan in which a program administrator contracts with a number of health care organizations. These organizations agree to provide treatment to subscribers in their own offices or clinics for a fixed capitation payment per month. Subscribers to IPA plans have limited or no choice of health care organization. IPA health care organizations continue to see their fee-for-service patients.

MATERNAL AND CHILD HEALTH PROGRAM

A **Maternal and Child Health Program (MCHP)** is a state and federal program for children who are younger than 21 years of age and have special health care needs. It assists parents with financial planning. The MCHP may assume part or all of the costs of treatment, depending on the child's condition and the family's resources.

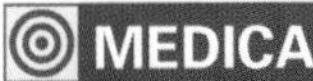

MEDICAID

Medicaid is a program sponsored jointly by federal, state, and local governments to provide health care benefits to medically indigent persons on public assistance, aged individuals who meet certain financial requirements, and the disabled. Some states have expanded coverage for other medically needy individuals who meet special state-determined criteria. Coverage and benefits vary widely from state to state.

MEDICARE

Medicare is a national four-part program. It consists of a hospital insurance system (Part A), supplementary medical insurance (Part B), Medicare Plus Choice Program (Part C), and the Medicare Prescription Drug benefits (Part D). It is for individuals who are at least 65 years of age. It was created by the 1965 Amendments to the Social Security Act and is operated under the provisions of the Act. Benefits are also extended to permanently disabled people and those with end-stage renal disease.

MEDICARE/MEDICAID

Medicare/Medicaid is a program that covers those persons eligible for both Medicare and Medicaid. In some areas of the country, dual coverage in both programs may be referred to as **Medi-Medi.**

POINT-OF-SERVICE PLAN

A **point-of-service (POS) plan** is a managed care plan consisting of a network of health care organizations and hospitals that provides an insurance company or employer with discounts on its services. Patients can refer themselves to a specialist or see an out-of-network health care organization for a higher copayment.

PREFERRED PROVIDER ORGANIZATION

A variation of a managed care plan is a **preferred provider organization (PPO).** This is a form of contract medicine by which a large employer, or any organization that can produce a large number of patients, contracts with a hospital or a group of health care organizations to offer medical care at a reduced rate.

STATE CHILDREN'S HEALTH INSURANCE PROGRAM

The **State Children's Health Insurance Program (SCHIP)** is a state-sponsored program that provides free or low-cost health coverage for low-income children.

TRICARE

A government-sponsored program called TRICARE provides military and non-military hospital and medical services. It covers spouses and dependents of active service personnel, retired service personnel and their dependents, and dependents of members who died on active duty. Active duty service members are not eligible for TRICARE but have benefits like TRICARE Prime, in which the Department of Defense covers all allowable charges for medically necessary care.

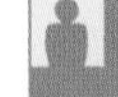

UNEMPLOYMENT COMPENSATION DISABILITY

Unemployment Compensation Disability (UCD) or **state disability insurance (SDI)** is insurance that covers off-the-job injury or sickness and is paid for by deductions from a person's paycheck. This program is administered by a state agency in only six states.

VETERANS HEALTH ADMINISTRATION

The **Veterans Health Administration** or Civilian Health and Medical Program of the Department of Veterans Affairs (**CHAMPVA**) is administered by the Department of Veterans Affairs (**VA**). This federal program covers medical bills for veterans with total, permanent, service-connected disabilities and their spouses and dependents. It also covers the surviving spouses and children of veterans who died as a result of service-connected disabilities.

> **WORKERS' COMPENSATION INSURANCE**
>
> **Workers' compensation insurance** is a contract that insures a person against on-the-job injury or illness. The employer pays the premium for his or her employees.

Examples of Insurance Billing

Sometimes it is difficult to comprehend the full scale of insurance billing. As an example of total medical billing, six cases are presented explain the entire billing picture from simple to complex.

CASE 1: A new patient comes in with complaints of a sore throat and an infected nail. The physician's office bills for:

Office visit, penicillin injection
Office surgery for infected nail
Sterile surgical tray (may or may not be billed, depending on third-party payer)

CASE 2: A patient comes in because of an accident and has complaints that require evaluation and management services, x-ray films, and laboratory studies (urinalysis) performed in the physician's office. The physician's office bills for:

Office visit
Office visit x-ray studies (including interpretation) and laboratory tests (urinalysis, including interpretation)

CASE 3: A patient is seen by the family physician after office hours in the hospital emergency department.

The physician's office bills for the visit to the hospital emergency department.
The hospital bills for hospital outpatient emergency department services (use and supplies).

CASE 4: A physician sends a patient's Papanicolaou (Pap) test to a private clinical laboratory. The physician's office bills for:

Office visit
Handling of specimen
The laboratory bills for the Pap test

CASE 5: A patient is sent to a local hospital for an upper gastrointestinal radiographic series. An x-ray technician obtains the films in the hospital and a privately owned radiologic group does the interpretation.

The hospital bills for the technical component of the upper gastrointestinal x-ray series (use of equipment).
The radiologic group bills for the professional component of the upper gastrointestinal x-ray series (the interpretation).

CASE 6: A patient is seen in the office and is immediately hospitalized for a hysterectomy.

The surgeon's office bills for initial hospital admission and surgical procedure.
The assistant surgeon bills for assisting the surgeon during hysterectomy.
The anesthesiologist bills for anesthesia administered during hysterectomy.
The hospital bills for hospital room, operating room, anesthesia supplies, medications, x-ray films, laboratory tests, and medica and surgical supplies (dressings, intravenous lines). The hospital might also bill for blood for transfusions, electrocardiogram, radiation therapy, and respiratory therapy.

In these scenarios, an insurance billing specialist in the offices of the attending physician, assistant surgeon, anesthesiologist, radiologic group, and private clinical laboratory submits an insurance **claim** form for reimbursement to the insurance payer. If the health care organization does not participate, he or she gives the patient the necessary information to submit his or her own claim to the insurance company

EXCEPTION

Medicare Patients by Federal Law May Not Submit Their Own Claims for Physician or Hospital Services.

In the hospital and hospital emergency department, a member of the hospital staff inputs services into a central computer system. This produces an itemized statement and completed insurance claim form via computer to be submitted to the third-party payer.

HANDLING AND PROCESSING INSURANCE CLAIMS

Most offices today are computerized and use practice management software (**PMS**) for scheduling, electronic health records, coding, billing, **accounts receivable management**, and other administrative functions. However, some smaller offices thrive in the paper environment and will continue to do so. A computerized office may still generate paper insurance claim forms and send them to the insurance payer. This chapter differentiates health care organizations that have computerized operations from those that are using paper ledgers and generating paper-only claims and do not use the computer for any administrative practice management functions. Use the icons as a guide to differentiate the methodologies of a computerized office and a paper-based office.

Different methods exist for processing insurance claims for the health care organization. The most common ones follow.

1. Posting charges and submitting to the insurance payer on the legacy paper CMS-1500 claim form. This form has been used in the industry since 1975. The CMS-1500 can be prepared manually by completing the claim information with a pen or electronically and transmitting it via computer.
2. Contracting with an outside billing service company to prepare and electronically transmit claims on behalf of the health care organization's office.
3. Direct data entry (DDE) in the payer's system. The billing specialist logs into the insurance company's system and keys in the data required to process the claim. Keep in mind that Health Insurance Portability and Accountability (HIPAA) regulations will determine whether a health care organization is a covered entity and whether it is required to submit claims electronically.

LIFE CYCLE OF AN INSURANCE CLAIM

The **life cycle** or **revenue cycle** of an insurance claim includes the administrative and clinical functions that are required to capture and collect payment for services provided by a health care organization.

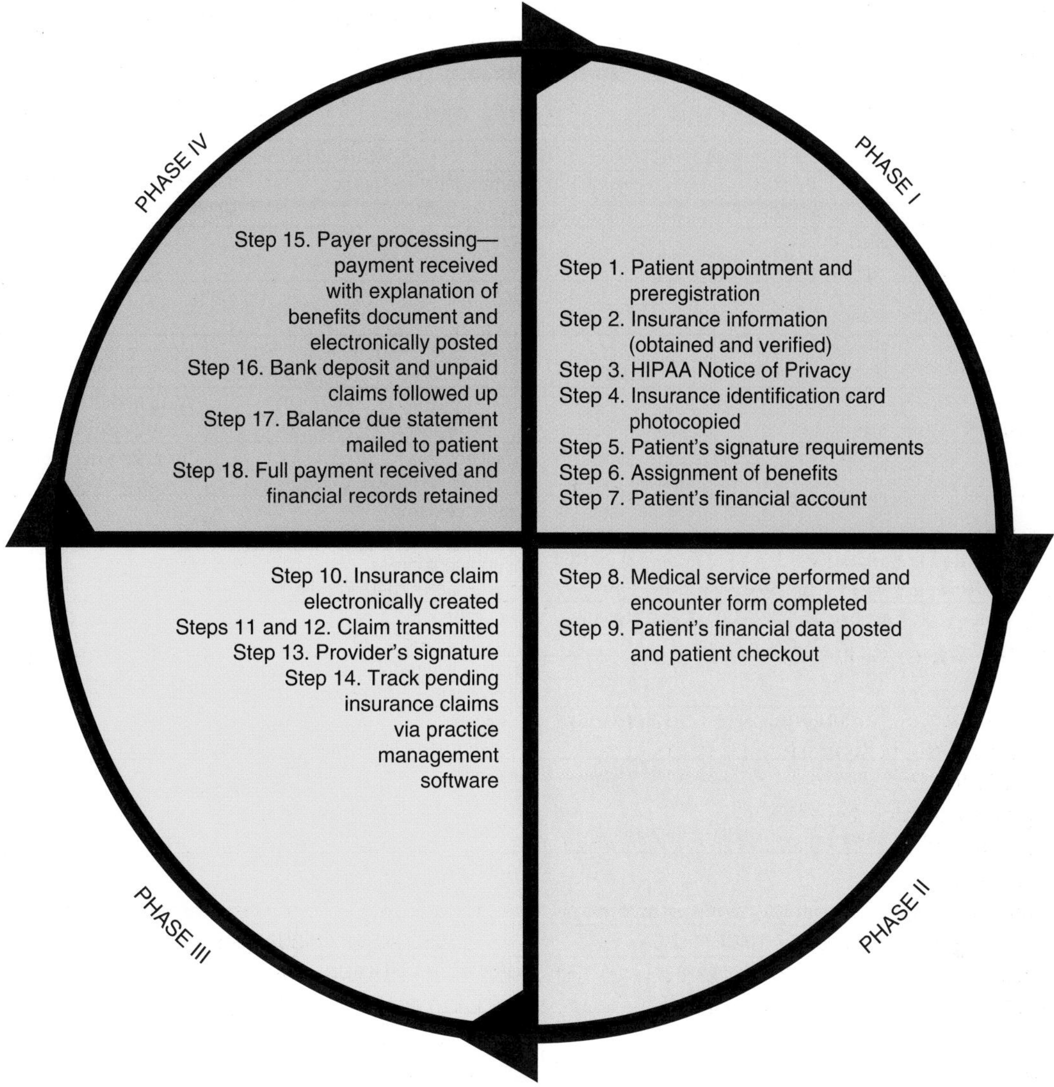

Fig. 4.5 Revenue cycle overview showing the basic steps in processing an insurance claim in a health care organization's office, to the third-party payer, and after payment is received.

The revenue cycle of an insurance claim outlines the basic steps (Fig. 4.5) in handling and processing insurance claims in a health care organization's office. The cycle begins when the patient makes an appointment and continues until payment is received.

1. **Preregistration:** Some health care organizations preregister a new patient during the initial telephone call. Some have a designated staff member contact the patient before the appointment time. Some send a letter confirming the appointment with an informative brochure about the health care organization and a patient registration form. This form may be printed off the organization's website, completed online, or completed when the patient arrives for his or her appointment.

   It is a good idea to have new patients arrive 15 to 20 minutes before the scheduled appointment. This allows time to collect vital statistics and insurance information and to discuss the patient's responsibility with respect to payment policies. A patient registration form also may be called a patient information form or intake sheet (Figs. 4.6 and 4.7).

   Instruct the patient to fill in all spaces and indicate not applicable (N/A) if an item does not apply. If the patient has a medical problem that makes it difficult to complete the form, such as rheumatoid arthritis of the hands or limited vision, then the insurance billing specialist should interview the patient and fill in the necessary data.

   Read the form carefully after completion to ensure that complete and accurate personal and financial information has been obtained from the patient. The patient registration form should contain the following facts:

   - Name: First, middle initial, and last. The name must match that shown on the insurance identification card. Some pediatric patients do not have the same last name as their parents or stepparents. Insurance payments show the policyholder's name, and it is time consuming to find and give credit to the patient's account without this information.
   - Practice management systems allow a cross-reference of the patient, subscriber, and guarantor's names, as well as Social Security number, so that when the policyholder's name is searched, the patient's name also appears.

Patient Registration

I was referred to this office by: Margaret Taylor City: Oxnard Date: 01/20/13

PATIENT INFORMATION			PRIMARY INSURED INFORMATION		
Name (Last) Fuhr	(First) Linda	(Middle) L	Name of insured (Last) Fuhr	(First) Gerald	(Middle) T
Name you like to be called Linda			Address (If different)		
Address 3070 Tipper street			City	State	Zip
City Oxnard	State CA	Zip 93030	Policyholder's birthdate 06-15-64	Sex ☒ M ☐ F	Home phone number 555-276-0101
Patient's birthdate 11-05-65	Sex ☐ M ☒ F	Home phone number 555-276-0101	SSN 545-XX-2771		Work phone number 555-921-0075
SSN 550-XX-5172		Work phone number 555-372-1151	Email address GFUHR64@AOL.COM		Cell phone number 555-243-2736
Email address LFUHR65@AOL.COM		Cell phone number 555-243-1777	Insurance name ABC Insurance Company		
Employer or school name Macys	Title Sales associate		Insurance address P.O. Box 12340, Fresno, CA 93765		
Patient status ☒ Employed	☐ Full time student		ID number H-550-XX-5172-02		Group number 17098
☐ Single	☒ Married	☐ Other	Primary insured's relationship to patient Spouse		
Ethnicity ☐ Hispanic	☐ Non-Hispanic	☒ Not specified	Employer Electronic Data Systems		
Race ☐ African American ☒ Caucasian or European American ☐ Native American	☐ Asian American ☐ Pacific Islander		Employer address 2700 West 5th Street Oxnard, CA 93030		
Preferred language English			Comments None		

EMERGENCY CONTACT INFORMATION		SECONDARY INSURANCE INFORMATION		
Name Hannah Gildea	Relationship Aunt	Name of insured (Last)	(First)	(Middle)
Address 4621 Lucretia St., Oxnard, CA 93030		Policy holder's birthdate	Sex ☐ M ☐ F	
Home phone number 555-274-0132	Cell phone number 555-243-1388	Insurance name None		
Email address GILDEAH@YAHOO.COM		Insurance address		
Does your emergency contact have power of attorney? ☐ Yes ☒ No	Advance health directive? ☒ Yes ☐ No	ID number		Group number

FOR WORK-RELATED PROBLEMS, PLEASE FILL OUT BELOW					
Workers' comp insurance	Policy number	Address	City	State	Zip
Claim number	Date of injury	Employer at time of injury			
Has this injury been reported to the employer? ☐ Yes ☐ No		Employer address			

INSURANCE SIGNATURE AUTHORIZATION

I authorize any holder of medical or other information about me to release to the insurance company any information needed for this or a related claim. I permit a copy of this authorization to be used in place of the original, and newest payment of medical insurance benefits to, (PHYSICIAN NAME OR PRACTICE NAME): ______________________

X *Linda Fuhr* Jan. 20, 20XX

ORDER # 58-8429 • © 2012 BIBBERO SYSTEMS, INC. • PETALUMA, CALIFORNIA
TO REORDER CALL TOLL FREE: (800) 242-2376 OR FAX (800) 242-9330 MFG IN U.S.A.

Fig. 4.6 Patient registration information form showing a comprehensive listing of personal and financial information obtained from the patient on his or her first visit to the office. (Courtesy Bibbero Systems, Inc., Petaluma, Calif. Telephone: 800-242-2376; fax: 800-242-9330; website: www.bibbero.com.)

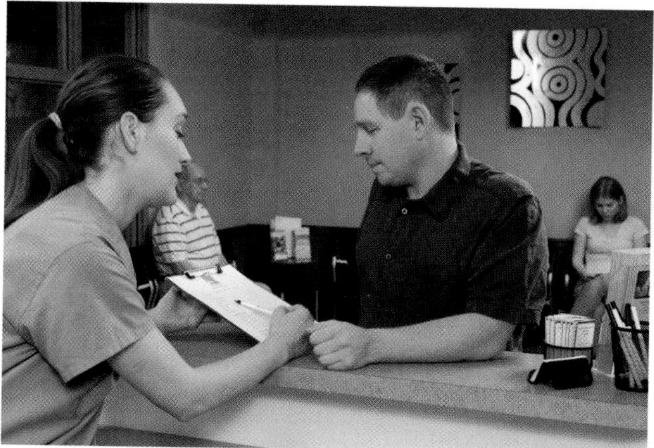

Fig. 4.7 Receptionist giving instructions to a patient on how to complete the patient registration form.

- Street address, including apartment number, zip code, and telephone numbers with area code (cell and landline)
- Business address, telephone number with extension, and occupation
- E-mail address
- Date of birth. HIPAA requires eight digits (year/month/day) to be submitted to payers; for example, the eight-digit format of January 2, 1936, is 19360102. A practice management system may collect these data in a different format but transmit in the required eight-digit format.
- Person responsible for account, either guarantor or insured's name
- Social Security number
- Spouse's name and occupation
- Referring physician's name or other referral source
- Driver's license number
- Emergency contact, such as a close relative or friend with name, address, and telephone number
- Insurance billing information: all insurance company names, addresses, policy numbers, and group numbers. This is important for the COBs. Medicare and Medicaid patients are given the option of joining managed care programs and are allowed to switch every 30 days. Always ask each older patient whether he or she is covered by traditional Medicare or a Medicare HMO. A good patient information sheet has space where this information can be written in by the patient.

2. **Verification of Insurance:** Verify insurance and all other information that may have changed since the last visit. This may be done by giving the patient a copy of the previously completed patient registration form and asking him or her to correct any incorrect data in red.
3. **Notice of Privacy Practices:** Each patient is given a Notice of Privacy Practices (NPP) that explains how his or her health information is used. Have the patient sign a form stating that they have received the NPP. If the patient refuses or is unable to sign, document this in his or her health record. An NPP is mandatory under federal law through HIPAA.
4. **Insurance Identification Card:** Photocopy both sides of all of the patient's insurance identification cards (Fig. 4.8). A copy produces error-free insurance data and can be used in lieu of completing the insurance section of the patient registration form. Ask for photo identification, such as a driver's license, to verify that the person has not used someone else's card. Call the insurance company to verify coverage and applicable deductible or copayment, and whether the insurance plan requires precertification for any services. On a return visit, ask to see the card and check it with the data on file (Fig. 4.9). If it differs, photocopy both sides and write the date on the copy, using this as the basis for revising data on file.

! COMPLIANCE ALERT

Release of Information

If the health care organization is submitting an insurance claim for the patient, the patient is not required to sign a release of information form for obtaining payment for services. However, some health care organizations prefer to operate at a higher level of privacy and continue to obtain patients' signatures on release of information forms.

5. **Patient's Signature Requirements:** Under HIPAA regulations, a patient's signed authorization is not required for treatment, payment, or routine health care operations (TPO). However, many organizations continue to have patients sign an authorization allowing the release of any medical or other information necessary to process the claim. If the patient is physically or mentally unable to sign, the person representing the patient may sign for the patient.

   Electronic environment: Electronic billers are permitted to obtain a lifetime authorization from the beneficiary to release health or other information necessary to process a claim. The signature should be retained in a file for future use on all electronic claims. This authorization allows the office to submit claims on the beneficiary's behalf. To use this procedure, the patient signs a brief statement that reads as follows: *(Name of Beneficiary) (Health Insurance Claim Number)*

   "I request that payment of authorized benefits be made either to me or on my behalf to (name of health care organization or supplier) for any services furnished me by health care organization or supplier. I authorize any holder of medical information about me to release to my insurance carrier and its agents any information needed to determine these benefits or the benefits payable for related services."

   Patient signature source codes are used on electronic claims to indicate the type of signatures on file for the patient. Under HIPAA Version 5010, adopted in 2013, they are no longer required, with the exception of a "P." This is reported when the signature is generated by the provider because the patient was not physically present for the service. If any other value is present on the electronic claim, it will be rejected. Most patient registration forms include a statement to sign regarding these two authorizations (see bottom of Fig. 4.6).

   Paper Environment: Since the enforcement of HIPAA regulations, a patient's signature for the release of information in Block 12 is no longer required. If a signature is obtained on a separate form, it should be filed in the patient's health record and the abbreviation SOF or the preferred spelled-out notation "signature on file" may be used on the insurance claim form.

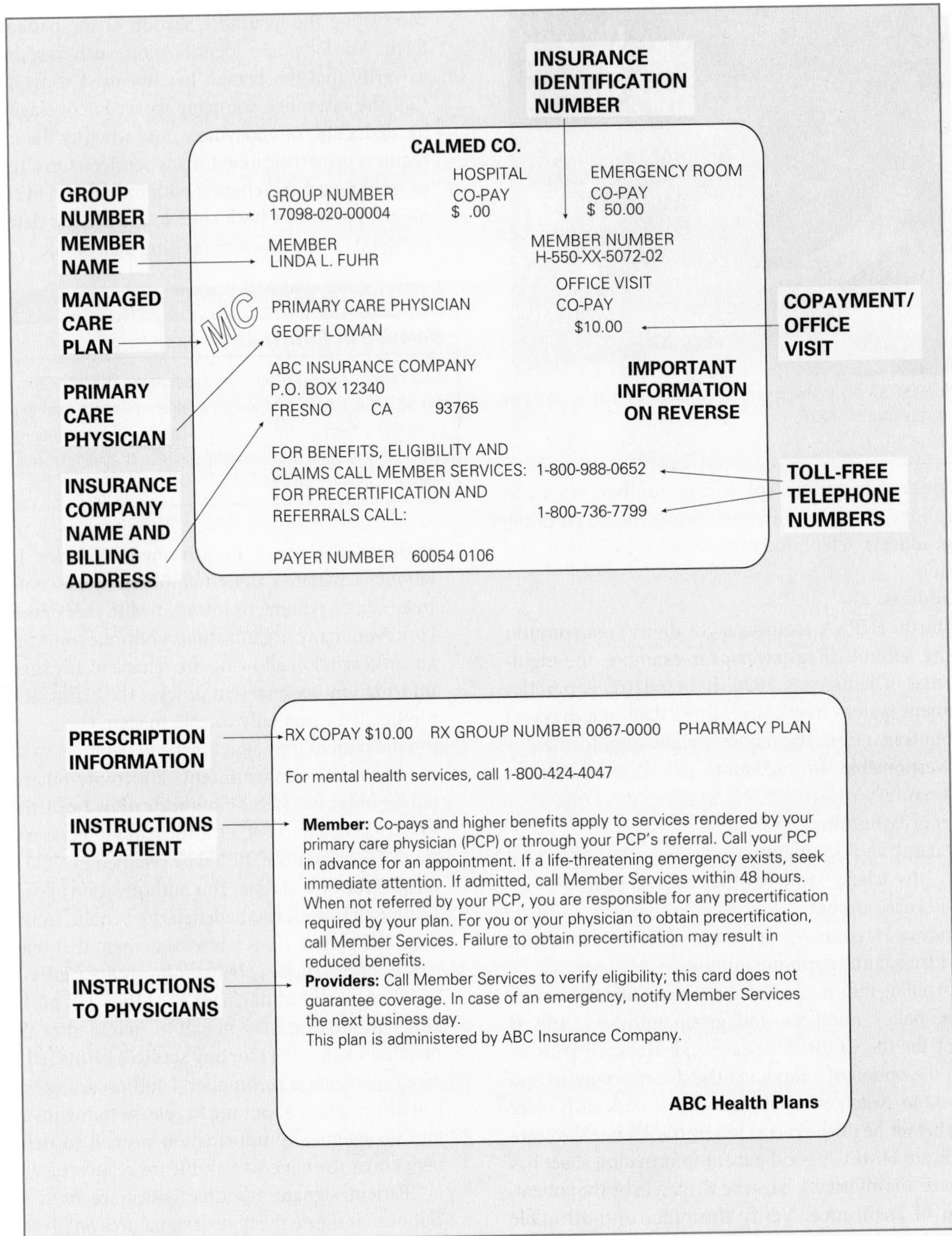

Fig. 4.8 Front *(top)* and back *(bottom)* sides of an insurance card.

6. **Assignment of Benefits:** The signature requirement for the **assignment** of benefits is included in Block 13 of the CMS-1500 insurance claim form (Fig. 4.10). For the health care organization to receive payment directly from the insurance payer, the patient must sign an assignment of benefits statement for each insurance company. However, before explaining an assignment, it is important to define the difference between **participating (par)** and **nonparticipating (nonpar) health care organizations or providers.**

A par health care organization has a contractual agreement with an insurance plan to render care to eligible beneficiaries and bill the third-party payer directly (Example 4.2). The third-party payer pays its portion of the allowed amount and the health care organization bills the patient for the balance after the disallowed portion is adjusted off of the account. Managed care plans also refer to par provider as member health care organizations. If the amount of the patient's responsibility can be determined, collect it at the time of the visit.

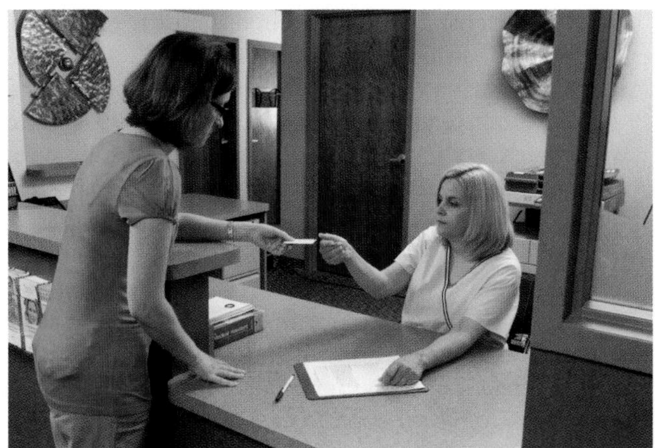

Fig. 4.9 Patient presenting an insurance identification card to the receptionist for photocopying.

13. INSURED'S OR AUTHORIZED PERSON'S SIGNATURE I authorize payment of medical benefits to the undersigned physician or supplier for services described below.

SIGNED ____________________

Fig. 4.10 Section 13 from the health insurance claim form CMS-1500, illustrating authorization for assignment of benefits.

EXAMPLE 4.2 Participating Provider

Dr. Gomez accepts assignment and is a par provider for the Liberty Health Insurance Plan. Pedro Nunez, a new patient, is seen in the office with complaints of a sore throat and infected nail, for which a $150 fee is charged for the office visit, office surgery, and penicillin injection. The patient has met his deductible for the year.

Provider fee (total billed amount)	$150
Provider contracted rate (allowable charge)	$140
Patient coinsurance or copayment amount	$10
Insurance claims payment	$130
Provider's adjusted (write-off) amount	$10

Dr. Gomez collects $10 from the patient and is paid a total of $140.

A nonpar provider is a health care organization without a contractual agreement with an insurance plan. It is not required to accept a contracted amount for care to eligible beneficiaries (Example 4.3). The health care organization may or may not file an insurance claim as a courtesy to the patient and may require full payment at the time of service. The patient should be made aware that his or her insurance plan will cover a considerable amount less on the claim when receiving services from a nonpar provider.

If a health care organization accepts assignment, the insurance carrier sends the payment directly to them. An agreement is obtained by having the patient sign an assignment of insurance benefits document that directs payment to the health care organization. The CMS-1500 claim form contains this provision as well. An assignment of benefits becomes a legally enforceable document but must refer to specific hospitalization, course of treatment, or office visits. Each course of treatment needs to have an assignment document signed by the patient unless an annual or lifetime signature authorization is maintained in the patient's file.

EXAMPLE 4.3 Nonparticipating Provider

Dr. Warner does not accept assignment and is a nonpar provider for the XYZ Health Insurance Plan. Estelle Cutter, an established patient, is seen in the office complaining that her ears are full of earwax that needs to be removed. A $60 fee is charged.

Provider fee (total billed amount)	$60
Usual, customary, and reasonable (UCR)	$55
Patient coinsurance or copayment amount	$10
Insurance claims payment	$44
Provider may bill patient over UCR	$6

Dr. Warner collects $16 from the patient and is paid a total of $60 because he can collect the difference between his fee and the patient's copayment plus the insurance payment.

PRIVATE CARRIERS

For private insurance companies with whom the health care organization does not have a contractual agreement, accepting assignment means that the claim will be paid to the health care organization's office instead of the patient. Because there is no signed agreement between the health care organization and the carrier, the difference between the billed amount and the carrier's allowed amount is not written off but collected from the patient as is any copayment or deductible. In private third-party liability cases, the health care organization needs to negotiate with the insurance company to make sure benefits are paid to him or her directly.

MANAGED CARE

In managed care plans, a par or preferred provider is a health care organization that has contracted with a plan to provide medical services to plan members. A nonpar provider refers to a health care organization that has not contracted with a managed care plan to provide medical services to plan members. The assignment is automatic for individuals who have signed with managed care contracts.

MEDICAID

For Medicaid cases, there is no assignment unless the patient has other insurance in addition to Medicaid. The Medicaid fiscal intermediary pays all providers directly.

MEDICARE

The words *participating, nonparticipating,* and *assignment* have slightly different meanings in the Medicare program. A health care organization that accepts assignment on Medicare claims is called a participating (par) health care organization. It may not bill or accept payment for the difference between the submitted charge and the Medicare allowed amount. However, an attempt must be made to collect the 20% coinsurance and any amount applied to the deductible.

A health care organization that does not participate is called a nonparticipating health care organization and has an option regarding assignment. The health care organization either may not accept assignment for all services or may exercise the option of accepting assignment for some services and collecting from the patient for other services performed at the same time and place. The health care organization collects the fee from the patient but may bill no more than the Medicare-limiting charge. The check is sent to the patient. When treating federal or state government employees or a Medicare recipient, the health care organization may lose the fee if government guidelines are not followed.

TRICARE

A health care organization that participates in TRICARE agrees to accept the allowable charge as the full fee and cannot charge the patient the difference between the health care organization's charge and the allowable charge. The exception to this is when the health care organization does not accept assignment on the claim.

A par or nonpar health care organization can submit a claim and choose to not accept assignment on a claim-by-claim basis. In the event the health care organization does not accept assignment, TRICARE sends the sponsor all payments. TRICARE does not communicate with the health care organization if the provider has questions about the claim. It is up to the health care organization to bill the sponsor for payment. The health care organization can collect 115% of the TRICARE allowable from the patient when a CMS-1500 claim form is marked "no" in the accepting assignment block.

WORKERS' COMPENSATION

There is no assignment for industrial cases. The workers' compensation carrier pays the fee for services rendered according to its fee schedule, and the check automatically goes to the health care organization. The patient is not responsible for payment of services for any work-related injury or illness.

7. **Patient's Financial Account:** Patient information is entered into the PMS program. Accuracy is crucial because the data will be used to construct the claim for transmission to the insurance company. If the health care organization is not computerized, a manual system includes paper daysheets and patient ledger cards.
8. **Encounter Form:** An encounter form (also called a charge slip, multipurpose billing form, patient service slip, routing form, superbill, or transaction slip) is attached to the patient's health record during the visit (Fig. 4.11). This contains the patient's name, the date, and in some instances the previous balance due. It also contains the procedural and diagnostic codes and the date the patient should return for an appointment. This two- or three-part form is a combination bill, insurance form, and routing document used in both computer- and paper-based systems. This also can be a computerized multipurpose billing form that may be scanned to input charges and diagnoses into the patient's computerized account. Time is saved and fewer errors occur because no keystrokes are involved.

   Health care organizations use the encounter form as a communications tool or routing sheet and as an invoice to the patient. When used as a routing sheet, it becomes a source document for insurance claim data. The encounter form is completed by the health care organization. Both a procedural code for services performed and a diagnostic code are chosen by the provider of services. In some situations, a certified coder may review the patient's health record to assign a proper code on the basis of the documentation.

   The encounter form's procedure and diagnostic code sections should be updated and reprinted biannually with correct descriptions because changes, additions, and deletions occur that may affect the organization. Remove all codes not used or seldom used and revise and add current, valid, commonly used codes for the organization. Because there is no grace period, update encounter forms twice a year: by October 1 for changes in diagnostic codes and by January 1 for changes in procedural codes.

   Some health care organizations develop encounter forms for different services (for example, surgical services, office services, and out-of-office services such as hospital visits, emergency, outpatient health care organization, nursing home, or house calls). The provider signs the encounter form and indicates whether the patient needs another appointment (Fig. 4.12).

   Some health care organizations may have patients carry the encounter form to the reception desk, where fees are determined and input for billing (Fig. 4.13). The patient is given the opportunity to pay and make a future appointment.
9. **Financial Accounting Record and Accounts Receivable Management:** The value of maintaining careful records of all insurance matters cannot be overemphasized. Accounts receivable (A/R) management breathes life into the organization's cash flow. *A/R management* refers to establishing the patient financial accounting record and carrying out the claims process. For compilation of claim data, services are entered into the computer by either front desk personnel or the in-office billing department. If the organization outsources this function, an off-site billing company retrieves the data and processes the claims. All charges and patient payments are posted to their respective accounts.

   Electronic Environment: A financial account is set up in the practice management system. Data obtained from the patient registration process are keyed into the program and a patient account is established. Usually an account number is automatically assigned by the program and used for tracking and reporting. All items posted to each patient account are housed in the computer database for accurate and easy retrieval.

   Using the encounter form, daily transactions are recorded by the billing staff. Professional fees, payments, adjustments, and balance due are also posted in the practice management software program. Accuracy is especially important when keying data into the computer because this is where the data begins to build an insurance claim.

   Paper Environment: In the paper environment, a ledger card or financial accounting record is maintained for each patient who receives professional services (Fig. 4.14). An established private patient who is injured on the job requires two ledgers, one for private care and one for workers' compensation services.

   At the end of each day, a daysheet is generated and printed. A daysheet, or daily record sheet, is a register for recording daily business transactions. The totals from this can be compared with the encounter forms to ensure that all charges, payments, and adjustments were properly posted. Also, the daysheet is a useful tool for checks and balances when assessing the bank deposit slip for accuracy.

   The paper environment allows transactions to be recorded on the patient ledger cards. All patients seen on one day have their charges (debits) recorded on the daysheet, along with all payments and adjustments (credits). Each day

STATE LIC.# C1503X
SOC. SEC. # 000-11-0000
PIN # ____________

College Clinic
4567 Broad Avenue
Woodland Hills, XY 12345-4700

Phone: 555-486-9002

☐ Private ☒ Bluecross ☐ Ind. ☐ Medicare ☐ Medi-cal ☐ Hmo ☐ Ppo

Patient's last name	First	Account #:	Birthdate	Sex	Today's date
Smith	Lydia	13845	09/ 13 / 92	☐ Male ☒ Female	09 / 17 / 20XX

Insurance company	Subscriber	Plan #	Sub. #	Group
Blue Shield of CA	Lydia Smith	0473	186-72-10XX	849-37000

ASSIGNMENT: I hereby assign my insurance benefits to be paid directly to the undersigned physician, I am financially responsible for non-covered services.
SIGNED: Patient,
or parent, if minor *Lydia Smith* Today's date 09 / 17 / 20XX

RELEASE: I hereby authorize the physician to release to my insurance carriers any information required to process this claim.
SIGNED: Patient,
or parent, if minor *Lydia Smith* Today's date 09 / 17 / 20XX

✓	DESCRIPTION		CODE	FEE	✓	DESCRIPTION	CODE	FEE	✓	DESCRIPTION	CODE	FEE
	OFFICE VISITS	NEW	EST.			Venipuncture	36415			OFFICE PROCEDURES		
	Blood pressure check		99211			TB skin test	86580			Anoscopy	46600	
	Level II	99202	99212			Hematocrit	85013			Ear lavage	69210	
	Level III	99203	99213			Glucose finger stick	82948			Spirometry	94010	
X	Level IV	(99204)	99214	70.92		IMMUNIZATIONS				Nebulizer Rx	94664	
	Level V	99205	99215			Allergy inj. X1	95115			EKG	93000	
	PREVENTIVE EXAMS	NEW	EST.			Allergy inj. X2	95117			SURGERY		
	Age 65 and older	99387	99397			Trigger pt. inj.	20552			Mole removal (1st)	17110	
	Age 40 - 64	99386	99396			Therapeutic inj.	96372			(2nd to 14th)	17003	
	Age 18 - 39	99385	99395			VACCINATION PRODUCTS				Flat warts (1st - 14th)	07110	
	Age 12 - 17	99384	99394			DPT	90701			15 or more	17111	
	Age 5 - 11	99383	99393			DT	90702			Biopsy, 1 lesion	11100	
	Age 1 - 4	99382	99392			Tetanus	90703			Addt'l. lesions	11101	
	Infant	99381	99391			MMR	90707			Endometrial Bx	58100	
	Newborn ofc		99432			OPV	90712			Skin tags to 15	11200	
	OB/NEWBORN CARE					Polio inj.	90713			Each addt'l. 10	11201	
	OB package		59400			Flu	90662			I & D abscess	10060	
	Post-partum visit N/C					Hemophilus B	90645			SUPPLIES/MISCELLANEOUS		
	LAB PROCEDURES					Hepatitis B vac.	90746			Surgical tray	99070	
	Urine dip		81000			Pheumovax	90670			Handling charge	99000	
	UA qualitative		81005			VACCINE ADMINISTRATION				Special report	99080	
X	Pregnancey urine		81025	20.00		Age: Through 18 yrs. (1st inj.)	90460			DOCTOR'S NOTES:		
	Wet mount		87210			Age: Through 18 yrs. (ea. addt'l. inj.)	90461					
	kOH prip		87220			Adult (1st inj.)	90471					
	Occult blood		82270			Adult (ea. addt'l. inj.)	90472					

DIAGNOSES	**ICD-10-CM**	Colitis/unspec.	K51.90	FUO	R50.9	Osteoarthritis (site)	M19._
Abdominal pain/unspec.	R10.9	Confusion	R41.0	Gastritis	K29.70	Otitis media	H66.9_
Absess	L02._	CHF	I50.9	Gastroenteritis (colitis)	K52.9	Parkinson's disease	G20
Allergic reaction	T78.40_	Constipation	K59.00	G.I. bleed	K92.2	Pharyngitis, acute	J02.9
Alzheimer's disease	G30	COPD	J44.9	Gout/unspec.	M10.9	Pleurisy	R09.1
Anemia/unspec.	D64.9	Cough	R05	Headache	R51	Pneumonia	J18.9
Angina/unspec.	I20.9	Crohn's disease/unspec.	K50.90	Health exam	200._	Pneumonia, viral	J12.9
Anorexia	R63.0	CVA	I63.9	Hematuria/unspec.	R31.9	Prostatitis/unspec.	N41.9
Anxiety/unspec.	F41.9	Decubitus ulcer	L89._	Herpes simplex	B00.9	PVD	I73.9
Apnea, sleep	G47.30	Dehydration	E86.0	Herpes zoster	B02.9	Radiculopathy	M54.1_
Arrhythmia, cardiac	I49.9	Dementia/unspec.	F03	Hiatal hernia	K44.9	Rectal bleeding	K62.5
Arthritis, rheumatoid	M06.9	Depression, major/unsp.	F32.9	HTN (HBP)	I10	Renal failure	N19
Asthma/unspec.	J45.909	Diab I, no complications	E10.0	Hyperlipidemia/unspec.	E78.5	Sciatica	M54.3_
Atrial fibrillation	I48.0	Diab II, no complications	E11.9	Hypothyroidism/unspec.	E03.9	Shortness of breath	R03.02
B-12 deficiency	E53.8	w/kidney complic.	E11.2_	Impotentce	N52._	Sinusitis, chr./unspec.	J32.9
Back pain, low	M54.5	w/ophthalmic compl.	E11.3_	Influenza, respiratory	J10.1	Syncope	R55
BPH	N40	w/neurolog.compl.	E11.4_	Insomnia	G47.0	Tachycardia/unspec.	R00.0
Bradycardia/unspec.	R00.1	w/circulatory cmpl.	E11.5_	IBS, diarrhea	K58.	Tachy., supraventric	I47.1
Bronchitis, acute	J20._	Insulin use	Z79.4	Lupus, systemic erythim.	M32.9	Tendinitis/unspec.	M77.9
Bronchitis, chronic	J42	Diarrhea/unspec.	R19.7	MI, acute	I21._	TIA	G45.9
Bursitis/unspec.	M71.9	Diverticulitis	K57.92	MI, old	I25.2	Ulcer, duodenal/unspec.	K26.9
CA, breast	C50._	Diverticulosis	K57.90	Migraine	G43.9	Ulcer, gastric/unspec.	K25.9
CA, lung	C34._	Dizziness	R42	Myalgia	M79.1	Ulcer, peptic/unspec.	K27.9
CA, prostate	C61	Dysuria	R30.0	Neck pain	M54.2	URI/unspec.	J06.9
Cellulitis	L03._	Edema/unspec.	R60.9	Neuropathy	G62.9	UTI	N39.0
Chest pain/unspec.	R07.9	Endocarditis	I38	Nausea	R11.1	Vertigo	R42
Cirrhosis, liver/unspec.	K74.60	Esophageal reflux	K21.0	X Nausea/vomiting	R11.0	Weight gain	R63.5
Cold, common	J00	Fatigue (lethargy)	R53.83	Obesity/unspec.	E66.9	Weight loss	R63.4

Diagnosis/additional description:
Pregnancy

Doctor's signature/date
Dr. B. Caesar 09-17-20XX

Return appointment information: -with whom (Self) other
Days Wks. (Mos.) 1 month

Rec'd. by:
☐ Cash
☐ Check
____

Total today's fee 90.92

Amount rec'd. today

PLEASE RMEMBER THAT PAYMENT IS YOUR OBLIGATION, REGARDLESS OF INSURANCE OR OTHER THIRD PARTY INVOLVEMENT.

Fig. 4.11 Encounter form: Procedural codes for professional services are taken from the Current Procedural Terminology (CPT) book and diagnostic codes are taken from the *International Classification of Diseases, Tenth Revision, Clinical Modification (ICD-10-CM)* book. (Courtesy Bibbero Systems, Inc., Petaluma, Calif. Telephone: 800-242-2376; fax: 800-242-9330; website: www.bibbero.com.)

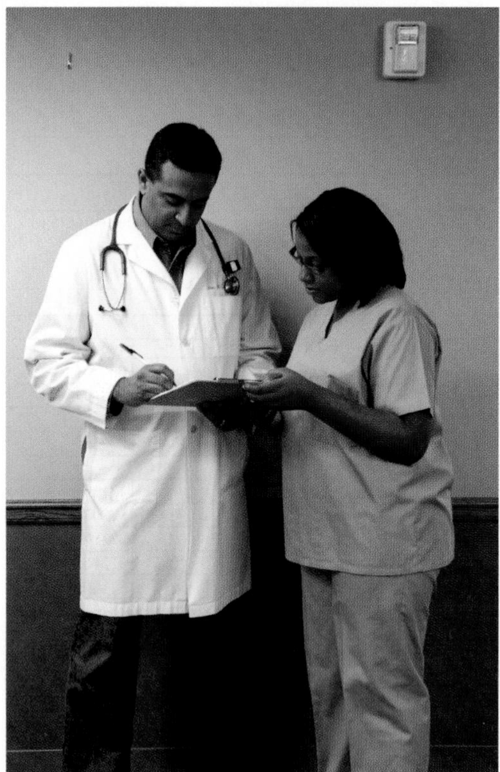

Fig. 4.12 Physician checking off procedures on the encounter form at the conclusion of a patient's office visit.

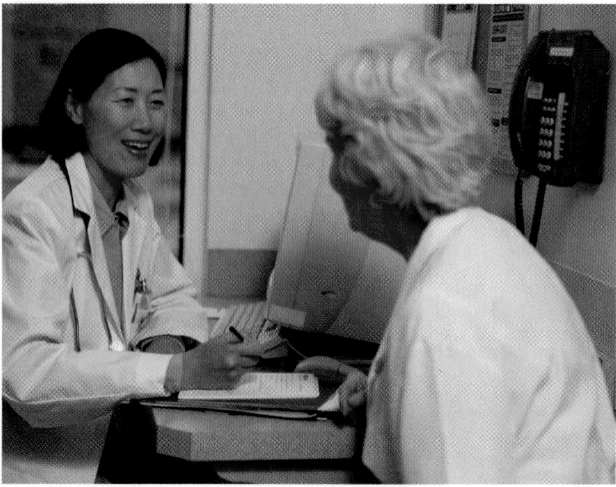

Fig. 4.13 Insurance billing specialist discussing the encounter form with the patient at the health care organization's checkout station.

the totals are carried forward and a new daysheet is set up to receive posting for that day (Fig. 4.15). The patient's ledger card should show an entry of the date an insurance claim is sent, including the date of services that were billed. Each service must be posted on its own line, and a running balance is calculated in the right column. When the ledger is completely filled, the account balance is carried over to a new card. Step-by-step instructions for completing a ledger card are given at the end of this chapter in Procedure 4.1.

10. **Insurance Claim:** Under HIPAA guidelines, health care organizations that are institutional organizations with more than 25 full-time employees or physicians with more than 10 full-time employees must send all claims electronically in the approved format. Generally, the insurance billing specialist in the health care organization's office completes the claim information for the following cases:
    - All hospitalized (both surgical and medical) patients
    - All claims in which the benefits are assigned to the health care organization
    - Special procedures (minor surgery or extensive testing)

    In these cases, the insurance billing specialist generates an accurate claim to be submitted by using exact procedural and diagnostic codes, including the use of any appropriate documents, such as operative report or invoice. It is then mailed or sent electronically to the correct third-party payer.

    The minimum information required by third-party payers is as follows:
    - What was done? *Services and procedures, using procedure codes and appropriate modifiers*
    - Why was it done? *Diagnoses*
    - When was it performed? *Date of service (DOS)*
    - Where was it received? *Place of service (POS)*
    - Who did it? *Provider name and identifying number*

    A helpful hint is to group together, or batch, all outstanding charges to the same type of insurance at one time. This cuts down on errors, makes claims easier to track, and in the paper environment makes manual completion of the forms less tedious.

    It is preferable to electronically transmit claims as soon as possible after services are rendered. Time limits for filing claims range from 30 days to 1½ years for from the DOS. This can vary depending on the commercial carrier, federal or state program, or whether the claim is for an illness or accident. Claims filed after the time limit will be denied and a detailed appeal process may be required to have the claim reconsidered.

    Financial losses from delays in processing can occur in the following instances. If a patient has had a long-term illness, insurance benefits can expire before a claim is processed. If several physicians treat the same patient, some insurance companies pay only one of them. Typically, whoever files the claim first is paid first. In this scenario, the other health care organizations may have to wait for disbursement by the health care organization that received the check. Submit hospitalized patients' insurance claim forms promptly on discharge or on a regular schedule. A good practice is to do this weekly or twice a month depending on the office protocol, regardless of the discharge date for long-term inpatients.

    Patients who pay at time of service and who wish to submit their own insurance claims are given two copies of the encounter form. The patient retains one copy for personal records and attaches the second copy to the insurance claim form and forwards it to the insurance company.

11. **Submitting the Paper Claim:** If a paper claim is submitted, a copy of the CMS-1500 form is placed in the office's pending file or the patient's health record chart, depending on office protocol. The date the claim is mailed is noted on the patient's ledger card and recorded on the insurance claims register. Mail claims in batches to each carrier to save on postage.

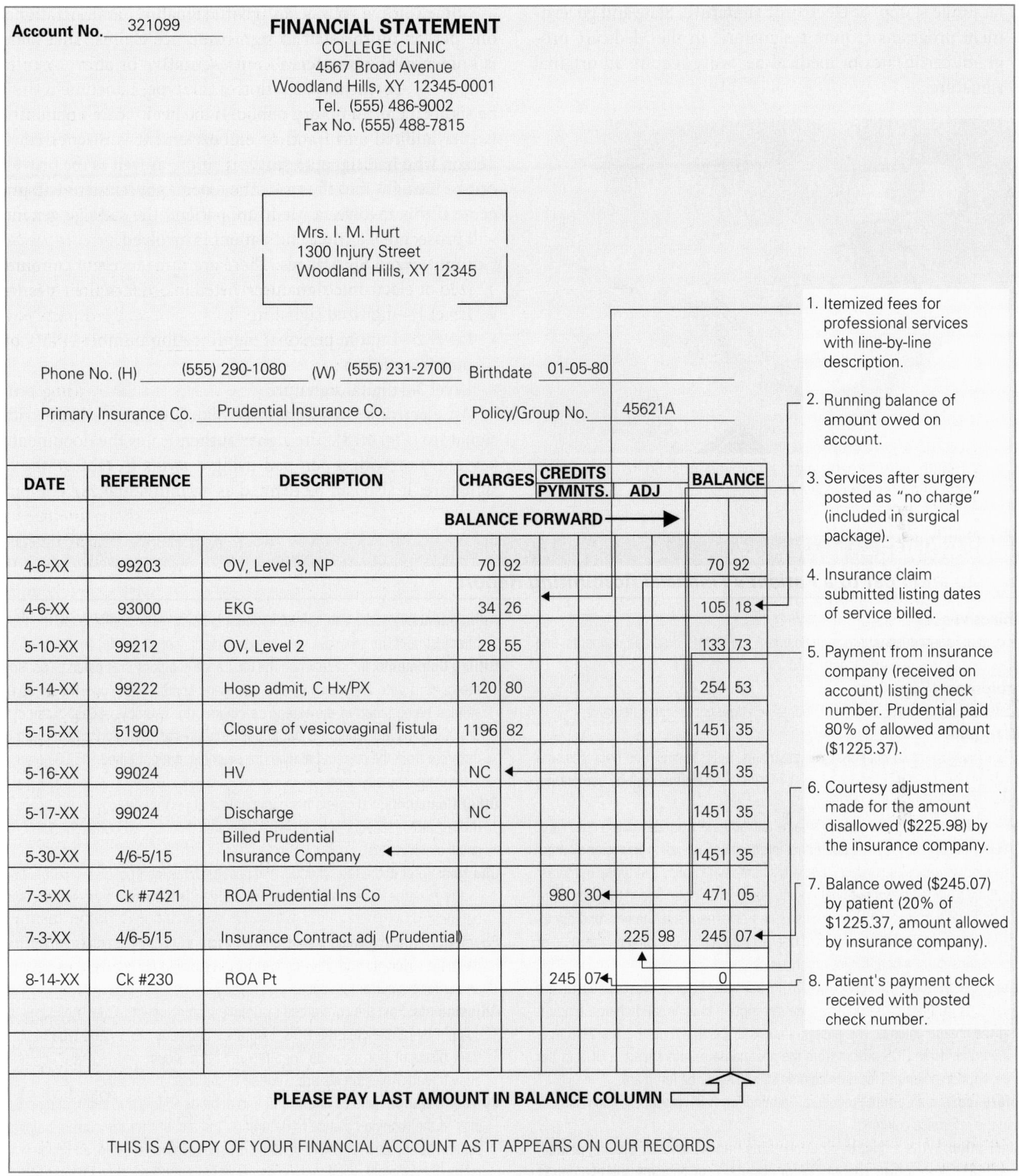

Account No. 321099

FINANCIAL STATEMENT
COLLEGE CLINIC
4567 Broad Avenue
Woodland Hills, XY 12345-0001
Tel. (555) 486-9002
Fax No. (555) 488-7815

Mrs. I. M. Hurt
1300 Injury Street
Woodland Hills, XY 12345

Phone No. (H) (555) 290-1080 (W) (555) 231-2700 Birthdate 01-05-80

Primary Insurance Co. Prudential Insurance Co. Policy/Group No. 45621A

DATE	REFERENCE	DESCRIPTION	CHARGES	CREDITS PYMNTS.	CREDITS ADJ	BALANCE
		BALANCE FORWARD →				
4-6-XX	99203	OV, Level 3, NP	70 92			70 92
4-6-XX	93000	EKG	34 26			105 18
5-10-XX	99212	OV, Level 2	28 55			133 73
5-14-XX	99222	Hosp admit, C Hx/PX	120 80			254 53
5-15-XX	51900	Closure of vesicovaginal fistula	1196 82			1451 35
5-16-XX	99024	HV	NC			1451 35
5-17-XX	99024	Discharge	NC			1451 35
5-30-XX	4/6-5/15	Billed Prudential Insurance Company				1451 35
7-3-XX	Ck #7421	ROA Prudential Ins Co		980 30		471 05
7-3-XX	4/6-5/15	Insurance Contract adj (Prudential)			225 98	245 07
8-14-XX	Ck #230	ROA Pt		245 07		0

PLEASE PAY LAST AMOUNT IN BALANCE COLUMN

THIS IS A COPY OF YOUR FINANCIAL ACCOUNT AS IT APPEARS ON OUR RECORDS

1. Itemized fees for professional services with line-by-line description.
2. Running balance of amount owed on account.
3. Services after surgery posted as "no charge" (included in surgical package).
4. Insurance claim submitted listing dates of service billed.
5. Payment from insurance company (received on account) listing check number. Prudential paid 80% of allowed amount ($1225.37).
6. Courtesy adjustment made for the amount disallowed ($225.98) by the insurance company.
7. Balance owed ($245.07) by patient (20% of $1225.37, amount allowed by insurance company).
8. Patient's payment check received with posted check number.

Fig. 4.14 Financial accounting record illustrating posting of professional service descriptions, fees, payments, adjustments, and balance due.

12. **Transmitting the Electronic Claim:** When filing claims electronically a batch is created and a digital file is stored in a predetermined directory. These files are either transmitted directly to the insurance payer or transmitted to a clearinghouse over a dial-up modem or digital subscriber line (DSL) modem or via the internet.

    Claims are transmitted either electronically as required by HIPAA or, in cases of exemption, on a paper CMS-1500 form. When sending paper claims, make a copy for office records and create an insurance claims register or spreadsheet to track and follow up claims. Refer to Fig. 4.16 for the phases of adjudication by the third-party payer for payment, partial payment, denial, or rejection.

13. **Provider's Signature:** Providers rarely sign the CMS-1500 insurance claim form. However, when a signature is required, it can be accepted in several formats—handwritten,

facsimile stamp, or electronic signature. State and government programs require a signature. In the Medicare program, certificates of medical necessity require an original signature.

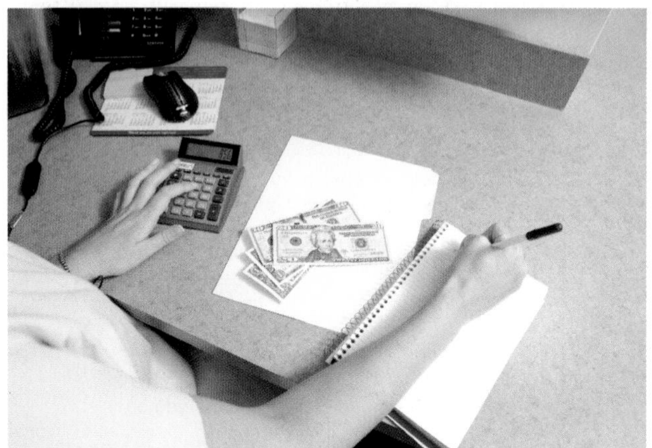

Fig. 4.15 Health care organization employee posting to a patient's financial accounting record or daysheet.

Sometimes a physician gives signature authorization to one person on the staff to sign insurance claims. That person is known as the physician's representative or attorney-in-fact (Fig. 4.17) . For an authorization of this type, a document should be signed before a notary public. If the health care organization is ever audited and fraud or embezzlement is discovered, the person who had signature authorization, as well as the provider, can be brought into the case. The federal government will prosecute if this involves a Medicare patient; the state government will prosecute if a Medicaid patient is involved.

Computerized Signatures: There are three levels of computerized or electronic signatures, listed in order of their strength.

- Level 1—digitized signature
- Level 2—button, personal identification number (PIN), biometric, or token
- Level 3—digital signature

An electronic signature looks like the signer's handwritten signature (Fig. 4.18). The signer authenticates the document by key entry or with a pen pad using a stylus to capture the live signature. It also can be defined as an individualized computer

PROCEDURE 4.1

Prepare and Post to a Patient's Financial Accounting Report

Objectives

To prepare; insert descriptions; and post fees, payments, credit adjustments, and balances due to a patient's ledger card

Equipment/Supplies

Typewriter or computer, patient accounts or ledger cards, and calculator

Directions

Follow these steps to post charges, payments, adjustments, and balances to a patient's ledger/account (see Fig. 4.14) and practice this skill by completing the assignments in the *Workbook*.

Personal Data: Insert the patient's name and address to prepare the ledger card. Some ledgers may require additional information (attending physician's name; type of insurance; insurance company's name with policy and group numbers; patient's home and work telephone numbers; birth date; Social Security number; driver's license number; spouse's and/or dependents' names; and name, address, and telephone number of nearest relative), depending on the style of card chosen for a health care organization.

Date: Post the date of service (DOS) in the date column, description of the services in the professional service description column, and charge amount in the charge column. The posting date is the actual date the transaction is recorded. If the DOS differs from the posting date, reference the DOS in the description column. This date column should never be left blank.

Reference: List a Current Procedural Terminology (CPT) procedure code number in the reference column.

Description: Write a brief description of the transaction that is being posted, such as *OV* for office visit or *HV* for hospital visit. Indicate the evaluation and management (E/M) service levels (1 through 5) using the last digit of the E/M code (for example, 9920**5** = Level **5**). List the name of other services or surgical procedures (for example, electrocardiogram, vaccination, tonsillectomy).

Charges: Add the charge to the running current balance and enter the current balance in the right column.

Payments: Post thze date the payment is received and indicate received on account **(ROA)** and who made the payment (for example, patient [pt] or name of insurance company) in the description column. List the type of payment (cash, check, debit card, money order, or credit card) and voucher or check number (for example, ck #430) in the reference column.

Adjustments: Post the date the adjustment is being made and indicate the type of adjustment (for example, insurance plan adj., contract adj., courtesy adj.).

Billing Comments: Indicate when the insurance company was billed by posting the current date and name of the insurance company. Include the dates of service being billed in the reference column (for example, 4/20/XX through 5/1/XX). Indicate when the patient statement was sent and amount due if different from the current balance (for example, patient billed $45.00 balance after insurance payment).

Other Comments: Indicate other comments that pertain directly to the account (for example, account sent to ABC Collection Agency, account scheduled for small claims court).

Charges: Refer to the fee schedule and post each fee (charge) on a separate line in the "Charge" column. Charges are debited (subtracted) from the account balance.

Payments: Enter the amount paid in the "Payment" column, credit (subtract) the payment received from the amount in the running current balance column, and enter the current balance.

Adjustments: Post the contracted insurance plan discount in the "Adjustment" column by referencing the DOS, insurance company name, and type of contract discount (for example, HealthNet PPO discount or Medicare courtesy adjustment). Adjustments are credited to the account balance.

Current Balance: Line by line, credit and debit by adding and subtracting postings to the running balance to determine the amount for the current balance column as shown in Fig. 4.14. If a line is used to indicate a date an action was taken (for example, insurance company or patient billed, account sent to collection), bring down the running balance from the previous line. This column must always contain an amount and should never be left blank. *Optional:* Post the adjustment on the same line as the payment.

Submit an itemized billing statement to the patient for the balance due.

Date	Description	Charge	Payment	Adjustment	Balance
					1346.17
7-3-XX	ROA Prudential Ins #7421		980.30	120.80	245.07

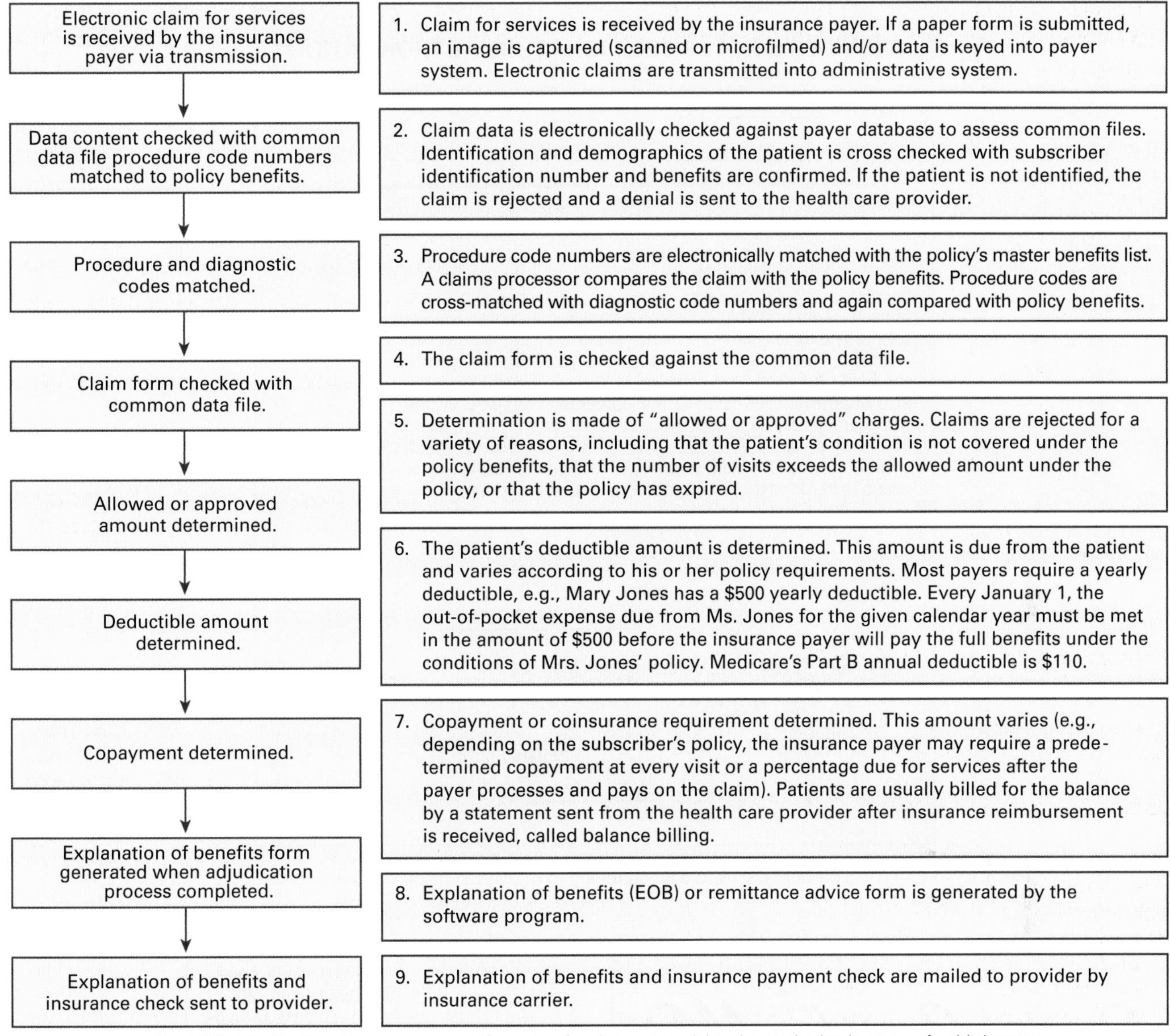

Fig. 4.16 Adjudication: Insurance payer life cycle of an insurance claim shows the basic steps of a third-party payer to pay an insurance claim and the documents generated.

access and identification system. Examples are a unique PIN, series of letters, electronic writing, voice, computer key, token, or fingerprint transmission (biometric system).

A digital signature may be lines of text or a text box stating the signer's name, date, and time and a statement indicating that a signature has been attached from within the software application (Fig. 4.19). Level 3 is the strongest signature because it protects the signature by a type of tamper-proof seal that breaks if the message content is altered.

Paper Environment: In the past, some health care organizations used a signature stamp so that the staff can process insurance forms and other paperwork without interrupting the provider and waiting for her or his signature. For an authorization of this type, a document must be signed before a notary (Fig. 4.17). Use of a signature stamp is not recommended. Most insurance carriers have updated signature policies advising providers that stamp signatures are no longer acceptable because of misuse or abuse. State laws may require that insurance claims or other related documents have an original signature. Billing specialists must follow state laws regardless of any carrier manual regulations. For information on state laws, contact the state legislature.

14. **Track Pending Insurance Claims:** In the computerized practice management system, a date is noted each time a claim is generated for submission, whether it is sent electronically or is printed on a paper claim form from the computer. An aging A/R report is used to determine outstanding balances. This can be generated using the date the claim was filed as a point to assess how many days old the claim is. The aging report is used to obtain the total A/R amount. This shows a snapshot of how much money is due to the organization from each patient or insurance carrier.

    Paper Environment: When submitting paper claims, keep a duplicate of the claim in the office pending file or in the computer system files. In the event payment is not received within a predetermined amount of time, the claim

PROVIDER'S NOTARIZED SIGNATURE AUTHORIZATION

State of Iowa)
)ss
County of Des Moines)

Know all persons by these presents:

That I John Doe, MD have made, constituted, and appointed and by these presents do make, constitute and appoint Mary Coleman my true and lawful attorney-in-fact for me and in my name place and stead to sign my name on claims, for payment for services provided by me submitted to the Blue Cross and Blue Shield of Iowa. My signature by my said attorney-in-fact includes my agreement to abide by the full payment concept and the remainder of the certification appearing on all CMS-1500 claim forms. I hereby ratify and confirm all that my said attorney-in-fact shall lawfully do or cause to be done by virtue of the power generated herein.

In witness whereof I have hereunto set my hand this 20th day of January 20XX.

John Doe, MD
(Signature)

Subscribed and sworn to before me this 20th day of January 20 XX

Notary Public

My commission expires ________.

Fig. 4.17 Example of a provider's signature authorization form that can be completed, notarized, and sent to the third-party payer after a copy is retained for the health care organization's records.

David Smith, MD

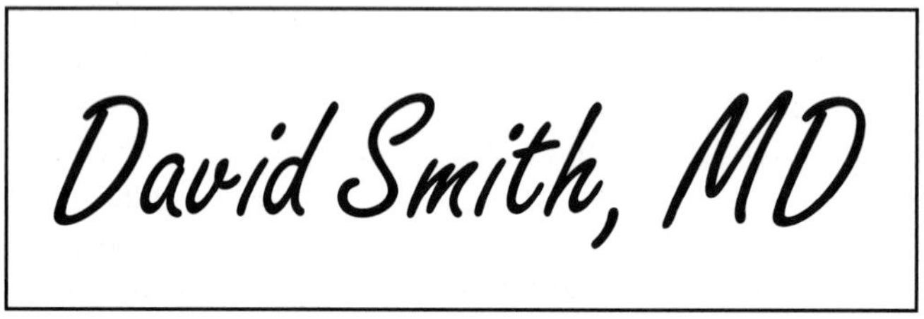

Fig. 4.18 Example of a provider's electronic signature.

Electronically signed:
David Smith, MD
07/12/2008 10:30:08

Fig. 4.19 Example of a provider's digital signature. This is an example of the strongest signature authentication.

must be followed up. This file also may be referred to as a suspense, follow-up, or tickler file. The term *tickler* came into existence because it tickles or jogs the memory at certain dates in the future.

If a computerized system is not being used, establish an insurance claims register or tracing file to keep track of the status of each case that has been billed. Record where and when the claim was sent on the insurance claims register and the patient's ledger card. The billing specialist handling the insurance forms can see at a glance which claims are becoming delinquent and the amounts owed to the organization. This is an efficient method used for 30- to 60-day follow-up. Fig. 4.20 Shows a document generated by a practice management system to assist in following up on electronically transmitted claims.

Keep two copies of each claim for the health care organization's records, one to be filed by patient name and the other by carrier name. Or simply record the name of the insurance company on each patient's ledger card and keep a file for each carrier by date of service. Filing by carrier allows all inquiries to be included in a single letter to the insurance company to eliminate having to write to the same company three or four times.

Whether claims are billed electronically or in paper format, a billing specialist should check with the insurance carrier to determine if their company features an online claim-tracking service on its website. This will allows a health care organization to follow up on unpaid claims and to check the status of a claim quickly using the insurance company's website.

15. **Insurance Payments:** After the claim is processed by the insurance payer, an EOB or remittance advice (RA) is generated and either sent on paper or transmitted electronically to the health care organization. Record of payment

Outstanding Claims
Primary Insurance
August 10, 20XX

Billing No.	Patient Name	Primary Insurance	Claim Sent	Bill Balance
1002	Simpson, Teri E	United Western Benefit		47.50
1003	Lee, Michael	United Western Benefit		83.55
1005	Bortolussi, Jabe	ABC Insurance Company	05/25/2007	465.00
1006	Blackwood, Crystal L	TRICARE	05/25/2007	16.07
1007	Helms, Clinton A	Medicare Health Systems Corporation	05/25/2007	33.25
1008	Jameson, Richard D	Royal Pacific Insurance Company	05/25/2007	41.07
1010	Kelsey, Ron	XYZ Insurance	06/09/2007	66.23
1011	Simpson, Teri E	United Western Benefit		16.07
1012	Simpson, Teri E	United Western Benefit		40.20
1013	Simpson, Teri E	United Western Benefit		16.07
1014	Simpson, Teri E	United Western Benefit		8.00
1015	Lee, Michael	United Western Benefit		16.07
1016	Lee, Michael	United Western Benefit		28.55
1017	Lee, Michael	United Western Benefit		40.20
1018	Martin, John R	Medicare Health Systems Corporation		149.86
1019	Jameson, Richard D	Royal Pacific Insurance Company		86.42
1020	Nunez, Margaret A	Aetna Health Plan		18.25
	Report Count: 17			1172.36

Fig. 4.20 Practice management software screen showing outstanding claims, patients' balances due, and names of insurance companies to follow up on claims.

or denial of the claim is posted to the patient's financial account.

Paper Environment: The payment is posted or credited to the patient's account and current daysheet indicating the date posted, name of insurance company, check or voucher number, amount received, contracted adjustment, and outstanding balance.

In both the electronic and paper environment, there may be claims that are not processed in a timely manner by the insurance payer. To follow up on these, a monthly review of outstanding claims, also known as an unpaid claims report or aged receivables, should be generated to determine further collection activity needed (Figure 4.20).

16. **Bank Deposit:** The health care organization should receive a payment from the third-party payer within 2 to 8 weeks from claim submission. The payment should accompany the RA sent by the insurance payer. Electronic funds transfer (EFT) may be used in place of a mailed paper check. EFT allows the automatic deposit of funds from the payer to the health care organization's bank account. In either electronic or paper office environments, all checks and cash are entered on the bank deposit slip and deposited at the bank.
17. **Monthly Statement:** The claim transaction is completed when the claim generated for each date of service has been processed by all responsible parties and the patient's financial account is at zero. For the patient who has insurance, a monthly statement for any outstanding balance should be sent indicating that insurance has been billed and the amount due is the patient's responsibility. The patient statement should always reflect the same fee as that submitted to the insurance company minus the amount paid by the patient copayment and/or the insurance amount paid or adjusted off. Patients who do not have insurance should receive a monthly statement indicating all outstanding balances due minus any payments or adjustments applied since the last billing statement.

    Some companies offer services to enable patients to pay their bills online securely through the health care organization's website. They also have electronic or eStatements that reduce processing and mailing costs by delivering patient statements securely or leave balance due reminders. Online bill payment may be set up to automatically draft patients' debit/credit cards; this eliminates checks and postage and speeds payments.
18. **Financial Records Retained:** Whether an office is computerized or still operates in a paper-based environment, a health care organization cannot escape the volumes of paperwork that business produces. Financial records must be retained and may include the following (not an all-inclusive list):
    - Copy of the completed patient information form, patient authorization or signature-on-file for assignment of benefits form, copies of insurance identification cards, responsible-party authorization, and insurance correspondence
    - Explanation of benefits or RA documents sent from insurance payers
    - Logs of all telephone conversations and actions taken regarding insurance disputes or collection activities. If these notes are not stored in the corresponding patient health record, the health care organization will likely have a master file set up where all logs are kept.
    - Encounter forms and referral and authorization slips
    - Daysheets and deposit slips

KEEPING UP TO DATE

- Make a folder or binder of pertinent insurance information. Obtain information booklets and policy manuals from the local offices of the various insurance companies. Obtain sample copies of all forms required for the insurance plans used most in the health care organization's office. Keep samples of completed claim forms.
- Changes occur daily and monthly, so keep well informed by reading Medicaid, Medicare, TRICARE, and local medical society bulletins. Maintain a chronologic file on each of these bulletins for easy reference, always keeping the latest bulletin on top.
- Attend any workshops on insurance in the health care industry offered in the area. Network with other insurance specialists to compare policies and discuss common problems. The American Association of Medical Assistants (AAMA) has chapters in many states that feature educational workshops and lectures.
- Become a member of one of the following professional organizations:
  - American Academy of Professional Coders (AAPC)
  - American Medical Billing Association (AMBA)
  - Medical Association of Billers (MAB)
  - Medical Group Management Association (MGMA)
  - Healthcare Financial Management Association (HFMA)
  - Healthcare Billing and Management Association (HBMA)
  - Professional Association of Health Care Office Management (PAHCOM)
  - American Health Information Management Association (AHIMA)
  - Each of these associations distributes journals or newsletters on a monthly basis featuring current information.
- Make good use of the internet.

KEY POINTS

This is a brief chapter review of the key issues presented. To further enhance your knowledge of the technical subject matter, review the key terms and key abbreviations for this chapter by locating the meaning for each in the Glossary at the end of this text, which appears in a section before the Index.

1. An insurance contract is a legal document in which the insured receives coverage that helps offset the cost of medical services. The four concepts of a valid insurance contract follow:
   a. The person must be a mentally competent adult and not under the influence of drugs or alcohol when signing the contract.
   b. The insurance company must make an offer (the signed application) and the person must accept the offer (issuance of the policy) without concealment or misrepresentation of facts on the application.
   c. An exchange of value (the first premium payment) submitted with the application, known as a *consideration,* must be present.
   d. A legal purpose must exist, which is an insurable interest in the case of a health insurance policy. This means that the policyholder expects to continue in good health but the insurance policy will provide something of value if an accident or illness strikes.
2. The insurance billing specialist must understand insurance terminology and policy provisions as they relate to billing and claims submission. An implied contract is created by the actions of the persons involved. On the other hand, an expressed contract can be verbal or written. However, most health care organization–patient contracts are implied.
3. There are many types of private and federal insurance programs, such as managed care, workers' compensation, Medicare, Medicaid, and TRICARE.
4. An aging accounts receivable report to determine outstanding balances can be generated using the date that the claim was filed as a point to assess how many days old the claim is. This report is used to understand how much money is due to the organization from each patient account.
5. Each type of insurance has different time limits for claims submission; if submitted after the designated time, claims will be denied.
6. Because federal program regulations have ongoing changes and new diagnostic and procedural codes are adopted annually, it is imperative that the insurance billing specialist keep up to date on technical information and have access to current reference books.
7. With the Affordable Care Act, Health Benefit Exchanges were created and changes occurred that affect the uninsured, preexisting conditions, prescription drugs, employers' responsibilities, and programs such as Medicare, Medicaid, and ERISA.

STUDENT ASSIGNMENT

- Study Chapter 4.
- Answer the fill-in-the-blank, multiple-choice, and true/false questions in the *Workbook* to reinforce the theory learned in this chapter and to help prepare for a future test.
- Complete the assignments in the *Workbook* to help reinforce the basic steps in submitting an insurance claim form.
- Turn to the Glossary at the end of this text for a further understanding of the key terms and key abbreviations used in this chapter.

5

The Blue Plans, Private Insurance, and Managed Care Plans

Linda M. Smith

OBJECTIVES

After reading this chapter, you should be able to:

1. Discuss the difference between a traditional indemnity insurance plan and a managed care plan.
2. State the provisions of the Health Maintenance Organization Act of 1973.
3. Explain the distinct types of managed care plans.
4. List features of an exclusive provider organization.
5. Define and discuss independent practice associations.
6. Name the features of preferred provider organizations.
7. Describe the features of a physician provider group.
8. Explain the features of a point-of-service plan.
9. Discuss triple-option health plans.
10. State the purpose of the Quality Improvement System for Managed Care.
11. Define a *carve out* and provide an example.
12. Discuss the patient information letter and its contents.
13. Identify four types of referrals for medical services, tests, and procedures.
14. State the purpose of creating an insurance and managed care plan reference guide.
15. Describe types of payment mechanisms used for managed care plans.

KEY TERMS

ancillary services
Blue Cross/Blue Shield Association
buffing
capitation
carve-out plans
churning
coinsurance
copayment
deductible
direct referral
disenrollment
exclusive provider organization
fee-for-service
formal referral
gatekeeper
group practice model
health maintenance organization
indemnity insurance plan
independent (or individual) practice association
managed care
managed care organizations
network HMO model
participating physician
per capita
physician provider group
point-of-service plan
preferred provider organization
prepaid group practice model
primary care physician
private health insurance
self-referral
staff model
stop-loss
tertiary care
traditional insurance plan
turfing
utilization review
verbal referral
withhold

KEY ABBREVIATIONS

copay
BCBSA
EPO
HMO
IPA
MCO
NCQA
PCP
POS
PPG
PPO
QISMC
UR

PRIVATE HEALTH INSURANCE

Private health insurance are plans marketed by the private health insurance industry rather than through government sponsored programs. Most private health insurance companies are publicly traded companies that operate to generate a profit for shareholders, although a smaller percentage operate as nonprofit organizations. Private insurance companies must meet the requirements of the state insurance agency in which they conduct business. Each state has different laws that dictate what services are mandated for coverage by private insurance companies and their obligations to beneficiaries. Private health insurance is generally offered through employers or other organizations. There are numerous private insurance companies across the United States who typically offer a variety of traditional and managed care plans.

Blue Cross/Blue Shield Plans

Blue Cross/Blue Shield (BCBS) is a pioneer in private insurance. It was founded in the 1930s as a not-for-profit organization. In 1994 the Blue Cross/Blue Shield Association (BCBSA) petitioned and was allowed to convert their status to for-profit corporations. The BCBSA developed into what is now a national association of approximately 36 independent, community-based, and locally operated BCBS companies. The BCBSA provides some form of health insurance in every state within the United States and has a program for US federal employees, retirees, and their families. They also act as administrators of Medicare in many states or regions of the United States. The BCBSA is the oldest and one of the largest insurance companies in the United States providing health care coverage to nearly one in three Americans.

Often referred to as the "Blues," the Blue Cross plans were developed to cover hospital expenses and the Blue Shield plans were established primarily to cover physician services. Each company is an independent franchise of the BCBSA and they often differ in corporate structure and policies. Each independent company offers local and national programs with several types of plans, including traditional indemnity plans and a broad range of managed care plans. Blue Cross/Blue Shield Companies also offer coverage through federal employee programs (FEPs), Medicare Advantage plans, Medicare supplemental plans, and Medicare Part D programs.

The patient's BCBS identification card is important in obtaining the correct information needed for billing purposes. The first step in obtaining the correct information is to identify the BCBSA trademark on the card and then locate the name and address of the BCBS home company that the patient is a member of. The address for claims submission should be identified on the back of the identification card. The BCBS card will also provide the type of plan the patient is enrolled in (for example, traditional, health maintenance organization, preferred provider organization, point-of-service plan . For specific examples of BCBS cards refer to https://www.bcbstx.com/provider/pdf/bav_id_card.pdf or https://www.bcbstx.com/provider/pdf/bca_id_card_sample.pdf.).

Health care organizations should have available for reference the current provider manual for its state's BCBS plans, which should provide the details needed for claim processing.

Fee-for-Service Plans

Until the early 1970s, most private health insurance companies offered only fee-for-service (FFS) plans. These are also referred to as traditional insurance plans or indemnity insurance plans. In an FFS plan, the insured pays a fixed monthly premium. The insured may obtain care from any health care organization and the organization is paid each time a service is rendered. The insured must meet an annual deductible. A deductible is a specific dollar amount that the patient must pay before an insurance plan begins covering health care costs. Once the annual deductible has been met, the insurance company will pay a percentage of the covered benefits. The remaining percentage is then paid by the insured; this referred to as the coinsurance amount.

MANAGED CARE

Through the 1960s and into the early 1970s, the financing and delivery of health care began to gain governmental attention. In an attempt to restrain the growth of health care costs for US citizens, legislators started to take notice of other models of health care coverage. They were interested in several types of prepaid group practice models that used a managed care approach to health care. Managed care refers to a group of techniques intended to reduce the cost of providing health care while improving the access to care and the quality of care. In a prepaid group practice model, the insurance carrier contracts with a network of providers to offer services to patients in their plan. The insurance carrier agrees to pay the providers in advance for the full range of services the patients in their plan are entitled to.

One of the earliest models was developed as far back as 1929, when an Oklahoma physician established a health cooperative for farmers in a small community. Participating farmers purchased shares for $50 each to raise money to establish a local hospital for the community and to bring several specialists into the area. In return the farmers received discounted medical care.

US legislators also noticed the work initiated in 1929 by two Los Angeles physicians, Donald Ross and Clifford Loos, who entered into a prepaid contract to provide comprehensive health services to 2000 employees of a local water company. Ross-Loos is now known as the *CIGNA Health Insurance Corporation*.

Another pioneer of modeled health care is the Kaiser Foundation Health Plans, which were started in 1937. The Kaiser construction company requested that Dr. Sidney R. Garfield and a few physicians working for him provide medical care for workers who were building a fresh-water aqueduct across the California desert to Los Angeles. Dr. Garfield charged the insurance carriers $1.50 per worker per month and the workers 5 cents per day. In return, he provided comprehensive health care. Then, in 1938, Henry J. Kaiser and his son, Edgar, started a joint venture to complete the Grand Coulee Dam in Washington and invited Dr. Garfield to form a medical group to furnish care to the workers for 7 cents per day prepaid by the employer. The group expanded to include the workers' wives and children. The *Kaiser Permanente Medicare Care Program* now has centers in 12 regions covering 16 states.

Health Maintenance Organization Act of 1973

The term **health maintenance organization (HMO)** originated in the 1970s by a policy advisor to the federal government on medical care whose name was Paul Ellwood. The term became institutionalized when Congress passed the Health Maintenance Organization Act of 1973 (Public Law 93-222), which began the movement to managed care in the United States. The emphasis of the movement was to do away with the FFS system, which rewarded health care providers for providing more services rather than for providing the appropriate services. The Health Maintenance Organization Act gave the federal government authority to assist HMO development in several ways, including (1) providing grants, loans, and loan guarantees to offset the initial operating deficits of new HMOs that meet federal standards (for example, are federally qualified) and (2) requiring most employers to offer an HMO to their employees as an alternative to traditional health insurance. Benefits under the HMO Act fall under two categories, basic and supplemental health service, and are listed in Box 5.1.

An HMO is a medical insurance group that provides coverage of health services for a prepaid, fixed annual fee. In an HMO, enrollees of the plan must seek services through a panel of providers who are members of the HMO network.

Over the past 20 years, HMOs have evolved into many types of managed care plans and have become the predominant form of health care in most parts of the United States. **Managed care organization (MCO)** is a generic term applied to a managed care plan. Although often criticized by disgruntled patients and consumer-advocacy groups, MCOs are credited with keeping down medical costs by reducing unnecessary hospitalizations, forcing providers to discount their rates, and causing the health care industry to become more efficient and competitive. Critics of managed care claim that managed care plans control costs by denying medically necessary services to patients, even in life-threatening situations, or by providing low-quality care. The criticism has led many states to pass laws mandating managed care standards.

BOX 5.1 Health Maintenance Organization Act Benefits of 1973

Basic Health Services

- Alcohol, drug abuse, and addiction medical treatment
- Dental services (preventive) for children younger than age 12 years
- Diagnostic laboratory, x-ray, and therapeutic radiology services
- Emergency health services in or out of the health maintenance organization (HMO) service area
- Family planning and infertility services
- Health education and medical social services
- Home health services
- Hospital services (inpatient and outpatient)
- Mental health services on an outpatient basis, short-term (not to exceed 20 visits) ambulatory, evaluative, and crisis intervention
- Physicians' services and consultant or referral services without time or cost limits
- Preventive health services (for example, physical examinations for adults, vision and hearing tests for children through age 17 years, well-baby care, immunizations, health education)

Supplemental Health Services

- Dental care not included in basic benefits
- Extended mental health services not included in basic benefits
- Eye examinations for adults
- Intermediate and long-term care (nursing facilities and nursing homes)
- Prescription drugs
- Rehabilitative services and long-term physical medicine (for example, physical therapy)

Accreditation

The National Committee for Quality Assurance (**NCQA**) is a not-for-profit organization that accredits managed care health plans. NCQA has built a rigorous set of standards to which health plans must attest and adhere. Receiving a seal of approval means that the health plan has met all key elements required by state and federal laws allowing them to participate in Medicaid and other managed care programs. NCQA is the most comprehensive evaluation in the industry and the only assessment that bases results of clinical performance and consumer experience.

Primary Care Physician

Most managed care plans use a **primary care physician (PCP)** as a gatekeeper. A **gatekeeper** is a physician who controls patient access to specialists and diagnostic testing services. Usually PCPs are physicians who practice in the fields of internal medicine, family practice, general practice, or pediatrics.

Identification Card

Each enrollee of a managed care plan is given an identification card. To see an example of a card from this type of plan, refer to Fig. 4.8. The card usually lists the patient's name, member number, group number, and primary care physician's name. The name of the MCO and type of plan with the amount of copayment for various outpatient services (for example, office visit, emergency department, urgent care center, and pharmacy) may be included by some plans.

Both sides of the patient's card should be photocopied because they contain important information such as the insurance companies address and telephone numbers used for inquiries and authorizations.

MANAGED CARE SYSTEMS

Managed care systems all have a network of physicians, hospitals and other health care providers contracted to provide services to their plan members at the lowest possible cost. However, not all managed care plans are alike. Some of the most common types of managed care plans are defined in this section.

Health Maintenance Organizations

The oldest of all prepaid health plans is the HMO. An HMO is a plan or program by which specified health services are rendered by providers to an enrolled group of persons. Fixed periodic payments on behalf of those enrolled in the plan are made in advance to providers of services.

Health Maintenance Organization Models

There are significant differences in the structure of various HMOs that influence the way health care organizations deliver services. Following are several types of HMO models.

Staff Model

The **staff model** is a type of HMO in which the physicians providing services are employed by the HMO. Physicians are usually paid on a salary basis and may also receive bonus or incentive payments based on their productivity and performance. Staff model HMOs must employ physicians of various specialties to meet the needs of their members.

Group Practice Model

In the **group practice model,** the HMO contracts with a multispecialty physician group practice to provide all physician services to its' members. The physicians are employed by the group practice and not by the HMO. For example, Kaiser Permanente is a group practice model wherein physicians form an independent group (Permanente) and contract with a health plan (Kaiser) to provide medical treatment to members enrolled by the plan. Although the physicians work for a salary, it is paid by their own independent group and not by the administrators of the health plan.

Network Health Maintenance Organization

In a **network HMO model,** the HMO contracts with two or more group practices to provide health services. These group practices may be broad-based, multispecialty groups or several small groups of primary care and specialty practices. Network physicians are typically paid using a capitation method. **Capitation** is a payment system used by managed care plans in which physician and hospitals are paid a fixed **per capita** (per person) amount for each patient enrolled over a stated period. The provider of services is paid a capitation amount for each HMO patient, regardless of whether the patient is actually seen by the physician in any given month.

Independent Practice Association Model

Independent (or individual) practice association (IPA) model HMOs contract with an association of physicians to provide services to their members. The physicians are members of the IPA, which is a separate legal entity. The IPA contract allows physicians to remain individual practitioners in their own separate offices and they are allowed to treat both HMO and non-HMO patients. Physicians are not employees and are not paid salaries. Instead, they are paid for their services on a capitation or FFS basis out of a fund drawn from the premiums collected from the subscriber, union, or corporation by an organization that markets the health plan. The IPA usually withholds a portion of the capitation to cover operating costs for risk sharing and incentive purposes.

Direct Contract Model

As the name implies, in direct contract models, the HMOs contracts directly with private physician practices in the community to provide services to their members. Direct contract model HMOs attempt to recruit broad panels of service providers, including primary care and specialist physicians. HMOs generally compensate physicians on either a FFS basis or a capitation basis.

Preferred Provider Organizations

A **preferred provider organization (PPO)** is another type of managed care plan. A PPO contracts with a group of providers (designated as "preferred") to deliver care to members. PPO members have the freedom to choose any physician or hospital for services, but they receive a higher level of benefits if the preferred providers are used. There are usually coinsurance requirements and deductibles. Occasionally the PPOs pay 100% of the cost of care but most do not. As with major medical policies, coinsurance requires the patient to pay 20% to 25% of the allowed amount up to a certain point and then the PPO pays 80% to 100% of the balance. Predetermination of benefits may be required, as well as fee limits, quality control, and utilization review.

Exclusive Provider Organizations

An **exclusive provider organization (EPO)** is a type of managed care plan that combines features of HMOs (for example, enrolled population, limited provider panel, gatekeepers, utilization management, capitated provider reimbursement, and authorization system) and PPOs (for example, flexible benefit design, negotiated fees, and FFS payments). It is referred to as exclusive because employers agree not to contract with any other plan. The member must choose medical care from network providers with certain exceptions for emergency or out-of-area services. If a patient decides to seek care outside the network, generally he or she is not reimbursed for the cost of the treatment. Technically, many HMOs can be considered EPOs. However, EPOs are regulated under insurance statutes rather than federal and state HMO regulations.

Point-of-Service Plans

The typical **point-of-service (POS) plan** combines elements of an HMO and a PPO while offering some unique features. It is basically an HMO consisting of a network of physicians and hospitals that provides an insurance company or an employer with discounts on its services. In a POS program, members choose a PCP who manages specialty care and referrals. A POS plan allows the covered individual to choose services from a participating or nonparticipating provider with different benefit levels. The POS program pays members a higher level of benefits when they use program (network) providers. The member may use providers outside the network, but higher deductibles and coinsurance percentages for out-of-network services act as incentives for members to stay within the network.

The POS plan may also provide nonparticipating benefits through a supplemental major medical policy. The key advantage of POS programs is the combination of HMO-style cost management and PPO-style freedom of choice.

Physician Provider Groups

A physician provider group (PPG) is a physician-owned business entity that has the flexibility to deal with all forms of contract medicine and still offer its own packages to business groups, unions, and the public. One division may function as an IPA under contract to an HMO. Another section may act as the broker or provider in a PPO that contracts with hospitals, as well as other physicians, to market services or medical supplies to employers and other third parties. Still another portion might participate in joint ventures with hospitals, freestanding imaging centers and laboratories, purchase of diagnostic equipment, retail medical equipment as a corporate subsidiary, and so on. The sideline businesses do not pay dividends but provide income to make future assessments to participating physicians unnecessary. The difference between an IPA and a PPG is that member physicians may not own an IPA, whereas a PPG is physician owned.

The ability of PPGs to combine services (joint purchasing, marketing, billing, collections, attorneys, and accountant fees) is an advantage because it cuts down on the cost of running a business and allows each physician to retain his or her own practice in addition to these joint ventures. The physicians turn over a small percentage of their income to the PPG for expenses. Patients call one telephone number to make appointments and the billing is done in one location.

Triple-Option Health Plans

Triple-option health plans allow members to select from three choices: HMOs, PPOs, or "traditional" indemnity insurance. Some of these plans allow the employee to change plans more often than traditional arrangements. They incorporate cost containment measures, such as precertification for hospital admission, hospital stays, and second surgical opinions.

Provider-Sponsored Organization

A *provider-sponsored organization (PSO)* is a managed care plan that is owned and operated by a health system, physicians group, or hospital instead of an insurance company. PSOs are gaining in popularity and growing in number. Many health systems are developing strategies to establish or expand their own health plans. They represent a move away from traditional FFS care to value-based care.

Consumer Directed Health Plans

Consumer directed health plans (CDHPs), also known as high-deductible plans (HDPs), are becoming more common as employers and individuals look for more economical health insurance options. CDHPs shift more of the payment responsibility to the plan member by requiring a large deductible that the family or patient is financially responsible for. Once the deductible is met, the insurance benefits will kick in.

Tables 5.1 and 5.2 give an overview or summary of five of the most common types of managed care plans.

MEDICAL REVIEW

Quality Improvement System for Managed Care

The federal government developed the Quality Improvement System for Managed Care (QISMC) program in 1996. The program was to provide oversight and ensure accountability of managed care plans using measurable standards. QISMC adopts a broad definition of "quality" to include the measurement of health outcomes, consumer satisfaction, accountability of MCOs for achieving ongoing quality improvement, the need for intervention to achieve this improvement, and the importance of data collection, analysis, and reporting.

Utilization Review of Management

Utilization management, also referred to as utilization review (UR), is a set of techniques used to manage health care costs. UR consists of a thorough case-by-case assessment of the appropriateness of care, medical necessity of health care services, and procedures according to evidence-based criteria or guidelines. The UR committee also watches over how providers use medical care resources. If medical care, tests, or procedures are denied, the patient must be informed of the need for the denied service and the risks of not having it. The written reasons for denial let the patient know his or her rights to receive the service and obligation to pay before obtaining such services.

Emphasis is placed on seeing a high volume of patients in a performance-based reimbursement system. Churning occurs when a physician sees a patient more than medically necessary, thus increasing revenue through an increased number of services. Churning may be seen in FFS practices as well as in some managed care environments. Turfing is the term used when the sickest high-cost patients are transferred to other physicians so that the provider appears to be a low utilizer. Buffing is the term for making this practice look justifiable to the plan. All of these situations may affect UR.

MANAGEMENT OF PLANS

Contracts

As an insurance billing specialist, you may be involved in negotiating contracts with private insurance and managed care companies. The health care organization must consider the financial implications that a contract with a private insurance company or a MCO will have on the organization's total revenue stream. Negotiated contracts should also have provisions that will lead to a positive working relationship with the payer, provide quality improvement strategies within the organization, and result in a higher level of patient satisfaction.

Although reimbursement is the key to finalizing most contracts, there are requirements in the billing process that should not be overlooked. The contract should identify the following:

- Authorization process for treatment
- Time limit for submitting claims and appealing denied claims
- How responsive the payer will be for processing claims and interest paid for overdue payment
- Process for adding new service lines

TABLE 5.1 Types of Managed Care Organizations and Their Characteristics

Plan Type	Member Advantages	Member Disadvantages
HMO	• Low cost for benefits • Preventive health care • No claim forms • Fixed, low copayments • Low monthly premium • Less out-of-pocket regardless of usage	• Restricted access to providers, tests, hospitals, and treatments except in emergencies or pay a penalty
Group	• Providers care only for plan members	• Must use gatekeeper, approved providers
Staff model	• Providers on staff of HMO	• Must use gatekeeper, approved providers
Network model	• Providers see plan and nonplan patients • Small copayment per office visit • Providers receive capitation fee	• Must use gatekeeper, approved providers
Direct contract model	• Contracted health care services to members by private practice physicians in the community	
IPA	Can use services from several affiliated providers, hospitals, or facilities Out-of-pocket expenses minor	Must use gatekeeper, approved providers
EPO	1. Flexible benefit design 2. Providers give negotiated discounts	• Must use gatekeeper, approved providers except in emergencies • Employer contracts only with one plan • Patient who seeks care outside the network is not reimbursed
POS	• Patients choose network or non-network providers • Providers give negotiated discounts • More flexible than basic HMO • Can bypass gatekeeper to see specialist	• Pay more if member sees non-network provider
PPO	1. More flexible than HMO 2. Does not require gatekeeper 3. Patients may choose network or non-network providers 4. Providers give negotiated discounts for each service and patients pay a small percentage 5. Pay less for network provider 6. Reduced costs for drugs	• Pay more if member sees non-network provider • Preventive services may not be covered • Patients pay a deductible • Claims must be filed • Possible predetermination of benefits • Pay fixed fees and patient pays the difference if bill is higher

EPO, Exclusive provider organization; *HMO,* health maintenance organization; *IPA,* independent (or individual) practice association; *POS,* point-of-service plan; *PPO,* preferred provider organization.

TABLE 5.2 Financial Systems of Managed Care Plans

Plan	NETWORK In	NETWORK Out	Copay Deductible	Payment Method	Authorization Required
HMO	X		Fixed copay	Capitated Fee-for-service (carve outs)	X
PPO	75%/25% 80%/20% 90%/10%	 60%/40% 70%/30%	 Fixed copay Deductible	 Fee-for-service	X
IPA	Limit Large group		Fixed copay	Capitated Fee-for-service (carve outs)	X
EPO	X		Fixed copay	Fee-for-service Capitated	X
POS	X	X	Fixed copay Deductible	Fee-for-service Capitated	X

EPO, Exclusive provider organization; *HMO,* health maintenance organization; *IPA,* independent (or individual) practice association; *POS,* point-of-service plan; *PPO,* preferred provider organization.

- Credentialing process for new providers
- Access to payer policies for all procedures
- How new policies and procedures imposed by the carrier will be communicated
- Noncovered services, excluded benefits, and **carve-out plans**

Carve-out plans refer to health insurance contracts that exclude specific diseases or injuries from coverage. For example, mental health services and chiropractic care are commonly carved out from coverage provided by an insurance plan. In those situations, mental health or chiropractic services are provided through a separately purchased contract at a higher premium. The insurance carrier may require that a specific group of health care providers be seen for related conditions and services that are usually reimbursed according to a different arrangement or rate formula than those services specified under the primary insurance contract.

PLAN ADMINISTRATION

Patient Information Letter

Inform patients what is expected from them and what they can expect in turn. The patient information letter should outline the names of the insurance plans that the health care organization is currently participating in. Outline any possible restrictions, noncovered items, and expectations for collection of deductibles, copayment, or coinsurance amounts. Note that if the patient neglects to notify the office of any change in eligibility status in the plan, such as **disenrollment**, the patient is then held personally responsible for the bill. Post a sign in the waiting room advising patients to check with the receptionist about participating plans.

Fig. 5.1 shows a sample letter of appropriate wording and content. File a copy of the letter given to the patient in the patient's medical record. If the patient refuses to agree with private insurance or managed care policy, document this in the medical record. Reimbursement may depend on the documentation.

! COMPLIANCE ALERT

Right to Audit Records

Many private insurance carrier and managed care organization (MCO) contracts contain a clause stating, "for quality care purposes, the insurance carrier or MCO has a right to access the medical records of their patients and for utilization management purposes." They have the right to audit those patients' financial records that relate only to the medical services provided to the member by the physician.

XYZ MEDICAL GROUP, INC.
1400 Avon Road, Suite 200
Woodland Hills, XY 12345

January 1, 20XX

TO: OUR PATIENTS

RE: PREFERRED PROVIDER ORGANIZATIONS

The following is a list of the PPOs and health insurance plans that we are members of and, therefore, will bill for you:

1. Georgia County Foundation
2. VIP Health Plan
3. Blue Cross Prudent Buyer Plan
4. Georgia County PPO
5. Northwest PPO
6. Blue Shield PPO

We are participating providers in several different PPOs. In order that we may maintain proper records for referrals and/or hospitalization, we request that each patient who is enrolled in a specific PPO keep our office currently informed regarding his or her eligibility status in that plan. Each time you are in the office for a visit, please verify with the receptionist that we have the correct coverage information.

If you have not informed us of changes in the status of your eligibility within the plan, you will be held responsible for any outstanding balance on your account due to that change.

Additionally, when your physician feels it is necessary to either hospitalize you or refer you to another physician outside this group, it is your responsibility to inform your physician that you belong to a specific PPO, as there may be restrictions imposed by that PPO regarding admission and referrals. If you fail to inform your physician at the time of referral or admission, our group may not be held responsible for noncoverage charges due to these restrictions.

If you have any questions regarding the above, please ask to speak to our insurance specialist.

I have read and understand the above text.

Signed: ______________________________ Date: ________________
Patient (subscriber)

Fig. 5.1 Letter to preferred provider organization *(PPO)* subscribers outlining restrictions and noncovered services.

Medical Records

When using an electronic medical record (EMR) system, the patient's account may be identified with a patient type that corresponds with the insurance plan the patient has joined.

Scheduling Appointments

Screen patients when they call for appointments to determine whether they belong to a health plan that the health care organization is participating with. Keep on hand an alphabetic list and profile of all plans with which the health care organization has a signed contract. If the patient is not in a participating plan, let the patient know and suggest that he or she locate a participating health care provider. If the patient still wishes to schedule services, advise him or her of your organization's policy for billing of nonparticipating insurances. Most organizations will require payment at time of service if the provider of services does not participate with their insurance.

Preauthorization or Prior Approval

Some managed care plans require preauthorization for certain services or referral of a patient to see a specialist. The following are several types of referrals that a plan may use.

- **Formal referral.** An authorization request is required by the MCO contract to determine medical necessity. This may be obtained via telephone or a completed authorization form (Fig. 5.2) mailed or transmitted by fax or e-mail.
- **Direct referral.** An authorization request form is completed and signed by the physician and handed to the patient. Certain services may not require completion of a form and may be directly referred (for example, obstetric care, dermatology).
- **Verbal referral.** The PCP informs the patient and telephones the referring service provider for an appointment.
- **Self-referral.** The patient refers himself or herself to a specialist. The patient may be required to inform the PCP.

Patients may be unaware of preapproval requirements. A good precaution is to ask the patient about insurance coverage at the time the appointment is made. If the patient is a member of a managed care plan, carefully review the patient's preauthorization requirements. If approval is necessary for certain situations, inform the patient of this before he or she sees the service provider. If a patient has obtained the written authorization approval, ask the patient to fax or mail you a copy because it may have an expiration date noted on it. Even if preapproved, the treatment must be medically necessary or payment may be denied after submission of a claim. If an authorization is delayed and the patient comes in for the scheduled services, the plan should be called to obtain a verbal authorization. The date, time, and name of the authorizing person should be documented; otherwise, the patient's appointment for services should be rescheduled. A referral recommendation must be documented in the patient's record and, if applicable, sent to the referring service provider.

A tracking system, such as a referral tracking log, should be in place for pending referrals so that care may be rendered in a timely manner and patients do not get "lost" in the system (Fig. 5.3). This log should include the date on which the authorization is requested, the patient's name, procedure or consultant requested, insurance plan, effective and expiration dates, dates of follow-up, name of person who approved or denied the request, and appointment date for consult or procedure. Sometimes authorization approvals are sent to the PCP and not to the referring or ordering physician. In these cases, follow-up must be made with the PCP. A maximum 2-week turnaround time should be allowed and all authorization requests should be tracked.

If a managed care plan refuses to authorize payment for recommended treatment, tests, or procedures, have the PCP send a letter to the plan that is worded similarly to that shown in Fig. 5.4. Include medical documentation, such as office and hospital visit notes, laboratory reports, and x-ray reports, to support the insurance claim. Then, after all efforts have been exhausted, send a letter such as the one shown in Fig. 5.5 to the patient informing him or her of this fact and asking the patient to appeal the denial of benefits.

In capitated managed care plans, when a PCP sends a patient for consultation to a specialist who is not in the managed care plan, the specialist bills the PCP. This is done because the PCP receives a monthly capitation check from the plan and any care for the patient must come from the capitation pool. This type of plan encourages PCPs not to refer patients so that they can retain profits.

If a specialist recommends referral to another specialist (**tertiary care**), ensure that the recommendation is provided in writing. Call the specialist at a later date to determine whether the recommendation was acted on. If the patient refuses to be referred, ensure that this is documented. If a referral form is necessary, do not telephone or write a letter. The managed care plan may refuse payment if the proper form is not completed.

When a referral authorization form is received, make a copy of the form for each approved office visit, laboratory test, or series of treatments. Then use the form as a reference to bill for the service. All copies being used indicates that all services that the patient's plan has approved are completed. Ask the PCP or the managed care plan for a new authorization to continue treatment on the patient. The request should be generated in a timely manner so that treatment is not delayed.

Diagnostic Tests

Many managed care plans require that patients have laboratory and radiology tests performed at plan-specified facilities. These are referred to as *network facilities.* Obtain the necessary authorizations for such services and allow sufficient time to receive the test or x-ray examination results before the patient's return appointment. When verifying benefits, ask if the deductible applies; that is, if a provider orders a radiology service that is on site, the deductible may not apply, but if the patient is sent to an outside facility, the deductible applies.

Inform the patient ahead of time when there is doubt about coverage for a test or the managed care plan indicates that a test is not covered. Disclose the cost and have the patient sign a waiver agreement to pay for the service, thus enabling the billing of the patient for the service. If an authorization is denied because a test is deemed "medically unnecessary" and the physician wishes to appeal, the physician can present clinical reasons

College Clinic
4567 Broad Avenue
Woodland Hills, XY 12345-0001
Telephone: (555) 486-9002
Fax: (555) 487-8976

MANAGED CARE PLAN AUTHORIZATION REQUEST

TO BE COMPLETED BY PRIMARY CARE PHYSICIAN OR OUTSIDE PROVIDER

☐ Health Net ☐ Met Life
☒ Pacificare ☐ Travelers
☐ Secure Horizons ☐ Pru Care
☐ Other

Member/Group No.: 54098XX

Patient Name: Louann Campbell Date: 7-14-20XX

☐ Male ☐ Female Birthdate: 4-7-1952 Home Telephone Number: (555) 450-1666

Address: 2516 Encina Avenue, Woodland Hills, XY 12345-0439

Primary Care Physician: Gerald Practon, MD Provider ID #: TC 14021

Referring Physician: Gerald Practon, MD Provider ID #: TC 14021

Referred to: Raymond Skeleton, MD Office Telephone number: (555) 486-9002

Address: 4567 Broad Avenue, Woodland Hills, XY 12345

Diagnosis Code: 724.2 Diagnosis Low back pain

Diagnosis Code: 722.10 Diagnosis Sciatica

Treatment Plan: Orthopedic consultation and evaluation of lumbar spine; R/O herniated disc L4-5

Authorization requested for: ☐ Consult only ☐ Treatment only ☐ Consult/Treatment ☐ Consult/Procedure/Surgery ☐ Diagnostic Tests

Procedure Code: 99244 Description: New patient consultation

Procedure Code: Description:

Place of service: ☒ Office ☐ Outpatient ☐ Inpatient ☐ Other Number of Visits: 1

Facility: Length of Stay:

List of potential future consultants (i.e., anesthetists, surgical assistants, or medical/surgical):

Physician's Signature: *Gerald Practon, MD*

TO BE COMPLETED BY PRIMARY CARE PHYSICIAN

PCP Recommendations: See above PCP Initials: *GP*

Date eligibility checked: 7-14-20XX Effective Date: 1-15-20XX

TO BE COMPLETED BY UTILIZATION MANAGEMENT

Authorized: Auth. No. Not Authorized

Deferred: Modified:

Effective date: Expiration date: Number of visits:

Fig. 5.2 A managed care plan treatment authorization request form completed by a primary care physician *(PCP)* for preauthorization of a professional service.

to the MCO's medical director to receive approval and bring attention to possible expansion of benefits for future patients.

Managed Care Guide

Creating a grid or matrix of all private insurance companies and MCOs with which the health care organizations has contracts with can help you to keep up with the many complexities of dealing with the various plans. Use a sheet of paper and list each plan with the billing address vertically in a column to the left. Then list significant data horizontally across the top. Suggested titles for column categories are as follows: eligibility telephone numbers, copayment amounts, preauthorization requirements, restrictions on tests frequently ordered, participating laboratories, participating hospitals, and the contract's time limit for promised payment. Referring

AUTHORIZATION REQUEST LOG								
Date requested	Patient name	Procedure/ consult	Insurance plan	1st F/U	2nd F/U	3rd F/U	Approved	Scheduled date
2/8/XX	Juan Percy	Bone scan- full body	Health Net	2/20			J. Smith	2/23/XX
2/8/XX	Nathan Takai	MRI-L-knee	Pru-Care	2/20	3/3			
2/9/XX	Lori Smythe	Consult Neuro G. Frankel MD	FHP	2/22			T. Hope	2/26/XX
2/10/XX	Bob Mason	Cervical collar	Secure Horizons	2/22	3/5	3/19		

Fig. 5.3 An authorization request log to be used as a system for tracing referral of patients for diagnostic testing, procedures, and consultations.

Ms. Jane Smith
Chairperson
Utilization Review Committee
ABC Managed Care Plan
111 Main Street
Anytown, XY 12345-0122

Dear Ms. Smith:

On ______________ I prescribed ______________ for ______________.
Date / List treatment, test, procedure / Patient's name

On ______________ you refused to authorize for that treatment. I find that I
Date
must take issue with your determination for the following reasons:

In my medical judgment, the treatment is a very important part of my overall care of ______________. This patient suffers from ______________. The treatment is
Patient's name / Describe condition
necessary to ______________. Failure to perform the treatment could
Describe why necessary
result in the following problem(s):

Enclosed are copies of the laboratory and radiological reports. For these reasons, I urge you to reconsider your refusal to authorize payment for the procedure I have prescribed.

By copy of this letter to ______________ I am reiterating my suggestion that
Patient's name
he/she obtain the treatment despite your refusal to authorize payment, for the reasons I have set forth in this letter and in prior discussions with ______________.
Patient's name

Yours truly,

John Doe, MD
Enclosures
cc: (Name of patient)

Fig. 5.4 A letter to a managed care plan when there is a refusal to authorize payment for a recommended treatment, test, or procedure.

to this grid can provide specifics about each plan's coverage and copayment amounts at a glance (Fig. 5.6). Some practices keep this information in a three-ring binder with dividers for each insurance plan. A good procedure is to include this information on each patient's data sheet when benefits are verified.

FINANCIAL MANAGEMENT

Payment

Private insurance companies, as well as federal and state programs, typically reimburse using an FFS payment schedule,

Mr. Avery Johnson
130 Sylvia Street
Anytown, XY 12345-0022

Dear Mr. Johnson:

On ______ (Date) I prescribed ______ (Treatment, test, procedure) for you. On ______ (Date), ______ (Name of Managed Care Plan) refused to authorize for same. On that basis, you have informed me of your decision to forego the treatment I have prescribed. I expressed my concerns regarding your decision during our discussion on ______ (Date) about the potential ramifications of your refusal to undergo the treatment.

The purpose of this letter is to recommend that you appeal ______ (Name of Managed Care Plan's) denial of benefits and reconsider your decision to forego the treatment in light of the potential consequences of your refusal.

Should you wish to discuss this further, please do not hesitate to contact me.

Sincerely yours,

John Doe, MD

Fig. 5.5 A letter sent by the provider to inform the patient about refusal of payment for treatment, test, or procedure by the managed care plan.

MANAGED CARE PLAN REFERENCE GUIDE

Plan name/address	Telephone eligibility	Copay	Preauthorization requirements	Test restrictions	Contracted lab(s) radiology	Contracted hospital(s)	Promised payment
Aetna PPO POB 43 WH XY 12345	555-239-0067	$5	hosp/surg/all dx tests	PE 1/yr	ABC Labs	College Hosp	30 days
Blue PPO POB 24335 WH XY 12345	555-245-0899	$8	referral specialist	PE 1/yr	Main St. Lab	St. John MC	30 days
Health Net POB 54000 WH XY 12345	555-408-5466	$5	hosp/surg see check list referrals	Mammo-gram 1/yr	Valley Lab	St. Joseph MC	45 days
Travelers MCO POB 1200 WH XY 12345	555-435-9877	$10	surg/hosp admit referrals	Pap >50 q3yr <50 q1yr	College Hosp Metro Lab	College Hosp	30 days

Fig. 5.6 Managed care plan quick reference guide to help keep track of specifics for each managed care plan in which the physician participates.

whereas managed care organizations have a multitude of payment methodologies.

Deductibles

Deductibles are generally associated with traditional or FFS insurance plans. Usually there is no deductible for a managed care plan. If the patient has a plan with a deductible, be sure to verify the amount of the deductible with the insurance company, ask patients if they have met their deductibles, and collect them in the early months of the year (January through April). Deductibles are applied to claims as they are received and processed by the plan.

Copayments

In a managed care plan, a copayment is a predetermined fee paid by the patient to the provider at the time service is rendered. It is commonly referred to as a copay and is a form of cost sharing because the managed care plan or insurance company pays the remaining cost. Remember to verify the copayment amount when inquiring about insurance plan benefits. Always collect the copay at the time of the patient's office visit. Billing for small amounts is not cost effective. Copays are commonly made for office visits, prescription drugs, inpatient mental health services, urgent care visits, and emergency department visits. However, the amount may vary according to the type of service. In some plans there may be a separate copayment for x-ray studies and durable medical equipment.

Payment Models and Mechanisms

Concierge medicine. Because insurance companies are paying less for services and there is an increase in documentation and paperwork, some health care organizations have opted to collect a monthly and/or annual retainer fee from patients. This system may be referred to as "concierge medicine" or "direct pay." A monthly fee for physician services can range from $50 to $150 or an annual fee can range from $1200 to $10,000. Services might include same-day appointments, more time for an office visit, and contact with physicians via telephone, e-mail, and text messaging. If the patient also has an insurance plan, the patient may have to do the paperwork and file the insurance claim.

Cash-only practices. Some health care organizations have decided not to join a network and prefer patients pay cash. If the patient has insurance, some service providers generate a completed claim form so that the patient can submit the claim to the insurance company.

Value-based reimbursement. Value-based reimbursement programs reward health care providers with incentive payments for the quality of care they provide. They are part of a larger quality strategy to reform how health care is delivered and paid for.

The Affordable Care Act instituted the Hospital Value-based Purchasing Program and the Hospital Readmission Reduction Program, which made a positive impact on the US health care system. As a result there is a greater movement from long-standing volume-based health care models toward value-based care models. For example, the FFS model rewards volume and intensity of service so that more procedures and hospital admissions give more money to the service provider versus value-based health care, which aligns payment and measures objectively the clinical quality of health care. Some of these value-based models are listed here.

Pay for performance. Health care organizations receive FFS payments and receive compensation or bonuses for complying with certain clinical goals. For example, a goal might be to immunize 80% of the organization's patients by age 2 using nationally approved guidelines. If the provider exceeds that goal, reaching a higher percentage, then health care organization receives a bonus.

Bundled payment/episode of care. Health care organizations agree to accept a single negotiated fee to deliver all medical services for one patient for a specified procedure or condition (for example, hip replacement surgery, pregnancy and birth, certain cardiac procedures). This can reduce costs for payers and increase payment to service providers. The service provider tries to improve efficiency and quality within episodes. However, one must watch that the costs of services for the procedures or conditions do not exceed the agreed-on reimbursement amount.

Patient-centered medical home (PCMH). The medical home consists of a single team managing with better coordination of medical care that agrees to provide more services. It is paid a negotiated FFS plus a monthly payment based on per-member-per-month (PMPM) and/or a pay-for-performance incentive. The team or group must show certain organizational and structural capabilities (for example, extended office hours, use of electronic health records, e-prescribing, patient disease registries).

Shared savings (one-sided risk). A combination of payment systems (FFS, pay for performance, bundled payments, global payments, or capitation) that rewards health care organizations that reduce total health care spending on their patients below an expected level set by the payer. The organizations receive a share of the savings.

Shared risk. Health care organizations receive performance-based incentives to share cost savings combined with disincentives to share the excess costs of health care delivery. There is an agreed-upon budget with the payer and the service provider must cover a portion of costs if savings targets are not achieved (for example, a percentage of premium or a set amount [50/50 sharing of excess costs]). If the payer wants the provider to accept more risk, the health care organization can either obtain stop-loss insurance or carve out certain patients or conditions. Another way of limiting risk would be to include a risk corridor arrangement. A corridor protects from high loss but at the same time obstructs opportunities for gains.

Provider-sponsored health plans (PSHPS). A large provider network or hospital system assumes 100% of the financial risk for insuring the patient population. It collects premiums from employers or individuals and directs how care is delivered to patients and how much is spent on giving that care. To set this up, the organization must have an insurance license and obtain approval as a health plan for the state in which it operates commercial, Medicare Advantage, or Medicaid plans. Such systems have responsibilities, such as claims payment, customer service, insurance reporting, and so on.

Full risk: capitation models. These are value-based systems involving managed care plans that can range from FFS and capitation to salaried physicians. Details about other payment mechanisms follow.

Contact capitation. Contact capitation is based on the concept of paying health care organizations for actual patient visits or "contacts." A scenario under this payment method occurs when a patient is referred to a specialist for care. A "contact" occurs when the patient visits the specialist for treatment. The patient is assigned to the specialist for a defined period called the *contact period.* The length of the contact period is set in advance for each type of specialty by the participating specialty physician panel and MCO and it may be tailored to the demographic and practice needs of the group. Each new patient visit during a contact period initiates a "contact point." Contact points determine how much to pay each physician. The average contact point value is determined by dividing the net specialty capitation pool or total amount of money set aside to be used for a particular specialty by the number of contacts in a certain period. The average contact value is used to determine the amount paid to each specialist during each month in the contact period.

Case rate pricing. For specialists, another payment method is case rate pricing. This means that the specialist contracts with the managed care plan for an entire episode of care. This may be done for certain high-volume, expensive surgical procedures (for example, knee surgery, cataracts, bypass surgery).

Stop-loss limit. Some contracts have a stop-loss section, which means that if the patient's services are more than a certain amount, the physician can begin asking the patient to pay (FFS). Monitor each patient's financial accounting record in those instances.

Contract Payment Time Limits

Usually state laws dictate the time limit within which a private insurance or managed care plan must pay. The contract may or may not state the terms of payment, time limits, and late payment penalties, all of which can vary from one plan to another. Prompt payment laws require payment within 30, 45, 55, or 60 days. To diminish late payment of claims, a contract can specify that late claims accrue interest (for example, 5% interest for claims paid after the payment time limit has elapsed). Some states have enacted laws enforcing interest penalties for late payment for either or both private payers, as well as managed care plans. Therefore know the laws for the pertinent state. A time limit payment provision is an important factor to consider when reviewing a contract before a medical practice participates.

Monitoring Payment

Monitor payments made from all private insurance and managed care plans and note whether the payment received is less than the agreed amount as stated in the contract. If payment has been reduced, send a letter to the plan citing, "As per contract, see page xx about the fee for the consultation."

Sometimes a procedure (for example, angioplasty with an assistant) may be done and the plan will not pay for an assistant, stating that it is not usual practice. However, perhaps the standard practice in a specific region is to always use an assistant for an angioplasty. When this is emphasized, the plan may remit additional payment.

Some states may have screening fees for emergency services and may or may not require prior approval for such services as defined by the Consolidated Omnibus Budget Reconciliation Act of 1985 (COBRA). Some states have adjudication laws with penalties if the plan does not pay promptly. The following steps should be taken if claims are not paid in a timely manner (30 days):

1. Write to the plan representative and list unpaid claims, claims paid after the payment time limit, and claims paid in error.
2. Send a statement to the director of the plan notifying him or her that if the bill is not paid, the employer's benefits manager or patient will be contacted and alerted to outstanding, slow-paying accounts. Explain that this will prevent the health care organization from renewing the plan's contract and ask the recipient to contact the plan's representative. The consumer has a choice of private and managed care plans; if the present plan does not fulfill his or her expectations, the plan loses members because of dissatisfaction.
3. Take examples and statistics to the next renegotiating session when health care organization's contract is expiring.

Statement of Remittance

Private insurance plans pay based on the services given to the patient (monthly check with a statement of remittance or explanation of benefits [EOB]). Many managed care plans pay using the same FFS basis. Other managed care plans may pay under a capitation system (monthly check for the number of patients in the plan).

In the capitation system, a monthly check arrives written out for the total amount of monthly capitation. The accompanying paperwork lists all eligible patients being paid for on a per capita basis divided into two groups: commercial and senior. Patients categorized as commercial are usually younger than age 65 and are paid at a lesser rate because their risk is lower (for example, they do not need to see the doctor frequently). The senior patient category includes those older than 65 years of age; these are paid at a higher rate because of the increased risk. Always verify the individual capitated amounts listed by each name on the accompanying paperwork against the monthly eligibility list to balance the amount of the check. Contact the MCO if an error appears. If a specialist is capitated, there may be thousands of patients on the capitation plan and a list of patients will not be provided. The capitation amount for a specialist may be only a few cents per month calculated according to the risk of the patient needing specialty services.

In the system where payment is based on services rendered and a statement of remittance or EOB is generated, such statements itemize services that have been rendered to patients and usually indicate the amount billed, amount allowed, amount paid, and any copayment to be made by the patient (Fig. 5.7).

Accounting

Managed care plans vary in their financial reimbursement structure and careful accounting procedures are required. Accounting can become a confusing issue because of a mixture of private and managed care patients with copayment requirements, coinsurance amounts, deductibles, and withholds. Good billing and accounts receivable management software is designed to handle each plan in the computer separately to eliminate mistakes.

Fee-for-Service

Some medical practices handle managed care patient accounts the same as FFS patient accounts. If coinsurance payment is necessary at the time of service, post first the charge and then the coinsurance prepayment, calculated based on either the percentage of the charge the plan allows or the flat copayment amount (for example, $15 for each office visit). After receiving the EOB document from the insurance plan, post an adjustment entry of the disallowed amount, which is calculated on a percentage of the MCO's allowable charge to balance the account (Fig. 5.8). An overpayment should be shown as a refund or credit to the account.

STATEMENT OF REMITTANCE

PATIENT NAME (ID NUMBER)	SERVICE DATE MO. DAY YR	POS	NO SVC	PROCEDURE NUMBER AND DESCRIPTION	AMOUNT BILLED	AMOUNT ALLOWED	RISK WITHHELD	CO PAY	AMOUNT PAID	ADJ. CODE
380224171-01 ALAN E.				CLAIM NO. 62730406 ACCOUNT NO.						
	092620XX	03	1	81000 URINALYSIS-ROUTINE	1000	1000	100	0	900	
	092620XX	03	1	82270 OCCULT BLOOD ANY S	1200	1200	120	0	1080	
	092620XX	03	1	99243 COMPRE RE-EXAM OR	6500	6500	650	0	5850	
	092620XX	03	1	36415 VENIPUNCTURE W/CEN	1700	1700	170	0	1530	
				CLAIM TOTALS =	10400	10400	1040	0	9360	
558700321-01 RONALD B.				CLAIM NO. 62730407 ACCOUNT NO.						
	092520XX	03	1	90050 LIM EXAM EVAL A/O	3000	3000	300	300	2400	
				CLAIM TOTALS =	3000	3000	300	300	2400	
473760096-01 DORMA L.				CLAIM NO. 62730408 ACCOUNT NO.						
	092520XX	03	1	90050 LIM EXAM EVAL A/O	3000	3000	300	300	2400	
				CLAIM TOTALS =	3800	3000	300	380	3120	

VENDOR SUMMARY: TOTAL AMOUNT PAID $1,638.96 TOTAL WITHHELD $194.39
AMOUNT PAID YEAR-TO-DATE: $42,411.95 AMOUNT WITHHELD YEAR-TO-DATE $5,109.94

Adjustment Code Legend
A = Adjusted: Billed amount exceeds VIP allowed.
O = Claim for service denied. Charges for this service included in other benefit payment. No patient liability.

Fig. 5.7 Statement of remittance or explanation of benefits for noncapitated patients or contracted fee-for-service indicating the amount billed, amount allowed, amount paid, and any copayment to be made by the patient.

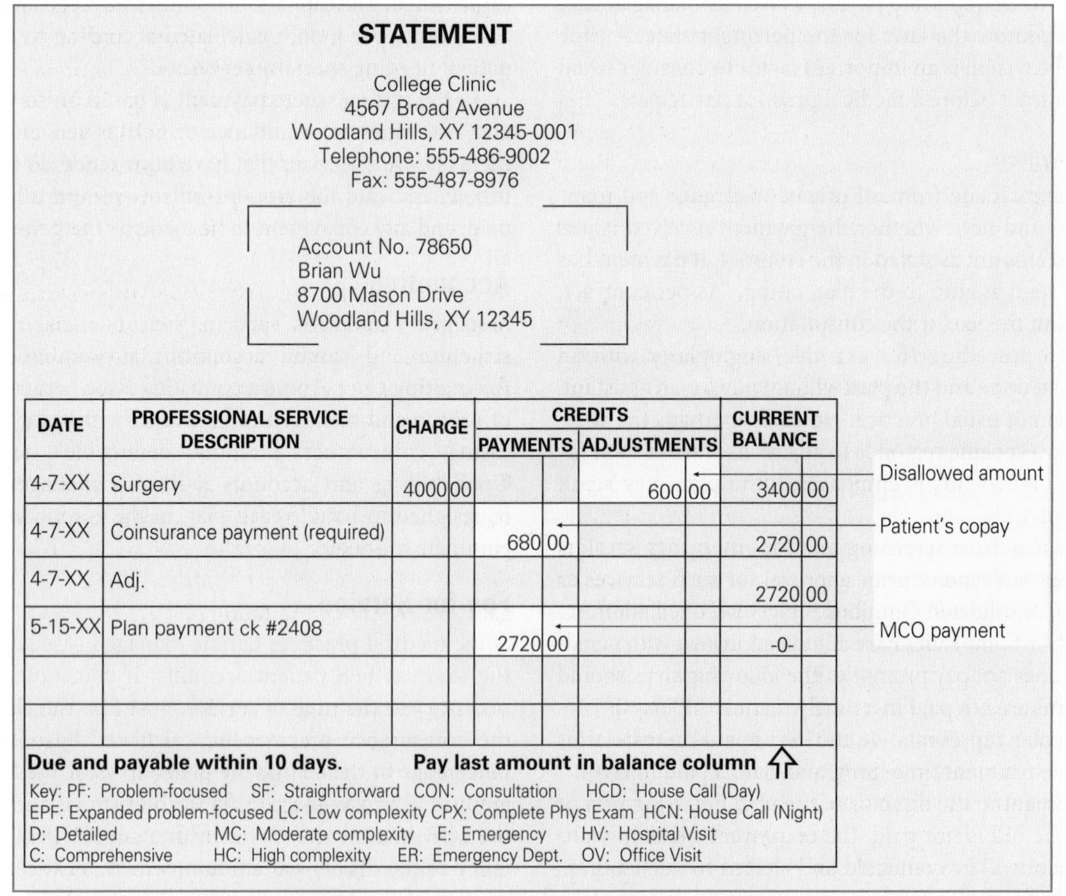

STATEMENT

College Clinic
4567 Broad Avenue
Woodland Hills, XY 12345-0001
Telephone: 555-486-9002
Fax: 555-487-8976

Account No. 78650
Brian Wu
8700 Mason Drive
Woodland Hills, XY 12345

DATE	PROFESSIONAL SERVICE DESCRIPTION	CHARGE	CREDITS PAYMENTS	CREDITS ADJUSTMENTS	CURRENT BALANCE
4-7-XX	Surgery	4000 00		600 00	3400 00
4-7-XX	Coinsurance payment (required)		680 00		2720 00
4-7-XX	Adj.				2720 00
5-15-XX	Plan payment ck #2408		2720 00		-0-

Due and payable within 10 days. **Pay last amount in balance column** ⇧

Key: PF: Problem-focused SF: Straightforward CON: Consultation HCD: House Call (Day)
EPF: Expanded problem-focused LC: Low complexity CPX: Complete Phys Exam HCN: House Call (Night)
D: Detailed MC: Moderate complexity E: Emergency HV: Hospital Visit
C: Comprehensive HC: High complexity ER: Emergency Dept. OV: Office Visit

Fig. 5.8 Posting to a patient's financial accounting record (ledger card) showing a charge of $4000. The plan allows $3400; therefore the patient's prepaid coinsurance amount is $680 (20% of $3400). The managed care plan sent a check for $2720 (80% of $3400) and the disallowed amount ($600) is adjusted off the account, which brings the account balance to zero.

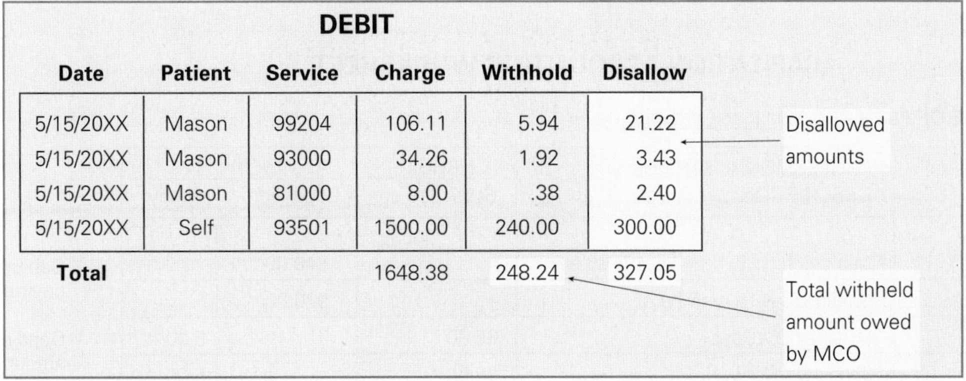

DEBIT

Date	Patient	Service	Charge	Withhold	Disallow
5/15/20XX	Mason	99204	106.11	5.94	21.22
5/15/20XX	Mason	93000	34.26	1.92	3.43
5/15/20XX	Mason	81000	8.00	.38	2.40
5/15/20XX	Self	93501	1500.00	240.00	300.00
Total			1648.38	248.24	327.05

Fig. 5.9 A managed care plan when payment is on a fee-for-service basis. Note the disallowed portion of the charge, which is based on the plan's allowable charge. A portion of the allowable charge is withheld.

Year-End Evaluation

Withhold

Depending on the contract, a managed care plan may retain a percentage of the monthly capitation payment or a percentage of the allowable charges to the health care organization until the end of the year to cover operating expenses. This is known as **withhold.** A statement of remittance from the MCO shows the risk amounts withheld for each patient's services in the eighth column of Fig. 5.7. The withhold plus interest is returned to the health care organization at the end of the plan year if the budgeted services for the plan are not overused. However, the withhold or a portion of it is retained by the plan if services are overused. Thus the health care organizations share in any surplus or pay part of any deficit at year's end. This risk sharing creates an incentive for limiting care by the gatekeeper and limiting referrals to specialists, thereby keeping medical costs down. The withhold can cover all services or be specific to hospital care, **ancillary services** (laboratory, x-ray use), or specialty referrals.

A managed care plan that withholds a percentage of the allowable charge must be tracked in the health care organization's accounts receivable so that it is not prematurely written off as a bad debt. To do this, develop a capitation accounting worksheet listing the dates of service, patients' names, Current Procedural Terminology (CPT) code for the service rendered, FFS charges, withheld amounts, and disallowed amounts (Fig. 5.9). Then total all columns. The total of the withheld column is a debit entry that indicates what the managed care plan owes to the health care organization pending its year-end reconciliation. When the withheld amount arrives, the accounting worksheet can be compared with the amount withheld during the year. The amount of withholds that are not returned to the health care organization is adjusted once withholds are settled. The total of the column for disallowed amounts shows the amount written off by the health care organization. Combine the withheld returned amount with the managed care payment for the year to determine whether it is worthwhile for the organization to participate in the plan. Some organizations can use the information to renegotiate increased fees when the managed care contract is to be renewed.

Capitation Versus Fee-for-Service

Financial management reports are generated via computer and are the responsibility of the manager or accountant in most health care organizations. However, it can be an asset for an insurance billing specialist to have some knowledge of the content of these reports. Most health care organizations monitor plan payments for profit or loss by comparing actual income from managed care patients with what would have been received from FFS plans. To do this, one designs a capitation accounting sheet for each capitated plan. This sheet shows a listing of dates of service and professional service descriptions (procedures, injections, and laboratory work) as well as charges and payments (Fig. 5.10). As managed care plan patients receive services, actual service fees are posted in a charge column from the service provider's fee schedule as if the patient were a private payer. In a payment column copayments, and the monthly capitation payment are posted. Then all columns are totaled. It is necessary to apply a discount to the total charged amount for a realistic comparison because the health care organization usually paid on an allowed amount rather than an actual charge. Calculate the difference between the actual charge and the average allowed amount to do this.

Compare the capitated payment amounts plus copayment amounts with the total discounted charges at the end of the year. This gives an accurate idea of whether the capitated payment received is adequate for the services the health care organization provided. Compiling monthly records and reviewing them at the end of the year helps a health care organization to assess the gain or loss of each capitation plan.

Bankruptcy

If a private insurance plan or an MCO declares bankruptcy, such as through a Chapter 11 filing, it is obligated to pay all bills incurred before the filing. However, in some situations, another entity may take over the plan and all services incurred after filing are paid by the new payer. If the patient had treatment before the filing, a delay in getting reimbursed may occur because the insurance plan cannot repay debts incurred before its filing until it has worked out a reorganization plan. Health care organizations under contract with the insurance plan are obligated to

CAPITATION ACCOUNTING WORKSHEET

NAME OF PLAN ABC Managed Care Plan

DATE OF SERVICE	PROFESSIONAL SERVICE DESCRIPTION	CHARGES	PAYMENTS	
		Services Fees	Capitation	Copay
20XX 1/15	Capitation (105 members) @ $8 ea		840.00	
2/15	Capitation (115 members)		920.00	
2/20	Sanchez OV/Copay	35.00		5.00
2/22	Jones OV/Copay	35.00		5.00
2/23	Davis OV/Copay	35.00		5.00
3/6	Evans OV/Copay	35.00		5.00
3/15	Capitation (130 members)		1040.00	
4/10	Wu OV/Copay	35.00		5.00
4/15	Capitation (135 members)		1080.00	
	May through December are not shown			
END OF YEAR TOTALS		3500.00	6880.00	500.00

Capitation payment

Copayment amount

Actual fee-for-service charge

Fig. 5.10 An accounting sheet for a capitation plan from January through April showing dates of service, professional service descriptions, members' charges, and capitation payments and copayments received by the medical practice. Charges and payments columns may be totaled at the end of the year to compare capitation with fee-for-service earnings.

honor their contractual commitments. If their contracts expire or if they have escape clauses, they may be required to continue accepting patients, depending on the contract provisions.

Some clauses allow a health care organization to withdraw from seeing patients or leave if the insurance plan is in bankruptcy proceedings for more than 4 months. However, bankruptcy courts have broad powers to prevent physicians from leaving insurance plans in bankruptcy proceedings if the court deems such actions to be detrimental to the rehabilitation of the debtor.

KEY POINTS

This is a brief chapter review, or summary, of the key issues presented. To further enhance your knowledge of the technical subject matter, review the key terms and key abbreviations for this chapter by locating the meaning for each in the Glossary at the end of this book, which appears in a section before the Index.

1. There are numerous private insurance companies across the United States who typically offer a variety of traditional and managed care plans. Private health insurance is generally offered through employers or other organizations. Plan benefits and coverage, as well as deductibles copayments and coinsurance amounts vary.
2. In a fee-for-service plan, the insured may obtain care from any health care organization.
3. *Managed care* refers to a group of techniques intended to reduce the cost of providing health care while improving the access to care and the quality of care.
4. Primary care physicians (PCPs) act as gatekeepers who control patient access to specialists and diagnostic testing services.
5. Health maintenance organizations (HMOs) have models, such as the prepaid group practice model, staff model, network HMO, and direct contract model.
6. Types of managed care plans are HMOs, exclusive provider organization (EPO), independent (or individual) practice association (IPA), preferred provider organization (PPO), physician provider group (PPG), point-of-service (POS) plan, triple-option health plan, and provider-sponsored organization (PSO).
7. Utilization review (UR) is a process based on established criteria for evaluating and controlling the medical necessity of services and providers' use of medical care resources to curb expenditures.

8. Some managed care plans may require prior approval for certain medical services or referral of a patient to a specialist. Four types of referrals are formal referral, direct referral, verbal referral, and self-referral.
9. Many private insurance carrier and managed care organization contracts provide them with the right to access the medical records of their patients for utilization management purposes.
10. If a contract has a stop-loss limit, it means that the health care organization can begin asking the patient to pay the fee for the service when the patient's services are more than a specific amount.
11. A managed care plan that has a withhold provision may retain a percentage of the monthly capitation payment or a percentage of the allowable charges to physicians until the end of the year to cover operating expenses.

STUDENT ASSIGNMENT

- Study Chapter 5.
- Answer the fill-in-the-blank, multiple-choice, and true/false review questions in the *Workbook* to reinforce the theory learned in this chapter and to help prepare you for a future test.
- Complete the assignments in the *Workbook* to give you hands-on experience in abstracting information from a medical record to complete treatment authorization forms.
- Turn to the Glossary at the end of this text for a further understanding of the key terms and key abbreviations used in this chapter.

6

Medicare

Linda M. Smith

OBJECTIVES

After reading this chapter, you should be able to:

- Explain the history of Medicare.
- Explain eligibility criteria for Medicare.
- Abstract important information from a patient's Medicare card.
- Identify the benefits of Medicare.
- List five federal laws adopted to increase health benefits for employed elderly individuals.
- Explain various Medicare programs and other insurance coverage combinations.
- Name the federal program that relates to utilization and quality control of health services.
- State the benefits for a participating versus nonparticipating provider.
- Explain the two different types of Medicare coverage policies that must be adhered to.
- Explain when to obtain a patient's signature on an Advance Beneficiary Notice of Noncoverage.
- Identify noncovered Medicare services.
- Define and discuss a Medicare prepayment screen.
- Discuss the different Medicare payment methodologies.
- Explain the resource-based relative value scale system that Medicare uses to establish fees.
- Explain how the Medicare Access and CHIP Reauthorization Act of 2015 have affected Medicare reimbursement.
- State the Medicare mandatory claim submission guideline.
- Define a Medicare Administrative Contractor and explain their responsibilities.
- Determine the time limit requirements for transmitting a Medicare claim.
- State the components of a Medicare remittance advice.
- Explain the importance of identifying Medicare overpayments.

KEY TERMS

adjudication
adjustment
Advance Beneficiary Notice of Noncoverage
Advanced Alternative Payment Model
approved charges
assignment
beneficiaries
benefit period
Centers for Medicare and Medicaid Services
Correct Coding Initiative
crossover claim
disabled
doughnut hole
durable medical equipment
end-stage renal disease
formulary
hospice
hospital insurance
jurisdiction
limiting charge
Local Coverage Determination
medical necessity
Medicaid
Medicare
Medicare Access and CHIP Reauthorization Act of 2015
Medicare administrative contractors
Medicare Advantage Plan
Medicare Beneficiary Identifier
Medicare Claims Processing Manual—Internet Only Manual
Medicare fee schedule
Medicare Improvements for Patients and Providers Act
Medicare/Medicaid
Medicare Part A
Medicare Part B
Medicare Part C
Medicare Part D
Medicare secondary payer
Medicare Summary Notice
Medigap
Merit-based Incentive Payment System
National Coverage Determination
national health insurance
national provider identifier
nonparticipating provider
nursing facility
participating provider
premium
prepayment screen
prospective payment system
Quality Improvement Organization
Recovery Audit Contractor Initiative
remittance advice
resource-based relative value scale
respite care
Supplemental Security Income
value-based programs

KEY ABBREVIATIONS

ABN	ICU	MIPS	par
APM	LCDs	MG	PFFS plan
CCI	LGHP	MMA	PPS
CMS	MA plan	MSA	PSO
DC	MAC	MSN	QIO
DHHS	MACRA	MSP	RA
DME	MBI	NCDs	RAC Initiative
ERA	Medi-Medi	NF	RBRVS
ESRD	MFS	nonpar	SSI
GPCIs	MIPAA	NPI	

BACKGROUND

National health insurance is a legally enforced system of health insurance that insures a countries' population against the costs of health care. It is usually established by national legislation but may be administered by the public sector, the private sector, or a combination of both.

The first move toward a national health insurance system began in Germany when the Sickness Insurance Law of 1883 was passed and industrial employers were mandated to provide insurance for their low-wage workers. Other countries such as the United Kingdom and most of Western and Central Europe began to follow suit to create other variations of national health insurance. At present, approximately 50 countries have legislation mandating universal or near-universal health coverage. National health insurance programs differ in both how money is collected and how services are provided.

The idea of a national health insurance system for Americans dates back to the presidency of Theodore Roosevelt in 1912. He envisioned a national health plan for the entire populations and individuals of all ages. Although his vision did not become reality during his term, he passed on his effort for a national health care program to President Harry Truman and President John F. Kennedy. Their presidencies also had significant impact in shaping the health plan. In 1965 Medicare legislation was signed by President Lyndon B. Johnson. It did not provide health coverage for the entire populations; however, it was established to provide national health coverage for Americans 65 years and older. Former President Truman attended the signing of this legislation and was issued the very first Medicare card.

POLICIES AND REGULATIONS

Medicare is administered by the Centers for Medicare and Medicaid Services (CMS), a federal agency within the US Department of Health and Humans Services (DHHS). The CMS is responsible for implementation of all rules, regulations, and health-related policies governing the Medicare program. The CMS is subdivided into three divisions:

1. The Center for Medicare Management oversees traditional fee-for-service (FFS) Medicare, which is health care coverage provided through the federal government. CMS oversees development of payment policy and management of FFS contractors.
2. The Center for Beneficiary Choices provides information on managed care options for individuals entitled to receive Medicare benefits. A Medicare managed care option is Medicare a health plan that is offered by a private company that contracts with the federal government to provide Medicare eligible individuals with health care coverage.
3. The Center for Medicaid and State Operations focuses on federal-state programs such as Medicaid, the State Children's Health Insurance Program, and insurance regulations.

The Medicare program consists of four parts.

- Part A (hospital insurance) covers inpatient care in hospitals, critical access hospital care, and nursing facility care. It also covers hospice care, some home health care, and certain blood services. A hospice is a public agency or private organization that is primarily engaged in providing pain relief, symptom management, and supportive services to terminally ill people and their families.
- Part B (medical insurance) covers physician care, outpatient hospital care, and other related health services that Part A does not cover, such as some of the services of physical and occupational therapists and some home health.
- Part C (Medicare Advantage) provides alternatives for Medicare beneficiaries through managed care plan options.
- Part D provides prescription drug coverage.

Eligibility Requirements

Medicare is a federal health insurance program for the following categories of people:

- People 65 years of age or older who receive Social Security benefits.
- People 65 years of age or older who are retired from the railroad or Civil Service
- Disabled individuals who are eligible for Social Security disability benefits and who are in the following categories:
  1. Disabled workers of any age
  2. Disabled widows of workers who are fully or currently insured through the federal government, Civil Service, Supplemental Security Income (SSI), or Railroad Retirement Act and whose husbands qualified for benefits under one of these programs. SSI is a program of income support for low-income aged, blind, and disabled persons established by the Social Security Act.
  3. Adults disabled before age 18 years whose parents are eligible for or retired on Social Security benefits

- Children and adults who have chronic kidney disease requiring dialysis or who have end-stage renal disease (ESRD). ESRD occurs when a patient who has chronic kidney disease has a gradual loss of kidney function and reaches an advanced state. In ESRD, kidneys are no longer able to work as they should to meet the body's needs.
- Kidney donors (All expenses related to the kidney transplantation are covered.)

Medicare Enrollment

The Social Security Administration (SSA) offices take applications for Social Security, control the Medicare eligibility process, and provide information about the Medicare program.

If an individual already receives Social Security or Railroad Retirement benefits, he or she is automatically enrolled in Medicare Parts A and B starting on the first day of the month that the individual turns 65 years of age with enough applicable work credits that are equal to 10 years of full-time employment. For those individuals who apply for Social Security benefits early (at age 62 years), they receive reduced Social Security retirement benefits; however, they do not receive Medicare benefits. If an individual is younger than 65 years of age and disabled, he or she will automatically get Medicare Parts A and B after getting Social Security disability or Railroad retirement benefits for 24 months.

All persons who meet eligibility requirements determined by SSA are eligible for Medicare Part A (hospital coverage) at no charge. Medicare Part B recipients pay annually increasing basic premiums to the SSA and some pay a Medicare surtax on federal income tax payments. This premium may be deducted automatically from the patient's monthly Social Security check if he or she wishes.

Illegal Immigrants

An illegal immigrant is an individual who is not a citizen or national of the United States but belongs to another country or people. In the Medicare program, an illegal immigrant may be eligible for Part A or B coverage. To be eligible, the applicant must have lived in the United States as a permanent resident for 5 consecutive years. It is usually not necessary to state on the claim form that the patient is an illegal immigrant when billing Medicare.

Health Insurance Card

Patients who are entitled to receive Medicare benefits are referred to as beneficiaries. On enrollment into the Medicare program the beneficiary is issued a red, white, and blue Medicare identification card. In the past, Medicare identified the patient by their name and their Social Security Number. However, the Medicare Access and CHIP Reauthorization Act of 2015 required removal of Social Security numbers from Medicare insurance cards to fight medical identity theft. Social Security numbers are currently being replaced by a Medicare Beneficiary Identifier (MBI), and the shift is expected to be complete by April 2019. During the transition period of April 1, 2018 through December 31, 2019 the patient's Social Security number or the MBI can be used for claim submission purposes. After the transition period ends on January 1, 2020, claims must be submitted with the patient's MBI. The MBI is 11 characters in length and is made up only of numbers and uppercase letters (Fig. 6.1). The patient's Medicare card will indicate the patient's MBI number, hospital and medical coverage status, and coverage start dates (Fig. 6.2).

Benefits

Medicare Part A: Hospital Benefits

Part A of Medicare is hospital insurance benefits for people 65 years of age or older, for people younger than age 65 with certain disabilities, or for people with ESRD. Funds for this health service come from special contributions from employees and self-employed persons, with employers matching contributions. These contributions are collected along with regular Social Security contributions from wages and self-employment income earned during a person's working years.

Medicare Part A provides benefits to applicants in any of the following situations:

1. A bed patient in a hospital (up to 90 hospital days for each benefit period). A benefit period begins on the day a patient enters a hospital and ends when the patient has not been a bed patient in any hospital or nursing facility (NF) (formerly called *skilled nursing facility*) for 60 consecutive days. It also ends if a patient has been in an NF but has not received skilled nursing care for 60 consecutive days. Hospital insurance protection is renewed every time the patient begins a new benefit period. There is no limit to the number of benefit periods a patient can have for hospital or NF care.
2. A bed patient in an NF receiving skilled nursing care (up to 100 extended care days for each benefit period). An NF offers nursing or rehabilitation services that are medically necessary to a patient's recovery. To be considered medically necessary, the medical services must be the appropriate care and generally accepted care to be reasonable and adequate for the diagnosis and treatment of the individual's illness or injury. Services would not be considered medically necessary if they are custodial. Custodial services are those that assist the patient with personal needs (e.g. dressing, eating, bathing, and getting in and out of bed).
3. A patient receiving home health care services.
4. A patient who needs care in a psychiatric hospital (up to 190 days in a lifetime).
5. A terminally ill patient diagnosed as having 6 months or less to live who needs hospice care.
6. A terminally ill patient who needs respite care. Respite care is a short-term inpatient stay that may be necessary for the terminally ill patient to give temporary relief to the person who regularly assists with home care. Inpatient respite care is limited to stays of no more than 5 consecutive days for each respite period.

Fig. 6.3 contains information on five major classifications of inpatient hospital cost-sharing benefits for Medicare Part A. Miscellaneous hospital services and supplies might consist of intensive care unit (ICU) costs, blood transfusions, drugs, x-ray and laboratory tests, medical supplies (casts, surgical dressings, and splints), use of wheelchair, operating room (OR) and recovery room costs, and therapy (physical, occupational, and speech language). There are no benefits for personal convenience items (television, radio, and telephone), private duty nurses, or a

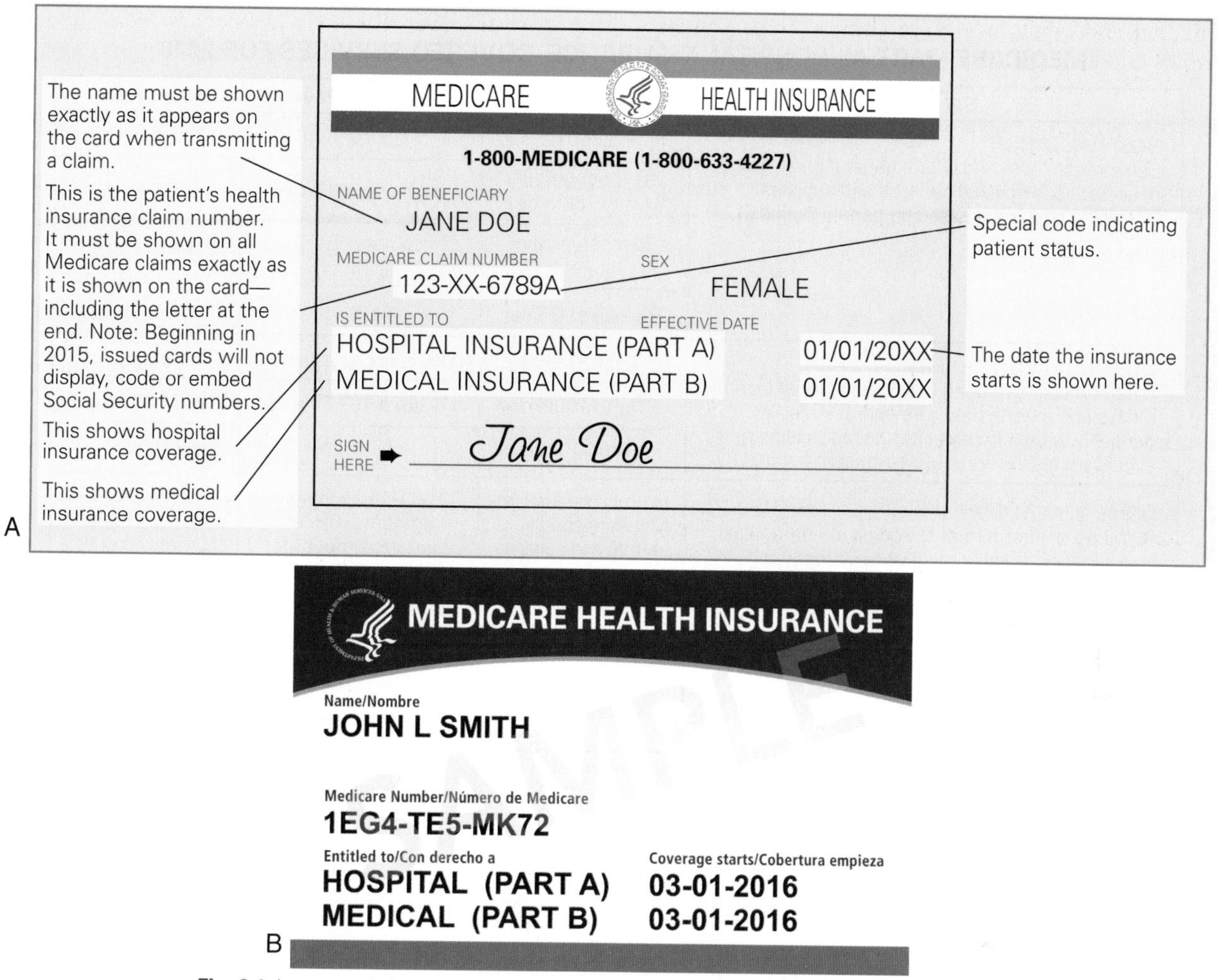

A

The name must be shown exactly as it appears on the card when transmitting a claim.

This is the patient's health insurance claim number. It must be shown on all Medicare claims exactly as it is shown on the card—including the letter at the end. Note: Beginning in 2015, issued cards will not display, code or embed Social Security numbers.

This shows hospital insurance coverage.

This shows medical insurance coverage.

MEDICARE HEALTH INSURANCE

1-800-MEDICARE (1-800-633-4227)

NAME OF BENEFICIARY
JANE DOE

MEDICARE CLAIM NUMBER
123-XX-6789A

SEX
FEMALE

IS ENTITLED TO
HOSPITAL INSURANCE (PART A)
MEDICAL INSURANCE (PART B)

EFFECTIVE DATE
01/01/20XX
01/01/20XX

SIGN HERE ➡ *Jane Doe*

Special code indicating patient status.

The date the insurance starts is shown here.

B

MEDICARE HEALTH INSURANCE

Name/Nombre
JOHN L SMITH

Medicare Number/Número de Medicare
1EG4-TE5-MK72

Entitled to/Con derecho a
HOSPITAL (PART A)
MEDICAL (PART B)

Coverage starts/Cobertura empieza
03-01-2016
03-01-2016

SAMPLE

Fig. 6.1 Important information on a patient's Medicare health insurance identification card.

private room unless the private room is determined medically necessary. Similar benefits also relate to nursing facilities.

Benefits for hospice and respite care consist of nursing and physicians' services, drugs, therapy (physical, occupational, and speech-language pathology), home health aide, homemaker services, medical social services, medical supplies and appliances, short-term inpatient care, and counseling.

Medicare Part B: Medical and Preventive Care Benefits

Part B of Medicare covers medical services and supplies that are medically necessary to treat the patient's health condition. Treatment can include outpatient care, preventive services (i.e., mammography screening, colon screening, annual wellness visit examinations), ambulance services, and durable medical equipment. It also covers part-time or intermittent home health and rehabilitative services such as physical therapy. Funds for this program come equally from those who sign up for it and the federal government. A medical insurance premium is automatically deducted from monthly checks for those who receive Social Security benefits, Railroad Retirement benefits, or a Civil Service annuity. Others pay the premium directly to the SSA. Table 6.1 contains specific information on medical and preventive care benefits for Medicare Part B. In addition to medical and surgical services by a doctor of medicine (MD), doctor of osteopathy (DO or MD), or a doctor of dental medicine or dental surgery (DDS), certain services by a doctor of podiatric medicine (DPM) and limited services by a doctor of chiropractic (DC) are paid for. Dental care is covered only for fractures or surgery of the jaw. Optometric examinations are provided if a person has aphakia (absence of the natural lens of the eye). In 2010 the Patient

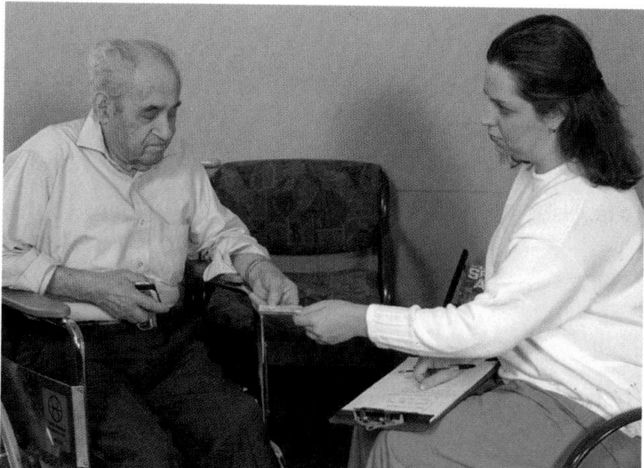

Fig. 6.2 Insurance billing specialist obtaining the identification card from a disabled Medicare patient.

MEDICARE (PART A): HOSPITAL INSURANCE–COVERED SERVICES FOR 2018

Services	Benefit	Medicare Pays	Patient Pays
HOSPITALIZATION Semiprivate room and board, general nursing and miscellaneous hospital services and supplies. (Medicare payments based on benefit periods.)	First 60 days	All but $ 1340	$ 1340 deductible
	61st to 90th day 91st to 150th day[1]	All but $ 335 a day	$ 335 a day
	60-reserve-days benefit	All but $ 670 a day	$ 670 a day
	Beyond 150 days	Nothing	All costs
NURSING FACILITY CARE Patient must have been in a hospital for at least 3 days and enter a Medicare-approved facility generally within 30 days after hospital discharge.[2] (Medicare payments based on benefit periods.)	First 20 days	100% of approved amount	Nothing
	21st to 100th day	All but $ 167.50 a day	Up to $ 167.50 a day
	Beyond 100 days	Nothing	All costs
HOME HEALTH CARE Part-time or intermittent skilled care, home health aide services, durable medical equipment and supplies, and other services.	Unlimited as long as Medicare conditions are met and services are declared "medically necessary."	100% of approved amount; 80% of approved amount for durable medical equipment.	Nothing for services; 20% of approved amount for durable medical equipment.
HOSPICE CARE Pain relief, symptom management, and support services for the terminally ill.	If patient elects the hospice option and as long as doctor certifies need.	All but limited costs for outpatient drugs and inpatient respite care.	Limited cost sharing for outpatient drugs and inpatient respite care.
BLOOD	Unlimited if medically necessary.	All but first 3 pints per calendar year.	For first 3 pints.[3]

[1] This 60-reserve-days benefit may be used only once in a lifetime.
[2] Neither Medicare nor private Medigap insurance will pay for most long-term nursing home care.
[3] To the extent the blood deductible is met under Part B of Medicare during the calendar year, it does not have to be met under Part A.

Fig. 6.3 Five major classifications of Medicare Part A benefits. (Updated from Medicare & You 2017, US Government Printing Office.)

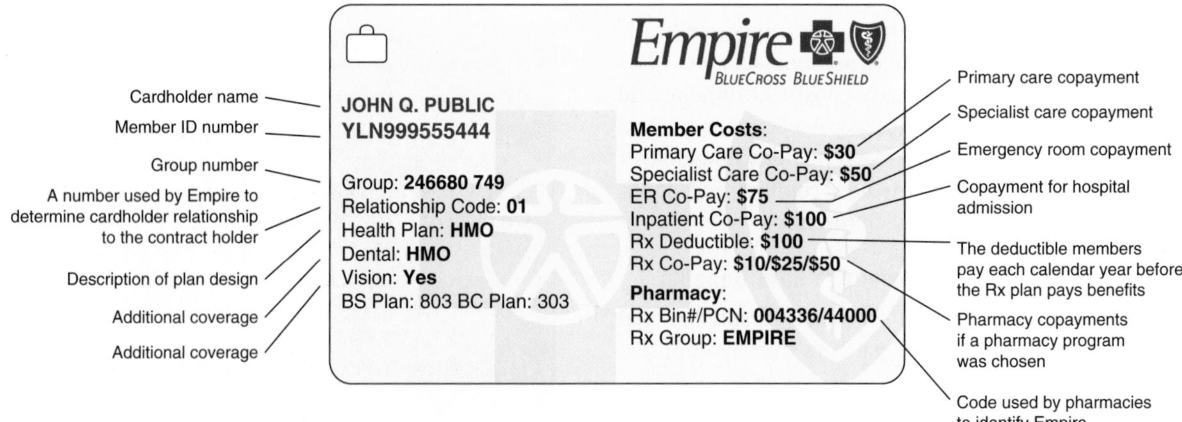

Fig. 6.4 A senior Medicare Advantage plan card.

Protection and Affordable Care Act (the Affordable Care Act) made preventive measures such as screenings for colon, prostate, and breast cancers free to Medicare beneficiaries.

Medicare Part C: Medicare Advantage Plan

Medicare Part C was created with the passing of the Balanced Budget Act of 1997. Under the Medicare Part C program, patients eligible for Medicare benefits, were given the option of choosing between traditional Medicare (described earlier) or a Medicare Advantage Plan (MA plan). Medicare Advantage Plans are offered by private insurance companies approved by Medicare. Medicare pays these companies to cover Medicare beneficiaries. This program was formed to increase the number of health care options, in addition to those that are available under Medicare Parts A and B (Fig. 6.4).

A Medicare beneficiary can join an MA plan if he or she has both Parts A and B and lives in the service area of the plan. Individuals who have ESRD must meet special situational requirements to join

TABLE 6.1 Medicare Part B: Medical Insurance—Covered Services and Preventive Care Benefits

Services	Coverage Requirements and Limitations	Medicare Pays	Patient Pays
Abdominal aortic aneurysm screening	One-time screening on referral	100% of approved amount	Nothing for screening test
Alcoholic misuse screening and counseling	One screening per adult per year	100% of approved amount if doctor accepts assignment	Nothing for screening or counseling in primary care setting
Ambulance services	For transportation to a hospital or skilled nursing facility	80% of approved amount after deductible	Current annual deductible* plus 20% of approved amount or limited charges†
Ambulatory surgery center	Facility fees are covered for approved services	80% of approved amount after deductible	Current annual deductible plus 20% of approved amount
Blood	Pints of blood as an outpatient or as part of a Part B–covered service	80% of approved amount	First three pints plus 20% of approved amounts for additional pints (after current annual deductible)‡
Bone mass measurement	Once every 24 months for qualified individuals and more often if medically necessary	100% of approved amount	Nothing for test
Cardiac rehabilitation	Includes exercise, education, and counseling	80% of approved amount after deductible	Current annual deductible plus 20% of approved amount
Cardiovascular disease (behavioral therapy)	One visit per year	100% of approved amount if doctor accepts assignment	Nothing for visit
Cardiovascular screening	Every 5 years to test cholesterol, lipid, and triglyceride levels for heart attack or stroke prevention	100% of approved amount	Nothing for test
Chemotherapy	In doctor's office	80% of approved amount after deductible	Current annual deductible plus 20% of approved amount
Chiropractic services	Limited services to correct subluxation using manipulation	80% of approved amount after deductible	Current annual deductible plus 20% of approved amount
Clinical laboratory services	Includes blood tests, urinalysis, and some screening tests	100% of approved amount	Nothing for tests
Clinical trials	Tests new types of medical care to prevent, diagnose, or treat diseases	80% of approved amount after deductible	Current annual deductible plus 20% of approved amount
Colorectal Cancer Screening (one or more of the following tests may be covered)§			
Fecal occult blood test	Once every 12 months	100% of approved amount	Nothing for test
Flexible sigmoidoscopy	Once every 48 months if age 50 or older or every 120 months when used instead of a colonoscopy for those not at high risk	100% of approved amount	Nothing for test
Screening colonoscopy	Once every 120 months (high risk every 24 months)	100% of approved amount	Nothing for test
Barium enema	Once every 48 months if age 50 or older (high risk every 24 months) when used instead of sigmoidoscopy or colonoscopy	80% of approved amount after deductible	Part B deductible does not apply; 20% of approved amount
Defibrillator (implantable automatic)	Outpatient setting	80% of approved amount after deductible	Current annual deductible plus 20% of approved amount
Depression screening	One screening per year	100% of approved amount if doctor accepts assignment	Nothing for screening
Diabetes screening	Twice a year for glucose monitors, test strips, and lancets	100% of approved amount	Nothing for screening
Diabetes self-management training	Provider must issue a written order	80% of approved amount after deductible	Current annual deductible plus 20% of approved amount
Diabetic supplies	Includes glucose testing monitors, test strips, lancet devices, lancets, glucose control solutions, and therapeutic shoes. Syringes and insulin covered if used with an insulin pump or if patient has Part D coverage	80% of approved amount after deductible	Current annual deductible plus 20% of approved amount
Doctor services	No coverage for routine physical examinations except for one-time "Welcome to Medicare" physical examination	80% of approved amount after deductible	Current annual deductible plus 20% of approved amount
DME	Oxygen, wheelchairs, walkers, and hospital beds for home use	80% of approved amount	20% of approved amount
Electrocardiogram screening	One-time screening	80% of approved amount	20% of approved amount

Continued

TABLE 6.1 Medicare Part B: Medical Insurance—Covered Services and Preventive Care Benefits—cont'd

Services	Coverage Requirements and Limitations	Medicare Pays	Patient Pays
Emergency department services	Bad injury or sudden illness when patient is in serious danger	80% of approved amount after deductible	Current annual deductible plus 20% of approved amount
Eyeglasses	One pair of glasses with standard frames after cataract surgery that implants an intraocular lens	80% of approved amount after deductible	Current annual deductible plus 20% of approved amount
Flu shots	Annually to prevent influenza or flu virus	100% of approved amount	Nothing for flu shots
Foot examinations and treatment	For diabetes-related nerve damage	80% of approved amount after deductible	Current annual deductible plus 20% of approved amount
Glaucoma screening	Once every 12 months	80% of approved amount after deductible	Current annual deductible plus 20% of approved amount
Hearing and balance examination	Ordered by a doctor to determine whether medical treatment is necessary; hearing aids and examinations for fitting hearing aids are not covered	80% of approved amount after deductible	Current annual deductible plus 20% of approved amount
Hepatitis B shots	Three shots for people with high or intermediate risk	100% of approved amount	Nothing for shots
Hepatitis C	Screening test for high-risk individuals	100% approved	Nothing for test
HIV screening	Once every 12 months	80% of approved amount for office visit	Nothing for test; 20% of approved amount for office visit
Home health services	Limited to reasonable and necessary part-time or intermittent skilled nursing care, home health aide services, physical therapy, and speech-language pathology; also includes DME	100% of approved amount; 80% of approved amount for DME	Nothing for services; 20% of approved amount for DME
Kidney dialysis services and supplies	In a facility or at home	80% of approved amount after deductible	Current annual deductible plus 20% of approved amount
Kidney disease education services	Six sessions of kidney disease education	80% of approved amount after deductible	Current annual deductible plus 20% of approved amount
Laboratory services	Certain blood tests, urinalysis, and some screening tests	100% of approved amount	Nothing for laboratory services
Mammogram screening[§]	Once every 12 months; also covers digital technologies	100% of approved amount	Nothing for screening
Medical nutrition therapy services	For people who have diabetes or renal disease not on dialysis or with a doctor's referral 3 years after a kidney transplantation	80% of approved amount after deductible	Current annual deductible plus 20% of approved amount
Mental health care (outpatient)	Certain limits and conditions apply	50% of approved amount after deductible	Current annual deductible plus 20% of approved amount
Obesity screening and counseling	Twenty-two face-to-face counseling sessions over 12 months	100% of approved amount if doctor accepts assignment	Nothing for counseling
Occupational therapy	To help patients return to usual activities after an illness (e.g., bathing)	100% of approved amount after deductible	Current annual deductible plus 20% of approved amount
Outpatient hospital services	When received as part of a doctor's care	Medicare payment to hospital based on hospital cost	Current annual deductible plus 20% of whatever the hospital charges
Outpatient medical and surgical services and supplies	For approved procedures	80% of approved amount after deductible	Current annual deductible plus 20% of approved amount
Papanicolaou (Pap) test/pelvic[§]	Once every 24 months (low risk) and once every 12 months (high risk)	100% of approved amount	Nothing for test
Physical examination	One-time "Welcome to Medicare" physical examination within first 12 months patient is on Part B	80% of approved amount after deductible	Current annual deductible plus 20% of approved amount
Physical therapy	Heat, light, exercise, and massage treatment of injuries and disease	100% of approved amount after deductible	Current annual deductible plus 20% of approved amount
PPV	Once in a lifetime	100% of approved amount	Nothing for flu and PPV if doctor accepts assignment
Practitioner services	Clinical social worker, physician assistant, and nurse practitioner	80% of approved amount after deductible	Current annual deductible plus 20% of approved amount
Prescription drugs	Certain injectable cancer drugs; drug coverage for patients who have Part D	80% of approved amount	Current annual deductible plus 20% after deductible of approved amount

TABLE 6.1 Medicare Part B: Medical Insurance—Covered Services and Preventive Care Benefits—cont'd

Services	Coverage Requirements and Limitations	Medicare Pays	Patient Pays
Prostate cancer screening§	Prostate-specific antigen test and digital rectal examination once every 12 months	100% of approved amount	Nothing for test
Prosthetic/orthotic items	Arm, leg, back, and neck braces; artificial eyes; artificial limbs and replacement parts; breast prostheses after mastectomy; prosthetic devices to replace an internal body part or function (includes ostomy supplies and parenteral and enteral nutrition therapy)	80% of approved amount after deductible	Current annual deductible plus 20% of approved amount
Pulmonary rehabilitation	Referral from doctor	80% of approved amount after deductible	Current annual deductible plus 20% of approved amount
Second surgical opinions	Covered in some cases; some third surgical opinions are covered for surgery that is not an emergency	80% of approved amount after deductible	Current annual deductible plus 20% of approved amount
Sexually transmitted infections screening and counseling	Once every 12 months or at certain times during pregnancy	100% of approved amount	Nothing for screening and counseling
Smoking cessation counseling	Eight face-to-face visits during a 12-month period if diagnosed with a smoking-related illness or if taking medicine that is affected by tobacco	100% of approved amount	Nothing for counseling sessions
Speech-language pathology services	To regain and strengthen speech skills	100% of approved amount after deductible	Current annual deductible plus 20% of approved amount
Surgical dressings	For surgical or surgically treated wound	80% of approved amount after deductible	Current annual deductible plus 20% of approved amount
Telemedicine	For some rural areas in a practitioner's office, hospital, or federally qualified health center	80% of approved amount after deductible	Current annual deductible plus 20% of approved amount
Tests	Radiographs, magnetic resonance imaging, computed tomography scans, electrocardiograms, and some other diagnostic tests	80% of approved amount after deductible	Current annual deductible plus 20% of approved amount
Transplant services	Heart, lung, kidney, pancreas, intestine, and liver transplants; bone marrow and corneal transplants; immunosuppressive drugs	80% of approved amount after deductible	Current annual deductible plus 20% of approved amount
Travel	Services in United States, District of Columbia, Puerto Rico, Virgin Islands, Guam, Northern Mariana Islands, American Samoa, and Canada, or on board a ship within US territorial waters	80% of approved amount after deductible	Current annual deductible plus 20% of approved amount
Urgently needed care	Treatment for sudden illness or injury that is not a medical emergency	80% of approved amount after deductible	Current annual deductible plus 20% of approved amount

*Once the patient has incurred expenses that match the amount of the deductible for covered services in the year, the Part B deductible does not apply to any further covered services received for the rest of the year. The Part B deductible amount for each year changes: 2012 is $140, 2013 is $147, 2014 is $147, 2015 is $147, 2016 is $166, 2017 is $183 and 2018 is $183.

†See Fig. 6.6 for an explanation of approved amount for participating providers and limited charges for nonparticipating providers.

‡To the extent that the blood deductible is met under Part A of Medicare during the calendar year, it does not have to be met under Part B.

§The Patient Protection and Affordable Care Act of 2010 made this preventive test free.

DME, Durable medical equipment; *PPV*, pneumococcal pneumonia vaccine.

an MA plan. Individuals who sign up for MA plans are issued an insurance card and do not use the Medicare Parts A and B cards. However, traditional Medicare cards are not forfeited, and an elderly patient may present with two cards. Special care should be taken when the patient presents for services to identify if the patient has the traditional Medicare or a MA plan and the effective date of the plan.

MA plans receive a fixed amount of money from Medicare to spend on their Medicare members. Some plans may require members to pay a premium similar to the Medicare Part B premium. There are many different types of Medicare Advantage plans. Plans available under this program may include the following: health maintenance organization (HMO), point-of-service (POS) plan, preferred provider organization (PPO), private fee-for-service (PFFS) plan, and provider-sponsored organization (PSO). These different types of managed care plans were outlined in Chapter 5.

A Medicare medical savings account (MSA) plan is another managed care option that may be offered. In an MSA plan, the patient chooses an insurance policy approved by Medicare that has a high annual deductible. Medicare pays the premiums for this policy and deposits the dollar amount difference between what it pays for the average beneficiary in the patient's area and the cost of the premium into the patient's MSA. The patient uses the MSA money to

EXAMPLE 6.1

Mr. Jones joins a Medicare medical savings account (MSA) plan and the plan deposits $2500 into his account. He has a yearly deductible of $4000. If he uses all of the money in his account for Medicare covered services, he'll have to spend $1500 out-of-pocket before he meets his deductible ($4000) and before the Medicare MSA plan will begin paying for his health care. Once Mr. Jones meets his deductible, the MSA plan will pay all his Medicare-covered health care services and he pays nothing. He must continue to pay the monthly Part B premium.

pay medical expenses until the high deductible is reached. If the MSA money becomes depleted, the patient pays out of pocket until the deductible is reached. Unused funds roll over for use in the following year. MSA plans vary, and the actual deposit and deductible amounts may be different from Example 6.1.

Another type of Medicare Advantage plan is a special needs plan (SNP), which provides focused and specialized health care for specific groups of people, like those who have both Medicare and Medicaid, live in a nursing home, or have certain chronic medical conditions.

Medicare Advantage plans must cover all the services that traditional Medicare covers except hospice care. Traditional Medicare covers hospice care even if you are in a Medicare Advantage plan. In all types of MA plans, the patient is always covered for emergency and urgent care. Many MA plans also offer extra benefits such as dental care, eyeglasses, or wellness programs.

Medicare Part D

Drug benefits started being offered to Medicare beneficiaries on January 1, 2006, under The Medicare Prescription Drug, Improvement, and Modernization Act (**MMA**). This legislation, known as **Medicare Part D,** offers seniors and people living with disabilities with a prescription drug benefit. It covers prescription drugs used for conditions not already covered by Medicare Parts A and B. It is a standalone prescription drug plan offered by insurance companies and other private companies providing drug coverage that meet standards established by Medicare. Other names for these plans are *Part D private prescription drug plans (PDPs)* and *Medicare Advantage prescription drug plans (MA-PDs).*

The two ways to get Medicare prescription drug coverage are as follows:

- Join a Medicare prescription drug plan that adds drug coverage to the original Medicare plan, some Medicare cost plans, some Medicare PFFS plans, and Medicare MSA plans.
- Join an MA plan, such as an HMO or PPO, that includes prescription drug coverage as part of the plan.

Individuals who enroll pay a monthly premium that varies depending on the plan. Those who decide not to enroll in a Medicare drug plan when they are first eligible may pay a penalty if they decide to join later. Enrollees pay an annual deductible that varies from plan to plan. The patient may also pay a percentage of the drug cost or a flat fee per prescription, referred to as a copayment. The amount of copayment required also varies from plan to plan.

Most Medicare drug plans have a coverage gap (also called the "**doughnut hole**"). This means that there is a temporary limit on what the drug plan will cover for drugs. The coverage gap begins after the patient and the drug plan together have spent a certain amount for covered drugs. Once the patient enters into the coverage gap, he or she pays a percentage of the plan's cost for covered brand-name drugs and a percentage of the plan's cost for covered generic drugs until he or she reaches the end of the coverage gap.

The DHHS estimates that more than a quarter of Part D participants stop following their prescribed regimen of drugs when they hit the doughnut hole. Provisions of the Affordable Care Act of 2010 have addressed this concern and will gradually phase out the coverage gap, eliminating it entirely by 2020. People who are eligible for Medicaid and Medicare pay no premium or deductible and have no gap in coverage. They pay a copayment of $1 per prescription for generics and $3 for brand names. Copayments are waived for those in nursing homes. In addition, several programs help people who have limited income and resources and the programs, qualifications, and copayments vary by area.

Each Medicare drug plan has its own list of covered drugs, referred to as a **formulary.** Many Medicare drug plans place drugs into different tiers on their formularies. Drugs in each tier have a different cost.

- Tier one represents generic drugs and generally cost less than a drug in a higher tier. Generics are equivalent to their brand-name counterparts and are ensured by the Food and Drug Administration to be as safe and effective. Generics drugs typically cost 30% to 70% less than brand-name drugs.
- Tier two covers preferred brand-name drugs and has a higher copayment than tier one. Preferred brand-name drugs do not have a generic equivalent available. They have been in the market for a time and are widely accepted.
- Tier three drugs are the nonpreferred drugs. Nonpreferred drugs are brand-name drugs that are not included on the plan's formulary and are higher-cost medications that have recently come on the market. In most cases an alternative preferred brand-name drug is available. If a brand-name drug is prescribed when a generic equivalent is available, the patient must pay the difference in cost in addition to the copayment. Nonpreferred drugs have higher copayments, or the patient may have to pay a higher percentage of the full drug cost.
- The fourth classification, identified as "S," represents specialty drugs. These are the most expensive drugs on the drug list. They are used to treat complex conditions like cancer and multiple sclerosis. They can be generic or brand name. Specialty drugs require a percentage of total cost of the drug.
- The following are several classes of drugs excluded from coverage under Medicare:
  - Drugs for cosmetic purposes
  - Drugs for symptomatic relief of cough and colds
  - Drugs for weight loss or gain
  - Erectile dysfunction drugs (unless there are medically accepted indications approved by the Food and Drug Administration)
  - Fertility drugs
  - Prescription vitamins or minerals, except prenatal

EXAMPLE 6.2 Prescription Note Clarifying Medical Use of Drug and Coverage Determination

Patient with psoriasis (autoimmune disorder) is prescribed methotrexate. Generally, this immunosuppressive drug is prescribed for transplant patients and is covered under Medicare Part B.

Added prescription note should read: "Psoriasis for Part D."

A provider who prescribes a drug that can be covered by either Part B or Part D must clarify the condition and part coverage on the prescription form (Example 6.2). When a patient has coverage under a Medicare Part D plan, obtain a photocopy of the patient's Medicare supplement or MA plan card. Then check whether the drug that the patient needs is covered by the plan, which generic drugs are available, and whether a drug needs prior authorization.

Medicare for Railroad Workers and Their Families

Patients who are receiving railroad retirement benefits or railroad disability checks will get Medicare from the Railroad Retirement Board. The Railroad Retirement Board automatically enrolls the patient in Medicare Parts A and B and medical insurance premiums are automatically deducted from their monthly Railroad Retirement benefit checks. Those who do not receive a monthly check pay their premiums directly or in some cases have premiums paid on their behalf under a state assistance program. Railroad Retirement beneficiaries generally are entitled to benefits for covered services received from a qualified facility in the United States. However, under certain circumstances a Medicare beneficiary may receive care in Canada or Mexico. Benefits and deductibles under Parts A and B are the same as for other Medicare recipients.

Some railroad retirees are members of a railroad hospital association or a prepayment plan. These members pay regular premiums to the plan and then receive health services that the plan provides without additional charges. In some plans, small charges are made for certain services such as drugs or home visits. Many prepayment plans make arrangements with Medicare to receive direct payments for services they furnish that are covered under Medicare Part B. Claims for services provided should be sent to the address of the Medicare railroad retiree center, listed on the back of the patient's Medicare card. After the claim is processed, a **remittance advice (RA)** document is generated to the service provider explaining the decision made on the claim and the services for which Medicare paid.

Employed Elderly Benefits

To understand various types of scenarios that may be encountered when transmitting claims for elderly individuals, one must know about several federal laws that regulate health care coverage of those aged 65 and older who are employed. Such individuals may have group insurance or a Medigap policy and may fall under billing categories of Medicare first payer or **Medicare secondary payer (MSP)** (all are discussed in detail later in this chapter). The federal laws that affect employed elderly individuals are shown in Box 6.1.

BOX 6.1 Federal Laws Affecting Employed Elderly Individuals

Omnibus Budget Reconciliation Act

The OBRA of 1981 required that in the case of a current or former employee or dependent younger than age 65 years and eligible for Medicare solely because of ESRD, the employer's group coverage is primary for up to 30 months. The Balanced Budget Act of 1997 mandated this change in the length of the coordination period. OBRA applies to all employers regardless of the number of employees. OBRA of 1986, effective in 1987, required that if an employee or dependent younger than age 65 years has Medicare coverage because of a disability other than ESRD, the group coverage is primary, and Medicare is secondary. This Act applies only to large group health plans (**LGHPs**) having at least 100 full- or part-time employees.

Tax Equity and Fiscal Responsibility Act

The TEFRA of 1982 established that an employee or spouse aged 65–69 years is entitled to the same health insurance benefits offered under the same conditions to younger employees and their spouses. The group insurance is primary and Medicare is secondary. TEFRA applies to employers with at least 20 full- or part-time employees.

Deficit Reduction Act

The DEFRA of 1984, effective in 1985, was an amendment to TEFRA and stated that a spouse age 65 to 69 years or an employee of any age is entitled to the same group health plan offered to younger employees and their spouses. The group's coverage is primary, and Medicare is secondary. DEFRA applies to employers with at least 20 full- or part-time employees.

Consolidated Omnibus Budget Reconciliation Act

The COBRA of 1985, effective in 1986, is another amendment to TEFRA eliminating the age ceiling of 69 years. An employee or spouse age 65 or older is entitled to the same group health plan offered to younger employees and their spouses. COBRA requires that third-party payers reimburse for certain care rendered in government-run veteran and military hospitals. The group's coverage is primary and Medicare is secondary. COBRA applies to employers with at least 20 full- or part-time employees.

Tax Reform Act

The Tax Reform Act was passed in 1986 and clarified certain aspects of COBRA. A spouse and dependents may elect to receive continued coverage even if the employee does not wish insurance coverage and terminates the plan. However, the spouse and dependents must have been covered under the plan before the covered employee terminates it. Spouses who are widowed or divorced while receiving continued coverage must report such changes to the benefit plan administrator within 60 days of the employee's death to determine how many additional months of coverage are available.

COBRA, Consolidated Omnibus Budget Reconciliation Act; *DEFRA*, Deficit Reduction Act; *ESRD*, end-stage renal disease; *OBRA*, Omnibus Budget Reconciliation Act; *TEFRA*, Tax Equity and Fiscal Responsibility Act.

ADDITIONAL INSURANCE PROGRAMS

Many Medicare recipients have Medicare in combination with other insurance plans. This section explains various coverage combinations.

Medicare/Medicaid

Medicaid is a joint federal and state program that helps pay medical costs if you have limited income and resources and meet other requirements. Some people qualify for both Medicare

The chart below shows basic information about the different benefits Medigap policies cover.
Yes = the plan covers 100% of this benefit
No = the policy doesn't cover that benefit
% = the plan covers that percentage of this benefit
N/A = not applicable

Medigap Benefits	Medigap Plans									
	A	B	C	D	F*	G	K	L	M	N
Part A coinsurance and hospital costs up to an additional 365 days after Medicare benefits are used up	Yes	Yes	Yes	Yes	Yes	Yes	Yes	Yes	Yes	Yes
Part B coinsurance or copayment	Yes	Yes	Yes	Yes	Yes	Yes	50%	75%	Yes	Yes***
Blood (first 3 pints)	Yes	Yes	Yes	Yes	Yes	Yes	50%	75%	Yes	Yes
Part A hospice care coinsurance or copayment	Yes	Yes	Yes	Yes	Yes	Yes	50%	75%	Yes	Yes
Skilled nursing facility care coinsurance	No	No	Yes	Yes	Yes	Yes	50%	75%	Yes	Yes
Part A deductible	No	Yes	Yes	Yes	Yes	Yes	50%	75%	50%	Yes
Part B deductible	No	No	Yes	No	Yes	No	No	No	No	No
Part B excess charge	No	No	No	No	Yes	Yes	No	No	No	No
Foreign travel exchange (up to plan limits)	No	No	80%	80%	80%	80%	No	No	80%	80%
Out-of-pocket limit**	N/A	N/A	N/A	N/A	N/A	N/A	$5,240	$2,620	N/A	N/A

* Plan F also offers a high-deductible plan. If you choose this option, this means you must pay for Medicare-covered costs up to the deductible amount of $2,240 in 2018 before your Medigap plan pays anything.

** After you meet your out-of-pocket yearly limit and your yearly Part B deductible, the Medigap plan pays 100% of covered services for the rest of the calendar year.

*** Plan N pays 100% of the Part B coinsurance, except for a copayment of up to $20 for some office visits and up to a $50 copayment for emergency room visits that don't result in inpatient admission.

Fig. 6.5 Medigap plans effective as of 2017 from a Medicare government publication.

and Medicaid and are called dual eligible. Patients designated as Medicare/Medicaid (Medi-Medi) are on both Medicare and Medicaid simultaneously. In these cases, Medicare processes the claims as the primary payer. Generally, the claim to Medicare can be completed in a manner that will allow for a crossover claim or claim transfer directly to the Medicaid program after Medicare payment has been made. Medicaid is always considered to be the payer of last resort and will process the payment as a secondary payer. If the Medicare payment exceeds the Medicaid fee schedule, little or no payment is made by Medicaid. If the beneficiary has not met his or her annual Medicare deductible, the Medicaid claim may result in payment of the Medicaid allowed amount.

Medicare/Medigap

Traditional Medicare pays for many, but not all, health care services and supplies. A Medigap (MG) policy is private insurance that helps pay some of the health care costs that traditional Medicare FFS Medicare plans don't cover. Coverage is commonly provided for copayments, coinsurance, and deductibles, all considered to be gaps in Medicare coverage. In some cases, a Medigap policy may also cover health care services that Medicare considers to be noncovered services. Patients pay monthly premiums to private insurance carriers for this supplemental insurance. Beneficiaries can elect not to enroll in a Medigap policy, and beneficiaries with a Medicare Advantage Plan do not need Medigap coverage. Every Medigap policy must follow federal and state laws designed to protect the Medicare patient, and it must be clearly identified as Medicare supplement insurance. All policies offer the same basic benefits, but some offer additional benefits. The patient can choose which one meets their needs. The policies are categorized by alpha letters A through N (Fig. 6.5). All policies are not available in all states, so individuals in some states have fewer options than others.

A slightly different variation of the MG policy is *Medicare Select*. This policy has the same coverage as regular MG policies, but there is a restriction in that the beneficiary must obtain medical care from a list of specified network doctors and providers.

The Medigap insurance carrier is usually billed after Medicare. If the beneficiaries' claim to Medicare has been submitted with the appropriate information, the Medicare contractor will automatically forward a crossover claim to the Medigap contractor for processing. This automation allows for faster claims processing.

Medicare Secondary Payer

Medicare secondary payer guidelines apply in situations when Medicare is not the beneficiary's primary health insurance coverage. In those cases, Medicare is considered the secondary payer. It is important that the billing specialist ensure that Medicare does not pay for services that the primary insurance carrier is responsible for. The MSP rules state that Medicare is the secondary payer when the patient falls into one of the following categories:

- Aged workers under group health plans with more than 20 covered employees
- Disabled individuals aged 64 and younger who are covered under a group health plan with more than 100 covered employees or covered under a family member's current employment
- Medicare beneficiaries under an employer-sponsored group health plan who have ESRD during the first 18 months of the patient's eligibility for Medicare
- Cases of workers' compensation when the injury or illness occurs at work
- Individuals with black lung disease either currently or formerly employed who fall under the Federal Black Lung Program
- Individuals receiving benefits under the Department of Veterans Affairs (VA) and Medicare
- Individuals covered under a federal research grant program

Automobile accident cases such as medical no-fault cases and third-party liability insurance cases. In these situations, Medicare is only billed after the primary insurance has processed the initial claim and has issued the service provider a remittance statement detailing the services that were billed and payment determination. The remittance statement must be forwarded with the claim to Medicare.

Follow the suggested steps in Procedure 6.1 at the end of the chapter to identify whether Medicare is primary or secondary and to determine what additional benefits the patient might have.

Managed Care and Medicare

Managed care plans were outlined in Chapter 5. When a patient's primary insurance is a managed care plan that requires fixed copayments at the time service is rendered, it is possible to obtain reimbursement from Medicare for those amounts. A claim must be filed with Medicare after the managed care organization (MCO) has paid. When Medicare's copayment reimbursement has been received, the provider must refund to the patient the copayment amount previously collected.

If the practice is paid a capitated amount by the managed care plan, they are paid a fixed per capita amount for each patient enrolled over a state period. There are no RA statements

PROCEDURE 6.1 Determine Whether Medicare Is Primary or Secondary and Determine Additional Benefits

1. Inquire whether the patient is covered under one or more of the following plans or situations:
   - Automobile liability insurance, no-fault insurance, or self-insured liability insurance. An individual injured or ill because of an automobile accident may be covered by liability insurance or no-fault insurance.
   - Disability insurance. Disability insurance coverage offered through an employer-sponsored large group health plan
   - Employee group health plan. Insurance policies for individuals 65 years of age or older who are still employed. Employers with 20 or more employees are required to offer workers and their spouses ages 65 through 69 years the same health benefits offered to younger workers. Workers may accept or reject the employer's health insurance plan. If they accept it, Medicare becomes the secondary insurance carrier.
   - Employer supplemental insurance. A Medicare beneficiary has this plan through a former employer. Some people are covered by employment plans even after retirement, as long as the plan allows it and the insured informs the insurance company that he or she wishes to maintain coverage. These are known as conversion policies. Complementary benefits can vary in these supplemental plans and these policies are not considered Medigap as defined by federal law. Note: When an employee retires, and Medicare becomes the primary coverage, the company's group health plan coordinates benefits with Medicare.
   - Federal Black Lung Act. This Act was formed to cover employees or former coal miner employees who have illness related to black lung disorder and have acceptable diagnoses that occur on the Department of Labor's list.
   - VA. A Medicare beneficiary is also receiving benefits from the VA. In this situation, there must be a decision made as to where to send the claim. Medicare is not secondary to the VA and the VA is not secondary to Medicare. The claim is sent where specified by the patient. The claim can be sent to Medicare, where if the claim is processed, the patient must satisfy his or her contractual requirement to pay any deductible and copayment amounts. If the patient asks that the claim be sent to the VA instead of Medicare, the claim is processed, and any payments issued are considered as payment in full. Many veterans want the claim sent to the VA.
   - Workers' compensation. An individual suffers a disease or injury connected with employment.

   These plans are billed as primary (first) payer and Medicare second. Payments for these types of policies may not necessarily go to the physician but may go to the insured.
2. Ask to see the Medicare card, as well as any other insurance cards, and make photocopies of both sides of each card.
3. Inquire of the patient whether the supplemental coverage was carried over (conversion policy) from his or her employer.
4. Call both carriers if the type of plan is not clearly identified.
5. Bill the correct insurance plan.

For MG cases, nonparticipating providers may collect copayments and deductibles up to their limiting charge (unless the state forbids collection of more than the allowed amount) from patients at the time of service. Participating providers may not collect copayments and deductibles from patients covered by MG if the patient requests that the physician submit the claim to the MG insurer. Collect copayments after receiving the Medicare/MG RA document.

For other secondary insurance, write the patient's group and policy (or certificate) numbers on the Medicare RA, attach it to either a new Medicare claim form or a copy of the original health insurance claim form, and electronically transmit or submit it to the secondary carrier. Then copy the physician's billing statement that shows date of treatment, description of services rendered, fees, and diagnosis.

MG, Medigap; *RA*, remittance advice; *VA*, Department of Veterans Affairs.

available from the managed care plan to forward to Medicare in these situations. Therefore the patient must sign a statement that explains the situation. Attach the statement and the copayment receipts to the claim. The statement may read as shown here.

> Patient Name ____________
> Medicare Number ____________
> There is no Explanation of Benefits documentation available for the attached billed services. I am currently enrolled with ____________ managed care plan for my health care. My physician, ____________ MD, is paid on a capitated basis, and the copayment that I pay is $ ____________ for each service or visit.
> Patient's signature____________
> Date ____________

Automobile or Liability Insurance Coverage

If the patient was involved in an automobile accident, the patient's automobile insurance is primary. Or, if it has been deemed that it is the legal responsibility of a person, business, or organization to pay for health care services, liability insurance coverage would be primary to Medicare. A physician who treats a Medicare patient who has filed a liability claim must bill the liability insurer first unless the insurer will not pay promptly (e.g., within 120 days after the liability insurance claim is filed). After 120 days have gone by without a payment from the liability insurer and if the services performed are covered Medicare benefits, a service provider or health care organization may seek **conditional payment** from Medicare. A conditional payment is a payment Medicare makes for services another payer may be responsible for so the patient does not have to use his or her own money to pay the bill. However, if a claim is filed with Medicare, the provider must drop the claim against the liability insurer.

If the payment made by the liability insurer is less than the physician's full charge, the physician may file a claim to Medicare. The provider cannot receive a higher combined reimbursement than what Medicare would have paid if they had been the primary payer.

For example:

Scenario 1:

- Patient received services; provider's full charge is $300.
- The liability insurance paid $200.
- The Medicare allowed amount for this service is $150.
- In this case a claim for the $100 balance would not be filed to Medicare because the liability insurance paid more than what Medicare would have allowed.
- The remaining balance of $100 will have to be written off by the service provider.

Scenario 2:

- Patient received services; provider's full charge is $300
- The liability insurance paid $100.
- The Medicare allowed amount for this service is $150.
- In this claim a claim for $50 may be filed to Medicare for the difference between what the liability insurance paid ($100) and what the Medicare allowed amount is ($150)
- The remaining balance of $150 will have be written off by the service provider.

UTILIZATION AND QUALITY CONTROL

Quality Improvement Organizations

DHHS has one of the largest federal programs dedicated to improving health quality for Medicare patients, the **Quality Improvement Organization (QIO)** program. The organization reviews for **medical necessity,** which CMS defines as the performance of services and procedures that are consistent with the diagnosis in accordance with standards of good medical practice, performed at the proper level, and provided in the most appropriate setting. QIO also reviews for reasonableness, appropriateness, and completeness and adequacy of care given in inpatient, outpatient, and emergency departments of hospitals; nursing facilities; home health agencies; PFFS plans; and ambulatory surgical centers.

It is extremely important that each patient's care be well documented from the treatment standpoint as well as for justifying maximum reimbursement. A physician who receives a letter from a QIO about quality of care should consult his or her attorney before responding by letter or personal appeal. A photocopy of the patient's health record can be used to substantiate the claim if there is detailed clinical documentation.

Medicare Billing Compliance Issues

Because Medicare is a federal program there is federal legislation that sets down the policies that must be followed. Therefore whoever participates in the program must comply with all regulations. General health care compliance has been discussed in Chapter 3; however, it is important to remind any staff member who may be involved in the health care organization of the issues they should be aware of. The following are issues that have been discussed in previous chapters or that will be outlined in later chapters of the textbook. The issues may include but are not limited to the following:

- Release of medical information
- Reassignment of payment
- Limiting charges for health care service providers
- Correct procedural code assignment and service utilization
- Accurate diagnostic code assignment
- Medical necessity of services performed
- Billing for ancillary employees (physician assistants and nurse practitioners), called "incident-to" billing
- Documentation related to selection of procedural codes for services performed
- Ancillary orders and supervision requirements
- Teaching physician and resident billing
- Routine waiver of copayments, deductibles, or professional courtesy discounts
- Stark I and II anti–referral and compensation regulations
- Overpayment refunds

PROGRAM FUNDAMENTALS

Provider

Healthcare providers are given the option to participate or not participate in the Medicare program. Most providers choose to participate in the Medicare program as there are payment incentives.

Participating Provider

In a **participating (par) provider** agreement, a service provider or health care organization agrees to accept payment from Medicare. Participating providers must accept **assignment** for all claims (Fig. 6.7). Accepting assignment means the patient has signed a statement to have Medicare send payment directly to the provider of services.

The fee that Medicare decides the medical service is worth is referred to as the **approved charge.** Medicare beneficiaries are required to meet their annual deductible, which is based on the calendar year January 1 through December 31 ($183 for calendar year 2017). Medicare will then reimburse 80% of the approved charges. The remaining 20% of the approved charge is paid by the patient (see Fig. 6.6).

PAYMENT EXAMPLES

	Actual charge	Medicare approved amount*	Deductible	Medicare pays	Beneficiary responsible for	Medicare courtesy adjustment†
Doctor A accepts assignment.	$480	$400	$147 already satisfied	$320 (80% of approved amount)	$80 (20% of approved amount)	$80 (difference between actual charge and approved amount)
Doctor B does not accept assignment and charges the limiting amount.	$437	$380	$147 already satisfied	$304 (80% of approved amount)	$133 (20% of approved amount [$76] plus difference between limiting charge [actual charge] and approved amount [$57] = $133)	None
Doctor C accepts assignment; however, the patient has not met the deductible amount.	$480	$253 ($400 minus the deductible)	$147 has not been met	$202.40 (80% of approved amount determined after subtracting the deductible)	$197.60 (deductible plus 20% of approved amount)	$80 (difference between actual charge and approved amount)

*The Medicare approved amount is less for nonparticipating physicians than for participating physicians.
†The courtesy adjustment is the amount credited to the patient's account in the adjustment column. The word "courtesy" implies that Medicare patients are treated well and is preferred to phrases like "not allowed."

Fig. 6.6 Payment examples for three physicians showing a physician accepting assignment versus one not accepting assignment and the amounts that the patient is responsible for paying with deductible satisfied and not met.

Nonparticipating Provider

Although there are few benefits, some healthcare providers may elect to not participate in the Medicare program. For instance, pediatric specialists rarely provide medical care to Medicare patients so they do not see a value in participation. A specialist in cosmetic surgery may choose to not participate as the services he provides would not be a covered benefit under Medicare.

A **nonparticipating (nonpar)** service provider or health care organization does not have a signed agreement with Medicare and has an option about assignment. The service provider may decline assignment for all services or accept assignment for some services and collect from the patient for other services performed at the same time and place. An exception to this policy is mandatory assignment for clinical laboratory tests and services by physician assistants.

Limiting charge is a percentage limit on fees, specified by legislation, that nonpar service providers may bill Medicare beneficiaries above the allowed amount. Nonpar service providers receive only 95% of the Medicare-approved amount. Nonpar providers may decide on a case-by-case basis whether to accept assignment. If the nonpar provider accepts assignment for a claim, Medicare pays 80% of the nonpar Medicare-approved amount directly to the provider and the provider collects the remaining 20% from the patient. If the nonpar provider does not take assignment on a particular claim, he or she may "balance bill" the patient 115% of the nonpar rate because Medicare will send the payment to the patient. For example, if the nonpar rate is $100, the provider can "balance bill" the patient for $115. However, in this case, even though the provider is required to transmit the claim to Medicare, the carrier pays the patient directly and the provider therefore must collect his or her entire fee from the patient; thus service providers must "chase

DRAFT - NOT FOR OFFICIAL USE

HEALTH INSURANCE CLAIM FORM

APPROVED BY NATIONAL UNIFOR MCLAIM COMMITTEE (NUCC) 02/12

PICA | PICA

CARRIER

1. MEDICARE (Medicare#) MEDICAID (Medicaid#) TRICARE (ID#DoD#) CHAMPVA (Member ID#) GROUP HEALTH PLAN (ID#) FECA BLK LUNG (ID#) OTHER (ID#)
1a. INSURED'S I.D. NUMBER (For Program in Item 1)
2. PATIENT'S NAME (Last Name, First Name, Middle Initial)
3. PATIENT'S BIRTH DATE MM DD YY SEX M F
4. INSURED'S NAME (Last Name, First Name, Middle Initial)
5. PATIENT'S ADDRESS (No., Street)
6. PATIENT RELATIONSHIP TO INSURED Self Spouse Child Other
7. INSURED'S ADDRESS (No., Street)
CITY STATE
8. RESERVED FOR NUCC USE
CITY STATE
ZIP CODE TELEPHONE (Include Area Code) ( )
ZIP CODE TELEPHONE (Include Area Code) ( )
9. OTHER INSURED'S NAME (Last Name, First Name, Middle Initial)
10. IS PATIENT'S CONDITION RELATED TO:
11. INSURED'S POLICY GROUP OR FECA NUMBER
a. OTHER INSURED'S POLICY OR GROUP NUMBER
a. EMPLOYMENT? (Current or Previous) YES NO
a. INSURED'S DATE OF BIRTH MM DD YY SEX M F
b. RESERVED FOR NUCC USE
b. AUTO ACCIDENT? YES NO PLACE (State)
b. OTHER CLAIM ID (Designated by NUCC)
c. RESERVED FOR NUCC USE
c. OTHER ACCIDENT? YES NO
c. INSURANCE PLAN NAME OR PROGRAM NAME
d. INSURANCE PLAN NAME OR PROGRAM NAME
10d. CLAIM CODES (Designated by NUCC)
d. IS THERE ANOTHER HEALTH BENEFIT PLAN? YES NO *If yes*, complete items 9, 9a, and 9d.

READ BACK OF FORM BEFORE COMPLETING & SIGNING THIS FORM.

12. PATIENT'S OR AUTHORIZED PERSON'S SIGNATUREI authorize the release of any medical or other information necessary to process this claim. I also request payment of government benefits either to myself or to the party who accepts assignment below.

SIGNED *Signature on File* DATE

13. INSURED'S OR AUTHORIZED PERSON'S SIGNATURE I authorize payment of medical benefits to the undersigned physician or supplier for services described below.

SIGNED

PATIENT AND INSURED INFORMATION

14. DATE OF CURRENT: ILLNESS, INJURY, or PREGNANCY(LMP) MM DD YY QUAL.
15. OTHER DATE QUAL. MM DD YY
16. DATES PATIENT UNABLE TO WORK IN CURRENT OCCUPATION FROM MM DD YY TO MM DD YY
17. NAME OF REFERRING PROVIDER OR OTHER SOURCE
17a. 17b. NPI
18. HOSPITALIZATION DATES RELATED TO CURRENT SERVICES FROM MM DD YY TO MM DD YY
19. ADDITIONAL CLAIM INFORMATION (Designated by NUCC)
20. OUTSIDE LAB? YES NO $ CHARGES
21. DIAGNOSIS OR NATURE OF ILLNESS OR INJURY Relate A-L to service line below (24E) ICD Ind.
A. B. C. D.
E. F. G. H.
I. J. K. L.
22. RESUBMISSION CODE ORIGINAL REF. NO.
23. PRIOR AUTHORIZATION NUMBER

24. A. DATE(S) OF SERVICE From MM DD YY To MM DD YY	B. PLACE OF SERVICE	C. EMG	D. PROCEDURES, SERVICES, OR SUPPLIES (Explain Unusual Circumstances) CPT/HCPCS MODIFIER	E. DIAGNOSIS POINTER	F. $ CHARGES	G. DAYS OR UNITS	H. EPSDT Family Plan	I. ID. QUAL.	J. RENDERING PROVIDER ID. #
1								NPI	
2								NPI	
3								NPI	
4								NPI	
5								NPI	
6								NPI	

25. FEDERAL TAX I.D. NUMBER SSN EIN
26. PATIENT'S ACCOUNT NO.
27. ACCEPT ASSIGNMENT? (For govt. claims, see back) X YES NO
28. TOTAL CHARGE $
29. AMOUNT PAID $
30. Rsvd for NUCC Use $
31. SIGNATURE OF PHYSICIAN OR SUPPLIER INCLUDING DEGREES OR CREDENTIALS (I certify that the statements on the reverse apply to this bill and are made a part thereof.)
SIGNED DATE
32. SERVICE FACILITY LOCATION INFORMATION
a. NPI b.
33. BILLING PROVIDER INFO & PH # ( )
a. NPI b.

PHYSICIAN OR SUPPLIER INFORMATION

NUCC Instruction Manual available at: www.nucc.org PLEASE PRINT OR TYPE OMB APPROVAL PENDING

Fig. 6.7 Block 12 of the CMS-1500 (02-12) claim form, where the patient signs to authorize that payment be sent to the physician, and Block 27 marked with an X, showing that the physician accepts Medicare assignment of benefits.

the money." Consequently, providers should evaluate whether the ability to balance bill and collect a higher fee from the patient is worth the potential extra billing and collection costs. Furthermore, some hospitals and states prohibit or limit balance billing, so health care organizations and service providers must ascertain whether these restrictions apply before making a Medicare participation or nonparticipation decision.

Prior Authorization

Prior authorization is a requirement for a health care provider to obtain approval from an insurance carrier to provide a medical service. Generally, traditional Medicare does not require prior authorization.

On the other hand, Medicare Advantage plans often require prior authorization for surgical procedures, diagnostic testing, out-of-network care, nonemergency hospital care, and referrals to specialists. Some of these procedures requiring authorization are on a mandatory list, whereas others are chosen by the regional carrier. The mandatory list is composed of procedures such as the following:

- Bunionectomy
- Carotid endarterectomy
- Cataract extractions
- Cholecystectomy
- Complex peripheral revascularization
- Coronary artery bypass graft surgery
- Hysterectomy
- Inguinal hernia repair
- Joint replacements (hip, shoulder, or knee)
- Transurethral prostatectomy

Each MA plan has different prior authorization requirements. To obtain prior authorization, the MA plans generally have a toll-free line to call for authorization or may require the completion of a preauthorization form. Check with the plan on its policy for preauthorization.

Medicare prescription drug (Part D) plans very often require prior authorization to obtain coverage for certain drugs. In many instances the health care provider must first contact the plan to determine if there is coverage for the drug and if a prior authorization is required. If the prescription is filled without prior authorization, the medical plan will probably not pay for the drug and the patient will be charged full-retail price for the drug.

National and Local Coverage Determinations

Although traditional Medicare does not generally require prior authorization of services to ensure payment, coverage policies have been developed that must be adhered to for assurance of payment.

National Coverage Determinations (NCDs) and **Local Coverage Determinations (LCDs)** are decisions by Medicare and its administrative contractors. The NCD/LCDs provide coverage information for medical services.

An NCD is mandated by CMS at the federal level, and all Medicare contractors must follow those guidelines. An LCD is mandated at the Medicare contractor level, and those guidelines are only applicable to that carrier's jurisdiction. Medicare contractors develop LCDs when there is no NCD or when there is a need to further define an NCD.

Both NCDs and LCDs are developed to decide whether to cover a particular service in accordance with CMS' definition of services that are medically necessary. The NCD and LCD are educational and administrative tools to assist physicians, providers, and suppliers in transmitting correct claims for payment. Typically, procedural and diagnosis codes describing what is covered and what is not covered can be part of the NCD/LCD. The NCD/LCD also specify under what clinical circumstances they consider a service to be reasonable and necessary. Coverage determinations also outline how contractors review claims to determine whether Medicare coverage requirements have been met.

NCD and LCD coverage policies are developed by CMS medical directors and staff with input from the public. CMS requires that local policies be consistent with national guidance. Use of NCDs and LCDs helps avoid situations in which claims are paid or denied without a full understanding of the basis for payment and denial. NCDs are available on the CMS website, whereas LCDs may be obtained from the Medicare contractor.

! COMPLIANCE ALERT

Advance Beneficiary Notice of Noncoverage

Medicare considers the appropriate use of an Advance Beneficiary Notice of Noncoverage (ABN) document as a compliance issue. Ask the patient to sign an ABN document if you know the service is not covered or if there is a possibility that a service may be denied for medical necessity or limitation of Medicare benefits. A step-by-step procedure of how to complete an ABN form is presented at the end of this chapter (Procedure 6.2).

PROCEDURE 6.2 Complete an Advance Beneficiary Notice of Noncoverage Form

There are 10 blanks for completion labeled A through J:

- Notifier(s): Enter the name, address, and telephone number of the provider.
- Patient Name: Enter the first and last name and middle initial of the Medicare beneficiary.
- Identification Number: Enter a number for the Medicare beneficiary that helps link the notice with a related claim. However, this field is optional and choosing not to enter a number does not invalidate the ABN. The beneficiary's Medicare health insurance claim number will no longer be used.
- Enter name of item(s), service(s), test(s), or procedure(s). If not enough space, use an attached sheet, noting it in the box.
- Reason Medicare May Not Pay: Explain the reason why you think the service may not be covered by Medicare (e.g., Medicare does not pay for this test for the condition or Medicare does not pay for these tests as often as this [denied as too frequent]).
- Estimated Cost: Enter a cost estimate for any item or service described in field D.
- Options: Patient should choose and check one of the three boxes. If the beneficiary cannot make a choice, the notice should be annotated.
- Additional Information: Insert more comments for clarification (e.g., provide context on Medicare payment policy applicable to a specific benefit or other payer information).
- Signature: Medicare beneficiary should sign the notice.
  - Date: Insert the date on which the beneficiary signed the ABN.

ABN, **Advance Beneficiary Notice of Noncoverage.**

Advance Beneficiary Notice of Noncoverage

NCDs and LCDs should be reviewed before furnishing services to ensure payment of them.

An advance beneficiary notice is a written notice you must issue to a FFS beneficiary before furnishing items or services that are usually covered by Medicare but are not expected to be paid. The ABN allows the beneficiary to make an informed decision about whether to get the item or service that may not be covered and accept financial responsibility if Medicare does not pay.

If you expect Medicare to deny payment (entirely or in part), instruct the patient to sign an **Advance Beneficiary Notice of Noncoverage (ABN),** also known as a *waiver of liability agreement,* as shown in Figs. 6.8 and 6.9. This form should not be given to someone who is in a medical emergency, confused, legally incompetent, or otherwise under great duress. It cannot be signed after a patient has received the service and must specifically state what service or procedure is being waived. Write the specific time frequency limitation for a particular service, such as screening colonoscopy once every 10 years. Each space on the ABN must be completed before providing the ABN to the patient. Blank or partially completed ABNs, even with the patient's signature, are not acceptable. An ABN may be mailed to a patient when presenting it face to face is not possible, but the patient must have an opportunity to ask questions. When the ABN is mailed, it should be sent with a cover letter explaining that the procedure will be denied by Medicare and include contact information so that the patient can ask questions before the procedure.

To determine which services require an ABN, refer to the NCDs and the LCDs from the insurance carrier. An office policy should be in place for handling patients who refuse to sign an ABN. When sending in a claim, the Healthcare Common Procedure Coding System (HCPCS) level II modifier *GA* (waiver of liability on file) must be added to pertinent codes to indicate that a patient has signed the waiver. The Medicare carrier then informs the patient that he or she is responsible for the fee. Keep this signed waiver with other patient financial documents and not with the patient's health record.

If the service was not reasonable because of Medicare guidelines but the patient thought it was covered and there is no advance notice given with signed waiver of liability agreement, the following apply:

- The provider cannot bill the patient.
- The patient does not have to pay the deductible or coinsurance.
- The patient is refunded any amount paid to the provider on the item or service.

If assignment is accepted and the physician and patient thought the service was covered under reasonable assumptions, the following apply:

- Medicare is billed to pay for the service.
- The patient must pay the deductible and coinsurance.
- Medicare will not seek a refund of money already paid to the physician.

Nonpar providers must refund any amount collected from the beneficiary when services are later found to be not reasonable and necessary.

Noncovered Services

Noncovered Medicare services are services that are never covered by Medicare. Some of the items or services that Medicare does not cover include the following:

- Long-term care
- Most dental care
- Eye examinations related to prescribing glasses
- Dentures
- Cosmetic surgery
- Acupuncture
- Hearing aids and exams for fitting them
- Routine foot care
- Routine physical examinations
- Services furnished outside the United States, except under certain limited services

Noncovered services are billed to the patient. It is not necessary to give a patient an ABN when a service is never covered by Medicare.

Prepayment Screens

Medicare **prepayment screens** or prepayment edits are put in place to prevent payment for noncovered and incorrectly coded services. Prepayment screens are also used to target claims for review before payment. The screens may be placed to target specific health care services that have high claim error rates or unusual billing practices that are considered to be a financial risk to Medicare.

The screens or edits are computer triggers that suspend claims processing. These screens are used to identify and review claims for medical necessity and determine compliance with other appropriate criteria. The suspended claim is held in a pended state until it is checked by a reviewer who decides whether the services are appropriate, medically necessary, or meet other specific criteria.

CMS requires Medicare contractors to implement prepayment screens or edits that include the following:

- *Procedure to procedure,* which screen for multiple services reported on a date of service to ensure they are not inclusive in the primary procedure. For example, an exploratory laparotomy is always inclusive in an open abdominal procedure when performed on the same date of service. Medicare implemented the **Correct Coding Initiative (CCI)** to identify procedures that are usually described by a single code or are inherent to another procedure. The CCI will be discussed further in Chapter 13.
- *Procedure to provider* permits selective screening of services that need review.
- *Frequency to time* allows screening for a certain number of services provided within a given period. For example, Medicare limits medically necessary routine foot care to one treatment every 60 days.
- *Diagnosis to procedure edits* allows screening for services submitted with a specific diagnosis. For example, vitamin B_{12} injections are only reimbursed if treatment is related to pernicious anemia, absence of the stomach, or distal ileum.
- *Procedure to specialty code* permits screening of services provided by a certain specialty or type of bill. For example, a physical therapist could not report a code for excision of tonsils.

A. Notifier: John Doe, MD, College Clinic, 4567 Broad Avenue, Woodland Hills, XY 12345 555-486-9002

B. Patient Name: Mary Judd **C. Identification Number:** 0920XX7291

Advance Beneficiary Notice of Noncoverage (ABN)

NOTE: If Medicare doesn't pay for **D.** B12 injections below, you may have to pay.
Medicare does not pay for everything, even some care that you or your health care provider have good reason to think you need. We expect Medicare may not pay for the **D.** B12 injections below.

D.	E. Reason Medicare May Not Pay:	F. Estimated Cost
B12 injections	Medicare does not usually pay for this injection or this many injections.	$35.00

WHAT YOU NEED TO DO NOW:

- Read this notice, so you can make an informed decision about your care.
- Ask us any questions that you may have after you finish reading.
- Choose an option below about whether to receive the **D.** B12 injections listed above.
  Note: If you choose Option 1 or 2, we may help you to use any other insurance that you might have, but Medicare cannot require us to do this.

G. OPTIONS: Check only one box. We cannot choose a box for you.

☑ **OPTION 1.** I want the **D.** B12 injections listed above. You may ask to be paid now, but I also want Medicare billed for an official decision on payment, which is sent to me on a Medicare Summary Notice (MSN). I understand that if Medicare doesn't pay, I am responsible for payment, but **I can appeal to Medicare** by following the directions on the MSN. If Medicare does pay, you will refund any payments I made to you, less co-pays or deductibles.

☐ **OPTION 2.** I want the **D.** ____________ listed above, but do not bill Medicare. You may ask to be paid now as I am responsible for payment. **I cannot appeal if Medicare is not billed.**

☐ **OPTION 3.** I don't want the **D.** ____________ listed above. I understand with this choice I am **not** responsible for payment, and **I cannot appeal to see if Medicare would pay.**

H. Additional Information:

This notice gives our opinion, not an official Medicare decision. If you have other questions on this notice or Medicare billing, call **1-800-MEDICARE** (1-800-633-4227/**TTY:** 1-877-486-2048).
Signing below means that you have received and understand this notice. You also receive a copy.

I. Signature:	J. Date:
Mary Judd	March 20, 20XX

According to the Paperwork Reduction Act of 1995, no persons are required to respond to a collection of information unless it displays a valid OMB control number. The valid OMB control number for this information collection is 0938-0566. The time required to complete this information collection is estimated to average 7 minutes per response, including the time to review instructions, search existing data resources, gather the data needed, and complete and review the information collection. If you have comments concerning the accuracy of the time estimate or suggestions for improving this form, please write to: CMS, 7500 Security Boulevard, Attn: PRA Reports Clearance Officer, Baltimore, Maryland 21244-1850.

Form CMS-R-131 (03/11) Form Approved OMB No. 0938-0566

Fig. 6.8 Advance Beneficiary Notice of Noncoverage, Form CMS-R-131, which is also referred to as a *responsibility statement* or *waiver of liability agreement.*

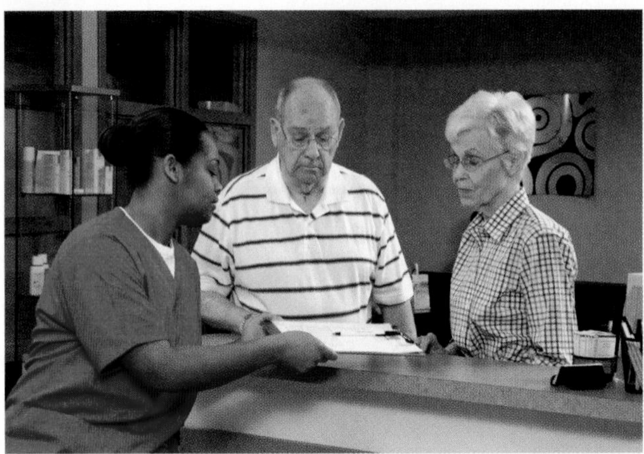

Fig. 6.9 Insurance billing specialist instructing an elderly patient to sign an Advance Beneficiary Notice of Noncoverage form for services not covered.

- *Procedure to place of service* allows selective screening of claims where the service was provided. For example, a nursing home admission must be performed in a nursing home. If it was reported with hospital as the place of service, the claim would be suspended.

MEDICARE REIMBURSEMENT

Traditional Medicare has different payment methodologies, depending on the type of services provided.

Medicare Fee Schedule

Since January 1992, CMS has reimbursed using a **Medicare fee schedule (MFS)** to pay doctors and other providers/suppliers. The fee schedule is a comprehensive listing of accepted charges or established allowances for specific medical procedures identified by procedural codes. CMS has developed fee schedules for physicians, ambulance services, clinical laboratory services, and durable medical equipment.

The **resource-based relative value scale (RBRVS)** is the system that Medicare uses for establishing fees. This system takes into account work value, overhead expense, and malpractice values for all Current Procedural Terminology (CPT) codes that are published in the *Federal Register* each November. These are adjusted for each Medicare local carrier by geographic practice cost indices (**GPCIs**) by using a formula that gives the total value for a code. This payment methodology will be discussed further in Chapter 13.

When using the MFS payment methodology, the approved amount is the amount that the amount that Medicare participating providers agree to accept. It is listed on the RA as an allowed charge for a procedure. This charge may be higher or lower than the fee the physician lists on the claim. When a physician accepts assignment, he or she may bill the patient only 20% of the Medicare-allowed charge. It is permissible to collect the deductible at the time of service if you know how much of the deductible has already been paid but the Medicare copayment should not be collected until Medicare pays.

Prospective Payment System

Since October 1983, CMS has used the **prospective payment system (PPS)** to reimburse hospitals. PPS is a method of reimbursement in which Medicare payment is made based on predetermined, fixed amounts. The payment amount for a particular service is derived based on the classification system of that system (e.g., diagnosis-related groups for inpatient hospital services). CMS uses separate PPS for reimbursement to acute inpatient hospitals, home health agencies, hospice, hospital outpatient, inpatient psychiatric facilities, inpatient rehabilitation facilities, long-term care hospitals, and skilled nursing facilities. These payment methodologies will be discussed further in Chapter 19.

Value-Based Programs

In an effort to lessen health care cost growth and to identify and encourage high quality of care to patients, legislation was passed in 2008 to change reimbursement methodologies. CMS has developed a multitude of programs since that time to transform to more affordable health care through value-based programs. **Value-based programs** are also known as pay-for-performance programs and are based on value-based purchasing (VBP) principles. Value-based programs reward health care organizations with incentive payments for the quality of care they give to people with Medicare. Payment are linked to the quality and efficiency of care provided with the shift away from paying providers based solely on their volumes of services (Fig. 6.10).

Medicare Improvements for Patients and Providers Act

One of the first value-based programs developed by Medicare was the ESRD Quality Incentive Program (QIP). Previously, ESRD care was paid through a bundled payment system. Under a bundled payment system, providers and/or health care organizations are paid a single payment for all the delivery of care within a specific period. Under the **Medicare Improvements for Patients and Providers Act (MIPAA)**, CMS was required to implement quality incentives into the ESRD bundled payment system. The ESRD-QIP was established to promote high-quality services to outpatient dialysis facilities treating patients with ESRD. This changed the way CMS pays for treatment of patients with ESRD by linking a portion of payment directly to facilities performance on quality of care measures. The ESRD-QIP reduces payments to ESRD facilities that do not meet or exceed certain performance standards. Payment reductions occur when the facility's score on applicable measures does not meet established standards. The ESRD-QIP now operates under a fully bundled, case-mix adjusted PPS and has implemented Medicare's first-ever mandatory pay-for-performance program.

Other programs that follow value-based program values are as follows:

- Hospital Value-Based Purchasing Programs (HVBP): A program to adjust payments to hospitals under the Inpatient Prospective Payment System (IPPS) based on the quality of care they provide.
- Hospital Readmissions Reduction Program (HRRP): A program implemented in 2012 that reduced payment to IPPS hospitals with excess readmissions.

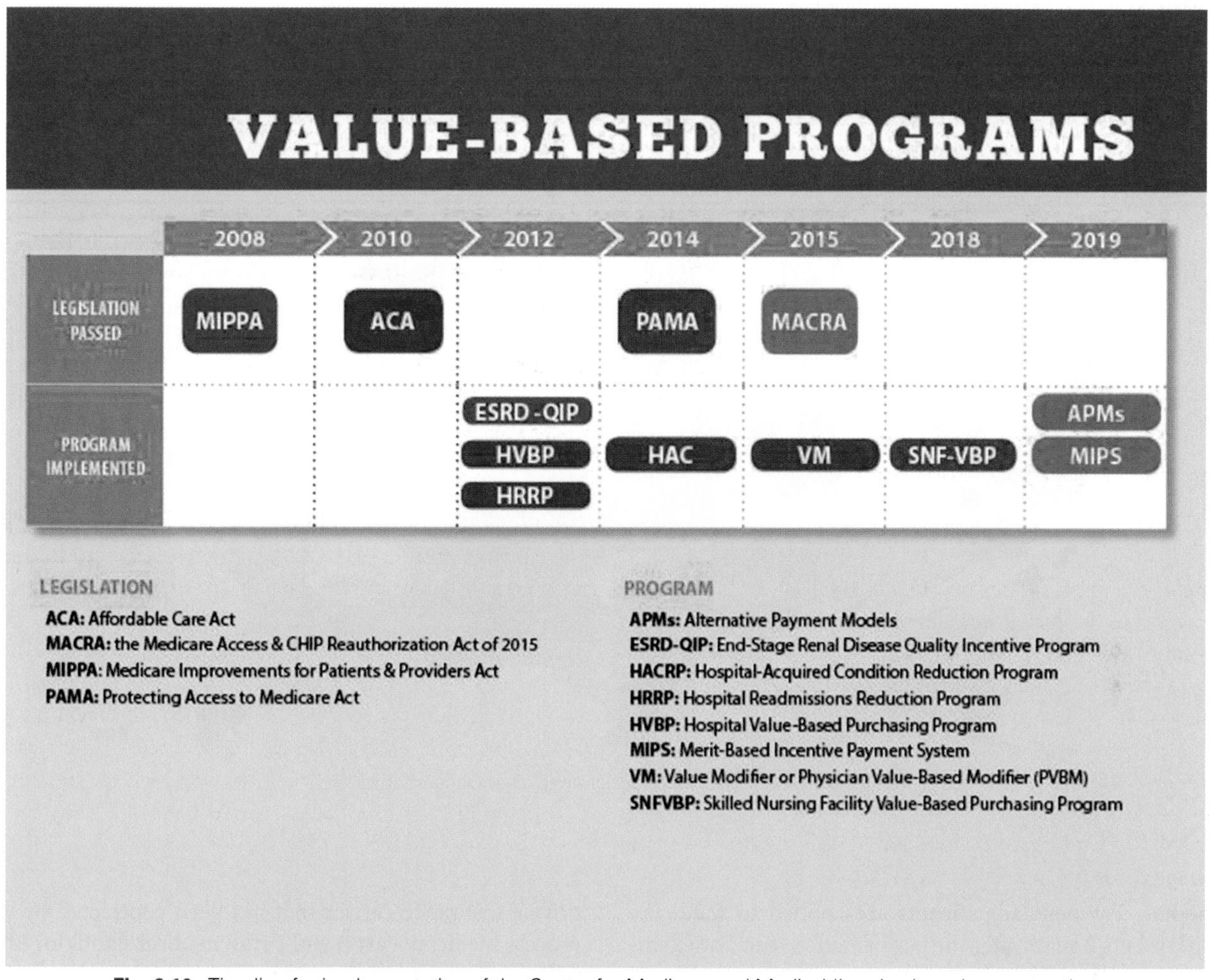

Fig. 6.10 Timeline for implementation of the Center for Medicare and Medicaid's value-based programs that will reform how healthcare is delivered and paid for. (https://www.cms.gov/Medicare/Qualityilnitiatives-Patient-Assessment-Instruments/Value-Based-Programs/Value-Based-Programs.html).

- Hospital-Acquired Condition Reduction Program (HACRP): A program established to provide an incentive for hospitals to reduce hospital-acquired conditions. The worst-performing hospitals are subject to a payment reduction.
- Value Modifier or Physician Value-Based Modifier (PVBM): This program provides for differential payment to a physician or group of physicians under the Medicare fee schedule based on the quality of care furnished compared with the cost of care during a performance period.
- Skilled Nursing Facility Value-Based Purchasing Program (SNFVBP): The SNFVBP program rewards skilled nursing facilities with incentive payments for the quality of care they give to people with Medicare.

Medicare Access and CHIIP Reauthorization Act of 2015

One of the most recent pieces of legislation to affect health care reimbursement is the Medicare Access and CHIP Reauthorization Act of 2015 (MACRA). MACRA established a quality payment program (QPP), which is a new way to pay providers. Under the QPP, which started on January 1, 2017, providers are rewarded for giving high-quality and high-value care through the Advanced Alternative Payment Model (APM) or the Merit-based Incentive Payment System (MIPS).

APM provides ways to pay health care providers for the care they give to Medicare beneficiaries by sharing the risk. Accountable care organizations (ACOs), patient-centered medical homes (PCMH), and bundled payment models are examples of APMs. From 2019 to 2024, health care providers who qualify for APMs will receive lump-sum incentive payments.

Most Medicare providers will fall under the MIPS payment adjustment option. MIPS defines the financial impact on providers by creating a composite score for each provider. The composite score will be between 1 and 100 and will be based on the following four components:

- Quality performance
- Advancing care information
- Cost
- Improvement activities

The health care organizations select measures from the categories described that fit their practice and then report on those measures. The health care organization must have a qualified electronic health record to report the measures.

The final score earned by a clinician for a given performance year then determines the MIPS payment adjustments to be incurred by that provider. Essentially, the composite score will lead to each provider having their own individual

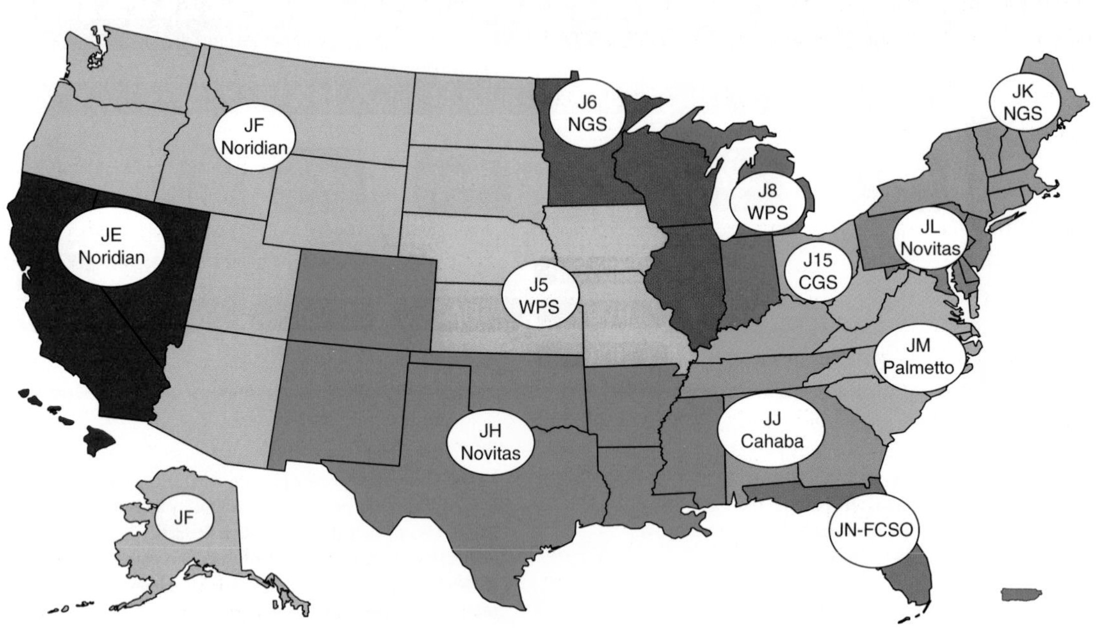

Fig. 6.11 Region A/B jurisdiction map as of December 2015.

fee schedule. Payment adjustments are applied to Medicare Part B payments 2 years after the performance year. For example, providers who report in the performance year 2017 will receive adjustments in 2019, which is referred to as the payment adjustment year.

CLAIM SUBMISSION

Medicare requires service providers to submit claims for their Medicare patients for services rendered. This mandatory claims submission requirement applies to all physicians and suppliers who provide covered services to Medicare beneficiaries. Violations to this requirement can lead to civil monetary penalties of up to $2000 per violation, a 10% reduction in future Medicare payments, and/or exclusion from the Medicare program. Medicare beneficiaries may not be charged for preparing or filing a Medicare claim. If the Medicare beneficiary submits a claim to Medicare, it will be returned to them with a letter explaining that the provider of services is required by law to submit a claim on behalf of the patient.

Initial claims for payment under Medicare must be submitted electronically unless the health care service provider qualifies for a waiver of exception. The waiver is a provision of the Administrative Simplification Compliance Act (ASCA) requirement for electronic submission of claims and will be discussed further in Chapter 15.

Medicare Administrative Contractors

Claims for traditional FFS Medicare services are sent to a **Medicare administrative contractor (MAC)**. A MAC is a private insurance carrier that has been contracted by CMS to process Medicare Part A and Part B medical claims for Medicare FFS beneficiaries. CMS relies on MACs to do the following:

- Process Medicare FFS claims
- Make and account for Medicare FFS payments
- Enroll providers in the Medicare FFS program
- Handle provider reimbursement services
- Process redetermination requests
- Respond to provider inquiries
- Educate providers about Medicare FFS billing requirements
- Establish local coverage policies
- Review medical records for selected claims
- Coordinate with CMS and other MACs

Currently, there are 12 Part A and Part B MACs contracted with CMS to process Medicare FFS claims (Fig. 6.11). Each MAC processes claims for a defined geographical area or **jurisdiction** that services institutional providers, physician, practitioners and suppliers. Some of those Part A and Part B MACs also process home health and hospice claims. Providers should send the Medicare claim to the MAC covering the jurisdiction where the services were furnished, rather than where the patient resides.

There are an additional four MACs that process claims for **durable medical equipment (DME)** suppliers. DME is any equipment that provides therapeutic benefits to a patient in need because of certain medical conditions and/or illnesses. Medicare covers medically necessary DME if it is prescribed and meets the following criteria:

- Can withstand repeat use (durable)
- Used for a medical reason

- Not usually useful to someone who isn't sick or injured
- Used in the patient's home
- Has an expected lifetime of at least 3 years

Examples of DME covered items include (but are not limited to) blood sugar monitors, canes, commode chairs, crutches, hospital beds, infusion pumps and supplies, nebulizers, patient lifts, traction equipment, and walkers.

Medicare beneficiaries who are enrolled in an MA plan should have claims submitted to the beneficiary's MA plan.

Provider Identification Numbers

Medicare claims must be submitted with the service provider's national provider identifier (NPI). The NPI is a unique 10-digit identification number issued to all covered health care providers. As outlined in the Health Insurance Portability and Accountability Act (HIPAA), service providers must also share their NPI with other providers that may need it for billing purposes. For additional information, refer to Chapter 2.

Time Limit

The Affordable Care Act (ACA) set the time limit policy for Medicare claims submission. Service providers must submit claims to traditional Medicare and Railroad Retirement within 12 months of the date of service. Medicare will deny claims if they arrive after the deadline date and they are not subject to appeal.

In limited circumstances, Medicare will allow for exceptions to the one calendar year time limit for filing FFS claims.

- Administrative error: If the deadline was not met because of administrative error, the MAC may extend the timely filing limit through the last day of the sixth month after the month in which the error was corrected.
- Retroactive Medicare entitlement: If the deadline was not met because patient was not entitled to benefits at time of service, and then was notified later that enrollment would be retroactive, the MAC will extend the timely filing limit through the last day of the sixth month after the beneficiary received notification of Medicare entitlement to benefits.
- Retroactive disenrollment from an MA plan: If the beneficiary was enrolled in a MA program but later disenrolled before the service was performed and the MA plan recoups payment from the service provider, Medicare will extend the timely filing limit through the last day of the sixth month after the month in which the MA plan recovered its payment from the service provider.

Instructions for Claims Submissions

Instructions for claims submissions can be found in the Medicare Claims Processing Manual—Internet Only Manual Publication (IOM Pub.) 100-04. The publication includes general billing requirements for various health care professionals and suppliers, as well as claims submission information specific to a health care professional or supplier type.

MACs are mandated to pay for services deemed medically necessary and reasonable for the diagnosis and treatment of illness and injury. Medicare is not required to pay for noncovered and undocumented services. Claims must be submitted accurately and in accordance with the current Medicare billing policies. Care must be taken to ensure that all documentation required to support the medical need for the service rendered is submitted when requested by the MAC.

AFTER CLAIM SUBMISSION

Remittance Advice

A RA is a notice of payment and explains any adjustments made to a payment during the Medicare adjudication process. Adjudication is the process of paying claims submitted or denying them after comparing the claim to benefit and coverage requirements. RAs provide itemizes claims processing decision regarding the following:

- Payments
- Deductible and copays
- Adjustments
- Denials
- Missing or incorrect data
- Refunds
- Claims withholding because of MSP or penalty situations

Health care service providers who accept assignment receive payment from the MAC for the claims they submitted as well as a RA. And although providers who do not accept assignment must submit a claim for services they provide Medicare beneficiaries, the payment for services will be sent to the patient. The provider of services will receive an informational RA to report the amount of payment and the adjustments the MAC made during adjudication. RAs can be sent in either electronic format (Electronic Remittance Advice [ERA]) or a paper format (Standard Paper Remittance Advice [SPR]). Both ERA and SPR have the same format; however, the advantage of an ERA is that it electronically posts payments and the billing specialist does not have to post them manually.

The RA provides detailed payment information about a health care claim and helps the billing specialist understand the actions the MAC took while processing the claim. Some RA codes may indicate a need to resubmit a claim with corrected information, whereas others may indicate whether the provider may appeal the payment decision. The RA also identified any adjustment to the claim. An *adjustment* refers to any change that related to how a MAC paid a claim differently than the original billing.

Claim Adjustment Reason Codes (CARCs) provide financial information about claim decision. CARCs communicate adjustments the MAC made and offer explanation when the MAC pays a particular claim or service line differently that what was on the original claim. If there is no adjustment to a claim, then there is no CARC. Examples of CARCs include the following:

4	The procedure code is inconsistent with the modifier used or a required modifier is missing.
5	The procedure code is inconsistent with the place of service.
6	The procedure code is inconsistent with the patient's age.

Remittance Advice Remark Codes (RARCs) further explain an adjustment or relay informational messages that CARCs cannot express. Additionally, there are some informational RARCs, starting with the work "alert" that MACS use to provide general adjudication information. These RARCs are not always associated with a CARC when there is no adjustment. Examples of RARCs include the following:

M51	Missing/incomplete/invalid procedure code.
M53	Missing/incomplete/invalid days or units of service.
M56	Missing/incomplete/invalid payer identifier.

Medicare Summary Notice

A patient is mailed a similar document called a **Medicare Summary Notice (MSN)** every 3 months. This document notifies the patient of Medicare Part A and Part B covered services that were paid on their behalf. Because many patients do not know what is meant by *amount charged, Medicare approved, deductible,* and *coinsurance,* it often becomes necessary for the insurance billing specialist to educate the patient (Fig. 6.12).

Posting Payments

The charge submitted by the service provider or health care organization will be higher than the charge approved by the MAC. This does not mean that his or her charges are unreasonable. However, the difference between the service provider's charge and the amount that is allowed under the Medicare fee schedule must be adjusted. This reduction is known as a contractual adjustment or may be referred to as a write-off. For example:

Service provider's charge is:	$200.00
Medicare approved/allowed amount is:	$150.00
Contractual adjustment is:	$50.00

Because some services may be disallowed or the payments on them may be lower than those charged by the physician, know how to post payments to the patient's financial accounting record card or computerized account. Fig. 6.13 illustrates how payments and contractual adjustments are posted.

Medicare does not allow for the standardized waiving of copayments. Medicare regulations require that a patient be billed for the copayment at least three times before the balance is adjusted off as uncollectable. Document this as further justification if the patient is suffering financial hardship.

When an RA is received, it may list many patients (Fig. 6.14). Do not post the entire payment made in a lump sum to the daysheet. Individually post each line item paid to the patient's financial accounting record card or computerized account and to the daysheet. To prevent funds from going astray, some offices prefer to post Medicare payments to a separate daysheet and deposit each multiple reimbursement check separately. The daysheet totals will then agree with the deposit slip totals and not get confused with other monies collected.

Fig. 6.15A, illustrates an example of a Medicare/Medicaid case after payment by Medicare. Medicare applied the patient's full $147 deductible amount to the Medicare-allowed amount, reducing payment to $26.40. The Medicaid RA (see Fig. 6.15B) shows reimbursement of the coinsurance and deductible amounts dual-billed to Medicaid.

Calculations are shown here:

Medicare		**Medicaid**	
$180	Allowed amount	$180	Medicare allowed amount
−147	Deductible	−32	Medicaid cutback
$ 33	Balance on which payment is calculated	$148	Medicaid allowed
× .80			
$26.40		26.40	Medicare paid
		$148.40	Medicaid payment

When referring to the Medicaid program, a *cutback* means a reduction, which is reducing Medicare's allowable charges to Medicaid's allowable charges. This would require an adjustment entry on the patient's financial accounting record. Cutbacks are common on Medicaid claims.

Medicare Overpayments

A Medicare overpayment is a payment you receive in excess of amounts properly payable under Medicare guidelines. Overpayments commonly occur because of insufficient documentation, medical necessity errors, and administrative and processing errors. Medicare overpayments can also occur in the following situations:

- The carrier processes the charge more than once.
- The physician receives duplicate payments from Medicare and a secondary payer.
- The physician is paid directly on an unassigned claim.
- The item is not covered but is paid.
- The payment is made on erroneous information.

After Medicare identifies an overpayment, it becomes a debt that the health care organization owes the federal government. Federal law requires the CMS to try to recover all identified overpayments. In fact, civil monetary penalties may be imposed if you know of an overpayment and do not report and return it.

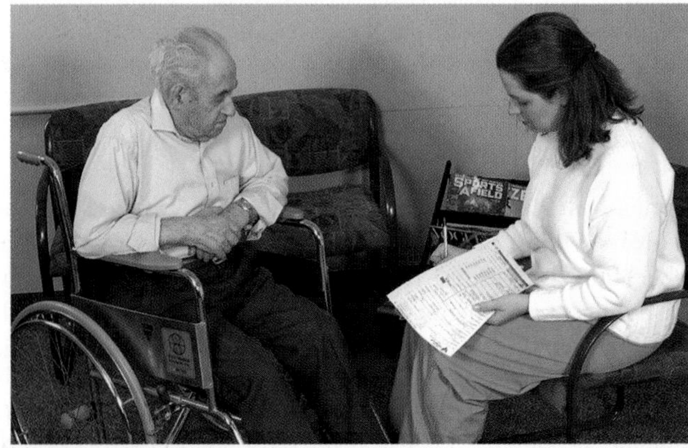

Fig. 6.12 Insurance billing specialist explaining a Medicare remittance advice document that the physician's office has received.

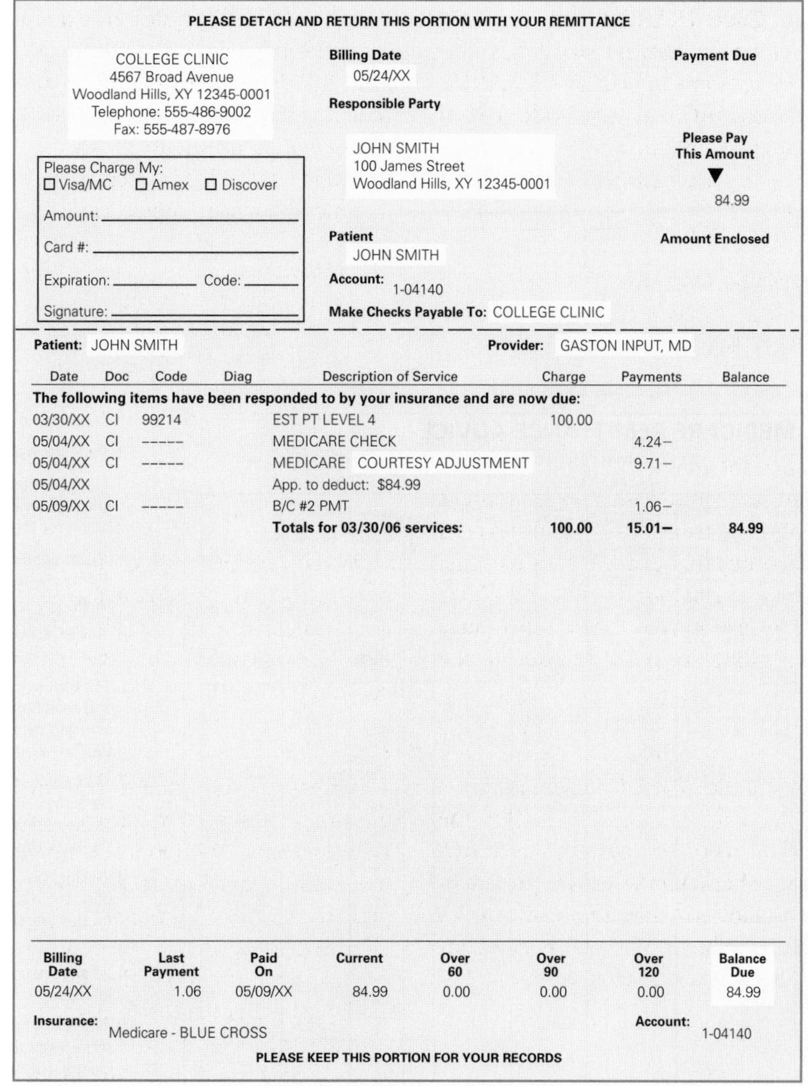

PLEASE DETACH AND RETURN THIS PORTION WITH YOUR REMITTANCE

COLLEGE CLINIC
4567 Broad Avenue
Woodland Hills, XY 12345-0001
Telephone: 555-486-9002
Fax: 555-487-8976

Billing Date 05/24/XX

Payment Due

Responsible Party
JOHN SMITH
100 James Street
Woodland Hills, XY 12345-0001

Please Pay This Amount ▼ 84.99

Please Charge My:
☐ Visa/MC ☐ Amex ☐ Discover
Amount: ______
Card #: ______
Expiration: ______ Code: ______
Signature: ______

Patient JOHN SMITH

Amount Enclosed

Account: 1-04140

Make Checks Payable To: COLLEGE CLINIC

Patient: JOHN SMITH **Provider:** GASTON INPUT, MD

Date	Doc	Code	Diag	Description of Service	Charge	Payments	Balance
The following items have been responded to by your insurance and are now due:							
03/30/XX	CI	99214		EST PT LEVEL 4	100.00		
05/04/XX	CI	-----		MEDICARE CHECK		4.24–	
05/04/XX	CI	-----		MEDICARE COURTESY ADJUSTMENT		9.71–	
05/04/XX				App. to deduct: $84.99			
05/09/XX	CI	-----		B/C #2 PMT		1.06–	
				Totals for 03/30/06 services:	**100.00**	**15.01–**	**84.99**

Billing Date	Last Payment	Paid On	Current	Over 60	Over 90	Over 120	Balance Due
05/24/XX	1.06	05/09/XX	84.99	0.00	0.00	0.00	84.99

Insurance: Medicare - BLUE CROSS **Account:** 1-04140

PLEASE KEEP THIS PORTION FOR YOUR RECORDS

Fig. 6.13 Electronically generated financial accounting record (ledger card) illustrating how payments and contractual or courtesy adjustments should be posted.

If an overpayment is identified, the health care organization has 60 days to report and return it. When Medicare identifies an overpayment of $25 or more, the MAC will initiate the overpayment recovery process by sending an initial demand letter requesting repayment. If overpayment is not repaid to the MAC in full within 30 days, interest will be charged. If the health care organization disagrees with an overpayment decision, an appeal can be filed with the MAC.

Review and Redetermination Process

Chapter 16 outlines in detail the steps to take to have a claim reviewed and the process of appealing a claim in the Medicare program.

Recovery Audit Contractor Program

The **Recovery Audit Contractor (RAC) Initiative** originally created a demonstration program that became permanently implemented when Congress enacted the Tax Relief and Health Care Act of 2006. This extended the RAC Initiative to all 50 states by 2010. Its goals are to identify Medicare underpayments and overpayments and recover overpayments using automated review and complex review. An automated review is done electronically without human review and a complex review is done using human review of the medical record. A single RAC will serve one of four geographic regions (regions A, B, C, and D) and perform recovery audit services for all Medicare claim types in that region. RACs may identify improper payments from claims they review that may show incorrect payment amounts, noncovered services, incorrectly coded services, miscoding, and duplicate services. RACs are paid a percentage of the incorrect payments they recover. When an underpayment is found, a RAC will communicate this to the MAC. If both underpayments and overpayments are found, the RAC will offset the underpayment from the overpayment. On overpayments, interest accrues from the date of the final determination. Claims identified as overpayments are subject to the Medicare appeals process.

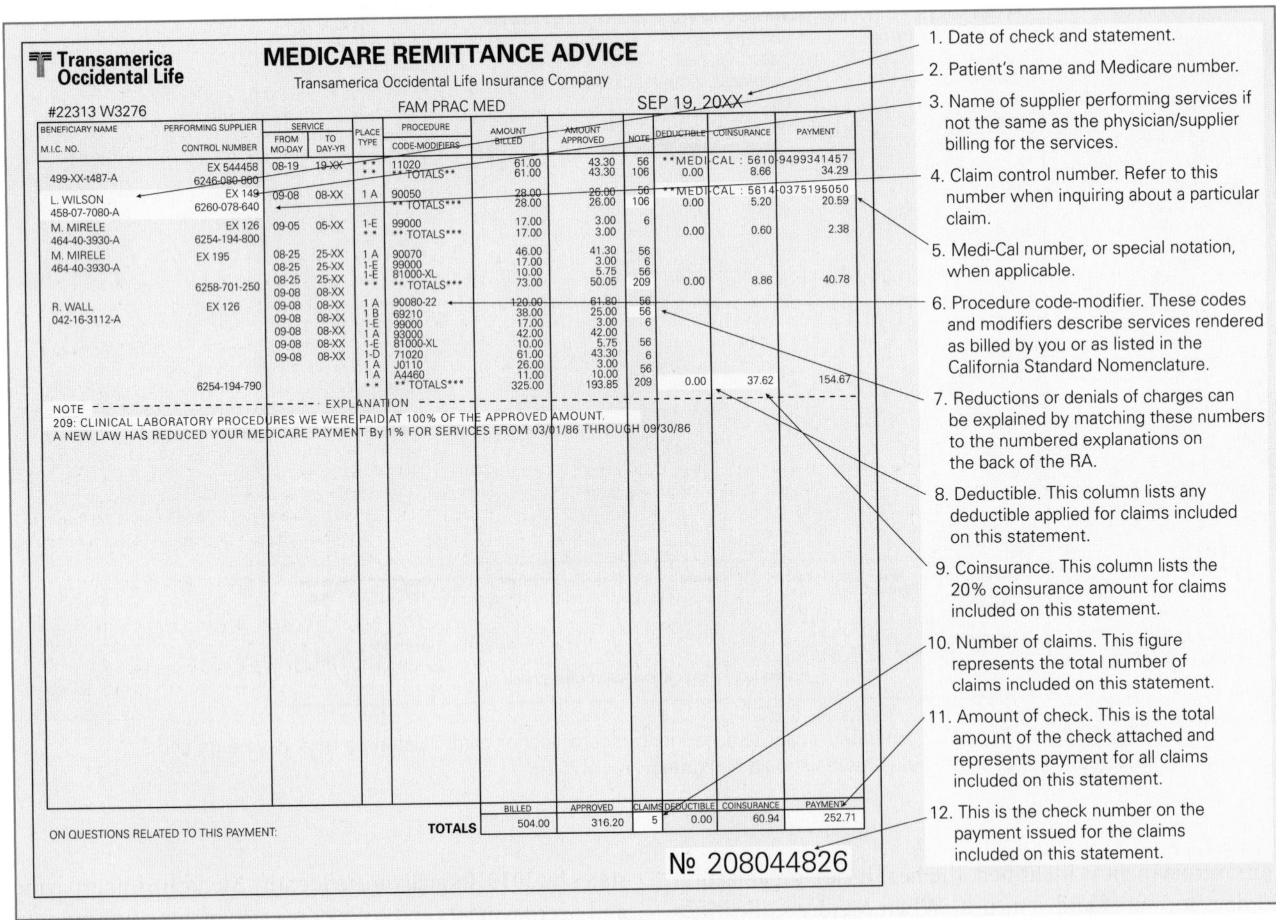

Transamerica Occidental Life

MEDICARE REMITTANCE ADVICE

Transamerica Occidental Life Insurance Company

#22313 W3276 FAM PRAC MED SEP 19, 20XX

BENEFICIARY NAME / M.I.C. NO.	PERFORMING SUPPLIER / CONTROL NUMBER	SERVICE FROM MO-DAY	SERVICE TO DAY-YR	PLACE TYPE	PROCEDURE CODE-MODIFIERS	AMOUNT BILLED	AMOUNT APPROVED	NOTE	DEDUCTIBLE	COINSURANCE	PAYMENT
	EX 544458	08-19	19-XX	* *	11020	61.00	43.30	56	**MEDI-CAL : 5610-9499341457		
499-XX-t487-A	6246-080-860			* *	** TOTALS**	61.00	43.30	106	0.00	8.66	34.29
L. WILSON	EX 149	09-08	08-XX	1 A	90050	28.00	26.00	56	**MEDI-CAL : 5614-0375195050		
458-07-7080-A	6260-078-640				** TOTALS***	28.00	26.00	106	0.00	5.20	20.59
M. MIRELE	EX 126	09-05	05-XX	1-E	99000	17.00	3.00	6			
464-40-3930-A	6254-194-800			* *	** TOTALS***	17.00	3.00		0.00	0.60	2.38
M. MIRELE	EX 195	08-25	25-XX	1 A	90070	46.00	41.30	56			
464-40-3930-A		08-25	25-XX	1-E	99000	17.00	3.00	6			
		08-25	25-XX	1-E	81000-XL	10.00	5.75	56			
	6258-701-250	09-08	08-XX	* *	** TOTALS***	73.00	50.05	209	0.00	8.86	40.78
R. WALL	EX 126	09-08	08-XX	1 A	90080-22	120.00	61.80	56			
042-16-3112-A		09-08	08-XX	1 B	69210	38.00	25.00	56			
		09-08	08-XX	1-E	99000	17.00	3.00	6			
		09-08	08-XX	1 A	93000	42.00	42.00				
		09-08	08-XX	1-E	81000-XL	10.00	5.75	56			
				1-D	71020	61.00	43.30	6			
				1 A	J0110	26.00	3.00				
				1 A	A4460	11.00	10.00	56			
	6254-194-790			* *	** TOTALS***	325.00	193.85	209	0.00	37.62	154.67

NOTE ---------------------- EXPLANATION ----------------------

209: CLINICAL LABORATORY PROCEDURES WE WERE PAID AT 100% OF THE APPROVED AMOUNT.

A NEW LAW HAS REDUCED YOUR MEDICARE PAYMENT By 1% FOR SERVICES FROM 03/01/86 THROUGH 09/30/86

ON QUESTIONS RELATED TO THIS PAYMENT:

TOTALS	BILLED	APPROVED	CLAIMS	DEDUCTIBLE	COINSURANCE	PAYMENT
	504.00	316.20	5	0.00	60.94	252.71

№ 208044826

A

Fig. 6.14 Medicare remittance advice (RA) document. **A,** Front. Insurance carriers are required to use Centers for Medicare and Medicaid Services messages for Medicare RA, but each carrier has its own code numbers to denote the messages. **B,** Back of Medicare RA document. (https://med.noridianmedicare.com/web/jddme/topics/ra/ra-tutorial).

EXPLANATION OF NOTES

Additional notes may be listed on the front of this form.

1 – See enclosed letter.
2 – Claim was filed after the time limit.
4 – These bills are handled by a special intermediary.
5 – This payment is for an adjustment of a previous claim.
6 – Charges over the maximum Medicare allowance are not covered.
7 – Services before Medicare entitlement are not covered.
8 – Services after Medicare entitlement ended are not covered.
10 – Other charges submitted with this claim may be on a separate statement which you have received or will receive soon.
12 – Routine examinations and related services are not covered.
13 – Immunizations or other routine and preventative services are not covered.
16 – We need an itemization of this charge. Please resubmit your claim with this information.
17 – Prescription drugs are not covered.
18 – Charges for this physician/supplier are not covered.
19 – We need a full description of the service or supply to consider this charge. Please resubmit your claim with this information.
23 – We need a written report for this service. Please resubmit your claim with this information.
26 – More than $312.50 annual psychiatric expense is not covered.
27 – We need from the prescribing physician the specific length of time this medical equipment is needed. Please resubmit your claim with this information.
30 – This charge was previously considered.
37 – Claims for these services will be made by a home health agency or hospital.
39 – Equipment that is not medically necessary is not covered. (See Note 89)
42 – These supplies or services are not covered.
45 – Over 62½% of psychiatric expenses is not covered.
46 – Routine foot care is not covered.
47 – Routine eye examinations or eye refractions are not covered.
48 – Partial payment of this claim was made to the beneficiary.
49 – This service cannot be considered until the hospital makes the necessary arrangement with the carrier for its processing.
50 – The beneficiary is not responsible for this reduction/denial under the assignment agreement.
54 – Care before and/or after surgery is included in the surgery benefit. (See Note 50)
56 – This is the full charge allowed based upon the prevailing or usual and customary rate.
62 – Payment has been reduced because this test is commonly part of an automated test group. (See Note 50)
66 – This service is not covered when done by this laboratory.
70 – There were no charges or bills with your claim form. Please resubmit your claim with this information.
72 – We need a signed and dated prescription showing medical necessity and specific length of time needed. Please resubmit your claim with this information.
73 – Before another month's payment can be made, we need a new signed and dated prescription showing further necessity of the medical equipment and specific length of time needed.
80 – We need to know the place of service to consider this charge. Please resubmit your claim with this information.
83 – SSA advises us that they are unable to verify the patient's eligibility for Part B Medical Insurance Plan. For this reason, no payment can be made on this claim.
84 – The patient's HIC number shown on this claim was incorrect. Please use the correct HIC number on all future claims.
85 – The patient's name shown on this claim was incorrect. Please use the correct name on all future claims.
86 – Over 62½% of the allowable charges for psychiatric services is not covered.
89 – If you did not know that Medicare does not pay for this medical service, you may request a review of this decision. See below paragraph entitled "Your right to review of a case."
90 – This service by a chiropractor is not covered.
93 – Over $500.00 annual expense billed by a physical therapist is not covered.
95 – These specific services by this supplier are not covered.
96 – Please verify the date of this service. Resubmit your claim with this information.
99 – We need a complete diagnosis before the claim can be considered. Please resubmit your claim with this information.
106 – The Medicare covered services on this claim have been forwarded for additional processing under Medi-Cal.
107 – This claim was not forwarded for Medi-Cal processing. Please bill Medi-Cal directly and attach a copy of this statement.
108 – The bills for these services have been transferred to Blue Shield of California Medicare Claims, Chico, CA 95976. You will hear from them.
129 – Payment for services prior to July 1 is based on the previous year's payment rate.
131 – Payment for this physician service in a hospital department is reduced since this service is commonly performed in the physician's office. (See Note 50)
138 – This amount is more than Medicare pays for maintenance treatment of renal disease.
147 – This charge is not covered because an allowance for purchase of the same equipment was previously made.
151 – Your claim was transferred to a Health Maintenance Organization for processing.
153 – These are more visits (treatments) for this diagnosis than Medicare covers unless there were unusual circumstances. (See Note 89)
154 – This service is not covered for your patient's reported condition. (See Note 89)
155 – Only one visit per month to a nursing home is covered unless special need is indicated. (See Note 89)
156 – This laboratory test for the reported condition and/or illness is not covered. (See Note 89)
158 – Procedures whose effectiveness has not been proven are not covered. (See Note 89)
161 – The frequency of services for this condition are not covered. (See Note 89)
162 – More than one visit per day for this condition are not covered. (See Note 89)
172 – This type of services billed by a psychologist are not covered.
179 – The amount for this service is included in the approved amount for the consultation/office/hospital visit.
181 – Payment for this service is included in the major surgical fee.
187 – We need the name and address of the individual doctor who performed this service. Please resubmit your claim with this information.
192 – Medicare benefits have been reduced because the patient's employer group health plan has paid some of these expenses.
198 – A claim must be sent to the patient's employer group health plan first. After the claim has been processed by that plan, resubmit this claim with the bills and the notice the other insurance company sent you.
203 – Clinical laboratory services. Blood Gas Studies and Rhythm Strips (1–3 leads) furnished in a hospital setting are reimbursed through the hospital.
205 – The date of this service is after the patient's expiration date provided to us by SSA. If service was rendered to this patient on this date, have the patient's estate contact the local Social Security Office for assistance.
206 – For payment, these services must be billed by the performing laboratory with the assignment accepted.
213 – We did not send this claim to Medicaid. Please send this statement and a copy of the claim to the agency that handles Medicaid in your area.
216 – This service or item cannot be processed until your application for a Medicare provider identification number is received and approved.
218 – Since you are Medicare participating, we have processed this claim as assigned. Future claims must be billed on assignment. If the bill was paid in full, you must immediately refund the amount due to the beneficiary.
219 – We need this charge submitted on your letterhead bill. Please resubmit your claim with this information.
221 – The name and Medicare number submitted on this claim do not match. Please verify for whom these services were rendered and provide the correct name and number on the claim and resubmit.
223 – We did not consider this for payment because you did not send the extra information we asked for. Payment can be requested again by sending us another claim form and all the information.
226 – Medicare will pay rent for the prescribed number of months or until the equipment is no longer needed, whichever occurs first. This is the first monthly rental payment.
227 – You will receive a notice each month when additional rental payments are paid.
231 – Medicare will no longer pay for rental on this item since the purchase price has been paid.
237 – The amount of this payment is the difference between the approved purchase allowance and the rental payments you have received.

YOUR RIGHT TO REVIEW OF A CASE

If you have a problem or question about the way a claim was handled or about the amount paid, please write Transamerica Occidental Life, Box 54905, Terminal Annex, Los Angeles, California 90054, within 6 months of the date of this notice. We will give your request full consideration.

Your Social Security office will help you file a request for review of a claim if it is more convenient for you.

WHERE TO SEND REFUNDS

When refunding a payment you should send a check with a letter of explanation. The letter should include your Transamerica Occidental/Medicare check number, beneficiary name and Medicare identification number (HICNo.), control number to which the payment relates, and any other information which may be pertinent to the refund. Send this information to:

Transamerica Occidental Life
C/O Check and Payment Control
Box 54905, Terminal Annex
Los Angeles, CA 90054-0905

KEY TO CODES FOR PLACE AND TYPE OF SERVICE

Place of service	Type of service
1. Office	A. Medical care
2. Home	B. Surgery (includes treatment of fractures)
3. Inpatient hospital	C. Consultation
4. Skilled nursing facility	D. Diagnostic X-ray
5. Outpatient hospital	E. Diagnostic laboratory
6. Independent laboratory	F. Radiation therapy
7. Other	G. Anesthesia
8. Independent kidney disease treatment center	H. Assistance at surgery
	I. Other medical service
	J. Whole blood or packed red cells

B

Fig. 6.14, cont'd.

MEDICARE REMITTANCE ADVICE
XYZ Insurance Company

Physician or supplier name	Dates of service From MMDD	To MMDDYY	See back serv typl	Sub code (alwcode)	Billed amount	Amount allowed	See ** act cde	Beneficiary obligation Deductible	Co-ins	Medicare payment to Beneficiary	provider
BENEFICIARY: BILL HUTCH				HIC NUMBER: 5432-112-34							
CONTROL NO.: 92106-30810-00			DE/MI: 2121D52								
John Doe MD	0310	0310XX	D 03	120101	245.00	180.00	101	147.00	1.00	0.00	26.40
CLAIM TOTALS:					245.00	180.00	101	147.00	1.00	0.00	26.40

A

MEDICAID REMITTANCE ADVICE

RECIPIENT NAME	RECIPIENT MEDICAID ID NO.	CLAIM CONTROL NUMBER	SERVICE DATE MO DAY YR	PROCEDURE CODE	PATIENT ACCT. NO.	QTY.	MEDICARE ALLOWED	MEDICAID ALLOWED	PATIENT LIABILITY	COMPUTED MCR AMT.	MEDICAID PAID	EOB MESSAGE
BILL HUTCH	521345678	4006984891200	03 10 XX	49555–80		001	180.00	148.00		26.40	.00	
		4006984891200	00 00 XX			000	180.00	148.00		26.40	148.00	
BLOOD DEDUCT 00 DEDUCTIBLE 147.00 COINSUR 1.00 CUTBACK 32.00												CUTBACK 443

B

Fig. 6.15 A, A Medicare/Medicaid case after payment by Medicare. **B,** The Medicaid remittance advice shows reimbursement of the coinsurance and deductible amounts dual billed to Medicaid.

KEY POINTS

This is a brief chapter review, or summary, of the key issues presented. To further enhance your knowledge of the technical subject matter, review the key terms and key abbreviations for this chapter by locating the meaning for each in the Glossary at the end of this book, which appears in a section before the index.

1. Medicare is administered by the Centers for Medicare and Medicaid Services (CMS).
2. Medicare is a health insurance program for people aged 65 or older, people younger than aged 65 with certain disabilities, and people of all ages with end-stage renal disease (ESRD).
3. Medicare Part A is for hospital insurance benefits and Medicare Part B is for medical insurance benefits.
4. Medicare Part C is referred to as *Medicare Advantage plan (MA plan)*. This plan offers a number of health care options in addition to those available under Medicare Part A and Part B.
5. Medicare Part D prescription drug plan is a standalone drug plan, presented by insurance and other private companies, that offers drug coverage that meets the standards established by Medicare.
6. On enrollment into the Medicare program, the Medicare beneficiary is issued an identification care.
7. Patients who received railroad retirement benefits will get Medicare from the Railroad Retirement Board.
8. Medigap is a specialized Medicare supplemental insurance policy whose predefined minimum benefits are regulated by the federal government and devised for the Medicare beneficiary.
9. Medicare secondary payer (MSP) is a primary insurance plan of a Medicare beneficiary who must pay for any medical care or services first before a Medicare fiscal intermediary is sent a claim.
10. The US Department of Health and Human Services' Quality Improvement Organization program is dedicated to improving the quality of services provided to Medicare beneficiaries.
11. Because Medicare is a federal program, providers that transmit claims to Medicare must comply with billing and coding regulations issued by CMS.
12. Participating providers and health care organizations agree to accept assignment on all Medicare claims and may bill the patient only for the Medicare deductible and coinsurance amounts.
13. National Coverage Determinations (NCDs) and Local Coverage Determinations (LCDs) are coverage policies that must be adhered to when determining if services to Medicare beneficiaries will be considered medically necessary and payable.

14. An Advance Beneficiary Notice of Noncoverage (ABN) is an agreement given to the patient to read and sign before rendering a service if the participating provider thinks that it may be denied for payment because of medical necessity or limitation of liability by Medicare. ABNs apply if the patient is in an original Medicare program and do not apply for patients in private fee-for-service (PFFS) or Medicare Advantage plans.
15. The Correct Coding Initiative (CCI) is federal legislation that attempts to identify services that are described by a single code or are inherent to another procedure.
16. A Medicare fee schedule (MFS) is a method of reimbursement for services provided by physicians, ambulance services, clinical laboratory services, and durable medical equipment (DME), agencies, hospice, hospital outpatient, inpatient psychiatric facilities, inpatient rehabilitation facilities, long-term care hospitals, and skilled nursing facilities.
17. The Medicare Access and CHIP Reauthorization Act of 2015 (MACRA) is legislation enacted to establish a new payment methodology to pay providers by rewarding high-quality and high-value care.
18. Medicare requites mandatory claims submission, which applies to all physician and suppliers who provide covered services to Medicare beneficiaries.
19. The time limit for sending in Medicare claims is within 12 months from the date of service.
20. Instructions for Medicare claims submission can be found in the Medicare Claims Processing Manual—Internet Only Manual Publication 100.04.
21. Medicare sends a payment check and a nationally standardized document to participating providers called a Medicare remittance advice (RA) and a similar document to the patient called a Medicare Summary Notice (MSN).

STUDENT ASSIGNMENT

- Study Chapter 6.
- Answer the fill-in-the-blank, multiple-choice, and true/false review questions in the *Workbook* to reinforce the theory learned in this chapter and to help you prepare for a future test.
- Complete the assignments in the *Workbook* to give you experience in computing Medicare in mathematic calculations, selecting Healthcare Common Procedure Coding System (HCPCS) code numbers, abstracting from patients' health records, preparing financial accounting record cards, and completing forms pertinent to the Medicare program.
- Turn to the Glossary at the end of this text for a further understanding of the key terms and key abbreviations used in this chapter.

7

Medicaid and Other State Programs

Linda M. Smith

OBJECTIVES

After reading this chapter, you should be able to:

1. Explain what the Medicaid program is.
2. Discuss the history of Medicaid.
3. Describe added benefits for Medicaid recipients afforded by the Patient Protection and Affordable Care Act and the Health Care and Education Reconciliation Act of 2010.
4. Discuss the different types of Medicaid programs.
5. Discuss how Medicaid is administered by state governments.
6. Identify those eligible for the Medicaid Qualified Medicare Beneficiaries program.
7. Name and describe the two Medicaid eligibility classifications.
8. Discuss a health care organization's responsibility as a participant in the Medicaid program.
9. List valuable information to abstract from the patient's Medicaid card.
10. Describe the Medicaid basic benefits.
11. Explain basic operations of a Medicaid-managed care system.
12. Explain basic Medicaid claim procedure guidelines.
13. File claims for patients who have Medicaid and other coverage.
14. Interpret and post a remittance advice.
15. Describe filing an appeal for a Medicaid case.
16. Explain the purpose of the Medicaid Fraud Control Unit.

KEY TERMS

categorically needy
Children's Health Insurance Program
coinsurance
copayment
covered services
Early and Periodic Screening, Diagnosis, and Treatment
federal poverty level
fiscal agent
Medicaid
Medi-Cal
medically needy
Medicare Savings Programs
payer of last resort
prior approval
recipient
share of cost
spousal impoverishment
Supplemental Security Income
Temporary Assistance for Needy Families

KEY ABBREVIATIONS

CHIP
DEFRA
EPSDT
FPL
MN
MSP
OBRA
OOY claims
POS machine
QI program
QMB
RA
SLMB
SSI
TANF

MEDICAID

Medicaid is not so much an insurance program as it is an assistance program. Medicaid is a government program for individuals and families whose income and resources are insufficient to pay for health care. The Medicaid program is jointly funded by the state and federal governments. On a federal level, the Centers for Medicare and Medicaid Centers (CMS) monitors the programs and establish requirements for service delivery, funding, quality and eligibility standards. The states are required to comply with all federal Medicaid laws.

Each state is allowed to administer and manage its own Medicaid program. This includes establishing eligibility requirements, determining the scope and types of services the state program will cover, and setting the rate of payment. Medicaid eligibility and benefits may vary from state to state.

History

Federal participation in providing medical care to needy persons began between 1933 and 1935 when the Federal Emergency Relief Administration made funds available to pay the medical expenses of the needy unemployed. The Social Security Act of 1935 created the public assistance programs. Although no special provision was made for medical insurance, the federal government paid a share of the monthly income assistance payments, which the individual could use to meet the costs of medical care. After the various attempts during the previous 30 years to provide medical care to the needy, in 1965 Title XIX of the Social Security Act became federal law and Medicaid legally came into being. Under the program, the federal government provided matching funds to states to enable them to provide medical assistance to individuals whose incomes and resources were insufficient to meet the costs of necessary medical services.

Since 1983, the trend in many states has been to expand Medicaid eligibility requirements and services. Changes in Medicaid eligibility allowing more people into the program were made by many states after the passage of the Deficit Reduction Act (DEFRA) of 1984 and the Child Health Assurance Program (CHAP) by the federal government. On July 1, 2006, as part of DEFRA, a federal law became effective requiring new applicants and current beneficiaries renewing their benefits (except seniors and people with disabilities) to submit birth certificates, passports, or other documents to establish their legal right to benefits as US citizens. If no documentation of citizenship can be found, sworn affidavits from the beneficiary and at least one or two other individuals can be used.

In 2002 and 2003, states across the nation faced steep budget shortfalls. A vast majority of them made cuts of some kind in their Medicaid programs by either instituting or boosting copayments for certain types of services or by eliminating some services. Copayment (copay) is a required specific dollar amount that must be collected at each office visit for medical services received by an individual. Under Medicaid, different copayment amounts may be set for each patient group as listed in Box 7.1 (which appears later in this chapter) and for certain medical procedures.

In 2010, health care reform legislation, known as the *Patient Protection and Affordable Care Act (PPACA)* and the *Health Care and Education Reconciliation Act (HCERA)*, was passed. These Acts affect the Medicaid program by expanding access for childless adults and nonelderly and nonpregnant individuals, and include preventive services and long-term care benefits. Additional funds were allocated for maternal and child health services.

PPACA created the Community First Choice Option, a plan that allowed state Medicaid plans to provide medical assistance for home- and community-based attendant services and support to eligible individuals. The Community First Choice Option became available in 2011.

PPACA created the opportunity for states to expand Medicaid to cover nearly all low-income Americans younger than 65. States were given the option to extend Medicaid eligibility to adults with incomes at or less than 133% of the federal poverty level (FPL). The FPL is a measure of income issued every year by the Department of Health and Human Services (HHS). As of January 1, 2017, 32 states have chosen to expand their programs; 19 states have not (Table 7.1).

MEDICAID PROGRAMS

As stated earlier, Medicaid programs vary from state to state. Some may have different names. For example, Medi-Cal is California's Medicaid health care program. New Jersey's Medicaid program is NJ Family Care. The state of Arizona has the Arizona Health Care Cost Containment System (AHCCCS) as their Medicaid agency, which offers health care programs to serve their residents.

BOX 7.1 Groups Eligible for Medicaid Benefits

Mandatory Eligibility Groups
- Low-income families
- TANF–related groups
- Non-TANF pregnant women and children
- Infants born to Medicaid-eligible pregnant women
- Recipients of adoption assistance or foster care assistance under Title IV-E of the Social Security Act
- Aged, blind, and disabled
- SSI–related groups
- Qualified Medicare beneficiaries
- Persons who receive institutional or other long-term care in nursing facilities and intermediate care facilities
- Medicare–Medicaid beneficiaries

Optional Eligibility Groups
- Low-income persons who are losing employer health insurance coverage (Medicaid purchase if person has Consolidated Omnibus Budget Reconciliation Act coverage)
- Infants up to age 1 and pregnant women not covered under the mandatory rules whose family income is not more than 185% of the federal poverty level (note that the percentage may be modified by each state)
- Children younger than age 21 who meet TANF income and resource requirements but who are otherwise not eligible for TANF
- Persons who would be eligible if institutionalized but receive care under home- and community-based service waivers
- Persons infected with tuberculosis who would be financially eligible for Medicaid at the SSI income level if they were within a Medicaid-covered category (limited coverage)
- Low-income children with the State Children's Health Insurance Program
- Low-income, uninsured women who are diagnosed through the Centers for Disease Control and Prevention's National Breast and Cervical Cancer Early Detection Program and who need treatment for breast or cervical cancer

Medically Needy Eligibility Group
- Medically indigent low-income individuals and families who have too much income to qualify under mandatory or optional eligibility Medicaid groups

SSI, Supplemental Security Income; *TANF*, Temporary Assistance for Needy Families.

Children's Health Insurance Program

The Children's Health Insurance Program (CHIP) is a partnership between the federal and state governments that provides low-cost health coverage to children in families that earn too much money to qualify for Medicaid. In some states, CHIP also covers care for pregnant women. Each state and certain other jurisdictions, including territories and the District of Columbia (56 programs total), operate a CHIP.

CHIP insures children from families whose income is less than 200% of the FPL or whose family has an income 50% higher than the state's Medicaid eligibility threshold. However,

TABLE 7.1 Department of Health and Human Services Federal Poverty Guidelines

Year	Annual Income for One Person	Annual Income for Four-Person Family
2017	$12,060	$24,600
2018	$11,880	$24,300
2015	$11,770	$24,250
2014	$11,670	$23,850
2013	$11,490	$23,550

Federal poverty levels used to determine eligibility for certain Medicaid programs as found in the *Federal Register*.

some states have expanded CHIP eligibility beyond the 200% FPL limit, and others are covering entire families and not just children. States have three options in designing their program. The state can do one of the following:

- Use CHIP funds to expand Medicaid eligibility to children who previously did not qualify for the program.
- Design a children's health insurance program that is entirely separate from Medicaid.
- Combine both the Medicaid and the separate program options.

Federal funds are granted to states, enabling them to do the following:

- Provide low-income mothers and children access to quality maternal and child health services.
- Reduce infant mortality and the incidence of preventable diseases and handicapping conditions among children.
- Increase the number of children immunized against disease and the number of low-income children receiving health assessments and follow-up diagnostic and treatment services.
- Promote the health of mothers and infants by providing prenatal, delivery, and postpartum care for low-income, at-risk pregnant women.
- Provide preventive and primary care services for low-income children.
- Provide rehabilitation services for the blind and disabled younger than age 16 years.
- Provide, promote, and develop family-centered, community-based, coordinated care for children with special health care needs.

CHIP programs may vary in name from state to state. For example, Michigan developed the Children's Special Health Care Services (CSHCS) program. CSHCS is a program for children and some adults with special health care needs. The state of Maryland has the Maryland Children's Health Program (MCHP), which provides access to health insurance coverage for higher-income uninsured children up to age 19, and Georgia has PeachCare for Kids, which is a comprehensive health program for uninsured children living in Georgia. Benefits of the program include primary, preventive, specialist, dental, and vision care. It also covers hospitalization, emergency room services, prescription medications, and mental health care.

Medicare Savings Programs

Medicare Savings Programs (MSPs) help low-income individuals with out-of-pocket costs for Medicare, including Medicare Part A and Part B premiums, deductibles, copayments, and coinsurance. There are four types of MSPs:

- Qualified Medicare Beneficiary program
- Specified Low-Income Medicare Beneficiary program
- Qualifying Individual program
- Qualified Disabled and Working Individuals program

All four types of MSP are run by state Medicaid programs. Each program addresses a different financial category, and the monthly income figures are adjusted each year. Eligibility for the programs may differ from state to state.

Medicaid Qualified Medicare Beneficiary Program

The Medicaid Qualified Medicare Beneficiary program was introduced in the Medicare Catastrophic Coverage Act of 1988 as an amendment to the Social Security Act. In 1990 the Omnibus Reconciliation Act (OBRA) of 1989 allowed for assistance to qualified Medicare beneficiaries (QMBs, pronounced "kwim-bees") who are aged and disabled, are receiving Medicare, and have annual incomes less than the FPL. Eligibility also depends on what other financial resources an individual might have.

Under this Act, states must provide limited Medicaid coverage for QMBs. They must pay Medicare Part B premiums (and Part A premiums if applicable), along with necessary Medicare deductibles and coinsurance amounts. Coinsurance is the portion of the Medicare allowed amount that the patient pays. When discussing Medicaid, the terms *copayment* and *coinsurance* do not have the same meaning that they do when talking about private insurance coverage issues. As discussed later in this chapter in the section titled "Copayment," there are two types of copayment for the Medicaid program depending on each state's established policy. QMB program coverage is restricted to Medicare cost sharing unless the beneficiary qualifies for Medicaid in some other way. Medicaid will not pay for the service if Medicare does not cover the service to the patient.

States are also required to pay Medicare Part A premiums but no other expenses for qualified disabled and working individuals. It is optional for states to provide full Medicaid benefits to QMBs who meet a state-established income standard.

Specified Low-Income Medicare Beneficiary Program

The Specified Low-Income Medicare Beneficiary (SLMB, pronounced "slim-bee") program was established in 1993 for elderly individuals whose income is 20% more than the FPL. It pays the entire Medicare Part B premium. The patient must pay the deductible and copay and must pay for noncovered items.

Qualifying Individual Program

The Qualifying Individual (QI) program was created in 1997 for qualifying individuals whose income is at least 135% but less than 175% of the FPL. This program pays for the Medicare

Part B premium and automatically qualifies them for prescription drug coverage assistance. Patients who qualify for Medicaid cannot receive QI benefits.

Qualified Disabled and Working Individuals Program

The Qualified Disabled and Working Individuals (QDWI) program is different from the other three Medicare Savings Programs in that it only pays for Medicare Part A premiums. Individuals may qualify for a QDWI Program if any the following apply:

- They returned to work and lost their premium-free Medicare Part A coverage.
- They are younger than 65, disabled, and currently working.
- They are not getting state medical assistance.
- They meet the income and resource requirements of their state.

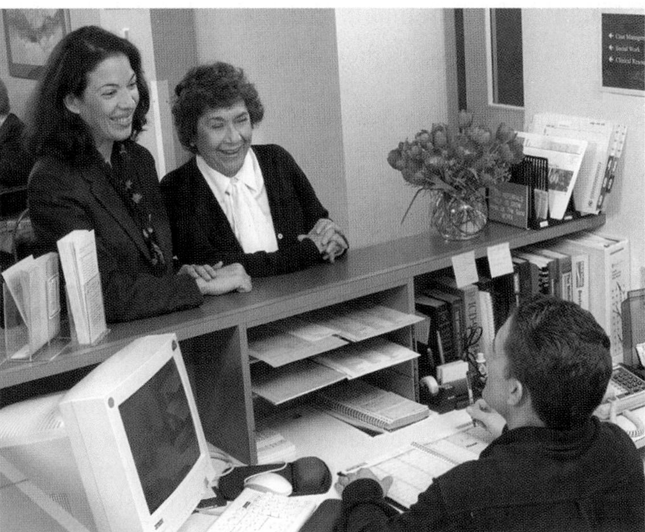

Fig. 7.1 Medicaid patient checking in with the receptionist.

MEDICAID ELIGIBILITY

Medicaid is available to certain needy and low-income people, such as those who are elderly (65 years or older), blind, or disabled and members of families with dependent children deprived of the support of at least one parent and financially eligible based on income and resources. In general, Medicaid is available only to US citizens and certain "qualified immigrants." Passports and birth certificates must be submitted for proof of citizenship.

Nonimmigrants and unauthorized aliens are not eligible for most federal benefits; however, states have the option to cover nonimmigrant and unauthorized aliens who are pregnant or who are children and can meet the definition of "lawfully residing" in the United States.

If a person may be eligible for Medicaid, he or she goes to the local public service welfare office, human service, or family independence agency and applies for benefits.

Verifying Eligibility

After acceptance into the program, the patient brings a form or card to the health care provider's office that verifies acceptance into the program (Fig. 7.1), but this does not indicate proof of eligibility. It is the provider's responsibility to verify at each visit that the person there to receive care is eligible on the date on which the service is rendered and is the individual to whom the card was issued.

Each state decides which services are covered and what the payments are for each service. There are two classifications—categorically needy and medically needy—that contain several basic groups of needy and low-income individuals.

Categorically Needy

The first classification, the categorically needy group, includes all cash recipients of Temporary Assistance for Needy Families. The Temporary Assistance for Needy Families (TANF) program is a federal assistance program that began on July 1, 1997. The program provides limited cash assistance to extremely low-income parents and their children. TANF assists families with children when the parents or other responsible relatives cannot provide for the family's basic needs. The federal government provides grants to states to run the TANF program. States may have different names for this program, and it can be called welfare, public assistance, temporary assistance, general assistance, or cash assistance.

Other individuals who may be considered categorically needy are most cash recipients of the Supplemental Security Income (SSI) program; other SSI-related groups; QMBs; and patients in institutional, long-term care, and intermediate care facilities (see Box 7.1). A recipient is an individual certified by the local welfare department to receive benefits of Medicaid under one of the specific aid categories.

Medically Needy

In states with medically needy (MN) Medicaid programs, individuals may qualify for Medicaid if they have medical expenses that significantly reduce their income. In these cases the patient makes a higher income than allowed to be eligible for Medicaid. However, assistance can be provided if patients' income minus their medical expenses fall below a certain limit. Most states have MN programs, allowing those with high medical expenses to still qualify for Medicaid.

States that choose to have MN programs may decide not to offer the MN option to all categories of Medicaid-eligible people. For example, a state may choose to offer the MN programs to elderly but not disabled people. However, states that offer any MN programs must offer them to most children and pregnant women.

A Medicaid recipient in this category may or may not pay a copayment or a deductible, which must be met within the eligibility month or other specified time frame before he or she can receive state benefits (also known as share of cost or *spend down*). Emergency care and pregnancy services are exempt by law from copayment requirements. This may be a component of a state's general assistance program for low-income people.

Spousal Impoverishment Protection Law

In 1988 Congress enacted provisions to prevent spousal impoverishment, which refers to leaving the spouse who is still living at home in the community with little or no income or resources. The Spousal Impoverishment Protection Law is federal legislation that affects special financial provisions in Medicaid for the elderly, blind, or disabled. Formerly, if one partner (institutionalized spouse) needed to be in a nursing facility, a couples' income and assets would become so depleted to qualify that the other spouse (community spouse) did not have a sufficient amount to live on. This protection counts assets, such as cash, checking and savings accounts, life insurance policies, and certificates of deposits. It does not count the couples' home, car, household furnishings, burial assets (insurance, trust funds, or plots), clothing, or other personal items. This prevents the community spouse from being impoverished by his or her spouse's institutionalization.

Accepting Medicaid Patients

Program Participation

A health care organization or provider must enroll for participation in the Medicaid program. The enrolling service provider must sign a written agreement with the fiscal agent as part of the application process. In the Medicaid program, a fiscal agent is an organization under contract to the state to process claims for a state Medicaid program.

Health care organizations and service providers have their own office procedures for handling Medicaid patients. The organization or provider may accept or refuse to treat Medicaid patients but must make the decision based on the entire Medicaid program, not an individual patient's personality, medical situation, or other discriminating factor. The patient must receive quality care and be treated the same as the paying patient. If the health care organization decides to take Medicaid patients, they must accept the Medicaid allowance as payment in full. The Medicaid allowance is the maximum dollar amount to be considered for payment for a service or procedure by the program.

A patient can be on Medicaid 1 month and then off it the following month, or the patient could be on the program for several months or years; each case is different. When obtaining personal information from the patient at the time of the first visit or a follow-up visit, always check and update the patient's name and address by asking for photo identification, such as a driver's license.

Identification Card

A plastic or paper Medicaid identification card (or coupons in some states) is usually issued monthly (Fig. 7.2). Under certain classifications of eligibility, identification cards are issued in some states on the first and fifteenth of each month, every 2 months, every 3 months, or every 6 months. Sometimes an unborn child can be issued an identification card that is used for services promoting the life and health of the fetus. Obtain a photocopy or scan of the front and back of the card. Carefully check the expiration date of the card each time the patient visits the health care office to see whether eligibility is indicated for the month of service. Note whether the patient has other insurance, copayment requirements, or restrictions, such as being eligible for only certain types of medical services. Remember that the presentation of an insurance ID card does not guarantee coverage. The items that must be abstracted from the card for claim submission are (1) the patient's name exactly as shown, (2) Medicaid identification number, (3) gender, and (4) date of birth.

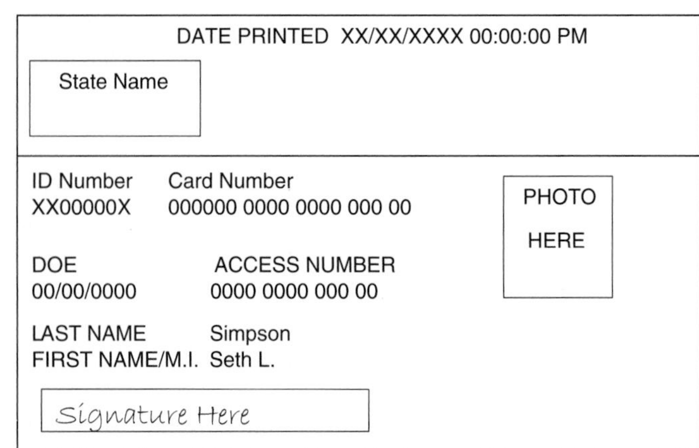
DATE PRINTED XX/XX/XXXX 00:00:00 PM

State Name

ID Number XX00000X
Card Number 000000 0000 0000 000 00

PHOTO HERE

DOE 00/00/0000
ACCESS NUMBER 0000 0000 000 00

LAST NAME Simpson
FIRST NAME/M.I. Seth L.

Signature Here

Fig. 7.2 Sample of information included on a state Medicaid card.

Point-of-Service Machine

When professional services are rendered, eligibility for that month must be verified. Verification is done if several ways, depending on how the state has developed their process. For example, the Nashville-based company Medifax provides internet Medicaid eligibility verification to California, North Carolina, New Jersey, and Georgia. Medifax provides real-time, online access to patient eligibility and benefit information for health care providers.

Some states provide their own electronic system for Medicaid verification via touchtone telephone, modem, or specialized Medicaid terminal equipment, such as a point-of-service (POS) machine (Fig. 7.3). New York State utilizes a POS verification device that uses basic analog telephone outlets to connect with their Medicaid Verification System (MEVS).

Retroactive Eligibility

Retroactive eligibility may be granted to a patient in some cases. In a situation where the patient has been referred to apply for Medicaid, the patient must ask for retroactive status; otherwise the approval effective date is the date of the application. When patients are seeking medical care, hoping to qualify for Medicaid but not accepted by the time of service, the account must be set up as a cash account until retroactive eligibility has been established. Retroactive eligibility status must be decided within 90 days of filing of the application. If the patient has documentation or a retroactive card confirming this and has paid for any services during the retroactive period, a refund must be made and Medicaid billed.

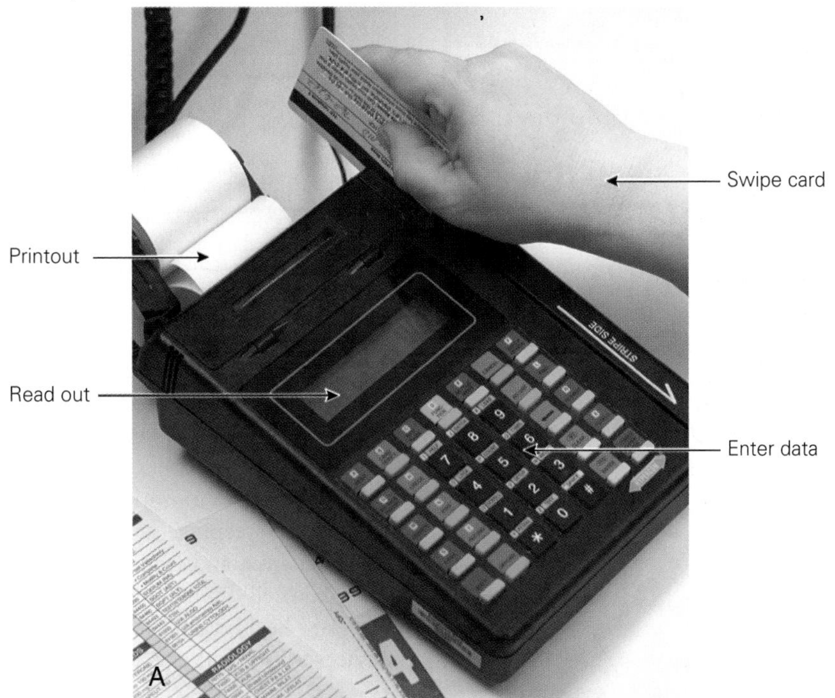

POS Device: Medi-Service Printout

EDS BROAD AVENUE TERMINAL T309006
XX-02-15
17:16:36

PROVIDER NUMBER:
12345F

TRANSACTION TYPE: MEDI-SERVICES

RECIPIENT ID:
5077534XX

YEAR & MONTH OF BIRTH:
1975-12

DATE OF ISSUE:
XX-02-15

DATE OF SERVICE:
XX-02-15

PROCEDURE CODE:
45339

LAST NAME: MORRISON MEDI SVC
RESERVATION APPLIED

B

POS Device: Share of Cost Printout

EDS BROAD AVENUE TERMINAL T309006
XX-02-15
17:16:36

PROVIDER NUMBER:
12345F

TRANSACTION TYPE: SHARE OF COST

RECIPIENT ID:
5077534XX

YEAR & MONTH OF BIRTH:
1984-10

DATE OF ISSUE:
XX-02-15

DATE OF SERVICE:
XX-02-15

CASE NUMBER:

PROCEDURE CODE:
90945

PATIENT APPLIED AMOUNT:
$50.00

TOTAL BILLED AMOUNT:
$100.00

LAST NAME: ADAMS
AMOUNT DEDUCTED: $50.00
SHARE OF COST HAS BEEN MET

C

Fig. 7.3 **A,** Insurance billing specialist using a point-of-service (POS) machine to check a patient's Medicaid eligibility. **B,** Printout from a POS machine for Medi-Service. **C,** Printout from a POS machine for share of cost.

BOX 7.2 Medicaid Basic Benefits

Inpatient hospital care
Outpatient hospital care
Early and Periodic Screening, Diagnostic and Treatment services
Nursing facility services
Home health services
Physicians' care
Rural health clinic services
Federally qualified health center services
Laboratory and x-ray services
Family planning services
Nurse midwife services
Certified pediatric and nurse practitioner services
Freestanding birth center services (when recognized by the state)
Transportation to and from medical care
Tobacco cessation counseling for pregnant women

In some states, additional services might include the following:

- Allergy care
- Ambulance services
- Certain medical cosmetic procedures
- Chiropractic care
- Clinic care
- Dental care
- Dermatologic care
- Diagnostic, screening, preventive, and rehabilitative services (e.g., physical therapy)
- Emergency department care
- Eyeglasses and eye refractions
- Hospice care
- Intermediate care
- Occupational therapy
- Optometric services
- Physical therapy
- Podiatric care
- Prescription drugs
- Private duty nursing
- Prosthetic devices
- Psychiatric care
- Respiratory care
- Speech, hearing, and language disorder services

MEDICAID BENEFITS

Covered Services

Under federal guidelines, states are required to provide mandatory Medicaid benefits to eligible recipients. Each state may have additional benefits that are offered beyond the basic, mandatory benefits. Covered services are reimbursable services under the state's Medicaid program. They consist of a combination of the mandatory basic benefits and optional services that the state may offer (Box 7.2).

Early and Periodic Screening, Diagnosis, and Treatment

Another benefit of the Medicaid program is the Early and Periodic Screening, Diagnosis, and Treatment (EPSDT) service. This is a program of prevention, early detection, and treatment of children who are under the age of 21 and enrolled in Medicaid (Table 7.2). In California (Medi-Cal) it is known as the *Child Health and Disability Prevention (CHDP) program* and in Ohio as *Healthchek*. Because many states are changing the name of EPSDT and the services offered under the program, check with the state Medicaid vendor.

TABLE 7.2 Explanation of Early and Periodic Screening, Diagnosis, and Treatment Benefits

Early	Identifying problems early, starting at birth
Periodic	Checking children's health at periodic, age-appropriate intervals
Screening	Doing physical, mental, developmental, dental, hearing, vision, and other screening tests to detect potential problems
Diagnosis	Performing diagnostic tests to follow up when a risk is identified
Treatment	Treating the problems found

The EPSDT guidelines include a medical history and physical examination; immunization status assessment; dental, hearing, and vision screening; developmental assessment; and screening for anemia and lead absorption, tuberculosis, bacteriuria, and sickle cell disease and trait. States are required to provide necessary health care, diagnostic services, treatment, and other services to correct any physical or mental defects found.

Disallowed Services

If a service is totally disallowed by Medicaid (denied claim), in many states the health care organization is within his or her legal rights to bill the patient; consult state regulations before deciding to bill. However, it is wise to have the patient sign a waiver of liability agreement if the service to be provided may be a denied service from known past claim submission experience. Write or telephone the state agency to obtain up-to-date information and details on the Medicaid program in a particular state.

MEDICAID MANAGED CARE

As early as 1967, some states began bringing managed care to their Medicaid programs. Over the past decade, many states adopted pilot projects to determine whether a managed care system would work and what benefits might be received. Mainly this was done to control escalating health care costs by curbing unnecessary emergency department visits and emphasizing preventive care.

When Arizona started its Medicaid program, it began with prepaid care rather than adhering to the way most states have structured their programs. By then, most states had been struggling with Medicaid for nearly 20 years. In these systems the Medicaid recipient enrolls in either an existing or a specifically formed plan similar to a health maintenance organization (HMO). The patient either may be assigned or may choose a gatekeeper (clinic or primary care physician [PCP]) who must approve all specialty care and inpatient or outpatient hospital treatment. Patients must use physicians, clinics, and hospitals that participate in their assigned plan. Some doctors prefer to operate on a contract-to-contract, per-patient basis rather than be a participating provider.

Patients can be cared for side by side with private-paying patients. Some states have adopted capitation (a flat fee per patient) rather than fee-for-service reimbursement. There may be a small copayment for services. It has been found that there is better access to primary health care and savings of monies in delivering the care if the Medicaid programs are well managed.

CLAIM PROCEDURES

Medicaid policies and claim procedures about identification cards, prior approval regulations, claim forms, and time limits vary from state to state. General guidelines for submitting claims are stated here.

For specific state guidelines, consult the current *Medicaid Handbook* online at the state fiscal agent's website.

Copayment

There are two types of copayment requirements that may apply to a state. Some states require a small fixed copayment paid to the provider at the time services are rendered. This policy was instituted to help pay some of the administrative costs of providers participating in the Medicaid program.

Another requirement is the share of cost or *spend down* copayment. Some Medicaid recipients must meet this copayment requirement each month before Medicaid benefits can be claimed. For example, if an individual's income is too high to qualify, some states allow deduction of certain medical expenses from his or her income so that the income may fall within Medicaid guidelines. These spend down programs are available in some states for the aged, the blind, or those who have a disability. Spend down eligibility is a monthly process and patients must submit proof of medical expenses that meet the spend down amount. Expenses covered by other insurance are not eligible to be used toward the spend down amount. For example, if the income is $150 more than the limit, the excess income is equal to the spend down amount and the patient must submit $150 of acceptable medical bills or pay in the spend down amount to receive Medicaid coverage for the remainder of the month. Because the amount may change from month to month, be sure to verify the copayment each time it is collected. Obtain this copayment amount when the patient comes in for medical care and report on the claim form that it has been collected.

Prior Approval

Many times, prior approval is necessary for various goods and services, except in a bona fide emergency. **Prior approval** is the evaluation of a provider's request for a specific good or service to determine the medical necessity and appropriateness of the care requested for the patient. In some states this may be referred to as *prior authorization*. Some of these goods and services are the following:

- Durable medical equipment
- Hearing aids
- Hemodialysis
- Home health care
- Inpatient hospital care
- Long-term care facility services
- Medical supplies
- Medications
- Prosthetic or orthotic appliances
- Some vision care
- Surgical procedures
- Transportation

Usually prior authorization forms are completed to obtain permission for a specific service or hospitalization (Fig. 7.4) and mailed or faxed to the Department of Health or a certain office in a region for approval. In some cases, time does not allow for a written request to be sent for prior approval, so an immediate authorization can be obtained via a telephone call to the proper department in any locale. Note the date and time that the authorization was given, the name of the person who gave authorization, and any verbal number given by the field office. Usually a treatment authorization form indicating that the service was already authorized must be sent in as follow-up to the telephone call.

Hospital-Acquired Condition

On July 1, 2012, under the Affordable Care Act, Medicaid implemented the provision to either make a payment adjustment or prohibit payment for any hospital-acquired condition (HAC), such as foreign object retained after surgery; air embolism; blood incompatibility; stages III and IV pressure ulcers; vascular catheter-associated infection; mediastinitis after coronary artery bypass graft; falls and trauma resulting in fractures, dislocations, intracranial injury, crushing injury, burn, and other unspecified effects of external causes; manifestations of poor glycemic control; surgical site infection after spine, neck, shoulder, or elbow orthopedic procedures; surgical site infection after bariatric surgery for obesity; deep vein thrombosis and pulmonary embolism after a total knee or hip replacement, except for pediatric (individuals younger than age 21) and obstetric populations; wrong surgical procedure; correct procedure performed on the wrong patient; or correct procedure performed on the wrong body part.

Time Limit

Each state has its own time limit for the submission of a claim. The time limit can vary from 2 months to 12 or 18 months from the date that the service was rendered. A bill can be rejected if it is submitted after the time limit unless the state recognizes some valid justification. Some states have separate procedures for billing over-one-year (**OOY**) **claims**. A percentage of the claim may be reduced according to the date of a delinquent submission. Prescription drugs and dental services are often billed to a different intermediary than are services performed by a physician or other health care provider, depending on the state guidelines.

Reciprocity

Most states have reciprocity for Medicaid payments if a patient requires medical care while out of state. Contact the Medicaid fiscal intermediary in the patient's home state and ask for the appropriate forms. If the case was an emergency, state this on the form. File the papers with Medicaid in the patient's home state. Reimbursement will be at that state's rate.

Claim Form

As of October 1, 1986, federal law has mandated that the CMS-1500 Insurance Claim Form be adopted for the processing of Medicaid claims in all states.

STATE USE ONLY | SERVICE CATEGORY

CONFIDENTIAL PATIENT INFORMATION
FOR F.I. USE ONLY

CCN

TYPEWRITER ALIGNMENT Elite Pica

TREATMENT AUTHORIZATION REQUEST
STATE OF CALIFORNIA DEPARTMENT OF HEALTH SERVICES

F.I. USE ONLY 40 41 42 43
TYPEWRITER ALIGNMENT Elite Pica

(PLEASE TYPE) FOR PROVIDER USE (PLEASE TYPE)

VERBAL CONTROL NO.

TYPE OF SERVICE REQUESTED: DRUG [ ] OTHER [X]

REQUEST IS RETROACTIVATE? YES [ ] NO [X]

IS PATIENT MEDICARE ELIGIBLE? YES [ ] NO [X]

PROVIDER PHONE NO. (555) 555-1111 AREA

PATIENT'S AUTHORIZED REPRESENTATIVE (IF ANY) ENTER NAME AND ADDRESS

PROVIDER NAME AND ADDRESS

PROVIDER NO. HSC12345F

PLEASE TYPE YOUR NAME AND ADDRESS HERE:
SMITH, SUSAN MD
727 ELM BLVD
ANYTOWN, CA 90101

30 83

FOR STATE USE
33 PROVIDER; YOUR REQUEST IS:
1 [X] APPROVED AS REQUESTED [ ] [ ] DEFERRED
2 [ ] APPROVED AS MODIFIED (ITEMS MARKED BELOW AS AUTHORIZED MAY BE CLAIMED) [ ] JACKSON VS RANK PARAGRAPH CODE

BY *John Doe*
MEDICAL CONSULTANT
I.D. # 34 0 7 DATE 35 0 8 2 0 X X
REVIEW COMMENTS INDICATOR 44

COMMENTS/ EXPLANATION

NAME AND ADDRESS OF PATIENT
PATIENT NAME (LAST, FIRST, M. I.) APPLEGATE, NANCY
MEDICAL IDENTIFICATION NO. 253971060 CD CHECK DIGIT
STREET ADDRESS 1515 RIVER ROAD
SEX F AGE 32 DATE OF BIRTH 06 18 70
CITY, STATE, ZIP CODE SACRAMENTO, CA 95822
PATIENT STATUS: [X] HOME [ ] BOARD AND CARE [ ] SNF/ICF [ ] ACUTE HOSPITAL
PHONE NUMBER (555) 545-1123
DIAGNOSIS DESCRIPTION: ENDOMETRIOSIS
ICD-9-CM DIAGNOSIS CODE 617.9
MEDICAL JUSTIFICATION: VISTA HOSPITAL - 1200 MAPLE ST., ANYTOWN, CA
UNCONTROLLABLE ENDOMETRIOSIS

RETROACTIVE AUTHORIZATION GRANTED IN ACCORDANCE WITH SECTION 51003 (B)
36 [ ]1 [ ]2 [ ]3 [ ]4 [ ]5 [ ]6

	AUTHORIZED YES	AUTHORIZED NO	APPROVED UNITS	SPECIFIC SERVICES REQUESTED	UNITS OF SERVICE	PROCEDURE OR DRUG CODE	QUANTITY	CHARGES
1	9 X		10 3	DAYS: 3 HOSPITAL DAYS REQUESTED		11	12	$
2	13 X		14 1	HYSTERECTOMY	1	15 5815070	16 1	$ $1300.00
3	17		18			19	20	$
4	21		22			23	24	$
5	25		26			27	28	$
6	29		30			31	32	$

TO THE BEST OF MY KNOWLEDGE, THE ABOVE INFORMATION IS TRUE, ACCURATE AND COMPLETE AND THE REQUESTED SERVICES ARE MEDICALLY INDICATED AND NECESSARY TO THE HEALTH OF THE PATIENT.

Susan Smith | *MD* | *8-10-XX*
SIGNATURE OF PHYSICIAN OR PROVIDER | TITLE | DATE

AUTHORIZATION IS VALID FOR SERVICES PROVIDED
37 FROM DATE 0 9 0 1 X X 38 TO DATE 0 9 3 0 X X

TAR CONTROL NUMBER
36 OFFICE 12 | SEQUENCE NUMBER 61240229 | PI 0

NOTE: AUTHORIZATION DOES NOT GUARANTEE PAYMENT. PAYMENT IS SUBJECT TO PATIENT'S ELIGIBILITY. BE SURE THE IDENTIFICATION CARD IS CURRENT BEFORE RENDERING SERVICE. SEND TO FIELD SERVICES (F.I. COPY)

SEE YOUR PROVIDER MANUAL FOR ASSISTANCE REGARDING THE COMPLETION OF THIS FORM. 50-1 12/87

Fig. 7.4 Completed treatment authorization request form used in California for the Medi-Cal program.

The health care provider of service must submit a claim form to the fiscal agent for the Medicaid program. In other cases, the provider of services may be directed to send a bill directly to the local public service welfare office, human service, or family independence agency. These agencies have different names in each state.

Chapter 14 includes general block-by-block instructions on how to complete the CMS-1500 claim form for the Medicaid program. Because guidelines for completing the form vary among all Medicaid intermediaries, refer to the local Medicaid intermediary for its directions.

To keep up to date, always read the current bulletins or program memos on the Medicaid state fiscal agent's website. Read and implement the rule changes and updates to avoid rejected claims.

Medicaid Managed Care

When filing a claim for a Medicaid managed care patient, send the bill or claim form to the managed care organization (MCO) and not to the Medicaid fiscal agent. The MCO receives payment for services rendered to eligible members via either the capitation or other managed care method.

Children's Health Insurance Program

Each state's jurisdiction operates its own CHIP with its own unique administrative characteristics. Thus each has its own system and forms for billing and related procedures. The official plans and documents are retained in the individual state offices and are not available on either a regional or a national office basis. For specific information about a state's policies, contact the state's local Department of Health.

Medicaid and Other Plans

It is possible that a person can be eligible for Medicaid and also have group health insurance coverage through an employer. When Medicaid and a third-party payer cover the patient, Medicaid is always considered the **payer of last resort.** The third-party payer (other insurance) is billed first.

After a remittance advice (**RA**) or check voucher is received from the primary carrier, Medicaid (the secondary carrier) is billed. A copy of the RA or check voucher is enclosed.

Government Programs and Medicaid

When a Medicaid patient has Medicare (sometimes referred to as a *crossover case* or *dual eligible case*), TRICARE, or Veterans Health Administration (CHAMPVA) coverage, always send the insurance claim first to the federal program fiscal agent servicing the region. Usually the Medicare fiscal agent automatically forwards the claim to the secondary payer, Medicaid. If this does not occur, bill Medicaid second and attach to the claim form the RA or check voucher that has been received from the federal program. Send in a claim only if the other coverage denies payment or pays less than the Medicaid fee schedule or if Medicaid covers services not covered by the other policy.

In the past, state Medicaid programs paid the Medicare deductibles and coinsurance for dual eligible cases at the full Medicare rate. However, the Balanced Budget Act of 1997 permits states to limit payment to the amount that the Medicaid program would otherwise pay for the service. Because of the health care reform legislation passed in 2010, many states have lowered their cost-sharing obligations for these cases to no more than the Medicaid payment amount for the same service. If the Medicare payment amount equals or exceeds the Medicaid payment rate, the state Medicaid program does not pay the Medicare deductible or coinsurance. The result is that the reimbursement becomes that of a Medicare-only patient even though it is crossed over to the Medicaid program.

AFTER CLAIM SUBMISSION

Remittance Advice

If a provider wants to receive an electronic RA, a form must be completed and submitted to the fiscal agent (Fig. 7.5). However, a provider that relies on the paper system is sent an RA or check voucher that accompanies all Medicaid payment checks. Sometimes five categories of adjudicated claims appear on an RA—adjustments, approvals, denials, suspends, and audit/refund (A/R) transactions—although this terminology may vary from one fiscal agent to another (Fig. 7.6). *Adjudication* or *claim settlement* is the processing of an insurance claim through a series of edits for final determination of coverage (benefits) for possible payment.

Adjustments occur from overpayments or underpayments by the fiscal agent. Approval is when an original claim or a previously denied claim is approved for payment. Denied claims are listed with a reason code on the RA. Claims in suspense for a certain period may be listed on the RA. Accounts receivable A/R transactions are miscellaneous transactions as a result of cost settlements, state audits, or refund checks received.

Appeals

The time limit to appeal a claim varies from state to state but is usually 30 to 60 days from the date listed on the RA. Most Medicaid offices consider an appeal filed when they receive it, not when it is sent. Usually appeals are sent on a special form or with a cover letter along with photocopies of documents applicable to the appeal (for example, claim form, RA, and preauthorization forms). Appeals go first to either the regional fiscal agent or Medicaid bureau, next to the Department of Social Welfare or Human Services, and then to an appellate court that evaluates decisions by local and government agencies. At each level, an examiner looks at the case and makes a decision. If not satisfied, the service provider may ask for further review at the next level.

! COMPLIANCE ALERT

Medicaid Fraud Control

Each state has a Medicaid Fraud Control Unit (MFCU), which is a federally funded state law enforcement entity usually located in the state attorney general's office. The MFCU employ teams of investigators, attorneys, and auditors who investigate and prosecute cases of fraud and other violations, including complaints of mistreatment in long-term care facilities. The Office of Inspector General (OIG) oversees and assess the MFCU for performance and compliance with federal requirements.

ELECTRONIC EXPLANATION OF PAYMENT (EOP) AGREEMENT

GROUP/BILLING PROVIDER NUMBER: HSC 11100F

GROUP/BILLING NAME: College Clinic

ADDRESS: 4567 Broad Avenue

CITY: Woodland Hills STATE: XY ZIP: 12345

CONTACT: Joan Biller PHONE NUMBER: 555-487-8976

SUBMITTER ID: 3664021CC

VENDOR NAME: United Billing Service

ADDRESS: 123 Main Street

CITY: Woodland Hills STATE: XY ZIP: 12346

VENDOR PHONE NUMBER: 555-218-4761

VENDOR CONTACT: Maria DeCortez

I (we) request to receive Electronic Explanation of Payment (EOP) information and authorize the information to be deposited in our electronic mailbox. I (we) accept financial responsibility for costs associated with receipt of Electronic EOP information.

I (we) understand that paper-formatted EOP information will continue to be sent to my (our) mailing address as maintained at EDS until I (we) submit an Electronic EOP Certification Request Form.

I (we) will continue to maintain the confidentiality of records and other information relating to recipients in accordance with applicable state and federal laws, rules, and regulations.

Authorized Signature: *Maria DeCortez* Date: 1-2-XX

Title: President Internet Address: DeCortez@UBS.net

Mail form to: EDS • Attn: ECS Department • P.O. Box 244035 • Montgomery, AL 36124
FAX form to: 334-215-4272 Attn: ECS Department

FOR EDS USE ONLY

BILLING MODE: ______ EOP MODE: ______ PROTOCOL: ______

CONTACT DATE: ______ SOFTWARE MAILED: ______

TEST DATE: ______ AGREEMENT DATE: ______ APPROVAL DATE: ______

BEGIN DATE: ______ END DATE: ______

NOTES: ______

Fig. 7.5 Electronic Explanation of Payment (EOP) Agreement used by the Medicaid program in Alabama. It must be completed by a provider and authorizes the fiscal agent to transmit EOPs to the physician's electronic mail box.

MEDICAID REMITTANCE ADVICE

TO: ANYBODY, FERNANDO G.
1000 ELM STREET
ANYTOWN, XY 12345-0001

REFER TO PROVIDER MANUAL FOR DEFINITION OF RAD CODES

PROVIDER NUMBER	CLAIM TYPE	WARRANT NO	EDS SEQ NO	DATE	PAGE 1 of 1 pages
00AX65800	MEDICAL	39248026	20000617	06/01/20XX	

RECIPIENT NAME	RECIPIENT MEDICAID I.D. NO.	CLAIM CONTROL NUMBER	SERVICE DATES FROM MMDDYY	TO MMDDYY	PROCED CODE MODIFIER	PATIENT ACCOUNT NUMBER	QTY	BILLED AMT	PAYABLE AMT			PAID AMT	RAD CODE
APPROVES (RECONCILE TO FINANCIAL SUMMARY)													
TORRES R	559978557	5079350917901	030720XX	030720XX	Z4802		0001	20.00	16.22			16.22	0401
		5079350917901	030720XX	030720XX	Z4802		0001	20.00	16.22			16.22	0401
						TOTAL		40.00	32.44			32.44	
CHAN B	561198435	5044351314501	020320XX	020320XX	Z4800		0001	30.00	27.03			27.03	0401
		5044351314501	020320XX	020320XX	Z4800		0001	20.00	16.22			16.22	0401
						TOTAL		50.00	43.25			43.25	
		TOTALS FOR APPROVES						90.00	75.69			75.69	
												75.69	AMT PAID
DENIES (DO NOT RECONCILE TO FINANCIAL SUMMARY)													
GOMEZ M	624163192	501134031900	122720XX	122720XX	Z4800		0001	30.00					0036
		TOTAL NUMBER OF DENIES					0001						
SUSPENDS (DO NOT RECONCILE TO FINANCIAL SUMMARY)													
HERN D	562416373	5034270703001	010520XX	010520XX	Z4800		0001	20.00					0602
MART E	623105478	5034270712305	010520XX	010520XX	Z4800		0001	20.00					0602
		5034270712305	010520XX	010520XX	Z4800		0001	20.00					0602
						TOTAL		40.00					0602
LOPEZ C	560291467	5034270712502	012420XX	012420XX	Z4800		0001	20.00					0602
		PAT LIAB 932.00 OTH COVG			0.00	SALES TX		0.00					
		TOTAL NUMBER OF SUSPENDS					0004	80.00					

EXPLANATION OF DENIAL/ADJUSTMENT CODES

0401 PAYMENT ADJUSTED TO MAXIMUM ALLOWABLE
0036 RESUBMISSION TURNAROUND DOCUMENT WAS EITHER NOT RETURNED OR WAS RETURNED UNCORRECTED, THEREFORE YOUR CLAIM IS FORMALLY DENIED.
0602 PENDING ADJUDICATION

OHC CARRIER NAME AND ADDRESS
N049 NORTHWESTERN NATIONAL LIFE 111 WASHINGTON AVE. FL 3 MINNEAPOLIS MN 55401

Fig. 7.6 Medicaid remittance advice form showing adjustments, cutbacks, denied claims, and claims in suspense.

KEY POINTS

This is a brief chapter review, or summary, of the key issues presented. To further enhance your knowledge of the technical subject matter, review the key terms and key abbreviations for this chapter by locating the meaning for each in the Glossary at the end of this book, which appears in a section before the Index.

1. Medicaid was established by Title XIX of the Social Security Act, a federally aided, state-operated, and state-administered program that provides medical benefits for certain low-income persons in need of health and medical care.
2. Medicaid is administered by each state's government with partial federal funding.
3. The Patient Protection and Affordable Care Act (PPACA) and the Health Care and Education Reconciliation Act (HCERA) passed in 2010 affect the Medicaid program by expanding access for childless adults and nonelderly and nonpregnant individuals and including preventive services and long-term care benefits.
4. Coverage and benefits vary widely from state to state.
5. Each state operates a children's health insurance program for children in families who earn too much money to qualify for Medicaid.
6. Some federal acts allow assistance to qualified Medicare beneficiaries (QMBs) and specified low-income Medicare beneficiaries (SLMBs) who are aged and/or disabled and receiving Medicare but have annual incomes below the federal poverty level (FPL).
7. A medically needy (MN) Medicaid classification may or may not pay a deductible, copayment, or share of cost (spend down) within a specific time frame before receiving state benefits.
8. Health care organizations and providers must enroll for participation in the Medicaid program with the fiscal agent.
9. Medicaid benefits identification cards are issued monthly to recipients.
10. Medicaid eligibility must be verified before providing medical services to patients. Some patients may have retroactive eligibility.
11. Sometimes prior approval is required for medical services and procedures.
12. Each state may have a different time limit for submitting a claim for reimbursement.
13. The CMS-1500 insurance claim form has been adopted for processing Medicaid claims in all states to a regional fiscal agent.
14. A remittance advice (RA) or check voucher accompanies all Medicaid payment checks sent by the fiscal agent to the provider of services.
15. Each state has a Medicaid Fraud Control Unit (MFCU) that investigates and prosecutes cases of fraud and other violations, including complaints of mistreatment in long-term care facilities.

STUDENT ASSIGNMENT

- Study Chapter 7.
- Answer the fill-in-the-blank, multiple-choice, and true/false review questions in the *Workbook* to reinforce the theory learned in this chapter and to help you prepare for a future test.
- Complete the assignments in the *Workbook* to give you hands-on experience in abstracting from case histories, posting to financial accounting record cards, and completing forms pertinent to the Medicaid program in your state. As an option, obtain Medicaid forms for your locale to use for your assignments.
- Turn to the Glossary at the end of this text for a further understanding of the key terms and key abbreviations used in this chapter.

8

TRICARE and Veterans' Health Care

Linda M. Smith

OBJECTIVES

After reading this chapter, you should be able to:

1. Discuss the history of TRICARE.
2. State who is eligible for TRICARE.
3. List the circumstances when a nonavailability statement is necessary.
4. Differentiate between authorized and nonauthorized providers.
5. Explain the benefits of the TRICARE Select government program.
6. State the TRICARE fiscal year.
7. State the managed care features of TRICARE Prime and discuss enrollment, Primary Care Managers, preauthorization, and payments.
8. Define individuals who may enroll in the TRICARE Prime Remote program and discuss enrollment, preauthorization, and payments.
9. Discuss the TRICARE Reserve Select, TRICARE Retired Reserve, and TRICARE Young Adult programs.
10. Explain TRICARE for Life benefits and those who are eligible individuals.
11. Name individuals eligible for TRICARE Plus and discuss enrollment, preauthorization, and payments.
12. Discuss the Supplemental Health Care Program, including enrollment and payments.
13. Discuss the TRICARE Hospice Program.
14. Identify individuals who are eligible for the Veterans Health Administration program (CHAMPVA) and discuss enrollments and preauthorization.
15. Describe how to process a claim for an individual who is covered by various types of TRICARE programs.
16. State the components of a TRICARE Summary Payment Voucher.
17. List the components of a Veterans Health Administration (CHAMPVA) Explanation of Benefits document.

KEY TERMS

active duty service member
allowable charge
authorized provider
beneficiary
catastrophic cap
catchment area
Civilian Health and Medical Program of the Department of Veterans Affairs
Civilian Health and Medical Program of the Uniformed Services
cooperative care
coordination of benefits
cost share
Defense Enrollment Eligibility Reporting System
Department of Veterans Affairs
emergency
health benefits advisor
health care finder
medically (or psychologically) necessary
Military Treatment Facility
network provider
nonavailability statement
nonparticipating provider
other health insurance
participating provider
partnership program
point-of-service option
preauthorization
Prime Service Area
primary care manager
regional contractor
service benefit program
service-connected injury
service retiree (military retiree)
sponsor
summary payment voucher
Supplemental Health Care Program
total, permanent service-connected disability
TRICARE
TRICARE Extra
TRICARE for Life
TRICARE Prime
TRICARE service center
TRICARE Select
TRICARE Standard
urgent care
veteran
Veterans Health Administration

KEY ABBREVIATIONS

ADSM	HCF	par	TMA
CHAMPUS	MHS	PCM	TPR
CHAMPVA	MTF	POS	TSC
COB	NAS	PSA	VA
DEERS	nonpar	SHCP	
HBA	OHI	TFL	

TRICARE

TRICARE is the health care program for active duty service members (ADSMs) of the United States military (Army, Navy, Air Force, Marines, Coast Guard) and their families. Retired military service members and their families and survivors of ADSMs are also eligible for TRICARE. TRICARE is a federally funded program that provides comprehensive health coverage to all its members including health plans, special programs, prescriptions and dental plans.

HISTORY OF TRICARE

The US Congress created Civilian Health and Medical Program of the Uniformed Services (CHAMPUS) in 1966 under Public Law 89-614. The purpose of the law was to assist individuals in the military who were finding it increasingly difficult to pay for the medical care required by their families In January 1994, TRICARE became the new title for CHAMPUS. The TRICARE program is managed and administered by the TRICARE Management Activity (TMA) office.

TRICARE is available worldwide and managed in separate regions. Previously, there were three US regions: Region West, Region North, and Region South. Effective January 1, 2018, these three US regions combined to become two. TRICARE North and South have combined to form TRICARE East and TRICARE West will remain the same (Fig. 8.1). Anywhere outside the United States is considered overseas, a separate region. Each area has their own regional contractor. A regional contractor is an insurance company under agreement with the federal government to handle claim processing within a particular state or country (Table 8.1).

Eligibility

An individual who qualifies for TRICARE is known as a beneficiary; the ADSM is called the sponsor. A person who is retired from a career in the armed forces is known as a service retiree (military retiree) and remains in a TRICARE program until age 65, at which time the individual becomes eligible for the Medicare program. If an individual served as an active duty military person for 4 to 6 years and gives up their military career and leaves, no further family benefits are provided.

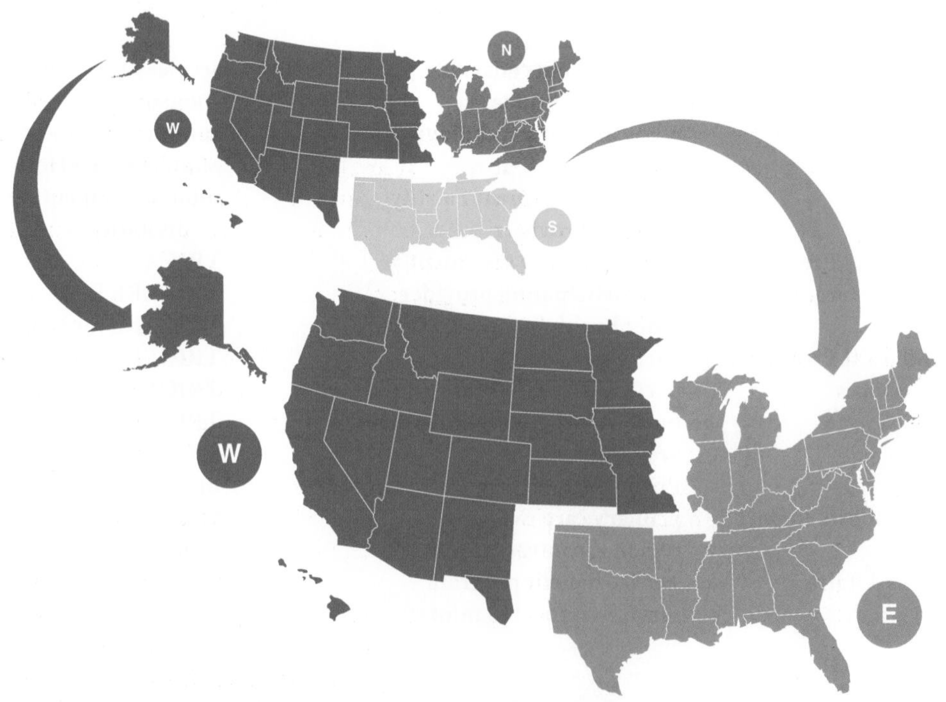

Fig. 8.1 Map of TRICARE effective January 2, 2018. TRICARE North and TRICARE South will combine to form TRICARE East. TRICARE West will remain unchanged. (From https://Tricare.mil/About/Regions.)

TABLE 8.1 Regional Contractors Effective January 1, 2018

Region	Regional Contractor
TRICARE West	Health Net Federal Services
TRICARE East	Humana Military

The following individuals are entitled to medical benefits under TRICARE:

- Active duty service members and their families
- National Guard/Reserve members and their families
- Retired service members and their families
- Surviving eligible family members of deceased, active, or retired service members
- Former spouses of active or retired service members who meet certain length-of-marriage rules and other requirements.
- Medal of Honor recipients and their families
- Others registered in the Defense Enrollment Eligibility Reporting System

Defense Enrollment Eligibility Reporting System

All TRICARE-eligible persons must be enrolled in the Defense Enrollment Eligibility Reporting System (DEERS) computerized database. Sponsors are automatically registered in DEERS; however, sponsors must register eligible family members. Only sponsors can add or remove family members.

TRICARE claims processors check DEERS before processing claims to verify beneficiary eligibility. A TRICARE beneficiary may check his or her status by contacting the nearest personnel office of any branch of the service or by calling the toll-free number of the DEERS center.

Nonavailability Statement

A nonavailability statement (NAS) is a certification from a military hospital stating that it cannot provide the care needed by the beneficiary. As of December 2003, this type of certification is no longer necessary for TRICARE and Veterans Health Administration beneficiaries for outpatient procedures or for those who wish to receive treatment as inpatients at a civilian hospital and who live within a catchment area surrounding a Military Treatment Facility (MTF). An MTF is a uniformed services hospital sometimes referred to as a *military hospital.* The only exception is that an NAS is still required for nonemergency inpatient mental health care services.

Catchment Area

The catchment area is a specific geographic region defined by zip codes and is based on an area of approximately 40 miles in radius surrounding each MTF in the United States. Individuals whose home address zip code falls outside the local military hospital's service area do not need an NAS before seeking civilian health care under TRICARE.

Identification Card

TRICARE patients are issued identification cards. Active duty uniformed service personnel are issued a common access card (CAC) to be used as standard identification. Military family members and retirees are issued a Uniformed Services Identification card to access health care benefits. Examples of the CAC and Uniformed Services ID card can be found on the TRICARE website. Essential information must be abstracted from the front and back of the card; therefore photocopy both sides to retain in the patient's health record.

Authorized Providers of Health Care

An authorized provider is a physician or other provider of care, a hospital or supplier approved by TRICARE to provide medical care and supplies. Providers must pass a credentialing process to be authorized by TRICARE.

Patients should verify that the health care organization or service provider they are seeking services from are authorized to treat TRICARE beneficiaries before receiving medical services. Regional TRICARE contractors will verify a provider's authorized status before they can pay for services. If the provider is not authorized, TRICARE cannot help with paying the bill. Beneficiaries who use nonauthorized providers may be responsible for their entire bill and there are no legal limits on the amounts these providers can bill beneficiaries.

A network provider is any TRICARE-authorized provider that has signed a contract with a regional TRICARE contractor. Network providers will file claims on behalf of the patient and will agree to accept the TRICARE-allowable charge as payment in full. The allowable charge is the maximum amount that TRICARE can pay a provider for a procedure or service. Patients are responsible for any deductibles or cost shares. By using a network provider, patients will pay less out-of-pocket and the provider will collect the rest of the amount directly from TRICARE.

Non-network providers are TRICARE-authorized civilian providers who have not established a contract with their regional TRICARE contractor. Non-network providers can determine whether they are participating or nonparticipating on a claim-by-claim basis.

- Participating providers (par) have signed a contractual agreement with TRICARE to give medical care to TRICARE beneficiaries. The provider agrees to accept assignment, agrees to accept the TRICARE-determined allowable charge as payment in full, and transmits claims to the regional contractor. The provider may bill the patient for their cost share, which is the portion of the allowable charges (20% to 25%) after the deductible has been met. Beneficiaries pay only a certain amount each year for the cost share and annual deductible. This amount is known as a catastrophic cap. After the cap is reached, TRICARE pays 100% of the allowable charges for the rest of the year. The cap does not apply to noncovered TRICARE services (Table 8.2).
- Nonparticipating providers (nonpar) do not agree to accept the TRICARE-allowable charge as payment in full. Nonparticipating providers may not bill the patient more than 115% of the allowable charge, which is referred to as the *limiting charge.* For example, if the TRICARE allowable charge for a procedure is $100, providers who decide not to participate in TRICARE may charge TRICARE patients no more than $115 for that procedure. The patient pays the deductible (20% or 25% of the charges determined to be

allowable) and any amount more than the allowable charge up to 115% when the physician or health care organization does not accept assignment (Fig. 8.2).

HEALTH PLANS

TRICARE offers several different health plans. Availability of the plans depend on the beneficiary's category and where they live. There are two primary TRICARE programs:

- TRICARE Select
- TRICARE Prime

TABLE 8.2 Catastrophic Cap

If Patient Is:	Catastrophic Cap
An active duty family	$1000 per family, per fiscal year
A family using TRICARE Reserve Select	$1000 per family, per fiscal year
All Others	$3000 per family per fiscal year

Catastrophic cap is the maximum amount paid by the patient each fiscal year. Cap amount depends on who the patient is. The TRICARE fiscal year begins October 1 and ends September 30.

Additional TRICARE programs include the following:

- TRICARE for Life
- TRICARE Reserve Select
- TRICARE Retired Reserve
- TRICARE Young Adult
- US Family Health Plan
- TRICARE Select Overseas

TRICARE Select

The **TRICARE Select** program is a new program that became effective January 1, 2018. TRICARE Select is a fee-for-service, self-managed, preferred provider network plan. Before January 1, 2018, TRICARE beneficiaries were offered the **TRICARE Standard**, **TRICARE Extra**, and TRICARE Standard Overseas programs. The TRICARE Select program replaced these three programs. Beneficiaries enrolled in TRICARE Select can choose any TRICARE authorized provider for services.

TRICARE Select is offered to the following:

- Active duty family members
- Retired service members and their families
- Family members of activated Guard/Reserve members

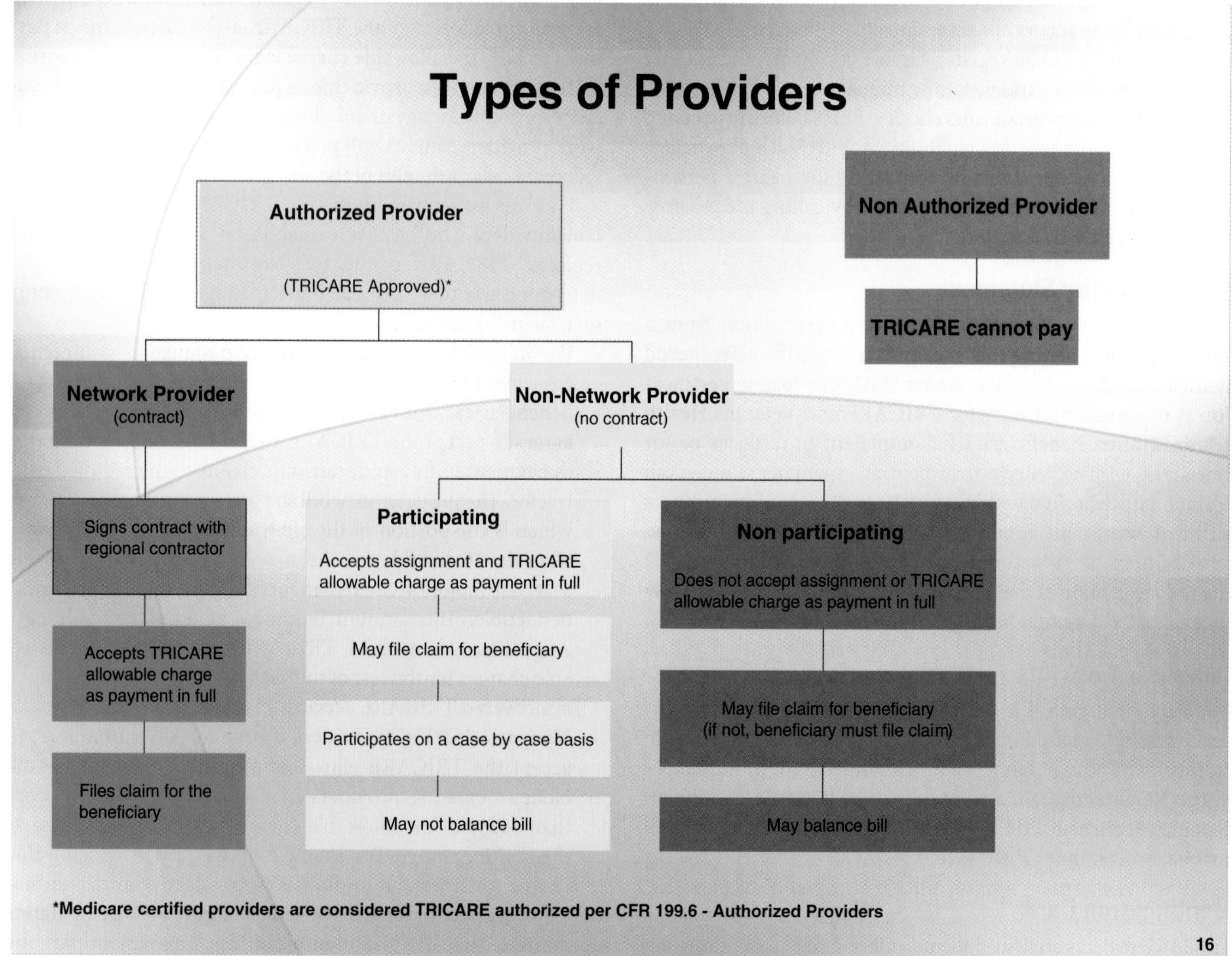

Fig. 8.2 Types of providers.

- Nonactivated Guard/Reserve members and their families who qualify for care under the Transitional Assistance Management Program (TAMP). TAMP is a premium-free transitional health care benefits after regular TRICARE benefits end.
- Retired Guard/Reserve members at age 60 and their families
- Survivors
- Medal of Honor recipients and their families
- Qualified former spouses

Enrollment

Those entitled to medical benefits under TRICARE are automatically enrolled in the TRICARE Select program. Beneficiaries who were previously using TRICARE Standard, Extra, or Standard Overseas programs were automatically enrolled in TRICARE Select.

Benefits

In the TRICARE Select program, beneficiaries may receive a wide range of civilian health care services with a significant portion of the cost paid by the federal government. Patients are not limited to using network providers and benefits include medical or psychological services or supplies that are considered appropriate care. Such services are generally accepted by qualified professionals to be reasonable and adequate for the diagnosis and treatment of illness, injury, pregnancy, and mental disorders or to be reasonable and adequate for well-baby care. These services are referred to as **medically (or psychologically) necessary.**

Beneficiaries also may receive urgent care and emergency care services. **Urgent care** is medically necessary treatment needed for an immediate illness or injury that would not result in further disability or death if not treated immediately. Treatment should not be delayed but should occur within 24 hours to avoid development of further complications. An **emergency** is a sudden and unexpected medical condition, or the worsening of a condition, that poses a threat to life, losing a limb, or sight and requires immediate treatment to alleviate suffering (for example, shortness of breath, chest pain, or drug overdose). Emergency care is usually obtained at a hospital emergency department.

TRICARE Select patients usually seek care from a military hospital near their home. The military physician may refer the patient to a civilian source if the service hospital that is managing the patient cannot provide a particular service or medical supplies. **Cooperative care** consists of services or supplies that may be cost-shared by TRICARE Select under certain conditions.

A **partnership program** is another option that allows TRICARE Select–eligible persons to receive inpatient or outpatient treatment from civilian providers of care in a military hospital or from uniformed services providers of care in civilian facilities. Whether a partnership program is instituted at a particular military hospital is up to the facility's commander, who makes the decision on the basis of economics.

In addition, there are times when there is no service hospital in the catchment area and a TRICARE Select beneficiary may seek care through a private physician's office or hospital. Delivery of care through the private physician is emphasized in this chapter.

Referrals and Preauthorization

Referrals are not required in the TRICARE Select program. However, some care may require preauthorization. **Preauthorization** is a requirement to obtain permission for a service or procedure before it is done to determine if the regional contractor considers it to be medically necessary.

When specialty care or hospitalization is necessary, the MTF must be used if services are available. If services are not available, the **health care finder (HCF)** can assist with the referral or preauthorization process. A TRICARE referral/authorization form is shown in Fig. 8.3. An HCF is a health care professional, usually a registered nurse, who helps the patient to work with his or her primary care physician (PCP) to locate a specialist or obtain a preauthorization for care. HCFs are found at a **TRICARE service center (TSC),** which is an office staffed by HCFs and beneficiary service representatives. All admissions, ambulatory surgical procedures, and other selected procedures require preauthorization. Certain types of health care services requiring prior approval from the TRICARE health contractor follow:

- Arthroscopy
- Breast mass or tumor removal
- Cardiac catheterization
- Cataract removal
- Cystoscopy
- Dental care
- Dilatation and curettage
- Durable medical equipment (DME) purchases
- Gastrointestinal endoscopy
- Gynecologic laparoscopy
- Hernia repairs
- Laparoscopic cholecystectomy
- Ligation or transection of fallopian tubes
- Magnetic resonance imaging (MRI)
- Mental health care
- Myringotomy or tympanostomy
- Neuroplasty
- Nose repair (rhinoplasty and septoplasty)
- Strabismus repair
- Tonsillectomy or adenoidectomy

TRICARE will only reimburse care received from authorized providers. For reduced cost, beneficiaries can use network providers.

Payment: Deductible and Copayment

TRICARE will pay authorized providers for covered services based on the allowable charge. TRICARE Select beneficiaries are subject to paying deductibles and copayments.

Patient Referral Authorization Form

TRICARE referrals should be submitted through www.humanamilitary.com (log on to Self-Service for Providers). If you do not have internet connection in your office, you may complete and submit this form by fax to 1-877-548-1547.

Humana. Government Business

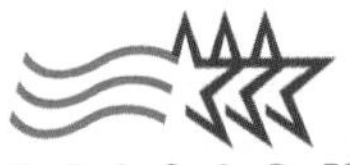

The Military Treatment Facility (MTF) in your area may have Right of First Refusal for this service.

TRICARE ID 9-11 Digits ☐☐☐☐☐☐☐☐☐☐☐ Patient Name ______

Patient DOB MM-DD-YYYY ☐☐-☐☐-☐☐☐☐ Patient Zip Code ☐☐☐☐☐-☐☐☐☐

Address ______ City ______ State ______

Other Health Insurance? ◯Yes ◯No Carrier ______ Phone ☐☐☐-☐☐☐-☐☐☐☐

Policy# ☐☐☐☐☐☐☐☐☐☐

Provider or Setting

☐ Physician's Office ☐ Allied Health Professional's Office ☐ Outpatient Facility ☐ Inpatient Facility

Date of Service (If known) MM-DD-YYYY ☐☐-☐☐-☐☐☐☐ Point of Contact ______

☐ Evaluate Only

☐ Evaluate and Treat

Ordering Provider ______ Phone ☐☐☐-☐☐☐-☐☐☐☐

Type of Service

☐ Office Visit List Specialty ______ Specialist Tax ID or NPI ______

☐ Surgical/Diagnostic Procedure ☐ Speech Therapy ☐ Hospice ☐ DME ☐ Other

☐ Observation ☐ Home Health ☐ PT/OT ☐ OP Behavioral Health

☐ Inpatient Admission: ☐ Acute Care ☐ Rehab ☐ SNF If inpatient, please provide a diagnosis code: ☐☐☐☐☐☐☐

Procedure or HCPC Code ☐☐☐☐☐ ☐☐☐☐☐ ☐☐☐☐☐ ☐☐☐☐☐ ☐☐☐☐☐

Facility ______ Tax ID or NPI ______ Address ______

City ______ State ______ Zip Code ☐☐☐☐☐-☐☐☐☐

Rendering Provider ______ Tax ID or NPI ______ Address ______

City ______ State ______ Zip Code ☐☐☐☐☐-☐☐☐☐

Presenting symptoms or reason for referral.

______

Pertinent history, findings and specials situations include known discharge needs if inpatient admission.

______

TP-2568.8 To assist with timely processing, please complete this form in its entirety. 08/15

Fig. 8.3 TRICARE Patient Referral Authorization Form. *ID*, Identification.

TRICARE Prime

TRICARE Prime is managed care, Health Maintenance Organization-style option available in Prime Service Areas that offers lower costs. Prime Service Areas (PSAs) are geographic areas that were created to ensure medical readiness of the active duty force by augmenting the capability and capacity of MTFs. Participation in TRICARE Prime is optional. Beneficiaries have the choice between TRICARE Prime or TRICARE Select. If the beneficiary elects to enroll in TRICARE Prime, the patient may no longer use the TRICARE Select program.

Primary Care Manager

On enrollment into the plan, the beneficiary has the option of choosing or being assigned a primary care manager (PCM). The PCM may be a civilian or military provider who provides the majority of patient care. The PCM is responsible for coordinating and managing the beneficiary's entire health care (except emergencies). The PCM may refer the beneficiary for additional services, when necessary, but specific referral and preauthorization requirements must be carried out. Referral patterns are evaluated to determine excessive or inappropriate referrals to specialists. A pattern of such referrals could result in termination of participation in TRICARE Prime. Enrolled beneficiaries may not use a non-network provider, except in emergencies or for pharmaceuticals, without a specific referral from an HCF.

Enrollment

An individual must complete an application and enroll for a minimum of 12 months to become a TRICARE Prime member. An annual enrollment fee is charged per person or family except for active duty families, who may enroll free. These members can use the local military and civilian provider network with necessary authorization.

Benefits

Covered services are the same as those for TRICARE Select patients plus there are additional preventive and primary care services. For example, periodic physical examinations are covered at no charge under TRICARE Prime but are not covered under TRICARE Select. Prime also covers certain immunizations and annual eye examinations for dependent children of retirees that are not a benefit under the Select plan. A dental plan is available for an additional monthly premium. An NAS is necessary only for nonemergency inpatient mental health care services if the beneficiary resides within the designated MTF catchment area.

Preauthorization

All admissions, ambulatory surgical procedures, and other selected procedures require preauthorization. Outpatient or ambulatory surgery must be on the approved procedure list before it is performed. The list is in the *TRICARE Handbook* available at www.tricare.mil.

The health benefits advisor (HBA) at the nearest military medical facility should be called to determine whether an NAS statement is necessary for the procedure before the surgery is scheduled in the approved facility. An HBA is a person at a military hospital or clinic who is there to help beneficiaries obtain medical care needed through the military and TRICARE. A point-of-service (POS) option is available if no authorization is obtained. This means that the individual can choose to get TRICARE-covered nonemergency services outside the Prime network of providers without a referral from the PCM and without authorization from the HCF.

Payments

Copayment. TRICARE Prime copayments for inpatient hospital services vary for active duty family members and for retirees and their family members and survivors. For outpatient services, copayments are the same for active duty family members and for retirees and their family members and survivors, but vary in amounts depending on the type of service received. Copayments should be collected at the time services are rendered.

TRICARE Prime Remote

TRICARE Prime Remote (TPR) is a health maintenance organization (HMO)–style managed plan that's available in remote areas in the United States. TPR can only be used if both the sponsor's home and work addresses are more than 50 miles or 1 hour's drive time from a military hospital or clinic.

TRICRE Prime Remote is available to ADSMs (including activated Guard/Reserve members) and certain family members. Retirees and their families can't enroll in TRICARE Prime Remote.

Beneficiaries are assigned a PCM who will provide most of the patient's care. Active duty and their family members pay no copay or cost share when seen by their PCM or referred specialist.

Identification Card

ADSMs must present their military identification card to receive care from providers. Photocopy the front and reverse sides of the card so that information is available for reference when completing the insurance claim form.

Benefits

TPR program benefits are similar to TRICARE Prime. Services may be received from an MTF when available or from any civilian provider. Primary routine care does not require prior authorization (for example, office visits, preventive health care). The HCF must be contacted to receive authorization for referrals, inpatient admissions, maternity, physical therapy, orthotics, hearing appliances, family planning (tubal ligation or vasectomy), outpatient and inpatient behavioral health services, and transplants. Table 8.3 provides a summary of the unique aspects of TPR.

Referral and Preauthorization

Routine primary care (for example, office visits, preventive health care) does not require prior authorization. The PCM must initiate all specialty referrals and coordinate requests through the HBA for certain outpatient services, all inpatient surgical or medical services, maternity services, physical therapy, orthotics, hearing appliances, family planning, transplants, and inpatient or outpatient behavioral health services. The HBA is a government employee who is responsible for helping all Military Health System (MHS) beneficiaries to obtain medical care.

TABLE 8.3 Summary of Unique Aspects of TRICARE Prime Remote Program and Supplemental Health Care Program

	TPR	SHCP
Plan description	TPR is a program for ADSMs who live and work more than 50 miles or 1 hour from an MTF. ADSMs must enroll.	SHCP is a program for • ADSMs • Inpatients at military treatment facilities who are not TRICARE eligible (e.g., eligible parents, parents-in-law) referred by an MTF to a civilian provider for care (usually for a specific test, procedure, or consultation) • Non–MTF-referred ADSMs (e.g., ROTC students, cadets/midshipmen, eligible foreign military)
Provider type	Any civilian provider	Any civilian provider
Beneficiary access to care	TPR ADSMs receive care from any civilian provider or from an MTF when available. Under TPR, ADSMs will have the same priority to care as other ADSMs at the MTF.	The beneficiary may receive services from any civilian provider in accordance with referral and preauthorization requirements (see later).
Beneficiary responsibility	TPR ADSMs have no annual deductible, cost shares, or copayments. The TPR ADSM must present his or her military ID card at the time care is received.	ADSMs and others eligible for SHCP referred to civilian providers have no copayment, deductible, or cost share. Beneficiary must present his or her military ID card at the time care is received.
POS	POS does not apply. If the ADSM receives care without a referral or preauthorization, the claim will be processed if it meets all other TRICARE requirements on a case-by-case basis.	The POS option does not apply.
Program benefits	Offers benefits similar to TRICARE Prime. Some benefits (including all behavioral health care) require preauthorization.	Offers benefits similar to TRICARE Prime. Some benefits (including all behavioral health care) require preauthorization.
Referrals and preauthorizations	*Primary care:* ADSMs can receive primary care from a provider without a referral or preauthorization. ADSMs with an assigned PCM will receive primary care from their PCM. ADSMs with no PCM can use any TRICARE-certified provider, or he or she can contact an HCF for assistance in locating a provider. *Specialty and inpatient care:* The SPOC will review requests for specialty and inpatient care.	*Specialty and inpatient care:* The MTF will review all requests for specialty and inpatient care for ADSMs. The MTF Commander or designee signature on a DD Form 2161 is required for designated patients referred for civilian care. Preauthorization for nonreferred ADSMs for specialty, inpatient, and behavioral health care must be obtained from the SPOC or the HCF.

ADSMs, Active duty service members; *HCF,* health care finder; *ID,* identification; *MTF,* Military Treatment Facility; *PCM,* primary care manager; *POS,* point-of-service; *ROTC,* Reserve Officers' Training Corps; *SHCP,* Supplemental Health Care Program; *SPOC,* service point of contact; *TPR,* TRICARE Prime Remote.

Payments

Those persons covered and receiving benefits under TPR are not responsible for any out-of-pocket costs. ADSM claims for services provided by a TRICARE network provider are paid at the same contracted rate as other TRICARE beneficiary claims.

TRICARE Prime Overseas

TRICARE Prime Overseas is an HMO-style managed plan available in overseas areas near military hospitals and clinics.

TRICARE Prime Overseas is only available to ADSMs (including activated Guard/Reserve members) and command sponsored family members. Retirees and their families cannot enroll in TRICARE Overseas Prime.

Beneficiaries are assigned a PCM who will provide most of the patient's care. Beneficiaries will be referred to specialists as needed. Active duty and their family members pay no copay or cost share when seen by the PCM or referred specialist.

TRICARE Prime Remote Overseas

TRICARE Prime Remote Overseas is an HMO-style managed plan available in designated remote overseas locations of Eurasia-Africa, Latin American, Canada, and the Pacific.

The program is only available to ADSMs, active Guard/Reserve members, and command sponsored family members. Retirees and their families cannot enroll in TRICARE Overseas Prime.

Beneficiaries are assigned a PCM who will provide most of the patient's care. Beneficiaries will be referred to specialists as needed. Active duty and their family members pay no copay or cost share when seen by the PCM or referred specialist.

US Family Health Plan

The US Family Health Plan is an additional TRICARE Prime option available through networks of community-based, not-for-profit health care systems in six areas of the United States. To enroll, beneficiaries must live in one of the designated US Family Health Plan service areas (Table 8.4). The beneficiary will receive all care (including prescription drug coverage) from a primary care provider that he or she selects from a network of private physicians and health care organizations affiliated with one of the not-for-profit health care systems (designated providers). Beneficiaries do not get care from military hospitals and clinics or from TRICARE network providers.

The plan is available to the following beneficiaries who live in a designated US Family Health Plan area:

- Active duty family members
- Retired service members and their families

TABLE 8.4 Designated US Family Health Plan Service Areas and Designated Providers

US Family Health Plan Service Area	Designated Provider
• Maryland • Washington, DC • Parts of Pennsylvania, Virginia, Delaware and West Virginia	• Johns Hopkins Medicine
• Maine • New Hampshire • Vermont • Upstate and Western New York • Northern Tier of Pennsylvania	• Martin's Point Health Care
• Massachusetts, including Cape Cod • Rhode Island • Northern Connecticut	• Brighton Marine Health Center
• New York City • Long Island • Southern Connecticut • New Jersey • Philadelphia and area suburbs	• St. Vincent Catholic Medical Centers
• Southeast Texas • Southwest Louisiana	• CHRISTUS Health
• Puget Sound area of Washington State	• Pacific Medical Centers (Pacmed Clinics)

- Family members of Activated National Guard/Reserve members
- Nonactivated National Guard/Reserve members and their families who qualify for care under the Transitional Assistance Management Program
- Retired National Guard/Reserve members at age 60 and their families
- Survivors
- Medal of Honor recipients and their families
- Qualified former spouses

TRICARE Reserve Select

TRICARE Reserve Select (TRS) is a premium-based health plan available worldwide for purchase by qualified members of the Selected Reserve and their families. TRS health care benefits are similar to TRICARE Select.

Members of the Selected Reserve and their families can participate in the program. Members can include the Army National Guard, Army Reserve, Navy Reserve, Marine Corps Reserve, Air National Guard, Air Force Reserve, and Coast Guard Reserve. Members must meet the following qualifications:

- Not on active duty orders
- Not covered under TAMP
- Not eligible for or enrolled in the Federal Employee Health Benefits (FEHB) program

TRICARE Retired Reserve

TRICARE Retired Reserve (TRR) is a premium-based health plan that qualified retired Reserve members and survivors may purchase. TRR offers coverage similar to TRICARE Select. Retired National Guard and Reserve personnel may qualify to purchase TRR coverage if they are members of the retired Reserve of a Reserve component of the armed forces, younger than age 60, and not eligible for or enrolled in the FEHB program. At age 60, TRR coverage is automatically terminated and the retiree becomes eligible for TRICARE Prime/Select and may enroll in one of those programs.

TRICARE Young Adult

The TRICARE Young Adult (TYA) program is a premium-based health care plan available for purchase by qualified dependents. TYA offers TRICARE Select or TRICARE Prime coverage based on the sponsor's status. It has medical and pharmacy benefits but no dental coverage. To join this program, the enrollee must be a dependent of an eligible uniformed service sponsor, unmarried, at least age 21, and not eligible to enroll in an employer-sponsored health plan. He or she can also enroll if under the age of 26 and enrolled in a full-time course of study at an approved institution of higher learning and if the sponsor provides at least 50% of his or her financial support.

TRICARE for Life

TRICARE for Life (TFL) is a Medicare-wraparound coverage for TRICARE-eligible beneficiaries who have Medicare Parts A and B. The program is available worldwide and offers additional TRICARE benefits as a supplementary payer to Medicare for uniformed service retirees, their spouses, and survivors age 65 or older. In overseas areas, TRICARE is the first payer.

When beneficiaries become entitled to receive Medicare Part A and Medicare Part B at age 65, they experience no break in TRICARE coverage. The only change is that TRICARE will pay secondary to Medicare beginning on the first day of the month in which they turn 65.

Enrollment

Enrollment is not required. Coverage is automatic if the beneficiary has Medicare Part A and B. The beneficiary must pay Medicare Part B premiums.

The DEERS notifies a beneficiary within 90 days before his or her 65th birthday that the medical benefits are about to change. It asks the beneficiary to contact the nearest Social Security Administration office about enrollment in Medicare. The beneficiary must elect to enroll in Medicare Part B to be eligible for TFL benefits. If the beneficiary is age 65 or older and has only Medicare Part A, he or she can enroll in Medicare Part B during the annual general enrollment period, which runs from January 1 to March 31 every year. Medicare Part B coverage then begins on July 1 of the year in which the beneficiary enrolls.

Identification Card

Beneficiaries who qualify for TFL do not need a TRICARE enrollment card. Beneficiaries will use the military identification as proof of coverage.

Benefits

Each beneficiary receives a matrix comparing Medicare benefits to TRICARE benefits. Certain benefits (for example, prescription medications) are covered under the TRICARE Senior Pharmacy Program. Pharmacy benefits provide Medicare-eligible retirees of the uniformed services, their family members, and survivors the same pharmacy benefit as retirees who are younger than age 65. This includes access to prescription drugs at MTFs and retail pharmacies and through the National Mail Order Pharmacy. Medicare Part B enrollment is not mandatory to receive TRICARE Senior Pharmacy Program benefits.

Referral and Preauthorization

There are no preauthorization requirements for the TFL program. All services and supplies must be benefits of the Medicare or TRICARE programs to be covered.

Payment

The following four scenarios represent most cases and explain the payment mechanism:

1. Services covered under both Medicare and TRICARE: Medicare pays first at the Medicare rate and the remaining amount is paid by TRICARE, which covers the beneficiary's cost share and deductible. No copayment, cost share, or deductible is paid by the TFL beneficiary.
2. Services covered under Medicare but not TRICARE: Medicare pays the Medicare rate and the beneficiary pays the Medicare cost share and deductible amounts. TRICARE pays nothing.
3. Services covered under TRICARE but not Medicare: TRICARE pays the allowed amount and Medicare pays nothing. The beneficiary is responsible for the TRICARE cost share and deductible amounts.
4. Services not payable by TRICARE or Medicare: The beneficiary is entirely responsible for the medical bill.

TRICARE Plus

TRICARE Plus is a primary care program offered at some military hospitals and clinics. The program allows patients to get primary care at their military hospital or clinic and pay nothing out of pocket. There is no enrollment fee, but beneficiaries must enroll to participate. Beneficiaries are limited to using only the hospital or clinic where they are enrolled. TRICARE Plus does not cover specialty care.

Enrollment

Beneficiaries are allowed to enroll in the program if they are TRICARE eligible and not enrolled in a TRICARE Prime Plan, the US Family Health Plan, or a civilian or Medicare HMO. Dependent parents or parent-in-laws are also eligible for enrollment; however, TRICARE will not pay for care by civilian providers, even if the military hospital or clinic refers the patient.

Identification Card

Persons enrolled in TRICARE Plus are issued an identification card and identified in the DEERS.

Benefits

The TRICARE Plus program is designed to function in the following ways:

- Enrollees use the MTF as their source of primary care; it is not a comprehensive health plan.
- Enrollees may seek care from a civilian provider but are discouraged from obtaining nonemergency primary care from sources outside the MTF.
- Enrollees are not guaranteed access to specialty providers at the MTF.
- Enrollees may not use their enrollment at another facility.
- The MTF's commander determines the enrollment capacity at each MTF.

Payment

TRICARE Plus offers the same benefits as TRICARE Prime when using an MTF. It has no effect on the enrollees' use or payment of civilian health care benefits.

Supplemental Health Care Program

The **Supplemental Health Care Program (SHCP)** provides coverage for civilian health care providers to ADSMs and non–TRICARE-eligible patients. This program is funded separately by the Department of Defense (DoD) and follows different rules than TRICARE. Authorizations and claims processing is administered by TRICARE regional contractors.

Referral and Preauthorization

The civilian or MTF provider must submit a request for TRICARE coverage. The request for services is reviewed against TRICARE coverage guidelines. The request is approved or denied based on the outcome of the review. The MTF initiates all referrals for ADSMs and other designated patients to civilian specialists when needed.

Enrollment

The SHCP covers both MTF-referred care and civilian health care provided to ADSMs. The MTF always administers routine care (for example, routine office visits, preventive health care).

Identification Card

ADSMs must present their military identification card to receive care from providers. The front and reverse sides of the card should be photocopied so that information is available for reference when the insurance claim form is completed.

Benefits

See Table 8.3 for a summary of the unique aspects of SHCP. SHCP enables beneficiaries to be referred to a civilian provider for care. The MTF must initiate all referrals to civilian providers. There is no deductible, copayment, or cost share for services provided by a civilian provider.

Payments

Those covered and receiving benefits under SHCP are not responsible for any out-of-pocket costs. ADSMs claims for services provided by a TRICARE network provider are paid at the same contracted rate as other TRICARE beneficiary claims.

TRICARE Hospice Program

The TRICARE hospice program is designed to provide care and comfort to patients who are terminally ill. Care may include physician service, nursing care, counseling, medical equipment, supplies, medications, medical social services, physical and occupational services, speech and language pathology, and hospice short-term acute patient care related to the terminal illness. To receive care under the hospice program, the patient, primary care physician, or an authorized family can initiate care, but the care will only start with a doctor's order. In addition, the patient must complete a statement electing to take hospice care and that must be filed with the regional contractor. Those persons who receive care under the hospice program cannot receive other services under the TRICARE basic programs (treatments aimed at a cure) unless the hospice care has been formally revoked. Many additional rules and limits apply to the hospice program; therefore the HBA at the nearest military medical facility should be called and a copy of the guidelines requested.

VETERANS HEALTH ADMINISTRATION PROGRAM

The Veterans Health Care Expansion Act of 1973 (PL93-82) authorized a CHAMPUS-like program called the **Civilian Health and Medical Program of the Department of Veterans Affairs (CHAMPVA)** (now known as the **Veterans Health Administration**), which became effective on September 1, 1973.

The Veterans Administration program is a comprehensive health care program for veterans. An individual is considered a **veteran** if they served in the active military service and were discharged or released under conditions other than dishonorable. The Veterans Health Administration is America's largest integrated health care system, providing care at 1243 health care facilities, including 170 medical centers and 1063 Veterans Health Administration outpatient clinics of varying complexity. The Veteran's Health Administration serves 9 million enrolled Veterans each year.

This program also serves the spouse and children of a veteran with a **total, permanent service-connected disability** or for the surviving spouse and children of a veteran who died as a result of a service-connected disability. Just as in the TRICARE program, individuals who qualify for the Veterans Health Administration (or CHAMPVA) program are known as *beneficiaries* and the veteran is called the *sponsor.*

Examples of total, permanent service-connected disabilities are an injury with paraplegic results, a bullet wound with neurologic damage, and loss of a limb. These contrast with a chronic or temporary service-connected disability, which might exist if an individual improperly lifts a heavy object while in the Navy, suffers a back injury with ongoing sporadic symptoms, and requires continuing medical care after leaving the service. Both scenarios involve service-connected disabilities; however, the first example illustrates a person permanently disabled, whereas the second illustrates what may be a chronic or temporary disability.

The Veterans Health Administration (or CHAMPVA) plan is not an insurance program in that it does not involve a contract guaranteeing the indemnification of an insured party against a specified loss in return for a premium paid. It is considered a **service benefit program**; therefore there are no premiums.

Eligibility

The following persons are eligible for Veterans Health Administration (or CHAMPVA) program benefits as long as they are not eligible for TRICARE Select and not eligible for Medicare Part A as a result of reaching age 65:

- The husband, wife, or unmarried child of a veteran with a total disability, permanent in nature, resulting from a **service-connected injury**
- The husband, wife, or unmarried child of a veteran who died as the result of a service-connected disability or who, at the time of death, had a total disability, permanent in nature, resulting from a service-connected injury
- The husband, wife, or unmarried child of an individual who died in the line of duty while in active service

Qualifying children are those unmarried and younger than age 18, regardless of whether dependent or not, or those up to age 23 who are enrolled in a course of instruction at an approved educational institution.

Determination of eligibility is the responsibility of the **Department of Veterans Affairs (VA),** the federal agency that oversees health care services to military veterans. The prospective beneficiary visits the nearest VA medical center and receives a VA identification card if eligible.

Enrollment

Dependents of veterans must have a Social Security number and must have contacted the local VA regional office to establish dependency on the veteran sponsor. The individual obtains and completes an application by telephone, fax, or downloading from the VA's website.

Identification Card

The Veterans Health Administration provides beneficiaries with an Veterans Health Identification Card (VHIC). The VHIC is for identification and check-in at VA appointments. It cannot be used as a credit card or an insurance card, and it does not authorize or pay for care at non-VA facilities. The VHIC will identify the member's name and a unique member identifier. This identifier is assigned by the DoD, and it is referred to as electronic data interchange personal identifier (EDIPI), which allows the VA to retrieve the Veteran's health record (Fig. 8.4).

Benefits

In general, the Veterans Health Administration (CHAMPVA) program covers most health care service and supplies that are medically necessary and psychologically necessary. The VA elected to provide these beneficiaries with benefits and cost-sharing plans similar to those received by dependents of retired and deceased uniformed services personnel under TRICARE Select. An overall picture of Veterans Health Administration benefits, which includes cost sharing (deductibles and copayments), can be seen in Table 8.5.

U.S. Department of Veterans Affairs
VA
Card Expires: 00/00/0000
VA HEALTHCARE ENROLLEE
SERVICE CONNECTED
MEDAL OF HONOR
PURPLE HEART
FORMER POW
U.S. AIR FORCE
Member ID
1234567890
Plan ID (80840)
1234 567 890
Member
JANE D SAMPLE
76637C003CP33293
877-222-VETS (8387)
Veterans Crisis Line: 1-800-273-8255
Foreign Medical Program 1-877-345-8179
In emergency call 911 or go to nearest medical facility
Report any emergency care to your VA treatment team within 72 hours.
For questions concerning non-health care VA benefits 1-800-827-1000
Property of the U.S. Government. If found, drop in nearest U.S. mail box.
POSTMASTER - RETURN TO:
Health Eligibility Center, 2957 Clairmont Road, Suite 200, Atlanta, GA 30329

Fig. 8.4 Veteran's health identification *(ID)* card.

TABLE 8.5 Veterans Health Administration (CHAMPVA) Service Benefits and Cost Share Summary Chart

	BENEFICIARY PAYS*		
Benefit (Covered Services)	**Deductible ($50/Individual or $100/Family per Calendar Year)**	**Cost Share†**	**Veterans Health Administration Pays**
Outpatient Services			
Ambulatory			
Family services	No	25% of allowable	75% of allowable
Professional services	Yes	25% of allowable	75% of allowable
Pharmacy services	Yes	25% of allowable	75% of allowable
DME			
Non-VA source	Yes	25% of allowable	75% of allowable
VA source	No	None	100% of VA cost
Inpatient Services			
Facility Services			
DRG based	No	Lesser of (1) per day amount × number of inpatient days, (2) 25% of billed amount, or (3) DRG rate	DRG rate less beneficiary cost share
Non-DRG based	No	25% of allowable	75% of allowable
Mental Health Services			
High-volume/RTC	No	Lesser of (1) per day amount × number of inpatient days or (2) 25% of billed amount	Balance of allowable *after* beneficiary cost share
Professional services	No		
No	25% of allowable	75% of allowable	

*Services received at VA health care facilities under the CHAMPVA In-house Treatment Initiative (CITI) program are exempt from beneficiary cost sharing.

†Under catastrophic protection plan (Cat Cap), annual beneficiary cost sharing is limited to $7500.

CHAMPVA, Civilian Health and Medical Program of the Department of Veterans Affairs; *DME*, durable medical equipment; *DRG*, diagnosis-related group; *RTC*, residential treatment center; *VA*, Department of Veterans Affairs.

Provider

The beneficiaries of the Veterans Health Administration (CHAMPVA) program have complete freedom of choice in selecting their civilian health care providers.

Preauthorization

Preauthorization is necessary for organ and bone marrow transplantation, hospice services, most mental health or substance abuse services, all dental care, and all DME with a purchase price or total rental cost of $300 or more. Preauthorization requests are made directly to Veterans Health Administration.

CLAIMS PROCEDURE

Regional Contractor

TRICARE Select is governed by the DoD. As such, it is not subject to those state regulatory bodies or agencies that control the insurance business. The DoD and the VA have agreed to use the Office of the Assistant Secretary of Defense and the TRICARE system of regional contractors and hospital contractors to receive, process, and pay Veterans Health Administration (CHAMPVA) claims, following the same procedures currently used for TRICARE Select.

A regional contractor, also known as a *fiscal intermediary (FI)* or *claims processor,* is an organization under contract to the government that handles insurance claims for care received under the TRICARE Select and Veterans Health Administration (CHAMPVA) programs.

TRICARE Select and Veterans Health Administration (CHAMPVA)

Remember to abstract the correct information from the front and back of the patient's identification card. Service members move often, and it is common for providers to have an old or temporary address on file. Always ask beneficiaries to update their information during each office visit. Refer to Chapter 14 and follow the TRICARE or Veterans Health Administration (CHAMPVA) instructions for completing the CMS-1500 claim form.

If the service provider is nonparticipating and does not accept assignment, the patient completes the top portion of the CMS-1500 claim form, attaches the service provider's itemized statement, and submits the claim. Alternatively, the patient may submit the claim on the white TRICARE claim DD Form 2642 Patient's Request for Medical Payment. Patients and providers of care for health services in foreign countries must use DD Form 2520. The Uniform Bill (UB-04) form is used for inpatient hospital billing.

Access to Health Records

Privacy Act of 1974

The Privacy Act of 1974 became effective on September 27, 1975, and established an individual's right to review his or her health records maintained by a federal medical care facility, such as a VA medical center or US Public Health Service facility, and to contest inaccuracies in such records. The Act directs each agency to make its own rules establishing access procedures. Agencies are allowed to adopt special procedures when it is believed that direct access could be harmful to a person. The Act requires that an individual from whom personal information is requested be informed of (1) the authority for the request, (2) the principal purpose of the information requested, (3) routine use of the information, and (4) the effect on an individual who does not provide the information.

Some federal agencies or federally funded institutions may be regulated by both the Privacy Act and Health Insurance Portability and Accountability Act (HIPAA) standards. Such entities are required to comply with both sets of regulations. Although HIPAA standards generally provide more restrictive regulations, entities are advised to revise their policies and procedures to comply with both HIPAA standards and the Privacy Act. Under certain situations, HIPAA standards are likely to prevail and require regulated entities to obtain individual authorization for some disclosures that they now make without authorization under the "routine uses" exception. HIPAA compliance managers should make a determination of the effects of the interplay between the federal laws and HIPAA standards, consult with legal counsel, and plan an entity's compliance initiatives accordingly.

Computer Matching and Privacy Protection Act of 1988

The Computer Matching and Privacy Protection Act of 1988 is specific to TRICARE. It permits the government to verify information by way of computer matches. By law, the provider must tell a TRICARE member that he or she is calling TRICARE, which is governed by the DoD, and only information to determine eligibility and to learn what services are covered is to be obtained.

Both these Acts are mentioned on the back of the CMS-1500 claim form. TRICARE patients must be made aware of this information by health care providers who treat them so that they are knowledgeable about routine use and disclosure of medical data. Providers must follow both HIPAA and the Computer Matching and Privacy Protection Act of 1988. Patients may make a Privacy Protection Act request in writing, in person, or by telephone. Individuals should call the facility to determine the required procedures to obtain access to the records and what to include in making a written request.

Time Limit

Effective January 1, 1993, claims must be filed within 1 year from the date a service is provided or (for inpatient care) within 1 year from the patient's date of discharge from the inpatient facility.

Claims Office

The insurance billing specialist must understand that when transmitting or sending the claim to TRICARE, the claim goes to the TRICARE claims office nearest to the residence of the military sponsor. For example, if the patient is a child who was treated in California, but the sponsor is an ADSM stationed in Florida, the claim should be transmitted to the TRICARE claims office in the South region and not a claims office in the West region. Refer to the TRICARE website to locate the address of the regional claims processor for submitting a TRICARE claim in each state.

The Veterans Health Administration (CHAMPVA) program is administered by the VA, Health Administration Center, PO Box 469063, Denver, CO 80206-9063.

TRICARE

The beneficiary does not file any claim forms under the TRICARE programs when using network providers. Providers must electronically transmit claims to TRICARE subcontractors for services given to beneficiaries. Referral and preauthorization numbers are required when applicable.

Time limit. For outpatient care, a claim must be transmitted to the state or region's TRICARE contractor within 1 year of the date that the provider rendered the service to the patient. For inpatient care, a claim must be received by the contractor within 1 year from the date that the patient was discharged from the facility. If a claim covers several different medical services or supplies that were provided at different times, the 1-year deadline applies to each item on the claim.

When a claim is electronically transmitted on time, but the contractor returns it for more information, the claim should be retransmitted with the requested information so that it is received by the contractor no later than 1 year after the medical services or supplies were provided or 90 days from the date the claim was returned to the provider, whichever is later.

A contractor may grant exemptions from the filing deadlines for several reasons. A request that includes a complete explanation of the circumstances of the late filing, all available documentation supporting the request, and the claim denied for late filing should be transmitted electronically to the contractor.

Claims office. See the TRICARE website to determine where claims should be transmitted electronically and to obtain more information about this program.

TRICARE Prime Remote and Supplemental Health Care Program

Outpatient professional services are electronically transmitted or paper claims may be submitted using a CMS-1500 claim form. Primary care service claims are processed and paid without a referral or preauthorization from a network or nonnetwork provider. A referral number provided by the HCF must be included for specialty medical or surgical care and for behavioral health counseling and therapy sessions. The POS option and NAS requirements do not apply to TPR and SHCP claims.

Time limit. A claim must be transmitted electronically within 1 year from the date on which a service is provided or (for inpatient care) within 1 year from the patient's date of discharge from the inpatient facility.

Claims office. Claims of ADSM patients should not be transmitted electronically to TRICARE. Claims for patients on active duty must be received by the specific branch of service (that is, Army, Navy, Air Force, or Marines). Claims are submitted to Palmetto Government Benefits Administrators (PGBAs) for processing and payment.

TRICARE for Life

If the beneficiary receives care from a civilian provider, the provider electronically transmits claims to Medicare. Medicare pays its portion and then electronically forwards the claim to TRICARE for the remaining amount. TRICARE sends its payment directly to the provider. The beneficiary receives a TRICARE **summary payment voucher** that indicates the amount paid to the provider.

TRICARE/Veterans Health Administration and Other Insurance

By law, TRICARE/Veterans Health Administration (CHAMPVA) is usually the second payer when a beneficiary is enrolled in **other health insurance (OHI).** OHI may be coverage through an employer, an association, a private insurer or any other nonmilitary organization. However, two exceptions are as follows:

- Bill TRICARE or Veterans Health Administration (CHAMPVA) claims first when the beneficiary is a recipient of the Medicaid program.
- Bill TRICARE or Veterans Health Administration (CHAMPVA) claims first when coverage is specifically designed to supplement TRICARE benefits (for example, Medigap [MG] health plan). When the patient has OHI that is primary, electronically transmit or send a paper claim using the CMS-1500 insurance claim form. Attach the explanation of benefits (EOB) from the primary carrier. If the patient is submitting his or her claim to the other insurance, take these steps:

1. Bill the other insurance carrier with the form it has supplied.
2. Bill TRICARE or Veterans Health Administration (CHAMPVA) by completing the top section of the CMS-1500 after receiving payment and an EOB from the other third-party payer. Submit the health care provider's itemized statement, which must contain the following:
   a. Provider's name
   b. Date on which the services or supplies were provided
   c. Description of each service or supply
   d. Place of treatment
   e. Number or frequency of each service
   f. Fee for each item of service or supply
   g. Procedure code number(s)
   h. Diagnostic code number(s) or description of condition(s) for which treatment is being received
   i. Billing statements showing only total charges, canceled checks, or cash register receipts (or similar-type receipts) are not acceptable as itemized statements.
   1. Attach a photocopy of the EOB from the other third-party payer.
   2. Electronically transmit the TRICARE or Veterans Health Administration (CHAMPVA) claim to the local contractor (claims processor/regional contractor).

Medicare and TRICARE

TRICARE is considered secondary to Medicare for persons younger than age 65 who have Medicare Part A as a result of a disability and who have enrolled in Medicare Part B. Those eligible for Medicare Part A are not covered by TRICARE unless disabled. Claims should be electronically transmitted to Medicare, then to TRICARE with a copy of the Medicare remittance advice. Services covered by TRICARE but not covered by Medicare (for example, prescriptions) are paid by TRICARE. Participating providers may obtain a TRICARE fee schedule by contacting their regional contractor.

Medicare and Veterans Health Administration (CHAMPVA)

The Veterans Health Administration (CHAMPVA) program is considered secondary to Medicare for persons younger than age 65 who are enrolled in Medicare Parts A and B. Claims first must be transmitted electronically to Medicare because the Veterans Health Administration (CHAMPVA) is a secondary payer.

Dual or Double Coverage

A claim must be filed if a patient has an additional private insurance policy that provides double coverage. Refusal by the beneficiary to claim benefits from OHI coverage results in a denial of TRICARE benefits. In double coverage situations, TRICARE pays the lower of the following:

- The amount of TRICARE-allowable charges remaining after the double coverage plan has paid its benefits
- The amount TRICARE would have paid as primary payer

When patients have double coverage and there are two insurance carriers providing benefits there must be coordination of benefits (COB). The insurance carriers must work together and coordinate the payment of their benefits so there is no duplication of payments between the primary and secondary insurance carrier.

Third-Party Liability

If the patient is in an automobile accident or receives an injury that may have third-party involvement, the following two options are available for reimbursement:

1. **Option 1:** TRICARE Form DD 2527 (Statement of Personal Injury, Possible Third-Party Liability) must be sent with the regular claim form for cost sharing of the civilian medical care. All five sections of the form should be completed by the patient. This form allows TRICARE to evaluate the circumstances of the accident and the possibility that the government may recover money for medical care from the person who injured the patient. If a CMS-1500 claim form is submitted without TRICARE Form DD 2527, a request is made to complete it. This form must be returned within 35 days of the request or the claims processor will deny the original and all related claims. Then the regional contractor submits a claim to the third party for reimbursement or files a lien for reimbursement with the liability insurance carrier, the liable party, or the attorneys or court involved.
2. **Option 2:** The provider can submit claims exclusively to the third-party liability carrier for reimbursement. Claims submitted with *International Classification of Diseases, Tenth Revision, Clinical Modification* (ICD-10-CM) diagnostic codes between S00 and T88 (Injuries, Poisonings, and External Causes) trigger the fact that there might be third-party litigation and the claims processor may request the completion of DD Form 2527.

Workers' Compensation

If a TRICARE or Veterans Health Administration (CHAMPVA) beneficiary is injured on the job or becomes ill because of his or her work, a workers' compensation claim must be filed with the compensation insurance carrier. TRICARE or the Veterans Health Administration (CHAMPVA) can be billed when all workers' compensation benefits have been exhausted.

In some situations, it must be decided whether a case that involves an accident or illness is work related and the claim might be transmitted electronically to the TRICARE or Veterans Health Administration (CHAMPVA) claims regional contractor. In those instances, the claims processor files a lien with the workers' compensation carrier for recovery when the case is settled.

AFTER CLAIM SUBMISSION

TRICARE Summary Payment Voucher

For each TRICARE claim, the claims processor issues a summary payment voucher (Fig. 8.5) that details the payment of the claim (that is, service or supplies received, allowable charges, amount billed, amount TRICARE paid, how much deductible has been paid, and patient's cost share amount). When the provider participates (accepts assignment), the voucher is sent to him or her with the check. The patient always receives a copy of the voucher, even if the provider receives payment directly from the regional contractor.

Veterans Health Administration (CHAMPVA) Explanation of Benefits Document

On completion of the processing of a claim, a payment check is generated and an EOB document is sent to the beneficiary (including the provider if the claim is filed by the provider). The EOB summarizes the action taken on the claim and contains information as illustrated and explained in Fig. 8.6.

Claims Inquiries and Appeals

Through the appeal process, providers may request reconsideration of a denial of certification for coverage or of the amount paid for a submitted claim. See Chapter 16 for inquiring about the status of a claim and to learn the procedures for how to file reviews and appeals.

Overview

Overview | Other Information | Reason Codes | Capital/Direct Medical Education |

How to Read Your TRICARE Summary Payment Voucher:

C(22)ndence Address:
...C
T...E CLAIMS ADMINISTRATOR
P.O. BOX XXXX
CAMDEN, SC 29020-XXXX

TRICARE SUMMARY PAYMENT VOUCHER

TRICARE

logo Prime Contractor Logo

Questions?
www.myTRICARE.com by PGBA
or 1-800-XXX-XXXX
or 1-800-XXX-XXXX

Date of Remittance: MAY 30, 2002 **Provider Number: 123456789010** **Check Number: 0010249692** **Page Number: 0001 of 0003**

Patient Account Number / Patient's Name	Rendering Provider or NABP	Sponsor's SSN	Dates of Service Begin	Dates of Service End	Procedure	# of Srvcs	Total Charges	Allowed Covered	Reason Code	Message Code	Patient's Cost Share	Patient's Copay	Patient's Deductible	TRICARE Payment
1234567890	1234567890	1234567890	042400	042400	99216	001	100.00	75.00	P7001	1	0.00	12.00	0.00	30.00
SMITH,	**TOTALS FOR CLAIM NUMBER 102331343-00-09**					>>>	100.00	75.00			0.00	12.00	0.00	30.00
JOHN	AMOUNT PAID BY PRIMARY INSURANCE					45.00					PATIENT'S RESPONSIBILITY			0.00
1234567890	1234567890	1234567890	020801	020801	87089	001	8.00	0.00	R5014		0.00	0.00	0.00	0.00
DOE,	**TOTALS FOR CLAIM NUMBER 102330178-00-00**					>>>	8.00	0.00			0.00	0.00	0.00	0.00
JOHN											PATIENT'S RESPONSIBILITY			0.00
1234567890	1234567890	1234567890	013001	013001	99125	001	60.00	52.00	P70001	1	10.40	0.00	0.00	41.60
SMITH,	**TOTALS FOR CLAIM NUMBER 102330223-00-00**					>>>	60.00	52.00			10.40	0.00	0.00	41.60
JANE											PATIENT'S RESPONSIBILITY			10.40

Example Only

Total Charges	Allowed Covered Charges	Cost Share	CoPay	Deductible	TRICARE Payment
168.00	127.00	10.40	12.00	0.00	71.60

TRICARE Payment	71.60
Interest	22.68
Federal Tax Withheld	-10.50
Offset	-20.00
Check Amount	**63.78**

CHECKS NOT ISSUED FOR AMOUNTS OF $.99 OR LESS

1. Correspondence address for PGBA, LLC, your region's TRICARE Claims Administrator.
2. The name and logo of the Prime contractor, the managed care support contractor for your TRICARE region.
3. The toll-free phone number/Web address for PGBA, your TRICARE Claims Administrator.
4. The date PGBA prepared this TRICARE payment voucher.
5. Social Security Number (SSN) or TIN of the provider who performed the services.
6. Number of the check issued as payment for the claim(s).
7. Number of this page followed by the total number of pages.
8. The patient's account number assigned by the provider's office and the patient's name.
9. SSN or TIN of the provider who performed the services or the provider's National Association of Boards of Pharmacy number.
10. The SSN of the military service member (active duty, retired or deceased).
11. Beginning and ending dates the services were performed.
12. CPT4 procedure code(s) or HCPCS equipment code(s) that identify the service(s) the provider performed.
13. The number of services the provider performed.
14. Total amount the provider billed for the services.
15. Amount TRICARE approves for the services.
16. This code corresponds to an explanation on the last page of how this claim was paid.
17. This code corresponds to a message on the last page that explains more about your claims payment.
18. Amounts subtracted from the total payment that are the patient's responsibility to pay.
19. Amount TRICARE has paid for the billed services.
20. If the claim was paid as DRG, the Diagnosis Related Group number would appear.
21. Total amounts for the claim and the amount other health insurance paid.
22. The amount the patient must pay the provider, including cost-shares, copayments, deductibles and non-covered charges.

Fig. 8.5 TRICARE summary payment voucher.

How to Read a CHAMPVA Explanation of Benefits

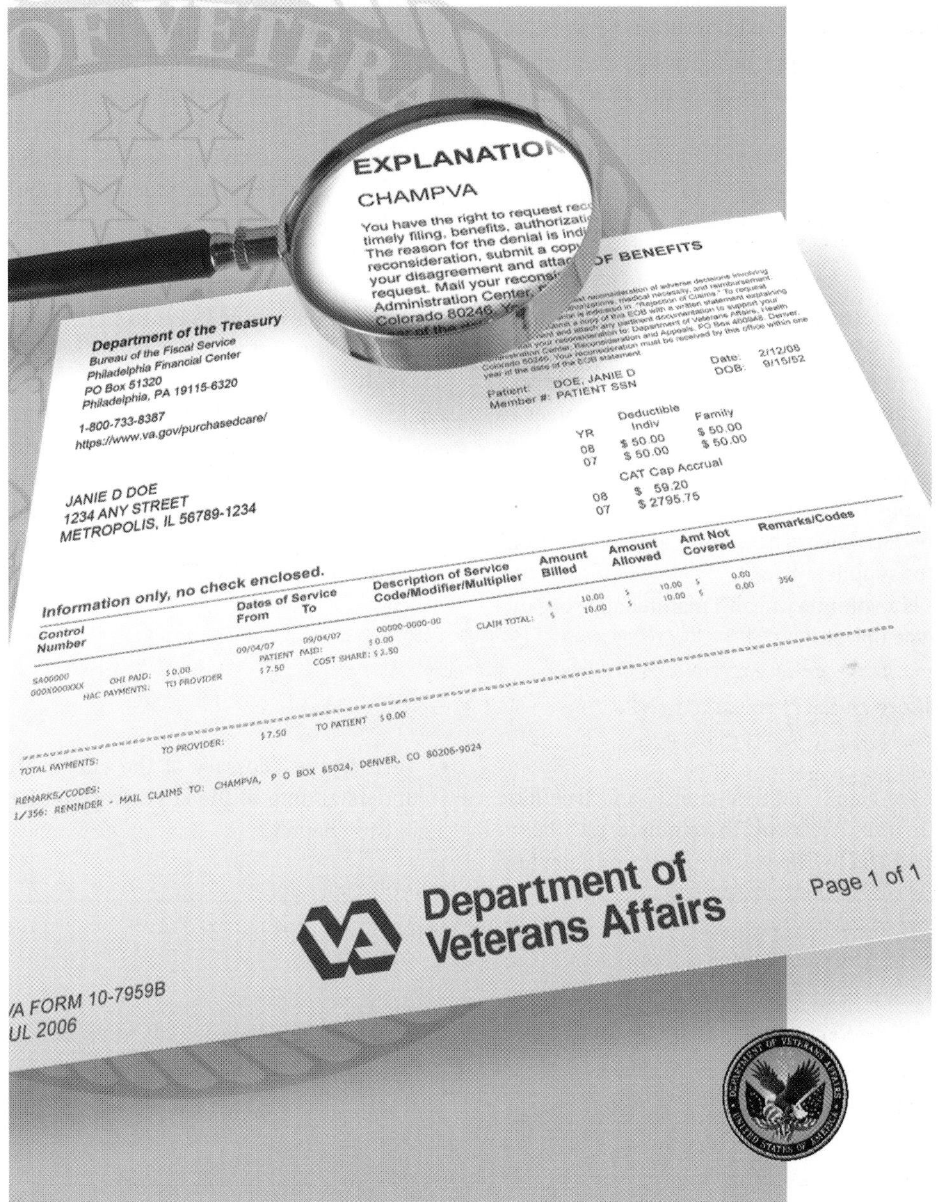

Fig. 8.6 Veterans Health Administration (Civilian Health and Medical Program of the Department of Veterans Affairs [CHAMPVA]) explanation of benefits document.

KEY POINTS

This is a brief chapter review, or summary, of the key issues presented. To further enhance your knowledge of the technical subject matter, review the key terms and key abbreviations for this chapter by locating the meaning for each in the Glossary at the end of this book, which appears in a section before the Index.

1. TRICARE is a health care program offered to spouses and dependents of service personnel with uniform benefits and fees implemented nationwide by the federal government. It also covers retirees, reservists on active duty after 30 days, widows, and widowers.
2. An electronic database called Defense Enrollment Eligibility Reporting System (DEERS) is used to verify beneficiary eligibility for those individuals in the TRICARE programs.
3. The TRICARE fiscal year begins October 1 and ends September 30.
4. There are certain referral and preauthorization requirements for TRICARE Select patients.
5. If the health care provider agrees to accept assignment in a TRICARE Select case, the participating provider agrees to accept the TRICARE-determined allowable charge as payment in full. The provider may bill the patient for his or her cost share or coinsurance (20% to 25% of the allowable charge after the deductible has been met) and for any noncovered services or supplies.
6. TRICARE Prime is a voluntary health maintenance organization (HMO)–type option.
7. TRICARE for Life (TFL) is a health care program that offers additional TRICARE benefits as a supplementary payer to Medicare for uniformed service retirees, their spouses and survivors age 65 or older, and certain former spouses.
8. TRICARE Prime Remote (TPR) is a program designed for active duty service members who work and live more than 50 miles or 1 hour from military treatment facilities (military hospitals and clinics).
9. The Veterans Health Administration (CHAMPVA) program is a service benefit program similar to TRICARE and is for veterans with total, permanent service-connected disabilities or surviving spouses and dependents of veterans who died of service-connected disabilities.
10. TRICARE and Veterans Health Administration (CHAMPVA) claims must be billed on the CMS-1500 claim form and submitted to the regional contractor for processing within 1 year from the date a service is provided or (for inpatient care) within 1 year from the patient's date of discharge from a facility.
11. The Computer Matching and Privacy Protection Act of 1988 permits the government to verify TRICARE patients' information by way of computer matches.
12. For each TRICARE claim, the claims processor issues a summary payment voucher that details the payment of the claim to the provider and sends a copy to the patient.

STUDENT ASSIGNMENT

- Study Chapter 8.
- Answer the fill-in-the-blank, multiple-choice, and true/false review questions in the *Workbook* to reinforce the theory learned in this chapter and to help you prepare for a future test.
- Turn to the Glossary at the end of this text for a further understanding of the key terms and key abbreviations used in this chapter.

9

Workers' Compensation

Linda M. Smith

OBJECTIVES

After reading this chapter, you should be able to:

1. Define key terms.
2. Discuss the history of workers' compensation, including statutes and reform.
3. State the purposes of workers' compensation laws.
4. Discuss workers' compensation program funding and the ways that premiums may be purchased by an employer.
5. Define and discuss *second-injury fund.*
6. Specify who is eligible for insurance coverage under federal workers' compensation laws.
7. Name persons entitled to be insured under state workers' compensation laws.
8. Determine the waiting period in each state before benefits begin.
9. Describe the types of compensation benefits.
10. Define *nondisability, temporary disability,* and *permanent disability claims.*
11. List signs of fraud and abuse involving employees, employers, insurers, medical providers, and lawyers.
12. State when to report fraud or abuse involving a workers' compensation claim.
13. Explain two ways in which depositions are used.
14. Explain the advantages of filing a lien.
15. Define and discuss third-party subrogation.
16. Describe workers' compensation health and financial record keeping in a medical practice.
17. Explain the procedure of completing the doctor's first report of occupational injury or illness.
18. Name the contents of a progress or supplemental medical report.
19. Complete workers' compensation forms properly and discuss fee schedules.
20. Discuss electronic claims submission and explain how to handle out-of-state claims.
21. Describe actions to take in following up on delinquent workers' compensation claims.

KEY TERMS

accident
adjudication
claims examiner
conversion factor
compromise and release
deposition
ergonomic
extraterritorial
Federal Employees' Compensation Act
injury
insurance adjuster
lien
medical service order
nondisability claim
occupational illness or disease
Occupational Safety and Health Administration
Office of Workers' Compensation Programs
permanent and stationary
permanent disability
petition
reexamination report
relative value scale
second-injury fund
sequelae
self-insure
state-run program
sub rosa films
subsequent-injury fund
temporary disability
third-party liability
third-party subrogation
waiting period
work hardening
Workers' Compensation Appeals Board
workers' compensation insurance

KEY ABBREVIATIONS

AME
C and R
ERISA
FECA
IME
LHWCA
ND
OSHA
OWCP
P and S
PD
QME
ROM
SIF
TD
WCAB
WP

Under state and federal workers' compensation laws, employers are required to purchase insurance that provides benefits to employees who suffer work-related injuries and illnesses. **Workers' compensation insurance** pays for medical services and wage replacement to employees injured in the course of employment or who have developed a work-related illness. If an employee dies, workers' compensation can cover funeral costs and benefits to the worker's family. Workers' compensation laws also protect employers from lawsuits by injured employees.

HISTORY

Before the establishment of a workers' compensation program in the United States, the employer was responsible for an employee's work-related medical bills or the employee paid for their own medical expenses. Employees are individuals employed by another, generally for wages, in exchange for labor or services. Originally the worker had to prove legally that injury was caused by negligence on the part of the employer. By the close of the nineteenth century, the number of accidents had increased and legal processes were uncertain; therefore federal and state legal provisions were required. In the early 1900s, employers' liability laws were adopted by many states, but there was still a great need for improvement. In 1911 the first workers' compensation laws that allowed injured employees to receive medical care without first taking employers to court were enacted. All states currently have workers' compensation laws.

Workers' compensation insurance is the most important coverage written to insure work-related injuries and illnesses. Previously this form of insurance was known as "workmens' compensation." The term *workmen* was changed to *workers* for a more generic title and to avoid sexual bias in language.

Workers' Compensation Statutes

There are two kinds of statutes under workers' compensation: federal compensation laws and state compensation laws. Federal laws apply to miners, maritime workers, and those who work for the government; they do not apply to state and private business employees. State compensation laws apply to employers and employees within each state. State laws vary from state to state.

The workers' compensation statutes relieve the employer of liability for injury received or illness contracted by an employee in a work situation, except in gross negligence cases. They also enable the employee to be more easily and quickly compensated for loss of wages and medical expenses. Most workers recover from their job injuries, but some continue to have problems. If the treating provider determines that the patient will never recover completely or will always be limited in the work they can do, this is considered a **permanent disability (PD)**. The workers' compensation laws assist the patient who is permanently disabled to receive disability income benefits without an extended delay.

Workers' Compensation Reform

By 1994, dysfunctional workers' compensation systems were costing companies more than $65 billion annually in many US cities. Some employers began moving their businesses to states requiring lower premiums. Other companies closed their doors because of the high cost of workers' compensation coverage. Widespread legal and medical corruption had evolved throughout the system in the form of record-high medical treatment and legal expenses. Reforms of the compensation of health care workers became necessary because of these problems. Reform laws have been introduced in a number of states that deal with the following issues:

- Antifraud legislation and increased penalties for workers' compensation fraud
    - Antireferral provisions (for example, restrictions of physicians referring patients for diagnostic studies to sites where the physician has a financial interest).
    - Proof of the medical necessity for treatment (or tests) as well as appropriate documentation. If guidelines are not adhered to, the carrier may refuse to pay the entire fee.
- Preauthorization for major operations and expensive tests
- Caps on vocational rehabilitation
- Use of a disabled worker in another division of the company where he or she was employed so that the worker may be gainfully employed while not using the injured part of the body
- Increase in occupational safety measures
- Employers offering a variety of managed care plans from which employees can choose, with some of these restricting their choice of provider
- Development of fee schedules specifically for workers' compensation claims
- Medical bill review to identify duplicate claims and billing errors
- Use of mediators instead of lawyers to reach agreement between employers and the injured employee
- Prosecution of health care organizations, physicians, lawyers, and employees who abuse the system

Although the system is far from perfect or complete, much progress has been made toward reducing high costs by trimming reimbursement for medical services and minimizing abuses of the system.

WORKERS' COMPENSATION LAWS AND INSURANCE

Purposes of Workers' Compensation Laws

Workers' compensation laws have been developed for a variety of reasons and accomplish much, including the following:

1. Provide the best available medical care necessary to ensure a prompt return to work of any injured or ill employee as well as achieving maximum recovery.
2. Provide income to the injured or ill worker or to his or her dependents, regardless of fault.
3. Provide a single remedy and reduce court delays, costs, and workloads arising out of personal injury litigation.
4. Relieve public and private charities of financial drains resulting from uncompensated work-related injuries and illnesses.
5. Eliminate payment of fees to attorneys and witnesses as well as time-consuming trials and appeals.

6. Encourage maximum employer interest in safety and rehabilitation through an appropriate experience-rating mechanism.
7. Promote the study of causes of accidents and reduce preventable accidents and human suffering rather than concealing fault.

Program Funding

Although workers' compensation systems vary from state to state, all workers' compensation benefits are paid for by the employer in some manner. There are typically three ways that workers' compensation premiums may be purchased by an employer:

- In most states, employers may purchase workers' compensation through a state-run program or insurance fund. The state's department of labor or industrial relations typically administer the program.
- Some states will allow employers to purchase workers' compensation insurance from private insurance companies such as Liberty Mutual, Chartis, and others.
- Employers who are large enough may be able to self-insure.

Self-Insurance

A large employer with sufficient capital can save money by self-insuring employees for work-related injuries and illnesses. The self-insuring employer does not pay insurance premiums. Instead the employer sets aside a state-mandated percentage of funding to cover medical expenses, wage compensation, death benefits and other benefits related to work injuries or illnesses. Employers who self-insure may also purchase a large deductible insurance policy for catastrophic problems. Benefits are variable from plan to plan and precertification for certain services may be required. Self-insured employers are governed by the Employee Retirement Income Security Act (ERISA). This federal law sets minimum requirements for group health plans and ensures that injured employees are taken care of in a fair manner. ERISA provides a safety net for injured workers by making sure their needs are met. Sometimes a self-insured plan may have stop-loss or reinsurance that becomes active on large claims or a set dollar limit per policy year or employee, depending on how it is structured. Such provisions give the insurer an excuse to delay claims until the reinsurer decides to fund the claim. In such cases it may be necessary to become aggressive and ask for the name, address, and telephone number of the reinsurer to learn the claim status. Prompt processing and payment should be demanded because delaying claims is a violation of federal laws and ERISA regulations.

A form of self-insurance designed to serve smaller or midsize companies is known as *captive insurance*. Captive insurance is owned by its policyholders. This is best for companies that have good safety records and those willing to implement worker safety programs to keep claims to a minimum. Members of captive self-insurance programs may hire an outside firm to process claims and purchase extra insurance for major claims. They share overhead expenses and investment income if any remains after paying expenses and claims.

Managed Care

Increasing numbers of employers are seeking managed care contracts with preferred provider organizations (PPOs) and health maintenance organizations (HMOs) to insure their workers against work-related accidents and illnesses. Some states have adopted laws authorizing managed care programs. Managed care contracts are not uniform and may limit the choice of providers, use fee schedule–based payments, require precertification for certain procedures, implement hospital and medical bill review, and incorporate utilization review of medical services.

Second-Injury Fund (Subsequent-Injury Fund)

The second-injury fund, also known as the subsequent-injury fund (SIF), was established to meet problems arising when an employee has a preexisting injury or condition and is subsequently injured at work. The preexisting injury combines with the second injury to produce disability that is greater than that caused by the latter alone.

Two functions of the fund are (1) to encourage hiring of the physically disabled and (2) to allocate more equitably the costs of providing benefits to such employees. Second-injury employers pay compensation related primarily to the disability caused by the second injury, even though the employee receives benefits relating to the combined disability. The difference is made up from the SIF.

SCENARIO: SECOND-INJURY FUND

Bob Evans lost his left thumb while operating machinery. Then, 2 years later, Bob lost his left index finger in a second work-related accident. A question could arise of whether the second injury added to a preexisting condition or was related to the prior injury. This case illustrates that the existence of the former injury or disability substantially increased (added to) the disability caused by the latter injury. The employer would pay compensation related to the second injury and funds would come from a second-injury fund to pay for the difference between the first and second injuries.

ELIGIBILITY

Individuals are entitled to workers' compensation insurance coverage if they are injured on the job or become ill or develop a disorder as a result of their work. Workers' compensation insurance also covers loss as a result of work-related injury or illness resulting in death. It is not always clear whether an injury that seems related to the job is actually covered under workers' compensation eligibility rules. For an injury to be considered work related, the individual must be injured while working within the scope of his or her job description or there must be a clear connection between the illness and the individual's employment. For example:

- An individual who amputates a finger while operating a drill press at work is considered a work-related injury.
- The posttraumatic stress disorder that a firefighter develops as a result of on-the-job experiences is considered work related.

- An employee who breaks his leg during an official company retreat at a ski resort would have an injury considered to be work related.
- An injury that occurs during the morning commute to work is *not* considered work related.

An independent contractor, who is not actually an employee, is not covered by the company he or she is contracted with.

Work-Related Accident

An **accident** is an unplanned and unexpected happening traceable to a definite time and place and causing **injury** (damage or loss).

Workers' compensation accidents do not necessarily occur at the customary work site. For example, an individual may be asked to obtain cash for the petty cash reserve during the lunch hour. He or she may misstep off the curb while walking to the bank and suffer a fractured ankle. This person is considered to be working, although not at the customary work site, and the injury is covered under workers' compensation insurance.

Occupational Illness

Occupational illness or disease is any abnormal condition or disorder caused by exposure to environmental factors associated with employment, including acute and chronic illnesses or diseases that may be caused by inhalation, absorption, ingestion, or direct contact. Occupational diseases usually become apparent soon after exposure. However, some diseases may be latent for a considerable amount of time. Therefore some states have extended periods during which claims may be filed for certain slowly developing occupational diseases. These diseases include silicosis, asbestosis, pneumoconiosis, berylliosis, anthracosilicosis, radiation disability, loss of hearing, cumulative trauma, and repetitive motion illnesses (for example, carpal tunnel syndrome).

COVERAGE

Federal Laws

Employees who work for federal agencies are covered by a number of federal workers' compensation laws. These programs are provided through an exclusive funding system and are administered through the **Office of Workers' Compensation Programs (OWCP)**. The mission of the OWCP is to protect the interests of workers who are injured or become ill on the job, their families, and their employees by making timely, appropriate, and accurate decisions on claims, providing prompt payment of benefits, and helping injured workers return to gainful work as early as is feasible.

- *Federal Coal Mine Health and Safety Act.* This Act, also referred to as the *Black Lung Benefits Act,* became effective on May 7, 1941. The Act provides compensation to coal miners who are totally disabled by pneumoconiosis arising out of coal mine employment and to survivors of coal miners whose deaths are attributable to the disease. The Act also provides eligible miners with medical coverage for the treatment of lung diseases related to pneumoconiosis. The Division of Coal Mine Workers' Compensation (DWMWC) administers claims filed under the Black Lung Benefits Act.
- *Federal Employees' Compensation Act.* The **Federal Employees' Compensation Act (FECA)** was instituted on May 30, 1908. The Act provides benefits for on-the-job injuries and occupational illnesses to any federal employee throughout the world. Federal employees include executive, legislative, and judicial branch employees; civilian defense workers; medical workers in veterans' hospitals; and employees of the US Postal Service.
- *Longshore and Harbor Workers' Compensation Act (**LHWCA**).* This Act became effective on March 4, 1927, and provides benefits for private or public employees engaged in maritime work nationwide. This includes occupations such as longshore workers, ship repairers, shipbuilders or ship breakers, and harbor construction workers. The injury must occur on the navigable waters of the United States or in the adjoin areas, including piers, docks, terminals, wharves, and areas used in loading and unloading vessels.
- *Energy Employees Occupational Illness Compensation Program Act (EEOICPA).* The EEOICPA became effective on July 31, 2001. This program provides compensation to current or former employees, or their survivors, of the Department of Energy (DOE), its predecessor agencies, and contractors and subcontractors who were diagnosed with diseases resulting from an exposure to radiation, beryllium, or silica while employed at covered facilities.
- An additional provision of the EEOICPA, enacted October 28, 2004, compensates DOE contractor and subcontractor employees, eligible survivors of such employees, and uranium miners, millers, and ore transporters, as defined by the Radiation Exposure Compensation Act (RECA), for any occupational illnesses that are causally linked to toxic exposures in the DOE or mining work environment. The OWCP oversees administration of claims for this program.

State Laws

State compensation laws cover those workers not protected by the previously mentioned federal statutes. Federal law mandates that states set up laws to meet minimum requirements. If an employer does not purchase workers' compensation insurance from a private insurance company, the employer must self-insure and have enough cash in reserve to cover the cost of medical care for all workers who suffer work-related injuries. An employer may be reluctant to file a workers' compensation report with the state in some instances, preferring to pay medical expenses out of pocket rather than have premium rates increase. It is illegal for an employer to fail to report a work-related accident when reporting is required by state law, and some states consider it a misdemeanor. Different penalties can be imposed, depending on state law, such as imprisonment or assessment of fines of $50 to $2500 or more.

Statutes require that employers have employers' liability insurance in addition to workers' compensation protection. The difference between workers' compensation insurance and employers' liability insurance is that the latter is coverage that protects against claims arising out of bodily injury to others (nonemployees) or damage to their property when someone is on business premises. It is not considered insurance coverage for someone who is working at a business site.

Workers' compensation requirements vary by state, by industry, and even by size and structure of businesses and payrolls (Table 9.1). State compensation laws are compulsory or elective, which may be defined as follows:

1. **Compulsory Law.** Each employer is required to accept its provisions and provide for specified benefits. Failure to carry compulsory workers' compensation insurance can face severe fines, a heavy lawsuit, or even criminal charges.
2. **Elective Law.** The employer may accept or reject the law. If the statute of the law is rejected, the employer loses the three common-law defenses, which are the following:
   a. Assumption of risk
   b. Negligence of fellow employees
   c. Contributory negligence

Minors

Every state requires children who are injured on the job to be entitled to the same workers compensation benefits as other injured workers. However, most states provide additional workers' compensation protection over and above the standard workers' compensation benefits paid to adults. For example, in some states, if a minor is injured on the job and is determined to be permanently disabled, the wage loss benefits may be calculated at a level higher than an adult worker to produce the maximum compensation rate.

Interstate Laws

Questions may arise as to which state's law determines payment of compensation benefits if a worker's occupation takes him or her into another state (for example, truck drivers). Most compensation laws are **extraterritorial,** which means they are effective outside the state, by either specific provisions or court decisions. When billing, follow the rules and fee schedule of the state in which the workers' compensation claim was originally filed. This may or may not be the same as the patient's current state of residence. The only exception is workers' compensation for federal employees, which has nationwide rules. For railroad workers, most states abide by nationwide rules, but some states have their own.

TABLE 9.1 Example of State Compensation Laws (Compulsory vs. Elective)

State	Law	Exceptions
Alabama	Compulsory for employers of 5 or more	Elective for partners, corporate affairs, and sole proprietors
Connecticut	Compulsory	Elective to officers and partners
Massachusetts	Compulsory	No exceptions
New York	Compulsory	Elective to partners, officers, self-employed
South Dakota	Compulsory	Elective to farm labor, employer
Texas	Not Compulsory	Elective
Vermont	Compulsory	Elective for officers, partners, sole proprietors

LLC, Limited liability corporation.

Volunteer Workers

Volunteers are not paid employees; therefore they are not typically covered under workers' compensation in most states. Instead the volunteer is more likely to be covered under the company's general liability insurance. Each state handles workers' compensation for volunteers differently. Therefore each state's law should be reviewed to determine whether a volunteer qualifies for workers compensation benefits. Several states have laws to compensate civil defense and other volunteer workers, such as firefighters who are injured in the line of duty.

Agricultural Workers

In some states there are workers' compensation exemptions for employers of agricultural or farm workers. This exemption is based on the historical concern that a small farming operation may not have the financial means to maintain the necessary records, insurance, and accounting to properly comply with the workers' compensation system. State exemptions vary widely and may be affected by the number of employees on the payroll, the average payroll wages, seasonal labor, or employment of family members. Each state's law should be reviewed to determine if agricultural workers qualify for workers compensation benefits.

Waiting Periods

There are no waiting periods for workers' compensation to pay for medical bills resulting from a workplace injury or illness. However, each state has a defined **waiting period (WP)** required for the injured employee to receive wage benefits. The WP is defined as the number of days an employee must be unable to work (as a result of a workplace injury or illness) before income benefits are payable. In most states the WP begins on the first day wages are lost. WPs were instituted to reduce paperwork for the claim administrator and ensure that wage benefits are not granted for a minor injury that typically should not keep an employee out of the workplace. If an injury results in disability that goes on for some time, the injured worker is retroactively paid wages that were lost during the waiting period. This is referred to as the retroactive period.

See Table 9.2 for the WP in each state.

TYPES OF STATE COMPENSATION BENEFITS

Workers' compensation pays for medical treatment and care for those who suffer a work-related illness or injury. It also provides additional benefits if the individual is disabled or the injury/illness results in death.

Five principal types of state compensation benefits that may apply in ordinary cases are the following:

1. *Medical treatment.* This includes hospital, medical and surgical services, medications, and prosthetic devices. Treatment may be rendered by a medical doctor, osteopath, dentist, or chiropractor.

TABLE 9.2 Waiting Period for Income and Medical Benefits*

Jurisdiction	Waiting Period (Days)	Jurisdiction	Waiting Period (Days)
Alabama	3	Nebraska	7
Alaska	3	Nevada	5
Arizona	7	New Hampshire	3
Arkansas	7	New Jersey	7
California	3	New Mexico	7
Colorado	3	New York	7
Connecticut	3	North Carolina	7
Delaware	3	North Dakota	5
District of Columbia	3	Ohio	7
Florida	7	Oklahoma	3
Georgia	7	Oregon	3
Hawaii	3	Pennsylvania	7
Idaho	5	Rhode Island	3
Illinois	3	South Carolina	7
Indiana	7	South Dakota	7
Iowa	3	Tennessee	7
Kansas	7	Texas	7
Kentucky	7	Utah	3
Louisiana	7	Vermont	3
Maine	7	Virgin Islands	0
Maryland	3	Virginia	7
Massachusetts	5	Washington	3
Michigan	7	West Virginia	3
Minnesota	3	Wisconsin	3
Mississippi	5	Wyoming	3
Missouri	3	FECA	3
Montana	4 days or 32 hours, whichever is less	LHWCA	3

FECA, Federal Employees' Compensation Act; *LHWCA*, Longshore and Harbor Workers' Compensation Act.
*These are statutory provisions for waiting periods (WPs). Statutes provide that a WP must elapse, during which income benefits are not payable. This WP affects only compensation because medical and hospital care are provided immediately.

2. *Temporary disability indemnity.* This is in the form of weekly cash payments for lost wages made directly to the injured or ill person.
3. *Permanent disability indemnity.* This may consist of either weekly or monthly cash payments for lost wages based on a rating system that determines the percentage of PD or a lump sum award. The payment amount depends on how much the individual earned before the injury/illness and is typically capped at two thirds of their wages.
4. *Death benefits for survivors.* This consists of cash payments to dependents of employees who are fatally injured. A burial allowance is also given in some states.
5. *Rehabilitation benefits.* Rehabilitation benefits may be offered to an individual who may be temporarily or permanently disabled. Although an ill or injured individual may not be able to return to his or her previous position, the purpose of rehabilitation (medical or vocational) is to retrain employees so they can return to the workforce in some capacity.

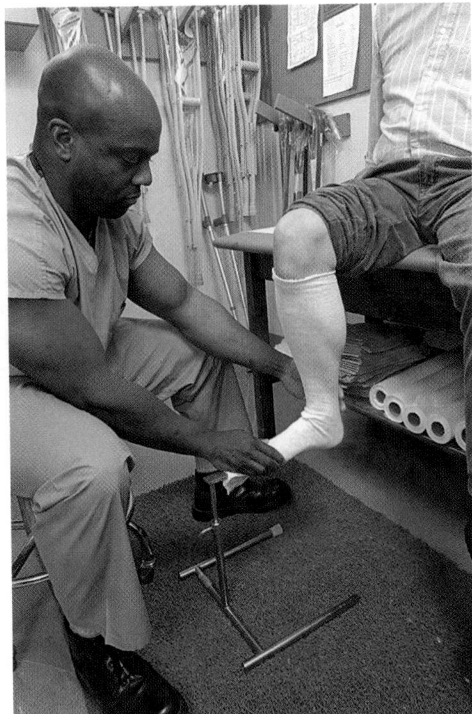

Fig. 9.1 Physician interacting with an injured worker in the examination room.

TYPES OF STATE WORKERS' COMPENSATION CLAIMS

There are three types of state workers' compensation claims: nondisability claims, temporary disability (TD) claims, and PD claims. Each type is discussed in detail to provide a clear definition and understanding of the determination process.

Nondisability Claim

The simplest type of claim is a **nondisability (ND) claim,** which generally involves a minor injury in which the patient is seen by the physician but is able to continue working (Fig. 9.1).

Temporary Disability Claim

Temporary disability occurs when a worker has a work-related injury or illness and is unable to perform the duties of his or her occupation for a specific time or range of time. The time period of TD can extend from the date of injury until the worker returns to full duty without residual ratable disability. TD may also occur when the patient returns to modified work or has ratable residual disability that the physician states is **permanent and stationary (P and S).** A condition is considered P and S when the patient reaches a point where their medical condition is not improving and not getting worse. This is referred to as the point in time when the patient has reached maximal medical improvement (MMI).

An **insurance adjuster** is the person at the workers' compensation insurance carrier who oversees the work-related injury or illness case. He or she is responsible for keeping in contact with the health care organization about the patient's ongoing progress. The insurance adjuster must evaluate the injury or illness, predict in advance the amount of money reserves needed to cover medical expenses, and calculate as accurate a reserve as possible for weekly TD payments to the injured. This is often a challenging task because a seemingly minor injury or illness can become very complex. For example, a simple back strain ultimately may require fusion or a small cut may become gangrenous and lead to an amputation. The insurance carrier wants to provide the best possible medical care for the patient. Usually workers' compensation weekly TD income payments are based on a percentage of the employee's earnings at the time of the injury. Compensation benefits are not subject to income tax.

Sometimes a patient is released from disability to light duty or a modified work program before returning to full duty, especially when heavy work is involved. Other times an employee is returned to the company and placed in a different department or division so that he or she is gainfully employed while not using the injured body part. This topic is further detailed in the next section.

Vocational Rehabilitation

Many states provide vocational rehabilitation in the form of retraining, education, job guidance, and placement to assist an injured individual in finding work before TD compensation benefits expire. In any successful rehabilitation program, the insurance carrier, health care organization, physician, physical therapist, employer supervisor, and personnel department must act as a team with the common goal of getting an injured employee back to light duty or regular work as soon as possible. It is believed that the longer a person remains out of work, the less chance there is that he or she will return to the workplace. The employer and insurance adjuster must remain in communication with rehabilitation center therapists to determine when the injured person will be able to resume some form of work. The physician may suggest a rehabilitation center that provides good care, or the employer may have an in-house program.

Work Hardening

Sports medicine therapy and physical medicine rehabilitation are often used to strengthen the injured worker. Another type of therapy, called **work hardening,** is an individualized program using simulated or real work tasks to build up strength and improve the worker's endurance toward a full day's work.

Ergonomics

Ergonomics is the applied science of designing and arranging things people use so they can interact more efficiently and safely. In some cases an ergonomic evaluation of the work site is performed and modifications may be instituted to the job or work site to lessen the possibility of future injury and to get the employee back to gainful employment. Injured individuals may also be retrained into another career field if their disability prevents them from returning to their former occupation.

Permanent Disability Claim

In a PD claim the patient or injured party is usually on TD benefits for a time and then concludes that he or she is unable to return to his or her former occupation. The physician states in the report that the patient has residual disability that will hamper his or her opportunity to compete in the open job market. Examples of residual disability include loss of a hand, an eye, or a leg and neurologic problems. Each patient who has PD is rated according to the severity of the injury, the age of the injured person, and the patient's occupation at the time of the injury. The older the person, the greater the PD benefit. One might think that a younger person deserves higher compensation because he or she will be disabled for a longer portion of his or her working career. However, the workers' compensation laws assume that a young person has a better chance of being rehabilitated into another occupation.

In a PD claim the physician's final report must include the words "permanent and stationary." The case is rated for PD, and a settlement, called a **compromise and release (C and R),** is made. This is an agreement between the injured party and the insurance company on a total sum. The case can then be closed.

Reasons that may delay closing a workers' compensation case include the following:

1. Unanswered questions or incomplete answers to data required on workers' compensation forms by the employee, employer, or physician
2. Vague terminology used by the physician or service provider in medical reports
3. Omitted signatures on forms or written reports by the employee, employer, or physician
4. Incorrect billing by the health care organization's office
5. Inadequate progress reports (for example, the physician or service provider fails to send in a medical report routinely to update the insurance carrier when the injured employee is seen in subsequent visits)

Rating

Final determination of the issues involving settlement of a work-related accident is known as **adjudication,** or the rating of a case. A physician does not rate disability but renders a professional opinion on whether the injured individual has TD or PD that prevents him or her from gainful employment. Rating itself is carried out by the state's industrial accident commission or workers' compensation board. Wage loss, earning capacity, and physical impairment are three categories that may be taken into consideration to rate temporary partial, permanent partial, or total disabilities.

In addition, permanent partial disabilities may be rated by using a scheduled or nonscheduled injury award system. This system is based on a set number of weeks of compensation for a specific loss, such as 288 weeks for the loss of a leg. Scheduled injuries may be loss of a body part, disfigurement, permanent hearing loss, and so on. Nonscheduled injuries are more general, such as disability caused by injury to the back or neck.

If an injured person is dissatisfied with the rating after the case has been declared P and S, he or she may appeal the case by submitting a formal request in writing. The request is referred to as a **petition** and is sent to the **Workers' Compensation Appeals Board (WCAB)** or the Industrial Accident Commission.

Surveillance

Sub rosa is a Latin term meaning "under the rose," which is a symbol of secrecy. In Workers' Compensation, the term *sub rosa* refers to the secret act of surveillance of a person. **Sub rosa films** are provided occasionally when rating a case to document the extent of a patient's PD. Videotapes are made over a period of 2 to 3 days without the patient's knowledge. This surveillance is expensive and is used as a last resort, especially in a case in which a person receiving workers' compensation benefits is suspected of making exaggerated complaints. It is also used in cases when a worker has been off work for a long time and supposedly is unable to perform any work activity, even light duty.

Investigators have been known to carry a camera in a gym bag and videotape a supposedly disabled claimant bench pressing at the gym. Patients also have been videotaped going into the physician's office for an appointment wearing a neck brace and removing the brace after returning to their car.

FRAUD AND ABUSE

Increases in the number of fraudulent workers' compensation claims were noted throughout many large metropolitan cities in the 1990s. These problems involved employers, employees, insurers, medical providers, and lawyers. An increasing number of states have enacted some kind of antifraud legislation and stiffened penalties for workers' compensation fraud, making it a felony. Some states require reporting suspected insurance fraud and have forms to incorporate wording in regard to fraudulent statements. An example is shown in Fig. 9.2.

Physicians are responsible for determining the legitimacy of work injuries and reporting findings accurately. If a report is prepared with the intent to use it in support of a fraudulent claim or if a fraudulent claim is knowingly submitted for payment under an insurance contract, the physician may be subject to fines or imprisonment and the revocation or suspension of his or her medical license. Some physicians sign and send a disclosure statement with the medical report certifying that they personally performed an evaluation. The physician may list the total time spent in reviewing records, face-to-face time with the patient, preparing a report, and other relevant activities.

It is the responsibility of all individuals who deal with workers' compensation cases to notify the insurance carrier of any suspicious situation. By doing so, action can be taken to have the case investigated further by personnel from the fraud divisions or referred to the district attorney's office. Perpetrators and signs of workers' compensation fraud and abuse are listed in Box 9.1.

LEGAL SITUATIONS

Medical Evaluator

Physicians who conduct medical–legal (ML) evaluations of injured workers must pass a complex medical examination. They are then certified by the Industrial Medical Council (IMC) and may be referred to as one of the following titles:

- Agreed medical evaluator (**AME**)
- Independent medical evaluator (**IME**)
- Qualified medical evaluator (**QME**)

The medical evaluator is hired by the insurance company or appointed by the referee or appeals board to examine an individual, independent from the attending physician, and render an unbiased opinion about the degree of disability of an injured worker. When the physician performs an evaluation on an injured worker, the workers' compensation fee schedule may have specific procedure codes to bill for the examination.

Depositions

When a case involves a medical evaluation, a deposition may be taken of the medical evaluator's testimony. A **deposition** is a proceeding in which an attorney asks a witness questions about a case and the witness answers under oath but not in open court. It may take place in the attorney's office or often in the physician's office. In PD workers' compensation cases, depositions are usually taken from the physician and the injured party by the attorney representing the workers' compensation insurance company. The injured party's attorney is also present if the witness is the defendant. Direct questioning and cross-examination may be done by both attorneys.

Exhibits may be entered into evidence. The witness is allowed to read the transcript and make corrections or changes. The witness may be asked to sign the transcript but can waive a signature if his or her attorney recommends against signing it. The deposition is used when the case comes to trial.

Depositions may be taken to find out additional information, the physician's version of the facts, the patient's version of the facts, what kind of witnesses the physician and patient will be, and so on. Another use for a deposition is to challenge the credibility of a witness on cross-examination. If the witness takes the stand and the testimony is inconsistent with the deposition, the attorney will make this known to the jury.

Medical Testimony

In a workers' compensation situation, a **third-party liability** claim is not made against a worker's employer, but against some separate person or company who may be responsible for the worker's injury. Third-party claims often arise when a worker is injured by a defective product or by someone other than the worker's boos or co-workers, such as a customer, a worker from another company, or a member of the public. In the instance of an accident case with third-party liability, the physician may have to testify as an expert witness, take time to give a deposition, or attend a pretrial conference. There should be a clear understanding of the terms of testimony and payment to eliminate future misunderstandings. A written agreement from the patient's lawyer should be obtained stating exactly what compensation the physician will receive for research (preparation), time spent waiting to testify (if appointments must be canceled), and actual testimony time (Fig. 9.3). In some cases the physician may want to ask for partial payment in advance. If the physician is subpoenaed, he or she must appear in court regardless of whether an agreement exists. This agreement should be signed by the physician and sent to the attorney. The attorney should return the original to the physician, retaining a copy for his or her files.

Liens

The word ***lien*** derives from the same origin as the word *liable,* and the right of lien expresses legal claim on the property of another for the payment of a debt. To file a lien, the health care organization must obtain permission from the patient (Fig. 9.4). An example of a complete lien can be found in Fig. 9.5. Liens sometimes are called *encumbrances* and may be filed for several reasons.

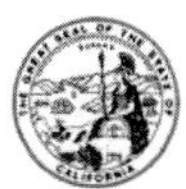

Workers' Compensation Claim Form (DWC 1) & Notice of Potential Eligibility

Formulario de Reclamo de Compensación de Trabajadores (DWC 1) y Notificación de Posible Elegibilidad

If you are injured or become ill, either physically or mentally, because of your job, including injuries resulting from a workplace crime, you may be entitled to workers' compensation benefits. Use the attached form to file a workers' compensation claim with your employer. **You should read all of the information below.** Keep this sheet and all other papers for your records. You may be eligible for some or all of the benefits listed depending on the nature of your claim. If you file a claim, the claims administrator, who is responsible for handling your claim, must notify you within 14 days whether your claim is accepted or whether additional investigation is needed.

To file a claim, complete the "Employee" section of the form, keep one copy and give the rest to your employer. Do this right away to avoid problems with your claim. In some cases, benefits will not start until you inform your employer about your injury by filing a claim form. Describe your injury completely. Include every part of your body affected by the injury. If you mail the form to your employer, use first-class or certified mail. If you buy a return receipt, you will be able to prove that the claim form was mailed and when it was delivered. Within one working day after you file the claim form, your employer must complete the "Employer" section, give you a dated copy, keep one copy, and send one to the claims administrator.

Medical Care: Your claims administrator will pay for all reasonable and necessary medical care for your work injury or illness. Medical benefits are subject to approval and may include treatment by a doctor, hospital services, physical therapy, lab tests, x-rays, medicines, equipment and travel costs. Your claims administrator will pay the costs of approved medical services directly so you should never see a bill. There are limits on chiropractic, physical therapy, and other occupational therapy visits.

The Primary Treating Physician (PTP) is the doctor with the overall responsibility for treatment of your injury or illness.

- If you previously designated your personal physician or a medical group, you may see your personal physician or the medical group after you are injured.
- If your employer is using a medical provider network (MPN) or Health Care Organization (HCO), in most cases, you will be treated in the MPN or HCO unless you predesignated your personal physician or a medical group. An MPN is a group of health care providers who provide treatment to workers injured on the job. You should receive information from your employer if you are covered by an HCO or a MPN. Contact your employer for more information.
- If your employer is not using an MPN or HCO, in most cases, the claims administrator can choose the doctor who first treats you unless you predesignated your personal physician or a medical group.
- If your employer has not put up a poster describing your rights to workers' compensation, you may be able to be treated by your personal physician right after you are injured.

Within one working day after you file a claim form, your employer or the claims administrator must authorize up to $10,000 in treatment for your injury, consistent with the applicable treating guidelines until the claim is accepted or rejected. If the employer or claims administrator does not authorize treatment right away, talk to your supervisor, someone else in management, or the claims administrator. Ask for treatment to be authorized right now, while waiting for a decision on your claim. If the employer or claims administrator will not authorize treatment, use your own health insurance to get medical care. Your health insurer will seek reimbursement from the claims administrator. If you do not have health insurance, there are doctors, clinics or hospitals that will treat you without immediate payment. They will seek reimbursement from the claims administrator.

Switching to a Different Doctor as Your PTP:

- If you are being treated in a Medical Provider Network (MPN), you may switch to other doctors within the MPN after the first visit.
- If you are being treated in a Health Care Organization (HCO), you may switch at least one time to another doctor within the HCO. You may switch to a doctor outside the HCO 90 or 180 days after your injury is reported to your employer (depending on whether you are covered by employer-provided health insurance).
- If you are not being treated in an MPN or HCO and did not predesignate, you may switch to a new doctor one time during the first 30 days after your injury is reported to your employer. Contact the claims administrator to switch doctors. After 30 days, you may switch to a doctor of your choice if

Si Ud. se lesiona o se enferma, ya sea físicamente o mentalmente, debido a su trabajo, incluyendo lesiones que resulten de un crimen en el lugar de trabajo, es posible que Ud. tenga derecho a beneficios de compensación de trabajadores. Utilice el formulario adjunto para presentar un reclamo de compensación de trabajadores con su empleador. **Ud. debe leer toda la información a continuación.** Guarde esta hoja y todos los demás documentos para sus archivos. Es posible que usted reúna los requisitos para todos los beneficios, o parte de éstos, que se enumeran dependiendo de la índole de su reclamo. Si usted presenta un reclamo, l administrador de reclamos, quien es responsable por el manejo de su reclamo, debe notificarle dentro de 14 días si se acepta su reclamo o si se necesita investigación adicional.

Para presentar un reclamo, llene la sección del formulario designada para el "Empleado," guarde una copia, y déle el resto a su empleador. Haga esto de inmediato para evitar problemas con su reclamo. En algunos casos, los beneficios no se iniciarán hasta que usted le informe a su empleador acerca de su lesión mediante la presentación de un formulario de reclamo. Describa su lesión por completo. Incluya cada parte de su cuerpo afectada por la lesión. Si usted le envía por correo el formulario a su empleador, utilice primera clase o correo certificado. Si usted compra un acuse de recibo, usted podrá demostrar que el formulario de reclamo fue enviado por correo y cuando fue entregado. Dentro de un día laboral después de presentar el formulario de reclamo, su empleador debe completar la sección designada para el "Empleador," le dará a Ud. una copia fechada, guardará una copia, y enviará una al administrador de reclamos.

Atención Médica: Su administrador de reclamos pagará por toda la atención médica razonable y necesaria para su lesión o enfermedad relacionada con el trabajo. Los beneficios médicos están sujetos a la aprobación y pueden incluir tratamiento por parte de un médico, los servicios de hospital, la terapia física, los análisis de laboratorio, las medicinas, equipos y gastos de viaje. Su administrador de reclamos pagará directamente los costos de los servicios médicos aprobados de manera que usted nunca verá una factura. Hay límites en terapia quiropráctica, física y otras visitas de terapia ocupacional.

El Médico Primario que le Atiende *(Primary Treating Physician- PTP)* es el médico con la responsabilidad total para tratar su lesión o enfermedad.

- Si usted designó previamente a su médico personal o a un grupo médico, usted podrá ver a su médico personal o grupo médico después de lesionarse.
- Si su empleador está utilizando una red de proveedores médicos (*Medical Provider Network- MPN)* o una Organización de Cuidado Médico *(Health Care Organization- HCO)*, en la mayoría de los casos, usted será tratado en la *MPN* o *HCO* a menos que usted hizo una designación previa de su médico personal o grupo médico. Una *MPN* es un grupo de proveedores de asistencia médica quien da tratamiento a los trabajadores lesionados en el trabajo. Usted debe recibir información de su empleador si su tratamiento es cubierto por una *HCO* o una *MPN*. Hable con su empleador para más información.
- Si su empleador no está utilizando una *MPN* o *HCO*, en la mayoría de los casos, el administrador de reclamos puede elegir el médico que lo atiende primero a menos de que usted hizo una designación previa de su médico personal o grupo médico.
- Si su empleador no ha colocado un cartel describiendo sus derechos para la compensación de trabajadores, Ud. puede ser tratado por su médico personal inmediatamente después de lesionarse.

Dentro de un día laboral después de que Ud. Presente un formulario de reclamo, su empleador o el administrador de reclamos debe autorizar hasta $10000 en tratamiento para su lesión, de acuerdo con las pautas de tratamiento aplicables, hasta que el reclamo sea aceptado o rechazado. Si el empleador o administrador de reclamos no autoriza el tratamiento de inmediato, hable con su supervisor, alguien más en la gerencia, o con el administrador de reclamos. Pida que el tratamiento sea autorizado ya mismo, mientras espera una decisión sobre su reclamo. Si el empleador o administrador de reclamos no autoriza el tratamiento, utilice su propio seguro médico para recibir atención médica. Su compañía de seguro médico buscará reembolso del administrador de reclamos. Si usted no tiene seguro médico, hay médicos, clínicas u hospitales que lo tratarán sin pago inmediato. Ellos buscarán reembolso del administrador de reclamos.

Cambiando a otro Médico Primario o *PTP*:

- Si usted está recibiendo tratamiento en una Red de Proveedores Médicos

Rev. 1/1/2016

Page 1 of 3

Fig. 9.2 Employee's claim form for workers' compensation benefits. Note the insert about fraudulent material.

your employer or the claims administrator has not created or selected an MPN.

Disclosure of Medical Records: After you make a claim for workers' compensation benefits, your medical records will not have the same level of privacy that you usually expect. If you don't agree to voluntarily release medical records, a workers' compensation judge may decide what records will be released. If you request privacy, the judge may "seal" (keep private) certain medical records.

Problems with Medical Care and Medical Reports: At some point during your claim, you might disagree with your PTP about what treatment is necessary. If this happens, you can switch to other doctors as described above. If you cannot reach agreement with another doctor, the steps to take depend on whether you are receiving care in an MPN, HCO, or neither. For more information, see "Learn More About Workers' Compensation," below.

If the claims administrator denies treatment recommended by your PTP, you may request independent medical review (IMR) using the request form included with the claims administrator's written decision to deny treatment. The IMR process is similar to the group health IMR process, and takes approximately 40 (or fewer) days to arrive at a determination so that appropriate treatment can be given. Your attorney or your physician may assist you in the IMR process. IMR is not available to resolve disputes over matters other than the medical necessity of a particular treatment requested by your physician.

If you disagree with your PTP on matters other than treatment, such as the cause of your injury or how severe the injury is, you can switch to other doctors as described above. If you cannot reach agreement with another doctor, notify the claims administrator in writing as soon as possible. In some cases, you risk losing the right to challenge your PTP's opinion unless you do this promptly. If you do not have an attorney, the claims administrator must send you instructions on how to be seen by a doctor called a qualified medical evaluator (QME) to help resolve the dispute. If you have an attorney, the claims administrator may try to reach agreement with your attorney on a doctor called an agreed medical evaluator (AME). If the claims administrator disagrees with your PTP on matters other than treatment, the claims administrator can require you to be seen by a QME or AME.

Payment for Temporary Disability (Lost Wages): If you can't work while you are recovering from a job injury or illness, you may receive temporary disability payments for a limited period. These payments may change or stop when your doctor says you are able to return to work. These benefits are tax-free. Temporary disability payments are two-thirds of your average weekly pay, within minimums and maximums set by state law. Payments are not made for the first three days you are off the job unless you are hospitalized overnight or cannot work for more than 14 days.

Stay at Work or Return to Work: Being injured does not mean you must stop working. If you can continue working, you should. If not, it is important to go back to work with your current employer as soon as you are medically able. Studies show that the longer you are off work, the harder it is to get back to your original job and wages. While you are recovering, your PTP, your employer (supervisors or others in management), the claims administrator, and your attorney (if you have one) will work with you to decide how you will stay at work or return to work and what work you will do. Actively communicate with your PTP, your employer, and the claims administrator about the work you did before you were injured, your medical condition and the kinds of work you can do now, and the kinds of work that your employer could make available to you.

Payment for Permanent Disability: If a doctor says you have not recovered completely from your injury and you will always be limited in the work you can do, you may receive additional payments. The amount will depend on the type of injury, extent of impairment, your age, occupation, date of injury, and your wages before you were injured.

Supplemental Job Displacement Benefit (SJDB): If you were injured on or after 1/1/04, and your injury results in a permanent disability and your employer does not offer regular, modified, or alternative work, you may qualify for a nontransferable voucher payable for retraining and/or skill enhancement. If you qualify, the claims administrator will pay the costs up to the maximum set by state law.

Death Benefits: If the injury or illness causes death, payments may be made to a

(Medical Provider Network- MPN), usted puede cambiar a otros médicos dentro de la MPN después de la primera visita.

- Si usted está recibiendo tratamiento en un Organización de Cuidado Médico (Healthcare Organization- HCO), es posible cambiar al menos una vez a otro médico dentro de la HCO. Usted puede cambiar a un médico fuera de la HCO 90 o 180 días después de que su lesión es reportada a su empleador (dependiendo de si usted está cubierto por un seguro médico proporcionado por su empleador).
- Si usted no está recibiendo tratamiento en una MPN o HCO y no hizo una designación previa, usted puede cambiar a un nuevo médico una vez durante los primeros 30 días después de que su lesión es reportada a su empleador. Póngase en contacto con el administrador de reclamos para cambiar de médico. Después de 30 días, puede cambiar a un médico de su elección si su empleador o el administrador de reclamos no ha creado o seleccionado una MPN.

Divulgación de Expedientes Médicos: Después de que Ud. presente un reclamo para beneficios de compensación de trabajadores, sus expedientes médicos no tendrán el mismo nivel de privacidad que usted normalmente espera. Si Ud. no está de acuerdo en divulgar voluntariamente los expedientes médicos, un juez de compensación de trabajadores posiblemente decida qué expedientes serán revelados. Si usted solicita privacidad, es posible que el juez "selle" (mantenga privados) ciertos expedientes médicos.

Problemas con la Atención Médica y los Informes Médicos: En algún momento durante su reclamo, podría estar en desacuerdo con su *PTP* sobre qué tratamiento es necesario. Si esto sucede, usted puede cambiar a otros médicos como se describe anteriormente. Si no puede llegar a un acuerdo con otro médico, los pasos a seguir dependen de si usted está recibiendo atención en una *MPN*, *HCO* o ninguna de las dos. Para más información, consulte la sección "Aprenda Más Sobre la Compensación de Trabajadores," a continuación.

Si el administrador de reclamos niega el tratamiento recomendado por su *PTP*, puede solicitar una revisión médica independiente *(Independent Medical Review-IMR)*, utilizando el formulario de solicitud que se incluye con la decisión por escrito del administrador de reclamos negando el tratamiento. El proceso de la *IMR* es parecido al proceso de la *IMR* de un seguro médico colectivo, y tarda aproximadamente 40 (o menos) días para llegar a una determinación de manera que se pueda dar un tratamiento apropiado. Su abogado o su médico le pueden ayudar en el proceso de la *IMR*. La *IMR* no está disponible para resolver disputas sobre cuestiones aparte de la necesidad médica de un tratamiento particular solicitado por su médico.

Si no está de acuerdo con su *PTP* en cuestiones aparte del tratamiento, como la causa de su lesión o la gravedad de la lesión, usted puede cambiar a otros médicos como se describe anteriormente. Si no puede llegar a un acuerdo con otro médico, notifique al administrador de reclamos por escrito tan pronto como sea posible. En algunos casos, usted arriesg perder el derecho a objetar a la opinión de su *PTP* a menos que hace esto de inmediato. Si usted no tiene un abogado, el administrador de reclamos debe enviarle instrucciones para ser evaluado por un médico llamado un evaluador médico calificado *(Qualified Medical Evaluator-QME)* para ayudar a resolver la disputa. Si usted tiene un abogado, el administrador de reclamos puede tratar de llegar a un acuerdo con su abogado sobre un médico llamado un evaluador médico acordado *(Agreed Medical Evaluator- AME)*. Si el administrador de reclamos no está de acuerdo con su *PTP* sobre asuntos aparte del tratamiento, el administrador de reclamos puede exigirle que sea atendido por un *QME* o *AME*.

Pago por Incapacidad Temporal (Sueldos Perdidos): Si Ud. no puede trabajar, mientras se está recuperando de una lesión o enfermedad relacionada con el trabajo, Ud. puede recibir pagos por incapacidad temporal por un periodo limitado. Estos pagos pueden cambiar o parar cuando su médico diga que Ud. está en condiciones de regresar a trabajar. Estos beneficios son libres de impuestos. Los pagos por incapacidad temporal son dos tercios de su pago semanal promedio, con cantidades mínimas y máximas establecidas por las leyes estales. Los pagos no se hacen durante los primeros tres días en que Ud. no trabaje, a menos que Ud. sea hospitalizado una noche o no puede trabajar durante más de 14 días.

Permanezca en el Trabajo o Regreso al Trabajo: Estar lesionado no significa que usted debe dejar de trabajar. Si usted puede seguir trabajando, usted debe hacerlo. Si no es así, es importante regresar a trabajar con su empleador actual tan

Rev. 1/1/2016 Page 2 of 3

Fig. 9.2, cont'd.

spouse and other relatives or household members who were financially dependent on the deceased worker.

It is illegal for your employer to punish or fire you for having a job injury or illness, for filing a claim, or testifying in another person's workers' compensation case (Labor Code 132a). If proven, you may receive lost wages, job reinstatement, increased benefits, and costs and expenses up to limits set by the state.

Resolving Problems or Disputes: You have the right to disagree with decisions affecting your claim. If you have a disagreement, contact your employer or claims administrator first to see if you can resolve it. If you are not receiving benefits, you may be able to get State Disability Insurance (SDI) or unemployment insurance (UI) benefits. Call the state Employment Development Department at (800) 480-3287 or (866) 333-4606, or go to their website at www.edd.ca.gov.

You Can Contact an Information & Assistance (I&A) Officer: State I&A officers answer questions, help injured workers, provide forms, and help resolve problems. Some I&A officers hold workshops for injured workers. To obtain important information about the workers' compensation claims process and your rights and obligations, go to www.dwc.ca.gov or contact an I&A officer of the state Division of Workers' Compensation. You can also hear recorded information and a list of local I&A offices by calling (800) 736-7401.

You can consult with an attorney. Most attorneys offer one free consultation. If you decide to hire an attorney, his or her fee will be taken out of some of your benefits. For names of workers' compensation attorneys, call the State Bar of California at (415) 538-2120 or go to their website at **www.californiaspecialist.org**.

Learn More About Workers' Compensation: For more information about the workers' compensation claims process, go to www.dwc.ca.gov. At the website, you can access a useful booklet, "Workers' Compensation in California: A Guidebook for Injured Workers." You can also contact an Information & Assistance Officer (above), or hear recorded information by calling 1-800-736-7401.

pronto como usted pueda medicamente hacerlo. Los estudios demuestran que entre más tiempo esté fuera del trabajo, más difícil es regresar a su trabajo original y a sus salarios. Mientras se está recuperando, su *PTP*, su empleador (supervisores u otras personas en la gerencia), el administrador de reclamos, y su abogado (si tiene uno) trabajarán con usted para decidir cómo va a permanecer en el trabajo o regresar al trabajo y qué trabajo hará. Comuníquese de manera activa con su *PTP*, su empleador y el administrador de reclamos sobre el trabajo que hizo antes de lesionarse, su condición médica y los tipos de trabajo que usted puede hacer ahora y los tipos de trabajo que su empleador podría poner a su disposición.

Pago por Incapacidad Permanente: Si un médico dice que no se ha recuperado completamente de su lesión y siempre será limitado en el trabajo que puede hacer, es posible que Ud. reciba pagos adicionales. La cantidad dependerá de la clase de lesión, grado de deterioro, su edad, ocupación, fecha de la lesión y sus salarios antes de lesionarse.

Beneficio Suplementario por Desplazamiento de Trabajo *(Supplemental Job Displacement Benefit- SJDB)*: Si Ud. se lesionó en o después del 1/1/04, y su lesión resulta en una incapacidad permanente y su empleador no ofrece un trabajo regular, modificado, o alternativo, usted podría cumplir los requisitos para recibir un vale no-transferible pagadero a una escuela para recibir un nuevo un curso de reentrenamiento y/o mejorar su habilidad. Si Ud. cumple los requisios, el administrador de reclamos pagará los gastos hasta un máximo establecido por las leyes estatales.

Beneficios por Muerte: Si la lesión o enfermedad causa la muerte, es posible que los pagos se hagan a un cónyuge y otros parientes o a las personas que viven en el hogar que dependían económicamente del trabajador difunto.

Es ilegal que su empleador le castigue o despida por sufrir una lesión o enfermedad laboral, por presentar un reclamo o por testificar en el caso de compensación de trabajadores de otra persona. (Código Laboral, sección 132a.) De ser probado, usted puede recibir pagos por pérdida de sueldos, reposición del trabajo, aumento de beneficios y gastos hasta los límites establecidos por el estado.

Resolviendo problemas o disputas: Ud. tiene derecho a no estar de acuerdo con las decisiones que afecten su reclamo. Si Ud. tiene un desacuerdo, primero comuníquese con su empleador o administrador de reclamos para ver si usted puede resolverlo. Si usted no está recibiendo beneficios, es posible que Ud. pueda obtener beneficios del Seguro Estatalde Incapacidad *(State Disability Insurance- SDI)* o beneficios del desempleo *(Unemployment Insurance- UI)*. Llame al Departamento del Desarrollo del Empleo estatal al (800) 480-3287 o (866) 333-4606, o visite su página Web en www.edd.ca.gov.

Puede Contactar a un Oficial de Información y Asistencia *(Information & Assistance- I&A)*: Los Oficiales de Información y Asistencia *(I&A)* estatal contestan preguntas, ayudan a los trabajadores lesionados, proporcionan formularios y ayudan a resolver problemas. Algunos oficiales de *I&A* tienen talleres para trabajadores lesionados. Para obtener información importante sobre el proceso de la compensación de trabajadores y sus derechos y obligaciones, vaya a www.dwc.ca.gov o comuníquese con un oficial de información y asistencia de la División Estatal de Compensación de Trabajadores. También puede escuchar información grabada y una lista de las oficinas de *I&A* locales llamando al (800) 736-7401.

Ud. puede consultar con un abogado. La mayoría de los abogados ofrecen una consulta gratis. Si Ud. decide contratar a un abogado, los honorarios serán tomados de algunos de sus beneficios. Para obtener nombres de abogados de compensación de trabajadores, llame a la Asociación Estatal de Abogados de California *(State Bar)* al (415) 538-2120, o consulte su página Web en www.californiaspecialist.org.

Aprenda Más Sobre la Compensación de Trabajadores: Para obtener más información sobre el proceso de reclamos del programa de compensación de trabajadores, vaya a www.dwc.ca.gov. En la página Web, podrá acceder a un folleto útil, "Compensación del Trabajador de California: Una Guía para Trabajadores Lesionados." También puede contactar a un oficial de Información y Asistencia (arriba), o escuchar información grabada llamando al 1-800-736-7401.

Fig. 9.2, cont'd.

State of California
Department of Industrial Relations
DIVISION OF WORKERS' COMPENSATION

Estado de California
Departamento de Relaciones Industriales
DIVISION DE COMPENSACIÓN AL TRABAJADOR

WORKERS' COMPENSATION CLAIM FORM (DWC 1)

PETITION DEL EMPLEADO PARA DE COMPENSACIÓN DEL TRABAJADOR (DWC 1)

Employee: Complete the **"Employee"** section and give the form to your employer. Keep a copy and mark it **"Employee's Temporary Receipt"** until you receive the signed and dated copy from your employer. You may call the Division of Workers' Compensation and hear recorded information at **(800) 736-7401.** An explanation of workers' compensation benefits is included in the Notice of Potential Eligibility, which is the cover sheet of this form. Detach and save this notice for future reference.

You should also have received a pamphlet from your employer describing workers' compensation benefits and the procedures to obtain them. You may receive written notices from your employer or its claims administrator about your claim. If your claims administrator offers to send you notices electronically, and you agree to receive these notices only by email, please provide your email address below and check the appropriate box. If you later decide you want to receive the notices by mail, you must inform your employer in writing.

Any person who makes or causes to be made any knowingly false or fraudulent material statement or material representation for the purpose of obtaining or denying workers' compensation benefits or payments is guilty of a felony.

Empleado: *Complete la sección* ***"Empleado"*** *y entregue la forma a su empleador. Quédese con la copia designada* ***"Recibo Temporal del Empleado"*** *hasta que Ud. reciba la copia firmada y fechada de su empleador. Ud. puede llamar a la Division de Compensación al Trabajador al* ***(800) 736-7401*** *para oir información gravada. Una explicación de los beneficios de compensación de trabajadores está incluido en la Notificación de Posible Elegibilidad, que es la hoja de portada de esta forma. Separe y guarde esta notificación como referencia para el futuro.*

Ud. también debería haber recibido de su empleador un folleto describiendo los benficios de compensación al trabajador lesionado y los procedimientos para obtenerlos. Es posible que reciba notificaciones escritas de su empleador o de su administrador de reclamos sobre su reclamo. Si su administrador de reclamos ofrece enviarle notificaciones electrónicamente, y usted acepta recibir estas notificaciones solo por correo electrónico, por favor proporcione su dirección de correo electrónico abajo y marque la caja apropiada. Si usted decide después que quiere recibir las notificaciones por correo, usted debe de informar a su empleador por escrito.

Toda aquella persona que a propósito haga o cause que se produzca cualquier declaración o representación material falsa o fraudulenta con el fin de obtener o negar beneficios o pagos de compensación a trabajadores lesionados es culpable de un crimen mayor "felonia".

Employee—complete this section and see note above ***Empleado—complete esta sección y note la notación arriba.***

1. Name. *Nombre.* ______ Today's Date. *Fecha de Hoy.* ______
2. Home Address. *Dirección Residencial.* ______
3. City. *Ciudad.* ______ State. *Estado.* ______ Zip. *Código Postal.* ______
4. Date of Injury. *Fecha de la lesión (accidente).* ______ Time of Injury. *Hora en que ocurrió.* ______a.m. ______p.m.
5. Address and description of where injury happened. *Dirección/lugar dónde occurió el accidente.* ______
6. Describe injury and part of body affected. *Describa la lesión y parte del cuerpo afectada.* ______
7. Social Security Number. *Número de Seguro Social del Empleado.* ______
8. ☐ Check if you agree to receive notices about your claim by email only. ☐ *Marque si usted acepta recibir notificaciones sobre su reclamo solo por correo electrónico.* Employee's e-mail. ______ *Correo electrónico del empleado.* ______.

You will receive benefit notices by regular mail if you do not choose, or your claims administrator does not offer, an electronic service option. *Usted recibirá notificaciones de beneficios por correo ordinario si usted no escoge, o su administrador de reclamos no le ofrece, una opción de servicio electrónico.*

9. Signature of employee. *Firma del empleado.* ______

Employer—complete this section and see note below. ***Empleador—complete esta sección y note la notación abajo.***

10. Name of employer. *Nombre del empleador.* ______
11. Address. *Dirección.* ______
12. Date employer first knew of injury. *Fecha en que el empleador supo por primera vez de la lesión o accidente.* ______
13. Date claim form was provided to employee. *Fecha en que se le entregó al empleado la petición.* ______
14. Date employer received claim form. *Fecha en que el empleado devolvió la petición al empleador.* ______
15. Name and address of insurance carrier or adjusting agency. *Nombre y dirección de la compañía de seguros o agencia adminstradora de seguros.* ______
16. Insurance Policy Number. *El número de la póliza de Seguro.* ______
17. Signature of employer representative. *Firma del representante del empleador.* ______
18. Title. *Título.* ______ 19. Telephone. *Teléfono.* ______

Employer: You are required to date this form and provide copies to your insurer or claims administrator and to the employee, dependent or representative who filed the claim within **one working day** of receipt of the form from the employee.

SIGNING THIS FORM IS NOT AN ADMISSION OF LIABILITY

Empleador: *Se requiere que Ud. feche esta forma y que provéa copias a su compañía de seguros, administrador de reclamos, o dependiente/representante de reclamos y al empleado que hayan presentado esta petición dentro del plazo de* ***un día hábil*** *desde el momento de haber sido recibida la forma del empleado.*

EL FIRMAR ESTA FORMA NO SIGNIFICA ADMISION DE RESPONSABILIDAD

☐Employer copy/*Copia del Empleador* ☐Employee copy/*Copia del Empleado* ☐Claims Administrator/*Administrador de Reclamos* ☐Temporary Receipt/*Recibo del Empleado*

Rev. 1/1/2016

Fig. 9.2, cont'd.

BOX 9.1 Perpetrators and Signs of Workers' Compensation Fraud and Abuse

Employee

- Symptoms are all subjective.
- Misses the first physician's visit or cancels or repeatedly reschedules appointments.
- Cannot describe the pain or is overly dramatic, such as an employee who comes to the physician's office limping on the left leg, suddenly starts limping on the right leg, and then goes back to limping on the left leg.
- Delays in reporting the injury.
- Does not report Friday's injury until Monday morning.
- First reports an injury to a legal or regulatory agency.
- Reports an injury after missing several days of work.
- Changes physicians frequently.
- Is a short-term worker.
- Has a curious claim history.
- Fabricates an injury.
- Exaggerates a work-related injury to obtain larger benefits, such as an injured employee who has a back pain and claims inability to bend over or lift. Surveillance cameras capture the individual at work on weekends repairing cars in the driveway at home—a task he is supposedly unable to perform.
- Blames an injury that occurred off the job on the employer.
- Adds symptoms in response to efforts to return the person to work.

Employer

- Misrepresents the annual payroll to get lower premium rates.
- Misrepresents the number of workers employed.
- Gives a false address with the least expensive premium rates.
- Falsely classifies the job duties of workers (as not hazardous), such as stating the job title as a clerical worker when in fact the employee is using a lathe every day.
- Conspires with the employee to defraud.
- Insurer.
- Refuses to pay valid medical claims.
- Forces the injured worker to settle by using unethical tactics. For example, an insurance agent tells an employee that he has a back sprain. Relying on that information, the worker settles the case. Later, a myelogram reveals a herniated intervertebral disk. The patient is left with a permanent partial disability.

Medical Provider

- Makes immediate referral for psychiatric care despite the worker's report of a trauma injury.
- Orders or performs unnecessary tests.
- Treatment dates fall on weekends and holidays.
- Renders unnecessary treatment.
- Lists a diagnosis that is not consistent with the course of treatment.
- Charges the insurance carrier for services never rendered.
- Prolongs treatment for what appears to be a minor injury.
- Participates in a provider mill scheme (see explanation under "Lawyer").
- Makes multiple referrals from a clinic practice regardless of type of injury.
- Sends medical reports that look photocopied with the same information typed in (for example, employer's address, description of injury) or that read almost identical to other reports.
- Sends in many claims in which injuries are of a subjective nature, such as stress, emotional distress, headaches, and inability to sleep.
- Sends in claims from one employer showing several employees with similar injuries, using the same physicians and/or attorneys.
- Bills both the workers' compensation carrier and the health insurer for the same service.

Lawyer

- Overbills clients.
- Participates in a medical provider mill scheme. For example, an individual is solicited while in the unemployment line by a recruiter known as a "capper." The capper tells the worker it is possible to obtain more money on disability than through unemployment. The worker is referred to an attorney and a "provider mill" clinic, which help the individual to fabricate a claim by claiming stress or an on-the-job injury. In some states, such acts may be considered a public offense and are punishable as a misdemeanor or felony.

The advantages of filing a lien are as follows:

- It is a written agreement and is recognized in court.
- It is a source of protection in the event of litigation.
- It ensures that payment for previously rendered medical services are received when the attorney and patient have reached a settlement with the insurance company in an accident case.
- It is an inexpensive method of collecting the fee. The health care organization can file suit and try to get a judgment against the patient, but this is relatively expensive compared with filing a lien.
- The health care organization will collect the full fee. If the delinquent account is turned over to a collection agency, the health care organization may lose as much as 50% of the fee when it is collected.
- If the health care organization wishes to bill more than what is allowed for a given service or services, a lien can be filed and the judge will determine whether it is reasonable.
- It avoids harassment in trying to collect the bill.

The chief disadvantage of not filing a lien is that there is no legal documentation if the case goes to court as far as collecting monies owed to the health care organization. A case could be settled, the attorney would get his or her fee, and the health care organization's fee may be placed last on the list for payment or remain unpaid.

A time limit should be specified when a lien form is completed; reaching a settlement may involve several years of litigation. Some patients may be persuaded to pay before a legal settlement is made or at least make payments until a settlement is reached. The lien becomes null and void at the end of the time limit. If the patient's financial status has changed, one might be able to collect because the patient can then be billed. If not, an amended or subsequent lien should be filed that states the actual balance of the patient's account. The word "amended" should be typed on the new lien below the WCAB case number.

The health care organization's fee should be protected by having the attorney sign the lien, thereby indicating that he or she will pay the service provider directly from any money received in a settlement. This makes the attorney responsible for the fee. The patient's file must be placed in a Hold for Settlement category until the case comes up in court. In some states the health care organization's fee owed by the patient constitutes a first lien against any such money settlement, and the attorney must first satisfy that lien before the patient or attorney receives any money from the settlement. State laws should be checked. The office of the patient's attorney should be called at least quarterly for an update.

MEDICAL TESTIMONY AGREEMENT

AGREEMENT made this ______ day of ________ 20XX, between ______________________
herein referred to as attorney, and ______________________________________,
of ______________________, ____________, ____________ ____________, a licensed ____________.
(street address) (city) (state) (ZIP code)

In consideration of their mutual covenants set forth herein, the parties agree as follows:

1. The doctor will give medical testimony in the case of:
____
as a treating physician or as an expert witness (delete the unwanted phrase).

2. The doctor agrees to appear promptly when called and to present his or her medical testimony in a well-prepared professional manner.

3. The doctor will be compensated for time away from the practice of his or her medical duties in accordance with the following:
(a) $________ per hour for reports and preparation of medical testimony.
(b) $________ per hour for pretrial conferences.
(c) $________ per hour for court appearance, including travel time to and from the office.
(d) $________ per hour for deposition.
(e) $________ per hour for being on call with cancellation of appointments but not appearing in court.

4. The doctor will appear in court on ______ hour's notice from the attorney, unless prior arrangements have been made for the exact time of appearance.

5. The doctor will be compensated on completion of his or her medical testimony, and payment will not be contingent upon the outcome of the case. However, if the case is settled before reaching the court, the doctor will be compensated for being on call as noted above.

This contract shall be binding upon the parties.

IN WITNESS WHEREOF, the said parties hereto have subscribed their respective signatures.

____
(physician)

____
(attorney)

Date: ______________________________

Fig. 9.3 Example of a medical testimony agreement between physician and attorney. This is signed by the physician and sent to the attorney for signature. A copy is retained by the attorney and the original is kept by the physician.

SCENARIO: FILING A LIEN

Problem 1: Suppose Attorney Blake advises client Roger Reed not to pay the physician until after the trial. Or what happens if payment is not made for Dr. Practon's courtroom testimony and the case is lost? Suppose that medical reports are ordered and Attorney Blake neglects to pay for them. What happens if Roger Reed forgets about the physician's bill?

Solution: If a lien had been signed, then once the case has been settled the money would be paid to the physician; otherwise, the settlement would belong to the patient, Roger Reed, and he could take any action with the money that he wanted.

Problem 2: Suppose that Dr. Practon had an oral agreement covering his fee. The patient, Katie Crest, was unable to pay for medical treatment except on legal monetary recovery. When Katie Crest settled her case, the proceeds went almost entirely to welfare agencies because she received retroactive Medicaid. Dr. Practon sued the patient's attorney and lost.

Solution: If Dr. Practon had gotten a written assignment of the proceeds, the lawyer could have been held liable for the fee.

If there is a third-party litigation involved in a workers' compensation case or a decision has not been reached as to whether an accident is work related, both a regular lien and a workers' compensation lien should be filed. In most states a special lien form for workers' compensation filing is available and should be used. A copy of the lien should be completed and sent to all concerned parties, including the following:

- Appeals board
- Employer of the patient
- Employee (the patient)
- Insurance carrier
- Health care organization or physician's files (lien claimant or one who is filing for the lien)

The patient/employee consents to the lien by his or her signature. Do not accept a lien form unless it is also signed by the patient's attorney. Check with the local Division of Industrial Accidents for forms pertinent to filing a lien and instructions on the formalities, number of copies required, and where they are to be sent.

REQUEST FOR ALLOWANCE OF LIEN
ASSIGNMENT AND AUTHORIZATION

WHEREAS, I have a right or cause of action arising out of personal injury, to wit:

I, ________________ hereby authorize ____________________,
patient's name physician's name

to furnish, upon request, to my attorney, ____________________, any and all medical records, or reports of examination, diagnosis, treatment, or prognosis but not necessarily limited to those items as set forth herein, in addition to an itemized statement of account for services rendered therefore or in connection therewith, which my attorney may from time to time request in connection with the injuries described above and sustained by me on the __________ day of ___________, 20XX.

I, hereby irrevocably authorize and direct my said attorney set forth herein to pay to ________________ all charges for attendance in court,
physician's name

if required as an expert witness whether he testifies or not; reports or other data supplied by him; depositions given by said doctor; medical services rendered or drugs supplied; and any other reasonable and customary charges incurred by my attorney as submitted by ________________ and in
physician's name

connection with said injury. Said payment or payments are to be made from any money or monies received by my attorney whether by judgment, decree, or settlement of this case, prior to disbursement to me and payment of the amount as herein directed shall be the same as if paid by me. This authorization to pay the aforementioned doctor shall constitute and be deemed as assignment of so much of my recovery I receive. It is agreed that nothing herein relieves me of the primary responsibility and obligation of paying my doctor for services rendered, and I shall at all times remain personally liable for such indebtedness unless released by the aforementioned doctor or by payment disbursed by my attorney.
I accept the above assignment:
Dated: ______________________ Patient: ____________________

As the attorney of record for the above-named patient, I hereby agree to observe the terms of this agreement, and to withhold from any award in this case such sums as are required for the adequate protection of Dr. _____
______________________.

Date: ______________________ Attorney: ____________________

Fig. 9.4 Patient's authorization to release information to an attorney and grant lien to the physician against proceeds of settlement in connection with a work-related injury/illness or third-party litigation cases.

Third-Party Subrogation

The legal term *subrogation* is the process of initiating a legal claim against either another individual, an individual's insurer, or, in the case of a car accident, one's own automobile insurance company to pay health insurance bills. **Third-party subrogation** means "to substitute" one party for another. When applied to workers' compensation cases, it means a transfer of the claims and rights from the original creditor (workers' compensation insurance carrier) to the third-party liability carrier. In a compensation case, the insurance carrier that is "subrogated" to the legal claims has a right to be paid all the monies it paid out for the injuries. That reimbursement is obtained from any money the injured collects from a legal claim, directly from the individual who caused the injury, or from another insurer.

SCENARIO: THIRD-PARTY SUBROGATION

Scenario: As Monica Valdez, a secretary, went to the bank to deposit some money for her employer, her car was rear-ended by another automobile and she was injured.

Subrogation Solution: In such a case there is no question of fault and no question of cause. Monica was hurt during the performance of her work and the workers' compensation insurance carrier is liable. The carrier must adjust the claim, provide all medical treatment, and pay all temporary disability and permanent disability benefits.

However, the insurance carrier does have legal recourse. It may send a representative to visit with Monica, explain to her that she has a good subrogation case, encourage her to seek the advice of an attorney and sue the third party (other automobile driver) in civil court. This is sometimes referred to as *litigation,* which is the process of carrying on a lawsuit. If Monica agrees to sue, the insurance carrier files a demand with the court for repayment of all money it has paid out. This is called a *lien,* which is discussed earlier in the chapter. When the case is settled, if an award is made to Monica, the insurance carrier is reimbursed for all that it has paid and Monica receives the balance. In some states, such as California, the patient is legally prevented from collecting twice.

STATE OF CALIFORNIA
DIVISION OF WORKERS' COMPENSATION
WORKERS' COMPENSATION APPEALS BOARD
NOTICE AND REQUEST FOR ALLOWANCE OF LIEN

Date Of Original Lien: 6-5-XX (MM/DD/YYYY) ☑ Original Lien ☐ Amended Lien

CA-46739-04
Case No.
(Choose only one)
☑ a specific injury on 4-3-XX (DATE OF INJURY: MM/DD/YYYY)

☐ a cumulative injury which began on ________ (START DATE: MM/DD/YYYY) and ended on ________ (END DATE: MM/DD/YYYY)

1. Must include case number and date of injury. Determine if the injury occurred on a specific date or over a period of time.

120XX6542
SSN (Numbers Only)

8-14-19XX
(DATE OF BIRTH: MM/DD/YYYY)

Injured Worker:

IMA — First Name
B — MI
HURT — Last Name

2. Patient demographic information.

300 EAST CENTRAL AVENUE
Address/PO Box (Please leave blank spaces between numbers, names or words)

WOODLAND HILLS — City
CA — State
12345 — Zip Code

Attorney/Representative for Injured Worker:

3. Information for patient's attorney.

I'M HERE FOR THE PATIENT LAWYERS FIRM
Name

232 NORTH RIVERSIDE DRIVE
Address/PO Box (Please leave blank spaces between numbers, names or words)

CALABASSAS — City
CA — State
12345 — Zip Code

Lien Claimant (Completion of this section is required):

4. The physician is the lien claimant.

RAYMOND SKELETON, MD
Name of Organization filing lien (for individual lien claimants, leave blank)

RAYMOND
First Name of Individual filing lien (organizational lien claimants, leave blank)

SKELETON, MD
Last Name of Individual filing lien (organizational lien claimants, leave blank)

4567 BROAD AVE
Address/PO Box (Please leave blank spaces between numbers, names or words)

WOODLAND HILLS — City
CA — State
12345 — Zip Code

(555) 486-9002
Phone

DWC/ WCAB Form 6 (Page 1) Rev(11/2008)

Fig. 9.5 Notice and request for lien. This form is used to file a lien on behalf of a physician who is providing services to a workers' compensation patient and has not been paid.

Lien Claimant's Attorney/Representative, if any

☑ Law Firm/Attorney ☐ Non-Attorney Representative ☐ Lien Claimant not represented

CORPORATE REPRESENTATIVE LAWYERS FIRM
Lien Claimant Law Firm/Representative

DANIEL
First Name

5. Attorney for the physician.

DIAMOND
Last Name

P.O. BOX 34285
Address/PO Box (Please leave blank spaces between numbers, names or words)

SIMI VALLEY	CA	17394
City	State	Zip Code

(555) 938-4930
Phone

Employer

6. Injured patient employer.

THE CONK OUT COMPANY
Name

45 SOUTH GORMAN ST.
Address/PO Box (Please leave blank spaces between numbers, names or words)

WOODLAND HILLS	CA	12345
City	State	Zip Code

Insurance Carrier or Claims Administrator

7. Workers' comp insurance company.

STATE COMPENSATION INSURANCE FUND
Name

P.O. BOX 28918
Address/PO Box (Please leave blank spaces between numbers, names or words)

FRESNO	CA	93729
City	State	Zip Code

Employer or Claims Administrator Attorney/Representative (if known)

8. Attorney for employer.

NONE
Name

Address/PO Box (Please leave blank spaces between numbers, names or words)

City	State	Zip Code

DWC/ WCAB Form 6 (Page 2) Rev(11/2008)

Fig. 9.5, cont'd.

The lien claimant hereby requests the Workers' Compensation Appeals Board to determine and allow as a lien the sum of $ 45,362.90 (Total Lien Amount) against any amount now due or which may hereafter become payable as compensation to the above-named employee on account of the above-claimed injury.

9. Amount of outstanding medical claims by this physician. If additional fees are incurred, an amended lien is filed with an updated amount.

This request and claim for lien is for (mark appropriate box):

- [x] A reasonable attorney's fee for legal services pertaining to any claim for compensation either before the appeals board or before any of the appellate courts, and the reasonable disbursements in connection therewith. (Labor Code § 4903 (a).)
- [ ] The reasonable expense incurred by or on behalf of the injured employee, as provided by Labor Code § 4600. (Labor Code § 4903 (b).)
- [ ] Reasonable expense incurred by or on behalf of the injured employee for medical-legal expenses. (Labor Code § 4903 (b).)
- [ ] The reasonable value of the living expenses of an injured employee or of his or her dependents, subsequent to the injury. (Labor Code § 4903 (c).)
- [ ] The reasonable burial expenses of the deceased employee. (Labor Code § 4903 (d).)
- [ ] The reasonable living expenses of the spouse or minor children of the injured employee, or both, subsequent to the date of the injury, where the employee has deserted or is neglecting his or her family. (Labor Code § 4903 (e).)
- [ ] The reasonable fee for interpreter's services performed on ___________ 20 __ . (Labor Code § 4600 (f).)
- [ ] The amount of indemnification granted by the California Victims of Crime Program. (Labor Code § 4903 (i).)
- [ ] The amount of compensation, including expenses of medical treatment, and recoverable costs that have been paid by the Asbestos Workers' Account. (Labor Code § 4903 (j).)

10. Various requests depending on the facts of the case.

- [ ] Other Lien(s): Specify nature and statutory basis.

NOTE: ITEMIZED STATEMENT JUSTIFYING THE LIEN MUST BE ATTACHED

11. This box should always be checked.

- [x] A copy of the lien claim and supporting documents was served by mail or delivered to each of the above-named parties.

Daniel Diamond	Raymond Skeleton, MD	6-5-XX
(Signature of Attorney/Representative for Lien Claimant)	(Signature of Lien Claimant)	Date (MM/DD/YYYY)
Physician's attorney	Physician's signature	

DWC/ WCAB Form 6 (Page 3) Rev(11/2008)

Fig. 9.5, cont'd.

MEDICAL REPORTS

Health Information Record Keeping

If a private patient comes to the office with a work-related injury or illness, a separate health record (chart) and financial record (ledger) should be set up for the work-related injury. A private health record should never be combined with a workers' compensation case record because separate disclosure laws apply to each and the workers' compensation case may go to court. Some medical practices use a colored file folder or tabs for the workers' compensation health record, which makes filing of all private and workers' compensation documents easier for the insurance billing specialist. If two charts are maintained, it is easy to pull the workers' compensation health record and financial accounting record quickly without having to go through the patient's previously unrelated private health records.

It is preferable that a patient not be scheduled to see a health care provider of services for a workers' compensation follow-up examination and an unrelated complaint during the same appointment. Separate appointments (back to back, if necessary) should be arranged. This allows for separate dictation without intermixing the required documentation for each chart.

! COMPLIANCE ALERT

Workers' Compensation and HIPAA Compliance

It is important to note that workers' compensation programs are not included under the definition of a "health plan" as identified in the Health Insurance Portability and Accountability Act (HIPAA). Therefore workers' compensation programs are not required to comply with HIPAA standards; however, it is beneficial to workers' compensation insurance payers and health care providers to use the adopted HIPAA Transaction and Code Set (TCS) to work harmoniously within the claims processing activities used throughout the industry.

! COMPLIANCE ALERT

Privacy and Confidentiality

The Health Insurance Portability and Accountability Act (HIPAA) Privacy Rule allows for the disclosure of protected health information (PHI) to workers' compensation insurers, state administrators, and employers to the extent necessary to comply with laws relating to workers' compensation. The HIPAA Privacy Rule recognizes the legitimate need of insurers and other entities involved in the workers' compensation systems to have access to individuals' health information as authorized by state or other law. Because of the significant variability among such laws, the HIPAA Privacy Rule permits disclosures of health information for workers' compensation purposes in several different ways.

1. *Disclosures without Individual Authorization.* The HIPAA Privacy Rule permits covered entities to disclose PHI to workers' compensation insurers, state administrators, employers, and other persons or entities involved in workers' compensation systems without the individual's authorization. This relates to workers' compensation injuries or illnesses and federal programs, such as Black Lung Benefits Act, Federal Employees' Compensation Act (FECA), the Longshore and Harbor Workers' Compensation Act (LHWCA), and Energy Employees Occupational Illness Compensation Program Act. The disclosure must comply with and be limited to what the state law requires. Disclosure is allowed for purposes of obtaining payment for any health care provided to the injured or ill worker.
2. *Disclosures with Individual Authorization.* Covered entities may disclose PHI to workers' compensation insurers and others involved in workers' compensation systems to which the individual has provided his or her authorization for the release of the information to the entity. For example, if a patient's attorney calls the physician's office for information, it is only ethical and legal to get a signed authorization from the patient and to ask permission from the insurance carrier before giving out any medical information. The contract exists between the physician and insurance carrier, not the physician and patient.
3. *Minimum Necessary.* Covered entities are required to limit the amount of PHI disclosed to the minimum necessary to accomplish the workers' compensation purpose. Under this requirement, PHI may be shared for such purposes to the full extent authorized by state or other law.

Documentation

In workers' compensation cases, it is important for the service provider to document how the injury occurred and where the injury occurred. Diagnosis codes will be assigned to relay this information on the claim form. For example, if a machinist receives a large cut on his hand because of operating a machine, this should be clearly documented; even the type of machine (saw, lathe, drill) should be specified. Where the injury occurred should also be documented in detail.

Terminology

Most workers' compensation cases involve accidents causing body injuries. Therefore one should become familiar with anatomic terms, directional and range-of-motion words, types of fractures, body activity terms, and words that describe pain and symptoms (Box 9.2). This terminology appears in progress chart notes and workers' compensation injury reports. The more knowledgeable one becomes about the meaning of the documentation, the more proficient one will be in knowing whether the procedure and diagnostic codes assigned are substantiated or if code selection is deficient and should be enhanced for better payment. One should learn how to spell the words and find the definitions of the words in the dictionary.

Directional terms are commonly used when a case is being rated for PD. A range-of-motion (**ROM**) test determines whether the body part can move to the full extent possible. Often, after an injury to an extremity or joint, there is restriction of motion and loss of strength (for example, grip). ROM can be improved with activity and therapy. It is measured with special measurement devices and documented each time a patient is examined. Fractures can occur from falling, blows, impact hits, a disease process, or direct violence, such as in an automobile accident. Healing may take months and depends on the location and severity of the injured part, associated injury, and complications or infections.

REPORTING REQUIREMENTS

Employer's Report

The laws clearly state that the injured person must promptly report the work-related injury or illness to his or her employer or immediate supervisor, which may be a safety officer in some businesses. By law in most states the employer must send an Employer's Report of Occupational Injury or Illness form

BOX 9.2 Terms that Describe Intensity of Pain and Frequency of Occurrence of Symptoms

Definitions that describe intensity of pain and frequency of symptoms were developed to assist the physician when documenting subjective complaints.

- A *severe* pain would preclude the activity causing the pain.
- A *moderate* pain could be tolerated but would cause marked handicap in the performance of the activity precipitating the pain.
- A *slight* pain could be tolerated but would cause some handicap in the performance of the activity precipitating the pain.
- A *minimal (mild)* pain would constitute an annoyance but would cause no handicap in the performance of the particular activity. It would be considered a nonratable permanent disability (PD).
- *Occasional* means approximately 25% of the time.
- *Intermittent* means approximately 50% of the time.
- *Frequent* means approximately 75% of the time.
- *Constant* means 90% to 100% of the time.

(Fig. 9.6) to the insurance company. The time limit for submission of this form varies from immediately to as long as 30 days in different states (Table 9.3). Many states have adopted the form shown in Fig. 9.6 to meet the requirements of the federal Occupational Safety Health Administration (OSHA) Act of 1970 and for state statistical purposes. OSHA was established to protect employees against on-the-job health and safety hazards. Work standards were designed to minimize exposure to on the job hazards, such as faulty machinery, noise, dust, and toxic chemical fumes. Employers are required by law to meet these health and safety standards. Failure to do so can result in fines against the employer.

Medical Service Order

In addition to the employer's report, the employer may complete and sign a medical service order, giving this to the injured employee to take to the health care organization or physician's office (Fig. 9.7). This authorizes the health care organization to treat the injured employee. The form should be photocopied and the copy retained by the health care organization. The original should be attached to the Doctor's First Report of Occupational Injury or Illness (preliminary report). An employer may prefer to write the service order on his or her business letterhead, on billhead, or simply on a piece of scratch paper.

Authorizations may also be obtained over the telephone. However, if a patient arrives for an appointment without written authorization, the employer can be telephoned and asked to have the authorization e-mailed or faxed to give permission for treatment. Subsequently, if payment is not received or the claim is disputed, it may be easier to collect if a copy of the written authorization is included when sending collection follow-up correspondence.

A copayment is not collected for a workers' compensation patient who submits a completed Employer's Report of Occupational Injury or Illness form (Fig. 9.8). If a patient was injured on the job but does not have this form, standard protocol is to bill the patient's primary health insurance and collect the appropriate copayment. The patient may decide to bring in the Employer's Report of Occupational Injury or Illness at a later time. The physician has the right to reevaluate the patient under the workers' compensation policy and submit a medical service order (Fig. 9.9).

If outside testing or treatment is necessary, authorization should be obtained from the employer or the adjuster for the insurance company. When this is done by telephone, the name of the procedure or test and the medical necessity for it should be stated. The name and title of the person giving authorization should be obtained and written in the patient's chart and on the order form along with the date. No authorization numbers are issued in workers' compensation cases.

The insurance adjuster handling the case should be contacted if a translator is necessary for a workers' compensation patient. He or she should make arrangements for an official translator to be present for all appointments. A member of the patient's family or the patient's friend should not be allowed to serve as a translator because there may be no legal recourse for the health care organization if miscommunicated information leads to a bad outcome.

SCENARIO: MULTIPLE INJURIES AND DATES OF INJURY

Problem: A patient has a workers' compensation claim for the left wrist and the right big toe. The patient needed to address pain in the left wrist on 10/4/20YY for carpel tunnel syndrome and was injured on 6/8/20YY when a steel bar crushed the patient's big toe.

Solution: Be sure to keep accurate records and file the medical claims for both injuries separately. If by chance the big toe injury was billed with the date of injury for the wrist, the claim will automatically be rejected. The insurance billing specialist should be accurate in posting the correct reimbursed amounts for the correct corresponding injury.

Physician's First Report

After the physician sees the injured person, he or she completes a medical evaluation of the patient and sends this medical report detailing the injury together with a CMS-1500 claim form (Fig. 9.10) and the Doctor's First Report of Occupational Injury or Illness form (used in California) (see Fig. 9.16). Time limits for filing the physician's first report vary from state to state but can range from 24 hours to 14 days of seeing the patient. Some states either have modified the CMS-1500 claim form, which allows for additional data so that an accompanying medical report may not be required, or have created a first treatment medical report form.

If the physician prefers to submit a narrative letter, the medical report should include the components, if relevant, shown in Table 9.4. The time limit for filing this report varies; state requirements are provided in Table 9.3. Failure to file the report can be a misdemeanor. Copies of the report form go to the insurance carrier and the state. Because the report is a legal document, each copy *must be signed in ink* by the physician. The insurance company waits for the physician's report and bill, then issues payment to the physician. The case can be closed if there is no further treatment or disability.

State of California
EMPLOYER'S REPORT OF OCCUPATIONAL INJURY OR ILLNESS

Please complete in triplicate (type if possible) Mail two copies to:
XYZ Insurance Company
P.O. Box 5
Woodland Hills XY 12345

OSHA CASE NO. # 18
FATALITY ☐

Any person who makes or causes to be made any knowingly false or fraudulent material statement or material representation for the purpose of obtaining or denying workers compensation benefits or payments is guilty of a felony.

California law requires employers to report within **five days** of knowledge every occupational injury or illness which results in lost time beyond the date of the incident **OR** requires medical treatment beyond first aid. If an employee subsequently dies as a result of a previously reported injury or illness, the employer must file within **five days** of knowledge an amended report indicating death. In addition, every serious injury, illness, or death must be **reported immediately** by telephone or telegraph to the nearest office of the California Division of Occupational Safety and Health.

EMPLOYER

		Please do not use this column
1. FIRM NAME The Conk Out Company	Ia. Policy Number B12345	CASE NUMBER
2. MAILING ADDRESS: (Number, Street, City, Zip) 45 South Gorman St. Woodland Hills, XY 12345	2a. Phone Number (555) 430-3488	OWNERSHIP
3. LOCATION if different from Mailing Address (Number, Street, City and Zip)	3a. Location Code	
4. NATURE OF BUSINESS; e.g.. Painting contractor, wholesale grocer, sawmill, hotel, etc. Plumbing Repair	5. State unemployment insurance acct.no	INDUSTRY
6. TYPE OF EMPLOYER: ☑ Private ☐ State ☐ County ☐ City ☐ School District ☐ Other Gov't, Specify: ______		OCCUPATION

INJURY OR ILLNESS

7. DATE OF INJURY / ONSET OF ILLNESS (mm/dd/yy) 04/03/20	8. TIME INJURY/ILLNESS OCCURRED ______ AM 2:00 PM	9. TIME EMPLOYEE BEGAN WORK 8:00 AM ______ PM	10. IF EMPLOYEE DIED, DATE OF DEATH (mm/dd/yy)	SEX
11. UNABLE TO WORK FOR AT LEAST ONE FULL DAY AFTER DATE OF INJURY? ☑ Yes ☐ No	12. DATE LAST WORKED (mm/dd/yy) 04/03/20	13. DATE RETURNED TO WORK (mm/dd/yy)	14. IF STILL OFF WORK, CHECK THIS BOX: ☑	AGE
15. PAID FULL DAYS WAGES FOR DATE OF INJURY OR LAST DAY WORKED? ☑ Yes ☐ No	16. SALARY BEING CONTINUED? ☐ Yes ☑ No	17. DATE OF EMPLOYER'S KNOWLEDGE /NOTICE OF INJURY/ILLNESS (mm/dd/yy) 04/03/20	18. DATE EMPLOYEE WAS PROVIDED CLAIM FORM (mm/dd/yy) 04/03/20	DAILY HOURS

19. SPECIFIC INJURY/ILLNESS AND PART OF BODY AFFECTED, MEDICAL DIAGNOSIS if available, e.g.. Second degree burns on right arm, tendonitis on left elbow, lead poisoning
Ankle Injury. Swelling, possible fracture.

20. LOCATION WHERE EVENT OR EXPOSURE OCCURRED (Number, Street, City, Zip): 45 Gorman St. Woodland Hills, XY 12345
20a. COUNTY:
21. ON EMPLOYER'S PREMISES? ☑ Yes ☐ No

22. DEPARTMENT WHERE EVENT OR EXPOSURE OCCURRED, e.g.. Shipping department, machine shop.
Stock Room
23. Other Workers injured or ill in this event? ☐ Yes ☑ No

24. EQUIPMENT, MATERIALS AND CHEMICALS THE EMPLOYEE WAS USING WHEN EVENT OR EXPOSURE OCCURRED, e.g.. Acetylene, welding torch, farm tractor, scaffold
6 Foot Ladder

25. SPECIFIC ACTIVITY THE EMPLOYEE WAS PERFORMING WHEN EVENT OR EXPOSURE OCCURRED, e.g.. Welding seams of metal forms, loading boxes onto truck.
Climbed ladder to remove a ream of paper from top shelf; Fell

26. HOW INJURY/ILLNESS OCCURRED. DESCRIBE SEQUENCE OF EVENTS. SPECIFY OBJECT OR EXPOSURE WHICH DIRECTLY PRODUCED THE INJURY/ILLNESS, e.g.. Worker stepped back to inspect work and slipped on scrap material. As he fell, he brushed against fresh weld, and burned right hand. USE SEPARATE SHEET IF NECESSARY
Worker climbed ladder to remove a ream of paper from the top shelf in stock room. She was descending and mis-stepped falling to the floor. She tried to land upright and her leg took the brunt of the fall.

27. Name and address of physician (number, street, city, zip)
Raymond Skeleton, MD 4567 Broad Ave., Woodland Hills, XY 12345
27a. Phone Number

28. Hospitalized as an inpatient overnight? ☐ No ☐ Yes If yes then, name and address of hospital (number, street, city, zip)
28a. Phone Number
29. Employee treated in emergency room? ☑ Yes ☐ No

Right column (Please do not use this column): DAYS PER WEEK; WEEKLY HOURS; WEEKLY WAGE; COUNTY; NATURE OF INJURY; PART OF BODY; SOURCE; EVENT; SECONDARY SOURCE; EXTENT OF INJURY

ATTENTION This form contains information relating to employee health and must be used in a manner that protects the confidentiality of employees to the extent possible while the information is being used for occupational safety and health purposes. See CCR Title 8 14300.29 (b)(6)-(10) & 14300.35(b)(2)(E)2.
Note: Shaded boxes indicate confidential employee information as listed in CCR Title 8 14300.35(b)(2)(E)2*.

EMPLOYEE

30. EMPLOYEE NAME: Ima B. Hurt
31. SOCIAL SECURITY NUMBER:
32. DATE OF BIRTH (mm/dd/yy):
33. HOME ADDRESS (Number, Street, City, Zip):
33a. PHONE NUMBER:
34. SEX ☐ Male ☒ Female
35. OCCUPATION (Regular job title, NO initials, abbreviations or numbers)
36. DATE OF HIRE (mm/dd/yy)
37. EMPLOYEE USUALLY WORKS ______ hours per day, ______ days per week, ______ total weekly hours
37a. EMPLOYMENT STATUS ☐ regular, full-time ☐ part-time ☐ temporary ☐ seasonal
37b. UNDER WHAT CLASS CODE OF YOUR POLICY WHERE WAGES ASSIGNED
38. GROSS WAGES/SALARY $ ______ per ______
39. OTHER PAYMENTS NOT REPORTED AS WAGES/SALARY (e.g. tips, meals, overtime, bonuses, etc.)? ☐ Yes ☐ No

Completed By (type or print)	Signature & Title	Date (mm/dd/yy)

* Confidential information may be disclosed only to the employee, former employee, or their personal representative (CCR Title 8 14300.35), to others for the purpose of processing a workers' compensation or other insurance claim; and under certain circumstances to a public health or law enforcement agency or to a consultant hired by the employer (CCR Title 8 14300.30). CCR Title 8 14300.40 requires provision upon request to certain state and federal workplace safety agencies.

FORM 5020 (Rev7) June 2002 FILING OF THIS FORM IS NOT AN ADMISSION OF LIABILITY

Fig. 9.6 Employer's Report of Occupational Injury or Illness. This form complies with Occupational Safety and Health Administration (OSHA) requirements and California State Workers' Compensation laws.

TABLE 9.3 Employers' or Physicians' Report of Accident

Jurisdiction	Time Limit	Injuries Covered
Alabama	Within 15 days	Death or disability exceeding 3 days
Alaska	Within 10 days	Death, injury, disease, or infection
American Samoa	Within 10 days of employer notification	Death, injury, or disease
Arizona	Within 10 days	All injuries
Arkansas	Within 10 days from notice of injury	Indemnity, injuries, or death[2]
		Controverted, medical only
California	Immediately (employer)	Death or serious injuries
	As prescribed	Disability of 1 day or more, other than first aid
	Within 5 days	Occupational diseases or pesticide poisoning
Colorado	Immediately 10 days[3]	Death
		Injuries causing lost time of 3 days or more or 3 shifts
		Any accident in which three or more employees are injured
		Occupational disease cases
		Cases of permanent physical impairment
Connecticut	Within 7 days or as directed	Disability of 1 day or more
Delaware	Within 48 hours[4]	Death or injuries requiring hospitalization
	Within 10 days	Other injuries
District of Columbia	Within 10 days	All injuries
Florida	Within 24 hours[5]	Death
	Within 7 days to carrier	All injuries requiring medical treatment
Georgia	Within 21 days[6]	All injuries requiring medical or surgical treatment or causing more than 7 days of absence
Hawaii	Within 48 hours	Death
	Within 7 working days	All injuries
Idaho	As soon as practicable but not later than 10 days after the accident[7]	All injuries requiring treatment by a physician or absence from work for 1 or more days
Illinois	Within 2 working days	Death or serious injuries
	Between the 15th and 25th of the month	Disability of more than 3 days
	As soon as determinable	Permanent disability
Indiana	Within 7 working days[8]	Disability of more than 1 day
Iowa	Within 4 days	Disability of more than 3 days, PP disability, or death
Kansas	Within 28 days of knowledge[9]	Death cases or disability of more than remainder of day or shift.
Kentucky	Within 7 days[10]	Disability of more than 1 day
Louisiana	Within 10 days of employer's actual knowledge of injury[11]	Lost time over 1 week or death
Maine	Within 7 days of ER's knowledge of lost time	Only injuries causing 1 day or more of lost time[13]
Maryland	Within 10 days	Disability of more than 3 days
Massachusetts	Within 7 days, except Sundays and holidays[12]	Disability of 5 or more calendar days
Michigan	Immediately	Death, disability of 7 days or more, and specific losses
Minnesota	Within 48 hours	Death or serious injury
	Within 14 days	Disability of 3 days or more
Mississippi	Within 10 days[13]	Death or disability of more than 5 days[14]
Missouri	Within 30 days[14]	Death or injury
Montana	Within 6 days	All injuries
Nebraska	Within 10 days[15]	All injuries or diagnosed occupational diseases that result in death, time away from work, restricted work, or termination of employment; loss of consciousness; or medical treatment other than first aid
Nevada	Within 6 working days after report from physician[16]	All injuries requiring medical treatment
New Hampshire	Within 5 calendar days	All injuries involving lost time or medical expenses
New Jersey	Within 3 weeks of learning of occupational disease	All injuries, other than those requiring first aid
New Mexico	Within 10 days of employer notification[17]	Any injury or illness resulting in 7 or more days of lost time
New York	Within 10 days[18]	Disability of 1 day beyond working day or shift on which accident occurred or requiring medical care beyond two first aid treatments
North Carolina	Within 5 days of knowledge of injury or allegation	Disability of more than 1 day or charges for medical compensation exceeding the amount set by the commission
North Dakota	Within 7 days	All injuries
Ohio	Within 1 week	Injuries causing total disability of 7 days or more
Oklahoma	Within 10 days of knowledge of death or injury	Fatalities; all injuries causing lost time or requiring treatment away from worksite
Oregon	Within 5 days after employer knowledge[19]	All claims or injuries that may result in compensable inquiry claims injuries
Pennsylvania	Within 48 hours	Death
	After 7 days but not later than 10 days	Disability of 1 day or more
Rhode Island	Within 48 hours	Death
	Within 10 days	Disability of 3 days or more and all injuries requiring medical treatment
		Any claim resulting in medical expense

TABLE 9.3 Employers' or Physicians' Report of Accident[1]—cont'd

Jurisdiction	Time Limit	Injuries Covered
South Carolina	Within 10 days	All injuries requiring medical attention costing more than $500, more than 1-day disability, or permanency
South Dakota	Within 7 days	Disability of 7 days or more, other than first aid or injuries requiring medical treatment
Tennessee	Within 14 days	Report of Injury must be filed when employee receives medical care outside of employer's premises
Texas	Within 8 days[20]	Lost time of more than 1 day or death/an occupational disease
Utah	Within 7 days	All injuries requiring medical attention
Vermont	Within 72 hours; Sundays and legal holidays excluded	Disability of 1 day or more requiring medical care
Virgin Islands	Within 8 days	Injury or disease
Virginia	Within 10 days[21]	All injuries
Washington	Immediately	Deaths and accidents resulting in workers' hospitalizations or inability to work
West Virginia	Within 5 days	All injuries
Wisconsin	Within 14 days	Disability beyond 3-day waiting period
Wyoming	Within 10 days	All injuries
Federal Employees' Compensation Act	Within 10 working days	All injuries involving medical expenses, disability, or death
Longshore and Harbor Workers' Compensation Act	10 days	Injuries that cause loss of one or more shifts of work or death

Time limits for filing the Report of Accident and the injuries covered, vary from state to state. Additional details related to time limits and injuries covered should be further investigated by the Medical Billing Specialist for the jurisdiction they are billing claims to.

WORKERS' COMPENSATION
MEDICAL SERVICE ORDER

To: Dr./Clinic Martin Feelgood, MD

Address 4567 Broad Avenue, Woodland Hills, XY 12345

We are sending Mrs. Ima Hurt

Address 300 East Central Ave., Woodland Hills, XY 12345

Social Security No. 120-XX-6542 Date of birth 3-4-1966
to you for treatment in accordance with the terms of the Workers' Compensation Laws. Please submit your report to the XYZ Insurance Company at once. Compensation cannot be paid without complete medical information.

Insurance carrier XYZ Insurance Company

Address P.O. Box 5, Woodland Hills, XY 12345 Telephone 555-271-0562

Employer The Conk Out Company

Address 45 S. Gorman St.,Woodland Hills, XY 12345 Telephone 555-430-3488

Signature J.D. HAWKINS, MD Date 4-3-20XX
If patient is able to return to work today or tomorrow, please show date and time below — sign and give to patient to return to employer. If there are any work restrictions indicate on the back of this form. Please submit your usual first report in any case.

Date/Time ____________ By ____________

Fig. 9.7 Medical service order.

State of California EMPLOYER'S REPORT OF OCCUPATIONAL INJURY OR ILLNESS	Please complete in triplicate (type, if possible). Mail two copies to: XYZ Insurance Company PO Box 5 Woodland Hills, XY 12345	OSHA Case No. # 18 ☐ Fatality

Any person who makes or causes to be made any knowingly false or fraudulent material statement or material representation for the purpose of obtaining or denying workers' compensation benefits or payments is guilty of a felony.

NOTICE: California law requires employers to report within **five days** of knowledge every occupational injury or illness which results in lost time beyond the date of the incident **OR** requires medical treatment beyond first aid. If an employee subsequently dies as a result of a previously reported injury or illness, the employer must file within **five days** of knowledge an amended report indicating death. In addition, every serious injury/illness, or death must be reported **immediately** by telephone or telegraph to the nearest office of the California Division of Occupational Safety and Health.

EMPLOYER

- 1. FIRM NAME: The Conk Out Company
- 1A. POLICY NUMBER: B12345
- 2. MAILING ADDRESS (Number and Street, City, ZIP): 45 South Gorman St. Woodland Hills, XY 12345
- 2A. PHONE NUMBER: 555-430-3488
- 3. LOCATION, IF DIFFERENT FROM MAILING ADDRESS (Number and Street, City, ZIP):
- 3A. LOCATION CODE:
- 4. NATURE OF BUSINESS, e.g., painting contractor, wholesale grocer, sawmill, hotel, etc.: Plumbing Repair
- 5. STATE UNEMPLOYMENT INSURANCE ACCT. NO.:
- 6. TYPE OF EMPLOYER: [X] PRIVATE ☐ STATE ☐ CITY ☐ COUNTY ☐ SCHOOL DIST. ☐ OTHER GOVERNMENT - SPECIFY ______

EMPLOYEE

- 7. EMPLOYEE NAME: Ima B. Hurt
- 8. SOCIAL SECURITY NUMBER: 120-XX-6542
- 9. DATE OF BIRTH (mm/dd/yy): 3-4-66
- 10. HOME ADDRESS (Number and Street, City, ZIP): 300 E.Central Ave. Woodland Hills, XY 12345
- 10A. PHONE NUMBER: 555-476-9899
- 11. SEX: ☐ MALE [X] FEMALE
- 12. OCCUPATION (Regular job title — NO initials, abbreviations or numbers): Clerk Typist
- 13. DATE OF HIRE (mm/dd/yy): 1-20-86
- 14. EMPLOYEE USUALLY WORKS: 8 hours per day; 5 days per week; 40 total weekly hours
- 14A. EMPLOYMENT STATUS (check applicable status at time of injury): X regular full-time ___ part-time ___ temporary ___ seasonal
- 14B. Under what class code of your policy were wages assigned? 7219
- 15. GROSS WAGES/SALARY: $ 700.00 per week
- 16. OTHER PAYMENTS NOT REPORTED AS WAGES/SALARY (e.g. tips, meals, lodging, overtime, bonuses, etc.)? ☐ YES $ ______ PER ______ [X] NO

INJURY OR ILLNESS

- 17. DATE OF INJURY OR ONSET OF ILLNESS (mm/dd/yy): 4-3-XX
- 18. TIME INJURY/ILLNESS OCCURRED: ______ A.M. 2:00 P.M.
- 19. TIME EMPLOYEE BEGAN WORK: 8:00 A.M. ______ P.M.
- 20. IF EMPLOYEE DIED, DATE OF DEATH (mm/dd/yy):
- 21. UNABLE TO WORK AT LEAST ONE FULL DAY AFTER DATE OF INJURY? [X] YES ☐ NO
- 22. DATE LAST WORKED (mm/dd/yy): 4-3-XX
- 23. DATE RETURNED TO WORK (mm/dd/yy):
- 24. IF STILL OFF WORK, CHECK THIS BOX [X]
- 25. PAID FULL WAGES FOR DAY OF INJURY OR LAST DAY WORKED? [X] YES ☐ NO
- 26. SALARY BEING CONTINUED? ☐ YES [X] NO
- 27. DATE OF EMPLOYER'S KNOWLEDGE/NOTICE OF INJURY/ILLNESS (mm/dd/yy): 4-3-XX
- 28. DATE EMPLOYEE WAS PROVIDED: 4-3-XX
- 29. SPECIFIC INJURY/ILLNESS AND PART OF BODY AFFECTED, MEDICAL DIAGNOSIS, if available, e.g., second degree burns on right arm, tendonitis of left elbow, lead poisoning.: ankle injury swelling, possible fracture
- 30. LOCATION WHERE EVENT OR EXPOSURE OCCURRED (Number, Street, City): 45 South Gorman St. Woodland Hills, XY 12345
- 30B. ON EMPLOYERS PREMISES? [X] YES ☐ NO
- 31. DEPARTMENT WHERE EVENT OR EXPOSURE OCCURRED, e.g., shipping department, machine shop.: stock room
- 32. OTHER WORKERS INJURED/ILL IN THIS EVENT? ☐ YES [X] NO
- 33. EQUIPMENT, MATERIALS AND CHEMICALS THE EMPLOYEE WAS USING WHEN EVENT OR EXPOSURE OCCURRED, e.g., acetylene, welding torch, farm tractor, scaffold.: 6 foot ladder
- 34. SPECIFY ACTIVITY THE EMPLOYEE WAS PERFORMING WHEN EVENT OR EXPOSURE OCCURRED, e.g., welding seams of metal forms, loading boxes onto truck.: climbed ladder to remove a ream of paper from shelf; fell
- 35. HOW INJURY/ILLNESS OCCURRED. DESCRIBE SEQUENCE OF EVENTS. SPECIFY OBJECT OR EXPOSURE WHICH DIRECTLY PRODUCED THE INJURY/ILLNESS, e.g., worker stepped back to inspect work and slipped on scrap material. As he fell, he brushed against fresh weld, and burned right hand. USE SEPARATE SHEET IF NECESSARY.: Worker climbed ladder to remove a ream of paper from top shelf in stock room. She was descending and mis-stepped falling to the floor. She tried to land upright, and her left leg took the brunt of the fall.
- 36. NAME AND ADDRESS OF PHYSICIAN (Number and Street, City, ZIP): Raymond Skeleton, MD 4567 Broad Ave., Woodland Hills, XY 12345
- 36A. PHONE NUMBER: 555-486-9002
- 37. IF HOSPITALIZED AS AN INPATIENT, NAME AND ADDRESS OF HOSPITAL (Number and Street, City, ZIP):
- 37A. PHONE NUMBER:

DO NOT USE THIS COLUMN: Case No. | Ownership | Industry | Occupation | Sex | Age | Daily Hours | Days per week | Weekly hours | Weekly wage | County | Nature of injury | Part of body | Source | Event | Sec. Source | Extent of injury

Completed by (type or print)	Signature	Title	Date
J.D. Hawkins	J. D. Hawkins	owner	4-3-XX

FILING THIS REPORT IS NOT AN ADMISSION OF LIABILITY

Fig. 9.8 Employer's Report of Occupational Injury or Illness. This form complies with Occupational Safety and Health Administration (OSHA) requirements and California State Workers' Compensation laws.

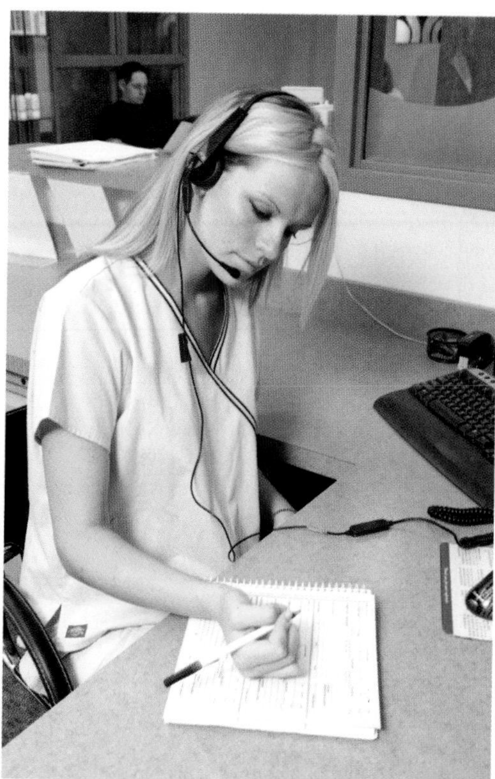

Fig. 9.9 Receptionist receiving a medical service order via telephone for the worker to receive medical services.

Progress or Supplemental Report

In a TD case, a supplemental report is sent to the insurance carrier after 2 to 4 weeks of treatment to give information on the status of the patient. If there is a significant change in the prognosis, a detailed progress report, referred to as a **reexamination report,** is sent to the insurance carrier. Subsequent progress or supplemental reports should be sent to the insurance carrier after each hospitalization and office visit to update the progress of a case (Fig. 9.11). Every evaluation and report submitted must be mailed promptly to the insurance company along with a CMS-1500 form. If the disability is ongoing over time, monthly progress reports should be submitted. A follow-up report must contain the following information:

Date of most recent examination
Present condition and progress since last report
Measurements of function
X-ray or laboratory report since last examination
Treatment (give type and duration)
Work status (patient working or estimated date of return to work if patient is still temporarily disabled)
PD to be anticipated

Final Report

TD ends when the physician tells the insurance carrier that the patient is able to return to work or if the disability is longer than 24 months. When the TD case is closing, the physician will submit a final evaluation report that provides an overview of the care provided and the patient's progress with the disability. When the patient resumes work, the insurance carrier closes the case and the TD benefits cease.

A physician's final report indicating any impairment or PD should be submitted with a CMS-1500 claim form.

CLAIM SUBMISSION

Financial Responsibility

The contract for treatment in a personal illness or injury case is between the health care organization and patient, who is responsible for the entire bill. However, when an individual is being treated as a workers' compensation case, the financial responsibility exists between the health care organization and the workers' compensation insurance company. As long as treatment is authorized by the insurance carrier, the insurance company is responsible for payment. A health care organization that agrees to treat a workers' compensation case must agree to accept payment in full according to the workers' compensation fee schedule. For workers' compensation cases, patients are not financially responsible so copayments or coinsurances cannot be collected.

An injured worker is under obligation to be evaluated by the employer's physician. However, the patient has the right to choose a different physician to seek care, but this request needs to be approved by the employer.

Some states have a medical program wherein employers can reduce their workers' compensation rates by paying the first $1000 in medical bills. This is similar to a deductible for the employer's policy. The physician will first file the insurance claim with the workers' compensation insurance plan. The explanation of benefits will then direct the physician to bill the employer for the deductible amount. The statement should be sent to the employer for payment in this situation; it should not be sent to the patient.

Health insurance information should always be obtained in case services provided are determined to be unrelated to work injury or illness. To assist in informing patients of financial responsibility for nonrelated illness, the worker should sign an agreement for nonrelated medical expenses, as shown in Fig. 9.12. If the workers' compensation carrier declares that the case is not work related, bill the patient's health insurance, attaching a copy of the refusal by the workers' compensation carrier.

When examining the injured or ill worker, the physician may discover a problem unrelated to the workers' compensation injury or illness. For example, the physician may determine that the patient has high blood pressure that is unrelated to the work injury or illness for which the patient is being examined. In that case the physician may bill the workers' compensation carrier for the examination but should code the claim carefully with regard to treatment of the injury. If treatment is initiated for the patient's high blood pressure, that portion of the examination becomes the financial obligation of the patient (or his or her private insurance plan) and not of the workers' compensation carrier.

DRAFT - NOT FOR OFFICIAL USE

CARRIER

HEALTH INSURANCE CLAIM FORM

APPROVED BY NATIONAL UNIFOR MCLAIM COMMITTEE (NUCC) 02/12

PICA PICA

PATIENT AND INSURED INFORMATION

1. MEDICARE (Medicare#) MEDICAID (Medicaid#) TRICARE (ID#DoD#) CHAMPVA (Member ID#) GROUP HEALTH PLAN (ID#) FECA BLK LUNG (ID#) OTHER [X] (ID#)

1a. INSURED'S I.D. NUMBER (For Program in Item 1): B785700

2. PATIENT'S NAME (Last Name, First Name, Middle Initial): Task, Lester, M

3. PATIENT'S BIRTH DATE MM DD YY: 05 06 1990 SEX M [X] F [ ]

4. INSURED'S NAME (Last Name, First Name, Middle Initial): Jonas Construction Company

5. PATIENT'S ADDRESS (No., Street): 5400 Holly Street

6. PATIENT RELATIONSHIP TO INSURED: Self [ ] Spouse [ ] Child [ ] Other [X]

7. INSURED'S ADDRESS (No., Street): 300 Main Street

CITY: Woodland Hills STATE: XY

8. RESERVED FOR NUCC USE

CITY: Woodland Hills STATE: XY

ZIP CODE: 12345-0000 TELEPHONE (Include Area Code): (555) 7833200

ZIP CODE: 12345-0000 TELEPHONE (Include Area Code): (555)3099800

9. OTHER INSURED'S NAME (Last Name, First Name, Middle Initial)

10. IS PATIENT'S CONDITION RELATED TO:

11. INSURED'S POLICY GROUP OR FECA NUMBER

a. OTHER INSURED'S POLICY OR GROUP NUMBER

a. EMPLOYMENT? (Current or Previous) [X] YES [ ] NO

a. INSURED'S DATE OF BIRTH MM DD YY SEX M [ ] F [ ]

b. RESERVED FOR NUCC USE

b. AUTO ACCIDENT? [ ] YES [X] NO PLACE (State)

b. OTHER CLAIM ID (Designated by NUCC)

c. RESERVED FOR NUCC USE

c. OTHER ACCIDENT? [ ] YES [X] NO

c. INSURANCE PLAN NAME OR PROGRAM NAME

d. INSURANCE PLAN NAME OR PROGRAM NAME

10d. CLAIM CODES (Designated by NUCC)

d. IS THERE ANOTHER HEALTH BENEFIT PLAN? [ ] YES [ ] NO *If yes*, complete items 9, 9a, and 9d.

READ BACK OF FORM BEFORE COMPLETING & SIGNING THIS FORM.

12. PATIENT'S OR AUTHORIZED PERSON'S SIGNATUREI authorize the release of any medical or other information necessary to process this claim. I also request payment of government benefits either to myself or to the party who accepts assignment below.

SIGNED ____ DATE ____

13. INSURED'S OR AUTHORIZED PERSON'S SIGNATURE I authorize payment of medical benefits to the undersigned physician or supplier for services described below.

SIGNED ____

PHYSICIAN OR SUPPLIER INFORMATION

14. DATE OF CURRENT: ILLNESS, INJURY, or PREGNANCY(LMP) MM DD YY: 08 11 20XX QUAL.

15. OTHER DATE QUAL. MM DD YY

16. DATES PATIENT UNABLE TO WORK IN CURRENT OCCUPATION FROM 11 08 20XX TO 12 08 20XX

17. NAME OF REFERRING PROVIDER OR OTHER SOURCE 17a. 17b. NPI

18. HOSPITALIZATION DATES RELATED TO CURRENT SERVICES FROM 11 08 20XX TO 11 10 20XX

19. ADDITIONAL CLAIM INFORMATION (Designated by NUCC)

20. OUTSIDE LAB? [ ] YES [X] NO $ CHARGES

21. DIAGNOSIS OR NATURE OF ILLNESS OR INJURY Relate A-L to service line below (24E) ICD Ind. 0

A. S82.001B B. C. D.
E. F. G. H.
I. J. K. L.

22. RESUBMISSION CODE ORIGINAL REF. NO.

23. PRIOR AUTHORIZATION NUMBER

	24. A. DATE(S) OF SERVICE From MM DD YY	To MM DD YY	B. PLACE OF SERVICE	C. EMG	D. PROCEDURES, SERVICES, OR SUPPLIES (Explain Unusual Circumstances) CPT/HCPCS	MODIFIER	E. DIAGNOSIS POINTER	F. $ CHARGES	G. DAYS OR UNITS	H. EPSDT Family Plan	I. ID. QUAL.	J. RENDERING PROVIDER ID. #
1	11 08 20XX		21		99222		A	125 00	1		NPI	46789377XX
2	11 08 20XX		21		27524		A	600 00	1		NPI	46789377XX
3											NPI	
4											NPI	
5											NPI	
6											NPI	

25. FEDERAL TAX I.D. NUMBER: 7544530XX SSN [ ] EIN [X]

26. PATIENT'S ACCOUNT NO.: 1577

27. ACCEPT ASSIGNMENT? (For govt. claims, see back) [ ] YES [ ] NO

28. TOTAL CHARGE: $ 725 00

29. AMOUNT PAID: $

30. Rsvd for NUCC Use: $

31. SIGNATURE OF PHYSICIAN OR SUPPLIER INCLUDING DEGREES OR CREDENTIALS (I certify that the statements on the reverse apply to this bill and are made a part thereof.)
Gregory Getwell MD
SIGNED *Gregory Getwell MD* DATE 110820XX

32. SERVICE FACILITY LOCATION INFORMATION
College Hospital
4500 Broad Ave
Woodland Hills XY 12345-0001
a. X950731067 b.

33. BILLING PROVIDER INFO & PH # (555)4590087
Gregory T Getwell MD
60 North State Street
Woodland Hills XY 12345-0001
a. 36644021CC b.

NUCC Instruction Manual available at: www.nucc.org PLEASE PRINT OR TYPE OMB APPROVAL PENDING

Fig. 9.10 Example of a completed CMS-1500 (02-12) Health Insurance Claim Form for a workers' compensation case. From National Uniform Claim Committee, NUCC Instruction Manual www.nucc.org

TABLE 9.4 Narrative Medical Report Issues, If Relevant

History	• Outline all specific details of accident, injury, or illness. • Physician should state whether there is a causal connection between the accident and conditions that may appear subsequently but are not obvious **sequelae** (diseased conditions following and usually resulting from a previous disease). If facts were obtained by reviewing prior records or x-ray films, the source should be mentioned. When a history is obtained through an interpreter, include that person's name.
Present complaints	Usually given as subjective complaints. *Subjective* refers to statements made by the patient about symptoms and how he or she feels. Subjective disability is evaluated by the following: • A description of the activity that produces the disability • The duration of the disability • The activities that are precluded by and those that can be performed with the disability • The means necessary for relief
Past history	Description of any previous, current, or subsequent medical information relevant to this injury or illness and whether there is a preexisting defect that might entitle the injured person to benefits from the subsequent injury fund or represent the actual cause of the present condition.
Examination findings	Usually given as objective findings. State all significant physical or psychiatric examination, testing, laboratory, or imaging findings.
Diagnostic impression	State all diagnostic findings and opinion as to relationship, if any, between the injury or disease and the condition diagnosed. Use diagnostic terminology that corresponds to the diagnostic code book.
Disability and prognosis	• Period during which the patient has been unable to work because of the injury or illness. • Opinion as to probable further temporary disability and a statement as to when the patient will be able to return to work or has returned to work. • Statement indicating whether the condition is currently permanent and stationary as well as the probability of future permanent disability. • Statement indicating that "All objective tests for organic pathology are negative. There is obviously a strong functional or emotional overlay," when a patient has multiple complaints but no clinical objective findings.
Work limitations	Description of any limitations to all activities.
Causation	Description of how the permanent disability is related to the patient's occupation and the specific injury or cumulative events causing the illness.

Fee Schedules

Each state has its own workers' compensation fee schedule. Some states have developed a workers' compensation fee schedule using a **relative value scale,** which is then adjusted with a **conversion factor.** The relative value scale considers the time, skills, and extent of the service provided by the health care provider of services. Each procedure is rated on how difficult it is, how long it takes, the training a health care provider must have to perform it, and expenses the health care organization incurs, including the cost of malpractice insurance. A conversion factor is then applied that sets a specific dollar amount for each of the sections of the fee schedule. Conversion factors may be adjusted to reflect regional differences and in some states are recalculated annually (Box 9.3).

Other states pay medical claims based on the Medicare fee schedule plus a certain percentage or have implemented managed care.

All claims are sent to the workers' compensation insurance, and no billing statements are sent to the patient. Fee schedules assist with the following:

1. They limit the amount that providers will be paid.
2. They make the allowable charges and procedures more consistent.
3. They provide follow-up procedures in case of a fee dispute.

Most workers' compensation fee schedules list the maximum reimbursement for all covered health care services, and service providers are expected to accept as payment in full. Service providers may ask for exceptions to the maximum reimbursement if any of the following factors can be supported:

- Provider's medical training, qualifications, and time in practice may warrant a higher reimbursement.
- Nature of services provided was more complex than what reimbursement allows for.
- Reimbursements for the same services in other regions are typically higher than what are allowed in the fee schedule.
- There are other relevant economic factors of the health care organization.
- Any unusual circumstances in the case.

The insurance carrier may pay the additional amount if documentation is sent validating the fee and noting any of the aforementioned considerations.

Reviews or audits may be performed by the following entities to enforce fee schedules:

- The state agency or state fund responsible for overseeing workers' compensation (bill review)
- The payer, employer, or insurance carrier (bill review)
- The payer (bill review) and state agency (compliance audit)

Helpful Billing Tips

The following are helpful hints for billing workers' compensation claims.

1. Ask whether the injury occurred within the scope of employment, and verify insurance information with the benefits coordinator for the employer. This will promote filing initial claims with the correct insurance carrier.
2. Obtain the date of injury. This date will be associated with the patient's care for the duration of patient care for the specific episode.

ATTENDING PHYSICIAN'S REPORT

Employee: Mrs. Ima B. Hurt Claim number: 120 XX 6542

Employer: The Conk Out Company Date of injury(ies): 4-3-20XX Date of next exam: 4-24-20XX

Date of this exam: 4-10-XX Patient Social Security No: 120 XX 6542

Current diagnosis: 824.6 closed fracture; L. trimalleolar ankle
(include ICD•9 code)

PATIENT STATUS

Since the last exam, this patient's condition has:

☒ improved as expected. ☐ improved, but slower than expected. ☐ not improved significantly.

☐ worsened. ☐ plateaued, no further improvement is expected. ☐ has been determined to be non-work related.

Briefly, describe any change in objective or subjective complaint: ______

TREATMENT

Treatment plan: (only list changes from prior status) ☐ No change ☐ Patient is/was discharged from care on ______

Est. discharge date: 5-18-20XX Medications: Tylenol for pain

Therapy: Type ______ Times per week ______ Estimated date of completion ______

Diagnostic studies: X-ray, L. ankle 3 views

Hospitalization/surgery: ______

Consult/other service: ______

WORK STATUS

The patient has been instructed to:

☐ return to full duty with no limitations or restrictions.

☐ remain off the rest of the day and return to work tomorrow:

______ with no limits or restrictions. ______ with limits listed below.

☐ return to work on ______

work limitations: ______

☒ remain off work until 5-17-20XX — discharge exam scheduled

Estimated date patient can return full duty: 5-18-20XX

DISABILITY STATUS

☐ Patient discharged as cured.

Please supply a brief narrative report if any of the below apply:

☐ Patient will be permanently precluded from engaging in his/her usual and customary occupation.

☐ Patient's condition is permanent and stationary.

☐ Patient will have permanent residuals

☐ Patient will require future medical care.

Physician name: Martin Feelgood, MD Address: 4567 Broad Avenue, Woodland Hills, XY 12345

Date: April 10, 20XX Telephone: (555) 482-9002

Signature: *Martin Feelgood, MD*

reference initials

Fig. 9.11 Physician's supplemental report form.

PATIENT AGREEMENT

Patient's Name James Doland Soc. Sec. # 431-XX-1942

Address 67 Blyth Dr., Woodland Hills, XY 12345 Tel. No. 555-372-0101

WC Insurance Carrier Industrial Indemnity Company

Address 30 North Dr., Woodland Hills Telephone No. 555-731-7707

Date of illness 2-13-20XX Date of first visit 2-13-20XX

Emergency Yes X No ____

Is this condition related to employment Yes X No ____

If accident: Auto ____ Other ____

Where did injury occur? Construction site

How did injury happen? fell 8 ft from scaffold suffering fractured right tibia

Employee/employer who verified this information Scott McPherson

Employer's name and address Willow Construction Company

Employer's telephone no. 555-526-0611

In the event the claim for workers' compensation is declared fraudulent for this illness or condition or it is determined by the Workers' Compensation Board that the illness or injury is not a compensable workers' compensation case, I James Doland, hereby agree to pay the physician's fee for services rendered.

I have been informed that I am responsible to pay any services rendered by Dr. Raymond Skeleton with regard to the discovery and treatment of any condition not related to the workers' compensation injury or illness. I agree to pay for all services not covered by workers' compensation and all charges for treatment and personal items unrelated to my workers' compensation illness or injury.

Signed *James Doland* Date 2-13-20XX

Fig. 9.12 Patient agreement to pay the physician's fees if the case is declared not work related or an illness is discovered and treated that is not work related.

BOX 9.3 2017 Conversion Factors of the Utah Labor Commission Industrial Accident Division Medical Fee Standards

$57/unit	Anesthesia
$62/unit	Surgery
$58/unit	Radiology
$56/unit	Pathology
$50/unit	Medicine
$50/unit	Restorative Services
$50/unit	Evaluation and Management

3. Either ask the employer the name of the claims adjuster or request that the patient obtain the claim number of his or her case when he or she comes in for the initial visit.
4. Educate the patient on the health care organization's billing policies for workers' compensation cases by having him or her complete the patient agreement form shown in Fig. 9.12.
5. Verify whether prior authorization is necessary before a surgical procedure is performed.
6. Document in the patient's record all data for authorization of examination, diagnostic studies, or surgery (for example, date, name of individual who authorizes, response).
7. Obtain the workers' compensation fee schedule for the relevant state.
8. Use appropriate procedural codes and modifiers to ensure prompt and accurate payment for services rendered.
9. Documentation should include a description of how the injury occurred and where it occurred.
10. Complete the Doctor's First Report of Occupational Injury or Illness form for the relevant state. Refer to the instructions in Procedure 9.1 at the end of this chapter. Submit the form within the time limit shown in Table 9.3.
11. Ask whether there is a state-specific insurance form or if the CMS-1500 form is acceptable.
12. Determine which procedural (*Current Procedural Terminology* [CPT]) and diagnosis (*International Classification of Diseases* [ICD]) coding manuals the insurance carrier uses. Some carriers use outdated coding manuals that do not reflect the deletion or addition of some procedure and diagnostic codes.

PROCEDURE 9.1 Completing the Doctor's First Report of Occupational Injury or Illness

The submission of this form (Fig. 9.16) has a deadline, from immediately to within 5 days after the patient has been seen by the physician, depending on each state's law. An original and three or four copies should be distributed as follows:

- Original to the insurance carrier (unless more copies are required)
- One copy to the state agency
- One copy to the patient's employer
- One copy retained for the physician's files in the patient's workers' compensation file folder

In some states, attending physicians may file a single report directly to the insurer or self-insured employer within a specified number of days from initial treatment. The insurer or self-insured employer, in turn, is required to send a report to the state agency. This reduces paperwork and postage. Table 9.3 provides the time limit in each state during which the physician must submit the initial report.

1. Enter the insurance carrier's complete name, street address, city, state, and zip code.
2. Enter the employer's full name and policy number if known. Some insurance carriers file by employer and then by policy number. Sometimes the employer's telephone number is necessary on this line.
3. Enter the employer's street address, city, state, and zip code.
4. Enter the type of business (for example, repairing shoes, building construction, retailing men's clothes).
5. Enter the patient's complete first name, middle initial, and last name.
6. Enter a check mark in the appropriate box to indicate the patient's gender.
7. Enter the patient's birth date and list the year as four digits.
8. Enter the patient's street address, city, state, and zip code.
9. Enter the patient's home telephone number.
10. Enter the patient's specific job title. Be accurate in listing the occupation with the job title so that the insurance carrier may be certain the patient was doing the job for which he or she was insured.
11. Enter the patient's Social Security number. Some insurance carriers use the Social Security number as the workers' compensation case number.
12. Enter the exact location where the patient was injured. Many times, the injury may occur off the premises of the company or factory, depending on the type of job on which the employee was working. List the county where the patient was injured.
13. Enter the date the patient was injured and time of the injury. List the year as four digits.
14. Enter the date the patient last worked. This date should coincide with the date the patient reported to work and worked any portion of his or her shift (workday). This may be the same date of injury. This item is important because it informs the insurance carrier of the working status of the patient or whether the patient has been disabled and cannot return to work. List the year as four digits.
15. Enter the date and hour of the physician's first examination. The insurance carrier should know how soon after the accident the patient sought medical attention. List the year as four digits.
16. Enter a check mark in the appropriate box indicating whether the physician or an associate treated the patient previously.
17. Have the patient complete this section if possible in his or her own words, stating how the illness or injury occurred. The physician also may dictate this information after obtaining it from the patient.
18. Enter the answers to these questions about the patient's complaints and medical findings, which may be found in the patient's health record. List all the patient's subjective complaints.
19. Enter all objective findings from physical examination.
20. Enter all x-ray and laboratory results. If none, state "none" or "pending."
21. Enter a check mark in "yes" or "no" to indicate if chemical or toxic compounds are involved. Enter the diagnosis and diagnostic code number. Specify etiologic agent and duration of exposure if occupational illness.
22. Enter a check mark in "yes" or "no" to indicate if the findings and diagnosis are consistent with the history of injury or onset of illness. Insert an explanation if "yes."
23. Enter a check mark in "yes" or "no" to indicate if there is any other current condition that will impede or delay the patient's recovery. Insert an explanation if "yes."
24. Enter a full description of what treatment was rendered.
25. Enter an explanation if further treatment is necessary and, if so, specify the treatment plan. Indicate if physical therapy is necessary and its frequency and duration.
26. Enter the name and location of the hospital, admission date, and estimated stay if the patient is to be hospitalized.
27. Enter a check mark in "yes" or "no" to indicate whether the patient is able to work as usual. If the answer is "no," give the date when it is estimated that the patient will be able to return to regular or modified work. List the year as four digits. Specify any work restrictions. It is very important for the insurance company to anticipate how long the patient will be off work so that money may be set aside for TD benefits, medical benefits, and, if necessary, PD benefits. If the estimated date of return to work should change after the form is submitted, a supplemental report or progress note should be sent to the insurance carrier to change the date of the disability.

Bottom of Form: If not preprinted, enter the physician's name and degree (for example, MD, DC), complete address, state license number, federal tax identification number, and telephone number. Indicate the date the report is submitted. The insurance billing specialist should type reference initials in the lower left-hand corner of the form. This form must be signed in ink by the physician. Any carbon copies or photocopies must be signed in ink, too. A stamped signature will not be accepted because sometimes these cases go into litigation or are presented for a PD rating. Only those documents considered original health records are acceptable; this means that a handwritten signature by the attending physician is necessary.

13. Clearly define any charges in excess of the fee schedule. Attach any x-ray reports, operative reports, discharge summaries, pathology reports, and any other medical reports that can clarify excess charges.
14. Itemize in detail and send invoices for drugs and dressings furnished by the physician.
15. Call the insurance carrier and talk with the **claims examiner.** The claims examiner may also be referred to as the claims adjuster or claims representative and would be familiar with the patient's case.
16. Search the internet for a website or write to the workers' compensation state plan office in each state for booklets, bulletins, forms, and legislation information.
17. Follow up and track the date on which the claim was filed. If no payment has been received or payment has been received beyond the 30- to 45-day deadline,

determine whether it meets eligibility requirements for interest.

Billing Claims

When the patient first seeks treatment for a work-related illness or injury, the claim for services will be submitted on a CMS-1500 form along with the first report of injury. Once the case has been established, a claim number will be assigned. The date of injury and the claim number should be included on all future CMS 1500-claim forms for services related to the work-related illness or injury.

Out-of-State Claims

Guidelines for billing for out-of-state claims vary from state to state. When billing for an out-of-state claim, insurance billing specialists must follow all workers' compensation regulations from the jurisdiction (state) in which the injured person's claim was originally filed.

Companies that have employees who travel to other states are required to obtain workers' compensation insurance in those states unless they have a policy that covers out-of-state employees. Sometimes a patient may seek care from a health care organization or physician in an adjacent state because he or she feels that the organization or physician provides a higher quality of care or the patient needs a specialized type of surgery, expensive diagnostic tests, or treatment. Referral requirements should be met before the patient is seen (for example, letter of referral or preauthorization from the managing doctor with a copy to the workers' compensation carrier). When a patient crosses a state line for treatment, he or she may be liable for some balance billing and the patient should be informed of this fact

When the claim is billed, the out-of-state fee schedule should be obtained to determine the proper procedure codes, modifiers, and amounts. It should be determined whether the claimant's jurisdiction accepts electronic submission of the CMS-1500 claim form or another form and whether other documents (for example, the operative report) are required to be submitted with the bill.

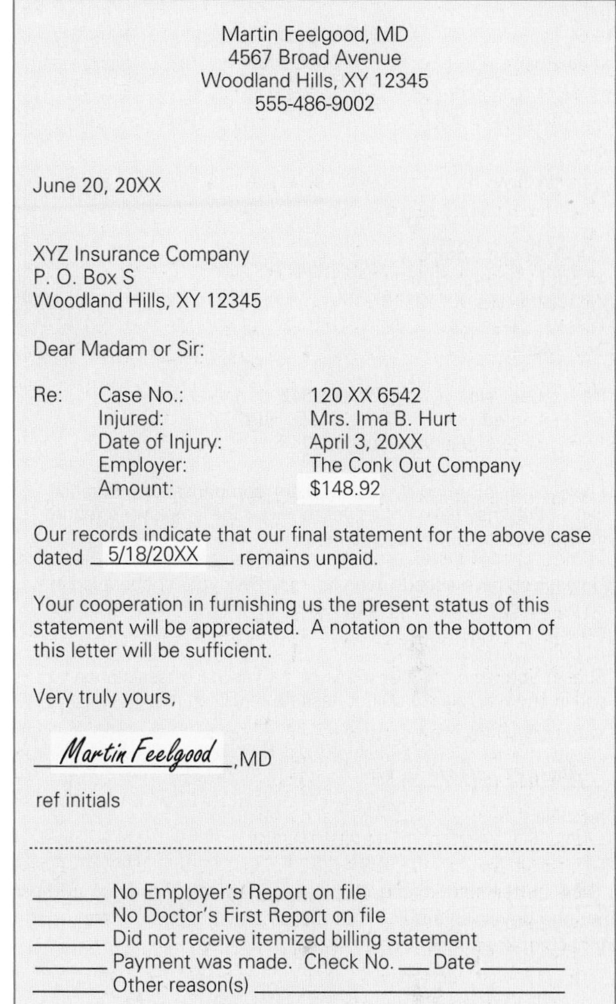

Martin Feelgood, MD
4567 Broad Avenue
Woodland Hills, XY 12345
555-486-9002

June 20, 20XX

XYZ Insurance Company
P. O. Box S
Woodland Hills, XY 12345

Dear Madam or Sir:

Re: Case No.: 120 XX 6542
Injured: Mrs. Ima B. Hurt
Date of Injury: April 3, 20XX
Employer: The Conk Out Company
Amount: $148.92

Our records indicate that our final statement for the above case dated 5/18/20XX remains unpaid.

Your cooperation in furnishing us the present status of this statement will be appreciated. A notation on the bottom of this letter will be sufficient.

Very truly yours,

Martin Feelgood, MD

ref initials

______ No Employer's Report on file
______ No Doctor's First Report on file
______ Did not receive itemized billing statement
______ Payment was made. Check No. ___ Date ______
______ Other reason(s) ______

Fig. 9.13 Letter sent to the insurance carrier when a workers' compensation claim becomes 45 days delinquent.

Delinquent or Slow Pay Claims

If payment of a workers' compensation claim is slow or the claim becomes delinquent (no payment for more than 45 days after the date of service), the insurance billing specialist should use an organized standard follow-up procedure.

1. Telephone the human resources department at the patient's employer. Note the name of the person with whom you speak; the name, address, and telephone number of the workers' compensation carrier; and the claim number. Verify the employer's address.
2. Send a copy of the claim form and the service provider's First Report of Occupational Illness or Injury form. Send a letter and include details of the accident if necessary (Fig. 9.13). For problem claims, it may be wise to obtain and complete a Certificate of Mailing form from the US Postal Service.
3. Telephone the insurance carrier after 45 working days, and request the expected date of payment.
4. Be reminded of the expected payment date by using a computer-automated reminder or a note on the desk calendar. If payment is not received on or before that day, call the carrier again and ask for payment on a day determined by the facility's expectations.
5. Telephone the patient's employer and explain that there is difficulty with the carrier. Ask the employer to contact the carrier and have the carrier send payment immediately. You also might talk to the patient and suggest that he or she discuss the problem with his or her employer to see if this will bring positive action.
6. Send the employer a copy of the financial account statement showing the outstanding balance. If the carrier is not paying, ask the employer for payment. An employer's legal obligation to pay may vary from case to case.
7. Contact the patient only if given information by the carrier or employer that the injury is not work related.
8. Develop office policies that address when an outstanding account should be reviewed (perhaps after 90 or 120 days),

Martin Feelgood, MD
4567 Broad Avenue
Woodland Hills, XY 12345
555-486-9002

June 20, 20XX

The Conk Out Company
45 South Gorman Street
Woodland Hills, XY 12345

Dear Madam or Sir:

Re: Case No.: 120 XX 6542
Injured: Mrs. Ima B. Hurt
Date of Injury: April 3, 20XX

I have been informed by your workers' compensation insurance carrier that they have not as yet received the employer's report in regard to the above injured person.

Unless you have already done so, may I ask your cooperation in completing and sending this report so that the case may be closed.

Should you have any questions or if I can be of assistance to you in any way, please do not hesitate to call on me.

Very truly yours,

Martin Feelgood, MD

ref initials

Fig. 9.14 Letter sent to the employer when the insurance company notifies the physician's office that the employer's preliminary report of injury has not been received.

whether to continue collection efforts internally, and at which point the account should be turned over to a collection agency.

It may be necessary to send subsequent letters to the employer after receiving a response from the insurance carrier. For example, a letter should be sent to the employer (Fig. 9.14) if the insurance company notifies the health care organization that the employer's preliminary report of injury has not been received.

Martin Feelgood, MD
4567 Broad Avenue
Woodland Hills, XY 12345
555-486-9002

July 15, 20XX

Division of Industrial Accidents
State Office Building
107 South Broadway, Room 4107
Woodland Hills, XY 12345

Dear Madam or Sir:

Re: Failure of employer to follow Section No. 3760

Your office is being solicited to help secure an Employer's Report of Work Injury from the employer listed below.

Case No.:	120 XX 6542
Name of Employer:	The Conk Out Company
Address:	45 South Gorman Street Woodland Hills, XY 12345
Name of Injured:	Mrs. Ima B. Hurt
Address:	300 East Central Avenue Woodland Hills, XY 12345
Date of Injury:	April 3, 20XX
Name of Insurance Carrier:	XYZ Insurance Company
Amount of Unpaid Bill:	$148.92

Your cooperation in this matter will be greatly appreciated. If you need further information, please feel free to contact my office.

Sincerely yours,

Martin Feelgood, MD

ref initials

Fig. 9.15 Letter sent to the Workers' Compensation Board or Industrial Accident Commission in your state if the employer does not respond to your letter requesting the Employer's Report of Work Injury after 30 days have elapsed from the date of the letter.

If 30 days have elapsed from the date on which the letter was sent requesting the Employer's Report of Work Injury and the employer has not responded, a letter should be sent to the state Workers' Compensation Board or Industrial Accidents Commission (Fig. 9.15).

STATE OF CALIFORNIA

DOCTOR'S FIRST REPORT OF OCCUPATIONAL INJURY OR ILLNESS

Within 5 days of your initial examination, for every occupational injury or illness, send two copies of this report to the employer's workers' compensation insurance carrier or the insured employer. Failure to file a timely doctor's report may result in assessment of a civil penalty. In the case of diagnosed or suspected pesticide poisoning, send a copy of the report to Division of Labor Statistics and Research, P.O. Box 420603, San Francisco, CA 94142-0603, and notify your local health officer by telephone within 24 hours.

	PLEASE DO NOT USE THIS COLUMN
1. **INSURER NAME AND ADDRESS** XYZ Insurance Company, P.O. Box 5, Woodland Hills, XY 12345	
2. **EMPLOYER NAME** The Conk Out Company Policy #B12345	Case No.
3. Address No. and Street: 45 So. Gorman St; City: Woodland Hills, XY; Zip: 12345	Industry
4. Nature of business (e.g., food manufacturing, building construction, retailer of women's clothes.) Plumbing Repair	County
5. **PATIENT NAME** (first name, middle initial, last name) Ima B. Hurt; 6. Sex ☐ Male ☒ Female; 7. Date of Birth Mo. Day Yr. 3-4-1966	Age
8. Address: No. and Street: 300 East Central Ave., City: Woodland Hills, XY Zip: 12345; 9. Telephone number (555) 476-9899	Hazard
10. Occupation (Specific job title) Clerk Typist; 11. Social Security Number 120-XX-6542	Disease
12. Injured at: No. and Street: 45 So. Gorman St.; City: Woodland Hills, XY 12345; County: Humbolt	Hospitalization
13. Date and hour of injury or onset of illness Mo. Day Yr. 4-3-20XX; Hour a.m. 2:00 p.m.; 14. Date last worked Mo. Day Yr. 4-3-20XX	Occupation
15. Date and hour of first examination or treatment Mo. Day Yr. 4-3-20XX; Hour a.m. 4:00 p.m.; 16. Have you (or your office) previously treated patient? ☐ Yes ☒ No	Return Date/Code

Patient please complete this portion, if able to do so. Otherwise, doctor please complete immediately, inability or failure of a patient to complete this portion shall not affect his/her rights to workers' compensation under the California Labor Code.

17. **DESCRIBE HOW THE ACCIDENT OR EXPOSURE HAPPENED.** (Give specific object, machinery or chemical. Use reverse side if more space is required.) I climbed a ladder in the stock room and while I was coming down I missed a step, lost my balance, and fell hurting my left ankle.

18. **SUBJECTIVE COMPLAINTS** (Describe fully. Use reverse side if more space is required.)
Pain in left ankle

19. **OBJECTIVE FINDINGS** (Use reverse side if more space is required.)
A. Physical examination
Pain, swelling and discoloration of L. ankle

B. X-ray and laboratory results (State if non or pending.) Ankle x-ray (left) 3 views

20. **DIAGNOSIS** (if occupational illness specify etiologic agent and duration of exposure.) Chemical or toxic compounds involved? ☑ Yes ☐ No
Trimalleolar ankle fracture (left) ICD-9 Code ___ ___ ___ - ___ ___

21. Are your findings and diagnosis consistent with patient's account of injury or onset of illness? ☑ Yes ☐ No If "no", please explain.

22. Is there any other current condition that will impede or delay patient's recovery? ☐ Yes ☑ No If "yes", please explain.

23. **TREATMENT RENDERED** (Use reverse side if more space is required.)
Examination, x-rays, closed treatment of trimalleolar ankle fracture (left) without manipulation.
Return in one week for recheck.

24. If further treatment required, specify treatment plan/estimated duration.

25. If hospitalized as inpatient, give hospital name and location Date admitted Mo. Day Yr. Estimated stay

26. WORK STATUS -- Is patient able to perform usual work? ☐ Yes ☐ No
If "no", date when patient can return to: Regular work 05 / 17 / 20XX
Modified work ___/___/___ Specify restrictions ___

Doctor's Signature *Martin Feelgood MD* CA License Number A 12345

Doctor Name and Degree (please type) Martin Feelgood, MD IRS Number 95-36640XX

Address 4567 Broad Avenue, Woodland Hills,XY 12345 Telephone Number (555) 486-9002

FORM 5021 (Rev. 4)
1992

Any person who makes or causes to be made any knowingly false or fraudulent material statement or material representation for the purpose of obtaining or denying workers' compensation benefits or payments is guilty of a felony.

Fig. 9.16 Doctor's First Report of Occupational Injury or Illness form, used in California.

KEY POINTS

This is a brief chapter review, or summary, of the key issues presented. To further enhance your knowledge of the technical subject matter, review the key terms and key abbreviations for this chapter by locating the meaning for each in the Glossary at the end of this book, which appears in a section before the Index.

1. Federal and state regulations require that employers have workers' compensation insurance coverage against on-the-job injury or illness and pay the premium for each of their employees.
2. Workers' compensation programs are not included under the definition of a health plan as identified in the HIPAA statutes.
3. Employees who work for federal agencies are covered by a number of federal workers' compensation laws.
4. The second-injury fund, also known as the *subsequent-injury fund,* was established to meet problems arising when an employee has a preexisting injury or condition and is subsequently injured at work.
5. Each state's legislation lists a waiting period (WP) that must elapse before income benefits are paid. However, medical and hospital care for work-related injuries or illnesses is provided immediately.
6. Workers' compensation benefits consist of medical treatment, temporary disability (TD) indemnity, permanent disability (PD) indemnity, death benefits for survivors, and rehabilitation benefits.
7. A nondisability (ND) claim involves a minor injury in which the patient is seen by the physician but is able to continue to work.
8. A TD claim occurs when a worker has a work-related injury or illness and is unable to perform the duties of his or her occupation for a specific time.
9. A PD consists of an illness or injury (impairment of the normal use of a body part) that is expected to continue for the lifetime of the injured worker and prevents the person from performing the functions of his or her occupation, therefore impairing his or her earning capacity.
10. In a PD case the physician's final report must contain the words "permanent and stationary" (P and S) so that the case can be adjudicated or rated, settlement can be reached (called a *compromise and release [C and R]*), and the case can be closed.
11. It is the responsibility of all individuals who handle workers' compensation cases to notify the insurance carrier of any fraudulent or suspicious situation.
12. The Occupational Safety and Health Administration (OSHA) is the federal agency that regulates and investigates safety and health standards at work sites for the protection of employees.
13. Depositions from the health care provider and the injured individual by the attorney representing the workers' compensation insurance company are usually taken in PD cases.
14. The health care organization should consider filing a lien in a workers' compensation case that has gone into third-party litigation or if there is a question whether the case is compensable.
15. A private health record should never be combined with a work-related injury/illness case record because separate disclosure laws apply to each and the workers' compensation case may go to court.
16. The first report of a work-related injury/illness must be completed by the employer and the physician and is required by law in most states.
17. A medical service order given to the employee by the employer authorizes the health care organization or physician to treat the injured worker.
18. In workers' compensation cases, all medical reports and forms are legal documents and must be signed in ink by the treating provider.

STUDENT ASSIGNMENT

- Study Chapter 9 .
- Answer the fill-in-the-blank, multiple-choice, and true/false review questions in the *Workbook* to reinforce the theory learned in this chapter and to help you prepare for a future test.
- Complete the assignments in the *Workbook* for hands-on experience in completing workers' compensation reports.
- Turn to the Glossary at the end of this text for a further understanding of the key terms and key abbreviations used in this chapter.

10

Disability Income Insurance and Disability Benefit Programs

Linda M. Smith

OBJECTIVES

After reading this chapter, you should be able to:

1. Discuss the history of disability income insurance.
2. Describe benefits and exclusions contained in individual and group disability income insurance.
3. Name and describe federal disability benefit programs.
4. Differentiate between Social Security Disability Insurance (SSDI) and Supplemental Security Income (SSI).
5. State eligibility requirements, benefits, and limitations of SSDI and SSI.
6. Explain disability benefit programs for disabled active military personnel, veterans, and their dependents.
7. Name states that have state disability insurance plans.
8. State eligibility requirements, benefits, and limitations of state disability plans.
9. Explain voluntary disability insurance plans.
10. Describe topics and contents of a medical report.
11. List guidelines for federal disability claims.
12. Explain procedures for state disability claims.
13. Recognize forms used for processing state disability plans.

KEY TERMS

accidental death and dismemberment
Armed Services Disability
benefit period
Civil Service Retirement System
consultative examiner
cost-of-living adjustment
Disability Determination Services
disability income insurance
double indemnity
exclusions
Federal Employees Retirement System
future purchase option
guaranteed renewable
hearing
long-term disability insurance
noncancelable clause
Non-VA Medical Care Program
partial disability
reconsideration
residual benefits
residual disability
short-term disability insurance
Social Security Administration
Social Security Disability Insurance program
State Disability Insurance
supplemental benefits
Supplemental Security Income
temporary disability
temporary disability insurance
total disability
Unemployment Compensation Disability
Veterans Affairs disability program
Veterans Affairs outpatient clinic card
voluntary disability insurance
waiting period
waiver of premium

KEY ABBREVIATIONS

AIDS
CE
COLA
CSRS
DDS
FERS
HIV
SDI
SSA
SSDI
SSI
TD
TDI
UCD
VA
WP

DISABILITY CLAIMS

This chapter introduces several types of **disability income insurance** is a form of insurance that provides reimbursement for lost income when the insured is unable to work because of illness, disease, or injury—not as a result of a work-related accident or condition. For example, a patient may have been diagnosed with pancreatic cancer and is unable to work because of the illness. This patient may be able to apply for disability income benefits.

This chapter will also introduce the insurance billing specialist to disability benefit programs that are administered by the federal government. The third part of the chapter deals with state disability programs. Five states and Puerto Rico currently have statutory state disability programs. Individuals in other states may have voluntary disability insurance plans that help individuals pay for daily living expenses while dealing with serious accidents or illnesses.

Disability insurance plays an important role in the financial planning and safeguarding of an individual's future. Efficiently and quickly completing the attending physician's portion of the disability insurance form assists the patient in obtaining disability income when he or she is unable to work because of a non-work-related illness or injury.

HISTORY

Before the late 1800s, disability income insurance provided only accident protection. Some life insurance contracts had disability income riders attached to them that offered limited benefits. In the early 1880s, insurance companies began selling disability income policies that offered coverage for accident and illness. The Paul Revere Life Insurance Company introduced the first "noncancelable" disability income policy in the early 1900s. The noncancelable clause guaranteed that the contract would be in force for a certain period and the premium would not be increased. By 1956, Congress had enacted legislation under the Social Security program that provided disability income protection to disabled individuals older than 50 years of age. This program was expanded in 1965 to cover workers without regard to age if certain eligibility standards were met.

Today, disability income insurance is available from private insurance companies (individual policies) and employer-sponsored plans (group policies). Government-funded and state benefit programs are also available for disabled persons. These plans and programs are discussed in this chapter, along with the role of the insurance billing specialist in dealing with this type of insurance.

DISABILITY INCOME INSURANCE

Individual

Individual disability income insurance is coverage that provides a specific monthly or weekly income when a person becomes unable to work, temporarily or totally, because of an illness or injury. Disability income policies do not provide medical expense benefits. The disability cannot be work related. As explained in the previous chapter, an illness or accident that is work related is covered by workers' compensation insurance.

For individuals who are self-employed, this insurance is particularly important because a business could not meet its financial obligations if the owner became injured or too ill to work. For example, if an individual is self-employed with a home-based business and faced with a repetitive stress injury (RSI), the condition would not allow that individual to use the computer for several months. He or she would have no income. The main purpose of these policies is to provide some benefits while the person is unable to work. To collect benefits, the individual must meet the policy's criteria of what constitutes partial, temporary, or total disability. These policies terminate when the individual retires or reaches a certain age, usually 65 years.

Waiting Period

The period from the beginning of disability to receiving the first payment of benefits is called an *elimination period* or waiting period (WP). During this initial period, a disabled individual is not eligible to receive benefits even though he or she is unable to work.

Benefit Period

A benefit period is the maximum amount of time that benefits will be paid to the injured or ill person for the disability (for example, 2 years, 5 years, to age 65, or lifetime).

Benefits

Compensation paid to the insured disabled person is called *indemnity benefits* and can be received daily, weekly, monthly, or semiannually, depending on the policy. Premiums and benefits depend on several risk factors, such as age, gender, health history and physical state, income, and occupational duties. Some policies include residual or partial disability income benefits. Benefits are not taxable if premiums are paid by the individual.

Residual benefits pay a partial benefit when the insured is not totally disabled. If one becomes partially disabled or can work only part time or in a limited capacity, the residual benefits make up the difference between what an individual can earn at present and what he or she would have earned working full time.

Supplemental benefits may consist of insurance provisions that will increase monthly indemnity, such as a future purchase option or a cost-of-living adjustment. Cost-of-living adjustment (COLA) means to increase monthly benefits in disability income benefit, pension benefit, or life income benefit to make up for a change in the cost of living. This is also known as future purchase option or cost-of-living rider. Provisions also distribute a percentage of the policy premiums if an individual keeps a policy in force for 5 or 10 years or does not file any claims.

An accidental death and dismemberment benefit is written into some contracts. This offers the insured person protection when loss of sight or loss of limb occurs. In some policies (for example, life insurance), a special provision known as double indemnity applies if an unintended, unexpected, and unforeseeable accident results in death. This feature provides for twice the face amount of the policy to be paid if death results from accidental causes.

Types of Disability

A disability may be partial, temporary, or total. There is no standard definition for total disability and the definition stated in each disability income policy varies. For example, a liberal definition might read as follows: "The insured must be unable to perform the major duties of his or her specific occupation." Social Security has a restrictive definition presented later in this chapter.

The terms *residual disability* and *partial disability* are defined as occurring "when an illness or injury prevents an insured person from performing one or more of the functions of his or her regular job"—in other words, when a person cannot perform all of their usual job duties.

Temporary disability (TD) exists when a person cannot perform all of the functions of his or her regular job for a limited period.

Clauses

With a guaranteed renewable policy, the insurer is required to renew the policy as long as premium payments are made for a specified number of years or to a specified age, such as 60, 65, or 70 years, or for life. However, the premium may be increased when it is renewed. When the policy has a noncancelable clause, the premium cannot be increased.

If a waiver of premium is included in the insurance contract, the policy pays all premiums while the employee is disabled; the employee does not have to pay. Usually, this provision is used as a total and permanent disability benefit and may be available in certain other cases.

Exclusions

Exclusions are provisions written into the insurance contract denying coverage or limiting the scope of coverage. Examples of preexisting conditions that may be written into a contract are disability because of war, riot, self-inflicted injury, or attempted suicide; mental or nervous conditions; disability while legally intoxicated or under the influence of narcotics (unless prescribed by a licensed physician); conditions arising from normal pregnancy; conditions arising during the act of committing a felony; or if benefits are being received under workers' compensation or a government program. The phrase "legally intoxicated" means intoxication in an individual whose blood alcohol level, when tested, exceeds limits set by state law.

Acquired Immunodeficiency Syndrome and Human Immunodeficiency Virus Infection

States have statutes governing questions that can and cannot be asked on insurance application forms about acquired immunodeficiency syndrome (AIDS) and human immunodeficiency virus (HIV) testing; therefore each state has developed its own forms. If a private insurance company wishes to test an applicant, a consent or notice form, including acceptance of pretest and posttest counseling, must be signed.

Group

Some employers elect to offer group disability income insurance as a fringe benefit. These contracts are drawn up between the insurer and employer. Premiums may be paid by the employer with or without contributions from the employee. Employees hold certificates of insurance and are covered under the employer's policy; therefore they are not called policyholders. When the employee leaves the company, the insurance terminates unless the employee is disabled. A few group policies allow conversion to a limited benefit individual policy.

Benefits

Benefits vary from one plan to another but are usually for short-term disability insurance (13 weeks to 24 months) or long-term disability insurance (to age 65). To qualify for benefits, an individual must be unable to perform the major duties of his or her occupation during the initial period of disability (for example, the first 2 years). Benefits cease when the employee returns to work, even part time. However, some of these policies offer the worker partial disability income benefits to motivate a disabled individual to return to work on a part-time basis. Monthly benefits are usually paid directly to the employee and are taxable if the employee is not making any contribution toward the premiums.

FEDERAL DISABILITY PROGRAMS

Workers' Compensation

The federal government has several programs that cover workers from loss of income because of work-related disability. These programs are mentioned in Chapter 9 because work-related disabilities fall under workers' compensation laws. When an individual is eligible under more than one program, coordination of benefits is used so that a worker cannot receive benefits that result in an amount greater than what the person receives when working. Coordination of benefits is a provision preventing double payment for expenses by making one of the programs the primary payer and ensuring that no more than 100% of the costs are covered.

Disability Benefit Programs

The government's major non–work-related disability programs are as follows:

- Social Security Disability Insurance (SSDI) program
- Supplemental Security Income (SSI)
- Civil Service Retirement System (CSRS)
- Federal Employees Retirement System (FERS)
- Armed Services Disability
- Veterans Affairs (VA) disability program

The Social Security Administration (SSA) is a United States federal agency that administers Social Security retirement benefits. It also manages two programs that pay monthly disability income benefits to people younger than age 65 who cannot work for at least 1 year because of a severe disability: Social Security Disability Insurance and Supplemental Security Income. Medical requirements are the same for both programs.

Social Security Disability Insurance Program

Social Security Disability Insurance (SSDI) is part of the Social Security program that also pays retirement benefits to older Americans. It is funded through payroll taxes that have been collected through workers' payroll deductions and matching employer contributions. SSDI is a long-term disability program that pays monthly income benefits to workers who are no longer able to work because of a significant illness or impairment that is expected to last at least a year or to result in death within a year.

Disability definition. *Disability* under Social Security has a strict definition: "inability to engage in any substantial gainful activity due to any medically determinable physical or mental impairment which can be expected to result in death or which has lasted or can be expected to last for a continuous period of not less than 12 months."

Eligibility. Individuals are eligible for SSDI if they have worked for a certain number of years and have made contributions to the Social Security trust fund in the form of Federal Insurance Contribution Act (FICA) Social Security Taxes.

The following is a list of individuals who meet eligibility requirements for SSDI:

- Disabled workers younger than age 65 years and their families
- Individuals who become disabled before age 22 years, if a parent (or in certain cases, a grandparent) who is covered under Social Security retires, becomes disabled, or dies
- Disabled widows or widowers, age 50 years or older, if the deceased spouse worked at least 10 years under Social Security
- Disabled surviving divorced spouses older than age 50 years, if the ex-spouse was married to the disabled person for at least 10 years
- Blind workers whose vision in the better eye cannot be corrected to better than 20/200 or whose visual field in the better eye, even with corrective lenses, is 20 degrees or less

Workers must be fully insured in accordance with standards set by the SSA in terms of age, number of quarters worked, and amount of wages earned per quarter. The processing of eligibility application forms may take up to 2 months.

Benefits. Monthly benefits are paid to qualified individuals. There is a 5-month WP for benefits, which means the individual will not receive SSA benefits for the first 5 months they become disabled. The amount of the monthly benefit will depend on the worker's past earning records. After 24 months of disability payments, the disabled individual also becomes eligible for Medicare. The benefits convert to retirement benefits when an individual reaches age 65.

Supplemental Security Income

The **Supplemental Security Income (SSI)** program pays monthly income benefits to people (adults and children) with limited income and resources who are disabled, blind, or age 65 or older. The SSI program is overseen and managed by the SSA and is funded by general fund taxes, not from the Social Security trust fund. The SSI program differs from the SSDI program in that it has nothing to do with work history. Eligibility for the SSI program is based strictly on financial need.

Eligibility. Eligibility for SSI benefits are based on income and assets.

No prior employment is necessary to receive SSI benefits. Many SSI recipients also qualify for Medicaid, a state assistance program. The following individuals may qualify for SSI disability payments:

- Disabled persons younger than 65 years who have limited income and resources
- Disabled children younger than age 18 years, if the disability compares in severity with one that would prevent an adult from working and has lasted or is expected to last at least 12 months or result in death
- Blind adults or children who have a visual acuity no better than 20/100 or have a visual field of 20 degrees or less in the better eye, with the use of corrective lenses

Disability determination process. Individuals applying for disability will initiate the process by applying in person, by telephone, or by completing an application online or to be sent through the mail. This information is usually processed through a network of local Social Security field offices. The field office is responsible for verifying eligibility requirements including factors such as income, age, employment, citizenship, and marital status. Once all information has been collected, the case is forwarded to **Disability Determination Services (DDS),** who will determine if the claimant is or is not disabled under the definition of the law. A physician may be involved in the determination process in one of three ways: (1) as a treating source who provides medical evidence on behalf of his or her patient, (2) as a **consultative examiner (CE)** who is paid a fee and examines or tests the applicant, or (3) as a full- or part-time medical or psychological consultant reviewing claims for a state or regional office.

Final determination of disability is made by a DDS team composed of a physician or psychologist and a disability examiner (DE), not by the applicant's physician. Upon making their disability determination, DDS will return the case to the field office. The field office will take appropriate action depending on whether the claim is allowed or denied.

Appeals evaluation process. If a claimant does not agree with the determination of disability, the following four-level appeals process is available:

1. A **reconsideration,** which is a complete review of the claim by a medical or psychological consultant or DE team who did not take part in the original disability determination.
2. The second level of appeals for a disability claim is a **hearing** before an administrative law judge who had no part in the initial or reconsideration determinations of the claim. The hearing is held within 75 miles of the claimant's home. The claimant and his or her representative are permitted to present their case in person and present a written statement. They are also permitted to review information the judge will use to make a decision and question any witnesses.
3. A review by the Appeals Council, which considers all requests for review but may deny a request if it believes that the decision by the administrative law judge was correct. If the Appeals Council decides that the case should be reviewed, it will make a decision on the case or return it to an administrative law judge for further review.
4. A review by the federal court for which the claimant may file an action where he or she resides.

Disability cases are reviewed from time to time to be sure that the individuals are still disabled. The frequency depends on the nature and severity of the impairment, the likelihood of improvement, rehabilitation, ability to work, and so on.

Benefits. Social Security disability programs are designed to give long-term protection and benefits to individuals totally disabled who are unable to do any type of work in the national economy. In contrast, **short-term disability** may be provided through workers' compensation, insurance, savings, and investments.

Work incentives. Special rules allow disabled or blind people presently receiving Social Security or SSI to work and still receive monthly benefits as well as Medicare or Medicaid (for example, an SSDI recipient who is given a 90-day trial of work and at the end of that time either continues to work and loses SSDI coverage or leaves the temporary employment and remains on SSDI). A limit exists as to how much the person can earn in a calendar year. These are referred to as "work incentives"; the rules are different for Social Security beneficiaries and SSI recipients. Occasionally a person may be working and receiving SSDI benefits, as illustrated by the earlier example.

Civil Service and Federal Employees Retirement Systems

Background. There are two types of federal retirement, Civil Service Retirement System (CSRS) and Federal Employees Retirement System (FERS). CSRS began in 1920, and a second system, FERS, was introduced in 1984. People who began working for the federal government in 1984 or later are covered by FERS instead of CSRS. Some workers who had been covered by the CSRS program changed to the FERS program when it became available.

Eligibility. Federal employees who work in civil service fall under the CSRS. This system has provisions for those who become totally disabled. This program is a combination of federal disability and Social Security disability. Both portions of the program must be applied for by the worker. The disability cannot be work related, and 5 years of service is necessary before benefits are payable. Eighteen months of service is necessary under the FERS.

Benefits. Those who qualify are entitled to benefits that are payable for life. For example, an individual who works for the Internal Revenue Service (IRS) performing clerical and filing job duties is involved in an automobile accident on the weekend. The head injuries are so severe that the person is unable to return to gainful employment at any job. He or she could apply for benefits under either CSRS or FERS, depending on his or her eligibility status.

Armed Services Disability

Eligibility. Individuals covered under the Armed Services Disability program must be members of the armed services on active duty who suffer a disability or illness.

Benefits. Monthly benefits are payable for life if a disability occurs or is aggravated while an individual is serving in the military. Benefit amounts are based on years of service, base pay, and severity of disability. This is also subject to review.

Veterans Affairs Disability

Eligibility. The VA is authorized by law to provide a wide range of benefits to both those who have served their country in the armed forces and those individuals' dependents. If a veteran who is honorably discharged files a claim for a service-connected disability within 1 year of sustaining that injury, he or she is eligible for outpatient treatment. Veterans with non–service-connected disabilities who are in receipt of housebound or aid-in-attendance benefits are eligible for treatment from a private physician if they are unable to travel to a VA facility because of geographic inaccessibility. Their identification cards, benefits, and claims procedures are identical to those of veterans with service-connected disabilities who receive outpatient medical care.

Benefits. A general list of veterans' medical benefits follows. Each benefit requires that certain criteria be met. These criteria are ever changing and are not mentioned here. A complete up-to-date booklet listing all benefits is available.

- Hospital care in a VA hospital
- Nursing home care in a VA facility
- Domiciliary care
- Outpatient medical treatment at a VA facility or by a private physician
- Emergency treatment in a hospital for a service-connected condition
- Prescription drugs and medications issued by a VA pharmacy or other participating pharmacy (only bona fide emergency prescriptions can be filled by a private pharmacy)
- Certain medical equipment, such as oxygen and prosthetics
- Travel expenses when receiving VA medical care
- Outpatient dental treatment (if the veteran files a claim within 90 days from the date that he or she was discharged from the service)
- Treatment for Agent Orange or nuclear radiation exposure
- Alcohol and drug dependence outpatient care
- Readjustment counseling services

The health care provider must accept what the VA pays as payment in full for treatment of a service-connected disability and cannot bill the patient for any additional charges, even if there is a balance after the VA pays the claim.

If the treatment is likely to cost more than $40 per month, the health care organization must obtain prior authorization from the nearest VA facility. A separate financial accounting record card must be prepared for VA benefits if the service provider is also treating the patient for ailments other than a service-connected disability. Any professional service that is not related to a service-connected disability must be paid for by the veteran out of his or her own pocket. For example, a Vietnam veteran who has a long history of stump pain at the site of an amputation or suffers from old shrapnel wounds as the result of stepping on a land mine during active duty is seen and treated for acute gastroenteritis. The VA disability benefits do not apply to the episode of acute gastroenteritis, and the veteran must personally pay for professional services related to that diagnosis.

Veterans with non–service-connected disabilities may have copayments when they seek treatment. For example, individuals on Medicare may be responsible for the deductible for the first 90 days of care during any 365-day period. For each additional 90 days of hospital care, the patient is charged half of the Medicare deductible, $10 a day for hospital care, and $5 a day for VA nursing home care. For outpatient care, the copayment is 20% of the cost of an average outpatient visit.

Outpatient treatment. Veterans eligible for outpatient treatment may obtain outpatient medical care by checking in with the Veterans Affairs outpatient clinic card (see Fig. 8.5), which is used for identification purposes. Usually a veteran seeks care at the nearest VA outpatient clinic. However, when a VA facility is not within reasonable distance, when the veteran is too ill to travel to the nearest location, or when the condition needs prompt attention, the veteran can apply for and be granted medical care by a private physician through the Non-VA Medical Care Program. This program permits medical care provided in the community that is paid by the Department of Veterans Affairs. The VA outpatient clinic must be notified within 15 days of the treatment rendered. In such cases the treating physician must submit evidence of medical necessity (for example, detailed justification on the invoice) to the VA outpatient clinic. Form 10-583, Claim for Payment of Cost of Unauthorized Medical Services (Fig. 10.1), generally used for hospital emergency care, can also be used for professional care if the doctor is billing after the 15-day period has elapsed. Some patients have both Medicare and medical

NOTE: Instructions are written for a multi-part form. Print additional copies as necessary.

OMB No: 2900-0080
Estimated Burden: 15 min.

Department of Veterans Affairs

CLAIM FOR PAYMENT OF COST OF UNAUTHORIZED MEDICAL SERVICES

The Paperwork Reduction Act of 1995 requires us to notify you that this information collection is in accordance with the clearance requirements of section 3507 of the Paperwork Reduction Act of 1995. We may not conduct or sponsor, and you are not required to respond to, a collection of information unless it displays a valid OMB number. We anticipate that the time expended by all individuals who must complete this form will average 15 minutes. This includes the time it will take to read instructions, gather the necessary facts and fill out the form. Comments regarding this burden estimate or any other aspect of this collection, including suggestions for reducing the burden, may be addressed by calling the Health Benefits Contact Center at 1-877-222-8387.

PRIVACY ACT INFORMATION: The information requested on this form is solicited under authority of Title 38, United States Code, "Veterans Benefits," and will be used to assist us in determining your entitlement to reimbursement for services rendered. It will not be used for any other purpose. Disclosure is voluntary. However, failure to furnish the information will result in our inability to process your claim. Failure to furnish this information will have no adverse effect on any other benefit to which you may be entitled. This form and relevant documents need to be sent to the VA Medical Facility where the Veteran is enrolled for medical care

PART I

1A. VETERAN'S NAME (Last, first, middle initial) (This is a mandatory field.)	1B. CLAIM NUMBER	1C. SOCIAL SECURITY NUMBER (Mandatory field.)
Thornberg, Joey T.	C-	421xx4182

1D. VETERAN'S ADDRESS (Include complete ZIP Code)
4628 Image St., Woodland Hills, XY 12345-0001

2A. NAME AND ADDRESS OF PERSON, FIRM OR INSTITUTION MAKING CLAIM (Leave blank if same as above)	2B. SOCIAL SECURITY NO. OR EMPLOYEE IDENTIFICATION NO.
Gerald Practon, MD 4567 Broad Ave., Woodland Hills, XY 12345-1290	

3. STATEMENT OF CIRCUMSTANCES UNDER WHICH THE SERVICES WERE RENDERED (Include diagnosis, symptoms, whether emergency existed, and reason VA facilities were not used)

Patient fell on sidewalk of home and suffered traumatic injury to right arm.
Symptoms: Localized pain, swelling and bruising of right arm near elbow.
AP and lateral x-rays of right elbow show anterior dislocation of right radius. Negative for fracture.
Medical care rendered in Emergency Dept. at College Hospital (99282)
Pt. unable to go to VA facility as this was 60 miles from patient's residence.
Treatment of closed elbow dislocation without anesthesia (23400)
Diagnosis: Anterior closed dislocation right radius (S32.014A)

4. AMOUNT CLAIMED	
$237.02	Attach bills or receipts showing services furnished, dates and charges

5. COMPLETE A OR B AS APPROPRIATE

A. Amount charged does not exceed that charged the general public for similar services. Payment has not been received.		B. I certify that the amount claimed has been paid and reimbursement has not been received.	
Gerald Practon, M.D.	05/XX/20XX		
SIGNATURE AND TITLE OF PROVIDER OF SERVICE AND DATE	(mm/dd/yyyy)	SIGNATURE OF VETERAN OR REPRESENTATIVE AND DATE	(mm/dd/yyyy)

PART II - FOR VETERANS AFFAIRS USE ONLY

6. ACTION		CLAIM MEETS THE REQUIREMENT OF VA REGULATION	
☐ APPROVED $	☐ DISAPPROVED	☐ 6080	☐ 6081

7. SIGNATURE OF CHIEF, MEDICAL ADMINISTRATION SERVICE	8. DATE	9. ADMINISTRATIVE VOUCHER NUMBER

VA FORM DEC 2010 **10-583**

Fig. 10.1 Veterans Affairs Form 10-583, Claim for Payment of Cost of Unauthorized Medical Services. From US Department of Veterans Affairs, Washington D.C.

coverage from the VA. In such cases, Medicare is not secondary to the VA and the VA is not secondary to Medicare. The claim is to be sent where specified by the patient. The claim can be sent to Medicare, where, if the claim is processed, the patient must satisfy his or her contractual requirement to pay any deductible and copayment amounts. If the patient asks that the claim be sent to the VA instead of Medicare, the claim is processed and any payments issued are considered as payment in full. Many veterans prefer to have the claim sent to the VA.

Veterans Affairs installations. For information on veterans' benefits or assistance in locating VA installations, go to the Evolve website http://evolve.elsevier.com/Fordney/handbook for a link to the VA home website.

STATE DISABILITY INSURANCE

Background

In 1944 Rhode Island began a **State Disability Insurance (SDI)** program that proved successful. This form of insurance is part of an employment security program that provides temporary cash benefits for workers suffering a wage loss because of off-the-job illness or injury. It can be referred to as **Unemployment Compensation Disability (UCD)** or **temporary disability insurance (TDI)**. California became the second state to add nonindustrial disability coverage to the Social Security protection afforded to its citizens by appending Article 10 to the Unemployment Insurance Act. This became law on May 21, 1946; when the legislation took effect on December 1, 1946, this article diverted the 1% tax formerly paid by workers for unemployment insurance to a disability insurance fund. New York and New Jersey soon followed with similar programs. Two decades later, in 1969, Puerto Rico and Hawaii passed nonindustrial disability insurance laws. To date, these five states (California, Hawaii, New Jersey, New York, Rhode Island) and Puerto Rico are the only non–work-related SDI Programs.

Funding

To fund SDI, a small percentage of wages is deducted from employees' paychecks each month, or the employer may elect to pay all or part of the cost of the plan as a fringe benefit for employees. The money is then sent in quarterly installments to the state and put in a special fund.

Eligibility

To receive SDI benefits, an employee must meet the following criteria:

- Employed full or part time or actively looking for work when disability begins
- Suffering a loss of wages because of disability
- Eligible for benefits, depending on the amount withheld during a previous period before disability began
- Under the care and treatment of a physician who certifies that the employee is disabled
- Disabled at least 7 calendar days
- Filing a claim within the time limit

If the worker was employed at the time of disability, benefits are not subject to federal income tax. An employee who retires is no longer eligible for the insurance. A worker may file a claim with the state seeking exemption from program participation on religious grounds.

Types of workers not covered are employees of school districts, community college districts, and churches; state workers; federal employees; interstate railroad workers; employees of nonprofit organizations; and domestic workers.

Benefits

Weekly benefits are determined by the wages earned in a base period or based on a percentage of average weekly wages (Table 10.1). Benefits begin after the seventh consecutive day of disability. There is no provision under the law for hospital or other medical benefits.

TABLE 10.1 State Disability Information Summary

State	Maximum Benefit Period (Weeks)	Waiting Period	2017 Employee Contribution from Salary (%)	Benefits
California	52	7-day waiting period Benefits begin on eighth day	0.9% of maximum annual taxable wage base: $110,902	55% of average weekly earnings in highest quarter of base period (maximum weekly benefit: $1173)
Hawaii	26	7-day waiting period Benefits begin on eighth day	0.5%; maximum weekly wage base: $1023	Based on 58% of average weekly wage (maximum weekly benefit: $594)
New Jersey	26	7-day waiting period Benefits begin on eighth day	0.24% of maximum annual employee contribution $80	66 2/3% of average weekly wage (maximum $633/week)
New York	26	7-day waiting period Benefits begin on eighth day	0.5% of weekly taxable wage base: $120	Based on 50% of average weekly wage (maximum $170/week)
Puerto Rico	26	7-day waiting period Benefits begin on eighth day	0.2% of annual taxable wage base: $9 per employee	Based on 65% of weekly earnings (maximum weekly benefit: $113)
Rhode Island	30	No waiting period Must be unemployed for at least 7 days because of non–job-related illness or injury	1.2% of annual taxable wage base: $68,100	4.62% of total high base period quarter wages (maximum weekly benefit: $817)

Statutory Disability Matrix by State, Effective January 1, 2017.

Limited Benefits

In some states a patient may qualify for benefits if he or she is a resident of an approved alcoholic recovery facility or an approved drug-free residential facility.

Reduced Benefits

An individual may be entitled to partial benefits if he or she is receiving certain types of income, such as the following:

- Sick leave
- Vacation
- Wages paid by employer
- Insurance settlement for the disability
- Workers' compensation benefits
- Unemployment benefits

Time Limits

A claim for SDI should be filed within the time limit of the state laws. There is usually a grace period of 7 or 8 days after the deadline. After the claim is approved, basic benefits become payable after the seventh day of disability. A person may continue to draw disability insurance for a maximum of 26 weeks in Hawaii, New Jersey, New York, and Puerto Rico; 30 weeks in Rhode Island; and 52 weeks in California for the same illness or injury or overlapping disabilities. An employee is also entitled to disability benefits 15 days after recovery from a previous disability or illness. For example, if a patient is discharged by the physician to return to work and is on the job 15 calendar days and then becomes ill with the same ailment, he or she may file a new claim.

Medical Examinations

The claimant may be required to submit to an examination or examinations by an independent medical examiner to determine any mental or physical disability. Fees for such examinations are paid by the state department that handles disability insurance. *Current Procedural Terminology* (CTP) code 99450 for billing these medical examinations may be found in the Special Evaluation and Management Services section of the CPT manual.

Restrictions

Disability insurance has many restrictions. A few of the major situations in which a claim could be denied are listed here.

1. Conditions covered by workers' compensation unless the rate is less than the disability insurance rate. In that case the state pays the difference between the two rates.
2. Applicants receiving unemployment insurance benefits that are more than a certain specified amount. *Exception:* If the applicant is on unemployment insurance and then becomes ill or injured, he or she is put on TDI until able to go on a job interview.
3. Disabilities beginning during a trade dispute. If an employee is on strike and is injured while walking a picket line, he or she is considered to still be employed. If injured while picketing, it may be considered workers' compensation. However, if the union is on strike and an individual member remains at home and then becomes ill or injured, he or she can claim disability and will receive benefits.
4. Confinement by court order or certification in a public or private institution as an alcoholic, drug addict, or sexual psychopath.
5. When the pursuit of legal custody of a child is the cause of inability to work.
6. When the employing company has a voluntary disability plan and is not paying into a state fund.
7. Religious exemption certificate on file by employee or company with no payment being made into a state fund.
8. Pregnancy-related disability, unless the pregnancy is complicated (for example, cases in which the patient has diabetes, varicose veins, ectopic pregnancy, or cesarean section). *Exceptions:* California, Hawaii, New Jersey, New York, and Rhode Island have maternity benefits that may be applied for at the time the physician tells the patient to stop working.

VOLUNTARY DISABILITY INSURANCE

Persons residing and working in states that do not have SDI programs may elect to contact a local private insurance carrier to arrange for coverage under a voluntary disability insurance plan. If these persons become ill or disabled, they receive a fixed weekly or monthly income, usually for approximately 6 months. If the disability or illness is permanent and the individual is unable to return to work, there is sometimes a small monthly income for the duration of the person's life. Some of the state laws provide that a "voluntary plan" may be adopted instead of the "state plan" if a majority of company employees consent to private coverage.

CLAIMS SUBMISSION GUIDELINES

Disability Income Claims

When the insurance billing specialist is handling disability income claim forms, he or she should note that the insured (claimant) is responsible for notifying the insurance company of the disability. A proof of loss form is completed to establish disability.

The necessary facts are as follows:

- Date on which the disability occurred
- Date on which the disabled person is expected to be well enough to return to work
- Description of how the disability occurred
- Name of treating physician
- Explanation of how the disability prevents the insured person from working

The report must show that the patient's disability meets the policy's definition of disability or benefits will be denied. Because the definition of disability varies among policies, the critical issues are the content and wording on the claim form.

A portion of this form is usually completed by the attending physician. The following data are necessary:

- Medical history
- Date on which patient became disabled
- Subjective symptoms (patient's own words about his or her chief complaints)

- Objective findings on physical examination (for example, rashes, lacerations, abrasions, or contusions)
- Severity of the illness or injury (range-of-motion [ROM] tests)
- Photocopies of laboratory tests, x-ray studies, or hospital discharge report
- Medication
- Treatment dates
- Diagnosis
- Prognosis (outcome of the disease or injury)
- Names of any other treating physician or service provider
- Date on which the patient is expected to return to work
- Description of job duties and patient's ability to perform work

Providing this information helps to verify the disability. In some cases, the physician may wish to dictate a medical report and attach it to the claim form instead of completing a portion of the form. The insurance billing specialist must be prepared to extract data from source documents, such as medical and financial records, to complete the claim form. In such situations, the physician should be asked to read the information carefully before signing the document. The patient should always be asked to sign an authorization form to release medical information. Reasons for denial of benefits often include improper choice of words or inadequate medical information.

The insurance company may request information from other places, such as employer's records, employee's wage statements or tax forms, or the patient's health records from the attending physician, to justify payment of benefits. A company representative may interview the insured if conflicting information exists.

If disability continues, additional claim forms should be completed monthly or more frequently by the insured and attending physician. Other sources of information may be requested, for example, records from medical specialists or Social Security records.

If the validity of the case is in question, an independent medical examiner may be asked by the insurance company to examine the disabled individual. If the claimant neglects to return claim forms, refuses telephone calls, misses appointments, or engages in questionable activities, the insurance company will discreetly engage in surveillance of the insured through the services of a professional investigation firm.

Federal Disability Claims

The SSA division called *Disability Determination Services* has a teledictation service so that the physician or psychologist can dictate the medical report over the telephone instead of completing a medical report form. The service is available at any time, including nights and weekends. A typed transcript is sent to the physician to review, sign, and return to the SSA state agency, or a report may be typed on the physician's stationery. The physician may photocopy relevant portions of the patient's chart and submit that information, but it should be legible. An authorization signed by the patient to release information should be on file. Copies of consultation reports and hospital summaries are also helpful. By law, only data no more than 1 year old are allowed.

A medical report must include the following:

- Relevant medical history, social history, or family history
- Subjective complaints (patient's symptoms)
- Objective findings on physical examination (for example, results of physical or mental status examination, blood pressure)
- Laboratory and x-ray findings
- Diagnostic studies (for example, treadmill tests, pulmonary function tests, and electrocardiogram [ECG] tracings)
- Diagnosis (statement of disease or injury based on signs and symptoms)
- Treatment prescribed, with patient's response and prognosis
- Medical prognosis about disability based on medical findings

A description of the individual's ability to perform work-related activities, such as standing, sitting, lifting, carrying, walking, handling objects, hearing, speaking, and traveling, is necessary. For cases of mental impairment, the statement should present the individual's capacity for understanding and remembering, sustained concentration and persistence, social interaction, and adaptation.

Veterans Affairs Disability Outpatient Clinic Claims

The processing of invoices from private physicians is a somewhat lengthy procedure as required by VA regulations and involves several steps. To keep the delay in payment to a minimum, private physicians and health care organizations are urged to bill the VA monthly. To ensure prompt processing, invoices should contain the following information:

- Patient's name as shown on the ID card, VA Form 10-1174 (see Fig. 8.5).
- Patient's Social Security number.
- Condition treated, shown on every invoice, because this is the basis for approval of payment.
- Diagnosis being treated must be listed on the ID card or authorized by the statement "for any condition." Abstract the diagnosis exactly as it is stated on the ID card.
- Treatment given and dates rendered.
- Physician's usual and customary fee for services rendered.
- Name and address of private physician and his or her Social Security or Federal Taxpayer ID number. If the ID number is assigned to a group and the physician wants to be paid individually, the VA outpatient clinic must be so advised.

Health care organizations and veterans are urged to read the instructions on the ID card carefully. This is sometimes neglected and can lead to misunderstanding.

If the health care organization does not wish to bill the VA outpatient clinic, the patient can pay the service provider and then be reimbursed, but the veteran must carefully follow the instructions on the back of the VA outpatient clinic card.

State Disability Claims

Residents of a state that provides state disability benefits may call or write to the nearest office that handles SDI to obtain a claim form and insurance pamphlet. See the state disability websites for detailed information about each state's benefits, claim procedures, and claim forms.

DB-450 9-17

New York State

NOTICE AND PROOF OF CLAIM FOR DISABILITY BENEFITS

Use this form if you became disabled **while employed** or if you became disabled **within four (4) weeks after termination of employment** OR if you became **disabled after having been unemployed for more than four (4) weeks**. Please answer all questions in Part A and questions 1 through 3 in Part B. Read all instructions on this form carefully. Health care providers must complete Part B on page 2.

PART A - CLAIMANT'S INFORMATION (Please Print or Type)

1. Last Name: ________ First Name: ________ MI: ___

2. Mailing Address (Street & Apt. #): ________

City: ________ State: ____ Zip: ________ Country: ______

3. Daytime Phone #: ________ 4. Email Address: ________

5. Social Security #: ____ - ___ - ____ 6. Date of Birth: ___ - ___ - ____ 7. Gender: ☐ Male ☐ Female

8. My disability is (if injury, also state how, when and where it occurred): ________

9. I became disabled or became ineligible for Unemployment Insurance because of this disability on: ___ / ___ / ____

I worked on that day: ☐ Yes ☐ No

Have you recovered from this disability? ☐ Yes ☐ No If Yes, what was the date you were able to work: ___ / ___ / ____

Have you since worked for wages or profit? ☐ Yes ☐ No If Yes, list dates: ________

10. Give name of last employer. If more than one employer during last eight (8) weeks, name all employers. Average Weekly Wage is based on all wages earned in last eight (8) weeks worked.

LAST EMPLOYER			PERIOD OF EMPLOYMENT		Average Weekly Wage (Include Bonuses, Tips, Commissions, Reasonable Value of Board, Rent, etc.)
Firm or Trade Name	Address	Phone Number	First Day	Last Day Worked	
			Mo. Day Yr.	Mo. Day Yr.	
OTHER EMPLOYER (during last eight (8) weeks)			**PERIOD OF EMPLOYMENT**		**Average Weekly Wage** (Include Bonuses, Tips, Commissions, Reasonable Value of Board, Rent, etc.)
Firm or Trade Name	Address	Phone Number	First Day	Last Day Worked	
			Mo. Day Yr.	Mo. Day Yr.	
			Mo. Day Yr.	Mo. Day Yr.	

11. My job is or was: ________ (Occupation) 12. Union Member: ☐ Yes ☐ No If "Yes": ________ (Name of Union or Local Number)

13. Were you claiming or receiving unemployment prior to this disability? ☐ Yes ☐ No

If you did **not** claim or if you claimed but did **not** receive unemployment insurance benefits after LAST DAY WORKED, explain reasons fully: ________

14. For the period of disability covered by this claim:

A. Are you receiving wages, salary or separation pay: ☐ Yes ☐ No

B. Are you receiving or claiming:

1. Workers' compensation for work-connected disability: ☐ Yes ☐ No
2. Paid Family Leave: ☐ Yes ☐ No
3. No-Fault motor vehicle accident (check box): ☐ Yes ☐ No or personal injury involving third party (check box): ☐ Yes ☐ No
4. Long-term disability benefits under the Federal Social Security Act for this disability: ☐ Yes ☐ No

IF "YES" IS CHECKED IN ANY OF THE ITEMS IN 14, COMPLETE THE FOLLOWING:

I have: ☐ received ☐ claimed from: ________ for the period: ___ / ___ / ____ to: ___ / ___ / ____

15. In the year (52 weeks) **before** your disability began, have you received disability benefits for other periods of disability? ☐ Yes ☐ No

If "Yes", fill in the following: Paid by: ________ from: ___ / ___ / ____ to: ___ / ___ / ____

16. In the year (52 weeks) **before** your disability began, have you received Paid Family Leave? ☐ Yes ☐ No

If "Yes", fill in the following: Paid by: ________ from: ___ / ___ / ____ to: ___ / ___ / ____

I hereby claim Disability Benefits and certify that for the period covered by this claim I was disabled. If my disability began while I was unemployed, I certify that I had been unemployed for more than four (4) weeks. I have read the instructions on page 2 of this form and that the foregoing statements, including any accompanying statements are, to the best of my knowledge, true and complete.

________ Claimant's Signature ________ Date

An individual may sign on behalf of the claimant only if he or she is legally authorized to do so and the claimant is a minor, mentally incompetent or incapacitated. If signed by other than claimant, print information below and complete and submit Form OC-110A, Claimant's Authorization to Disclose Workers' Compensation Records.

________ On behalf of Claimant ________ Address ________ Relationship to Claimant

DB-450 (9-17) Page 1 of 2

Fig. 10.2 Form DE 2501, Claim for Disability Insurance (DI) Benefits. The first four pages of this seven-page form are completed by the claimant. *From New York State Workers' Compensation Board*

In some states the claim form is in three parts and must be completed by the claimant, employer, and physician. In other states, the form is in two parts and is completed by the claimant and physician (Fig. 10.2). In either instance the case must be substantiated by a physician before the applicant may begin receiving benefits. All information from the SDI office should be read carefully and the directions followed precisely. The data requested should be provided and the physician and patient should sign the forms. The form should be submitted within the stated time limits.

PART B - HEALTH CARE PROVIDER'S STATEMENT (Please Print or Type)

THE HEALTH CARE PROVIDER'S STATEMENT MUST BE FILLED IN COMPLETELY. THE ATTENDING HEALTH CARE PROVIDER SHALL COMPLETE AND RETURN TO THE CLAIMANT WITHIN SEVEN (7) DAYS OF RECEIPT OF THIS FORM. For item 7-d, you must give estimated date. If disability is caused by or arising in connection with pregnancy, enter estimated delivery date in item 9. **INCOMPLETE ANSWERS MAY DELAY PAYMENT OF BENEFITS.**

1. Last Name: ______ First Name: ______ MI: __

2.Gender: ☐ Male ☐ Female 3. Date of Birth: ___ / ___ / ___

4. Diagnosis/Analysis: ______ Diagnosis Code: ______

a. Claimant's symptoms: ______

b. Objective findings: ______

5. Claimant hospitalized?: ☐ Yes ☐ No From: ___ / ___ / ___ To: ___ / ___ / ___

6. Operation indicated?: ☐ Yes ☐ No a. Type ______ b. Date ___ / ___ / ___

7. ENTER DATES FOR THE FOLLOWING	MONTH	DAY	YEAR
a Date of your first treatment for this disability			
b. Date of your most recent treatment for this disability			
c. Date Claimant was unable to work because of this disability			
d. Date Claimant will again be able to perform work (Even if considerable question exists, estimate date. Avoid use of terms such as unknown or undetermined.)			
e. If pregnancy related, please check box and enter the date ☐ estimated delivery date OR ☐ actual delivery date			

8. In your opinion, is this disability the result of injury arising out of and in the course of employment or occupational disease?: ☐ Yes ☐ No If "Yes", has Form C-4 been filed with the Board? ☐ Yes ☐ No

I certify that I am a:

(Physician, Chiropractor, Dentist, Podiatrist, Psychologist, Nurse-Midwife) | **Licensed or Certified in the State of** | **License Number**

Health Care Provider's Printed Name | **Health Care Provider's Signature** | **Date**

Health Care Provider's Address | **Phone #**

CLAIMANT: READ THESE INSTRUCTIONS CAREFULLY

PLEASE NOTE: Do not date and file this form prior to your first date of disability. In order for your claim to be processed, Parts A and B must be completed.

1. If you are using this form because you became disabled **while employed** or you became disabled **within four (4) weeks after termination of employment**, your completed claim should be mailed **within thirty (30) days to your employer or your last employer's insurance carrier**. You may find your employer's disability insurance carrier on the Workers' Compensation Board's website using Employer Coverage Search.

2. If you are using this form because you became **disabled after having been unemployed for more than four (4) weeks**, your completed claim should be mailed to: **Workers' Compensation Board, Disability Benefits Bureau, 328 State Street, Schenectady, NY 12305.** If you answered "Yes" to question 14.B.3, please complete and attach Form DB-450.1.

If you have any questions about claiming disability benefits, you may contact the Board's Disability Benefits Bureau at (800) 353-3092. Additional information may be obtained at the Board's website: www.wcb.ny.gov, or you may write to the Disability Benefits Bureau at the address listed above.

Notification Pursuant to the New York Personal Privacy Protection Law (Public Officers Law Article 6-A) and the Federal Privacy Act of 1974 (5 U.S.C. § 552a). The Workers' Compensation Board's (Board's) authority to request that claimants provide personal information, including their social security number, is derived from the Board's investigatory authority under Workers' Compensation Law (WCL) § 20, and its administrative authority under WCL § 142. This information is collected to assist the Board in investigating and administering claims in the most expedient manner possible and to help it maintain accurate claim records. Providing your social security number to the Board is voluntary. There is no penalty for failure to provide your social security number on this form; it will not result in a denial of your claim or a reduction in benefits. The Board will protect the confidentiality of all personal information in its possession, disclosing it only in furtherance of its official duties and in accordance with applicable state and federal law

HIPAA NOTICE - In order to adjudicate a workers' compensation claim or disability benefits claim, WCL 13-a(4)(a) and 12 NYCRR 325-1.3 require health care providers to regularly file medical reports of treatment with the Board and the insurance carrier or employer. Pursuant to 45 CFR 164.512 these legally required medical reports are exempt from HIPAA's restrictions on disclosure of health information.

Disclosure of Information: The Board will not disclose any information about your case to any unauthorized party without your consent. If you choose to have such information disclosed to an unauthorized party, you must file with the Board an original signed Form OC-110A, Claimant's Authorization to Disclose Workers' Compensation Records, or an original signed, notarized authorization letter. You may telephone your local WCB office to have Form OC-110A sent to you, or you may download it from our website, www.wcb.ny.gov. It can be found under Forms on the 'List of All Common Workers' Compensation Board Forms' web page. Mail the completed authorization form to the address listed above.

An employer or insurer, or any employee, agent, or person acting on behalf of an employer or insurer, who KNOWINGLY MAKES A FALSE STATEMENT OR REPRESENTATION as to a material fact in the course of reporting, investigation of, or adjusting a claim for any benefit or payment under this chapter for the purpose of avoiding provision of such payment or benefit SHALL BE GUILTY OF A CRIME AND SUBJECT TO SUBSTANTIAL FINES AND IMPRISONMENT.

DB-450 (9-17) Page 2 of 2

Fig. 10.2, cont'd.

After the claim has been completed by all parties concerned, it is submitted to the nearest local office for processing. The most important items on the claim form are the following:

- The claimant's Social Security number; without it the claim cannot be researched properly to establish wages earned in the base period.
- The first day on which the patient was too sick to perform all of his or her regular work duties (item 3). This cannot be the same day the patient worked, even if the patient went home sick.
- The last day the patient worked (item 4). List the last day on which the patient worked even if for only part of the day.

NOTE: The two dates listed in items 3 and 4 cannot be the same; for example, if the patient went home sick on October 4, that would be considered the last day worked; October 5 would be the first day the patient was unable to work.

California has been selected as the model state for examples of the different forms used in the processing of disability insurance. To establish a claim, the Claim for Disability Insurance Benefits, Form DE 2501, must be completed by both the patient (see Fig. 10.2) and the attending physician. If an extension of disability is necessary, the Physician/Practitioner's Supplementary Certificate, Form DE 2525XX, must be completed by the physician. This accompanies the last check issued to the patient.

All follow-up correspondence should include the patient's name and Social Security number. The insurance billing specialist should promptly report any change of address, telephone number, or return-to-work date to the SDI office. Patients must report any income received to the SDI office because income received may affect benefits.

CONCLUSION

This chapter ends with a bit of levity. The following errors were taken from actual disability insurance application forms, completed by employees, that came across the desk of a claims adjuster.

Spelled as:	Should have been:
yellow "jonders"	yellow jaundice
"goalstones"	gallstones
"limp glands"	lymph glands
"falls teeth"	false teeth
"high pretension"	hypertension
"Pabst smear"	Pap smear
"wrecktum"	rectum

KEY POINTS

This is a brief chapter review, or summary, of the key issues presented. To further enhance your knowledge of the technical subject matter, review the key terms and key abbreviations for this chapter by locating the meaning for each in the Glossary at the end of this book, which appears in a section before the Index.

1. Disability income insurance is a type of insurance that provides periodic wage replacement payments under certain conditions when the insured is unable to work because of illness, disease, or injury, not as a result of a work-related accident or condition.
2. While disabled, benefits begin after an elimination or waiting period (WP).
3. The types of disability are temporary, residual or partial, and total.
4. Disability policies may be guaranteed renewable for a specific number of years to a certain age.
5. The Social Security Administration (SSA) manages two programs that pay monthly disability benefits to people younger than age 65 who cannot work for at least 1 year because of a severe disability: Social Security Disability Insurance (SSDI) program and Supplemental Security Income (SSI) program.
6. Federal employees who have put in a certain number of years of service and who become disabled not by work-related means may be eligible for Civil Service Retirement System (CSRS) and Federal Employees Retirement System (FERS) programs.
7. Individuals on active duty fall under the Armed Services Disability program if they become disabled while serving in the military.
8. The Veterans Affairs (VA) disability program provides benefits for veterans who have suffered a service-connected disability.
9. Five states plus Puerto Rico have a State Disability Insurance (SDI) program for those who suffer a wage loss because of off-the-job illness or injury.
10. Claims for SDI must be filed within the time limits of each state's laws.
11. For disability income claims, the insured must file a proof of loss form, and the attending physician must also complete a section to verify the disability.
12. For federal disability cases, the physician must submit details about the individual's disabled condition.
13. State disability claim forms must be completed by the attending physician to substantiate the claimant's condition to receive benefits.

STUDENT ASSIGNMENTS

- Study Chapter 10.
- Answer the fill-in-the-blank, multiple-choice, and true/false review questions in the *Workbook* to reinforce the theory learned in this chapter and to help prepare you for a future test. Complete the assignments in the *Workbook*. These assignments will provide you with hands-on experience in working with patient histories and completing disability insurance claim forms described in this chapter.
- Turn to the Glossary at the end of this text for a further understanding of the key terms and key abbreviations used in this chapter.

UNIT 3

Documentation and Coding for Professional Services

11

Medical Documentation and the Electronic Health Record

Cheryl Fassett

OBJECTIVES

After reading this chapter, you should be able to:

1. Identify the most common documents found in the health record.
2. Discuss health record systems and list the advantages and disadvantages of an electronic health record system.
3. Define the various titles of physicians as they relate to health record documentation.
4. Explain the reasons that legible documentation is required.
5. Describe common billing errors found in health records and define medical necessity.
6. Discuss various billing patterns that could cause possible audit.
7. Define common terminology related to medical, diagnostic, and surgical services.
8. Abstract information from the health record to complete a life or health insurance application.
9. Describe the difference between prospective and retrospective review of records.
10. Respond appropriately to the subpoena of a witness and records.
11. Identify principles for retention of health records.
12. Formulate a procedure for termination of a case.
13. Discuss in-depth documentation requirements for evaluation and management services, including documentation guidelines for medical services, as well as the documentation of history, examinations, and medical decision making.

KEY TERMS

acute
attending physician
back up
chief complaint
chronic
clinical documentation improvement
cloned note
comorbidity
comprehensive
concurrent care
consultation
consulting physician
continuity of care
counseling
critical care
degaussing
detailed
documentation
electronic health record
emergency care
eponym
established patient
expanded problem focused
external audit
family history
health record
high complexity
history of present illness
internal review
legible
low complexity
medical decision making
medical necessity
moderate complexity
morbidity
mortality
new patient
non-physician practitioner
ordering physician
past history
physical examination
prepayment audit
primary care physician
problem focused
prospective review
query
referral
referring physician
resident physician
retrospective review
review of systems
social history
straightforward
subacute
subpoena
subpoena duces tecum
teaching physician
treating, or performing, physician
zeroization

KEY ABBREVIATIONS

ARRA
C level of history or examination
CC
CDI
CCU
D level of history or examination
dx or Dx
ED or ER
EHR
E/M service
EMR
EPF level of history or examination
FH
HC medical decision making
HIM
HIV
HPI
ICU
LC medical decision making
LLQ
LUQ
MC medical decision making
MDM
PCP
PE or PX
PF level of history or examination
PFSH
PH
POMR system
RCU
RLQ
ROS
RUQ
SF medical decision making
SH
SOAP style
SOR system
WNL

THE DOCUMENTATION PROCESS

Health Record

The **health record** is the most important tool in clinical care and communication. **Documentation** is the process of chronologically recording pertinent facts and observations about the patient's health. A health record is the written or graphic documentation of facts and events during the patient care visit. It may be kept in either a paper or an electronic format. Some health care organizations use different terminology when referring to the health record, such as medical information, medical report, progress or chart note, facility record, or health care record.

Contents of a health record vary from case to case, but some of the most common health care organization documents are as follows:

- Patient demographic information
- Medication record
- History and **physical examination** notes or report
- Progress or chart notes
- **Consultation** reports
- Imaging and x-ray reports
- Laboratory reports
- Immunization records
- Consent and authorization forms
- Operative reports
- Pathology reports

In a health care facility setting there will also be attending physician's orders, discharge summaries, and dates of admission and discharge dates. Supporting **documentation** is the key to substantiating procedure and diagnostic code selections for claim submission and to ensuring appropriate reimbursement. Proper documentation can prevent penalties and refund requests in the event that the health care organization is reviewed or audited.

Health Record Systems

An **electronic health record (EHR)** can be organized using a problem-oriented medical record (**POMR**) system, or as a source-oriented record (**SOR**) system.

The POMR system is designed to organize patient information by the presenting problem. This allows the provider to obtain a quick and structured overview of the patient's history when the patient presents for care. The record consists of flow sheets, charts, or graphs that allow a service provider to quickly locate information and compare evaluations. These data sheets are commonly used to record blood sugar levels, blood pressure readings, weight, immunizations, medication refills, and so on. Using this type of system assists the provider in focusing on the patient's problems, his or her evolution, and the relationship between clinical events.

In the SOR system, documents are arranged according to type of document. For example, history and physical sections, progress notes, laboratory tests, radiology reports, or surgical operations are grouped together. Documents are typically filed in reverse chronological order.

Electronic Health Records

Paper-based offices are becoming a thing of the past. The electronic format has grown in popularity as the ability to share patient health records among care team members has become increasingly important.

An EHR is a collection of medical information about the past, present, and future of a patient that resides in a centralized electronic system. This system receives, stores, transmits, retrieves, and links data from many information systems. This enables information such as laboratory test results, radiology reports and x-ray images, pathology reports, and financial documents to be shared between various departments.

The terms *EHR* and *EMR* may be used interchangeably; however, they are not the same. The electronic medical record (**EMR**) is an individual physician's record for the patient, including medical history, allergies, and appointment information. In comparison, the EHR is all patient medical information from many information systems, including all components of the EMR.

In an EHR system, medical information software may allow the service provider to type or dictate (free-text) the entire record for each encounter. Software may also allow providers to use built-in templates. Templates are a sample document that has some of the details already in place but requires the service provider a fill-in-the-blank approach either by hand or through an automated iterative. Templates help structure documentation through a process of answering a series of questions and entering data.

Electronic Health Records in the Billing Process

Many EHR programs allow the insurance billing specialist to perform insurance verification automatically during the preregistration process. The electronic verification then becomes part of the health record.

Selection of procedure and diagnostic codes by the provider may be computer assisted before final review by a medical coder. These codes are then used for interpretation by the insurance company when processing a claim. When billing the insurance company, the date of service (DOS), place of service (POS), diagnosis (dx or Dx), and procedures are recorded and transmitted in electronic format per Health Insurance Portability and Accountability Act (HIPAA) standards. Electronic signatures are applied to documents when they are reviewed and authenticated by the creator. Insurance claims are generated and transmitted to a clearinghouse or to the insurance carrier. In this way the revenue cycle is managed completely online.

Advantages of Electronic Health Records

An EHR system has several advantages over a paper-based system. The greatest advantage of the EHR is the accessibility of health records between providers and health care organizations. Providers have full access to a patient's complete record in an EHR system. For example, most EHR systems have a built-in system that will alert health care providers about potential problems with medications and allergies. This type of access can improve quality of care and patient safety.

Cost savings and decreasing workplace inefficiencies are other advantages of the EHR. The EHR system requires less physical space because the files remain in an electronic database and are available online. The health record is accessible from remote sites, and retrieval of information at almost any work site is nearly immediate. Chart chasing is eliminated. The EHR can decrease charting time and charting errors, thus increasing the productivity and effectiveness of providers.

The need for staff to select information from a patient's EHR for completion of an insurance claim is often eliminated because data may be captured automatically from various documents via dictation or templates. The EHR is expected to increase patient safety through built-in safety features by use of medical alerts and reminders that can capture things such as medication allergies. The EHR reduces the likelihood of errors, since there is no illegible handwriting to decipher.

Disadvantages of Electronic Health Records

The greatest drawback to EHRs is startup costs, which can be extremely high. Usability can also be a major obstacle in implementation of an EHR. Learning curves vary depending on the user's technical abilities and knowledge.

With increased accessibility comes greater concern with confidentiality and security issues. These issues are the primary focus of the HIPAA Privacy and Security Rules. As discussed in Chapter 2, health care organizations must maintain a higher level of integrity in these areas.

Although EHR is designed to save providers time and improve the quality and legibility of their documentation, the use of EHR has also led to a new problem with the medical record, related to copied and templated documentation. These are referred to as cloned notes. The process may also be referred to as "cut and paste" or "carried over." The Centers for Medicare and Medicaid Services (CMS) considers documentation to be cloned when each entry in the health record for a patient is worded exactly the same as or similar to the previous entries. Cloning also occurs when medical documentation is exactly the same from patient to patient.

Cloned notes increase the risk for medical errors and can result in the loss of crucial clinical details that may be omitted from a patient's assessment or treatment plan. All documentation in the health record must be specific to the patient and his or her situation at the time of the encounter. Payers are refusing to pay for services that appear to be cloned, and this process has come under increased scrutiny by the Office of Inspector General (OIG). It is a red flag for fraud investigations.

INCENTIVE PROGRAMS FOR ADOPTION OF ELECTRONIC HEALTH RECORDS

Federal legislation established by the American Recovery and Reinvestment Act of 2009 (ARRA) created programs to help the health care industry change to electronic health records. Legislation affecting Medicare and Medicaid programs was established to provide more than $27 billion in payout of incentives to eligible providers who implement electronic health records. The programs provided a reimbursement incentive for health care organizations who adopted, implemented, upgraded, and demonstrated meaningful use (MU) of certified EHR technology. It was anticipated that compliance with MU would result in the following:

- Better clinical outcomes
- Improved population health outcomes
- Increased transparency and efficiency
- Empowered patients
- More robust research data on health systems

Starting in 2015, these incentive programs began transitioning from incentives into reimbursement penalties for those who have not adopted EHR. Medicare payments were reduced by 1% for those who were not using EHR in the previous year. Penalties rose to 2% in 2016 and 3% in 2017.

During the last decade, Medicare implemented additional programs such as the Physician Quality Reporting System (PQRS) and the Merit-based Incentive Payment System (MIPS). These programs link reimbursement directly to documentation of quality measures. Similar to the MU incentives, failure to adopt these documentation and reporting measures will result in reimbursement penalties.

Further legislation in the Medicare Modernization Act created the Commission on Systemic Interoperability to develop a strategy to make health care information available at all times to patients and providers. To reach a goal of having electronic records for all Americans, adoption of health information standards and increased funding for these projects has begun.

It is important for insurance billing specialists to be familiar with all incentive programs. They will be involved in submission of qualifying data, collection of incentive payments, and analysis of incentive program outcomes as they affect the organization's accounts receivable.

GENERAL PRINCIPLES OF HEALTH RECORD DOCUMENTATION

Documentation is the core of the revenue cycle in any health care organization. To bill for any health care services, the medical billing specialist will refer to the documentation to identify the services provided and to complete the claim form. Documentation must be accurate and complete. Supporting documentation is critical to ensure accurate and timely payment of services furnished.

Additionally, clear and concise documentation of health records is critical to providing patients with quality care. Documentation of health records assists health care professionals in evaluating and planning the patient's immediate treatment and monitoring the patient's health care over time.

Documenters

All individuals providing health care services may be referred to as documenters because they record pertinent facts and observations about the patient's health. Documentation (charting) may be electronically handwritten, dictated and transcribed, or downloaded from a personal digital assistant (PDA) or smartphone using an electronic template. It is the health care provider's responsibility to either handwrite the medical information or dictate it for transcription.

Some documenters use a speech recognition system. These computerized voice recognition systems make it possible for a computer system to respond to spoken words. There are two basic categories of speech recognition systems:

- Navigation or command control systems allow an individual to launch and operate software applications with spoken directions.
- Dictation software systems make it possible for a computer system to recognize spoken words and automatically convert them into text.

When a dictation software speech recognition system is used, many health care organizations use a medical editor or correctionist who proofreads and edits the computer-generated documents. Some organizations use printed checklists for typical examinations. The health care provider notes his or her findings on the checklists and gives this document to an employee for input to the EMR system.

Health care service providers are not the only documenters in a health care organization. The receptionist obtains the first document completed by the patient, called the patient registration information form. The medical assistant or a front desk staff member is often the one who records entries for no-show appointments, prescription refills, and telephone calls. The insurance billing specialist uses the information in the health record for billing purposes. It is his or her responsibility to bring any substandard documentation to the provider's or office manager's attention, depending on office policy. In the health care facility setting, a trained health information management (HIM) professional maintains the health record for completeness.

When referring to guidelines for documentation of the health record and completion of the insurance claim form, a service provider's role and title may change, depending on the circumstances of each patient encounter. This can get confusing at times. To clarify the various roles, some of these titles are defined as follows:

- *Attending physician* refers to the facility staff member who is legally responsible for the care and treatment given to a patient.
- Consulting physician is a provider whose opinion or advice regarding evaluation or management of a specific problem is requested by another provider.
- Non-physician practitioner is a nurse practitioner, clinical nurse specialist, licensed social worker, nurse midwife, physical therapist, speech therapist, audiologist, or physician assistant who furnishes a consultation or treats a patient for a specific medical problem. Non-physician practitioners are also known as *physician extenders.*
- Ordering physician is the individual in the health care organization directing the selection, preparation, or administration of tests, medication, or treatment.
- Primary care physician (PCP) oversees the care of patients in a managed health care plan and refers patients to see specialists for services as needed.
- Referring physician is a provider who sends the patient for tests or treatment.
- Resident physician is a physician who has finished medical school and is performing one or more years of training in a specialty area on the job at a health care facility. A resident performs the elements required for an evaluation and management (E/M) service or another service in the presence of or jointly with the teaching physician. The resident documents the service.
- Teaching physician is a doctor who has responsibilities for training and supervising medical students, interns, or residents and who takes them to the bedsides of patients in a teaching facility to review course and treatment. Teaching physicians must document that they supervised and were physically present during key portions of the service provided to the patient when performed by a resident.
- Treating, or performing, physician is the provider who renders a therapeutic or evaluation service to a patient.

Clinical Documentation Improvement

Clinical documentation improvement (CDI) is the process of creating accurate and effective patient health records. CDI programs were developed in response to CMS's transition to quality-based reimbursement systems. The goal of any CDI program is to improve patient outcomes, provide accurate data for quality measurement reporting, and ensure proper reimbursement. Different techniques can be used to achieve this. For example, concurrent and retrospective reviews of health records may flag incomplete or conflicting documentation.

A query is a tool used by the CDI specialist to request additional clarification from the provider. Queries should include the clinical indicators that prompted the request, and should not be leading. The query should not introduce new information not contained in the medical record. Queries and query forms often become part of the permanent health record. It is beneficial if a CDI program has a physician advisor who can provide education to the CDI specialist and serve as a liaison between them and the medical staff.

Often service providers are unfamiliar with the documentation requirements for proper coding. On the other hand, many coders lack the clinical knowledge that explains procedures and tests. A CDI specialist links the two, providing documentation education to both. For those interested in pursuing a career focusing on this area, the American Health Information Management Association (AHIMA) offers a clinical documentation improvement practitioner (CDIP) certification. The American Association of Professional Coders (AAPC) also offers a clinical documentation expert outpatient (CDEO) certification.

! COMPLIANCE ALERT

Legible Documentation

If handwritten, entries in the patient's record must be legible. Illegible entries should be returned to the health care provider for clarification or to be rewritten.

LEGIBLE DOCUMENTATION

Health record documentation details pertinent facts, findings, and observations about an individual's health history, examinations, tests, treatments, and outcomes. It enables the health care professional to evaluate and plan the patient's immediate treatment and monitor the patient's health care over time. It also helps health care providers communicate with each other regarding a patient's diagnosis and treatment. A health record also acts as a legal document for evidence if the need arises. It is a basic and important element in providing the highest level of quality of care.

The documentation guidelines issued by CMS state that the health record should be complete and **legible**. The CMS definition of legible is that the data must be easily recognizable by someone outside the health care organization who is unfamiliar with the handwriting. It is important that providers have comprehensive and legible documentation describing what occurred during the patient's visit for the following reasons:

- To avoid denial or delay of payments by insurance carriers
- To avoid misdiagnosing patients
- To avoid dispensing incorrect medications
- To ensure proper treatments are given
- To ensure continuity of care
- To comply with insurance carrier payment policies requiring documentation to support procedural and diagnostic codes submitted on claims
- For subpoena of health records by state investigators or the court for review
- For defense of any professional liability claims
- For execution of the health care provider's written instructions to the patient or the caregiver
- To avoid charges of negligence and malpractice

Common Documentation Errors

Understandably, health care providers put patient care first. The documentation process is secondary and is often times hurried and treated as an afterthought. Providing excellent patient care is often used as an excuse for poor documentation. It is important to help health care provider's understand the link between quality care and documentation.

The following is a list of common errors found in health records:

- Medication lists are not updated with new or discontinued medications.
- Incorrect dosages of prescription medications are documented.
- Duplicate prescriptions are documented for both brand-name and generic medications.
- Over-the-counter medications the patient is taking are not documented.
- Information related to medication allergies is not documented.
- Treatment outcomes are often incorrect. For example, a condition is noted as being resolved when it is still being treated.
- Laboratory information is missing or not updated.
- Important information related to the patient's illness and symptoms, as stated by the patient, are not documented.
- There are inaccuracies in diagnosis and incomplete documentation related to the plan of care for the condition.
- Information from other providers is missing.

! COMPLIANCE ALERT

Medically Necessary

Third-party payers and federal programs have a responsibility to ensure that professional services provided to patients were medically necessary. Documentation must support the level of service and each procedure rendered.

Medical Necessity

Payment for services may be delayed, downcoded, or denied if the **medical necessity** of a treatment is questioned. As a rule, medical necessity is a criterion used by insurance companies, as well as federal programs such as Medicare, when making decisions to limit or deny payment. Some health care organizations use electronic medical necessity software that verifies that the medical services or procedures are justified by the patient's symptoms and diagnosis. Medical treatment must be done in accordance with standards of good medical practice and the proper level of care provided in the most appropriate setting. However, insurers differ on this definition and may or may not cover the services depending on the benefits of the plan. Inform the patient of this situation with a letter, as shown in Fig. 11.1. As discussed in Chapter 6, if the patient has Medicare coverage, an Advance Beneficiary Notice of Noncoverage (ABN), also known as a waiver of liability agreement or responsibility statement, is required in this type of situation.

Legalities of Health Record Billing Patterns

Insurance carriers have become stricter in enforcing accurate coding substantiated by documentation. It is not uncommon for carriers to perform random prepayment and postpayment

COLLEGE CLINIC
4567 Broad Avenue
Woodland Hills, XY 12345-0001
Phone: 555/486-9002
Fax: 555/487-8976

September 20, 20XX

Dear ABC Managed Care Plan Participant:

This is a quick fact sheet to help our patients understand that some services may not be paid by ABC Managed Care Plan unless there is a *medical* reason to perform them.

The coverage provided by ABC Managed Care Plan, in most instances, includes payment for medically necessary services provided to treat a problem or illness. However, patients who wish their health care providers to perform services outside of those considered a "medical necessity" will be responsible for paying for those services out-of-pocket.

For example, many patients come to our office for the purpose of removing noncancerous facial moles. Although this procedure may be desired by the patient, ABC Managed Care Plan will not pay for the removal without a medical reason for it.

The patient's cost for noncancerous facial mole removal at our practice is approximately $75.

Please understand that, legally, we are required to submit our bill to ABC Managed Care Plan using accurate information about all of the services you received. Using a false medical reason to try to get insurance to pay for a service it otherwise would not cover is considered fraud, and our doctors will not do this. We regret that ABC Managed Care Plan may not wish to pay for a service you desire, but we must follow insurance regulations.

If you would like additional information about payment coverage for these services, you may refer to your ABC Managed Care Plan benefits handbook or call your ABC Managed Care Plan customer service representative at 555-271-0311.

Thank you for choosing us to assist you with your health care needs. As always, providing high-quality health care to you is and remains our primary purpose. If you have any questions about this information, please do not hesitate to telephone and ask our front office staff for more information.

Sincerely,

Mary Anne Mason, CPC

Fig. 11.1 Letter to a patient who is a member of a managed care plan that provides important information about medical procedures or services that are not covered for payment unless there is a medical necessity.

audits or for carriers to monitor the accuracy of providers' use of medical services and procedure codes. Medicare administrative contractors and other carriers have "walk-in rights" that they may invoke to conduct documentation reviews, audits, and evaluations. This means that they have access to a health care organization without an appointment or search warrant.

Fraudulent or abusive billing patterns that may draw attention to a health care organization for possible audit are as follows:

- Billing intentionally for unnecessary services
- Billing incorrectly for services of physician extenders, such as nurse practitioner, midwife, physician assistant
- Billing for diagnostic tests without a separate report in the health record
- Changing dates of service on insurance claims to comply with policy coverage dates
- Waiving copayments or deductibles or allowing other illegal discounts
- Ordering excessive diagnostic tests, such as laboratory tests or x-ray studies
- Using two different provider numbers to bill the same services for the same patient
- Misusing provider identification numbers, resulting in incorrect billing
- Using improper modifiers for financial gain
- Failing to return overpayments made by the Medicare program

Termination of a Case

A health care provider may wish to withdraw formally from further care of a patient because of patient noncompliance. There are many reasons for this, such as the following:

- The patient discharged the health care provider.
- The patient did not follow instructions.
- The patient did not take the recommended medication.

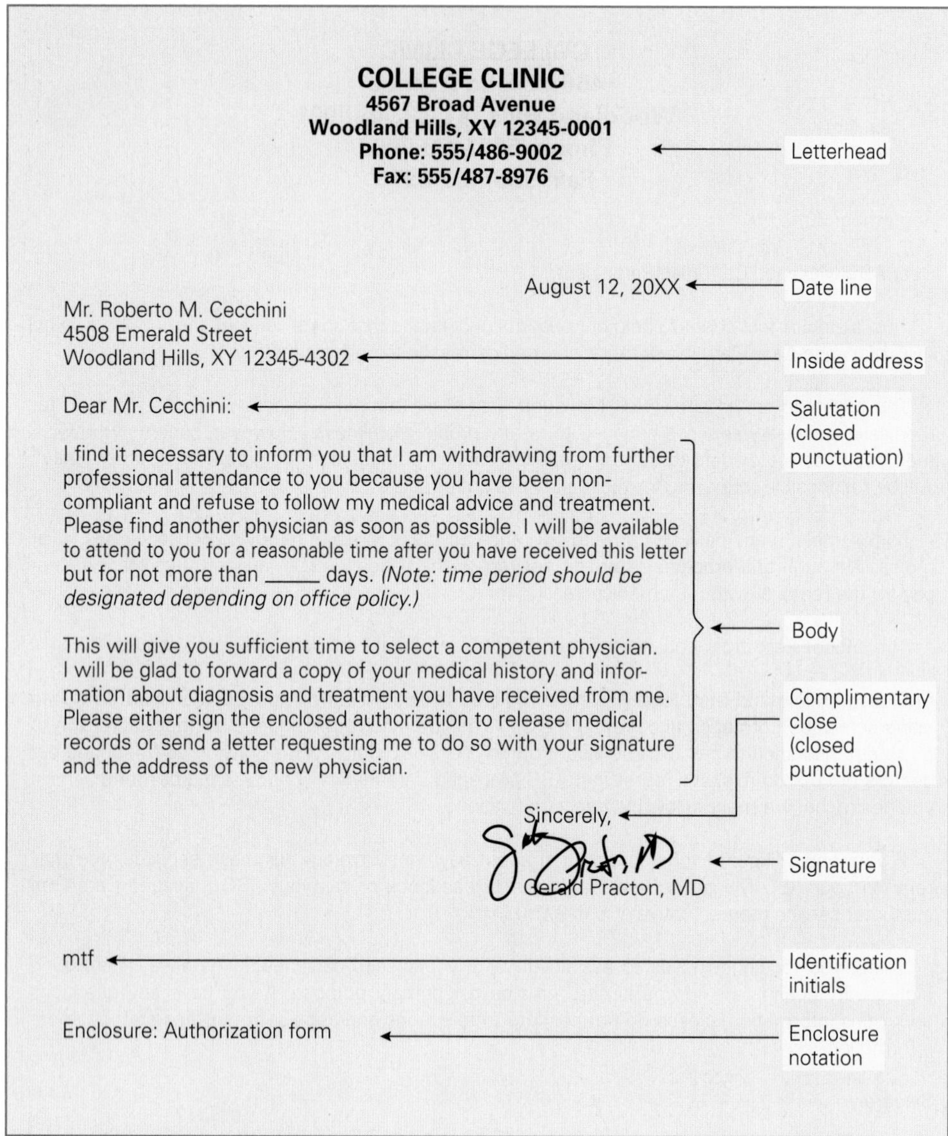
COLLEGE CLINIC
4567 Broad Avenue
Woodland Hills, XY 12345-0001
Phone: 555/486-9002
Fax: 555/487-8976

August 12, 20XX

Mr. Roberto M. Cecchini
4508 Emerald Street
Woodland Hills, XY 12345-4302

Dear Mr. Cecchini:

I find it necessary to inform you that I am withdrawing from further professional attendance to you because you have been non-compliant and refuse to follow my medical advice and treatment. Please find another physician as soon as possible. I will be available to attend to you for a reasonable time after you have received this letter but for not more than _____ days. *(Note: time period should be designated depending on office policy.)*

This will give you sufficient time to select a competent physician. I will be glad to forward a copy of your medical history and information about diagnosis and treatment you have received from me. Please either sign the enclosed authorization to release medical records or send a letter requesting me to do so with your signature and the address of the new physician.

Sincerely,

Gerald Practon, MD

mtf

Enclosure: Authorization form

Fig. 11.2 Example of letter of withdrawal from a case.

- The patient failed to return for an appointment.
- The patient discontinued payment on an overdue account.

Termination of patient care should always be made in writing. If the health care provider is terminating the relationship, he or she should send a letter of withdrawal to the patient by certified mail with return receipt so that proof of termination is in the patient's health record (Fig. 11.2).

If the patient terminates the relationship, the health care provider should send a letter of confirmation of discharge when the patient states that he or she no longer desires care (Fig. 11.3). This should also be sent certified mail with return receipt requested.

If the patient leaves a health care facility against medical advice, the provider should send a letter confirming this. If there is a signed statement in the patient's facility records to this effect, it is not necessary to send a letter. If a letter is sent, a copy of the letter and return signature card from the post office must be filed with the patient's records.

If a noncompliant patient refuses a certified dismissal letter and it is returned unopened, file the returned letter and refusal notice in the patient's chart. Then, in a plain envelope, send another copy of the letter to the patient. Document the date and time it was posted and the location of the mailbox used. Place these data in the patient's chart and initial them. After 10 days, telephone the patient to confirm receipt of the correspondence. If the patient denies receiving it, read it over the telephone. In most regions, this will provide immunity against medical abandonment of a case, which is the discontinuance of medical care by a provider without proper notice. All record of notification attempts should be maintained in the patient's health record. This record should be retained per the health care organization's records retention policy.

DOCUMENTATION TERMINOLOGY

Terminology for Evaluation and Management Services

While learning the complexities of medical documentation and how important it is as it relates to coding and billing, a billing specialist must have a good foundation of medical terminology.

COLLEGE CLINIC
4567 Broad Avenue
Woodland Hills, XY 12345-0001
Phone: 555/486-9002
Fax: 555/487-8976

September 3, 20XX

Mrs. Gregory Putnam
4309 North E Street
Woodland Hills, XY 12345-4398

Dear Mrs. Putnam:

This will confirm our telephone conversation today during which you discharged me from attending you as your physician in your present illness. In my opinion, your medical condition requires continued treatment by a physician. If you have not already obtained the services of another physician, I suggest you do so without further delay.

You may be assured that, upon your written authorization, I will furnish your new physician with information regarding the diagnosis and treatment you have received from me.

Very truly yours,

Gerald Procton, MD

mtf

Fig. 11.3 Letter to confirm discharge of a patient.

A solid foundation of language, abbreviations, and symbols is important to using the diagnostic and procedure code books efficiently.

In the early 1990s the American Medical Association (AMA) modified the term *office visits* and replaced this phrase with *office and other outpatient services*. The AMA also adopted the phrase *evaluation and management (E/M)* for the name of the section of *Current Procedural Terminology* (CPT) in which those procedure codes appear. This wording better reflects the components involved when performing an office visit. However, E/M services are also performed in other settings, such as inpatient health care facilities and nursing homes.

New versus Established Patient

In coding E/M services, two categories of patients are considered: the new patient and the established patient. A **new patient** is one who has not received any professional services within the last 3 years from the physician or another physician of the same specialty who belongs to the same group practice. An **established patient** is one who has received professional services within the last 3 years from the physician or another physician of the same specialty who belongs to the same group practice. Refer to the decision tree in Fig. 11.4 to help decide whether a patient is considered new or established.

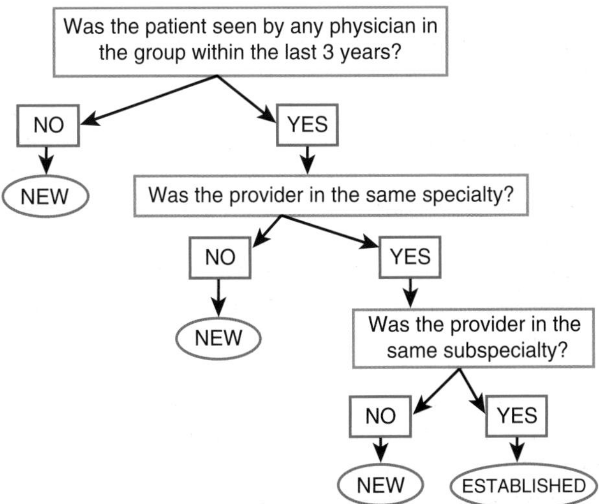

Fig. 11.4 Decision tree for new patient versus established patient when selecting a *Current Procedural Terminology* evaluation and management code.

A physician may provide a course of action to evaluate and manage a patient who is seeking medical care. Some of the options include the following:

- Refer to a specialist for consultation
- See a referral from another physician
- Give concurrent care as one of several physicians
- Render continuity of care for a doctor who is out of town
- Administer critical care
- Direct emergency care
- Furnish counseling discussion to a patient's family

Consultation

A **consultation** occurs when a physician is asked to provide an opinion or advice in the evaluation or treatment of a patient's illness or a suspected problem. The requesting physician must document the request in the patient's health record and the consulting physician should state: "Patient is seen at the request of Dr. John Doe for a … reason." Consultations may occur in a home, office, hospital, extended care facility, or other location. A consulting physician recommends diagnostic or therapeutic services and may initiate these services if requested by the referring physician. The opinion must be in writing, documented in a consultation report, and communicated to the referring physician. The consulting physician may order a diagnostic or therapeutic service to formulate the opinion at an initial or subsequent visit.

Referral

A **referral** is the transfer of the total or specific care of a patient from one provider to another for known problems. It is not a consultation. For example, a patient is sent by a PCP to an orthopedist for care of a fracture.

However, when dealing with managed care plans, the term *referral* is also used when requesting an authorization for the patient to receive services elsewhere (for example, referral for laboratory tests, radiology procedures, or specialty care). In most cases, the PCP must obtain authorization for the referral to ensure that the managed care plan will pay for the specialist's services. Appropriate documentation of the referral and authorization is needed to substantiate approval of the referral.

Concurrent Care

Concurrent care occurs when one or more service providers deliver similar services to the same patient on the same day. For example, two internists, a general internist and a cardiologist, see the same patient in the hospital on the same day. The general internist admits the patient for diabetes and requests that the cardiologist also follow the patient's periodic chest pain and arrhythmia. If the second physician is not identified in carrier records as a different type of specialist, the claim may be denied. This is because the services appear to be duplicated by physicians of the same specialty.

When billing insurance companies, physicians providing concurrent care may be cross-referenced on the claim form. Medicare has a list that includes 62 specialties and subspecialties to help carriers more accurately judge whether concurrent care is necessary. Periodically, the physician should check with the carrier's provider service representative to determine whether the provider has updated its subspecialty status so that claims for concurrent care are not denied.

Continuity of Care

If a case involves **continuity of care,** there are two service providers who are both treating the patient's condition. For example, if a PCP refers a patient to a cardiologist, both physicians should provide the other with a copy of the patient's records of care. In this way, the two physicians will be aware of the treatments and medications being prescribed by the other. If the patient received treatment in a health care facility, the facility's health records department should provide copies of reports after treatment or after the patient's discharge to the patient's primary care physician.

Critical Care

Critical care refers to the intensive care provided for a variety of acute, life-threatening conditions requiring constant full attention by a physician. Critical care may sometimes, but not always, be rendered in a critical care area, such as a coronary care unit (**CCU**), intensive care unit (**ICU**), respiratory care unit (**RCU**), or emergency department (**ED**), also called an emergency room (**ER**). A critical illness or injury acutely impairs one or more vital organ systems. There is a high probability of imminent or life-threatening deterioration in the patient's condition. Examples of vital organ system failure include, but are not limited to, the following:

- Central nervous system failure
- Circulatory failure
- Shock
- Renal, hepatic, metabolic, or respiratory failure

Emergency Care

Emergency care is care provided to acutely ill patients that may or may not involve organ system failure but does require immediate medical attention. An emergency may take place in any medical setting, not just an ED. In physician-directed emergency care advanced life support, the physician is located in a hospital emergency or critical care department and is in two-way voice communication with ambulance or rescue personnel outside the hospital. The physician directs the performance of necessary medical procedures.

According to CMS, an emergency medical condition is one that manifests itself by acute symptoms of sufficient severity. It is one that without immediate medical attention could lead to impairment of body functions, dysfunction of any body organ or part, or death. Examples of a medical emergency are as follows:

- Severe pain
- High fever
- Difficulty breathing
- Uncontrolled bleeding
- Chest pain
- Poisoning
- Broken bones
- Sudden facial drooping, slurred speech, or weakness in limbs
- Severe trauma such as a gunshot wound or crush injury from a car accident
- Loss of consciousness

Counseling

Counseling is a discussion with a patient, family, or both. Counseling may concern diagnostic results, impressions, or

TABLE 11.1 Do Not Use Abbreviations

Do Not Use	Potential Problem	Use Instead
U, u (unit)	Mistaken for "0" (zero), the number 4 (four), or "cc"	Write "unit"
IU (International Unit)	Mistaken for IV (intravenous) or the number 10 (ten)	Write "International Unit"
Q.D, QD, q.d., qd (daily)	Mistaken for each other. Period after the Q mistaken for "I" and the "O" mistaken for "I"	Write "daily"
Q.O.D., QOD, q.o.d., qod (every other day)		Write "every other day"
Trailing zero (X.0 mg)	Decimal point is missed	Write X mg
Lack of leading zero (.X mg)		Write 0.X mg
MS	Can mean morphine sulfate or magnesium sulfate.	Write "morphine sulfate"
MS04 and MgS04	Confused for one another	Write "magnesium sulfate"

From "Facts About the Official 'Do Not Use' List of Abbreviations," Joint Commission, June 9, 2017, https://www.jointcommission.org/facts_about_do_not_use_list/.

recommended diagnostic studies. A service provider may also counsel a patient or family about the prognosis, risks and benefits of treatment options, instructions for treatment or follow-up, or the importance of compliance with chosen treatment options. Counseling may also provide education, particularly in discussing lifestyle risk factors. For example, a physician may counsel a patient regarding weight loss or smoking cessation.

Diagnostic Terminology and Abbreviations

Problems can occur with documentation because of missing or misused essential words. Consider these two phrases: "heart failure due to diastolic dysfunction" or "diastolic dysfunction." The first statement gives more complete documentation of the medical condition. Always query the service provider if in doubt about the documentation to obtain the most specific, accurate terminology for the record.

Some providers document "imp" for impression or "Dx" for diagnosis, which usually serves as the diagnosis when completing the claim. If the diagnosis is not in the health record or there is doubt about the diagnosis, always ask the provider to review it. If the patient has been in a health care facility, request the electronic file of the discharge summary, which contains the admitting and discharge diagnoses.

The health care field uses many abbreviations and acronyms that can save time and aid in communication. However, they may be confusing in their interpretation. Often an abbreviation can be translated into several meanings. Official American Hospital Association (AHA) policy states that "abbreviations should be totally eliminated from the more vital sections of the health record, such as final diagnosis, operative notes, discharge summaries, and descriptions of special procedures." Many providers are not aware of this policy, and the final diagnosis may appear as an abbreviation in the patient's record.

The Joint Commission is an agency that provides accreditation status to health care organizations that comply with their standards of patient care. The Joint Commission has made it a mission to research what practices provide the best health care to patients and has hundreds of performance standards with which organizations must comply. Its National Patient Safety Goal was initiated to improve communication between caregivers and has stated that health care facilities must take reasonable approaches to standardizing abbreviations, acronyms, and symbols. For example, facilities can develop a standardized list of abbreviations or use a published reference source. When providers use multiple abbreviations, symbols, or acronyms for the same term, the facility must identify what they should use to eliminate any ambiguity.

EXAMPLE 11.1 Eponyms and Medical Terms

Eponym	Comparable Medical Term
Buerger disease	Thromboangiitis obliterans
Graves' disease	Exophthalmic goiter
Wilk's syndrome	Myasthenia gravis
Hartmann's procedure	Proctosigmoidectomy

In 2004 the Joint Commission created its "do not use" list of abbreviations (Table 11.1) for all organizations accredited with it. Use a medical dictionary to interpret an abbreviation or ask the provider when clarification is necessary. Most list abbreviations alphabetically with the unabbreviated words.

Most health care organizations create and retain a list of acceptable abbreviations with translations in their office policy manual to avoid misinterpretation.

If a lay term appears in a patient record, the correct medical term should be substituted to locate the correct diagnostic code. For example, use the term *contusion* when coding for bruise.

An **eponym** is a term including the name of a person, such as Graves' disease. Eponyms should not be used when a comparable anatomic term can be used in its place. A few examples of eponyms that describe medical conditions and their more appropriate documentation are included in Example 11.1.

The word ***acute*** refers to a condition that runs a short but relatively severe course. Acute conditions typically last 3 to 5 days. The word ***chronic*** means a condition persisting over a long period, often more than 3 months. ***Subacute*** refers to a condition that is both acute and chronic. When the terms *acute* and *chronic* are listed in the diagnostic statement, always search for these terms in the code description.

An abnormal or unexpected finding without elaboration in the health record is insufficient documentation and should be described. For example, if the provider documents that "the patient presents for review of abnormal labs," this would be insufficient. The provider should document more specifically, such as "the patient presents today for abnormally high blood sugar test results."

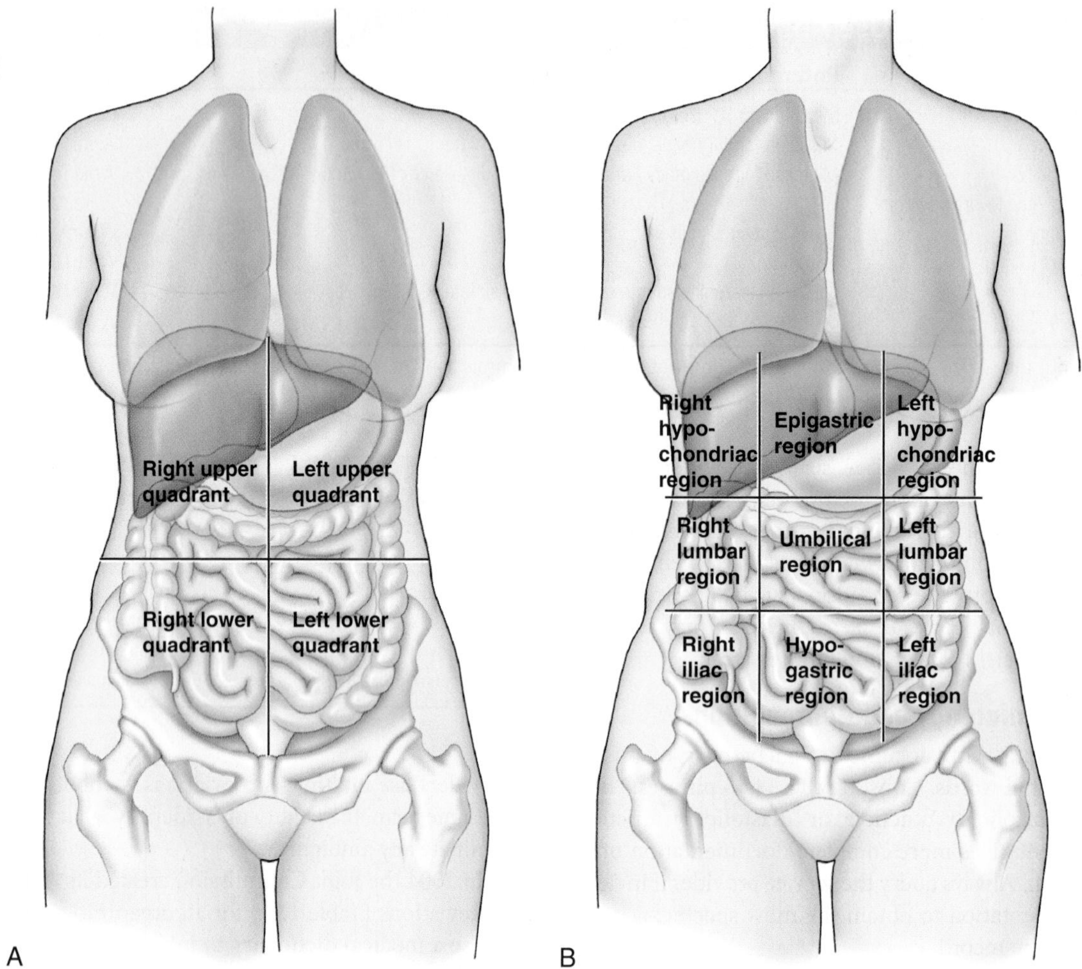

Fig. 11.5 Regions of the abdomen. **A,** Four quadrants. **B,** Nine regions. (From Herlihy B, Maebius NK: *The human body in health and illness,* ed 4, St. Louis, 2011, Elsevier.)

Commonly used phrases or abbreviations that may not support billing of services are "WNL" (within normal limits), "noncontributory," "negative/normal," "other than the above, all systems were normal," and so on. For example, phrases used to document findings, such as "all extremities are within normal limits," do not indicate how many extremities or which ones were examined. Documentation must indicate exactly which limb was examined. Providers who document that the patient's family history is "noncontributory" do not give any family background at all. Abbreviated wording will not pass an external audit. If it is determined that such phrases are copied from a template, it can mean that no assessment was actually performed. This is fraud.

Another word commonly used when a patient is examined and the findings are within normal limits is "negative." The note may contain phrases like "ears, nose, and throat negative," or "chest x-rays negative." The physician needs to document that there were no abnormalities in the system being examined. Detailed documentation justifies billed services by providing verification and provides supporting documentation when an external audit is performed.

Directional Terms

The following terms are commonly used to describe the location of pain and injuries to areas of the abdomen, as shown in Fig. 11.5, *A* (four quadrants) and *B* (nine regions):

Right upper quadrant (RUQ) or right hypochondriac: Liver (right lobe), gallbladder, part of the pancreas, parts of the small and large intestines

Epigastric: Upper middle region above the stomach

Left upper quadrant (LUQ) or left hypochondriac: Liver (left lobe), stomach, spleen, part of the pancreas, parts of the small and large intestines

Right and left lumbar: Middle, right, and left regions of the waist

Umbilical: Central region near the navel

Right lower quadrant (RLQ) or right inguinal: Parts of the small and large intestines, right ovary, right uterine (fallopian) tube, appendix, and right ureter

Hypogastric: Middle region below the umbilical region contains urinary bladder and female uterus

Left lower quadrant (LLQ) or left inguinal: Parts of the small and large intestines, left ovary, left uterine tube, and left ureter

Surgical Terminology

Two commonly used terms are *preoperative* and *postoperative. Preoperative (preop)* pertains to the period before a surgical procedure. Commonly the preoperative period begins with the first preparation of the patient for surgery and ends with the introduction of anesthesia in the operating suite, whereas *postoperative* pertains to the period after surgery. It begins with the patient's emergence from anesthesia and continues through the time required for the acute effects of the anesthetic and surgical procedures to decrease.

Surgical procedures of the integumentary system, such as repair of lacerations, are listed in the procedure code book as *simple, intermediate,* or *complex* repairs. Simple lacerations are superficial, requiring one-layer closure. Intermediate lacerations require layered closure of one or more of the deeper layers of the skin and tissues. Complex lacerations require more than layered closure and may require reconstructive surgery. Documentation should list the length in centimeters of all incisions and layers of involved tissues (subcutaneous, fascia, muscle, and grafts) so that correct procedure codes for excision of lesions and type of repair can be determined.

If time is a factor in coding for reimbursement, documentation should clearly state time. For example:

- For anesthesia services, start and stop times are required documentation.
- For critical care services, time spent providing critical care must be documented.
- For psychiatry visits, time spent with the patient must be documented.
- For E/M visits, time must be documented if more than 50% of the time spent was counseling and coordinating care.
- If unusual circumstances cause a surgery caused a surgery to take longer than usual and additional reimbursement is requested, time must be documented.

If state-of-the-art instruments or equipment are used, document the equipment as well as the time spent using it.

Therapeutic or cosmetic surgical procedures should be broken down into two categories—state how much of the procedure was functional and how much was cosmetic or therapeutic. Generally the insurance carrier pays for the functional portion of the procedure even if there is no coverage for cosmetic or therapeutic procedures. For example, if a physician provides anesthesia services for a patient who is having an abdominoplasty (cosmetic) and an inguinal hernia, he will need to indicate how much of the time was dedicated to each procedure. Most insurance companies will not pay for cosmetic procedures and the physician will need to collect his reimbursement for the abdominoplasty from the patient.

A billing specialist may type reports to be submitted with insurance claims to help justify the claims. Being familiar with the terms for various operational incisions is helpful (Fig. 11.6).

Terms such as *undermining* (cut in a horizontal fashion), *take down* (to take apart), or *lysis of adhesions* (destruction of scar tissue) appear in many operations but should not be coded separately. Note the position of the patient during the operation. Some examples of positional terms would be *dorsal* or *lateral.* The surgical approach should also be noted. Examples of surgical approach would be *vaginal* or *abdominal.* These help to determine the proper code selection. Major errors can occur when an insurance biller is not familiar with the medical terms being used. Ask the provider to clarify the case if there is a question because medical terminology is technical and can puzzle even the most knowledgeable insurance billing specialist.

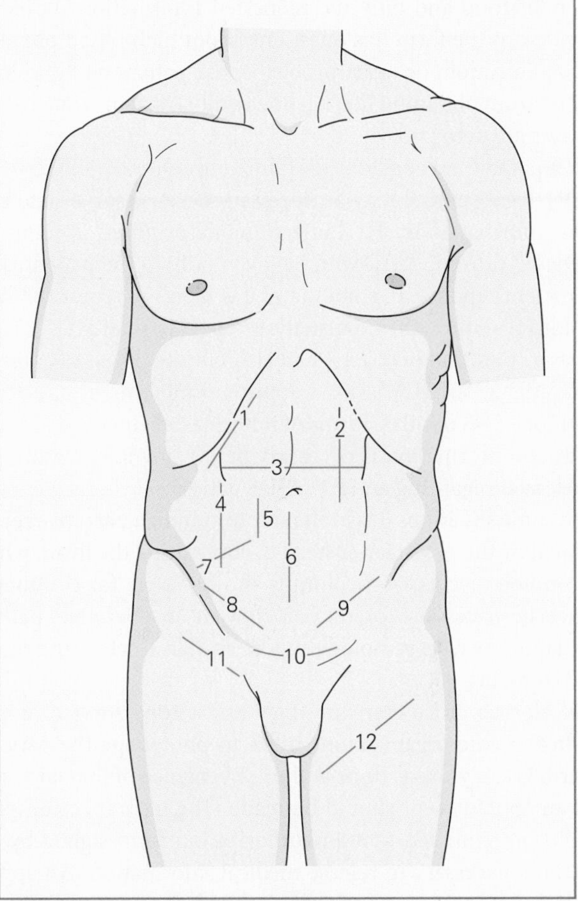

Fig. 11.6 Operational incisions. Anterior (front) view: *1,* Subcostal incision; *2,* paramedian incision; *3,* transverse incision; *4,* upper right rectus incision; *5,* midrectus incision; *6,* midline incision; *7,* lower right rectus incision; *8,* McBurney or right iliac incision; *9,* left iliac incision; *10,* suprapubic incision, *11,* hernia incision; *12,* femoral incision.

ABSTRACTING FROM HEALTH RECORDS

The insurance billing specialist may be required to abstract information from health records. Abstraction of technical information from patient records may be requested for three situations:

1. To complete insurance claim forms
2. When sending a letter to justify a health insurance claim form after professional services are rendered
3. When a patient applies for life, mortgage, or health insurance

Life or Health Insurance Applications

When a patient applies for insurance, the insurance company may request information from the patient's physician, require a physical examination, or both. Before completing the forms, the patient must sign a release of information form. Insurance companies will typically include a check when requesting medical information. The amount of the check may vary, depending on how much information is requested. If no payment is included, the health care organization should request fee payment before sending in the completed report form. Be sure the service provider checks the documentation thoroughly before signing it to ensure that the information is accurate and properly stated.

Be extremely accurate when abstracting medical information from the patient's record. Abbreviations on the chart must be understood and only the requested information should be provided. If the form has questions about high blood pressure, kidney infection, or heart problems, the patient could be prohibited from obtaining life, health, or mortgage insurance if the answers are derogatory.

If a patient tests positive for human immunodeficiency virus (HIV), legal counsel may be necessary because some state laws allow information on HIV infection and acquired immunodeficiency syndrome (AIDS) to be given only to the patient or to the patient's spouse. In some states it is illegal to require a blood test for HIV antibodies, a urinalysis for HIV, or an HIV antigen test as a condition of coverage. It also may be illegal to question applicants about HIV status or prior symptoms of and treatment for AIDS or other forms of immune deficiency. A separate release of information is necessary before any information can be released regarding an HIV/AIDS patient.

In some situations it is preferable to submit a narrative report dictated by the physician instead of completing the form, which has numerous check-off columns and no space for comments. It may be necessary to attach a copy of an operative, pathology, laboratory, or radiology report and an electrocardiogram (ECG) tracing.

A life insurance company may ask a copy service to visit the health care organization's office to photocopy the patient's record. Usually this is done at the convenience of the office staff and an appointment should be made. The insurance company should be reminded that an authorization form signed by the patient is necessary to release medical information. An appropriate fee for this service is charged and quoted at the time of the telephone request. The physician should review the records in advance to ensure that they are in proper order.

REVIEW AND AUDIT OF HEALTH RECORDS

Internal Reviews

Prospective Review

The first type of internal review is a prospective review, also termed *prebilling audit* or *review,* which is done before billing is submitted. This may be done by some health care organizations daily, weekly, or monthly.

Stage 1 of a prospective review is done to verify that completed encounter forms match patients seen according to the appointment schedule and have been posted on the daysheet. A prospective review is begun by obtaining the encounter forms and locating the dates in question for the review in the appointment schedule, printing the schedule as verification. The appointment schedule is then compared with the encounter forms to match patients for the date in question. Next, check to see if all procedures or services have been posted and the charges on the daysheet are complete.

Stage 2 of a prospective review is done to verify that all procedures or services and diagnoses listed on the encounter form match data on the insurance claim form. To perform this stage, use the completed claim form or print an insurance billing worksheet. Match the information on the claim or worksheet with the date of service, procedure or service, and diagnosis on the encounter form. It is possible that one or more diagnoses may not match. A common reason is because an active diagnosis has not been entered in the computer system, the computer defaults to the last diagnosis given for an established patient. Another problem occurs when the diagnosis is not linked to the procedure. Such problems must be found before billing and corrected before claims are printed.

Retrospective Review

The second type of internal review is called a retrospective review, which is done after billing insurance carriers. A coder or insurance billing specialist may be asked to perform a retrospective review to determine whether there is a lack of documentation. To accomplish this, pull 15 to 20 health records per provider from the past 2 to 4 months at random. The following are recommended internal audit tools:

- Internal record review worksheets
- CPT code book
- Current *International Classification of Diseases, Tenth Revision, Clinical Modification* (ICD-10) code book
- Current Healthcare Common Procedure Coding System (HCPCS) code book
- Medical dictionary
- Abbreviation reference book
- Drug reference book (for example, *Physicians' Desk Reference* or drug reference for nurses)
- Laboratory reference book
- Provider's manual for insurance program or plan
- Insurance carrier's newsletters

Forms similar to the Internal Record Review Form shown in Figs. 11.11 to 11.16 may be used as tools to gather information from the patient's record, laboratory reports, pathology reports, radiology reports, operative reports, and other diagnostic tests. If the health care provider's documentation is inadequate, errors or deficiencies will appear as the review is being conducted. Doing an internal review of this type is not an exact science, and critical thinking skills are needed. Because documentation guidelines and code policies are updated and refined periodically, it is extremely important to read and keep bulletins from all insurance carriers, especially those from the local Medicare Administrative Contractor. An audit should only be performed using the most up-to-date policies. Advise the service provider of any new requirements. This resource may be the only notification of changes unless health care employees routinely attend local or national workshops.

External Reviews

An external review is an audit of medical and financial records by an outside contractor or by an external reviewer. The external audit may be performed by an insurance carrier, a Medicare Administrative Contractor, or other Centers for Medicare and Medicaid Services (CMS) representative to investigate suspected fraud or abusive billing practices.

Health care organizations and facilities may initiate their own external review and request an outside contractor to perform an audit as part of its compliance program. This is a way to pinpoint areas needed for education and training. External reviews will also provide a third-party opinion for claims processing and may help an organization appeal trends in denials. An external audit may also be requested by a health care organization to evaluate the policies and procedures related to a particular service to ensure proper guidelines and regulations are being adhered to. This will point out areas for improvement and prepare the organization for an external audit by Medicare or another insurance company.

External audits can be performed as **prepayment audits** (prospective) or as retrospective audits. When a health care provider is placed on a prepayment audit review by an insurance company, each time the provider submits a claim, the claim is pended by the insurance carrier. The health care provider must submit a copy of his or her patient's health record to support the claim. On receipt of the health record, the insurance carrier will review the record and determine whether the claim should be paid or not. This process can be very time consuming and can have a significant impact on the health care organization's cash flow.

Retrospective audits are performed by insurance carriers after a claim has been paid. If it is determined that incorrect payment was made, a request will be made for monies to be refunded. Most insurance companies perform routine audits on unusual billing patterns, such as the same diagnosis code for every visit or billing the same procedure code repeatedly. Additional red flags to auditors include the following:

- Lack of documentation for health care facility admissions
- Canned template documentation
- Illegible documentation
- Blank documentation
- Tests documented but not performed

Insurance companies have computer software programs capable of editing and screening insurance claims to identify billing excesses or potential abuses before payment is rendered. Insurance carriers may hire undercover agents who visit health care provider's offices if overuse and abuse of procedure codes are suspected. Health care organizations who charge fees that are higher than others in their geographic area are routinely audited by most carriers. Insurance carriers spot-check claims by sending questionnaires to patients and asking them if they received medical care from a provider and, if so, to verify the services rendered. The answers are then compared with what the service provider billed.

Many insurance companies have installed antifraud telephone hotlines for patients. Investigations can result from such calls, depending on the circumstances. Tips also come from peer review organizations, state licensing boards, whistle-blowing providers and physicians, former staff members, and patients. If there is any suspicion of fraud, the insurance company will notify the health care organization, specify a date and time at which they will come to the office, and indicate which records they wish to audit.

Investigators question the patient, look at the documentation in the health record, and interview the staff and all health care providers who have participated in the care of the patient. Auditors also look at appointment books and add up the hours the health care provider sees patients on any given day when a health care organization uses time-based procedure codes when submitting insurance claims.

Software Edit Checks

An edit check is a good audit prevention measure to have in place. Many software programs have edits in their software programs that automatically screen insurance claims for errors and conflicting code entries prior to submission of them. For example, if the diagnosis does not match the service provided, the claim will be thrown out by the edit and it can be corrected before being billed incorrectly.

RELEASE AND RETENTION OF HEALTH RECORDS

Subpoena

Subpoena literally means "under penalty." In legal language, it is a writ requiring the appearance of a witness at a trial or other proceeding. Strictly defined, a ***subpoena duces tecum*** requires the witness to appear and bring or send certain records in his or her possession. For a *subpoena duces tecum* for health information to be valid under the HIPAA Privacy Rule, it must be accompanied by a court order. If there is no court order, the covered entity must receive satisfactory assurance from the party seeking the information that reasonable efforts have been made to ensure that the patient or legal guardian was given notice of the request. If no notice was given, the party must show that reasonable efforts were made to secure a qualified protective order that meets the requirements of the HIPAA Privacy Rule. A subpoena is a legal document signed by a judge or an attorney in the name of a judge. If an attorney signs it, he or she must attest it in the name of a judge, the court clerk, or other proper officer. In some states in which a pretrial of evidence or deposition is set up, the subpoena may be issued by a notary public, in which event it is called a *notary subpoena.*

It is possible for a state investigator to subpoena patient records and then file administrative charges against the provider or health care organization, not because of the practice of shoddy medicine but rather because the case was inadequately documented for the treatment provided. Health records also may be subpoenaed as proof in a medical malpractice case. Complete documentation and well-organized patient records help to establish a strong defense in a medical professional liability claim.

Subpoena Process

A subpoena must be personally served or handed to the prospective witness or keeper of the health records. The acceptance of a document by someone authorized to accept it is the equivalent of personal service. The subpoena cannot be left on a counter or desk. Never accept a subpoena or give records to anyone without the provider's prior authorization. The medical office should designate one person as keeper of the health records. If the subpoena is only for health records or financial data, the representative for the specific doctor can usually accept it and the provider will not be called to court.

If a service provider is on vacation and there is no designated keeper of the records, tell the deputy that the provider is not in and cannot be served. Suggest that the deputy contact the provider's attorney and relay this information.

The health care organization is given a prescribed time in which to produce the records. It is not necessary to show them at the time the subpoena is served unless the court order so states. The attorney usually employs a person or copy service to copy records that are under subpoena. At the time the subpoena is served, a date is usually agreed upon when the representative will return and copy the portion of the record that is named in the subpoena. Often only the portion of the health record requested is removed from the original chart and put in a copy folder. Items such as the patient registration information sheet, encounter form, and explanation of benefits should not be included. The attorney who sent the subpoena can be called to see whether the records can be mailed. If so, mail them by certified mail with a return receipt requested. Retain a copy of the records released. A billing specialist will have to appear in court if specified in the subpoena. Verify with the court that the case is actually on the calendar. Failing to appear places the employee in contempt of court and subject to a penalty, possibly several days in jail.

Retention of Records

In an electronic system, health records are stored in the computer. Paper-based records either are stored in color-coded file folders containing a collection of paper documents or reside in multiple electronic databases displayed in a variety of formats via computer access. Many health care organizations have a combination of both paper records and electronic records to consider when they are creating a records retention policy. Regardless of the system used, general guidelines must be followed to record information correctly, use it according to law, and retain it. A sample retention policy is shown in Table 11.2.

Financial Documents

According to income tax regulations on record retention, accounting records should be kept for a minimum of 4 to 7 years after the due date for filing the tax return or the date the tax is paid, whichever is later. Always contact an accountant before discarding records that may determine tax liability.

A federal regulation mandates that assigned claims for Medicaid and Medicare be kept for 7 years; the health care organization is subject to auditing during that period. The federal False Claims Amendments Act of 1986 allows a claim of fraud to be made up to 10 years from the date a violation was committed. Documentation must be available for inspection and copying by the investigator of the false claim (31 US Code §3729-3733).

Health Records

Preservation of health records is governed by federal and state laws. Under federal legislation, the HIPAA Administrative Simplification Rules require a covered entity to retain required documentation for 6 years from the date of its creation or the date when it last was in effect, whichever is later. However, individual states have their own laws for health record retention. Whichever law is more stringent (federal or state) is the law that should be adhered to.

CMS maintains that the health record needs to be in its original form or in a legally reproduced form, which may be electronic, so that health records may be reviewed and audited by authorized entities. Providers must have a record system that ensures that the record may be accessed and retrieved promptly. Guidance concerning record retention after these time periods should be obtained through legal advice based on laws applicable to the state in which the health care organization resides.

Effective December 1, 2006, changes to the Federal Rules of Civil Procedure make requests for electronic data a standard part of the discovery process during federal lawsuits. This includes health records, accounting documents, cellphone records, instant messaging, and electronic mail that might be needed for future litigation.

Under the federal False Claims Act, a claim may be filed 7 to 10 years after a date of service. Cases that involve radiologic injury claims (for example, leukemia from radiation) may begin running the statute of limitations after discovery of the injury, which may occur 20 or 30 years after radiation exposure.

A person's health record may be of value not only to himself or herself in later years but also to the person's children. In some states a minor may file suit after he or she has attained legal age for any act performed during childhood that the person believes to be wrong or harmful. Sometimes a suit may be permitted even 2 to 3 years after the child has reached legal age. Thus it is important to keep records until patients are 3 to 4 years beyond the age of majority.

Many factors must be considered when developing a retention policy for health records. Different types of health care facilities may have different retention requirements. For example, research facilities are required to maintain patient records permanently. All record retention policies should be reviewed and approved by a health care attorney who would be most knowledgeable of the laws in their state.

TABLE 11.2 Sample Records Retention Schedule

Record	Retention Period	Reference
Accounts receivable (patient ledger)	7 years	IRS
Appointment sheets	3 years	False Claims Amendment Act
Bank deposit slip (duplicate)	1 years	IRS
Bank statements and canceled checks	7 years	IRS
Cash receipt records	6 years	IRS
Contracts (expired)	7 years	IRS
Correspondence, general	6 years	IRS
Correspondence, legal	retain indefinitely	IRS
Daysheets (balance sheets and journals)	5 years	False Claims Amendment Act
Health records (active patients)	retain indefinitely	False Claims Amendment Act
Health records (inactive patients)	retain indefinitely	False Claims Amendment Act
Health records (expired patients)	5 years	HIPAA
Income tax returns and documents	retain indefinitely	IRS
Insurance policies and records	retain indefinitely	IRS
Inventory records	3 years	IRS
Invoices	6 years	IRS
Medicare financial records	7 years	CMS
Remittance advice documents	10 years	False Claims Amendment Act
Payroll records	7 years	IRS
X-ray films	retain indefinitely	False Claims Amendment Act

CMS, Centers for Medicare and Medicaid Services; *HIPAA,* Health Insurance Portability and Accountability Act; *IRS,* Internal Revenue Service.

Data Storage

A paperless office requires an organized and efficient system for keeping files that have been saved to the hard drive protected from accidental destruction. Keep financial records on computer disks or tapes and store them in an area that does not have temperature extremes or magnetic fields.

When data are entered into a computer system, it is wise to **back up** (save data) frequently, preferably daily. Automated backup is possible, and the computer regularly initiates the process. Most financial software programs display a screen prompt instructing the operator to back up before quitting the program. If there is no automated backup, always back up files at the end of the day or several times a week so that information is not lost during a power outage or computer breakdown.

About once a week, a verification process should be done that compares the original records with the copies. This can take 20% to 30% longer than ordinary backup, but if a comparison is not made, there is no way to ensure that the data have been backed up. Store backup copies away from the office in case of fire, flood, or theft.

Maintain a log of the documents on computer disks or CDs with an index located at the front of the book. The log enables the health care organization to keep track of files and should list when the files were backed up last so that they can be located quickly. Be sure that another employee knows where the log is kept and is familiar with how to track down files through this system. Note the code for accessing these documents and date revisions when updating old documents. Do not put anything related to protected health information (PHI) in this log.

Data Disposal

In a paper-based system, it is recommended that documents that are no longer needed be shredded. Electronic storage media, such as CD-ROMs, floppy disks, or flash drives, containing confidential or sensitive information may be disposed of only by approved destruction methods. These methods should be outlined in the health care organization's HIPAA Security Plan and may include burning, shredding, pulverizing, or some other approach that renders the media unusable. Two methods of destroying electronic storage media are **degaussing**, which uses electromagnetic fields to erase data, or **zeroization**, which is a process of writing repeated sequences of ones and zeros over the information. CD-ROMs and other media storage devices must be physically destroyed.

Some health care organizations prefer to use health record storage companies. When records are disposed of by a professional company, be sure to obtain a certificate of destruction verifying the method of disposal. This document should be indefinitely retained in the office. Permanently retain a log of destroyed records showing the patient's name, Social Security number, date of last visit, and treatment.

HIPAA's security rule is the establishment of policies and procedures for final disposal of electronic PHI (ePHI) and the hardware or electronic media on which it is stored. It is easy to recover ePHI from hard drives, CD-ROMs, and other media storage devices if it is not properly erased or destroyed. Simply deleting files or formatting drives is not sufficient to keep ePHI from being accessed. Covered entities must implement reasonable safeguards when disposing of information. Some acceptable methods are as follows:

- Reformat and overwrite the disk media several times to sanitize the hard drive.
- Reinitialize the storage space of the computer hardware, if possible.
- Break, incinerate, crush, or destroy the storage device.
- Shred audiotapes, microfilm, or microfiche.

Electronic Power Protection

Plug equipment into power surge suppressors or, better yet, receptacles with an uninterruptible power supply (UPS) to prevent computer and data file damage. In addition, the entire office should be protected by a surge suppressor installed near the electric circuit breaker panel. This device is called an *all-office* or *whole-office surge suppressor*.

Prevention of Legal Problems

Throughout this text, there are many instances in which an insurance billing specialist must be careful in executing job duties to avoid the possibility of a lawsuit. Potential legal issues may arise from confidentiality issues to outright fraud. A summary of guidelines for prevention of lawsuits is shown in Box 11.1. It is best to err on the side of caution if a potential legal situation is encountered. Always consult the health care organization's manager if there is a concern.

DOCUMENTATION GUIDELINES FOR EVALUATION AND MANAGEMENT SERVICES

Earlier in this chapter, E/M services were introduced. The following information is a more extensive look at the documentation requirements for those services. More experienced billing specialists may be given the additional task of auditing E/M services to ensure that the guidelines for the services are met. Understanding the documentation requirements for E/M services is essential in effectively carrying out that task.

BOX 11.1 Prevention of Lawsuits: Guidelines for Insurance Billing Specialists

1. Keep information about patients strictly confidential.
2. Obtain proper instruction and carry out responsibilities according to the employer's guidelines.
3. Keep abreast of general insurance program guidelines, annual coding changes, and medical and scientific progress to help when handling insurance matters.
4. Secure proper written consent in all cases before releasing a patient's protected health information (PHI) for purposes other than treatment, payment, or routine health care operations (TPO).
5. Do not refer to consent or acknowledgment forms as "releases." Use the word "consent" or "authorization" forms as required by law. This also produces a better understanding of the document to be signed.
6. Ensure that documentation of patient care in the health record corresponds with billing submitted on the insurance claim.
7. Exercise good judgment in writing and wording e-mails because they do not give security against confidentiality.

continued

BOX 11.1 Prevention of Lawsuits: Guidelines for Insurance Billing Specialists—cont'd

8. Make every effort to reach an understanding with patients in the matter of fees by explaining what services will be received and what the "extras" may be. For health care facility cases, it is advisable to explain that the fee the physician charges is for his or her services only and that charges for the bed, operating room, laboratory tests, and anesthesia will be billed separately in addition to the physician's charges.
9. Do not discuss other physicians or health care providers with the patient. Patients sometimes invite criticism of the methods or results of former providers.
10. Tell the health care provider immediately if a new patient is still under treatment by another physician and did not give this information to the provider during the initial interview.
11. Do not compare the respective merits of various forms of therapy and refrain from discussing patients' ailments with them. Patients come to talk to the physician about their symptoms; nonclinical personnel may give the patient incorrect information. Let the physician make the diagnosis.
12. Report a health care provider who is doing something illegal. Health care workers can be held responsible for being silent and failing to report an illegal action.
13. Say nothing to anyone except as required by the attorney of the health care organization or by the court if litigation is pending.
14. Be alert to hazards that may cause injury to anyone in the office and report such problems immediately.
15. Consult the physician or service provider before turning over a delinquent account to a collection agency.
16. Be courteous in dealing with patients and always act in a professional manner.

The AMA and CMS developed documentation guidelines for CPT E/M services. These were released to Medicare carriers by CMS in 1995 and then modified and released again in 1997. The guidelines were developed because Medicare has an obligation to its beneficiaries to ensure that services paid for have been provided and are medically necessary. Auditors determined that some health care organizations needed to improve their quality of documentation.

CMS is considering a modification of the 1997 guidelines, but it has not been released as of this edition. The modification will focus on changing the guidelines for the history and physical exam. It will also revamp the medical decision-making component.

Until the new revisions are in place, insurance claims processors and auditors may use either the 1995 or 1997 guidelines when coding a service or performing an internal or external chart audit. An audit assists the health care organization to determine whether the reported services were actually rendered and the level of service was warranted. When significant irregular reporting patterns are detected, a review is conducted.

The following is a brief overview of documentation guidelines for medical services.

1. The health record should be accurate, complete, and legible.
2. The documentation of each patient encounter should include or provide reference to the following:
   a. **Chief complaint** or reason for the encounter
   b. Relevant history
   c. Examination
   d. Findings
   e. Prior diagnostic test results
   f. Assessment, clinical impression, or diagnosis
   g. Plan for care
   h. Date and legible identity of the health care professional
3. The reason for the encounter or chief complaint should be stated and the rationale should be documented or inferred for ordering diagnostic and other ancillary services, such as x-rays or laboratory tests.
4. Past and present diagnoses, including those in the prenatal and intrapartum period that affect the newborn, should be accessible to the treating or consulting physician.
5. Appropriate health risk factors should be identified.
6. The patient's progress, response to, and changes in treatment, planned follow-up care and instructions, and diagnosis should be documented.
7. Patient refusal to follow medical advice should be documented and a letter sent to the patient about this noncompliance.
8. Procedure and diagnostic codes reported on the health insurance claim form or billing statement should be supported by the documentation in the health record and be at a level sufficient for a clinical peer to determine whether services have been coded accurately.
9. The confidentiality of the health record should be fully maintained, consistent with the requirements of medical ethics and the law.
10. Each health record entry must have a date and signature or electronic validation, including the title or position of the person verifying the documentation. If a signature log has been established for paper-based records, initials are acceptable, because these would be defined in the log (Fig. 11.7). A signature log is a list of all staff members' names, job titles, signatures, and initials. In regard to paperless documents, if passwords are used for restricted access, electronic or digital signatures may be acceptable.
11. Charting procedures for progress notes should be standardized. For office visits, the majority of health care providers in a paper-based system use a method called the **SOAP** (*s*ubjective, *o*bjective, *a*ssessment, *p*lan) **style** of documentation (Fig. 11.8). Some providers prefer to document using a narrative or more detailed descriptive style when creating a medical report such as history and physical report, operative report, radiologic report, or pathology report. Whatever method is used, the provider must ensure that it is detailed enough to support current documentation requirements.
12. Treatment plans should be written. Include patient and family education and specific instructions for follow-up. Treatment must be consistent with the working diagnosis.
13. Medications prescribed and taken should be listed, specifying frequency and dosage.
14. Request for a consultation from the attending or treating physician and the need for consultation must be documented. The consultant's opinion and any services ordered or performed must be documented and communicated to the requesting physician. Remember the four Rs: There must be a requesting physician and the consultant must render an opinion and send

SIGNATURE LOG

Name	Position	Signature or Initials	
Ann M. Arch	Receptionist	Ann M. Arch	AMA
John Bortolonni	Office manager	John Bortolonni	JB
Gerald Practon, MD	Provider	Gerald Practon, MD	GP
Rachel Vasquez, CPC	Insurance billing specialist	Rachel Vasquez, CPC	RV
Mary Ann Worth	Clinical medical assistant	Mary Ann Worth	MAW

Fig. 11.7 Example of a signature log for paper-based records.

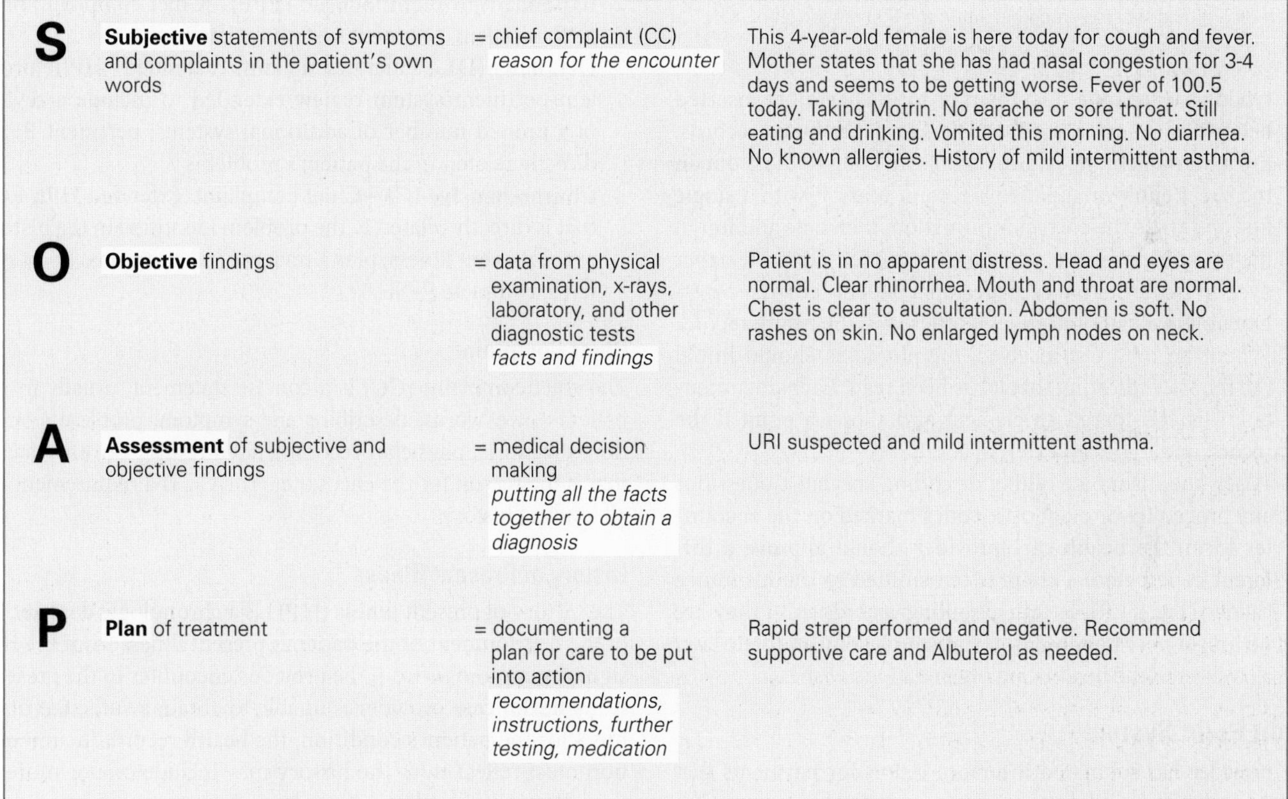

S	**Subjective** statements of symptoms and complaints in the patient's own words	= chief complaint (CC) *reason for the encounter*	This 4-year-old female is here today for cough and fever. Mother states that she has had nasal congestion for 3-4 days and seems to be getting worse. Fever of 100.5 today. Taking Motrin. No earache or sore throat. Still eating and drinking. Vomited this morning. No diarrhea. No known allergies. History of mild intermittent asthma.
O	**Objective** findings	= data from physical examination, x-rays, laboratory, and other diagnostic tests *facts and findings*	Patient is in no apparent distress. Head and eyes are normal. Clear rhinorrhea. Mouth and throat are normal. Chest is clear to auscultation. Abdomen is soft. No rashes on skin. No enlarged lymph nodes on neck.
A	**Assessment** of subjective and objective findings	= medical decision making *putting all the facts together to obtain a diagnosis*	URI suspected and mild intermittent asthma.
P	**Plan** of treatment	= documenting a plan for care to be put into action *recommendations, instructions, further testing, medication*	Rapid strep performed and negative. Recommend supportive care and Albuterol as needed.

Fig. 11.8 Explanation of the acronym SOAP used as a format for progress notes defining subjective and objective information, the assessment, and the treatment plan.

a report. The requesting physician must document the reason for a consult in the patient's health record. A possible fifth R of consultations is *return*. The consulting physician must return the patient to the requesting physician for treatment of the problem so that no transfer of care is shown.

! COMPLIANCE ALERT

Signature Requirements

Ensure that all health record entries are signed or electronically verified by the health care provider with his or her title or position. This provides clear evidence that the physician reviewed the note and ensures that he or she is aware of all test results, both normal and abnormal. Documented physician review of test results can be factored when determining appropriate coding levels for service.

15. Record a patient's failure to return for needed treatment by noting it in the health record, in the appointment book, and on the financial record or ledger card. Follow up with a telephone call or send a letter to the patient advising him or her that further treatment is indicated.
16. For electronic health records, the software program should make an electronic record entry permanent when originally completed and authenticated. To make a correction, note that a section is in error with the date and time and enter the correct information with a notation of when and why the health care provider changed the entry. Authenticate the correction via electronic signature and date. Never delete or key over incorrect data in a computerized file. Another method for correcting a health record is to flag it as amended or obsolete and create an addendum either

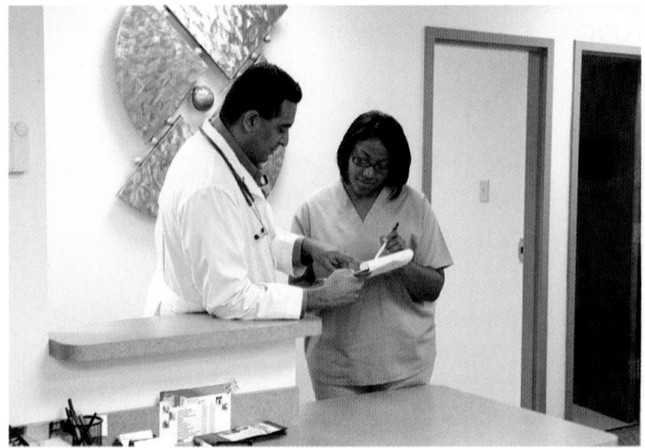

Fig. 11.9 Insurance billing specialist checking information with the health care provider before recording it on the insurance claim.

typed as a separate document or for a chart note inserted below in the next space available. For paper-based records, use a permanent, not water-soluble, ink pen to cross out an incorrect entry on a patient's record. Mark it with a single line and write the correct information, then date and initial the entry. Never erase, white out, or use self-adhesive paper over any information recorded on a patient record.

17. Document all laboratory tests ordered in the health record. When the report is received, the physician should initial the report, indicating that it has been read. Each documentation is considered an element and allows a point if the record undergoes an external audit.
18. When the insurance billing or coding specialist questions any procedure or diagnostic codes marked on the encounter form, the health care provider should approve a different code before a claim is transmitted to the insurance carrier (Fig. 11.9). Retain all billing records until they are no longer necessary by conforming to federal and state laws as well as to the health care organization's wishes.

Audit Point System

If a provider has submitted insurance claims for payments that are deemed to be fraudulent or inappropriate by the government, an investigation may be conducted in the form of an audit of the health care organization's financial records. A point system is used while reviewing each patient's health record during the performance of an audit. Points are awarded only if documentation is present for elements required in the health record. When sufficient points have been reached within a section for the level of code used in billing, no further documentation is counted for audit purposes, even though there may be additional comments for other body systems. This point system is used to show where deficiencies occur in health record documentation. It is also used to evaluate and substantiate proper use of diagnostic and procedural codes.

Both private and government health insurance carriers have the right to claim refunds in the event of accidental or intentional miscoding. However, Medicare has the power to levy fines and penalties and exclude providers from the Medicare program. If improper coding patterns exist and are not corrected, the provider of service will be penalized. Insurance carriers go by the rule "If it is not documented, then it was not performed" and they have the right to deny reimbursement.

Documentation of History

The following documentation information for the history and physical examination is based on the 1997 Medicare guidelines. The history includes the chief complaint (CC); **history of present illness** (HPI); **review of systems** (ROS); and past, family, or social history (PFSH).* The extent of the history depends on clinical judgment and the nature of the presenting problems. Each history includes some or all of the elements shown in Fig. 11.10.

The types of E/M services for the history are based on four levels of history. The four levels of history may be defined as follows:

1. **Problem focused (PF)**—Chief complaint; brief HPI or problem
2. **Expanded problem focused (EPF)**—Chief complaint; brief HPI; problem-pertinent system review
3. **Detailed (D)**—Chief complaint; extended HPI; problem-pertinent system review extended to include a review of a limited number of additional systems; pertinent PFSH directly related to the patient's problems
4. **Comprehensive (C)**—Chief complaint; extended HPI; ROS that is directly related to the problem identified in the history of the present illness, plus a review of all additional body systems; complete PFSH

Chief Complaint

The chief complaint (CC) is a concise statement, usually in the patient's own words, describing the symptom, problem, condition, diagnosis, physician-recommended return, or other factor that is the reason for the encounter. The CC is a requirement for all levels of history.

History of Present Illness

The history of present illness (HPI) is a chronologic description of the development of the patient's present illness from the first sign or symptom or from the previous encounter to the present. If the health care provider is unable to obtain a sufficient diagnosis for the patient's condition, the health record documentation must reflect this. The history may include one or more of the following eight descriptive elements:

1. Location—Area of the body where the symptom is occurring
2. Quality—Character of the symptom or pain. Examples of this may be burning, gnawing, stabbing, fullness.
3. Severity—Degree of symptom or pain on a scale from 1 to 10. Severity also can be described with terms such as *severe, slight,* and *persistent.*
4. Duration—How long the symptom or pain has been present and how long it lasts when the patient has it
5. Timing—When the pain or symptom occurs. For example, symptoms may occur in the morning or evening, or after or before meals.
6. Context—The situation associated with the pain or symptom. For example, a patient may have pain after he ingests

*These abbreviations in the history portion of the report may vary, depending on the physician who is dictating (for example, PI for present illness, PH for past history, FH for family history).

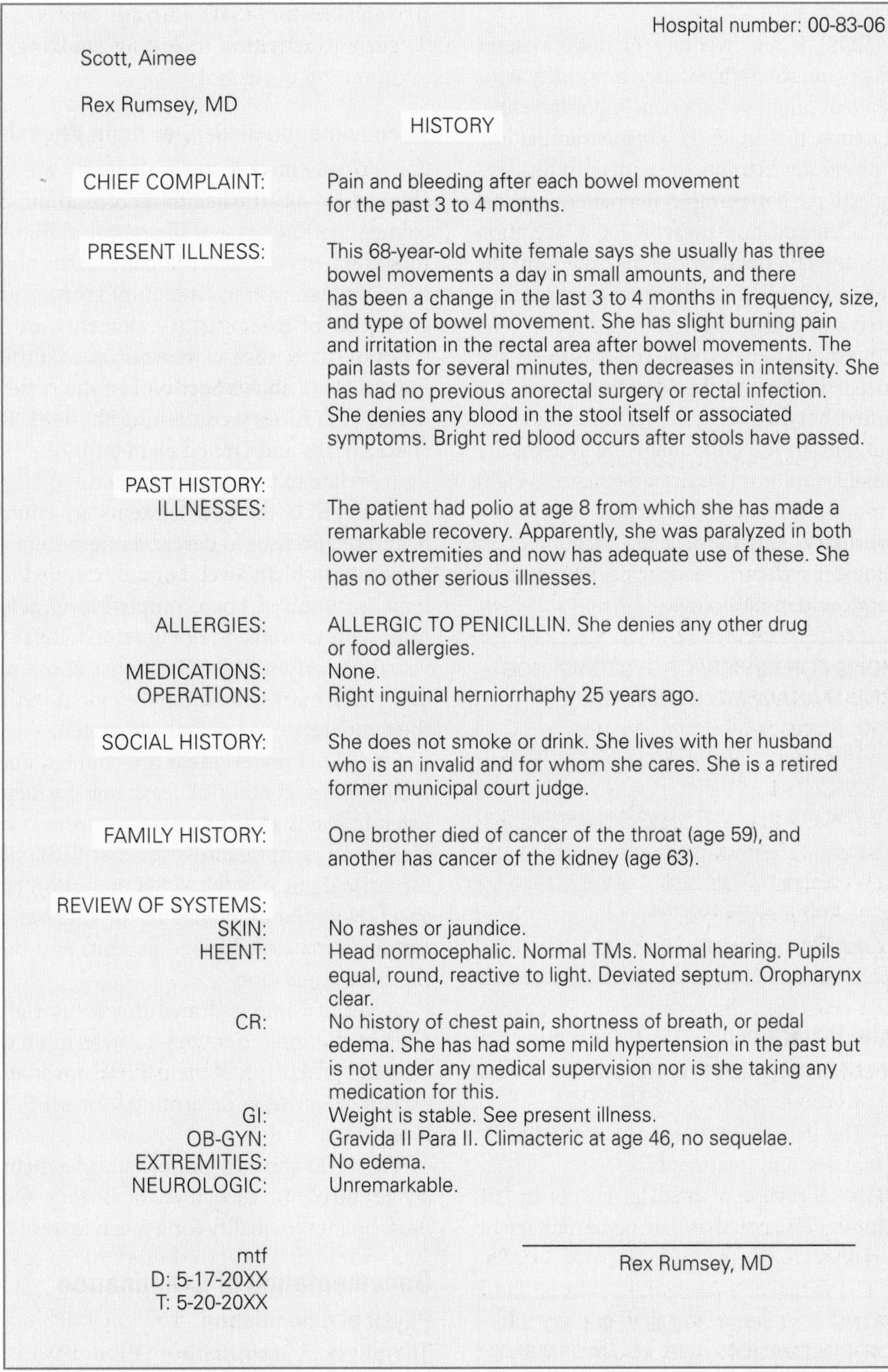

Hospital number: 00-83-06

Scott, Aimee

Rex Rumsey, MD

HISTORY

CHIEF COMPLAINT: Pain and bleeding after each bowel movement for the past 3 to 4 months.

PRESENT ILLNESS: This 68-year-old white female says she usually has three bowel movements a day in small amounts, and there has been a change in the last 3 to 4 months in frequency, size, and type of bowel movement. She has slight burning pain and irritation in the rectal area after bowel movements. The pain lasts for several minutes, then decreases in intensity. She has had no previous anorectal surgery or rectal infection. She denies any blood in the stool itself or associated symptoms. Bright red blood occurs after stools have passed.

PAST HISTORY:
ILLNESSES: The patient had polio at age 8 from which she has made a remarkable recovery. Apparently, she was paralyzed in both lower extremities and now has adequate use of these. She has no other serious illnesses.

ALLERGIES: ALLERGIC TO PENICILLIN. She denies any other drug or food allergies.
MEDICATIONS: None.
OPERATIONS: Right inguinal herniorrhaphy 25 years ago.

SOCIAL HISTORY: She does not smoke or drink. She lives with her husband who is an invalid and for whom she cares. She is a retired former municipal court judge.

FAMILY HISTORY: One brother died of cancer of the throat (age 59), and another has cancer of the kidney (age 63).

REVIEW OF SYSTEMS:
SKIN: No rashes or jaundice.
HEENT: Head normocephalic. Normal TMs. Normal hearing. Pupils equal, round, reactive to light. Deviated septum. Oropharynx clear.
CR: No history of chest pain, shortness of breath, or pedal edema. She has had some mild hypertension in the past but is not under any medical supervision nor is she taking any medication for this.
GI: Weight is stable. See present illness.
OB-GYN: Gravida II Para II. Climacteric at age 46, no sequelae.
EXTREMITIES: No edema.
NEUROLOGIC: Unremarkable.

mtf
D: 5-17-20XX
T: 5-20-20XX

Rex Rumsey, MD

Fig. 11.10 Example of medical report showing the six components of a history.

dairy products or big meals, or at times of increased activity.

7. Modifying factors—Things done to make the symptom or pain worse or better. For example, a patient may state "If I eat spicy foods I get heartburn, but if I drink milk afterward the pain is not as bad."
8. Associated signs and symptoms—The symptom or pain and other things that happen when the symptom or pain occurs. For example, a patient may note that her chest pain leads to shortness of breath.

MEDICARE CONDITIONS FOR HISTORY OF PRESENT ILLNESS (HPI) FOR EVALUATION AND MANAGEMENT SERVICES

Brief HPI		Documentation of one to three of the eight elements
Extended HPI	**1995**	Documentation of four or more elements
	1997	Documentation of four or more elements or the status of at least three chronic or inactive conditions

Review of Systems

A review of systems (ROS) is an inventory of body systems obtained through a series of questions that is used to identify signs or symptoms that the patient might be experiencing or has experienced. It is important to note that an ROS is not an examination. The provider does not physically examine the patient in this section, but merely asks questions. For example, if a patient has lost his or her balance and fallen and now presents for a laceration of the head as a result of the fall, the provider may question the patient as to whether he or she has had any dizziness or headaches. This would be considered a neurologic review of symptoms. The provider is asking the questions to determine the reason for the fall, to identify any associated or underlying conditions.

Checklists are permitted, but if a body system is not considered, it should be crossed out. For an ROS, the following systems are recognized: constitutional symptoms (for example, fever, weight loss), eyes, ears, nose, mouth, throat, cardiovascular, respiratory, gastrointestinal, genitourinary, musculoskeletal, integumentary (skin or breast), neurologic, psychiatric, endocrine, hematologic and lymphatic, and allergic and immunologic.

MEDICARE CONDITIONS FOR REVIEW OF SYSTEMS (ROS) FOR EVALUATION AND MANAGEMENT SERVICES

Problem-pertinent ROS		Positive and pertinent negatives for the system related to the problem
Extended ROS		Positive and pertinent for two to nine systems
Complete ROS	**1995**	Review 10 or more systems or a problem-pertinent ROS plus a notation that all other systems appear negative
	1997	Review of at least 10 systems

Past, Family, and Social Histories

The past, family, and social histories (PFSH) consists of a review of three areas:

1. Past history (PH)—The patient's past experiences with illnesses, operations, injuries, and treatments
2. Family history (FH)—A review of medical events in the patient's family, including diseases that may be hereditary or place the patient at risk
3. Social history (SH)—An age-appropriate review of past and current activities, including smoking, drug use, and consumption of alcohol

MEDICARE CONDITIONS FOR PAST, FAMILY, OR SOCIAL HISTORY (PFSH) FOR EVALUATION AND MANAGEMENT SERVICES

Pertinent PFSH		Specific information for one of the history areas directly related to the problem identified in the history of present illness (HPI)
Complete PFSH	**1995**	Specific information for two or three history areas
	1997	Specific information for one specific item from two of the three history areas for established patient services (office, home care) and emergency room services. One specific item from each of the three history areas for new patient services (office, home care); hospital observation, inpatient services, initial care; consults; comprehensive nursing facility assessments

Documentation Review or Audit Worksheet

The documented history elements are counted and totaled (Fig. 11.11, *A*). The health record should describe one to three elements of the present illness for a brief level of HPI. At least four elements of the HPI or the status of at least three chronic or inactive conditions is required for the extended level of HPI. Only two of three history elements are required for certain types of cases, such as newborns or subsequent hospital care. Fig. 11.11, *B*, shows Section I of the review or audit sheet that depicts the history containing the HPI, ROS, and PFSH. The check marks and circled element in the HPI (Section I) of the figure relate to the case illustrated.

In the ROS the body systems are counted and totaled. The health record should describe one system of the ROS for a pertinent to problem level. For an extended level, two to nine systems are required. For a complete level, at least 10 organ systems must be reviewed and documented. Refer to Fig. 11.11, *B*, for a visual understanding of Section I of the review or audit sheet. The check marks and circled element in the ROS (Section I) of the figure relate to the case illustrated.

The PFSH review areas are counted and totaled. The health record must contain at least one history area for a detailed extended level and specific items from two of the three history areas for a comprehensive level of PFSH. Refer to Fig. 11.11, *B*, for a visual guide of the PFSH in Section I of the review or audit sheet. Note the difference in the number of required elements for new versus established patients and the circled element for the case in question.

A vertical line is drawn down the right four columns that contain the most elements to determine the history level. The elements of HPI, ROS, and PFSH must at least be met or may exceed the criteria determined for a PF, EPF, D, or C history level.

Fig. 11.12 shows a gradual advancement of the elements that are required for each level of history. One to three elements must be met to qualify for a given level of history.

Documentation of Examination

Physical Examination

The physical examination (PE or PX) is objective in nature; that is, it consists of the health care provider's findings by examination or test results. Fig. 11.13 is an illustration of a multiorgan system examination from the CMS Documentation Guidelines for 1997 that shows the details (elements) of examination for each body area within the genitourinary system. The three circled elements of the genitourinary system and one circled element of the gastrointestinal system relate to the case shown in Fig. 11.11, *A*. For purposes of examination, the following body areas and organ systems are recognized.

Organ Systems and Body Areas—Elements of Examination

Constitutional (vital signs, general appearance)
Eyes
Ears, nose, mouth, and throat

10-21-20XX

HISTORY OF PRESENT ILLNESS: This new patient is an 80-year-old white male who has had problems with voiding difficulty since 9-5 2000. During the night, the patient had only 50 cc output and was catheterized this morning because of his poor urinary output (200 cc). He was thought to have a distended bladder. He has not had any gross hematuria. He has voiding difficulty, especially when lying down and voiding in the supine position. His voiding pattern is improved while standing and sitting, however, the patient has developed a wound to his left lateral malleolus and is only able to ambulate with assistance.

PAST MEDICAL HISTORY: Unremarkable. He does have some slowing of his urinary stream and nocturia three to five times.

MEDICATIONS: He was on amitriptyline which may affect his bladder.

ALLERGIES: He has no known allergies.

PHYSICAL EXAMINATION: Shows the abdomen to be soft, nontender, and not distended. His bladder was nonpalpable and nondistended.

GENITOURINARY: Normal penis. Testes descended bilaterally. His prostate is 10 gm and benign in feeling.

IMPRESSION: Benign prostatic hypertrophy with some mild voiding difficulty exacerbated by the patient's poor ambulatory status.

I suspect that as his ambulatory status improves, that his voiding pattern will also improve. I will try him on Hytrin 5 mg/day by mouth. I will follow him as needed.

mtf Gene Ulibarri, MD

A

Annotations: Severity; Genitourinary (ROS); Integumentary (ROS); Location; Duration; Context; Genitourinary (ROS); Modifying factor

Notice that there is no family or social history for this new patient.

Notice that the examination of the wound is missing.

Chief Complaint ____________________

History				
HPI Elements Location Severity Timing Modifying Factors Quality Duration Context Associated signs and symptoms **(OR STATUS OF 3 CHRONIC CONDITIONS = EXTENDED)**	**Brief** **1-3 elements**	**Brief** **1-3 elements**	**Extended** **4 or more elements**	**Extended** **4 or more elements**
ROS (review of systems): Constitutional ENMT GI Integumentary/Breast Endo Eyes Cardio GU Neuro Hem/Lymph Resp MS Psych All/Imm "All others negative"	**None**	**Pertinent to problem** **1 system**	**Extended** **2-9 systems**	**Complete** **10 OR MORE SYSTEMS**
PFSH Past History (patient's past illnesses, surgeries, injuries & treatments) Family History (a review of medical events & diseases in patient's family) Social History (an age appropriate review of past & current activities) No PFSH required for Subsequent Hospital Care or Subsequent Nursing Facility Care	**None**	**None**	**Pertinent** **New= 1** **Est - 1**	**Complete** **New = 3** **Est - 2**
Final Total for Level of History	Problem Focused	Expanded Problem Focused	Detailed	Comprehensive

PFSH Requirements:
Established Patient (Office/OP/Domiciliary, Home) and ED:
- Pertinent = 1 history area; Complete = 2 history areas

New patient (Office/OP, Domiciliary, Home), Consults, Initial Hospital, Hospital Observation, Comprehensive Nursing Facility Assessment:
- Pertinent = 1 history area; Complete = 3 history areas

If a physician is unable to obtain history, the record should describe circumstances which preclude obtaining it.

B

Fig. 11.11 A, Documentation from a health record highlighting elements required for the history. **B,** Review or audit sheet Section I with check marks and circled elements shows how the history in the example is declared as detailed. This shows two of three history components *(arrow)* used for the purpose of determining the assignment of a procedure code at the appropriate level of service.

Elements Required for Each Level of History			
Present History	**Review of Systems**	**Past, Family, or Social History**	**Levels of History**
Brief	N/A	N/A	Problem focused
Brief problem	Problem pertinent	N/A	Expanded focused
Extended	Extended	Pertinent	Detailed
Extended	Complete	Complete	Comprehensive

Fig. 11.12 Elements required for each type of history. One to three elements must be met to qualify for a given level of history.

Neck
Respiratory
Cardiovascular
Chest, including breasts and axillae
Gastrointestinal (abdomen)
Genitourinary (male)
Genitourinary (female)
Lymphatic
Musculoskeletal
Skin
Neurologic
Psychiatric

Note: In addition, any reasons for not examining a particular body area or system should be listed.

Types of Physical Examination

When performing a review of a patient's health record, the number of elements identified by bullets are counted for each system and a total is obtained. The total is circled on Section II of the review or audit sheet as shown in Fig. 11.14 for the case illustrated.

The levels of E/M services are based on four types of PE:

1. **Problem focused (PF)**—A limited examination of the affected body area or organ system. The health record should describe one to five elements identified by a bullet in Fig. 11.14 for a problem-focused level of PE.
2. **Expanded problem focused (EPF)**—A limited examination of the affected body area or organ system and other symptomatic or related organ systems. At least six elements identified by a bullet in Fig. 11.14 are required for an expanded problem focused level of PE.
3. **Detailed (D)**—An extended examination of the affected body areas and other symptomatic or related organ systems. At least two elements identified by a bullet in Fig. 11.14 from each of six areas and body systems or at least 12 elements identified by a bullet in two or more areas and body systems are required for a detailed level of PE.
4. **Comprehensive (C)**—A general multisystem examination or complete examination of a single organ system. For a comprehensive level of PE, all elements must be identified by a bullet in Fig. 11.14 and documentation must be present for at least two elements identified by a bullet from each of nine areas and body systems.

1995 MEDICARE CONDITIONS FOR THE PHYSICAL EXAMINATION FOR EVALUATION AND MANAGEMENT SERVICES

Problem focused (PF)	Documentation of only one body area or organ system
Expanded problem focused (EPF) or detailed	Documentation of up to seven systems (the affected body area or system plus up to six additional systems)
Comprehensive	Documentation of eight or more systems

1997 MEDICARE CONDITIONS FOR GENERAL MULTISYSTEM EXAMINATION

Problem focused (PF)	One to five elements identified by a bullet in one or more body or system areas
Expanded problem focused (EPF)	At least six elements identified by a bullet in one or more body or system areas
Detailed	At least two elements identified by a bullet from each of six body areas or systems or at least 12 elements in two or more body or system areas
Comprehensive	Perform all elements for each selected system or body area; document at least two elements identified by a bullet from each of at least nine body or system areas

The extent of the examination and what is documented range from limited examinations of single body areas to general multisystem or complete single-organ system examinations, depending on clinical judgment and the nature of the presenting problem.

Documentation of Medical Decision Making

Medical decision making (MDM) is a health care management process done after performing a history and PE on a patient that results in a plan of treatment. It is based on establishing one or more diagnoses and/or selecting a management or treatment option, amount or complexity of data reviewed, and risk of complications or associated morbidity or mortality. ***Morbidity*** is a diseased condition or state, whereas ***mortality*** refers to death.

Number of diagnoses or management options is based on the number and types of problems addressed during the visit, the complexity of establishing a diagnosis, and the number of management options that must be considered by the physician. For the case illustrated, the number of problems is 1, which equals 3 points (Fig. 11.15, *top section*).

Amount or complexity of data to be reviewed is based on the types of diagnostic tests ordered or reviewed. A decision to obtain and review old health records or obtain history from sources other than the patient increases the amount and complexity of data to be analyzed. For the case illustrated, no points apply (see Fig. 11.15, *middle section*).

Risk of complications, morbidity, or mortality is based on other conditions associated with the presenting problem known as the risk of complications, morbidity, or mortality as well as

MULTIORGAN SYSTEM EXAMINATION REQUIREMENTS (SHADED)

CONTENT and DOCUMENTATION

Level of Exam	Perform and Document
Problem Focused	**One to five** elements identified by a bullet.
Expanded Problem Focused	**At least six** elements identified by a bullet.
Detailed	**At least twelve** elements identified by a bullet.
Comprehensive	Perform all elements identified by a bullet; document every element in every shaded box and at least one element in every unshaded box.

Genitourinary

System/Body Area	Elements of Examination
Constitutional	• Measurement of **any three of the following seven** vital signs: 1) sitting or standing blood pressure, 2) supine blood pressure, 3) pulse rate and regularity, 4) respiration, 5) temperature, 6) height, 7) weight (may be measured and recorded by ancillary staff) • General appearance of patient *(e.g., development nutrition, body habitus, deformities, attention to grooming)*
Neck	• Examination of neck *(e.g., masses, overall appearance, symmetry, tracheal position, crepitus)* • Examination of thyroid *(e.g., enlargement, tenderness, mass)*
Respiratory	• Assessment of respiratory effect *(e.g., intercostal retractions, use of accessory muscles, diaphragmatic movement)* • Auscultation of lungs *(e.g., breath sounds, adventitious sounds, rubs)*
Cardiovascular	• Auscultation of heart with notation of abnormal sounds and murmurs • Examination of peripheral vascular system by observation *(e.g., swelling, varicosities)* and palpation *(e.g., pulses, temperature, edema, tenderness)*
Chest (breasts)	See genitourinary (female)
Gastrointestinal (abdomen)	⦿ Examination of abdomen with notation of presence of masses or tenderness • Examination for presence or absence of hernia • Examination of liver and spleen • Obtain stool sample for occult blood test when indicated
Genitourinary (male)	• Inspection of anus and perineum Examination (with or without specimen collection for smears and cultures) of genitalia including: • Scrotum *(e.g., lesions, cysts, rashes)* • Epididymides *(e.g., size, symmetry, masses)* ⦿ Testes *(e.g., size, symmetry, masses)* • Urethral meatus *(e.g., size, location, lesions, discharge)* ⦿ Penis *(e.g., lesions, presence or absence of foreskin, foreskin retractability, plaque, masses, scarring, deformities)* Digital rectal examination including: ⦿ Prostate gland *(e.g., size, symmetry, nodularity, tenderness)* • Seminal vesicles *(e.g., symmetry, tenderness, masses, enlargement)* • Sphincter tone, presence of hemorrhoids, rectal masses
Genitourinary (female) Includes at least seven of the eleven elements to the right identified by bullets:	• Inspection and palpation of breasts *(e.g., masses or lumps, tenderness, symmetry, nipple discharge)* • Digital rectal examination including sphincter tone, presence of hemorrhoids, rectal masses Pelvic examination (with or without specimen collection for smears and cultures) including: • External genitalia *(e.g., general appearance, hair distribution, lesions)* • Urethral meatus *(e.g., size, location, lesions, prolapse)* • Urethra *(e.g., masses, tenderness, scarring)* • Bladder *(e.g., fullness, masses, tenderness)* • Vagina *(e.g., general appearance, estrogen effect, discharge, lesions, pelvic support, cystocele, rectocele)* • Cervix *(e.g., general appearance, lesions, discharge)* • Uterus *(e.g., size, contour, position, mobility, tenderness, descent or support)* • Adnexa/parametria *(e.g., masses, tenderness, organomegaly, nodularity)* • Anus and perineum

Genitourinary (continued)

System/Body Area	Elements of Examination
Lymphatic	• Palpation of lymph nodes in neck, axillae, groin and/or other location
Skin	• Inspection and/or palpation of skin and subcutaneous tissue *(e.g., rashes, lesions, ulcers)*
Neurological/ psychiatric	Brief assessment of mental status including: • Orientation to time, place, and person • Mood and affect *(e.g., depression, anxiety, agitation)*

Skin

System/Body Area	Elements of Examination
Constitutional	• Measurement of **any three of the following seven** vital signs: 1) sitting or standing blood pressure, 2) supine blood pressure, 3) pulse rate and regularity, 4) respiration, 5) temperature, 6) height, 7) weight (may be measured and recorded by ancillary staff) • General appearance of patient *(e.g., development, nutrition, body habitus, deformities, attention to grooming)*
Eyes	• Inspection of conjunctivae and lids
Ears, nose, mouth, and throat	• Inspection of lips, teeth and gums • Examination of oropharynx *(e.g., oral mucosa, hard and soft palates, tongue, tonsils, and posterior pharynx)*
Neck	• Examination of thyroid *(e.g., enlargement, tenderness, mass)*
Gastrointestinal (abdomen)	• Examination of liver and spleen • Examination of anus for condyloma and other lesions
Lymphatic	• Palpation of lymph nodes in neck, axillae, groin and/or other location
Extremities	• Inspection and palpation of digits and nails *(e.g., clubbing, cyanosis, inflammation, petechiae, ischemia, infections, nodes)*
Skin	• Palpation of scalp and inspection of hair of scalp, eyebrows, face, chest, pubic area (when indicated) and extremities • Inspection and/or palpation of skin and subcutaneous tissue *(e.g., rashes, lesions, ulcers, susceptibility in and presence of photo damage)* in **eight of the following ten areas:** 1) head including face, 2) neck, 3) chest including breasts and axilla, 4) abdomen, 5) genitalia, groin, buttocks, 6) back, 7) right upper extremity, 8) left upper extremity, 9) right lower extremity, 10) left lower extremity Note: For the comprehensive level, the examination of all eight anatomic areas must be performed and documented. For the three lower levels of examination, each body area is counted separately. For example, inspection and/or palpation of the skin and subcutaneous tissue of the head and neck extremities constitutes two areas. • Inspection of eccrine and apocrine glands of skin and subcutaneous tissue with identification and location of any hyperhidrosis, chromhidroses or bromhidrosis
Neurological/ psychiatric	Brief assessment of mental status including: • Orientation to time, place and person • Mood and affect *(e.g., depression, anxiety, agitation)*

Fig. 11.13 Review or audit worksheet of a general multiorgan system physical examination that shows the elements of examination for each body area and system. Circled bullets relate to the example case shown in Fig. 11.11, *A*. (Audit Tool format developed by Iowa Medical Society, IMS Services, West Des Moines, Iowa, 1998.)

comorbidities, the diagnostic procedures, or the possible management options (treatment rendered—surgery, therapy, drug management, services, and supplies). *Comorbidity* means underlying disease or other conditions present at the time of the visit. In determining the level of risk, the element (presenting problem, diagnostic procedure ordered, or management options selected) that has the highest level (minimal, low, moderate, or high) is used.

To discover whether the level of risk is minimal, low, moderate, or high, bulleted elements are marked on the review or audit sheet (Fig. 11.16). For the case illustrated, the elements fall within the moderate level of risk category.

To conclude the internal review of a patient's health record, a level must be determined by the health care provider from one of four types of MDM: **straightforward (SF)**, **low complexity (LC)**, **moderate complexity (MC)**, and **high complexity (HC)**. The bottom portion of Fig. 11.15 shows the results obtained from Parts A, B, and C highlighted. For the case illustrated, the number of diagnoses is declared multiple, there are no data to review, and the risk of complications is moderate; therefore a moderately complex level of decision making has been assigned to be used for coding and billing purposes.

Examination

1995 Organ Systems (OS)						1995 Body Areas (BA)	
Constitutional	Respiratory	Integumentary				Head/face	Genitalia/groin/buttock
Eyes	GI	Neurologic				Neck	Back/spine
ENMT	GU	Psych				Chest/breast/axillae	Each extremity
Cardiovascular	MS	Hem/Lymph/Immuno				Abdomen	

Description	1995 Guidelines	Exam Level
Limited to affected body area or organ system.	1 BA or OS	Problem Focused Exam
Limited exam of the affected body area or organ system & other symptomatic or related organ systems. (95: Minimal detail for areas and/or systems examined; check list type documentation without any expansion of findings.	2-7 BA or OS	Expanded Problem Focus
Extended exam of affected body area or organ system & other symptomatic or related organ systems. (95: Expanded documentation of areas and/or systems examined; requires more than checklists; needs to have normal/abnormal findings expanded upon.)	2-7 BA or OS	Detailed Exam
A general multi-system examination or complete examination of a single organ system and other symptomatic or related body area(s) or organ systems(s).	8 or more OS	Comprehensive Exam

Fig. 11.14 Review or audit worksheet Section II for a general multisystem physical examination and single organ system examination. The circled item relates to a problem-focused examination for the example case (see Fig. 11.11, A) for coding purposes. (Audit Tool format developed by Iowa Medical Society, IMS Services, West Des Moines, Iowa, 1998.)

A **Number of Diagnoses or Treatment Options:**

Identify each problem or treatment option mentioned in the record.
Enter the number in each of the categories in column below

Problem to Exam Physician	Number	Points	Result
Self-limited or minor (stable, improved or worsening)		1	Max=2
Est. problem; stable, improved		1	
Est. problem; worsening		2	
New problem; no additional workup planned	1	3	Max-3 3
New problem; additional workup planned		4	
		Total	3

Bring total to **line A** in Final Result for Complexity.

B **Amount and/or Complexity of Data to Be Reviewed:**

For each category, circle the number in the points column. Total the points.

Data To Be Reviewed	Points
Review and/or order of clinical lab tests	1
Review and/or order of tests in the radiology section of CPT	1
Review and/or order of tests in the medicine section of CPT	1
Discussion of test results with performing physician	1
Decision to obtain old records and/or obtain history from someone other than patient	1
Review and summarization of old records and/or obtaining history from someone other than patient and/or discussion of case with another health care provider	2
Independent visualization of image, tracing or specimen itself (not simply review of report)	2
Total	0

Bring total to **line B** in Final Result for Complexity.

Final Result for Complexity:

Hi-lite the results from Figure 11.15.A, 11.15.B and II.16 to identify the type of decision making in that column.
After completing this table, which classifies complexity, hi-lite the type of MDM.

A	Number or Diagnosis or Treatment Options	< or = 1 Minimal	2 Limited	3 Multiple	> or = 4 Extensive
B	Amount and/ or Complexity of data	< or = 1 Min. to Low	2 Limited	3 Moderate	> or = 4 Extensive
C	Highest Risk	Minimal	Low	Moderate	High
	MDM	**Straight-forward**	**Low Complexity**	**Moderate Complexity**	**High Complexity**

Fig. 11.15 Section III of the review or audit worksheet. *Part A:* Number of diagnoses or treatment options. *Part B:* Amount or complexity of data to be reviewed. *Lower one third:* Used to compile the results obtained from Parts A, B, and C (see Fig. 11.14) to determine the level of medical decision making (MDM). In Fig. 11.11, *A* and *B*, for the example case, circled points and words relate to a moderately complex level of decision making for coding and billing purposes. (Audit Tool format developed by Iowa Medical Society, IMS Services, West Des Moines, Iowa, 1998.)

SECTION III

C

RISK OF COMPLICATIONS AND/OR MORBIDITY OR MORTALITY			
Level of risk	**Presenting problem(s)**	**Diagnostic procedure(s) ordered**	**Management options selected**
MINIMAL	• One self-limited or minor problem *(e.g., cold, insect bite, tinea corporis)*	• Laboratory tests requiring venipuncture • Chest x-rays • KOH prep • EKG/EEG • Urinalysis • Ultrasound *(e.g., echo)*	• Rest • Gargles • Elastic bandages • Superficial dressings
LOW	• Two or more self-limited or minor problems • One stable chronic illness *(e.g., well-controlled hypertension, non-insulin dependent diabetes, cataract, BPH)* • Acute uncomplicated illness or injury *(e.g., cystitis, allergic rhinitis, simple sprain)*	• Physiologic test not under stress *(e.g., pulmonary function tests)* • Non-cardiovascular imaging studies with contrast *(e.g., barium enema)* • Superficial needle biopsies • Clinical laboratory tests requiring arterial puncture • Skin biopsies	• Over-the-counter drugs • Minor surgery with no identified risk factors • Physical therapy • Occupational therapy • IV fluids without additives
MODERATE	• *One* or more *chronic illnesses* with mild exacerbation, progression or side effects of treatment • Two or more stable chronic illnesses • Undiagnosed new problem with uncertain prognosis *(e.g., lump in breast)* • Acute illness with systemic symptoms *(e.g., pyelonephritis, pneumonitis, colitis)* • Acute complicated injury *(e.g., head injury with brief loss of consciousness)*	• Physiologic test under stress *(e.g., cardiac stress test, fetal contraction stress test)* • Diagnostic endoscopies with no identified risk factors • Deep needle or incisional biopsy • Cardiovascular imaging studies with contrast and no identified risk factors *(e.g., arteriogram, cardiac cath)* • Obtain fluid from body cavity *(e.g., lumbar puncture, thoracentesis, culdocentesis)*	• Minor surgery with identified risk factors • Elective major surgery (open percutaneous or endoscopic) with no identified risk factors • *Prescription drug management* • Therapeutic nuclear medicine • IV fluids with additives • Closed treatment of fracture or dislocation without manipulation
HIGH	• One or more chronic illnesses with severe exacerbation, progression or side effects of treatment • Acute or chronic illnesses or injuries that may pose a threat to life or bodily function *(e.g., multiple trauma, acute MI, pulmonary embolus, severe respiratory distress, progressive severe rheumatoid arthritis, psychiatric illness with potential threat to self or others, peritonitis, acute renal failure)* • An abrupt change in neurological status *(e.g., seizure, TIA, weakness, sensory loss)*	• Cardiovascular imaging studies with contrast with identified risk factors • Cardiac electrophysiological tests • Diagnostic endoscopies with identified risk factors • Discography	• Elective major surgery (open, percutaneous, or endoscopic) with identified risk factor • Emergency major surgery (open, percutaneous, or endoscopic) • Parenteral controlled substances • Drug therapy requiring intensive monitoring for toxicity • Decision not to resuscitate or de-escalate care because of poor prognosis

Fig. 11.16 Section III, Part C, of the review or audit worksheet used for determining the level of risk. The highlighted areas relate to a moderate level of risk for the example case (see Fig. 11.11, *A*) for coding purposes. (Audit Tool format developed by the Iowa Medical Society, IMS Services, West Des Moines, Iowa, 1998.)

PROCEDURE 11.1 How to Abstract Data From a Health Record

Objective

To abstract data from a health record for composing a letter or completing an insurance claim form or other related billing document

Equipment/Supplies

Patient's health record, form to insert abstracted data, and pen or pencil

Directions

Follow these steps, including rationales to learn this skill, and practice it by completing the *Workbook* assignment.

1. What is the patient's diagnosis? This gives the reason for the visit.
2. What professional services were provided?
3. Did the patient undergo surgery? What surgical procedure was performed?
4. Read and review the patient's health record thoroughly to learn all parts of the case. In the *Workbook* assignment, use the check-off list and answer the questions to assist you in understanding all aspects of the patient's health record.
5. What medication was prescribed, if any?
6. Does the patient have any past history (PH) indicating anything of importance?
7. Does the patient have any food or drug allergies? If so, what are they?
8. What is the etiology (cause) of the present disease, injury, or illness?
9. What is the prognosis (prediction) for this patient's medical condition?
10. What laboratory tests were ordered or performed?
11. What x-rays were ordered or obtained?
12. Define every abbreviation listed in the patient's chart notes or history and physical examination.
13. What documents assisted you in locating the answers to these questions?

KEY POINTS

This is a brief chapter review of the key issues presented. To further enhance your knowledge of the technical subject matter, review the key terms and key abbreviations for this chapter by locating the meaning for each in the Glossary at the end of this text, which appears in a section before the Index.

1. The key to substantiating procedure and diagnostic code selection for appropriate reimbursement is supporting documentation in the health record.
2. Paper-based offices are becoming a thing of the past. The electronic health record (EHR) is becoming the norm as the ability to share patient health records among other professionals who constitute the patient's health care team has become increasingly important.
3. Federal legislation has established programs to help the health care industry change to electronic health record (EHR) and has offered incentives to those who participate in the programs. These incentive programs will transition to reimbursement penalties for organizations that have not adopted EHRs.
4. Every patient seen by a service provider must have comprehensive legible documentation about what occurred during the visit for the following reasons: (1) avoidance of denied or delayed payments by insurance carriers investigating the medical necessity of services; (2) enforcement of health record-keeping rules by insurance carriers requiring accurate documentation that supports procedure and diagnostic codes; (3) subpoena of health records by state investigators or the court for review; (4) defense of a professional liability claim.
5. Consultation and referral are not the same. A consultation service is rendered at the request of opinion or advice by another physician, whereas a referral is the transfer of the total or specific care of a patient for a known problem.
6. External and internal audit of health records shows where deficiencies occur in health record documentation and substantiates proper use of diagnostic and procedural codes.
7. Health record abbreviations should be eliminated from the more vital sections, such as final diagnosis, operative notes, discharge summaries, and descriptions of special procedures.
8. An eponym should not be used when a comparable anatomic term can be used in its place.
9. Abstraction of technical information from patient records may be requested to complete insurance claim forms; when sending letters to justify a health insurance claim form; or when a patient applies for life, mortgage, or health insurance.
10. The two types of internal and external review of records are (1) prospective (prepayment) review and (2) retrospective review (after payment).
11. An edit check is a good audit prevention measure because the software program automatically screens transmitted insurance claims and electronically examines them for errors and conflicting code entries.
12. When health records are subpoenaed, produce only the records requested and nothing more. Retain a copy of the records released.
13. The Health Insurance Portability and Accountability Act (HIPAA) requires documents to be retained for 6 years from the date of creation or the date when it was last in effect, whichever is later. However, if the state requires a longer retention period, the law that is most stringent should be adhered to.
14. When a patient does not comply with a health care organization's office policy, the service provider may wish to withdraw formally from further care of the patient. The service provider must send a formal letter of termination, or withdrawal, by certified mail with return receipt to the patient.
15. In 1995 and 1997, the Centers for Medicare and Medicaid Services (CMS) introduced documentation guidelines to Medicare carriers to ensure that services paid for have been

provided and were medically necessary. Documentation must support the level of service and each procedure rendered.

16. The levels of evaluation and management (E/M) services selected by the provider must be supported through documentation of the chief complaint, history of present illness (HPI); review of systems (ROS); past, family, or social history (PFSH); examination; and medical decision making (MDM).

STUDENT ASSIGNMENT

- Study Chapter 11.
- Answer the fill-in-the-blank, multiple-choice, and true/false questions in the *Workbook* to reinforce the theory learned in this chapter and help prepare you for a future test.
- Complete the assignments in the *Workbook* to give you experience in reviewing patients' medical reports and records.
- Turn to the Glossary at the end of this text for a further understanding of the key terms and key abbreviations used in this chapter.

12

Diagnostic Coding

Cheryl Fassett

OBJECTIVES

After reading this chapter, you should be able to:

1. Explain the reasons for and importance of coding diagnoses.
2. Describe the importance of matching the correct diagnostic code to the appropriate procedural code.
3. Differentiate between primary (first listed), principal, and secondary diagnoses and discuss admitting diagnoses.
4. Describe how medical necessity is supported by the diagnosis code.
5. Discuss the history of diagnostic coding.
6. Discuss the benefits of the ICD-10 coding system and differentiate between ICD-10-CM and ICD-10-PCS.
7. Identify and describe the Alphabetic and Tabular Index of the ICD-10-CM coding manual.
8. Define and demonstrate an understanding of diagnostic code conventions, symbols, and terminology.
9. Apply general coding guidelines to translate written descriptions of conditions into diagnostic codes.
10. Apply chapter-specific coding guidelines to reporting of specific illnesses and conditions.
11. Relate additional coding guidelines specific to reporting of outpatient services.
12. Describe methods of becoming more familiar with codes commonly encountered in a specific health care organization and discuss computer-assisted coding.
13. Anticipate future changes to the diagnosis coding system, known as ICD-11.

KEY TERMS

adverse effect
benign tumor
carcinoma in situ
chief complaint
combination code
complication
computer-assisted coding
conventions
eponym
essential modifiers
etiology
Excludes 1
Excludes 2
external causes of morbidity
International Classification of Diseases, Tenth Revision, Clinical Modification
International Classification of Diseases, Tenth Revision, Procedure Coding System
intoxication
late effect
laterality
malignant tumor
manifestation
medical necessity
metastasis
morbidity
mortality
neoplasm
nonessential modifiers
not elsewhere classifiable
not otherwise specified
Official Guidelines for Coding and Reporting
ordinality of encounter
placeholder
poisoning
primary diagnosis
principal diagnosis
prophylaxis
residual subcategories
rule out
secondary diagnosis
sequela
sequencing
syndrome
Uncertain Behavior
Z codes

KEY ABBREVIATIONS

AHA
AHIMA
CAC
CC
CPT
DM
ICD-10-CM
ICD-10-PCS
ICD-11
GEMS
HIV
MRI
NCHS
NEC
NOS
WHO

DIAGNOSIS CODING OVERVIEW

This chapter deals with diagnostic coding for outpatient professional services. The rules for coding inpatient cases can differ and are covered more thoroughly in Chapter 19 of this text. Health care providers and outpatient facilities use diagnostic codes on insurance claims to explain the reason the patient has sought health care services. Using a code eliminates the need to write out the diagnostic description on the claim form.

Diagnostic codes must be used on all claims and must be accurately assigned. Appropriate diagnosis coding can mean the financial success or failure of a health care organization. To assign diagnosis codes accurately, the billing and coding specialist must have knowledge of the current approved coding guidelines and a working knowledge of medical terminology. This includes having knowledge of anatomy and physiology, clinical disease processes, and medical terminology. There are many consequences of inaccurate assignment of diagnostic codes. For example, claims can be denied, fines or penalties can be levied, sanctions can be imposed, and the service provider's level of reimbursement for claims may be affected.

Assigning a Diagnosis Code

All documented diagnoses that affect the current status of the patient must be assigned a code. This includes conditions that exist at the time of the patient's initial contact with the service provider as well as conditions that develop subsequently and affect the treatment received. Diagnoses that relate to a patient's previous medical problem but have no bearing on the patient's present condition are not coded. The Centers for Medicare and Medicaid Services (CMS) and the National Center for Health Statistics (**NCHS**), departments within the Department of Health and Human Services (DHHS), provide a set of Official Guidelines for Coding and Reporting. These guidelines are a set of rules that have been developed to provide instructions. Adherence to the guidelines when assigning diagnosis codes is required under the Health Insurance Portability and Accountability Act (HIPAA).

Sequencing of Diagnostic Codes

Diagnosis codes must be sequenced correctly on an insurance claim so that the reason for medical services and the severity of the disease can be understood. **Sequencing** codes means listing them in the appropriate order as outlined in the *International Classification of Diseases* (ICD) guidelines. The correct diagnostic code must be matched to the appropriate surgical or medical procedure code for third-party reimbursement.

When submitting insurance claims for a health care provider or outpatient service, the **primary diagnosis** is the main reason for the encounter and should be listed first on the claim. In an evaluation and management (E/M) service, this is related to the **chief complaint (CC)**. The **secondary diagnosis**, listed subsequently, may contribute to the condition or define the need for a higher level of care but is not the underlying cause. The underlying cause of a disease is referred to as the **etiology** and is sequenced in the first position. The **principal diagnosis**, used in inpatient hospital coding, is the diagnosis that prompted the hospitalization. It is possible for the primary and principal diagnosis codes to be the same. The concept of a "principal diagnosis" is only applicable to inpatient hospital claims or cases. Box 12.1 outlines important differences between a primary and a principal diagnoses.

BOX 12.1 Primary Versus Principal Diagnosis

	Primary Diagnosis	Principal Diagnosis
Definition	Main reason (diagnosis, condition, chief complaint) for the encounter/visit in the health record that is responsible for services provided.	Condition established after study that prompted the hospitalization.
Location	Outpatient setting only (physician office visits and hospital-based outpatient services).	Inpatient setting only.
"Probable," "suspected," "questionable," "rule out," or "working diagnosis"	May not report "probable," "suspected," "questionable," "rule out," or "working diagnosis." Codes that describe symptoms and signs, as opposed to diagnoses, are acceptable for reporting purposes when a related definitive diagnosis has not been established (confirmed) by the provider.	Code the condition as if it existed or was established at the time of discharge if it is documented on the final diagnostic statement as "probable," "suspected," "questionable," "rule out," or "working diagnosis."

Admitting Diagnoses

Some diagnostic codes are considered problematic when used as the first diagnosis on admission of a patient to the hospital. Examples of questionable admitting diagnoses are obesity, benign hypertension, or controlled diabetes. The inpatient admission diagnosis may be expressed as one of the following:

1. One or more significant findings, symptoms or signs representing patient distress, or abnormal findings on examination.
2. A diagnosis established on an ambulatory care basis or previous hospital admission.
3. An injury or poisoning.
4. A reason or condition not classifiable as an illness or injury, such as pregnancy in labor or follow-up inpatient diagnostic tests.

When a physician makes hospital visits, code the reason for the visit, which might not necessarily be the reason the patient was admitted to the hospital (Example 12.1).

Medical Necessity

CMS defines **medical necessity** as the services or supplies needed to diagnose and treat a medical condition. Most health plans will not pay for health care services that they deem to be not medically necessary. The most common example is a cosmetic procedure, such as the injection of Botox to decrease facial wrinkles or tummy-tuck surgery. In those cases a health

EXAMPLE 12.1 Coding Physician Hospital Visits

A patient is admitted to the hospital with chest pains and is being monitored in the cardiac telemetry unit. On examination, it is noted that the patient has an enlarged thyroid and an endocrinologist is asked to see the patient in consultation.

Reason for Hospital Admission	Reason for Hospital Visit by Endocrinologist
Chest pain	Enlarged thyroid

plan may deny payment because of lack of medical necessity. In addition to certain surgical procedures, other services may have medical necessity restrictions. These include the following:

- Most imaging services (for example, radiography, computed tomography, or magnetic resonance imaging [MRI])
- Cardiovascular services (for example, electrocardiograms, Holter monitors, echocardiography, Doppler imaging, or stress testing)
- Neurologic services (for example, electroencephalography, noninvasive ultrasonography)
- Many laboratory services
- Vitamin B_{12} injections

It is important to know exactly which diagnosis relates to the procedure being billed. A reference book may be helpful in this situation and a number of manuals are available from commercial publishers. For cases dealing with CMS, consult the regional fiscal intermediary's website for local coverage determinations (LCDs) and the federal government's website for national coverage determinations (NCDs), or download the manual that is updated quarterly.

INTERNATIONAL CLASSIFICATION OF DISEASES

Diagnosis coding is performed using the World Health Organization's (WHO's) *International Classification of Diseases* (ICD). The coding system classifies morbidity and mortality information for (1) statistical purposes, (2) indexing of hospital records by disease and operations, and (3) data storage and retrieval. *Morbidity* refers to disease, and *mortality* refers to death. These are important to track in terms of how they affect a population.

History

From the earliest days of medical treatment, people have tried to name and classify diseases. The ICD had its beginning in England during the seventeenth century.

In 1948 the WHO developed the official version of the ICD in Geneva, Switzerland. The system was designed to compile and present statistical data on morbidity and mortality rates and frequency. WHO assumed responsibility for preparing and publishing revisions to the coding system every 10 years. The United States began using the ICD to report causes of death and prepare mortality statistics in the latter half of the twentieth century. Hospitals began using the ICD in 1950 to classify and index diseases.

The eighth revision of the ICD was constructed in 1966 and was adapted for use in the United States in 1968 by the United States Public Health Service. This became known as ICDA-8 and served as the basis for coding diagnostic data for both official morbidity and mortality statistics in the United States.

EXAMPLE 12.2 Transition and Mapping From ICD-9-CM to ICD-10-CM

ICD-9-CM	ICD-10-CM
461.9 Acute sinusitis, unspecified	J01.80 Other acute sinusitis J01.90 Acute sinusitis, unspecified J01.91 Acute recurrent sinusitis, unspecified
470 Deviated nasal septum	J34.2 Deviated nasal septum

Because of the higher specificity of the ICD-10-CM, crosswalks were not exact and did not always provide a one-to-one correlation but assisted in finding appropriate code ranges for reporting purposes.

ICD-9-CM, International Classification of Diseases, Ninth Revision, Clinical Modification; ICD-10-CM, International Classification of Diseases, Tenth Revision, Clinical Modification.

In 1979 the ninth revision of the *International Classification of Diseases* (ICD-9) was published by the WHO. Passage of the Medicare Catastrophic Coverage Act in 1988 then placed requirements on providers and health care organizations to submit appropriate diagnosis codes on all claims when billing for services provided to Medicare beneficiaries on or after April 1, 1989. The CMS designated *International Classification of Diseases, Ninth Revision, Clinical Modification (ICD-9-CM)* as the coding system physicians must use.

In 1992 the WHO published the tenth revision of the *International Classification of Diseases* (ICD-10). The NCHS further developed a clinical modification to the WHO's system, which is referred to as *International Classification of Diseases, Tenth Revision, Clinical Modification (ICD-10-CM).* On January 16, 2009, the DHHS published the final rule in the *Federal Register* for adoption of the ICD-10-CM code set with an implementation date of October 1, 2015.

The implementation date for the shift from ICD-9-CM to ICD-10-CM was repeatedly delayed in the United States due to the cost concerns for providers, payers, and health information professionals. Updating the EHR, coding, billing, and payment systems to handle the new code format and additional specificity was a monumental task. Although this may seem like the United States is lagging behind the rest of the world in diagnosis coding, it is important to note that many countries do not use ICD-10 for billing purposes. Rather, ICD-10-CM is used strictly for cause of death reporting and statistics.

Transition From ICD-9-CM to ICD-10-CM

During the transition period between the ICD-9-CM and ICD-10-CM, CMS provided crosswalks called GEMS (general equivalency mappings) that mapped old codes to the newer versions (Example 12.2). Because of the increased number of codes and higher degree of specificity in ICD-10-CM, there was rarely a one-to-one translation.

Noncovered entities, such as workers' compensation or no fault insurance companies, were not required to implement

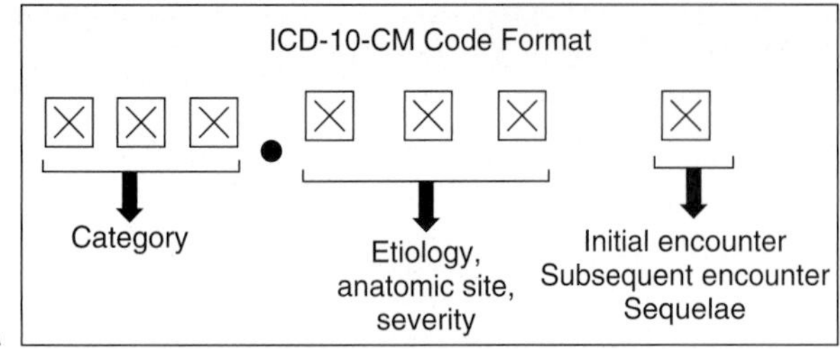

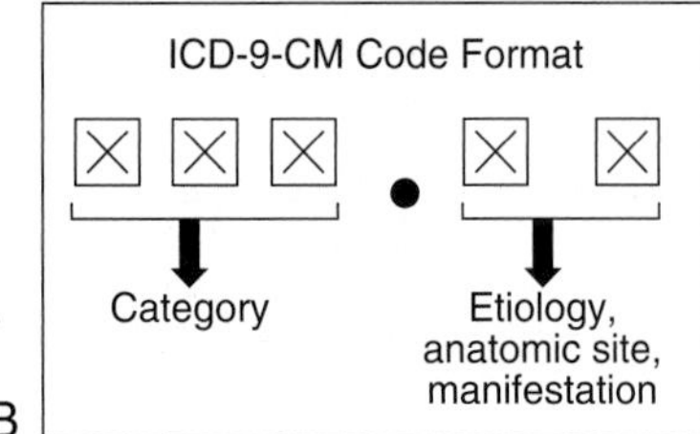

Fig. 12.1 *International Classification of Diseases, Tenth Revision, Clinical Modification* (ICD-10-CM) versus ICD-9-CM diagnostic code format. (From Fordney, M. T. (2010). *Fordney's medical insurance dictionary for billers and coders.* St. Louis: Elsevier.)

ICD-10-CM. However, it is in the noncovered entities' best interest to use the ICD-10-CM coding system because of the significant value of the increased detail of diseases. Because of this, many states have adopted ICD-10-CM for workers' compensation claims processing (Table 12.1). Coding and billing specialists should check with their state to determine which code set to use.

The ICD-10-CM coding system exceeds previous versions of the ICD in the number of concepts and codes provided. The disease classification was expanded to include health-related conditions and to provide greater specificity through reporting at a sixth-digit level with a seventh-digit extension. The sixth and seventh characters are not optional and are required for use in recording the information documented in the clinical record. ICD-10-CM allows more code choices and requires greater documentation in the health record (Fig. 12.1). Many of the conventions and guidelines are the same for both coding systems; however, there are more extensive guidelines for ICD-10-CM.

ICD-10 Diagnosis and Procedure Codes

There are many benefits associated with the adoption of the ICD-10 coding system. Benefits include the following:

- Much greater specificity, including laterality, which defines the side of the body is affected, or ordinality of encounter, which determines whether the care encounter is the patient's first for the condition
- Expansion of clinical information and reduced cross-referencing
- Flexibility and ease of expandability of the coding system
- Updated medical terminology and classification of diseases
- The ability to compare mortality and morbidity data
- Fewer nonspecific codes than in ICD-9-CM

The ICD-10 coding system consists of two code sets, ICD-10-CM and ICD-10-PCS.

ICD-10-CM

The Clinical Modification (CM) provides the specifics that the United States needs for collecting data on health status. This became known as the *International Classification of Diseases, Tenth Revision, Clinical Modification* (ICD-10-CM). It is used for reporting of diagnoses treated during encounters in all health care settings. Additional information on using ICD-10-CM is included in this chapter.

ICD-10-PCS

The *International Classification of Diseases, Tenth Revision, Procedure Coding System (ICD-10-PCS)* was developed in mid-1992 by 3M Health Information Systems under contract with the CMS. This replaced Volume 3 of ICD-9-CM. ICD-10-PCS is used by hospitals to report inpatient procedure codes. Additional information on using ICD-10-PCS is included in Chapter 19.

! COMPLIANCE ALERT

ICD-10-CM and Its Compliance With HIPAA

ICD-10-CM meets HIPAA criteria by

- providing specific information for outpatient and inpatient procedures;
- describing medical services using terminology in today's environment;
- expanding injury and disease codes and categories; and
- giving a more precise, clear, and clinical picture of the patient.

Organization and Format of ICD-10-CM

ICD-10-CM contains a Tabular List of Diseases (Volume 1), in which each disease has an assigned number (Fig. 12.2), and an Alphabetic Index to Diseases and Injuries (Volume 2) (Fig. 12.3). The systematized arrangement in these books makes it possible to encode, computerize, store, and retrieve large volumes of information from the patient's health record. ICD-10-CM is used by hospitals, physicians, and other health care providers to code and report diagnostic information. This information is necessary for participation in various government programs such as Medicare, Medicaid, quality improvement organizations, and professional review organizations.

Annual updates of ICD-10-CM are published in three publications: *Coding Clinic,* published by the American Hospital Association (AHA); *American Health Information Management Association Journal,* published by American Health Information Management Association (AHIMA); and the *Federal Register,* published by the US Government Printing Office. Coding from an out-of-date manual can delay payment, result in denied claims, or cause costly mistakes that can lead to financial disaster. Annual ICD-10-CM code revisions must be in place and in use by October 1 each year.

! COMPLIANCE ALERT

ICD-10-CM Standard Code Set

A code set is any set of codes with their descriptions used to encode data elements, such as tables of terms, medical concepts, medical diagnostic codes, or medical procedure codes. Each transaction must include the use of medical and other code sets. The *International Classification of Disease, Tenth Revision, Clinical Modification* (ICD-10-CM) official guideline for coding and reporting is the standard code set outlined under the Health Insurance Portability and Accountability Act (HIPAA) and must be used when assigning diagnostic codes. HIPAA does not require health insurance plans to change their business rules regarding payment based on the codes. However, insurance payers cannot reject an insurance claim because it includes a valid HIPAA standard code that the payer system does not yet recognize.

D55 **PART III / Tabular List of Diseases and Injuries** D57.1

HEMOLYTIC ANEMIAS (D55-D59)

● **D55 Anemia due to enzyme disorders**

Excludes 1 drug-induced enzyme deficiency anemia (D59.2)

D55.0 Anemia due to glucose-6-phosphate dehydrogenase [G6PD] deficiency
Favism
G6PD deficiency anemia

D55.1 Anemia due to other disorders of glutathione metabolism
Anemia (due to) enzyme deficiencies, except G6PD, related to the hexose monophosphate [HMP] shunt pathway
Anemia (due to) hemolytic nonspherocytic (hereditary), type I

D55.2 Anemia due to disorders of glycolytic enzymes
Hemolytic nonspherocytic (hereditary) anemia, type II
Hexokinase deficiency anemia
Pyruvate kinase [PK] deficiency anemia
Triose-phosphate isomerase deficiency anemia
Excludes 1 disorders of glycolysis not associated with anemia (E74.8)

D55.3 Anemia due to disorders of nucleotide metabolism

D55.8 Other anemias due to enzyme disorders

■ **D55.9 Anemia due to enzyme disorder, unspecified**

D56.3 Thalassemia minor
Genetic disorders that have in common defective production of hemoglobin
Alpha thalassemia minor
Alpha thalassemia silent carrier
Alpha thalassemia trait
Beta thalassemia minor
Beta thalassemia trait
Delta-beta thalassemia minor
Delta-beta thalassemia trait
Thalassemia trait NOS
Excludes 1 alpha thalassemia (D56.0)
beta thalassemia (D56.1)
delta-beta thalassemia (D56.2)
hemoglobin E-beta thalassemia (D56.5)
sickle-cell trait (D57.3)

D56.4 Hereditary persistence of fetal hemoglobin [HPFH]
Persistent production of hemoglobin

D56.5 Hemoglobin E-beta thalassemia
Excludes 1 beta thalassemia (D56.1)
beta thalassemia minor (D56.3)
beta thalassemia trait (D56.3)
delta-beta thalassemia (D56.2)
delta-beta thalassemia trait (D56.3)
hemoglobin E disease (D58.2)
other hemoglobinopathies (D58.2)
sickle-cell beta thalassemia (D57.4-)

Diagnosis code verified
Complete description

Fig. 12.2 Excerpt from the Tabular List of *International Classification of Diseases, Tenth Revision, Clinical Modification* (ICD-10-CM), Volume 1.

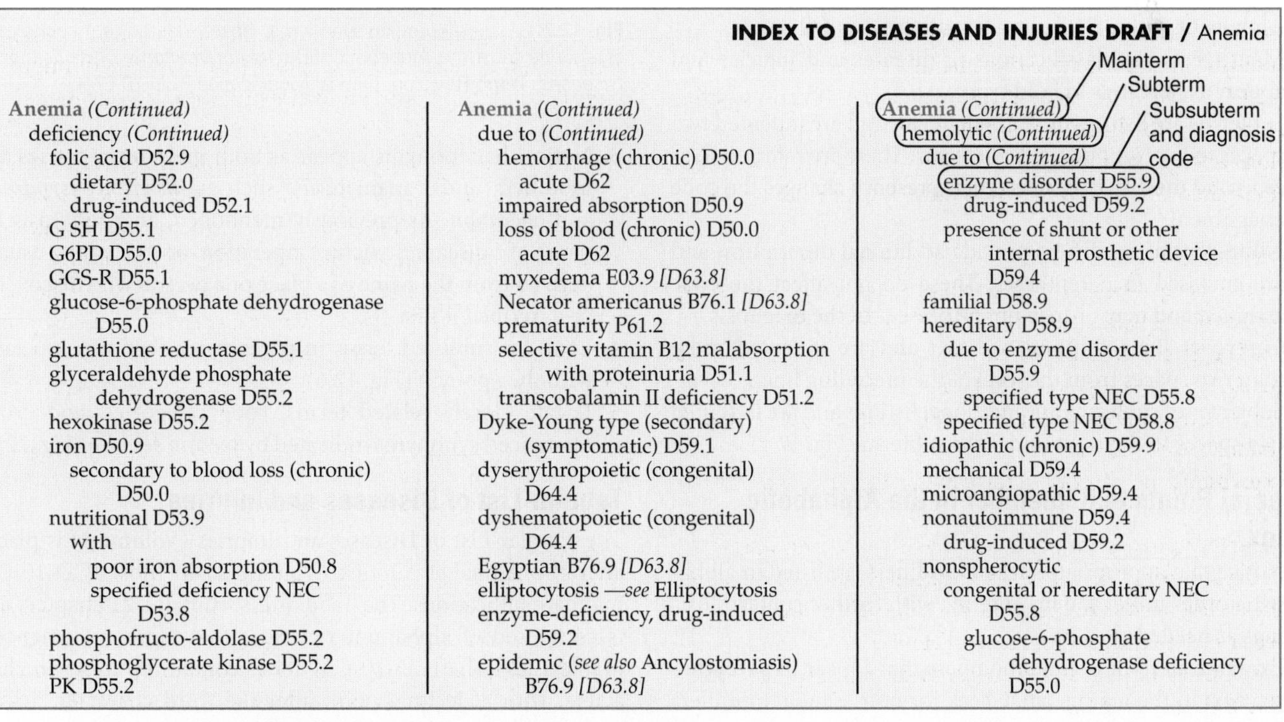

INDEX TO DISEASES AND INJURIES DRAFT / Anemia

Anemia *(Continued)*
deficiency *(Continued)*
folic acid D52.9
dietary D52.0
drug-induced D52.1
G SH D55.1
G6PD D55.0
GGS-R D55.1
glucose-6-phosphate dehydrogenase D55.0
glutathione reductase D55.1
glyceraldehyde phosphate dehydrogenase D55.2
hexokinase D55.2
iron D50.9
secondary to blood loss (chronic) D50.0
nutritional D53.9
with
poor iron absorption D50.8
specified deficiency NEC D53.8
phosphofructo-aldolase D55.2
phosphoglycerate kinase D55.2
PK D55.2

Anemia *(Continued)*
due to *(Continued)*
hemorrhage (chronic) D50.0
acute D62
impaired absorption D50.9
loss of blood (chronic) D50.0
acute D62
myxedema E03.9 *[D63.8]*
Necator americanus B76.1 *[D63.8]*
prematurity P61.2
selective vitamin B12 malabsorption with proteinuria D51.1
transcobalamin II deficiency D51.2
Dyke-Young type (secondary) (symptomatic) D59.1
dyserythropoietic (congenital) D64.4
dyshematopoietic (congenital) D64.4
Egyptian B76.9 *[D63.8]*
elliptocytosis —*see* Elliptocytosis
enzyme-deficiency, drug-induced D59.2
epidemic (*see also* Ancylostomiasis) B76.9 *[D63.8]*

Anemia *(Continued)*
hemolytic *(Continued)*
due to *(Continued)*
enzyme disorder D55.9
drug-induced D59.2
presence of shunt or other internal prosthetic device D59.4
familial D58.9
hereditary D58.9
due to enzyme disorder D55.9
specified type NEC D55.8
specified type NEC D58.8
idiopathic (chronic) D59.9
mechanical D59.4
microangiopathic D59.4
nonautoimmune D59.4
drug-induced D59.2
nonspherocytic
congenital or hereditary NEC D55.8
glucose-6-phosphate dehydrogenase deficiency D55.0

Fig. 12.3 Excerpt from the Alphabetic Index of Diseases and Injuries of *International Classification of Diseases*, Tenth Revision, Clinical Modification (ICD-10-CM).

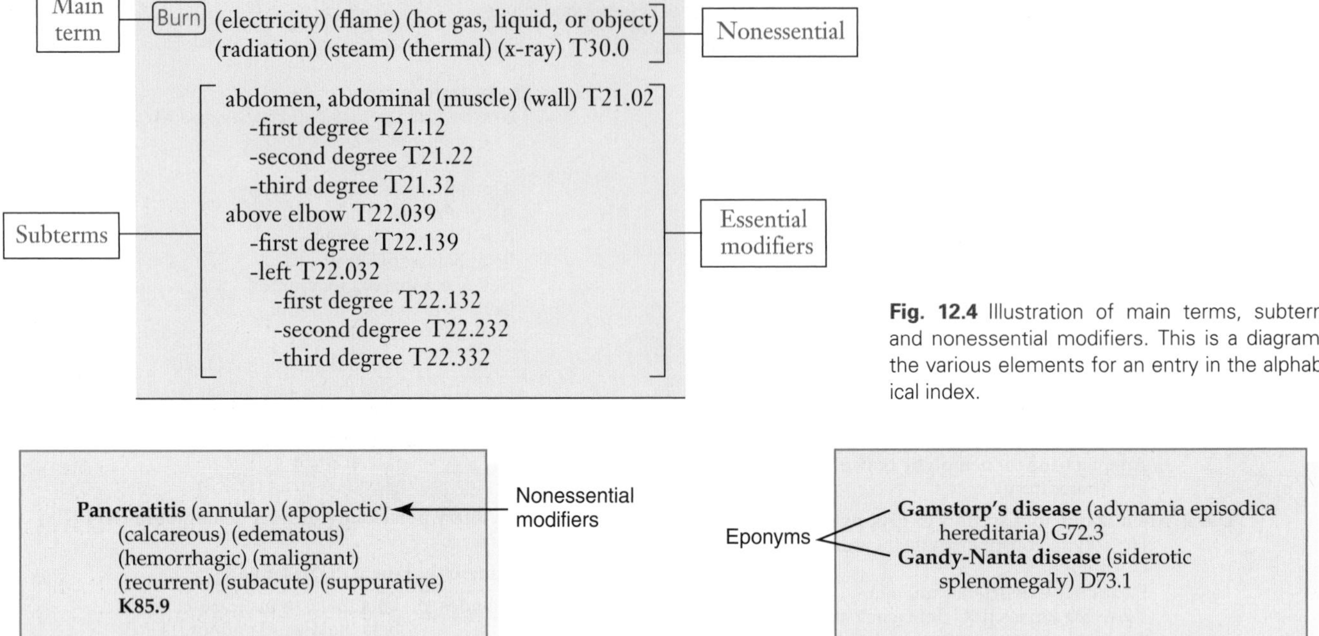

Fig. 12.4 Illustration of main terms, subterms, and nonessential modifiers. This is a diagram of the various elements for an entry in the alphabetical index.

Pancreatitis (annular) (apoplectic) ← Nonessential modifiers
(calcareous) (edematous)
(hemorrhagic) (malignant)
(recurrent) (subacute) (suppurative)
K85.9

Fig. 12.5 Coding with modifiers in parentheses.

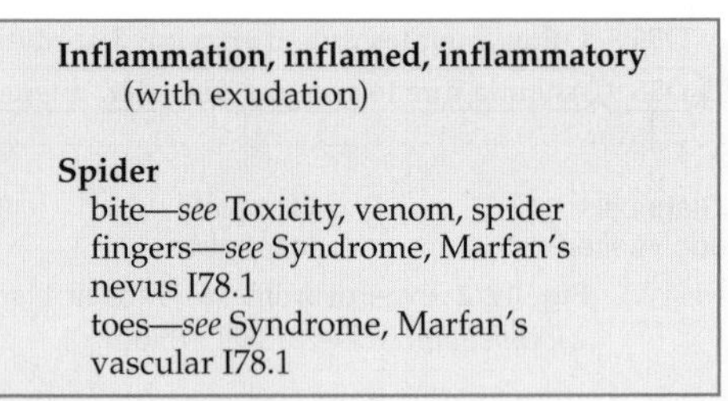

Fig. 12.6 Coding diagnoses associated with an eponym.

Alphabetic Index to Diseases and Injuries

The Alphabetic Index to Diseases and Injuries (Volume 2) is placed first in most ICD-10-CM coding manuals. The Alphabetic Index contains the Neoplasm Table, Tables of Drugs and Chemicals, and Index to External Cause. Main code descriptor items are in alphabetic order and indented subterms, and applicable additional qualifiers, descriptors, or modifiers are beneath the main terms.

Alphabetic Index elements are structured as follows:

- Main terms are classifications of diseases and injuries and appear as headings in bold type.
- Subterms are listings under main terms and are indented two spaces to the right under main terms. These are referred to as **essential modifiers** because their presence changes the code assignment.
- **Nonessential modifiers** provide additional description and are enclosed in parentheses. These do not affect the code assigned and may or may not be present in the diagnosis.
- Carryover lines continue the text and are indented more than two spaces from the level of the preceding line.
- Subterms of subterms are additional listings and are indented two spaces to the right under the subterm (Fig. 12.4).

Special Points to Remember in the Alphabetic Index

1. Notice that appropriate sites or modifiers are listed in alphabetic order under the main terms with further subterm listings as needed.
2. Examine all nonessential modifiers that appear in parentheses next to the main term. Check for nonessential modifiers that apply to any of the qualifying terms used in the statement of the diagnosis found in the patient's health record (Fig. 12.5).

Inflammation, inflamed, inflammatory
(with exudation)

Spider
bite—*see* Toxicity, venom, spider
fingers—*see* Syndrome, Marfan's
nevus I78.1
toes—*see* Syndrome, Marfan's
vascular I78.1

Fig. 12.7 Cross-referencing synonyms, closely related terms, and code categories from the Alphabetic Index of *International Classification of Diseases,* Tenth Revision, Clinical Modification (ICD-10-CM).

3. Notice that eponyms appear as both main term entries and modifiers under main terms such as *disease* or *syndrome* and *operation.* As previously mentioned, an **eponym** is the name of a disease, structure, operation, or procedure, usually derived from the name of a place or a person who discovered or described it first.
4. Look for sublisted terms in parentheses that are associated with the eponym (Fig. 12.6).
5. Locate closely related terms, code categories, and cross-referenced synonyms indicated by *see* and *see also* (Fig. 12.7).

Tabular List of Diseases and Injuries

The Tabular List of Diseases and Injuries (Volume 1) is placed after the Alphabetic Index (Volume 2) in most ICD-10-CM manual publications. The Tabular List contains 21 chapters and is composed of alphanumeric codes that represent diagnoses (Table 12.2). The ICD-10-CM codes contain up to seven characters, with a decimal point after the third character. This is shown as digit 1 (alpha character), digits 2 and 3 (numeric character), and digits 4 to 7 (alpha or numeric character). The first three characters are placed to the left of the decimal point and

TABLE 12.1 State Decisions Regarding Workers' Compensation and ICD-10 as of 2016*

ICD-10 Adopted	ICD-10 Not Adopted	ICD-10 Adopted Only for Certain Claim Types	ICD-10 Pending
Alabama	Arizona	Maine (inpatient)	Alaska
California	Arkansas	South Carolina (inpatient)	Tennessee
Delaware	Hawaii	Colorado (inpatient)	Wyoming
Florida	Iowa	Nebraska (trauma surgery)	
Georgia	Kansas		
Idaho	Kentucky		
Illinois	Missouri		
Louisiana	Mississippi		
Maryland	Oklahoma		
Massachusetts	Rhode Island		
Minnesota	Utah		
North Carolina	Vermont		
New Hampshire	Wisconsin		
Nevada			
New York			
Ohio			
Oregon			
Pennsylvania			
South Dakota			
Texas			
Washington			
US Department of Labor for federal workers' compensation claims			

*Coding and billing specialists in states listed as not adopting or pending ICD-10 should check with their state labor department to determine the current status of the transition.
Data from Wilson, S. ICD-10's impact to the worker's compensation industry, *ICD10 Monitor*, March 28, 2016. Retrieved from https://www.icd10monitor.com.

TABLE 12.2 Outline of Tabular List and Alphabetic Index of ICD-10-CM

Tabular List	Chapter Headings	Codes
1	Certain Infectious and Parasitic Diseases	A00-B99
2	Neoplasms	C00-D49
3	Diseases of the Blood and Blood-Forming Organs and Certain Disorders Involving the Immune Mechanism	D50-D89
4	Endocrine, Nutritional, and Metabolic Diseases	E00-E89
5	Mental and Behavioral Disorders	F01-F99
6	Diseases of the Nervous System	G00-G99
7	Diseases of the Eye and Adnexa	H00-H59
8	Diseases of the Ear and Mastoid Process	H60-H95
9	Diseases of the Circulatory System	I00-I99
10	Diseases of the Respiratory System	J00-J99
11	Diseases of the Digestive System	K00-K95
12	Diseases of the Skin and Subcutaneous Tissue	L00-L99
13	Diseases of the Musculoskeletal System and Connective Tissue	M00-M99
14	Diseases of the Genitourinary System	N00-N99
15	Pregnancy, Childbirth, and the Puerperium	O00-O9A
16	Certain Conditions Originating in the Perinatal Period	P00-P96
17	Congenital Malformations, Deformations, and Chromosomal Abnormalities	Q00-Q99
18	Symptoms, Signs, and Abnormal Clinical and Laboratory Findings, Not Elsewhere Classifiable	R00-R99
19	Injury, Poisoning, and Certain Other Consequences of External Causes	S00-T88
20	External Causes of Morbidity	V00-Y99
21	Factors Influencing Health Status and Contact with Health Services	Z00-Z99
Alphabetic Index		
Section 1	Index to Diseases, Alphabetic	
Section 2	Table of Drugs and Chemicals	
Section 3	Alphabetic Index to External Causes	

indicate the category. The remaining digits to the right of the decimal point indicate the etiology, anatomic site, and severity. The sixth character can signify the following:

- Laterality
- Intent of a drug poisoning (intentional self-harm, assault)
- "With" or "without" a given manifestation
- Trimester of a pregnancy
- Depth of a skin ulcer
- Nature of an injury

An X is used as a placeholder to save a space for future code expansion and/or to meet the requirement of coding to the highest level of specificity (Fig. 12.8).

Special Points to Remember in the Tabular List

1. Use two or more codes when necessary to describe a given diagnosis completely. For example, for arteriosclerotic cardiovascular disease with congestive heart failure, use I25.10 with I50.9.
2. Search for one code when either two diagnoses or a **manifestation** or a **complication** is present. A manifestation is an associated secondary process or disease. A complication is an evolution or consequence of a disease. There are instances when two diagnoses are classified with a single code number called a ***combination code.*** An example of a combination code is diabetic retinopathy E11.319.
3. Use category codes only if there are no subcategory codes. An example of a category code that is appropriately used as a complete diagnostic code is hypertension I10.
4. Read all instructional notes provided.

OFFICIAL GUIDELINES FOR ICD-10-CM

The **Official Guidelines for Coding and Reporting** is a set of rules developed to accompany and complement the official conventions and instructions provided in the ICD-10-CM coding manual. The guidelines include definitions, standards, rules, general coding guidelines, and 21 chapter-specific coding guidelines. Adherence to the guidelines when assigning an ICD-10-CM diagnosis code is required under HIPAA and has

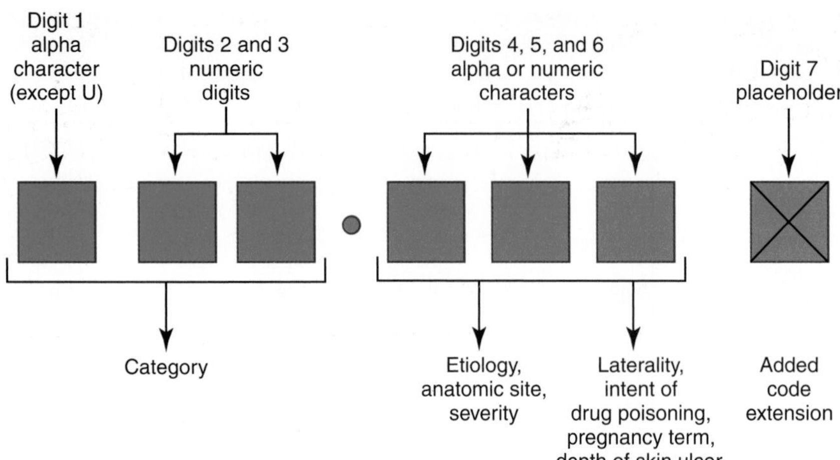

Fig. 12.8 Explanation of the seven character positions in the *International Classification of Diseases, Tenth Revision, Clinical Modification* (ICD-10-CM).

been adopted for all health care settings. It is important that the health care provider and the billing/coding specialist work together to achieve complete and accurate documentation, code assignment, and reporting of diagnosis codes.

Selection of a Coding Manual

Many companies publish the ICD-10-CM coding manuals. Publishers very often use different styles and formats, so it is important to study and compare the features of several books before making a decision to purchase. When choosing a book, the following questions should be asked:

- Are colors used for emphasis in locating items quickly?
- Are definitions or notes included to help one interpret and gain a better understanding of difficult medical terms and phrases?
- Are coding guidelines boxed for easy reference?
- Are icons or symbols used?
- Are fonts and type styles used that can be read easily?
- Is print large enough to allow accurate coding?

All of these benefit the coder.

Diagnostic Code Book Conventions

To become a proficient coder, it is important to develop an understanding of the conventions and terminology related to the ICD-10-CM coding system. **Conventions** are rules or principles for determining a diagnostic code when using diagnostic code books such as each space, typefaces, indentations, punctuation marks, symbols, instructional notes, abbreviations, cross-reference notes, and specific usage of the words *and, with,* and *due to*. These rules assist in the selection of correct codes for the diagnoses encountered. Some of the conventions for ICD-10-CM are listed in Box 12.2; however, the billing/coding specialist should read all the information included in the introduction section of the coding manual, which will provide a complete outline of all conventions used in the manual.

Placeholder Character

As mentioned, ICD-10-CM uses the **placeholder** character X when reporting certain codes to allow for future expansion of the code. When a placeholder is indicated, the X must be used in order for the code to be valid (Example 12.3).

Seventh Characters

Certain ICD-10-CM codes require seventh characters. If a code that requires a seventh character is not six characters, placeholder Xs must be used to fill the empty characters (Example 12.4).

Other and Unspecified Codes

The abbreviation **NEC** represents codes that are **"not elsewhere classifiable."** The Alphabetic Index will direct the coder to an "other specified" code in the Tabular List. Alphabetic Index entries with NEC in the line designate "other" codes in the Tabular List. These Alphabetic Index entries represent specific disease entities for which no specific code exists, so the term is included within an "other" code (Example 12.5).

The abbreviation **NOS** represents **"not otherwise specified"** and means unspecified. In ICD-10-CM, a code with a fourth digit 9 or fifth digit 0 for diagnosis codes labeled "unspecified" is used when the information in the health record is insufficient to assign a more specific code. For those categories for which an unspecified code is not provided, the "other specified" code may represent both other and unspecified. "Other specified" and "unspecified" subcategories are referred to as *residual subcategories* (Example 12.6).

Residual subcategories are used for conditions that are specifically named in the health record but not specifically listed under a code description. If there is a lack of details in the record and a specific subdivision cannot be matched, look for a qualifying statement in the provider's progress notes or history and physical examination report that indicates a more specific diagnostic code.

Punctuation and Symbols

ICD-10-CM's Alphabetic Index and Tabular List make use of certain abbreviations, punctuation, symbols, and other conventions, as shown in Box 12.2.

Brackets, [ ], are used in the Tabular List to enclose synonyms or alternative wording or to provide explanatory phrases (Example 12.7).

BOX 12.2 Official ICD-10-CM Code Book Conventions

Punctuation

[ ]	Brackets are used in the Tabular List to enclose synonyms, alternative wording, or explanatory phrases. **Example: J95.85**- Mechanical complication of respirator **[**ventilator**]**
:	Colons are used in the Tabular List after an incomplete term, which needs one or more of the modifiers following the colon to make it assignable to a given category. **Example: L99** Other disorders of skin and subcutaneous tissue in diseases classified elsewhere Code first underlying disease, such as: amyloidosis (E85.-)
-	Dashes are used in both the ICD-10-CM Indexes and the Tabular List. The Indexes use the dash to show the level of indentation. A symbol (-) at the end of an index entry indicates an incomplete code, so additional characters are needed. Locate the referenced category or subcategory elsewhere in the Tabular List, review the options, and assign the code. **Example:** **Excludes 2:** cellulitis of fingers (L03.01**-**)
( )	Parentheses are used in the Tabular List to enclose supplementary words (nonessential modifiers) that may be present or absent in the statement of a disease or condition without affecting the code number to which it was assigned. **Example: N39.3** Stress incontinence **(**female**)** **(**male**)**
Abbreviations	
NEC	Not elsewhere classifiable (NEC) in the Tabular List under a code identifies it as an "other specified" code. **Example: A85** Other viral encephalitis, not elsewhere classifiable **Includes:** specified viral encephalomyelitis **NEC**
NOS	Not otherwise specified (NOS) is equivalent to an unspecified code. **Example: Q66.89** Other congenital deformities of feet Congenital clubfoot **NOS**
Cross-Reference Terms	
and	This word represents and/or when used in a narrative statement. **Example: B35.0** Tinea barbae **and** tinea capitis
with/without	When a condition may have two versions—*with* or *without* a specific sign, symptom, or manifestation—this is indicated by a change in one of the code characters. These words in the Alphabetic Index are sequenced after the main term, not in alphabetical order. **Example:** Epilepsy, epileptic, epilepsia intractable G40.91-**with** status epilepticus G40.911 **without** status epilepticus G40.919
see	Instruction that follows a main term in the Index indicating that another term should be referenced. Go to the main term referenced with the "see" note to find the correct code. **Example:** Postphlebitic syndrome—**see** Syndrome, postthrombotic
see also	Instruction after a main term in the Index to indicate that there is another main term that may also be referenced and may provide additional index entries that may be useful. It is not necessary to follow the "see also" note when the original main term gives the code. **Example:** Preterm delivery (**see also** Pregnancy, complicated by, preterm labor) O60.10
Instructional Notes	
Code first/use additional code	Notes that certain conditions have both an underlying etiology and multiple body system manifestations due to the underlying etiology. Manifestation code titles have a phrase, "in diseases classified elsewhere." The underlying condition must be sequenced first followed by the manifestation. **Example: E08** Diabetes mellitus due to underlying condition **Code first** the underlying condition, such as: Congenital rubella (P35.0) **Use additional code** to identify any insulin use (Z79.4), oral antidiabetic drugs or oral hypoglycemic drugs (Z79.84).
Code also	Note instructions that two codes may be needed to completely describe a condition dependent on the severity of the conditions and the reason for the encounter. **Example: S85** Injury of blood vessels at lower leg level **Code also** any associated open wound (S81.-)
Includes	*Includes* appears under certain categories to add to the definition or give an example of the content of the category. **Example: S93** Dislocation and sprain of joints and ligaments at ankle, foot, and toe level **Includes:** avulsion of joint or ligament of ankle, foot, and toe
Inclusion terms	List of terms included under some codes, such as conditions for which that code is to be used, synonyms, or various specified conditions assigned to "other specified" codes. **Example: C46.1** Kaposi's sarcoma of soft tissue **Kaposi's sarcoma of blood vessel** **Kaposi's sarcoma of connective tissue** **Kaposi's sarcoma of fascia** **Kaposi's sarcoma of ligament**

Continued

BOX 12.2 Official ICD-10-CM Code Book Conventions—cont'd

Punctuation

Excludes 1 An *Excludes 1* note very simply indicates "not coded here." An Excludes 1 note should never be used at the same time as the code above the Excludes 1 note. It is used when two conditions cannot occur together, such as a congenital form versus an acquired form of the same condition.
Example: E20 Hypoparathyroidism
Excludes 1: Di George's syndrome (D82.1)

Excludes 2 An *Excludes 2* note very simply indicates "not included here." An Excludes 2 note indicates that the condition excluded is not part of the condition represented by the code but that a patient may have both conditions at the same time. When an Excludes 2 note appears under a code, use both the code and the excluded code together.
Example: I10 Essential (primary) hypertension
Excludes 2: Essential (primary) hypertension involving vessels of brain (I60-I69)

ICD-10-CM, International Classification of Diseases, Tenth Revision, Clinical Modification.

EXAMPLE 12.3 Placeholder Character

T55.0X1A	Toxic effects of soap, unintentional; Initial encounter

EXAMPLE 12.4 Seventh Characters

S01.312A	Laceration without foreign body of left ear; Initial encounter
T36.0X2A	Poisoning by penicillin, intentional, self-harm; Initial encounter

EXAMPLE 12.5 Other Specified Codes

K63.0	Abscess, intestine, intestinal, NEC

EXAMPLE 12.6 Unspecified Codes

J32.9	Chronic sinusitis, unspecified Sinusitis (chronic) NOS

EXAMPLE 12.7 Brackets

B01-	Varicella [chickenpox]

EXAMPLE 12.8 Parentheses

E05.90	Hyperthyroidism (latent) (pre-adult) (recurrent)

Parentheses, ( ), are used in the Alphabetic Index and Tabular List to enclose supplementary words that may further define the condition but do not affect the code number assigned. These are referred to as *nonessential modifiers* (Example 12.8).

Colons, :, are used in the Tabular List after an incomplete term that requires additional modifiers to appropriately assign the code (Example 12.9).

Includes Notes

A note appears immediately under the three-character code title in the Tabular List and provides further definition and examples of additional content to the category (Example 12.10).

EXAMPLE 12.9 Colons

D59.3	Hemolytic-uremic syndrome
Use additional code to identify associated:	*E. coli* infection (B96.2-)
	Pneumococcal pneumonia (J13) *Shigella dysenteriae* (A03.9)

EXAMPLE 12.10 Includes Notes

R18.- Ascites	Includes: fluid in the peritoneal cavity

EXAMPLE 12.11 Excludes Notes

R07.- Pain in throat and chest	Excludes 1: epidemic myalgia (B33.0)
	Excludes 2: jaw pain (R68.84) pain in breast (N64.4)

EXAMPLE 12.12 Default Code

K37	*Unspecified* appendicitis

Excludes Notes

There are two types of excludes notes used in the Tabular List of ICD-10-CM. An **Excludes 1** note indicates certain codes that should never be used at the same time as the code selected. It is used when two conditions could not possibly occur at the same time. **Excludes 2** notes indicate that the condition selected is not part of the excluded condition; however, it is possible for the patient to have both conditions at the same time. It is acceptable to report both the code and the excluded code together, when applicable (Example 12.11).

Default Code

A default code is shown next to a main term in the Alphabetic Index and represents the condition that is commonly associated with the main term or is the unspecified code for the condition. For example, if the electronic health record (HER) documents appendicitis but does not list acute or chronic, then the default code should be assigned (Example 12.12).

EXAMPLE 12.13 Gender and Age Codes

C50.411	Malignant neoplasm of upper-outer quadrant of right *female* breast
C50.421	Malignant neoplasm of upper-outer quadrant of right *male* breast
P70.2	*Neonatal* diabetes mellitus

PROCEDURE 12.1 Basic Steps in Selecting Diagnostic Codes From ICD-10-CM

Objective

Accurately choose and insert diagnostic codes for electronic transmission of an insurance claim

Equipment/Supplies

ICD-10-CM diagnostic code book, medical dictionary, and pen or pencil.

Directions

Use a standard method and establish a routine for locating a code. Follow these steps for coding the first diagnosis. For each subsequent diagnosis in a patient's health record, repeat these steps.

1. Read the patient's health record to find the main term. To identify the main term, ask what is wrong with the patient.
2. Next, locate the main term (disease or condition), not the anatomic site, in the Alphabetic Index. The Alphabetic Index is organized by main terms and has three sections:
   - Section 1—Index to Diseases and Nature of Injury includes Neoplasm Table and Table of Drugs and Chemicals
   - Section 2—Index to External Causes of Injury
   - Section 3—Table of Drugs and Chemicals
3. Read any notes under the main term. Select and write down the code.
4. Next, go to the Tabular List, review how it is organized for the subclassification, read and be guided by any instructional terms, and then verify that the selected code gives the highest level of specificity (up to seven alphanumeric characters). Possible errors may occur when using the Tabular List and when coding diseases or conditions that begin with categories "O" and "I." These can look like the numbers "zero" and "one" (for example, I00 and O99 are correct—not 100 and 099). In these categories, special attention must be given. Always read the specific chapter guidelines and refer to the general guidelines in the code book for certain diagnoses and/or conditions in the classification before choosing a code.
5. Assign the code.

ICD-10-CM, International Classification of Diseases, Tenth Revision, Clinical Modification.

Gender and Age Codes

Diagnostic codes must match the age and gender of the patient. If an adult male patient with breast cancer is seen, a code that matches gender must be used (Example 12.13).

General Coding Guidelines

Locating a Code in the ICD-10-CM

To select a code that corresponds to a diagnosis or reason for a medical service, the coder should first locate the term in the Alphabetic Index and then verify the code in the Tabular List. Step-by-step procedures for selecting ICD-10-CM diagnostic codes are presented at the end of this chapter in Procedure 12.1.

EXAMPLE 12.14 A Dash

Conjunctivitis, acute, unspecified	H10.3-

EXAMPLE 12.15 No Precise Diagnosis

The patient has an enlarged liver and further diagnostic studies may or may not be done. **Use code R16.0 for hepatomegaly.**

A dash (-) at the end of an Alphabetic Index entry indicates that an additional character is required and can be determined by referencing the Tabular List. Even if a dash is not present, the coder must always consult the Tabular List to refer to all additional instructional notes (Example 12.14).

Level of Detail in Coding

ICD-10-CM codes are composed three, four, five, six, or seven characters. Some conditions may be reported with a three-character code. However, if the code is further subdivided, it should be reported at the highest number of characters assigned. This is commonly referred to as coding to the highest level of specificity. A code is invalid if it has not been coded to the full number of characters required for that condition.

Signs and Symptoms

Codes that describe signs and symptoms are acceptable for reporting purposes when a related definitive diagnosis has not been established. This is reported using codes from Chapter 18 of the ICD-10-CM coding manual. Examples of codes found in this section are symptoms, signs, and abnormal clinical and laboratory findings, not elsewhere classified. When coding for professional or outpatient services, if the final diagnosis at the end of the encounter is qualified by any of the following terms:

- *Apparent*
- *Likely*
- *Might*
- *Possible*
- *Probably*
- *Questionable*
- *Rule Out*
- *Suspected*
- *Suspicion Of*

Do not code these conditions as if they existed or were established. Instead, document the condition to the highest degree of certainty and code the chief complaint, sign or symptom, abnormal test result, or other reason for the encounter.

This is contrary to coding practices used by hospital health information management departments for coding the diagnoses of hospital inpatients. For example, if a patient is admitted and is suspected of having a heart attack, this would be coded as a confirmed case of myocardial infarction.

The following are instances in which sign and symptom codes can be used for professional or outpatient services.

- No precise diagnosis can be made (Examples 12.15 and 12.16).
- Signs or symptoms are transient and a specific diagnosis was not made (Example 12.17).

EXAMPLE 12.16 No Precise Diagnosis

The patient complains of painful urination and urinalysis is negative. **Use code R30.0 for dysuria.**

EXAMPLE 12.17 Transient Sign and Symptom Code

The patient complains of chest pain on deep inspiration. On examination, the physician finds nothing abnormal and tells the patient to return in 1 week. When the patient returns, the pain has ceased. **Use code R07.1 for painful respiration.**

EXAMPLE 12.18 Provisional Diagnosis

On examination, the physician documents abnormal percussion of the chest. The patient is sent for a chest x-ray examination and is asked to return for a recheck. The patient does not have the x-ray examination and fails to return. **Use code R09.89 for abnormal chest sounds.**

EXAMPLE 12.19 Sign and Symptom Code Before Definite Diagnosis

A patient complains of nausea and vomiting and is referred to a gastroenterologist. **Use code R11.2 for nausea with vomiting.**

EXAMPLE 12.20 Conditions That Are an Integral Part of a Disease Process

The provider documents asthma with wheezing. Wheezing is a sign and symptom typically associated with asthma; therefore the code for asthma is all that should be reported.

The provider documents nausea and vomiting due to gastroenteritis. Nausea and vomiting are signs and symptoms typically associated with gastroenteritis; therefore only the code for gastroenteritis should be reported.

- Provisional diagnosis is made for a patient who does not return for further care (Example 12.18).
- A patient is referred for treatment before a definite diagnosis is made (Example 12.19).

Conditions That Are an Integral Part of a Disease Process

Signs and symptoms that are typically associated with a disease process should not be assigned as additional codes (Example 12.20).

Conditions That Are Not an Integral Part of a Disease Process

Signs and symptoms that are not typically associated with a disease process should be reported when documented (Example 12.21).

Multiple Coding for a Single Condition

In some cases, two codes will be required to describe a single condition. "Use additional code" notes from the Tabular List will guide the coder as to when it is appropriate to report a secondary code. When determining which code to sequence first, the additional code would be reported as secondary code (Example 12.22).

EXAMPLE 12.21 Conditions That Are Not an Integral Part of a Disease Process

The provider documents diverticulosis with abdominal pain. Patients can have diverticulosis without having abdominal pain. By reporting abdominal pain in addition to diverticulosis, the severity of the condition is better described. Medical necessity for further study is also supported by reporting abdominal pain with diverticulosis.

The provider documents benign prostatic hypertrophy with urinary frequency. Patients can have benign prostatic hypertrophy without urinary frequency. By reporting urinary frequency in addition to benign prostatic hypertrophy, the severity of the condition is better described. Medical necessity for further study is also supported by reporting urinary frequency with benign prostatic hypertrophy.

EXAMPLE 12.22 Multiple Coding for a Single Condition

Alzheimer's disease (G30.-)	Use additional code to identify: Delirium, if applicable (F05) Dementia with behavioral disturbance (F02.81) Dementia without behavioral disturbance (F02-80)

EXAMPLE 12.23 "Code First" Notes

Maternal care for abnormality of pelvic organ (O34.-)	Code first any associated obstructed labor (O65.5)

EXAMPLE 12.24 Acute, Subacute, and Chronic Conditions

Appendicitis (pneumococcal) (retrocecal) K37
 Acute (catarrhal) (fulminating) (gangrenous) (obstructive) (retrocecal) (suppurative) K35.80
 Subacute (adhesive) K36
 Chronic (recurrent) K36

"Code first" notes are also indicated in the Tabular List and are typically used to identify an underlying condition. The underlying condition is always reported as the primary code (Example 12.23).

Acute, Subacute, and Chronic Conditions

When the documentation mentions that a condition is both acute (subacute) and chronic and separate codes exist in the Alphabetic Index, both are coded with the acute (subacute) sequence first followed by the code for the chronic condition (Example 12.24).

For documentation to support chronic conditions, the provider must discuss the chronic condition and state that the condition is pertinent to the patient's current treatment. For example, if a physician states "controlled diabetes," he or she is stating a fact. If the physician asks the patient about his blood sugar level and diet and documents the findings, then something specific has been identified about the chronic condition. This would be considered proper documentation.

EXAMPLE 12.25 Combination Code

J44.0	Chronic obstructive pulmonary disease with acute lower respiratory infection Use additional code to identify the infection.
G03	Meningitis due to other and unspecified causes Includes: arachnoiditis NOS Excludes 1: meningomyelitis (G04.-)

NOS, Not otherwise specified.

EXAMPLE 12.26 Sequela

R13.1-	Dysphagia
I69.991	Dysphagia due to late effect (sequela) of cerebrovascular disease (Instructional note states: "Use additional code to identify the type of dysphagia, if known [R13.1-]".)

EXAMPLE 12.27 Impending or Threatened Condition

I20.0	Impending myocardial infarction
O20.0	Threatened abortion

Combination Code

A **combination code** is a situation in which a single code is used to classify two diagnoses or a diagnosis with an associated secondary process (manifestation) or a diagnosis with an associated complication. Identify a combination code by referring to subterm entries in the Alphabetic Index and by reading the inclusion and exclusion notes in the Tabular List. If the combination code does not specifically describe the manifestation or complication, use a secondary code (Example 12.25).

Sequela

A **sequela** is a **late effect** or condition produced after the acute phase of an illness. There is no time limit on when a late effect code can be used. Coding of sequela generally requires two codes. The nature of the sequela is sequenced first; the sequela code is sequenced second (Example 12.26).

Impending or Threatened Condition

Codes that are described as impending or threatened should be referenced as such in the Alphabetic Index and reported accordingly. If there is no subterm under impending or threatened for the condition described, report the existing underlying condition(s) (Example 12.27).

Reporting the Same Diagnosis Code More Than Once

Each unique ICD-10-CM diagnosis code may be reported only once for an encounter. This applies to bilateral conditions where there are no distinct codes to identify laterality or two different conditions are classified to the same diagnosis code.

Laterality

When reporting bilateral sites, the final character of the code in ICD-10-CM should be selected to indicate laterality. The right side is always character 1 and the left side character 2. In those situations when a bilateral code is given, the bilateral character is always 3. If the side is not identified, an unspecified code is provided, which is either 0 or 9, depending on whether it is a fifth or sixth character (Example 12.28).

EXAMPLE 12.28 Laterality

S67.0-	Crushing injury of thumb
S67.00-	Crushing injury of thumb of unspecified side
S67.01-	Crushing injury of right thumb
S67.02-	Crushing injury of left thumb

EXAMPLE 12.29 Syndrome

Q90.9	Down syndrome
I45.9	Adams-Stokes syndrome

EXAMPLE 12.30 Complications of Care

T88.59-	Complication of anesthesia
K94.00	Complication of colostomy

Documentation for Body Mass Index and Pressure Ulcer Stages

Information documented by clinicians who are not the patient's provider in the health record to indicate body mass index (BMI) or pressure ulcer stage codes can be coded. However, the patient's provider must document the associated diagnosis such as obesity or pressure ulcer.

Syndromes

A **syndrome** is another name for a symptom complex, which is a set of signs, symptoms, or other manifestations resulting from a common cause or appearing in combination, presenting a distinct clinical picture of a disease or inherited abnormality. Syndromes should be reported by following the Alphabetic Index (Example 12.29).

Documentation of Complications of Care

Complications of care codes are assigned based on provider's documentation of the relationship between the condition and the care or procedure (Example 12.30).

Chapter-Specific Coding Guidelines

In addition to general diagnosis coding guidelines, there are guidelines specific to the 21 chapters of the Tabular Index. Some of the most commonly referenced chapter-specific coding guidelines are provided in this text; however, the billing/coding specialist must be familiar with the entire contents of the Official Guidelines for Coding and Reporting and refer to them when reporting all conditions. The chapter-specific guidelines are located in Section I, Subsection C of the Official Guidelines.

Human Immunodeficiency Virus

Human immunodeficiency virus (**HIV**) is a disease of the immune system characterized by increased susceptibility to

TABLE 12.3 Coding for Neoplasms

	MALIGNANT					
	Primary	Secondary	Carcinoma in Situ	Benign	Uncertain Behavior	Unspecified
Neoplasm, neoplastic	C80.1	C79.9	D09.9	D36.9	D48.9	D49.9
Abdomen, abdominal	C76.2	C79.8-	D09.8	D36.7	D48.7	D49.89
Cavity	C76.2	C79.8-	D09.8	D36.7	D48.7	D49.89
Organ	C76.2	C79.8-	D09.8	D36.7	D48.7	D49.89
Viscera	C76.2	C79.8-	D09.8	D36.7	D48.7	D49.89
Wall	C44.509	C79.2-	D04.5	D23.5	D48.5	D49.2
Connective tissue	C49.4	C79.8-	—	D21.4	D48.1	D49.2
Abdominopelvic	C76.8	C79.8-	—	D36.7	D48.7	D49.89
Accessory sinus—see Neoplasm, sinus						
Acoustic nerve	C72.4-	C79.49	—	D33.3	D43.3	D49.7
Adenoid (pharynx) (tissue)	C11.1	C79.89	D00.08	D10.6	D37.05	D49.0
Adipose tissue (see also Neoplasm, connective tissue)	C49.4	C79.89	—	D21.9	D48.1	D49.2
Adnexa (uterine)	C57.4	C79.89	D07.39	D28.7	D39.8	D49.5
Adrenal	C74.9-	C79.7-	D09.3	D35.0-	D44.1-	D49.7
Capsule	C74.9-	C79.7-	D09.3	D35.0-	D44.1-	D49.7
Cortex	C74.0-	C79.7-	D09.3	D35.0-	D44.1-	D49.7
Gland	C74.9-	C79.7-	D09.3	D35.0-	D44.1-	D49.7
Medulla	C74.1-	C79.7-	D09.3	D35.0-	D44.1-	D49.7
Ala nasi (external)	C44.301	C79.2-	D04.39	D23.39	D48.5	D49.2
Alimentary canal or tract NEC	C26.9	C78.80	D01.9	D13.9	D37.9	D49.0

NEC, Not elsewhere classifiable.

opportunistic infections, certain cancers, and neurologic disorders. Specific guidelines for reporting HIV infections are provided in Section Ia, Chapter 1, Subsection C of the Chapter-Specific Coding Guidelines. Only confirmed cases of HIV infection or illness should be reported. The provider's documentation that the patient is HIV positive would serve as confirmation. The diagnosis code B20 is used to report HIV disease, whereas an asymptomatic HIV infection status is reported as Z21. Patients who present for testing for HIV are coded as Z11.4, encounter for screening for HIV. Once a patient is given a confirmed diagnosis of HIV, it should be coded for every subsequent admission or encounter thereafter. Sequencing is determined by the reason for the encounter.

Neoplasms

Section I, Chapter 2, Subsection C of the Chapter-Specific Coding Guidelines provides guidelines for neoplasm coding. A **neoplasm** is a spontaneous new growth of tissue forming an abnormal mass that is also known as a *tumor.* It may be benign or malignant. A table is provided in the Alphabetic Index to look up the condition using the main entry "Neoplasm." The table has the column headings Malignant, Benign, Uncertain Behavior, and Unspecified (Table 12.3).

First, check the index; if the term for the area in active treatment is not listed, then go to the table. Often the index entry will produce the correct code and indicate what area of the table to look in. If a coder searches the table first, an incorrect code may be obtained. Code numbers for neoplasms are given by anatomic site. For each site, there are six possible code numbers, indicating whether the neoplasm in question is malignant (primary, secondary, or carcinoma in situ), benign, of uncertain behavior, or of unspecified nature. The description of the neoplasm often indicates which of the six code numbers is appropriate. For example, a melanoma of skin is malignant, a fibroadenoma of breast is benign, and a carcinoma in situ of cervix uteri is malignant by definition of the type of neoplasm (Example 12.31).

EXAMPLE 12.31 Adenocarcinoma of the Breast With Metastases to the Pelvic Bone

Step 1 Look up adenocarcinoma in the Alphabetic Index. Notice it states: "*see also* Neoplasm, by site, malignant."

Step 2 Locate neoplasm in the table in the Alphabetic Index. At the top of the page, notice the Malignant heading with the subheadings Primary, Secondary, and Ca In Situ. *Primary* means the first site of development of the malignancy. *Secondary* means metastasis from the primary site to a second site. *Ca In Situ* means cancer confined to the epithelium of the site of origin without invasion of the basement membrane tissue of the site.

Step 3 Find the site of the adenocarcinoma (in this case the breast) and look under the Malignant and Primary headings. Note that the code given is C50.919.

Step 4 Next, find bone as a subterm in the Neoplasm Table and look for the subterm *pelvic.* Then look at the three columns under Malignant and using the Secondary column, find the correct code number C79.51. In listing these diagnoses on the insurance claim, give the following: C50.919 and C79.51.

A **benign tumor** is one that does not have the properties of invasion and **metastasis** or spread or transfer of tumor cells from one organ to another site. It is usually surrounded by a fibrous capsule. It is important to note that cysts and lesions are not neoplasms. A neoplasm is not necessarily cancer or malignant.

EXAMPLE 12.32 Primary and Secondary Cancerous Tumors

Primary	C64-	Malignant neoplasm of kidney, except renal pelvis
	C65-	Malignant neoplasm renal pelvis
Secondary	C79.0-	Secondary malignant neoplasm of kidney and renal

EXAMPLE 12.33 Uncertain Behavior

Congenital giant pigmented nevus (D48.5)	See also Neoplasm, skin, uncertain behavior

A **malignant tumor** has the properties of invasion and metastasis. The term *carcinoma* refers to a cancerous or malignant tumor. **Carcinoma in situ** means cancer confined to the site of origin without invasion of neighboring tissues. A *primary malignancy* means the original malignant neoplastic site. A *secondary neoplasm* or malignancy is the site or location to which the original malignancy has spread or metastasized. If the diagnosis does not mention metastasis, code the case as a primary neoplasm (Example 12.32). Lymphomas and leukemias are not classified using the primary and secondary terminology.

The diagnostic statement "metastatic from" indicates primary stage carcinoma whereas "metastatic to" indicates secondary stage carcinoma. If the diagnostic statement is "malignant neoplasm spread to," code it as the primary site spread to the secondary site. The phrase "recurrent malignancy" is coded as a primary neoplasm.

The column of the neoplasm table labeled **Uncertain Behavior** is used when the lesion's behavior cannot be predicted. The pathologist has examined the specimen and found it to be benign at the present time but there is a chance it could undergo malignant transformation over time. These are well-defined neoplasms, the subsequent behavior of which cannot be predicted from the present appearance. These codes should be reported only if the pathology reports the neoplasm as "Uncertain Behavior" or an instructional note in the Alphabetic Index points toward an "Uncertain Behavior" code (Example 12.33).

If a neoplasm has been excised but no pathology report is available, it is not reported as uncertain behavior; it would be reported using the "Unspecified Behavior" column of the table. Reporting a lesion of unknown diagnosis as a lesion of uncertain behavior is a common coding error. It is always recommended that the coder wait for the final pathology report after excision of a neoplasm. Although waiting for the final diagnosis may mean a delay in submission of the bill for payment, it is preferable to submit with the correct diagnosis.

Coding of Diabetes Mellitus

Diabetes mellitus (**DM**) is an endocrine disease; guidelines for coding DM are found in Section 1, Subsection C, Chapter 4 of the Chapter-Specific Coding Guidelines. DM is categorized as either type 1 or type 2 and should be identified in the provider's documentation for accurate reporting of the condition. Table 12.4 outlines the clinical features important in the classification of diabetes.

TABLE 12.4 Features of Type 1 and Type 2 Diabetes

Type 1 Diabetes	Type 2 diabetes
Insulin-dependent diabetes mellitus	Non–insulin-dependent diabetes mellitus
Patients must be treated with insulin	Patients may be treated with insulin
Insulin levels are very low	Insulin levels may be high, "normal," or low
Ketosis prone	Non–ketosis prone
Patients usually are lean	Patients usually are obese
Usually "juvenile onset" (peak onset at early puberty)	Usually "adult onset," although occasionally seen in children
Often little family history of diabetes mellitus	Often strong family history of diabetes mellitus

EXAMPLE 12.34 Complications Related to Diabetes

E11.40	Diabetic neuropathy
E11.36	Diabetic cataracts

Type 1 DM is also known as juvenile diabetes, which commonly develops before the individual reaches puberty; however, the age of the patient is not the sole determining factor for this diagnosis. In type 1 diabetes, the patient's pancreas does not function properly and does not produce insulin. Thus this patient's body is dependent on insulin. Do not assume that because a patient is taking insulin, he or she has an insulin-dependent diabetes; look to the service provider's documentation for clarification.

Type 2 DM used to be referred to as adult-onset diabetes. In type 2 diabetes, the patient's pancreas produces some insulin but the insulin is ineffective in doing its job, which is to remove sugar from the bloodstream. This type of diabetes may be controlled with diet, oral medication, or insulin. If the type of diabetes is not documented in the health record, the default is E11.-, type 2 diabetes.

Patients with DM often encounter complications that affect other body systems. The diabetes codes are combination codes that include the type of diabetes, the body system affected, and the complications affecting that body system. The coder should assign as many codes from categories E08-E13 as needed to identify all the associated conditions the patient has. They should be sequenced based on the reason for the particular encounter (Example 12.34).

Diabetes code categories (E08, E09, E11, and E13) have an associated instructional note in the Tabular Index that advises the coder to "Use additional code to identify any insulin use (Z79.4), oral antidiabetic drugs or oral hyperglycemic drugs (Z79.84)." If the patient routinely takes insulin, use diagnosis code Z79.4, long-term (current) use of insulin, but do not use this code if the patient takes insulin temporarily to control blood sugar.

If the patient receives an underdose because of pump failure, assign a code from subcategory T85.6, mechanical complication of other specified internal and external prosthetic devices, implants and grafts, followed by code T38.3X6-, with the appropriate code for the type of DM and any associated complications. If the pump failure causes an insulin overdose, the second diagnosis code should be T38.3X1-, poisoning by insulin and oral hypoglycemic drugs, accidental, with the appropriate code for the type of DM and related complications.

Diabetes is a significant complicating factor in pregnancy. When coding DM in pregnancy, assign a code from category O24, DM in pregnancy, childbirth, and the puerperium, as the primary code. The appropriate diabetes code from the category E08-E13 should be reported as a secondary code. Gestational diabetes occurs when the diabetes was induced by the pregnancy. This can occur during the second or third trimester of pregnancy in women who were not diabetic before pregnancy. Codes from subcategory O24.4, gestational DM, are reported when this condition is documented.

Circulatory System Conditions

Diseases of the circulatory system are difficult to code because of the variety and lack of specific terminology used by service providers in stating the diagnoses. The billing/coding specialist should refer to Section 1, Subsection C, Chapter 9 of the Chapter-Specific Coding Guidelines for assistance in coding circulatory system conditions. When selecting codes, carefully read all inclusion, exclusion, and "use additional code" notations contained in the Tabular List.

Hypertension

The lay term *high blood pressure* is medically termed *hypertension.* Hypertension may be documented as malignant, which has nothing to do with tumor formation. Malignant hypertension is a condition of very high blood pressure with poor prognosis. It is a symptom complex of markedly elevated blood pressure where the diastolic pressure greater than 140 mm Hg and is associated with papilledema. In this disease, the term *malignant* denotes that it is life threatening. *Benign hypertension* refers to high blood pressure that runs a relatively long and symptomless course. In ICD-10-CM, hypertension is reported with the code I10, regardless of whether the hypertension is documented as benign or malignant.

Hypertension can cause various forms of heart and vascular disease or it can accompany some heart conditions. There are code categories used to report these conditions as combination codes.

Code Category I11	Hypertensive heart disease
Code Category I12	Hypertensive chronic kidney disease
Code Category I13	Hypertensive heart and chronic kidney disease

When the diagnostic statement indicates a cause by stating "heart condition *due to* hypertension" or "hypertensive heart disease," assign a code from category I11. If the diagnostic statement reads "*with* hypertension" or "cardiomegaly *and* hypertension," two separate codes are needed.

Elevated blood pressure without mention of hypertension is coded R03.0. If a patient has a single high blood pressure reading, it does not indicate there is a problem or the need for medical intervention. Sometimes, a patient simply gets nervous when seeking medical evaluation or treatment. This is referred to as *white coat syndrome.*

Secondary hypertension is due to an underlying condition and is reported from the code category I15. An additional code is required to report secondary hypertension to identify the cause of the hypertension when specified.

Myocardial Infarctions

A myocardial infarction (MI) is commonly referred to as a heart attack. During an MI, there is death to a segment of heart muscle caused by a blood clot in the coronary artery that interrupts the heart's blood supply. An MI that is equal to, or less than, four weeks old is considered acute and is reported with codes from category I21. If the patient is still receiving care related to the MI after the 4-week time frame, the appropriate aftercare code should be assigned. If the patient suffers an acute MI during the 4-week time frame, the incident should be reported with a code from category I22 to indicate a subsequent acute MI. The code I25.2 is reported for old or healed myocardial infarctions that do not require further care.

Pregnancy, Delivery, or Abortion

Section 1, Subsection C, Chapter 15 of the Chapter-Specific Coding Guidelines provides guidelines for reporting pregnancy, delivery, or abortion cases. Chapter 15 codes have sequencing priority over codes from other chapters. When the provider has treated a condition unrelated to the pregnancy but the pregnancy has been documented as incidental to the encounter, code Z33.1, pregnant state, incidental, should be used in place of a Chapter 15 code.

The following main sections are included:

O00-O08 Pregnancy with abortive outcome
O09 Supervision of high-risk pregnancy
O10-O16 Edema, proteinuria, and hypertensive disorders in pregnancy, childbirth, and the puerperium
O20-O29 Other maternal disorders predominately related to pregnancy
O30-O48 Maternal care related to the fetus and amniotic cavity and possible delivery problems
O60-O77 Complications of labor and delivery
O80-O82 Encounter for delivery
O85-O92 Complications predominantly related to the puerperium
O94-O9A Other obstetric conditions, not elsewhere classifiable

An entire section of the Chapter-Specific Coding Guidelines is devoted to reporting obstetric cases, which are not limited to but include the following:

1. Chapter 15 codes are reported only on the maternal record, never on the newborn record.
2. Codes in Chapter 15 have a final character to indicate the trimester of pregnancy. Trimesters are counted from the first day of the last menstrual period and defined as first trimester (less than 14 weeks, 0 days), second trimester

EXAMPLE 12.35 Complications Related to Pregnancy

O10.919	Preexisting hypertension complicating pregnancy, unspecified trimester
O36.5910	Pregnancy complicated by poor fetal growth, third trimester, unspecified number of gestations

(14 weeks, 0 days to less than 28 weeks, 0 days), and third trimester (28 weeks, 0 days until delivery). Assignment of the final character should be based on the provider's documentation of the trimester. If documentation in the record is insufficient to clarify trimester, report the final character for "unspecified trimester."

3. When reporting complications in pregnancy or childbirth, a seventh character may be required in some instances to identify the fetus affected by the complications. A seventh character of "0" is reported for single gestations when the document in the record is insufficient or when it is not possible to clinically determine which fetus is affected (Example 12.35).
4. Routine outpatient prenatal visits are reported with a code from category Z34 when no complications are present.
5. Outpatient prenatal visits for high-risk patients are reported with a code from category O09.
6. Full-term uncomplicated vaginal delivery should be reported with code O80. Code O80 is always a principal diagnosis and is not reported with any other code from Chapter 15.
7. A code from category Z37 is reported on every maternal record to report the outcome of delivery.

Injury, Poisoning, and Other Consequences of External Causes

Section 1, Subsection C of Chapter 19 of the Chapter-Specific Coding Guidelines is a large section of rules for coding of the following:

- Injuries
- Fractures
- Burns
- Poisoning
- Adult and child abuse
- Complications of care

Most categories in Chapter 19 require a seventh character extension to indicate whether the encounter is an initial encounter (identified with an A), a subsequent encounter (identified with a D), or a sequela or late effect (identified with an S).

Injuries and Late Effects

Diagnostic codes for injuries are listed in the Alphabetic Index by the type of injury and are broken down by anatomic site. To code multiple injuries, a separate code should be assigned for each injury, unless a combination code is assigned. List the diagnosis for the conditions treated in order of importance, with the diagnosis for the most severe problem listed first. If surgery is involved, the diagnostic code for the surgical problem should be listed first unless there is a severe injury of another part of the body (Example 12.36).

EXAMPLE 12.36 Injuries

Case: An intracranial injury, managed medically, and a fractured middle phalanx of the right hand, managed surgically

S06.9X0A	Intracranial injury, Initial encounter (first-listed primary diagnosis)
S62.602A	Fractured right middle phalanx, Initial encounter (secondary diagnosis)

TABLE 12.5 Common Injury Medical Terms

Main Term	Explanation
Contusion	Bruise and hematoma without a fracture or open wound.
Crush	Crushing injury not complicated by concussion, fractures, injury to internal organs, or intracranial injury.
Dislocation	Displacement and subluxation. Dislocation may be open or closed. Closed dislocation may be complete, partial, simple, or uncomplicated. Open dislocation may be compound, infected, or with foreign body. A dislocation not indicated as closed or open is classified as closed.
Fracture	Fractures may be open or closed. A fracture not indicated as open or closed is classified as closed. An injury described as fracture dislocation is coded as a fracture. Open fractures may be described as compound, infected, missile, puncture, or with foreign body. Closed fractures may be described as comminuted, depressed, elevated, fissured, greenstick, impacted, linear, march, simple, slipped, epiphyseal, or spiral.
Injury, blood vessel	Described as arterial hematoma, avulsion, laceration, rupture, traumatic aneurysm, or traumatic fistula.
Injury, internal	Includes all injuries to internal organs such as the heart, lung, liver, kidney, and pelvic organs. Types of injuries to internal organs include laceration, tear, traumatic rupture, penetrating wound, blunt trauma, crushing, blast injury, or open wound to internal organs with or without fracture in the same region.
Injury, intracranial	Includes concussion, cerebral laceration and contusion, or intracranial hemorrhage. These injuries may be open or closed. Intracranial injuries with skull fractures may be found under fracture.
Injury, superficial	Includes abrasion, insect bite (nonvenomous), blister, or scratch.
Sprain or strain	Injury to the joint capsule, ligament, muscle, or tendon described by the following terms: avulsion, hemarthrosis, laceration (closed), rupture, or tear. Open laceration of these structures should be coded as open wounds.
Wound, open	Includes open wounds not involving internal organs. Wounds may be to skin, muscle, or tendon, described as animal bite, avulsion, cut, laceration, puncture wound, or traumatic amputation. Open wounds may be complicated or uncomplicated. Complicated includes injuries with mention of delayed healing, delayed treatment, foreign body, or major infection.

The most difficult part of assigning injury codes is to know what main terms to look for in the Alphabetic Index. Codes S00-T88 include fractures, dislocations, sprains, and other types of injury. Injuries are coded according to the general type of injury and broken down within each type by anatomic site. A list of common injury medical terms and the types of injuries included for each is shown in Table 12.5.

EXAMPLE 12.37 Current Injury

S82.92XA	**Current injury:** Fracture, left ankle; Initial encounter
	or
M12.572 and S82.92XS	**Late effect:** Traumatic arthritis, due to old fracture, left ankle

EXAMPLE 12.38 Late Effects

A Unilateral posttraumatic osteoarthritis (M17.31), **due to crushing injury of right knee (S87.01XS)**
B Osteoporosis (M81.8), **due to late effect of calcium deficiency (E64.8)**
C Anemia of the puerperium (O90.81), **sequela of pregnancy, childbirth and the puerperium (O94)**

Use the following guidelines for coding injuries:

1. Decide whether a diagnosis represents a current injury or a late effect of an injury (Example 12.37).
2. Fractures are coded as "closed" if there is no indication of whether the fracture is open or closed.
3. The word *with* indicates involvement of both sites and the word *and* indicates involvement of either one or two sites when multiple injury sites are given.

As discussed, a sequela describes the residual effect or condition produced after the acute phase of an illness or injury has terminated. An injury may have a residual effect, which must be coded in a different fashion. An effect is considered to be a sequela if the diagnosis includes any of the following terms or descriptions:

- "due to an old injury"
- "late"
- "due to"
- "following (previous illness or injury)"
- "due to" an injury or illness that occurred 1 year or more before the current admission of encounter

Residual effects can be found under the main term "sequelae." The condition or nature of the residual effect is sequenced first and the sequela is listed second (Example 12.38).

Use the following guidelines for coding a sequela:

1. Refer to the main term "sequelae—*see also* condition" in ICD-10-CM's Alphabetic Index when coding a case with a sequela.
2. Look for the condition.
3. The Tabular Index will provide instructional notes that may indicate that two codes must be reported; code first the condition resulting from the sequela.

Burns and Corrosions

Burn codes are used for reporting thermal burns, except sunburns, that come from a heat source, such as a fire or hot appliance, or those that result from electricity or radiation. Corrosions are defined as burns caused by chemicals.

Burns are classified by depth, extent, and agent. When multiple burns are reported, a separate code for each burn site is reported. The degrees of a burn are defined as follows:

- First degree: erythema
- Second degree: blistering
- Third degree: full thickness involvement

It is important to note that burns of the eye and internal organs are coded by site, not depth. The code that reflects the highest degree of burn should be sequenced first using a code from the range T20 to T25.

An additional code from category T31 or T32 should be reported to identify the total body surface area (TBSA) for all sites. Think of the body as a whole and not the body parts as a whole. The adult body is divided into regions: head, 9%; arms, 9% each; trunk, 18% front and 18% back; legs, 18% each; and perineum, 1% (Fig. 12.9). Children's and infants' bodies have different regional percentages.

Adverse Effects, Poisoning, Underdosing, and Toxic Effects

Adverse effects, poisoning, underdosing, and toxic effects are reported using combination codes from the range T36 to T65. No additional external cause code is required.

The Table of Drugs and Chemicals is found after the Alphabetical Index, Section 2, and contains a classification of drugs and other chemical substances for identifying poisoning states and external causes of adverse effects.

Adverse effect is defined as an adverse or pathologic reaction to a drug that occurs when appropriate doses are given to humans for **prophylaxis** or prevention of disease, diagnosis, and therapy (Example 12.39). When an adverse effect occurs, such as a drug reaction, hypersensitivity, drug intolerance, or idiosyncratic reaction, a code is assigned to the diagnosis that classifies the specific reaction or symptom. For example, dermatitis, syncope, tachycardia, or urticaria can all be adverse effects. The specific reaction or symptom from use of the drug is reported as the primary code, followed by a code from the table for the correct code assignment for the adverse effect of the drug (T36–T50). The code for the drug should have a fifth or sixth character.

Poisoning is defined as a condition resulting from an intentional overdose of drugs or chemical substances or from the drug or agent given or taken in error. The following situations occur and are documented in the health record to indicate poisoning:

- Taking the wrong medication
- Receiving the wrong medication
- Taking the wrong dose of the right medication
- Receiving the wrong dose of the right medication
- Ingesting a chemical substance not intended for human consumption
- Overdose of a chemical substance (drug)
- Prescription drug taken with alcohol
- Mixing prescription drugs and over-the-counter medications without the physician's advice or consent

Each of the substances listed in Table 12.6 is assigned a code according to the poisoning classification (categories T36–T50). These adverse effect codes are used when there is a state of poisoning, overdose, wrong substance given or taken, or **intoxication.** Intoxication is defined as an adverse effect rather than a poisoning when drugs such as digitalis and steroid agents are involved. However, whenever the term *intoxication* is used, the billing/coding specialist should clarify with the service provider the circumstances surrounding the administration of the drug

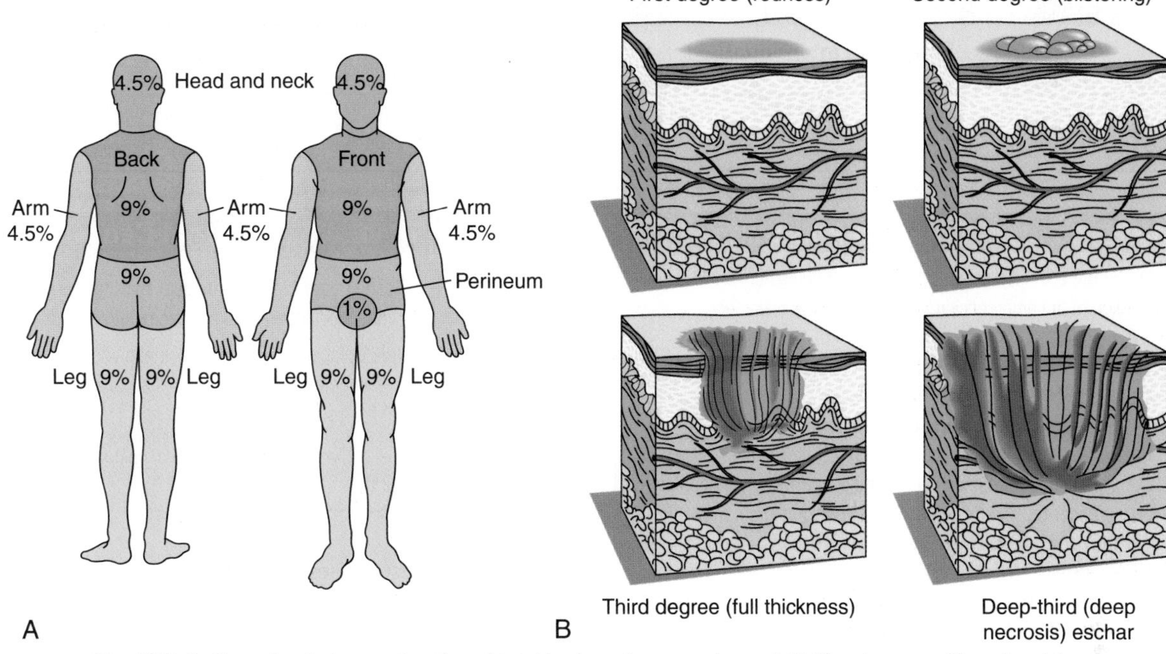

Fig. 12.9 A, The rule of nines estimation of total body surface area burned. **B,** The degrees of burn involving the layers of the skin: first-degree burns include the epidermis (redness), second-degree burns include the epidermis and dermis (blistering), third-degree burns include the first two layers and the subcutaneous tissues (full thickness), and deep-third burns involve all layers of the skin with resulting eschar (deep necrosis).

EXAMPLE 12.39 **Coding an Adverse Effect**

An inpatient had an adverse effect (ventricular fibrillation) to the medication digoxin, which was prescribed by her physician and taken correctly.

Step 1	Refer to the Table of Drugs and Chemicals in the Alphabetic Index and look up **digoxin.**
Step 2	Because this medication was for therapeutic use, locate the correct code number under the adverse effect column.
Step 3	The correct number is **T46.0X5.**
Step 4	Verify the code number T46.0X5 in the Tabular List. Note that a seventh character is required to indicate initial encounter **T46.0X5A.**
Step 5	Locate the main term **fibrillation** in the Alphabetic Index to Diseases and Injuries.
Step 6	Find the subterm **ventricular.**
Step 7	The correct code number is **I49.01.**
Step 8	Verify the code number I49.01 in the Tabular List.
Sequencing	**I49.01 Ventricular fibrillation (chief complaint)** **T46.0X5A Therapeutic use, Digoxin**

or chemical before assigning the appropriate code. This must be documented in the health record. If a diagnosis is stated as possible or suspected suicide attempt, go to the column titled "Undetermined" and not to "Suicide Attempt."

Example 12.40 shows the steps for coding a case that involves poisoning.

External Causes of Morbidity

External causes of morbidity codes are a classification of codes that describe external causes of injury rather than disease. The code description refers to the circumstances that caused an injury rather than the nature of the injury. The codes are also used in coding adverse reactions to medications (Fig. 12.10).

External cause codes are listed in a separate section of the Tabular List and are included in the code range V01-Y99. The external cause codes are also in a separate section, Index to External Causes of Injury and Poisoning, which follows the regular Alphabetic Index. To look up external cause codes, use Section III in the Alphabetic Index.

Use of an external cause code after the primary or other acute secondary diagnosis explains the mechanism for the injury. For example, if a patient falls and fractures a finger, the fracture code is primary and an external cause code after it helps explain how the accident or injury occurred (Example 12.41). This can help to speed the reimbursement process because a payer will see an acute injury code and know that a third party is responsible for payment, as in a workers' compensation injury or motor vehicle accident. External cause codes also play a role in gathering data, such as in statistical reporting, credentialing, utilization, review, and state injury prevention programs.

On the negative side, however, many payers require that chart notes accompany external cause code claims, which means generating a paper claim rather than sending it electronically. External cause codes often trigger a questionnaire that is sent to the beneficiary. This may lead to a delay in reimbursement.

Although external cause codes do not generate revenue, it is recommended that they be reported in addition to the appropriate procedural and diagnostic codes. This ensures that the most specific information possible is provided regarding the patient's injury. External cause codes are billed by the initial entity seeing the patient. If the patient visits the physician's office after hospitalization for injuries sustained in a motor vehicle accident, the hospital assigns an

TABLE 12.6 Table of Drugs and Chemicals

Substance	Poisoning, Accidental	Poisoning, Intentional Self-Harm	Poisoning, Assault	Poisoning, Undetermined	Adverse Effect	Underdosing
Acetylsalicylic acid (salts)	T39.011	T39.012	T39.013	T39.014	T39.015	T39.016

EXAMPLE 12.40 Coding a Poisoning

Baby Kathy got into the kitchen cabinet and ingested liquid household ammonia. She was taken to the emergency room for immediate treatment.

Step 1	Refer to the Table of Drugs and Chemicals in the Alphabetic Index and look up **ammonia.**
Step 2	Find the subterm **liquid (household).**
Step 3	Because this is a case of ingesting a chemical substance not intended for human use, locate the correct code number under the **Accidental Poisoning** column.
Step 4	The correct number is **T54.3X1.**
Step 5	Verify the code number T54.3X1 in the Tabular List. Note that a seventh character is required to indicate initial encounter **T54.3X1A.**
Sequencing	Codes in categories T36–T65 are combination codes that include the substances related to the poisoning as well as the external cause. No additional external cause code is required for poisoning. The code from categories T36 to T65 are sequenced first, followed by any codes that specify any outcomes of the poisoning (for example, nausea and vomiting).

INDEX TO EXTERNAL CAUSES

Fall, falling (accidental) W19
  building W20.1
    burning (uncontrolled fire) X00.3
  down
    embankment W17.81
    escalator W10.0
    hill W17.81
    ladder W11
    ramp W10.2
    stairs, steps W10.9
  due to
    bumping against
      object W18.00
        sharp glass W18.02
        specified NEC W18.09
        sports equipment W18.01
      person W03
        due to ice or snow W00.0
        on pedestrian conveyance — *see* Accident, transport, pedestrian, conveyance
    collision with another person W03
      due to ice or snow W00.0
      involving pedestrian conveyance — *see* Accident, transport, pedestrian, conveyance

Fig. 12.10 External cause coding.

external cause code and there is no requirement for repeating it for the office visit. An external cause code may never be sequenced as the primary diagnosis in the first position. When using external cause codes, be sure to list them last on the claim form.

EXAMPLE 12.41 External Cause Codes

26720	Closed treatment of phalangeal shaft fracture, proximal phalanx, finger; without manipulation, each
S62.649A	Nondisplaced fracture of proximal phalanx of finger, Initial encounter
W10.1XXA	Fall from sidewalk curb

Note: Code 26720 is a *Current Procedural Terminology* (**CPT**) code; CPT is discussed in Chapter 13.

External cause codes must be reported with appropriate seventh character (initial encounter, subsequent encounter, or sequela) for each encounter for which the injury or condition is being treated. As many external cause codes as are necessary to fully explain each cause should be reported.

Codes from category Y92, place of occurrence, should be reported to identify the location of the patient at the time of injury or other condition. The place of occurrence code is reported only at the initial encounter for treatment. It should not be reported if not stated in the provider's documentation.

Factors Influencing Health Status and Contact With Health Services

Factors influencing health status and contact with health services are reported with the code range Z00-Z99 and are referred to as **Z codes.** All guidelines for reporting Z codes can be found in Section 1, Subsection C of Chapter 21 of the Chapter-Specific Coding Guidelines.

Z codes are included in the major section of the Alphabetic Index to Diseases and Injuries. They are used for the following four primary circumstances:

1. When a person who is not currently sick encounters health services for some specific purpose, such as to act as a donor of an organ or tissue, receive a vaccination, discuss a problem that is not in itself a disease or injury, seek consultation about family planning, request sterilization, or obtain supervision of a normal pregnancy (Example 12.42).
2. When a person with a resolving disease or injury, such as a chronic, long-term condition that needs continuous care, seeks aftercare (Example 12.43).
3. When a circumstance influences an individual's health status but the illness is not current (Example 12.44).
4. When it is necessary to indicate the birth status of a newborn (Example 12.45).

These types of encounters are among the more common services for hospital outpatients and patients of private practitioners, health clinics, and others. Certain Z codes may appear only as a primary code and others only as secondary codes.

EXAMPLE 12.42 Supervision of First Pregnancy, Normal, First Trimester

Step 1 Find the heading **Pregnancy** in the Alphabetic Index.

Step 2 Look for the subheading **supervision.**

Step 3 Look for the second subheading **normal** and a further subheading **first,** which indicates the code Z34.0-.

Step 4 Find **Z34.0-** in the Tabular List. By Tabular List, it indicates **"Encounter for Supervision of Normal First Pregnancy."**

Step 5 Find **Z34.01** in the Tabular List, which indicates **"Encounter for Supervision of Normal First Pregnancy, First Trimester."**

EXAMPLE 12.43 Aftercare

Z47.81 Encounter for orthopedic aftercare following surgical amputation
Instructional note: Use additional code to identify the limb amputated. (Z89.-)

EXAMPLE 12.44 Personal History

Z85.3 Personal history of malignant neoplasm of breast

EXAMPLE 12.45 Newborn Birth Status

Z38.00 Single liveborn infant, delivered vaginally, born in hospital

EXAMPLE 12.46 Routine Annual Adult Physical Examination, Without Abnormal Findings

Step 1 Look up **examination,** and notice **annual (adult)** as a subterm and the code **Z00.00.**

Step 2 Find **Z00.00** in the Tabular List and the wording **"Encounter for general adult medical examination without abnormal findings."**

Some key words in patient care that indicate that a Z code might be necessary include the following:

- *Exposure*
- *Routine annual examination*
- *Admission*
- *History of*
- *Encounter*
- *Vaccination*

Z codes also are used when some circumstance or problem is present that influences the person's health status but is not in itself a current illness or injury, such as when the person is known to have an allergy to a specific drug. In this instance, the Z code cannot be used as a stand-alone code and should be used only as a supplementary code.

Additional code numbers are given for occupational health examinations and routine annual physical examinations; therefore select specific codes depending on the circumstances (Example 12.46).

Encounters for Reproductive Services

Z codes are used to report family planning, contraceptive or procreative management, and counseling. Codes from the category Z30 are used only when the encounter is for contraceptive management and must be specific to the type of contraceptive managed.

Z30.011	Encounter for initial prescription of contraceptive pills
Z30.012	Encounter for prescription of emergency contraception
Z30.013	Encounter for prescription of injectable contraceptive
Z30.014	Encounter for initial prescription of intrauterine contraceptive device
Z30.018	Encounter for initial prescription of other contraceptives
Z30.019	Encounter for initial prescription of unspecified contraceptive
Z30.02	Counseling and instruction in natural family planning to avoid pregnancy
Z30.09	Encounter for other general counseling and advice on contraception

Codes from the category Z30.4, encounter for surveillance of contraceptives, are available for reporting encounters for continued management. The codes from category Z30.4 are also specific to the type of contraceptive being used. When sterilization is performed for the major purpose of contraception rather than being an incidental result of the treatment of a disease, code Z30.2 is reported.

Diagnostic Coding and Reporting Guidelines for Outpatient Services

Section IV of the Official Guidelines contains a set of rules specific to reporting of outpatient services with which the billing/coding specialist should be familiar. The guidelines are approved for use for reporting hospital-based outpatient services and provider-based office visits. The guidelines are used in conjunction with the general and disease-specific guidelines.

Outpatient Surgery

When patients present for outpatient surgery, the first-listed diagnosis should be the reason for the surgery. If the postoperative diagnosis is different and is confirmed, select the more specific postoperative diagnosis code.

Uncertain Diagnosis

When reporting hospital-based outpatient services and provider-based office visits, if the provider has documented a condition as "probable," "suspected," "questionable," "rule out," or "working diagnosis," do not code as if the patient has the condition. An uncertain diagnosis, or a "rule out" diagnosis is often documented to keep an open mind about the possibility of that diagnosis. For example, a patient may have fallen and injured their wrist. The emergency room provider may request an x-ray examination to rule out a fracture. It has not been confirmed yet that the patient has a fracture; however, the provider is keeping

EXAMPLE 12.47 Code All Documented Conditions That Coexist

A patient is seen by her primary care physician (PCP) for management of chronic hypertension. The physician also performed a completed skin assessment, based on the patient's history of malignant melanoma in situ, which was previously excised in full.	Hypertension: I10 Personal history of malignant neoplasm, skin: Z85.820

EXAMPLE 12.48 Patients Receiving Diagnostic Services Only

Patient seen in the emergency room for pain in the left leg is sent to x-ray. The x-ray is read and is negative.	Report as: Left leg pain M79.605

an open mind about the possibility of that diagnosis. In cases such as this, code for the symptom, sign, or reason for the visit. In the example given, it would be best to report the diagnosis as "wrist injury" until a more definitive diagnosis has been documented. This guideline is different for health record coders in the inpatient hospital setting.

Chronic Disease

Chronic diseases that are treated on an ongoing basis may be reported as long as E/M of the condition are documented.

Code All Documented Conditions That Coexist

All conditions that coexist at the time of the visit that are evaluated and managed and affect patient care should be reported. If the condition was previously treated but no longer exists, it should be reported as a history code (Z80–Z87) if the condition has an impact on the current plan of care (Example 12.47).

Patients Receiving Diagnostic Services Only

Sequence first the diagnosis, condition, problem, or other reason for the visit for patients receiving diagnostic services. For routine laboratory or radiology testing in the absence of any signs or symptoms, assign Z01.89, encounter for other specified special examination (Example 12.48).

Preoperative Evaluations

Sometimes a patient receives a consultation for a preoperative medical evaluation as an inpatient or outpatient (Example 12.49) and the majority of the results are negative for chronic or current illness. A good-health diagnosis code will trigger a rejection by the third-party payer unless the insurance company allows or requires it. When reporting, sequence first a code from subcategory Z01.81-, encounter for preprocedural examination, to describe the preoperative consultation, followed by a code for the condition describing the reason for the surgery. Any additional findings related to the preoperative evaluation should also be reported.

EXAMPLE 12.49 Preoperative Examination

A patient to have surgery for gallstones is sent to a cardiologist for a preoperative examination to evaluate the patient's suspected cardiovascular disease.

Step 1 In the Alphabetic Index, look up **examination** and notice **preprocedural (preoperative)** and **cardiovascular** as subterms and the code **Z01.810.** Verify it in the Tabular List.

Step 2 Code the reason for the surgery—K80.20, cholelithiasis.

EXAMPLE 12.50 General Medical Examinations

Z00.00	Encounter for general adult medical examination without abnormal findings
Z00.01	Encounter for general adult medical examination with abnormal findings
Z00.121	Encounter for routine child health examination with abnormal findings
Z00.129	Encounter for routine child health examination without abnormal findings

General Medical Examinations With Abnormal Findings

General medical examinations are reported with the category of codes Z00.0-. Subcategories provide codes for examinations with and without abnormal findings. A general medical examination that results in an abnormal finding should be reported with the code for general medical examination with abnormal finding assigned as the first-listed diagnosis. A secondary code for the abnormal finding should also be reported (Example 12.50).

Handy Hints for Diagnostic Coding

If the ICD-10-CM code books are not color coded, identify important references with a colored highlighter pen. Also add tabs to main sections of the Alphabetic Index, Tabular List, and Drug and Chemical Table. Refer to the end of this chapter to learn how to locate and select diagnostic codes step by step.

Many times a cross-referenced code in the Alphabetic Index is the same when verified in the Tabular List. In some cases, indicating these codes in Volume 2 with a different-colored highlighter pen will remind a billing/coding specialist that this code is correct as described in the Alphabetic Index, which saves time. However, keep in mind that the Tabular List has many instructional notes that are not indicated in the Alphabetic Index and must be followed for accurate coding.

Keep a list of diagnostic codes commonly encountered by the office. Some insurance companies publish lists of diagnostic codes that support medical necessity and are acceptable for specific procedures. Consult payer guidelines by calling the insurance company or managed care plan to determine whether certain procedures are a covered benefit for certain diagnoses and, if not, have the patient sign a waiver. Reference books that show codes that link diagnostic and procedure codes are available. The American Medical Association (AMA) publishes a list of the most common diagnostic codes at the end of each of its mini–specialty code books.

In the past, some health care organizations have developed an encounter form that is an all-encompassing billing document and reference page and that acts as a shortcut to locating diagnostic codes for conditions commonly seen by a physician specialist. Although these may have served a good purpose under the previous ICD-9 coding system, it is no longer recommended that these types of billing documents be used. Most often these types of documents are found to lack the specificity necessary to infer diagnosis details needed for accurate coding. Continuing their use in ICD-10-CM will only prevent reporting of the increased detail now required.

Computer-Assisted Coding

Computer-assisted coding (CAC) is computer software that automatically generates a set of medical codes for review, validation, and use based on clinical documentation provided by health care practitioners. Many factors have pushed health care organizations to adopt CAC. Some of these factors are as follows:

- Shortage of coders throughout the United States
- Financial need to reduce the cost of filing insurance claims
- Increased complexity of coding systems with implementation of the ICD-10-CM coding system
- Adoption of EHRs
- Advancement in natural language processing (NLP) technology
- Frequent changes in code numbers and coding rules and regulations
- Compliance liability for increased erroneous claims

CAC uses two technology options: structured input and NLP. In structured input, the health care provider inputs information on a data entry screen that has point-and-click fields, pull-down menus, or structured templates. The system prompts the health care provider for detailed information. Words and phrases selected are linked to diagnostic and procedural codes that are automatically generated when all fields are completed. Input of the detailed information results in a completed document with the appropriate level of detail. Recommended diagnostic and procedural codes are then checked and edited by a coder.

The NLP system uses artificial medical intelligence. The health care provider dictates a report, handwrites a note, or inputs a picture file. The document is sent to an NLP engine that scans the health record, chooses important, relevant words, and converts them into suggested codes. A coder searches and validates the diagnostic and procedural codes and makes any changes, and then the codes are transmitted to billing. NLP systems must be updated regularly to address new medical terminology and conform to changes in coding guidelines.

Automated coding software uses a statistics-based method, rules-based method, or both methods to assign codes. In a statistics-based program, also called a *data-driven method,* the software predicts the code for a word or phrase based on statistics from the past. A rules-based or knowledge-driven method applies coding rules, such as those used in logic- or rules-based encoders, and imaged coding applications, to electronic clinical documents. The codes are processed through associated established rules for refinement and code assignment.

Another feature of CAC is the use of crosswalks or *data mapping,* which gives a coder the ability to input a discontinued code and find a new replacement code.

Sometimes professional coders disagree about which codes to apply to a specific case; thus checking and editing codes may be needed when using CAC. Usually, repetitive procedures are quick for coders to approve but complex procedures may need more time for validation. CAC technology helps coders to do their jobs faster and more efficiently and does not diminish the need for coders.

THE FUTURE OF DIAGNOSIS CODING

The ICD is constantly under revision to better reflect progress in health sciences and medical practices. Development of the next edition of ICD (ICD-11) for diagnosis coding began in April 2007 and included some very specific goals:

- To improve on the ability to function in an electronic environment
- To allow for collaborative web-based editing by interested parties while under peer review
- To incorporate international multilingual reference standards for scientific comparability

ICD-11 is alphanumeric, building on the structure of ICD-10, and will be similar in appearance. It will be a digital product that will link with terminologies (such as SNOMED CT) and support EHRs and information systems. SNOMED CT is a comprehensive health care database that incorporates terminology and clinical content with diagnostic standards in EHRs.

ICD-11 was scheduled for dissemination by 2012; however, the timeline was extended given the size of the task, the technical complexity of the system, and the limited funding and human resources for the project. The beta version of ICD-11 was produced in September 2013 and will undergo field trials and final review. According to the WHO, ICD-11 is expected to be unveiled to the world in 2018.

KEY POINTS

This is a brief chapter review of the key issues presented. To further enhance your knowledge of the technical subject matter, review the key terms and key abbreviations for this chapter by locating the meaning for each in the Glossary at the end of this text, which appears in a section before the Index.

1. Accurate diagnostic coding can mean the financial success or failure of a health care organization.
2. Payment for outpatient services is related to procedure codes but must be supported and justified by the diagnosis.
3. Diagnostic coding was developed for the following reasons: (a) tracking of disease processes, (b) classification of causes of mortality, (c) medical research, and (d) evaluation of hospital service use.

4. When submitting insurance claims for patients seen in a physician's office or an outpatient hospital setting, the primary diagnosis, which is the main reason for the encounter, is listed first.
5. For services provided after October 1, 2015, always use the *International Classification of Diseases, Tenth Revision, Clinical Modification* (ICD-10-CM) Alphabetic Index and then go to the Tabular (numerical) List before assigning a diagnostic code.
6. Always code to the highest degree of specificity. The more digits a code has, the more specific the description is.
7. Always code the underlying disease, the etiology, or the cause first; subsequently list the secondary diagnosis.
8. Z codes in ICD-10-CM are used when a person who is not currently sick encounters health services for some specific purpose, such as to receive a vaccination.
9. External cause codes in ICD-10-CM are used to report the causes of injury rather than the nature of the injury or disease and to code adverse reactions to medications. In ICD-10-CM, these codes begin with V, W, X, and Y.
10. Always follow coding conventions because they assist in the selection of correct codes for the diagnoses encountered. These conventions are rules or principles for determining a diagnostic code when using diagnostic code books, such as each space, typefaces, indentations, punctuation marks, symbols, instructional notes, abbreviations, cross-reference notes, and specific usage of the words *and, with,* and *due to.*

STUDENT ASSIGNMENTS

- Study Chapter 12.
- Answer the fill-in-the-blank, multiple-choice, and true/false review questions in the *Workbook* to reinforce theory learned in this chapter and to help prepare for a future test.
- Complete the assignments in the *Workbook* to gain hands-on experience in diagnostic coding.
- Turn to the Glossary at the end of this text for a further understanding of the key terms and key abbreviations used in this chapter.

13

Procedural Coding

Cheryl Fassett

OBJECTIVES

After reading this chapter, you should be able to:

1. Explain the purpose and importance of coding for professional services.
2. Define terminology used in *Current Procedural Terminology* (CPT).
3. Demonstrate an understanding of CPT code conventions.
4. Discuss the format and content of the HCPCS and CPT code books, including category I, II, and III codes.
5. Interpret the meaning of CPT code book symbols.
6. Identify and discuss the complexity of evaluation and management (E/M) services codes.
7. Explain the surgical global package.
8. Discuss the sections of the CPT book.
9. Explain correct usage of modifiers in procedure coding.
10. Explain various types of code edits.
11. Explain how to choose accurate procedure codes for descriptions of services and procedures documented in a patient's health record, including discussions on bundled codes, unbundling, downcoding, upcoding, and code monitoring.
12. Describe various methods of payment by insurance companies and state and federal programs.

KEY TERMS

bilateral
bundled codes
comprehensive code
conversion factor
Current Procedural Terminology
customary fee
downcoding
durable medical equipment
emergency department
fee schedule
global surgery policy
Healthcare Common Procedure Coding System
modifiers
mutually exclusive code edits
National Correct Coding Initiative
never event
physical status modifiers
procedure code numbers
professional component
qualifying circumstances
reasonable fee
relative value studies
relative value unit
resource-based relative value scale
surgical package
technical component
unbundling
upcoding
usual, customary, and reasonable

KEY ABBREVIATIONS

CF
CPT
DME
ECG
ED
E/M
EOB
FTC
GAF
GPCIs
HCPCS
NCCI
PC
PS
QC
RBRVS
RVS
RVU
TC
UCR

UNDERSTANDING THE IMPORTANCE OF PROCEDURAL CODING SKILLS

The health care provider documents his or her care in the patient's health record. Procedure coding is the translation of these written descriptions of procedures and professional services to numeric designations or code numbers. This translation may be done by the health care provider or a billing or coding specialist. Electronic health record (EHR) systems are often sold as a method to improve billing and coding. However, removing the human element from the coding process is not recommended. Certain features in EHR systems make it too easy for health care providers to use auto-fill and auto-prompt tools that can result in coding above the services provided (upcoding) and cloned records.

With the implementation of computer technology and stricter adherence to federal regulations, more emphasis is being placed on correct procedural coding. Coding must be correct if claims are to be paid promptly and optimally. Every procedure or service must be assigned correct and complete code numbers. Because of the complexity of procedural coding, a working knowledge of medical terminology, including anatomy and physiology, is essential.

Procedure codes are a standardized method used to precisely describe the services provided by physicians and allied health care professionals, such as chiropractors and nurse practitioners. They allow claim forms to be optically scanned by insurance companies. The general acceptance of the codes by third-party payers and government agencies assures the health care provider who uses a standardized coding system that the services and procedures they perform can be objectively identified and priced.

The Health Insurance Portability and Accountability Act of 1996 (HIPAA) requires the use of standardized code sets. The *Current Procedural Terminology* (CPT) and Healthcare Common Procedure Coding System are the standard code sets designated for coding for professional services, equipment, and supplies.

A CODING SPECIALIST'S TOOLS

CPT and HCPCS are updated annually, as is the *International Classification of Diseases, Tenth Revision* (ICD-10). Health care organizations should always strive to use the current manuals to ensure correct codes are used. Coding and billing specialists should obtain their own manuals whenever possible, so they may customize them. This can aid in code selection and make their jobs easier.

Some coding and billing specialists choose to break apart the manual into as many sections as needed on the basis of their specialty, three-hole punch it, and place it in a binder. Index tabs may be added to frequently used section. Coding edits, Medicare updates, and notes may also be placed in the binder. Color coding any codes that typically need modifiers or that should not be chosen without reviewing criteria will also help. Customizing the CPT book annually will familiarize a coding specialist with any changes and reduce coding errors.

HEALTHCARE COMMON PROCEDURE CODING SYSTEM

The **Healthcare Common Procedure Coding System (HCPCS)** (pronounced "hick-picks") was developed for the Medicare program by the Health Care Financing Administration, who later became CMS. The Medicare HCPCS consists of the following two levels of coding:

- Level I: The American Medical Association (AMA) CPT codes and modifiers. CPT is used to report professional services and procedures performed.
- Level II: The CMS-designated codes and alpha modifiers. Table 13.1 lists the Level II HCPCS national code content and code ranges with details of each alphanumeric code category.

TABLE 13.1 Level II HCPCS National Code Content

Code Category	Contents	Code Ranges
	New/revised/deleted codes and modifiers	
Index	Alphabetically arranged	
	Table of drugs	
	Level II national modifiers	
A codes	Transportation services, including ambulance (medical and surgical supplies, administrative, and miscellaneous and investigational services and supplies)	A0000-A9999
B codes	Enteral and parenteral therapy	B4000-B9999
C codes	Temporary codes for hospital outpatient Prospective Payment System	C1000-C9999
D codes		D0000-D9999
E codes	Durable medical equipment (canes, crutches, walkers, commodes, decubitus care, bath and toilet aids, hospital beds, oxygen and related respiratory equipment, monitoring equipment, pacemakers, patient lifts, safety equipment, restraints, traction equipment, fracture frames, wheelchairs, and artificial kidney machines)	E0100-E9999
G codes	Procedures and professional services (temporary) under review before inclusion in the CPT code book	G0000-G9999
H codes	Alcohol and drug abuse treatment services	H0001-H9999
J codes	Drugs administered other than oral method (chemotherapy drugs, immunosuppressive drugs, inhalation solutions, and miscellaneous drugs and solutions)	J0100-J9999
K codes	Temporary codes (durable medical equipment and drugs)[†]	K0000-K9999
L codes	Orthotic procedures and devices (prosthetic devices, scoliosis equipment, orthopedic shoes, and prosthetic implants)	L0100-L4999
P codes	Pathology and laboratory services	P0000-P9999
Q codes	Miscellaneous temporary codes	Q0000-Q9999
R codes	Diagnostic radiology services codes	R0000-R9999
S codes	Temporary national codes (non-Medicare; replaced many of Level III (local) codes, which have been phased out)	S0009-S9999
T codes	National T codes established for state Medicaid agencies and not valid for Medicare	T1000-T9999
V codes	Vision, hearing, and speech-language pathology services	V0000-V2999

*Dental procedures (diagnostic, preventive, restorative, endodontic, periodontic, prosthodontic, prosthetic, orthodontic, and surgical)
These codes have been removed from the official HCPCS list but remain available from and are maintained by the American Dental Association.
[†]When these codes are approved for permanent inclusion in HCPCS, they become A, E, or J codes.
Contents in HCPCS books will vary by edition. It is a good idea to compare editions to see which one is more user friendly. For example, the Professional Edition has appendices not included in the Standard Edition.
CPT, Current Procedural Terminology; HCPCS, Healthcare Common Procedure Coding System.

EXAMPLE 13.1 *Current Procedural Terminology* Procedure Code Numbers

A 45-year-old woman is seen for an initial office visit for evaluation of recurrent right shoulder pain. The patient's condition warranted a detailed history and physical examination (D HX & PX) with low complexity medical decision making (LCMDM). The patient complains of pain radiating down her right arm. A complete radiographic study of the right shoulder is obtained in the office and read by the physician. A corticosteroid solution is injected into the shoulder joint.

CPT Code	Description of Services
99203	Office visit, new patient (E/M service)
73030	Radiologic examination, shoulder, two views (Diagnostic service)
20610	Arthrocentesis inj.; major joint, shoulder (Therapeutic service)

CPT, Current Procedural Terminology; E/M, evaluation and management.

Level I: *Current Procedural Terminology* Codes

The primary coding system used for professional services and procedures is *Current Procedural Terminology (CPT),* published and updated annually by the AMA. CPT uses a basic five-digit system for coding professional services and two-digit add-on **modifiers** to indicate circumstances in which a procedure as performed differs in some way from that described in the code. **Procedure code numbers** represent diagnostic and therapeutic services on medical billing statements and insurance forms (Example 13.1).

The first edition of CPT appeared in 1966. It is now updated and revised annually on October 1. Code numbers are added or deleted as new procedures are developed or existing procedures are modified. These changes are shown in each edition by the use of symbols, which are described and shown later in this chapter (Fig. 13.1). The symbols with their meanings are located at the bottom of each page of code numbers in the CPT code book.

! COMPLIANCE ALERT
Coding Compliance Plan

Because the government is more involved in health care, each health care organization should construct and maintain a policy and procedure manual regarding coding guidelines so that it is in compliance with Health Insurance Portability and Accountability Act (HIPAA). Establishing coding and billing policies and procedures helps health care organization and their staff to address potential risk areas for fraud and abuse. A plan should include the health care organization's basic ethical philosophy, outline policies, detail coding procedures, and create an environment of confidentiality. Billing and coding specialists should sign a statement annually indicating that they have read, understood, and agreed with the health care organization's standards of conduct. The plan should provide coders with the framework for correct coding and indicate that health record documentation must support the codes billed. An internal audit should be done on a regular basis, and action should be taken to correct the offense if noncompliance is discovered. Such plans must have a compliance officer or a committee that oversees the audits, monitors compliance issues, and trains employees in compliance issues.

CPT content will be discussed in further detail in this chapter. Procedure 13.1 at the end of this chapter gives step-by-step directions on how to use a CPT code book for billing purposes.

Level II: HCPCS Codes

HCPCS Level II codes include those for the following:

- Ambulance
- Medical and surgical supplies
- Enteral and parenteral therapy
- Outpatient Prospective Payment System (PPS)
- Dental procedures
- Durable medical equipment
- Procedures/professional services
- Alcohol and drug abuse treatment services
- Drugs administered other than oral method
- Orthotic procedures
- Prosthetic procedures
- Other medical services
- Pathology and laboratory services
- Casting and splinting supplies
- Diagnostic radiology services
- Temporary non-Medicare codes
- T codes for state Medicaid agencies
- Vision and hearing services.

The CPT code should be used when both a CPT and Level II code have the same description. The Level II code should be used if the descriptions are not identical. For example, if the CPT code narrative is generic and the HCPCS Level II code is specific, code from the HCPCS Level II.

Several companies annually publish Level II HCPCS code books. Content, numbers of the appendices, color-coded coverage instructions, notes, and unlisted procedures vary between the editions. Notes or special instructions may appear in or following subsections or headings or as part of the description in a heading or code.

! COMPLIANCE ALERT
Durable Medical Equipment

Durable medical equipment (DME) is any equipment that provides therapeutic benefits to a patient in need because of certain medical conditions and/or illnesses. Medicare covers medically necessary DME if prescribed and meets the following criteria:

- Can withstand repeated use (durable)
- Used for a medical reason
- Not usually useful to someone who isn't sick or injured
- Used in the patient's home
- Has an expected lifetime of at least 3 years

The HCPCS is updated each January 1, with periodic updates made throughout the year as needed. In some states, the TRICARE and Medicaid programs accept HCPCS codes. Most commercial insurance companies have adopted the Level I (CPT) and Level II (HCPCS) code systems.

Procedure 13.2 at the end of this chapter gives step-by-step directions on how to use a HCPCS code book for billing purposes.

! COMPLIANCE ALERT
HIPAA Diagnostic and Procedural Code Guidelines

Under HIPAA, providers and medical facilities are responsible for using ICD-10-CM diagnostic codes to document why patients are seen and CPT-4 and HCPCS codes for what is done to patients during their encounter. They are also responsible for implementing the updated codes in a timely manner, using the HIPAA-mandated transaction code set codes, and deleting old or obsolete codes.

CPT, Current Procedural Terminology; HCPCS, Healthcare Common Procedure Coding System; *HIPAA, Health Insurance Portability and Accountability Act; ICD-10-CM, International Classification of Diseases, Tenth Revision, Clinical Modification.*

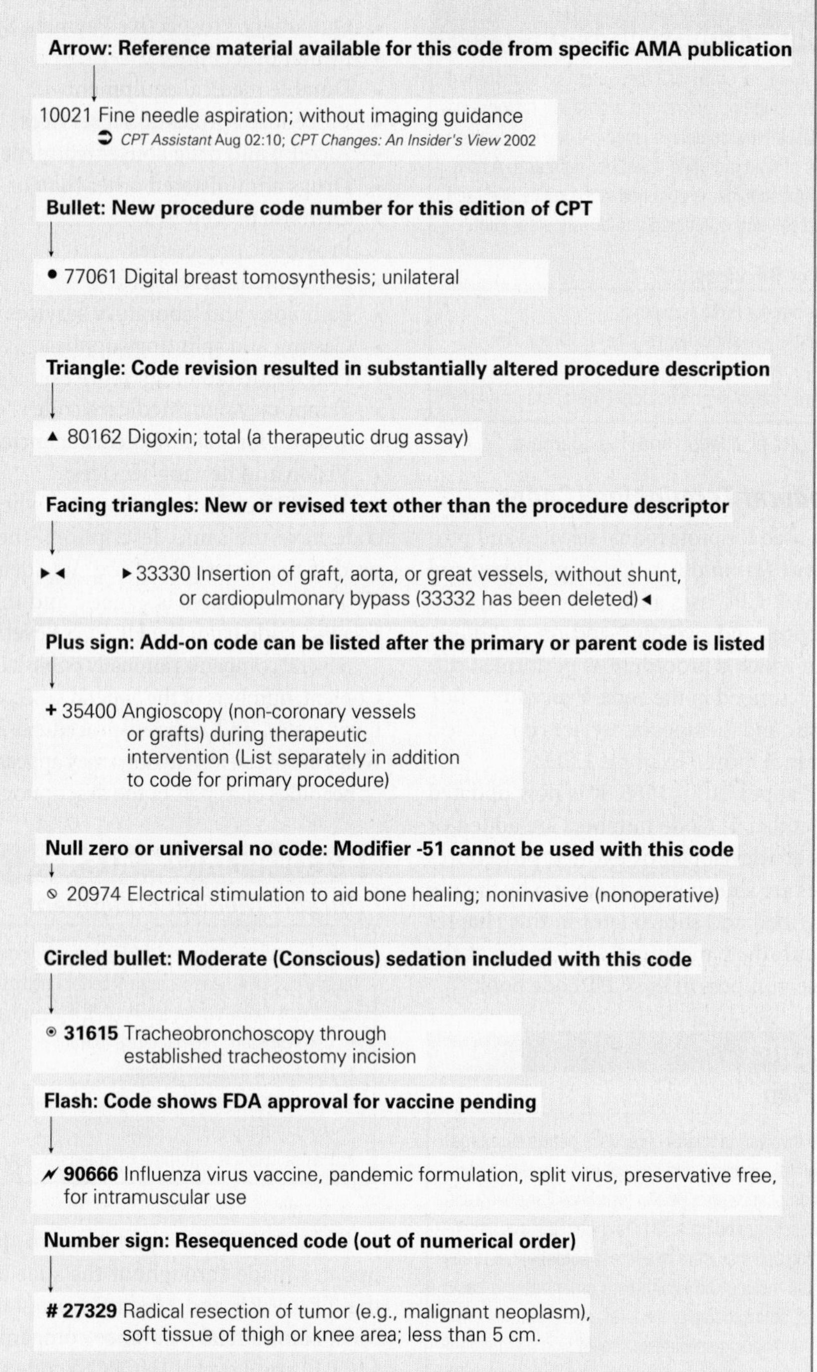

Fig. 13.1 Symbols that appear in the 2018 *Current Procedural Terminology (CPT)* code book and a brief explanation of what they tell the coder. These symbols and their meanings appear at the bottom of each page of codes in the CPT code book. *AMA,* American Medical Association; *FDA,* Food and Drug Administration.

PROCEDURE 13.1 Choose Correct Procedural Codes for Professional Services

Objective

Accurately locate and select procedural codes for professional services

Equipment/Supplies

Current Procedural Terminology (CPT) code book, medical dictionary, and pen or pencil

Directions

Follow these step-by-step procedures, which include rationales, to practice this job skill. Fig. 13.12 will explain how to search and choose correct CPT codes for a procedure, eponym, and acronym.

1. Read the patient's health record and identify the main term by asking what is wrong with the patient.
2. Always read the Introduction section at the beginning of the code book, which may change annually with each edition.
3. Use the Index at the back of the book to locate a specific item by generalized code numbers, not by page numbers. Never code from the Index. Listings may be looked up according to names of procedures or services, organs, conditions, synonyms, eponyms, and abbreviations; for example, some primary entries might be as follows:
   - Procedure or service (for example, anastomosis, endoscopy, splint)
   - Organ or other anatomic site (for example, salivary gland, tibia, colon)
   - Condition (for example, abscess, entropion, tetralogy of Fallot)
   - Synonyms, eponyms, and abbreviations (for example, electroencephalogram [EEG], Bricker operation, Clagett procedure)

   If the procedure performed is not listed, check for the organ involved. If the procedure or organ is difficult to find, look up the condition. Key words, such as synonyms or eponyms, and abbreviations, will help to find the appropriate code.
4. Locate the code number in the code section for the code range given in the Index.
5. Turn to the beginning of the section for the code range given in the Index and read the Guidelines at the beginning of the section. This gives general information and instructions on coding certain procedures within the section, defines commonly used terms, explains classifications within the section, and gives instructions specific to the section.
6. Turn to the correct section, subsection, category, or subcategory and read through the narrative description to locate the most appropriate code to apply to the patient's procedure. Some code books have color-coded titles, making this determination easier. In the surgery section, each subsection is further divided into categories based on anatomic site. Within each category are subcategories listed by type of procedure (for example, excision, repair, destruction, graft) or condition (burn, fracture). Read the notes and special subsection information throughout the section.
7. Notice punctuation and indenting. Descriptions for standalone codes begin at the left margin and have a full description. No matter how many indented codes are listed, always go back to the standalone code to begin reading the description. A semicolon (;) separates common portions from subordinate designations; subterms are indented (Fig. 13.13). Any terminology after the semicolon has a dependent status, as do the subsequent indented entries. In Fig. 13.13, the procedure code number 11044 should read as follows: Debridement; skin, subcutaneous tissue, muscle, and bone. Fig. 13.14 shows an insurance claim for a patient who has had six corns pared.
8. When trying to locate an evaluation and management (E/M) code, identify the place or type of service rendered. Then identify whether the patient is new or established and locate the category or subcategory. Review any guidelines or instructions pertaining to the category or subcategory. Read the descriptors of the levels of E/M service. Identify the requirements necessary for code assignment. Ensure that the components necessary were performed by the physician and documented in the chart for the assigned E/M code. Commercial templates are available to aid in E/M code selection and help tremendously when verifying a code that has been selected by the physician.
9. For a code that has been assigned, note the following:
   - Parentheses, ( ), further define the code and tell where other services are located (Fig. 13.15).
   - Measurements throughout the code book are based on the metric system (Fig. 13.16).
   - All anesthesia services are reported by use of the five-digit anesthesia code plus a physical status modifier. Physical status modifiers describe the overall health of the patient by referencing patients who are healthy or those who have mild or severe systemic diseases. Example: Patient is a healthy 23-year-old Caucasian woman. Anesthesia is given for a vaginal delivery. The procedure code with modifier is 01960-P1. The P-1 identifies the patients as "a normal healthy patient."
   - The Surgery section is the largest segment of the code book. It has many subsections and subheadings. Learn to break down a procedure and identify various terms that will aid in choosing the correct code. Blocks 24A through 24J of the revised CMS-1500 insurance claim form show placement of the code on Line 2 (Example 13.29).
10. Determine whether one or more modifiers are necessary to give a more accurate description of the services rendered or the circumstances in which they were performed.
11. Enter the five-digit code number and modifier to the proper field on the insurance claim form exactly as given for each procedure or service rendered. Be careful not to transpose code numbers.

PROCEDURE 13.2 Locate Correct Level II HCPCS Codes for Professional Services

Objective

Accurately locate and select Level II Healthcare Common Procedural Coding System (HCPCS) codes for professional services

Equipment/Supplies

HCPCS code book, medical dictionary, and pen or pencil

Directions

Follow these step-by-step procedures, which include rationales, to practice this job skill.

1. Read the patient's health record for items or services that might be covered under Level II HCPCS codes.
2. Go to the Index that is arranged alphabetically and locate the name of the supply, drug, or service. This will point to the proper code. Never code from the Index.
3. Turn to the code number in the section and verify that it is the proper code for the item or service the provider supplied to the patient.
4. Select the code.
5. Determine whether a modifier is necessary to give a more accurate description of the service or item.
6. Enter the code number and modifier (if needed) to the proper field on the insurance claim form exactly as given for each service or item. Be careful not to transpose code numbers.

CURRENT PROCEDURAL TERMINOLOGY CONTENT AND FORMAT

The AMA is responsible for creating and maintaining the official CPT code set. The CPT content is outlined in Table 13.2, with three categories of codes.

Category I Codes

Category I contains five-digit code numbers with no decimal. It is divided into categories and subcategories according to anatomic body systems, procedure, condition, description, and specialty. Fig. 13.2, *A*, illustrates the format of the Index, and Fig. 13.2, *B*, illustrates the format of the CPT section.

Example of Category I codes:

10060	Incision and drainage of abscess
42825	Tonsillectomy, younger than age 12

Category II: Performance Measurement Codes

Category II codes describe clinical components that typically may be included in evaluation and management (E/M) services or clinical services and do not have a relative value associated with them. They also describe results from clinical laboratory or radiology tests and other procedures, identified processes intended to address patient safety practices, or services reflecting compliance with state or federal laws. These codes are used for optional performance tracking.

Category II also have an alphanumeric identifier with a letter in the last field (for example, 0502F, Subsequent prenatal care visit) to distinguish them from category I codes. Four modifiers in this section are used to indicate that a service specified by a performance measure was considered but because of either medical or patient circumstance(s) documented in the health record, or as a result of system issues, the service was not provided. The modifiers are 1P, 2P, 3P, and 8P. Use of these codes is optional for correct coding.

Examples of category II codes:

0500F	Initial prenatal care visit
0502F	Subsequent prenatal care visit

Category III: New and Emerging Technology Codes

Category III codes are a temporary set of tracking codes used to code emerging technologies that do not yet have any procedure code assignment in category I. They are intended to expedite data collection and assessment of new services and procedures to substantiate widespread use and clinical effectiveness. A category III code may become a category I code. When it is deleted from category III and adopted as a category I code, the CPT code book provides clear indication of this change by inserting a cross reference in place of the former category III code; for example, ▸(0024T has been deleted. To report use 93799)◂. The AMA website posts updates to this category in January and July of every year.

TABLE 13.2 *Current Procedural Terminology* Book Content Outline

Category I Codes	(99201–99607)
Evaluation and Management (E/M)	99201 to 99499
Anesthesia	00100 to 01999
Surgery	10021 to 69990
Radiology, Nuclear Medicine and Diagnostic Ultrasound	70010 to 79999
Pathology and Laboratory	80047 to 89398
Medicine	90281 to 99607
Category II Codes	0001F to 7025F
Category III Codes	0019T to 0290T
Appendices	
A—Modifiers	
B—Summary of Additions, Deletions, and Revisions	
C—Clinical Examples	
D—Summary of CPT Add-On Codes	
E—Summary of CPT Codes Exempt From Modifier 51	
F—Summary of CPT Codes Exempt From Modifier 63	
G—Summary of CPT Codes That Include Moderate (Conscious) Sedation	
H—Alphabetical Clinical Topics Listing	
I—Genetic Testing Code Modifiers	
J—Electrodiagnostic Medicine Listing of Sensory, Motor, and Mixed Nerves	
K—Product Pending FDA Approval	
L—Vascular Families	
M—Renumbered CPT Codes—Citations Cross-Walk	
N—Summary of Resequenced CPT Codes	
O—Multianalyte Assays With Algorithmic Analyses	
Index	

CPT, Current Procedural Terminology; FDA, Food and Drug Administration.

Examples of category III codes:

0329T	Monitoring of intraocular pressure for 24 hours or longer, unilateral or bilateral, with interpretation and report
0331T	Myocardial sympathetic innervation imaging, planar qualitative and quantitative assessment.

Code Book Symbols

CPT is published each year with deletions, new codes and description changes. Coding and billing specialists should become familiar with the new codes and any description changes or deleted codes related to codes that may exist on the health care organization's fee schedule. Fig. 13.1 shows how to identify new codes and description changes by following the symbols that are used. The symbols placed below many codes throughout the code book indicate that the AMA has published reference material on those particular codes. The reference citation is also provided. All these symbols are also located at the bottom of each page of codes in the CPT code book.

When using a new code, marked with a bullet (•), it may take as long as 6 months before a third-party payer has a mandatory value assignment; therefore reimbursements are received in varying amounts during that time. An exception is in the Medicare program, which has a value assignment published annually each fall in the *Federal Register.*

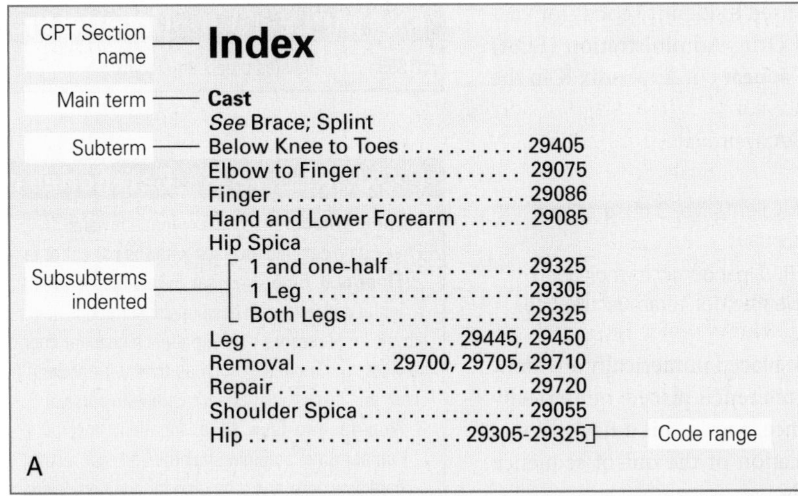

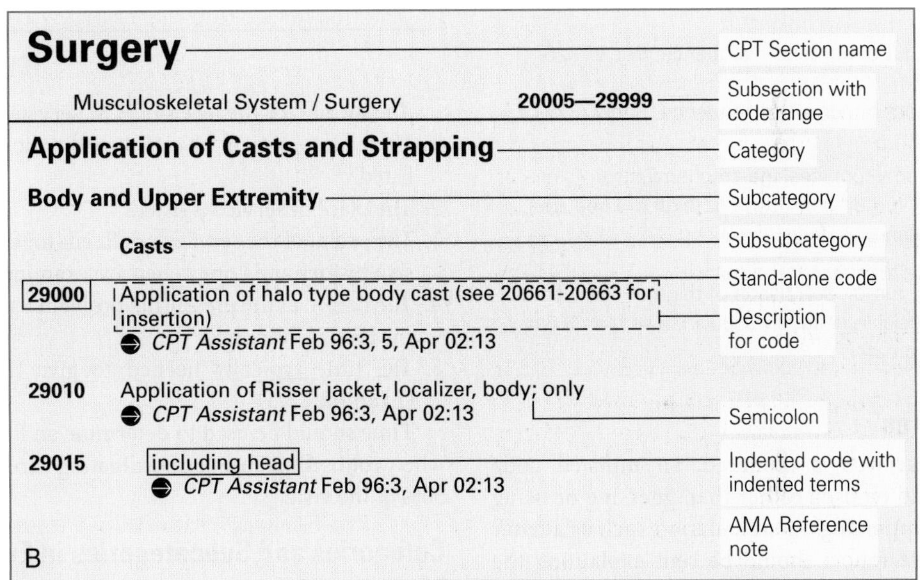

Fig. 13.2 A, *Current Procedural Terminology* (CPT) format illustrating conventions of the Index and a section. **B,** CPT format illustrating conventions of the Index and a section.

Revised codes or revised text, marked with a triangle (▲) or (▸◂), highlight what is new or deleted. This saves time in trying to figure out what was changed and prevents using these codes incorrectly. Appendix B in the CPT code book provides a summary of code additions, deletions, and revisions.

Add-on codes, shown with a plus sign (+), indicate that the code can *only* be listed after the primary or parent code has been listed. Add-on codes always reference the appropriate primary codes. Add-on codes are always exempt from using Modifier -51 to indicate an additional procedure.

Examples of add-on codes:

+49568 Implantation of mesh or other prosthesis for open incisional or ventral hernia repair or mesh for closure of debridement for necrotizing soft tissue infection (List separately in addition to code for the incisional or ventral hernia repair) (Use 49568 in conjunction with 11004-11006, 49560-49566)

+59525 Subtotal or total hysterectomy after cesarean delivery (List separately in addition to code for primary procedure)
(Use 59525 in conjunction with 59510, 59514, 59515, 59618, 59620, 59622)

Modifier -51 exempt codes, shown with a symbol Ø, means that the modifier cannot be used with this code. Codes with this symbol are not Add-on codes; they can be stand-alone procedures. They are typically exempt from multiple procedure reductions in payment. These codes are listed in Appendix E.

Examples of Modifier -51 exempt codes:

Ø 20974 Electrical stimulation to aid bone healing; noninvasive (nonoperative)
Ø 20975 invasive (operative)
Ø 31500 Intubation, endotracheal, emergency procedure

A lightning bolt symbol (Ø) is used to identify codes for vaccines that are pending Food and Drug Administration (FDA) approval. A complete list of these appears in Appendix K in the CPT code book.

Examples of codes pending FDA approval:

90587	Dengue vaccine, quadrivalent, live, 3 dose schedule, for subcutaneous use
90666	Influenza virus vaccine (IIV), pandemic formulation, split virus, preservative free, for intramuscular use

Resequenced codes that are not placed numerically are identified with the # symbol and a reference placed numerically ("Code is out of numerical sequence. See ...") is a navigational alert to direct the user to the location of the out-of-sequence code. A list appears in Appendix N.

Examples of codes that are out of sequence:

27337	Code is out of numerical sequence. See 27326-27331
27339	Code is out of numerical sequence. See 27326-27331
27326	Neurectomy, popliteal (gastrocnemius)
27327	Excision, tumor, soft tissue of thigh or knee area,
#27337	subcutaneous; less than 3 cm
27328	3 cm or greater
#27339	Excision, tumor, soft tissue of thigh or knew area; subfascial (e.g., intramuscular); less than 5 cm
	5 cm or greater

Unlisted Procedures

When an unusual service is rendered, an unlisted code (Example 13.2) should be used rather than guessing or using an incorrect code. Supporting documentation such as a letter and copy of operative report should be sent explaining the service.

Since the development of category III codes, it is important to double check that section of the CPT code book to verify whether a code exists before using an unlisted code. Unlisted codes generally end in -99 and are found at the end of each section or subsection. A comprehensive list of unlisted codes is found at the beginning of each section. Some Medicare Administrative Contractors (MACs) do not pay for any of the special -99 adjunct or unlisted codes.

Evaluation and Management Services (99201–99499)

The E/M section is divided into office visits, hospital visits, and consultations and other types of patient management services. Two subcategories of office visits exist: new patient and established patient. Hospital visits also have two boldfaced subcategories: initial and subsequent. Each subcategory has levels of E/M services identified by specific codes. This classification is based on the nature of the physician's work, such as type of service, place of service, and the patient's status. The documentation chapter introduced several terms and concepts pertinent to this section and explained how to level an E/M visit.

EXAMPLE 13.2 Unlisted Procedure Code

31599 Unlisted procedure, larynx

EXAMPLE 13.3 Categories of Time

1. **Face-to-face:** Office and outpatient visits
(Physician meets face-to-face with the patient or family.)
2. **Floor/unit time:** Hospital observation services, inpatient hospital care, initial and follow-up hospital consultations, and nursing facility services
(Physician is present on the patient's hospital floor or unit providing bedside services to the patient, such as time with patient, time working on patient's chart, and discussing patient's care with nurses.)
3. **Non–face-to-face time:** Inpatient hospital preencounter and postencounter time, obtaining records and test results, talking with other health care providers, and arranging for additional services
(Physician does work related to the patient before or after face-to-face time or floor/unit time.)

The format for the levels of E/M service is as follows:

1. Under new patient or established patient, a code number is listed.
2. The place of service is listed.
3. The extent of the service is defined (for example, comprehensive history and comprehensive examination).
4. The nature of the presenting problem usually associated with the level is described.
5. The time typically needed to give the service is stated (Example 13.3).

Time should be used to determine an E/M service level only when counseling and/or coordinating care takes up more than 50% of the visit.

Categories and Subcategories in Evaluation and Management

The E/M section of CPT has categories and subcategories that have from three to five levels for reporting purposes. These levels are based on key components, contributory factors, and face-to-face time with the patient or family. To begin the coding process, the provider of service must identify the category such as office, hospital inpatient, outpatient, or consultation, and then select the subcategory of new patient or established patient. The description should be read thoroughly to note the key components of history, examination, and medical decision making and the contributory factors such as counseling and coordination of care. Review the sample in Fig. 13.3 illustrating an E/M code for a new patient seen in the office or in an outpatient or ambulatory setting.

Because key components are clinical in nature, the physician must document these factors in the patient's record. In a case in which counseling and coordination of care make up more than 50% of the face-to-face physician–patient encounter, time is considered the key component to qualify for a particular level of E/M services.

Many physicians refer to the E/M codes as level 5 for the most complex to level 1 for the least complex. These levels coincide with the fifth or last digit of the CPT code (for example, 99205).

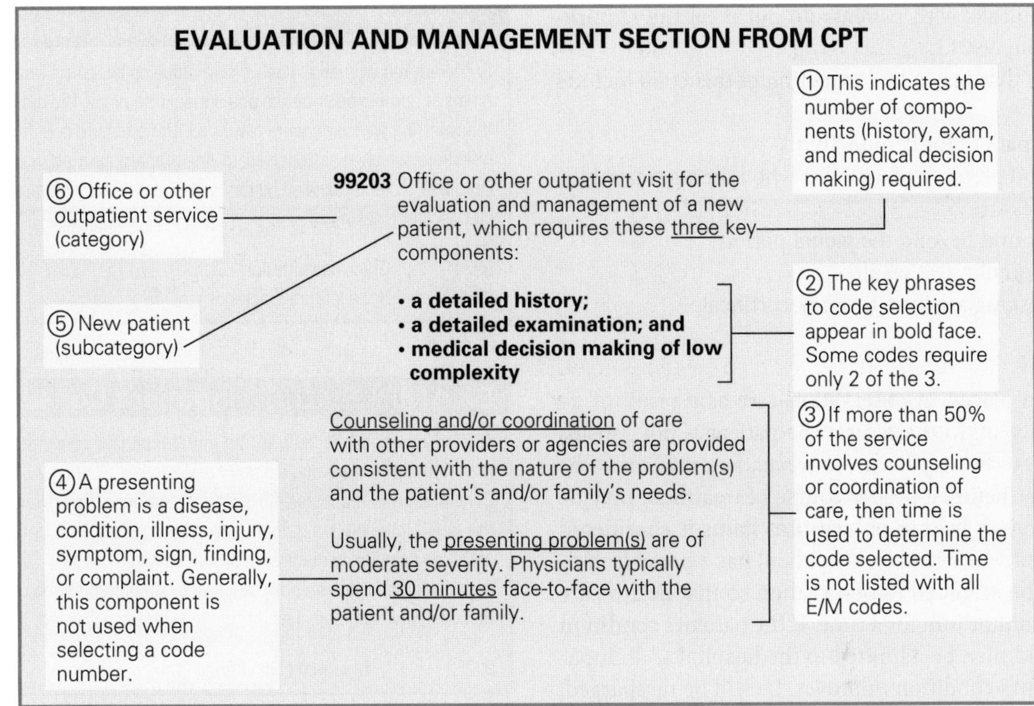

Fig. 13.3 Evaluation and management code 99203 defining the main words and phrases. This code is used for a new patient seen in the office or in an outpatient or ambulatory setting.

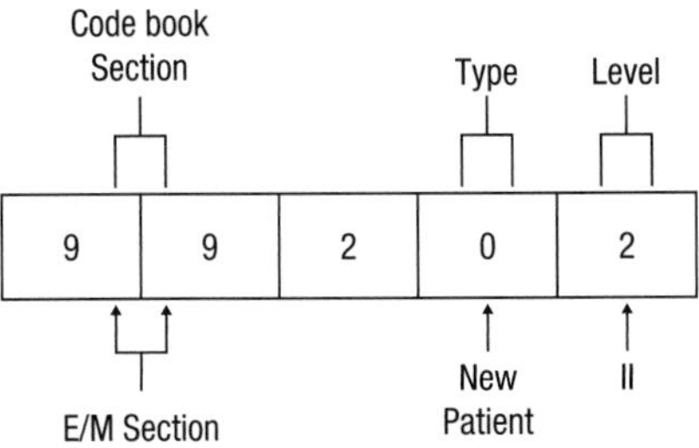

Fig. 13.4 *Current Procedural Terminology* code digit analysis.

TABLE 13.3 Levels With Code Numbers

	OFFICE VISITS		CONSULTATIONS	
	New	**Established**	**Office**	**Hospital**
Level 1	99201	99211	99241	99251
Level 2	99202	99212	99242	99252
Level 3	99203	99213	99243	99253
Level 4	99204	99214	99244	99254
Level 5	99205	99215	99245	99255

It is common to hear a physician say, "Ted Brown was seen for a level 5 today." This terminology may appear on encounter forms with five-digit CPT code numbers and be referred to as levels 1 through 5 (Fig. 13.4).

Alternatively, this terminology may be seen abbreviated as L-1, L-2, and so on, but this usage is not preferred because it can be confused with the nomenclature for the sections of the lumbar vertebrae. The level also may be written out as level one, level two, and so on, depending on the complexity of the case. A breakdown of the E/M levels with code numbers is shown in Table 13.3.

Office or Other Outpatient Services

For office or other outpatient services, there are seven elements when selecting an E/M code to bill. Providers consider them in the following order:

1. History
2. Examination
3. Medical decision making
4. Nature of presenting problem
5. Counseling
6. Coordination of care
7. Time

History, examination, and medical decision making are considered to be key components. A service must meet three out of three key components to qualify for a service level for a new patient; two out of three key components must be met for an established patient. Nature of presenting problem, counseling, coordination of care, and time are contributing factors.

Consider the decision tree discussed in Chapter 11, Documentation, when determining if a patient is new or established.

E/M code 99211 for established patients is often called a "nurse visit" and does not always require the presence of a physician. However, the patient must be established, and the physician must have initiated the service. To report a nurse visit, Medicare requires that the nurse must be following a plan of care that was established by the physician in a previous visit. Medicare also requires that patient encounter must be face-to-face and the physician must be on-site in the immediate suite of offices. Telephone calls with patients do not meet the requirements for reporting 99211.

Some services that may allow reporting of this code include the following:

- Rechecking a patient for conjunctivitis
- Checking blood pressure of a patient who is being treated for high blood pressure
- Checking a wound beyond the global period
- Reading a tuberculin test result
- Recheck for issuing a return-to-work certificate

Observation Care

Patients are often placed in observation care as a result of an emergency room visit. In these cases the patient is not considered well enough to be sent home; however, he or she must be monitored further before a proper course of treatment may be determined. A patient held in observation status is considered to be an outpatient. For example, if a patient has a possible concussion, he may be admitted to observation so that health care providers may monitor him for a time. If the patient's condition worsens, he would then be admitted to the hospital as an inpatient. If the patient's condition improves, he will be discharged. A patient may be placed in observation for up to 3 days before being admitted or discharged.

Codes reflect admission to observation, subsequent observation care, and discharge from observation. These codes do not distinguish between new and established patients. It is not necessary for the patient to be in a designated observation area of the hospital. An admission and a discharge may be reported on the same day. If a patient is admitted to the hospital from observation, the observation services are not coded.

Hospital Inpatient Services

The hospital inpatient service codes include subcategories for Initial Hospital Care, Subsequent Hospital Care, and Discharge Services. They do not differentiate between new and established patients. Similar to the outpatient codes, Initial Care codes require three of three key components and Subsequent Care requires two of three key components.

Only the admitting physician reports an Initial Hospital Care code. Any other provider seeing the patient should report initial inpatient consultation codes or subsequent care codes, as appropriate. If a patient is seen in the emergency department (ED) and is subsequently admitted to the hospital by the same physician on the same date of service as the ED visit, it is billed as initial hospital care. The physician includes the services related to the admission that he or she provided in the other hospital service departments as well as in the inpatient setting.

Discharge Services are time-based codes. These services include final examination, continuing care instructions, discharge paperwork, prescriptions, and referrals.

Consultations

As previously discussed in the documentation chapter, a consultation includes services rendered by a physician whose opinion or advice is requested by another physician or agency in the evaluation or treatment of a patient's illness or a suspected problem.

EXAMPLE 13.4 Outpatient Consultation

A 20-year-old woman is seen for an office consultation for cystitis. She complains of burning on urination and urinary frequency. The patient's records from the referring physician were reviewed. Urine culture confirmed a urinary tract infection, which was reported to her primary care physician for treatment. Obtained problem-focused history and examination with straightforward medical decision making.

99241 Office consultation
87086 Urine culture, bacterial

EXAMPLE 13.5 Inpatient Consultation

A 50-year-old man is seen for an initial inpatient consultation with a status post–left hip fracture and a history of well-controlled type 2 diabetes mellitus. Consultation is requested for surgical clearance. Reviewed medical data on the unit. Obtained a detailed history and performed a detailed examination with low complexity medical decision making (LCMDM). Discussed diagnosis and treatment options with patient and completed health record documentation. Will give ongoing consultation to referring physician.

99253 Inpatient consultation

A consulting physician must submit a written report containing his or her findings and opinions to the requesting physician. In contrast, a referral is the transfer of the total or specific care of a patient from one physician to another for known problems.

Effective January 1, 2010, the CMS no longer allows consultation codes (ranges 99241 through 99245 and 99251 through 99255) for inpatient and office or outpatient settings and for various places of service. An exception would be for telehealth consultation (HCPCS G-codes). CMS indicates that the initial hospital care codes 99221 through 99223 should be used when billing a consultation on a hospital inpatient. The attending physician must append with HCPCS Level II modifier AI (A-eye) *principal physician of record* to the code.

For non-Medicare cases, codes for consultations are as follows:

- Office or other outpatient consultations (new or established patient): 99241 through 99245 (Example 13.4)
- Inpatient consultations (new or established patient): 99251 through 99255 (Example 13.5)

In the office setting, use the appropriate consultation code for the initial encounter; if a follow-up visit is required for additional diagnostic testing or examination, then use the appropriate established patient code. In a hospital setting, use the appropriate inpatient hospital consultation code; if a follow-up is required for additional services, then use subsequent hospital care codes. Remember the four Rs of consultations: There must be a *requesting* physician and the consultant must *render* an opinion and send a *report*. The requesting physician must document the *reason* on the health record.

Emergency Department Services

Codes 99281 through 99285 describe various levels of emergency care provided in an emergency department. An emergency department is defined as an organized hospital-based facility for the provision of unscheduled episodic services to patients who present for immediate medical attention. An ED must be open 24 hours, 7 days per week. CPT codes 99281 through 99285 should not to be used to report emergency care provided in an office setting.

Code 99288 is used when advanced life support is necessary during emergency care and the physician is located in a hospital emergency or critical care department and is in two-way voice communication with ambulance or rescue personnel outside the hospital.

Miscellaneous service codes 99050 through 99058 can be used depending on the hour at which the patient is seen as an emergency either in the physician's office or if taken to the ED of a hospital (24-hour facility). Most payers, including Medicare, do not pay for these codes. Some payers might pay for these codes and require documentation from the provider to support the code. Other codes under Miscellaneous Services in the Medicine section may be applicable for a patient receiving emergency care, so these should be scrutinized carefully.

Critical Care

According to CPT guidelines, critical care is the direct delivery of medical care by a physician for a critically ill or injured patient. A critical illness or injury acutely impairs one or more vital organ systems and makes an imminent or life-threatening deterioration in the patient's condition highly probable. Critical care involves highly complex decision making to assess, manipulate, and support vital system functions to treat single or multiple vital organ system failure or prevent further life-threatening deterioration of the patient's condition. Examples of vital organ system failure include but are not limited to central nervous system failure; circulatory failure; shock; and renal, hepatic, metabolic, or respiratory failure. Critical care may be provided on multiple days, even if no changes are made in the treatment rendered to the patient, as long as the patient's condition supports it.

Critical care is not always given in a critical care area, such as the coronary care unit, intensive care unit, pediatric intensive care unit, respiratory care unit, or emergency care facility. It could occur in the patient's room or in the ED. Also, it is important to note that a service that takes place in an intensive or critical care unit is not automatically coded as critical care. Services for a patient who is not critically ill but is in a critical care or intensive care unit are reported by use of other appropriate in-hospital E/M codes.

Critical care codes 99291 and 99292 are used to report the total duration of time spent by a physician providing critical care services to a critically ill or injured patient. For any given period spent providing critical care services, the physician must devote his or her full attention to the patient and therefore cannot provide services to any other patient during the same period.

Time spent with the individual patient must be recorded in the patient's record. Time spent engaged in work directly related to the individual patient's care, whether that time was spent at the immediate bedside or elsewhere on the floor or unit (even if not continuous), is reported as critical care. For example, time spent on the unit or at the nursing station on the floor reviewing test results or imaging studies, discussing the critically ill patient's care with other medical staff, or documenting critical care services in the health record is reported as critical care, even though it does not occur at the bedside.

Time spent in activities that occur outside of the unit or off the floor may not be reported as critical care because the physician is not immediately available to the patient. Time spent in activities that do not directly contribute to the treatment of the patient may not be reported as critical care, even if they are performed in the critical care unit. Time spent performing separately reportable procedures or services should not be included in the time reported as critical care time.

Code 99291 is used to report the first 30 to 74 minutes of critical care on a given date. It should be used only once per date, even if the time spent by the physician is not continuous on that date. Critical care of less than 30 minutes total duration on a given date should be reported with the appropriate E/M code. Code 99292 is used to report additional blocks of time, up to 30 minute each, beyond the first 74 minutes. This code has a plus sign (+) and is an "add-on" code. It is never used alone.

Critical care and other E/M services may be provided to the same patient on the same date by the same physician. Some services are included in critical care codes used to report critical care when performed during the critical period by the physician providing critical care. They are not coded in addition to critical care codes. These services are as follows:

- Interpretation of cardiac output measurements (93561, 93562)
- Chest radiographs (71045, 71046)
- Pulse oximetry (94760, 94761, 94762)
- Blood gases and information data stored in computers (e.g., electrocardiograms, blood pressures, hematologic data [99090])
- Gastric intubation (43752, 43753)
- Temporary transcutaneous pacing (92953)
- Ventilator management (94002 through 94004, 94660, 94662)
- Vascular access procedures (36000, 36410, 36415, 36591, 36600)

Any services performed in excess of those listed earlier should be reported separately.

Inpatient critical care services provided to neonates and infants 29 days through 24 months of age are reported with pediatric critical care codes 99468 through 99476. The pediatric critical care codes are reported as long as the infant or young child qualifies for critical care services during the hospital stay. Inpatient critical care services provided to neonates (28 days of age or younger) are reported with the neonatal critical care codes 99468 and 99469. The neonatal critical care codes are reported as long as the neonate qualifies for critical care services through the 28th postnatal day. The reporting of the pediatric and neonatal critical care services is not based on time or on the type of unit (for example, pediatric or neonatal critical care unit), nor is it dependent on the type of provider delivering the care. For additional instructions on reporting these services, see the section on Inpatient Neonatal and Pediatric Critical Care in the Evaluation and Management section of CPT.

There are subcategories for critical care for neonates, infants 29 days through 24 months of age, and various ages of children, as well as those subcategories for adults. A coding specialist must be sure to read the age categories carefully when choosing the appropriate subcategory of codes.

Nursing Facilities, Prolonged Services, Case Management

The Nursing Facilities subcategory is for services provided to patients in nursing facilities or psychiatric residential treatment facilities. Like some of the previous categories, initial visits for patients require three of three key components, while established patients require two of three key components.

Preventive Medicine

Preventive medicine is composed of services provided to prevent the occurrence of illness, injury, and disease, such as vaccine immunizations, routine physical examinations, and screening programs for detection of signs of disorders. Codes 99381 through 99397 describe initial or periodic comprehensive preventive medicine examination and are based on the age of the patient. Codes 99401 through 99412 should be used for reporting counseling given at an encounter separate from the preventive medicine examination.

Sometimes a patient may have an annual checkup, but while having the examination, he or she tells the health care provider of another issue. The physician provides both preventive and problem-focused services at the same time. Both services may be billed with the modifier -25 to indicate a separately identifiable service. When this occurs with Medicare patients, only the Medicare covered screenings or services (for example, problem-focused E/M, Papanicolaou (Pap) test, colon/rectal cancer screening, or prostate cancer screening) may be billed to the insurance. Noncovered services must be "carved out" to be billed to the patient. For preventive medicine when billing a Medicare case, an Advance Beneficiary Notice of Noncoverage (ABN) is not required.

Prolonged Services and Standby

Codes 99354 through 99359 should be used to indicate prolonged services with direct face-to-face patient contact; for example, the physician has spent time beyond the usual amount allotted for the service. There are specific codes for services with face-to-face contact and without face-to-face contact. Prolonged service that is less than 30 minutes should not be billed using these codes because the time is included in the E/M code. Time should be documented in the health record to justify use of these codes. Reimbursement for prolonged attendance in the hospital is higher than payment for many other types of care and reimbursement for critical care is even higher.

Physician standby services over the first 30 minutes are billed using code 99360. Some insurance programs or plans like Medicare do not pay for physician standby services, so be sure to check before billing to see whether the commercial payer will pay. The charge for this type of service is based on what the physician believes to be the value of 1 hour of his or her time. An example of this might be when a pediatrician is on standby during a high-risk cesarean section performed on a pregnant woman.

Other Evaluation and Management Codes

Other subcategories in this section cover home health care, case management, care plan oversight, telephone and online services, transitional care management, and advance care planning.

Anesthesia Services (00100-01999)

Anesthesia services are usually provided by an anesthesiologist, certified registered nurse anesthetist (CRNA), or a team of both. When a physician overseas one or more teams of CRNAs, it is required that the physician be present for specific portions of the procedure including the following:

- Providing a preanesthetic examination
- Outlining the anesthesia plan
- Participating in induction and emergence
- Monitoring at frequent intervals
- Being present and immediately available for emergencies
- Handling postanesthetic care

Anesthesia codes are grouped anatomically. Because the anesthesia code is directly related to the type of surgery a patient has, it is important for coding specialists to have a good knowledge of terminology from many different specialties.

All anesthesia codes include the following:

- Standard preoperative and postoperative visits
- Anesthesia care during the procedure
- Administration of fluids and/or blood products
- Usual monitoring services, such as electrocardiogram (ECG), temperature, blood pressure, pulse oximetry, and mass spectrometry

Anesthesia billing is made of two components: a base unit and a time unit. Anesthesia codes are assigned base units by the American Society of Anesthesiology based on the difficulty of the procedure. Time units are determined by the length of the procedure. The start time begins when the anesthesiologist prepares the patient for anesthesia. This does not include the pre-anesthesia visit and assessment. The anesthesia time ends when the patient is safely transferred to the care of the post anesthesia care unit or equivalent area.

Medicare requires that time is report per minute. Other payers may require a time unit be equal to 15 minutes or any increment thereof. It is important that coding and billing specialist check with each insurance payer to determine their requirements.

When multiple procedures are performed on a patient during anesthesia, the surgery that represents the most complex procedure is reported as it will have a higher base unit. The total anesthesia time for all procedures is reported.

Anesthesia codes should include a physical status (PS) modifier to indicate the health status of the patient and the potential issues with anesthesia they may pose. Some payers such as Medicare will not pay additional units for these modifiers, but some will. They are as follows:

- P1: Patient is normal and healthy (+0 units)
- P2: Patient has a mild systemic disease (+0 units)
- P3: Patient has a severe systemic disease (+1 unit)
- P4: Patient has a severe systemic disease that is a constant threat to life (+2 units)
- P5: Patient is not expected to survive without the operation (+3 units)

- P6: Patient is brain dead and organs are being removed for donor purpose (+0 units)

To arrive at a fee for anesthesia, a billing specialist must understand the following formula: Base units + Time units + PS + QC = Total units.

Case example for calculating anesthesia fee:

A 36-year-old patient receives anesthesia services by an MD for carpal tunnel surgery. The procedure starts at 0800 and ends at 0856. Code 01810 is allotted 3 base units. 1 time unit = 15 minutes or any increment thereof. The provider charges $100.00 per unit.	To determine the anesthesia fee: 3 base units (for procedure) + 4 time units = 7 total units × $100.00 per unit = $700.00

Qualifying circumstances (QC) are add-on codes for anesthesia services. They are used when a patient's age or status has a significant effect on the service provided. Although these are not paid by Medicare, many third-party payers do cover them.

- 99100, Anesthesia for patient of extreme age, younger than 1 year and older than 70 (+1 unit)
- 99116, Anesthesia complicated by utilization of total body hypothermia (+5 units)
- 99135, Anesthesia complicated by utilization of controlled hypotension (+5 units)
- 99140, Anesthesia complicated by emergency conditions (must specify) (+2 units)

Anesthesia teams often provide other services such as endotracheal intubation, central venous catheters, and arterial catheterization for monitoring, as well as various nerve blocks for postoperative and chronic pain management.

Surgical anesthesia codes always include a two-letter modifier that indicates the provider who performed the service. Some examples are included here. AA indicates an anesthesiologist working solo on the case. When anesthesia is provided by a physician and CRNA team, the charge is split in half and billed with a QX to indicate the CRNA, and a QK to indicate the physician (Example 13.6). In some states, CRNAs are able to provide their own anesthesia with no physician oversight. This would be indicated with a QZ modifier.

Surgery Guidelines

Coding From an Operative Report

It is best to obtain a copy of the patient's operative report from the hospital when coding surgery. A photocopy can be used so the coding specialist can make notes right on the document. When reviewing the report, use a ruler or highlighter pen. Use the ruler to read the report line by line. Highlight words that could indicate that the procedure performed may be altered by specific circumstances and to indicate that a code modifier may be necessary. Look up any unfamiliar terms using a medical dictionary or anatomic reference book and write the definitions in the margin.

Assign the code for the postoperative diagnosis shown at the beginning of the operative report. Also search for additional diagnoses in the body of the report that can be added as secondary diagnostic codes to support medical necessity, especially if the case is complex.

If the complex surgical procedure is not accurately described in the procedure code nomenclature, include an operative report and list "Attachment" in Block 19 of the insurance claim form so that the claims adjuster clearly understands the case and generates maximum payment.

Code numbers that describe a part of the body treated render higher reimbursement, depending on their location (for example, suturing of a facial laceration pays a higher rate than suturing of an arm laceration).

Remember the rule: Not documented, not done. Code only the procedures that are actually documented in the report.

Do not code using only the name of the procedure as it is given in the heading of the operative report. Read the report thoroughly before coding to see whether additional procedures were performed and whether they were part of the main procedure, performed independently, or unrelated. If the surgical position is noted, this can help to identify the right approach code. All codes include approach and closure except some skull base surgery codes.

Check to see how many surgeons were involved in the operative procedure and their roles (assistant surgeon, co-surgeon, team surgeon).

Look for unusual details, such as special instruments used, unusually long or complex procedures, rare approach techniques, reoperation, or extensive scarring encountered. These conditions may need one or more modifiers appended to the code.

Surgical code descriptions may define a correct coding relationship wherein one code is part of another based on the language used in the description (Example 13.7). An explanation

EXAMPLE 13.6 Anesthesia Teams and Modifiers

Anesthesia for Total Knee Replacement

Anesthesiologist working alone:	01402AA	$1000.00
Anesthesiologist and CRNA working as a team:	01402QX	$500.00
	01402QK	$500.00

CRNA, Certified registered nurse anesthetist.

EXAMPLE 13.7 Integral Code

Partial and complete, which means the partial procedure is included in the complete procedure.

56620	Vulvectomy simple; partial
56625	complete

Partial and total, which means the partial procedure is included in the total procedure.

58940	Oophorectomy, partial or total, unilateral or bilateral

Unilateral and bilateral, which means the unilateral procedure is included in the bilateral procedure.

58900	Biopsy of ovary, unilateral or bilateral

Single and multiple, which means the single procedure is included in the multiple procedure.

49321	Laparoscopy, surgical, with biopsy (single or multiple)

of how to read a description for stand-alone codes and indented codes can be found in Procedure 13.2 at the end of this chapter.

Confirm that the report findings agree with the procedure codes on the claim.

Global Surgical Package

Global **surgical package** is a phrase commonly encountered when billing. Generally a surgical procedure includes the standard preoperative, intraoperative, and postoperative services, with the preoperative service component depending on whether it is a minor or major surgery.

The majority of surgical procedures, including fracture care, are handled in this manner. Typical postoperative follow-up care includes only care that is usually a part of the surgical service. Complications, exacerbations, recurrence, or the presence of other diseases or injuries that require additional services should be reported separately. Table 13.4 lists what is and is not included in a global package.

Medicare defines the postoperative global periods of 0, 10, or 90 days and most third-party insurance companies apply the same criteria. Procedures shown in the *Federal Register* may show one of the three-digit or three-alpha codes in the global period column. These codes are not used on the claim form. They give information related to billing rules and regulations that indicate whether a global time period is part of a CPT code. This is particularly important when a patient comes in for a visit after surgery and helps in deciding whether the visit can be billed or is included in the surgical fee. These codes appear are outlined in Table 13.5.

TABLE 13.4 What Is and Is Not Included in a Global Package

Services Included in Global Package	Services Not Included in Global Package
Preoperative visits on the day before of day of a major procedure (090), an preoperative visits on the day of a minor procedure (010)	Initial evaluation, regardless of when it occurs, to decision for surgery (see modifier -57)
Intraoperative services that are a usual and necessary part of the surgical procedure	Postoperative visits unrelated to the diagnosis for which the surgical procedure was performed (see modifier -24)
Complications after surgery that do not require additional trips to the operating room (medical and surgical services)	Treatment necessary to stabilize seriously ill patient before surgery
Postoperative visits, including hospital visits, discharge and office visits for appropriate postoperative periods (10 or 90 days)	Diagnostic tests and procedures
Writing orders	Related procedure for postoperative complications requiring a return trip to the operating room (see modifier -78)
Evaluating the patient in the recovery area	Immunosuppressive therapy after transplant surgery
Normal postoperative pain management	An additional, more extensive procedure if a less extensive procedure fails

Note: A CMS proposal to discontinue the Medicare Global Package beginning in 2017 was put on hold because of the initiation of Medicare Access and CHIP Reauthorization Act (MACRA) quality reporting. This change would eventually eliminate both the 10-day and 90-day follow-up periods. Be sure to check CMS updates.

! COMPLIANCE ALERT

HIPAA and Medicare Global Billing Guidelines

Understanding which services are included, what constitutes the global surgical period, and how to code related or unrelated services in the global surgical package for Medicare patients is critical in ensuring correct payment and meeting compliance guidelines.

Never Event

Effective January 15, 2009, Medicare will not cover certain surgical never events and some insurance companies have stopped payment to hospitals for never events. A **never event** is an occurrence related to a surgical procedure that involves the following:

- Performed on the wrong side, wrong site, wrong body part, or wrong person
- Retention of a foreign object in a patient after a procedure
- Patient death or disability associated with the use of contaminated drugs, devices, or biologics provided by the health care facility
- Patient death or serious disability associated with a medication error
- Stage 3 or 4 pressure ulcers acquired after admission to the health care facility
- Patient death or disability associated with a fall while being cared for at the health care facility

Such occurrences should never happen in a health care organization and are usually preventable. Medicare will not cover hospitalization and other services related to these noncovered procedures. After discharge, reasonable and necessary services are covered whether they are or are not related to the surgical error.

TABLE 13.5 Global Package Status Indicators

000	No global package. Endoscopies and some minor procedures.
010	Minor procedures with expected normal follow-up in a 10-day period.
090	Major surgery with a 1-day preoperative period and a 90-day postoperative period included in the fee.
MMM	No global period. Uncomplicated maternity cases, which include prenatal care, delivery, and postnatal care.
XXX	No global period. Visits, procedures, and follow-up services may be billed separately.
YYY	The global period will be determined by the local Medicare fiscal agent because the code is for an unlisted procedure.
ZZZ	The code is part of another service and falls within that service's global period.

From Medicare and Medicaid Services: Global surgery, https://www.cms.gov/Outreach-and-Education/Medicare-Learning-Network-MLN/MLNProducts/downloads/GloballSurgery-ICN907166.pdf.

Supplies

When billing for office surgery and supplies used, checklists for the items used on the sterile tray (Fig. 13.5, *A*) and for determining complete and incomplete records (Fig. 13.5, *B*) should be used. These items can be charged only if the surgery required the use of additional items not normally used for this type of surgery. Medicare pays for trays with some procedure codes but not with others.

Integumentary System (10030–19499)

Procedure codes in the integumentary system involve skin, hair, nails, sebaceous glands, subcutaneous tissue and breasts. There are codes for debridement, skin tags, and biopsies, as well as treatment of burns and pressure ulcers. The breast section includes various types of biopsies and lumpectomy and mastectomy procedures, as well as cosmetic procedures such as augmentation, lifts, and reductions.

MINOR OPERATING ROOM INSTRUMENT TRAY SUPPLY CHECKLIST

1 Adson Brown tissue forceps _____
1 Adson tissue forceps with teeth _____
1 long tissue forceps _____
2 mosquito clamps _____
1 Peck Joseph dissecting scissors _____
1 Kahn dissecting scissors _____
1 Reynolds dissecting scissors _____
1 Stratte needle holder _____
1 Webster needle holder _____
4 small piercing towel clips _____
2 double-skin hooks _____
2 single-skin hooks _____
1 knife handle _____
1 #15 blade _____
10 4 x 4s _____
2 cotton-tipped applicators _____
1 small basin _____
3 sterile towels (drapes) _____
1 Bovie pencil _____
Sutures: _____ _____ _____
Dressings: 1/2-inch Steri-strips _____

A

OFFICE SURGERY MEDICAL RECORD CHECKLIST

Patient information sheet _____
H and P or progress note _____
Consent form _____
Diagnostic studies _____
Pathology report(s) _____
Anesthesia record _____
Circulating nurse's note _____
Doctor's orders _____
Discharge note _____
Operative report _____
Signature/operative report _____

B

Fig. 13.5 A, Checklist to document supplies used when billing for office surgery. This list can be kept with the patient's health record. **B,** Checklist for identifying complete and incomplete health records used for a patient receiving office surgery. As each item or document is completed, it is checked off so that the person reviewing the chart can see at a glance what needs to be finalized.

Multiple Lacerations

If multiple lacerations are repaired with the same technique and are in the same anatomic category, the insurance billing specialist should add up the total length of all lacerations and report one code to obtain maximum reimbursement. However, always read the notes and directives from the CPT manual when assigning these codes because these sites and sums can be confusing. Anatomic categories are the scalp, neck, axillae, external genitalia, trunk, extremities (hands or feet), face, ears, eyelids, nose, lips, and mucous membranes. If the patient had three repairs and each was listed with a different code, the second and third codes are downcoded (coded down one level) by the third-party payer so that a smaller payment is generated. If a patient has lacerations on both sides of the face, the lengths of all lacerations should be combined because the anatomic region is the same, and a claim should be submitted for the total length. No modifier is used and the right and left sides of the face are not billed separately (Example 13.8).

Multiple Lesions

The descriptions for the surgical codes that relate to accessory structures (for example, scalp, arms, and legs) and lesions found in the integumentary system (pertaining to the skin) can cause confusion. Code descriptions, including indentations, should be read completely with attention paid to terms such as *complex, complicated, extensive,* and *multiple.* Lesion excision code selection is based on the lesion's clinical diameter plus margin before excision and the character of the lesion—benign or malignant. Measurements should be taken before excision because a specimen subject to pathologic examination may shrink. Do not refer to a pathology report because the diameter of the mass may be measured after shrinkage or fragmentation of the specimen. Example 13.9 is a guide to obtain maximum reimbursement for the paring of seven corns.

EXAMPLE 13.8 Repair of Multiple Lacerations

Three lacerations of the face totaling 8.2 cm.

Incorrect Coding

12011	Repair 2.5-cm laceration of face
12013	Repair 2.7-cm laceration of face
12013	Repair 3-cm laceration of face

Correct Coding

12015	Repair 8.2-cm laceration of face

EXAMPLE 13.9 Paring of Seven Corns

Incorrect Coding

11055	Paring; single lesion
11056-51	Two to four lesions
11057-51	More than four lesions
or	
11055 ×7	Paring; single lesion (× seven corns)

Correct Coding

11057	Paring; more than four lesions (seven corns)

If possible, delay submission of the insurance claim for removal of a lesion or lesions until the pathology report is received. Usually a malignant lesion is reimbursed at a higher rate because of the more detailed nature of the procedure.

Repairs, Flaps, and Tissue Transfers

Wound repairs are divided into three types: simple, intermediate, and complex. Simple repairs require a single layer closure and suture. Intermediate is a layered closure or a heavily contaminated single layer closure with extensive cleaning and removal of debris. A complex repair includes extensive undermining. Wounds must be measured and reported in centimeters.

Many times a wound repair may involve tissue transfers and rearrangements to restore appearance and maintain proper healing. Tissue transfers and flaps are coded by type, location, and size of the wound.

Flaps are another type of tissue rearrangement where the flap is formed in another area of the body and moved to the wound. They are often completed in stages.

Musculoskeletal System (20005–29999)

The Musculoskeletal System section is the longest section of the CPT book. Procedures in this section address joints, muscles, bones, ligaments, tendons, and cartilage. Codes are grouped by anatomic site with the exception of sections for casting/strapping and arthroscopies.

Fractures

One of the first distinctions that must be made in coding a fracture is whether it is open or closed treatment. Closed fracture treatment is one where no incision is made at the fracture site. Open treatment occurs when an incision is made and the bones are held together with some type of internal fixation. The type of fracture does not necessarily indicate the type of treatment. For example, a closed fracture of the elbow may require an open treatment if the elbow is shattered. The global fracture code typically includes the first cast and its later removal. It also includes standard setting and care of a closed fracture.

Arthroscopies

An arthroscopy is used to diagnosis and treat a joint. It is less invasive than an open surgical approach and heals faster. If a procedure begins as a diagnostic arthroscopy and turns into a surgical arthroscopy, the diagnostic portion of the procedure would be included in the surgical portion and not coded separately. If an arthroscopic procedure turns into an open procedure, it is appropriate to code both procedures and attach the appropriate modifier on the arthroscopic code.

Respiratory (30000–32999)

The respiratory anatomic sections begin with the nose and sinuses, continue through the larynx and trachea, and end in the lungs and pleura. Many types of endoscopy codes appear in this section.

Laryngoscopies and Bronchoscopies

Laryngoscopies can be either direct or indirect. It is important to determine this before choosing a code. An indirect laryngoscopy uses mirrors and lights to visualize the larynx by reflection; whereas a direct laryngoscopy examines the back of the throat and the vocal cords directly.

Bronchoscopies help a health care provider visualize the airway using an instrument called a bronchoscope. Similar to the endoscopic joint procedures, a diagnostic bronchoscopy that leads to a surgical bronchoscopy would be included in the surgical portion and not billed separately. However, if a diagnostic bronchoscopy prompts the surgeon to perform an open procedure, both may be billed.

Video-Assisted Thoroscopic Surgery

Many procedures in the lungs may be performed with video-assisted thoroscopic surgery (VATS). This is a minimally invasive method of treating lung diseases. Often patients who have VATS are more likely to have less pain, quicker healing time, and shorter hospital stays than those having open procedures. VATS uses a small video camera introduced into the chest cavity. A surgical VATS code always includes the diagnostic VATS as well. If a diagnostic VATS prompts an open procedure, both may be billed, using the appropriate modifier.

Cardiovascular System (33010–37799)

Cardiovascular procedure codes encompass catheters, pacemakers, and bypass surgeries, among many others. Other procedures described in this section include, shunts, valve repairs, aneurysms, noncardiac bypass grafts, and angioplasty. Many codes in this section will require additional codes from the medicine or radiology sections as well.

Pacemakers

A pacemaker is made up of a pulse generator and one or more electrodes or leads. There are many different procedures described in this section, so read the descriptors carefully. More than one code may be needed to fully describe the procedure. To choose the correct code, a coding specialist must know the following information:

- What type of system is it?
- Is it temporary or permanent?
- How many leads?
- Where will the electrodes be placed?
- What is being done (removal, replacement or insertion)?

Coronary Artery Bypass Graft

A coronary artery bypass graft (CABG) is performed to redirect blood flow around a blockage in the artery or vein. Other veins and arteries in the patient's body are harvested for the grafts. Harvesting of most arteries and the saphenous vein are included in the CABG codes and not reported separately. Only endoscopic harvesting is reported separately. To accurately code a CABG, consider the following questions:

- How many grafts were performed?
- How many were from arteries? Which ones?
- How many were from veins? Which ones?

- Were the grafts harvested endoscopically or in an open procedure?
- Did the patient have a previous CABG?
- Is the whole system being worked on or just a component?

Vascular Injection Procedures

Vascular injection procedures are sometimes referred to as *interventional radiology*. Catheters are introduced through vessels for diagnostic and therapeutic purposes. Catheterization should be coded to the highest level accessed. Appendix L in the CPT book explains the vascular families and is helpful in choosing the appropriate code.

Hemic and Lymphatic Systems (38100–38999)

Codes in this section focus on bone marrow and stem cell procedures. Lymph node procedures are limited to biopsies, removal, and imaging procedures.

Digestive System (40490–49999)

Digestive system codes range from diagnostic and therapeutic procedures from the lips to the anus. It also includes the accessory organs used in digestion, the pancreas, liver, and gallbladder. Some procedures found here are gastric bypasses, appendectomies, and colon resections.

Colonoscopies and Upper Gastrointestinal Endoscopies

Endoscopic procedures of the colon and the upper gastrointestinal (GI) tract allow health care providers to visualize organs to diagnose and treat various conditions such as bleeding, infections, ulcers, and tumors. Similar to endoscopic procedures in the respiratory system, a diagnostic endoscopy that converts to a surgical endoscopy is not coded separately. More than one surgical endoscopy may be billed for the same date of service. For example, if more than one polyp is removed with more than one technique, each type of removal may be reported.

Hernias

A hernia is a protrusion of one body part into another. To choose the correct code in this section, a coding specialist must know the following:

- Site of the hernia
- Type of repair performed (laparoscopic or open)
- Age of the patient
- If the hernia is new or recurrent
- Clinical aspects of the hernia (incarcerated, strangulated, reducible)
- If mesh was used in the repair

Urinary System (50100–53899)

Codes in the Urinary System section address procedures in the kidneys, ureters, bladder, and urethra. They include incisions, excisions, endoscopies, removals, and repairs, as well as some procedures involving the prostate.

Male Genital System (54000–55899)

Procedures in the Male Genital System section include those done on the penis, testis, epididymis, scrotum, spermatic cord, and prostate. The codes describe excisions, repairs, penile implants, and prostatectomies, to name a few.

Female Reproductive System (56405–58999)

Codes in the Female Reproductive System section include not only repairs and treatments for the reproductive organs but also obstetric codes for prenatal care, delivery, and postnatal care. As with other sections, there are endoscopy procedures that aid in the diagnosis and treatment of various disease and disorders.

Endocrine System (60000–60699)

The majority of codes for the endocrine system describe excisions. In some cases the excision is for a tumor or cyst, but many codes describe excising the endocrine gland itself.

Nervous System (61000–64999)

The nervous system codes include the skull and brain, spine and spinal cord, and nerves. When coding spinal surgery, it is important to note the approach, such as transpedicular or anterior, as well as the number of vertebral levels.

Nerve Injections

Nerve blocks are reported based on the nerve targeted. When coding nerve injections, consider the following questions:

1. What is being injected? Was it an anesthetic agent or a neurolytic agent?
2. Which nerve is being injected?
3. Is it single or multiple injections? Unilateral or bilateral?
4. What is the duration of the infusion? Was it a single injection or continuous infusion?
5. Was their imaging guidance?

Eye and Auditory Systems (65091–69979)

The Eye and Auditory Systems sections describe surgical procedures for repair and treatment of the various parts of the ocular and auditory systems. Eye examinations and services for glasses or contact lens are not in this section but may be found in the Medicine section. The same is true for hearing tests and hearing aid fittings.

Radiology (70010–79999)

Radiology procedures can be done on any part of the body. They can be a separate procedure like a radiograph (x-ray examination) of the knee or part of another procedure such as guidance to place a nerve block. It is important to understand directional terms like those discussed in the documentation chapter, as well as the different types of radiologic procedures.

Diagnostic radiology includes radiographs, computed tomography (CT), and magnetic resonance imaging (MRI). An x-ray examination uses ionizing radiation to take a picture. It is particularly useful in imaging bones. CT produces cross-sectional pictures and are used to diagnose internal injuries and vascular disease. MRIs are useful in diagnosing cancers and various disorders of soft tissue. MRI may also be used to analyze blood vessels.

Diagnostic ultrasound uses sound waves to visualize internal structures. One of the most common uses is to visualize the fetus during pregnancy. This noninvasive test allows health care providers to measure and observe the fetus.

Breast mammography is a method of looking at breast tissue. It may be unilateral or bilateral. Screening mammography is considered to be part of preventive care and is covered by most health insurance without being applied to the deductible.

Other types of procedures found in the radiology section include bone and joint studies, radiation oncology, and nuclear medicine.

Pathology and Laboratory (80047–89398)

The Pathology and Laboratory section of CPT describe tests that can be performed on tissue, blood, urine, tumors and so on. It is important to understand the difference between the different types of tests.

Presumptive tests assume that there is a disease or infection. In these tests, a culture is grown to prove or disprove this. Qualitative tests determine only the presence of a virus, infection, or bacteria. Quantitative tests will determine not only the presence of a virus or bacteria but the exact amount of it present. Semi-quantitative tests will determine the amount of bacteria or virus within a given range, but not the exact amount.

Medicine Section (90281–99607)

The Medicine section contains codes describing a multitude of noninvasive or minimally invasive procedures. This section covers many areas including but not limited to the following:

- Immunizations and vaccines
- Psychiatry
- Biofeedback
- Dialysis
- Gastroenterology
- Ophthalmology
- Vestibular function and audiologic function tests
- Therapeutic cardiovascular procedures
- Allergy testing
- Noninvasive vascular diagnostic studies
- Pulmonary management and diagnostic tests
- Neurology and neuromuscular tests
- Genetic counseling
- Hydration and chemotherapy
- Physical and rehabilitative therapy
- Acupuncture, osteopathic and chiropractic services

Drugs and Injections

Reporting of drugs and injections generally requires two codes. One code is reported for the administration of the drug. CPT codes for immunization administration for vaccines are 90460 through 90474 and for therapeutic or diagnostic injections are 96372 through 96379.

A second code is reported to identify the product being administered, either immune globulin codes 90281 through 90399, vaccine/toxoid codes 90476 through 90479, or Level II HCPCs national alphanumeric codes J0000–J9999.

Documentation in the patient's health record must identify the name of the drug, amount of dosage, strength, and how it was administered. This information will be reported in Block 19 of the claim form. If the drug is experimental, you may need to attach a copy of the invoice.

CODE MODIFIERS

The use of a CPT code's two-digit add-on **modifier** permits the health care providers to indicate circumstances in which a procedure is performed differs in some way from that described by its usual five-digit code (Example 13.10). It may be necessary when using a modifier to include an operative, pathology, x-ray, or special report to justify its use to a third-party payer. A modifier can indicate the following:

- A service or procedure has either a professional component or a technical component.
- A service or procedure was performed by more than one health care provider, in more than one location or in the case of anesthesia, a physician alone, or as a team with a CRNA.
- A service or procedure has been increased or reduced.
- A service or procedure was provided more than once.
- Only part of a service was performed.
- An adjunctive service was performed.
- A bilateral procedure was performed.
- Unusual events occurred.

Common *Current Procedural Terminology* Modifiers

Any modifier that fits the situation being coded may be used, except when the modifier definition restricts the use of specific codes; for example, modifier -51, Multiple Procedures, states that -51 is to be appended for "multiple procedures, other than Evaluation and Management Services…." Discussion of the most commonly used modifiers follows. A complete listing of CPT modifiers may be found in Appendix A of the CPT.

Modifier -22: Increased Procedural Services

Modifier -22 is used when the service provided is substantially greater than that typically required for the listed procedure. If modifier -22 is added, the documentation in the health record, such as operative reports and/or chart notes, must support the substantial additional work. The reasons for use of this modifier are that the work encompasses increased intensity, time, technical difficulty of procedure, severity of the patient's condition, and physical and mental effort needed. This modifier may not be used with E/M services. Most third-party payers send an insurance claim to medical review before payment is made if modifier -22, indicating unusual services, appears on the claim. Because payments may be delayed, be cautious when using this modifier. An operative report should be submitted with the claim. If the third-party payer routinely denies the claim with modifier -22, an appeal for review should be made.

EXAMPLE 13.10 How to Report a Modifier on a Claim Form

Add a two-digit modifier to the five-digit code number.

Single line item:

12345-22 OR 1234522

Modifier -25: Significant, Separately Identifiable Evaluation and Management Service

Modifier -25 is defined as "significant, separately identifiable evaluation and management service by the same physician on the same day of the procedure or other service." The industry standard is to use -25 when a diagnostic procedure or minor procedure is involved. Typically, E/M services that are modified with -25 are office visits performed on the day of a minor procedure for an established patient.

Modifier -26: Professional Component

Certain procedures are a combination of a professional component (PC) and a technical component (TC) and are considered a global service. Usually these involve radiology and pathology procedures. The PC is a portion of a test or procedure that the physician does, such as interpreting an ECG, reading an x-ray film, or making an observation and determination using a microscope. The TC refers to the use of the equipment, the supplies, and the operator who performs the test or procedure, such as ECG machine and technician, radiography machine and technician, and microscope and technician. The TC is billed by the entity that owns the equipment. Do not modify procedures that are either 100% technical or 100% professional or when the physician performs both the PC and the TC. Modifier -26 represents the PC only. Use of this modifier alerts the insurance company to expect a separate claim from another provider or facility for the TC.

In Example 13.11, the physician is performing only one of two services—he or she is interpreting the results of bilateral hip x-ray films.

The facility where the patient had the x-ray film taken bills only for the TC by using either 73525 or 73521 with modifier -TC. If the physician owns the equipment and reads the x-ray film, there is no need to modify the x-ray code (73521) because both the PC and the TC were done in the office. Modifier -TC is assigned at the carrier's discretion.

Modifier -51: Multiple Procedures

Multiple procedures occur when more than one surgical service and/or related surgical service is performed on the same day or at the same surgical session by the same physician. In such cases, first report the primary service or procedure, which can be determined easily by the highest dollar value. Identify all additional services or procedures by appending codes with modifier -51 (Example 13.12).

The operative report should clearly state which procedures were done through separate incisions and which were done through the same incision. There are many circumstances when multiple procedures are performed. Modifier -51 may be used to identify the following:

- Multiple surgical procedures performed at the same session by the same provider
- Multiple related surgical procedures performed at the same session by the same provider
- Surgical procedures performed in combination at the same session, whether through the same or another incision or involving the same or different anatomy
- A combination of medical and surgical procedures performed at the same session by the same provider

The primary surgical procedure code must always be listed first on the claim form for full reimbursement and the secondary procedures must be listed in succession. Usually, payment by third-party payers for the primary code is 100% of the allowable charge, for the second code is 50%, for the third code is 25%, and for the fourth and remaining codes is 10%. However, under Medicare guidelines, Medicare pays 100% of the allowable charge for the primary code, pays 50% for two to five secondary procedures. Some computer systems can determine code order and automatically make the code adjustment.

Many carriers no longer require modifier -51 because they process claims electronically and the software program recognizes when multiple procedures are performed and automatically makes the reduction in payment. Contact insurance carriers and ask which method is preferred when reporting multiple surgical procedures. Then note this for each payer's policy to refer to for future billings. Always bill the full amount and let the third-party payer make the payment adjustments for percentage considerations. A decision flow chart is provided for reference to help simplify the modifier decision process (Fig. 13.6, *A* and *B*).

Do not use the -51 modifier with add-on codes designated with a "+" (see Appendix D in CPT) or codes listed as exempt to modifier -51 (see Appendix E in CPT). Add-on codes are codes that cannot stand alone. When billing with add-on codes, first

EXAMPLE 13.11 Professional and Technical Components

73521-**26**	**Professional component** only for a radiograph of both hips. Use to bill physician's fee for interpretation of x-ray film.	$
73521-**TC** or **73525**	**Technical component** only for a radiograph of both hips. Use to bill fee for facility that owns equipment and employs technician. Modifier -TC is at carrier's discretion.	$
73521	**Global service:** Radiologic examination, hips, bilateral. Minimum of two views of each hip. Use to bill complete fee when physician owns equipment, employs technician, and interprets x-ray film.	$

EXAMPLE 13.12 Multiple Procedure Modifier -51

Excision of 2.0-cm benign lesion on the nose and at the same session a biopsy of the skin and subcutaneous tissue of the forearm.

Code	RVU	Description of Services
11442	$	Excision, other benign lesion including margins, face, ears, eyelids, nose, lips, mucous membrane; excised diameter 1.1–2.0 cm
11100-**51**		Biopsy of skin, subcutaneous tissue, or mucous membrane (including simple closure), unless otherwise listed; single lesion **(second; multiple procedure)**

RVU, Relative value unit.

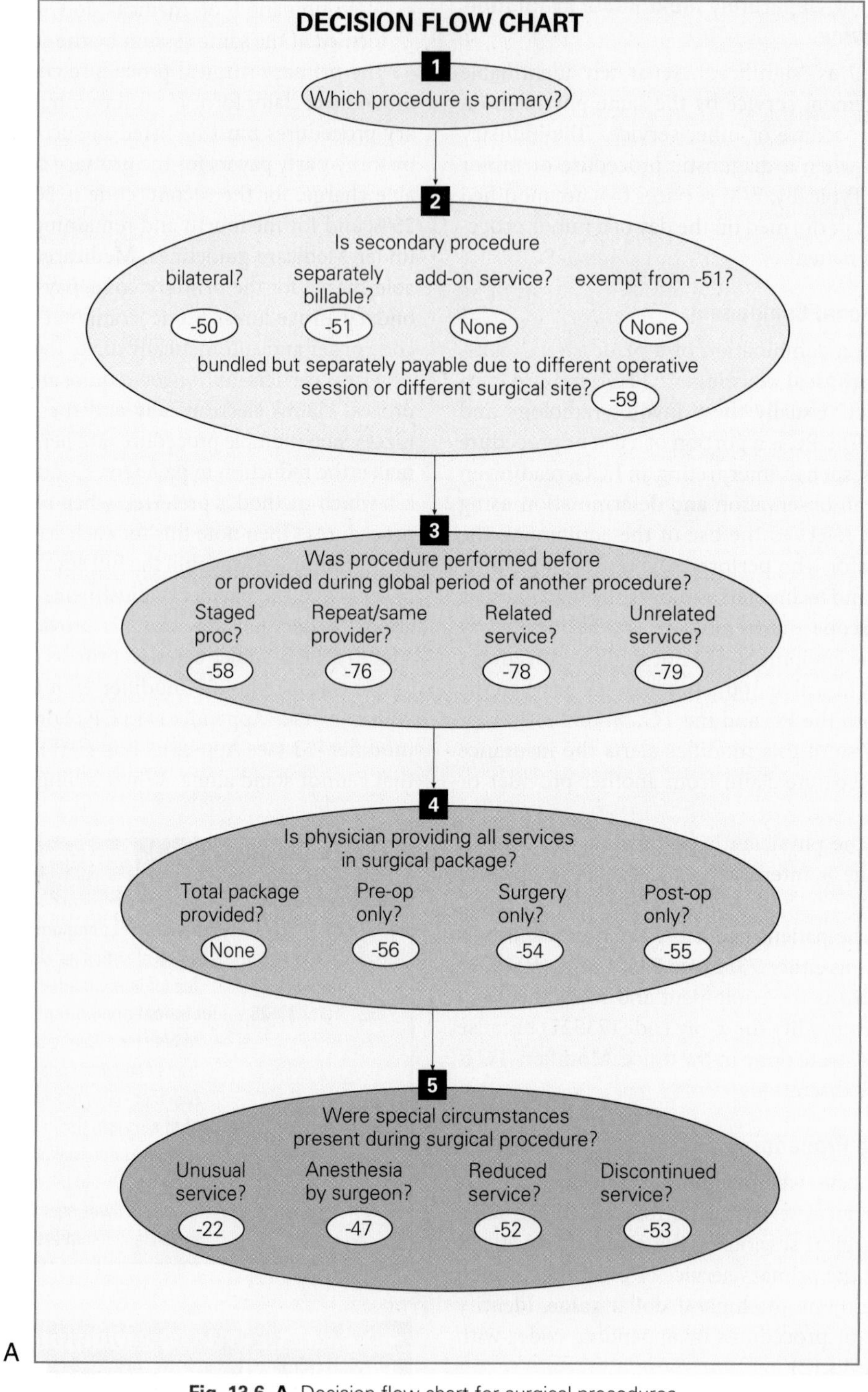

Fig. 13.6 A, Decision flow chart for surgical procedures.

list another code referred to as the "parent code" to give a full description for service billed (Example 13.13).

Modifier -52: Reduced Services

Use of the modifier -52 indicates that under certain circumstances a service or procedure is partially reduced or eliminated at the physician's discretion. It is wise to provide an explanation of why the service was reduced. A cover letter or a copy of the operative report should not accompany these claims because usually they are not sent to medical review and attached documents may impede processing. Never use this modifier if the fee is reduced because of a patient's inability to pay.

Modifier -57: Decision for Surgery

The modifier -57 is used strictly to report an E/M service that resulted in the initial decision to perform a major surgical procedure within 24 hours of the office visit; see Examples 13.14 and 13.15. A -57 modifier may be used for inpatient or outpatient

MULTIPLE SURGICAL PROCEDURES

Multiple services must be related to:
- Same patient
- Same provider
- Same date of service

1

- List all procedures in order of reimbursement, highest to lowest.
- Most comprehensive service brings greatest reimbursement and is considered primary.
- Check all procedures to make sure there is no unbundling (i.e., using two codes when one code describes procedure).
- Decision making expands at this point. Follow numbered question to determine correct modifier usage.

2

-50 Bilateral procedure, not described by code
-51 Not bundled, separately billable
-59 Ordinarily bundled, separately payable due to special circumstance

3

- The term "primary procedure" can also refer to the first procedure initiating a global surgical period

-58 Current service was planned prospectively at time of first service
-76 Physician repeats procedure subsequent to original procedure
-78 Return to operating room for subsequent procedure, complication relating to original procedure
-79 Unrelated procedure performed during global period of previous surgery

4

- Surgical package means one fee covers the whole package, surgical procedure, and postoperative care.

5

-22 An extremely difficult procedure due to altered anatomy or unusual circumstances (add 10% to 30% reimbursement)
-47 When the surgeon administers regional or general anesthesia
-52 Procedure/service reduced or eliminated at the discretion of the physician
-53 Procedure is discontinued due to extenuating circumstances or because of threat to the patient

B

Fig. 13.6, cont'd B, Guidelines and description of modifiers for multiple surgical procedures.

EXAMPLE 13.13 Add-On Code

Parent code	11100	Biopsy of skin … single lesion each separate/ additional lesion (list separately in addition to code for primary procedure)
Add-on code	+11101	

EXAMPLE 13.14 Decision for Surgery

A new patient is seen in the office complaining of a great deal of pain. Cholangiography is done and reveals blocked bile ducts. The patient is scheduled for surgery the next day.

8-1-20XX	99204-**57**	New patient office visit	$00.00
8-2-20XX	47600	Cholecystectomy	$000.00

SELECTING E/M MODIFIER WITH SURGICAL PROCEDURE

When a surgical procedure is performed within 24 hours of an office visit, choose the appropriate modifier for Evaluation and Management Service.

–57	–25
• New/established patient • *Major* procedure (90-day global period) • *Initial* decision for surgery made • Procedure within 24 hours	• New/established patient • *Minor* procedure (10-day global period) • Significant, separately identifiable E/M service • Procedure/service same day

Fig. 13.7 Two selections, with criteria to evaluate them, when choosing the appropriate code or modifier for evaluation and management *(E/M)* services when a surgical procedure is performed within 24 hours of an office visit.

consultations, inpatient hospital visits, and new or established patient visits that occur the day of or the day before surgery. Do not attach modifier -57 to a hospital visit code for the day before surgery or the day of surgery when a decision for a major surgical procedure was made a week before surgery. Think of -57 as telling the insurance company that the office visit is not part of the global fee.

Modifier -57 is often confused with modifier -25. Consult Fig. 13.7 when making the decision about which modifier to use for a surgical procedure that is performed within 24 hours of an office visit.

Modifier -58: Staged or Related Procedure

The modifier -58 is used to indicate that the performance of a procedure or service during the postoperative period was as follows:

- Planned (staged) at the time of the original procedure
- More extensive than the original procedure
- For therapy after a surgical procedure

Such circumstances should be reported by adding modifier -58 to the staged or related procedure. The use of this modifier requires accurate documentation of events leading up to the initial surgery and any subsequent surgery. It is only possible to modify procedures if the coder has all of the relevant facts and circumstances. In Example 13.15 the fracture is considered surgery because it is in the surgery section of the CPT book. All fracture codes have 90-day postoperative periods.

Modifiers -62, -66, -80, -81, and -82: More Than One Surgeon

If more than one surgeon is involved, the appropriate modifier will clarify who is billing the service:

- 62, Co-surgeon: Two surgeons work together as primary surgeons performing distinct parts of a procedure. Each physician reports his or her distinct operative work by adding this modifier.
- 66, Team surgery: A group of surgeons work together. Each participating physician adds this modifier to the basic procedure number for the service.
- 80, Assistant at surgery: Used when the surgery is not performed in a teaching hospital (Example 13.16).

EXAMPLE 13.15 Decision for Surgery

A new patient comes to the office after sustaining a fall while in-line skating. She is in distress, complaining of right wrist pain and swelling of the joint. The injury is evaluated **(1)** with an x-ray film. **(2)** It is determined that the patient has a Smith fracture and manipulation is performed. A long-arm cast is applied **(3)** using fiberglass (Hexcelite) material **(4).**

(1)	99203-57	Initial office evaluation (detailed) with decision for surgery
(2)	73100-RT	Radiologic examination, right wrist, anteroposterior (AP) and lateral (lat) views
(3)	25605	Closed treatment of distal radial fracture (for example, Colles or Smith type), with manipulation
(4)	99070	Supplies: Casting material (third-party payer) Medicine section code *or* Supplies: Hexcelite material (Medicare fiscal agent)
	A4590	HCPCS Level II code

The patient returns in 4 weeks for follow-up care **(1).** The wrist is radiographed again **(2),** the long-arm cast is removed **(3),** and a short-arm cast is applied **(4)** using plaster material **(5).**

(1)	No code	Follow-up care included in global fee
(2)	73100-RT	Radiologic examination, right wrist, AP and lat views
(3)	No code	Cast removal included in original fracture care (25605)
(4)	29075-58	Application, plaster, elbow to finger (short arm) staged procedure
(5)	99070	Supplies: Casting material (third-party payer) Medicine section code *or* Supplies: Plaster material (Medicare fiscal agent)
	A4580	HCPCS Level II code

HCPCS, Healthcare Common Procedural Coding System.

EXAMPLE 13.16 Assistant at Surgery

Closure of Intestinal Cutaneous Fistula

Operating surgeon bills	44640	**No modifier**
Assistant surgeon bills	44640-**80**	**With modifier**

- 81, Minimum assistant surgeon.
- 82, Assistant surgeon: Used for surgeries performed in a teaching hospital when a qualified resident surgeon is not available to act as an assistant at surgery.

The assisting doctor is paid a reduced fee of 16% to 30% of the allowed fee the primary surgeon receives for performing the surgery on the basis of the patient's contract. The assisting physician uses the same surgical code as the primary surgeon and adds the -80 modifier to it. Some payers require the billed fee reflect the reduced percentage. Others prefer to have the full fee listed and make the reduction themselves. Under some insurance contracts, there may be some surgical procedures that restrict payment for an assistant surgeon.

EXAMPLE 13.17 Multiple Modifiers

A physician sees a patient who is grossly obese. The operative report documents that a bilateral sliding-type inguinal herniorrhaphy was performed and the procedure took 2 hours, 15 minutes.

49525-**99** Bilateral repair sliding inguinal hernia requiring 2 hours 15 minutes

-50
-22

EXAMPLE 13.18 HCPCS Modifiers

When taking x-ray films of both feet, the billing portion of the insurance claim appears as follows.

05/06/XX	73620 **RT**	Radiologic examination, foot—right
05/06/XX	73620 **LT**	Radiologic examination, foot—left

HCPCS, Healthcare Common Procedural Coding System.

Modifier -99: Multiple Modifiers

If a procedure requires more than one modifier code, use the two-digit modifier -99 after the usual five-digit CPT code number, all typed on one line; then list each modifier on a separate line (Example 13.17). Some insurance companies require -99 with a separate note in Block 19 of the CMS-1500 claim form or in the freeform area of electronic submissions, indicating which two or more modifiers are being used.

HCPCS Modifiers

In addition to CPT modifiers, HCPCS Level II modifiers are used by Medicare and may be used by some commercial payers. HCPCS Level II modifiers may be two alpha digits (Example 13.18), two alphanumeric characters (Fig. 13.8), or a single alpha digit used for reporting ambulance services or results of positron emission tomography scans. A comprehensive list of HCPCs Level II modifiers can be found in an HCPCS national Level II code book.

Use the two-digit HCPCS modifiers whenever they are necessary. HCPCS modifiers further describe the services provided and can increase or decrease the health care provider's fee. If not used properly, they can drastically affect the physician's fee profile by reducing future payments to the provider.

CORRECT CODING EDITS AND PRACTICES

National Correct Coding Initiative Edits

In 1996 the Medicare program implemented the National Correct Coding Initiative (NCCI). This initiative involves a code editing system consistent with Medicare policies to eliminate inappropriate reporting of CPT codes. *Code editing* is a

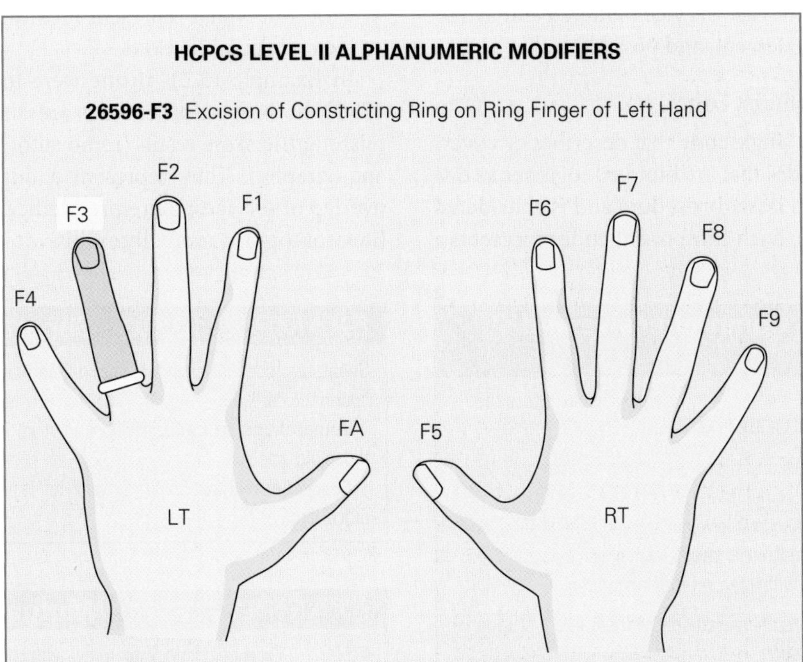

Fig. 13.8 Healthcare Common Procedural Coding System *(HCPCS)* Level II alpha modifiers (*LT* and *RT* used to identify left and right hands) and alphanumeric modifiers (*FA* through *F9*) used to identify digits (fingers) of left and right hands.

computer software function that performs online checking of codes on an insurance claim to detect improper code submissions. Some coders refer to this process as *code screening.* NCCI edits are updated quarterly. Such software is used by private payers, federal programs, and state Medicaid programs.

> Medicare's Correct Coding initiative is implemented by the Centers for Medicare and Medicaid Services (CMS) in an attempt to eliminate unbundling or other inappropriate reporting of *Current Procedural Terminology* (CPT) codes. As you will recall, **unbundling** is coding and billing numerous CPT codes to identify procedures that usually are described as a single code. Coding conflicts are picked up and claims are reviewed, suspended, or denied when conflicts occur. Software is available to give physicians, private insurance companies, and billing services access to the same government database used in auditing physicians for improper use of CPT codes. It is currently available on the CMS website at no charge. See https://www.cms.gov/Medicare/Coding/NationalCorrectCodInitEd/index.html?redirect=/nationalcorrectcodinited/.

Some code pairs in the NCCI edits are followed by a 0 and others by a 1. If the superscript 0 appears with a code pair, it means that Medicare never allows a modifier to be used with the codes, so the code pair could never be reported together. The superscript 1 means that a modifier may be used under certain circumstances with appropriate documentation to have both codes reimbursed.

Because every health care organization has billing problems and questions unique to its specialty, coding and billing specialists must become detectives and discover how to obtain maximum reimbursements in the appropriate specialty. The best way is to telephone the third-party payer to inquire about new coding options and to note improvements in reimbursement. Coding takes expertise. It is an art, not an exact science. The following explanations of various ways of coding claims assist in obtaining maximum reimbursement for each service rendered and avoiding denials, lowered reimbursement, and possible audit.

Comprehensive and Component Edits

A **comprehensive code** is a single code that describes or covers two or more component codes that are bundled together as one unit. A component code is a lesser procedure and is considered part of the major procedure. Each component code represents a portion of the service described in the comprehensive code and should be used only if a portion of the comprehensive service was performed (Example 13.19).

Under the Medicare program, NCCI component code edits involve procedures that meet any of the following criteria:

1. Code combinations that are specified as "separate procedures" by CPT
2. Codes that are included as part of a more extensive procedure
3. Code combinations that are restricted by the guidelines outlined in CPT
4. Component codes that are used incorrectly with the comprehensive code

If any one of these restricted code combinations is billed, Medicare allows payment for only the procedure with the highest relative value (Example 13.20).

For example, when performing an inguinal hernia repair, the surgeon makes an incision in the groin and dissects tissue to expose the hernia sac, internal oblique muscle, and spermatic cord. If a lesion is excised from the spermatic cord, it is considered a component of the comprehensive hernia repair procedure and is not separately billable. Medicare will deny code 55520 (lesion excision) as a component of procedure code 49505 (hernia repair) when performed during the same operative session.

Mutually Exclusive Code Edits

Mutually exclusive code edits relate to procedures that meet any of the following criteria:

1. Code combinations that are restricted by the guidelines outlined in CPT
2. Procedures that represent two methods of performing the same service
3. Procedures that cannot reasonably be done during the same session
4. Procedures that represent medically impossible or improbable code combinations

In Example 13.21, if one were to submit codes 47605 and 47563, both these procedures are different methods of accomplishing the same result (removal of the gallbladder with cholangiography). They represent a duplication of effort and an overlap of services; therefore Medicare would deny code 47563 (laparoscopy) as mutually exclusive to code 47605 (the excision).

EXAMPLE 13.19 Comprehensive and Component Codes

Comprehensive code	93015	Cardiovascular stress test
Component codes	93016, 93017, 93018	
93015	Cardiovascular stress test using maximal or submaximal treadmill or bicycle exercise, continuous electrocardiographic monitoring, or pharmacologic stress; with physician supervision, with interpretation and report	
93016	Physician supervision only, without interpretation and report	
93017	Tracing only, without interpretation and report	
93018	Interpretation and report only	

EXAMPLE 13.20 Separate Procedure

Separate procedure example: Inguinal hernia repair with lesion excised from spermatic cord

Comprehensive code: 49505 Repair initial hernia age 5 years or older; reducible

Component code: 55520 Excision of lesion of spermatic cord (separate procedure)

EXAMPLE 13.21 Mutually Exclusive

47605	Excision, cholecystectomy; with cholangiography
47563	Laparoscopy, surgical; cholecystectomy with cholangiography

Note: Different methods of accomplishing the same procedure.

Bundling

For insurance claim purposes, **bundled codes** means to group related codes together. To completely understand bundled codes, one must have a thorough knowledge of the service or procedure that is being provided or use an unbundling book as a reference guide.

Example 13.22 illustrates one type of bundling found in the CPT code book. Because code 19272 (excision of chest wall tumor with plastic reconstruction; with mediastinal lymphadenectomy) includes mediastinal lymphadenectomy, a separate code for mediastinal lymphadenectomy (38746) should not be billed in addition to it on the same date of service.

In the Medicare program, a number of services may be affected because CMS considers the services to be bundled. Because many commercial third-party payers may follow Medicare guidelines, an understanding of this bundling concept is necessary. When dealing with private insurance, an explanation of benefits (**EOB**) document may print out with the statement "Benefits have been combined," which means the same thing as bundling.

For example, when listing a sterile tray for an in-office surgical procedure, the tray is bundled with the procedure unless supplies are necessary in addition to those usually used. CPT code 99070 (supplies and materials) is not reimbursed by Medicare; however, HCPCS level II alphanumeric codes may be used in such cases. The cost of some services and supplies is bundled in E/M codes. For example, telephone services and reading of test results are not separately billable. However, Medicare pays for slings, splints, rib belts, cast supplies, Hexcelite and light casts, pneumatic ankle-control splints, and prosthetics, but a supplier number is necessary to bill for take-home surgical supplies and DME.

Some coding reference books also include a comprehensive list of codes that CMS considers bundled for the Medicare program. When appealing a claim, a great deal of time may be spent on paperwork only to discover that the code is bundled and denial is imminent. When in doubt about whether or not services are combined, contact the third-party payer and ask.

Unbundling

Unbundling is coding and billing numerous CPT codes to identify procedures that usually are described by a single code. It is also known as *exploding* or *a la carte* medicine.

Some health care organizations do this unwittingly, but it is considered fraud if it is done intentionally to gain increased reimbursement. Unbundling can lead to downward payment adjustments and possible audit of claims.

EXAMPLE 13.22 Bundled Code

Component code	19271	Excision of chest wall tumor involving ribs, with plastic reconstruction; without mediastinal lymphadenectomy
Comprehensive code	19272	with mediastinal lymphadenectomy

Types of unbundling are as follows:

- Fragmenting one service into component parts and coding each component part as if it were a separate service (Example 13.23)
- Reporting separate codes for related services when one comprehensive code includes all related services (Example 13.24)
- Coding **bilateral** (both sides of the body) procedures as two codes when one code is proper (Example 13.25)
- Separating a surgical approach from a major surgical service that includes the same approach (Example 13.26)

EXAMPLE 13.23 Unbundled Code

Incorrect Coding

12011 Simple repair of superficial wounds of face, ears, eyelids, nose, lips and/or mucous membranes 2.5 cm or less.
12014 5.1 cm to 7.5 cm

Correct Coding

12015 7.6 cm to 12.5 cm

EXAMPLE 13.24 Unbundling (Comprehensive Code)

Unbundled Claim

58150 Total abdominal hysterectomy (corpus and cervix) with removal of tubes and with removal of ovary ($1200)
58700 Salpingectomy ($650)
58940 Oophorectomy ($685)
Total Charge: $2535

Claim Coded Correctly

58150 Comprehensive code for all three services
Total Charge: $1200

EXAMPLE 13.25 Unbundling (Bilateral)

Incorrect Coding

77065-RT Right mammography
77065-LT Left mammography

Correct Coding

77066 Mammography, bilateral

EXAMPLE 13.26 Bundling (Surgical Approach)

Incorrect Coding

49000 Exploratory laparotomy
44150 Colectomy, total, abdominal

Correct Coding

44150 Colectomy, total, abdominal (correct because it includes exploration of the surgical field)

To avoid this problem, always use a current CPT code book. The use of outdated codes often inadvertently results in unbundling. A new technology or technique may have its own code when it is developed but may be bundled with another code as it becomes commonplace. If the health care organization uses a billing service, request in writing that the service's computer system include no unbundling programming.

! COMPLIANCE ALERT

HIPAA and Procedural Coding Guideline

Always submit current *Current Procedural Terminology* (CPT) codes. If outdated codes are used, this could red flag a provider with Medicare as being in noncompliance.

Downcoding

Downcoding at the health care organization level typically occurs when there is not enough documentation to support the correct code or to code the diagnosis to the optimal level of specificity. It may also occur because a provider mistakenly hopes to avoid audits by staying within a lower payment range.

This also occurs at the payer level when the coding system used on a claim submitted to a third-party payer does not match the coding system used by the company receiving the claim. The computer system converts the code submitted to the closest code in use, which is usually down one level from the submitted code. Therefore the payment that is generated is usually less.

In many states it is illegal for an insurance company to downcode a claim. Insurance commissioners have published bulletins warning payers to cease this claims adjudication practice. When a payer receives a claim, the payer is allowed to pay or deny the claim. If additional information is necessary to adjudicate the claim, it should be requested from the patient or provider. The payer is limited by the number of days it has to review the claim. At completion of the review, the payer must pay or deny the claim (Example 13.27).

! COMPLIANCE ALERT

HIPAA Documentation Guideline

Make sure that the documentation from the provider supports the code that is being submitted to prevent downcoding.

EXAMPLE 13.27 Downcoding

Document states: Excision of bone tumor from anterior tibial shaft.
Pathology report states: Tibia bone tumor; benign

Incorrect Coding

11400 Excision of benign lesion including margins except skin tag, trunk, arms or legs; excised diameter 0.5 cm or less

Correct Coding

27635 Excision of bone tumor of tibia, benign

Upcoding

The term *upcoding* is used to describe deliberate manipulation of CPT codes for increased payment. This practice can be spotted by Medicare fiscal agents and third-party payers using prepayment and postpayment screens or "stop alerts," which are built into most computer coding software programs. An example of intentional upcoding might be a physician who selects one level of service code for all visits with the theory that the costs even out, such as always using code 99213. This opens the door to audits and in the end may cost the health care organization money. Upcoding may occur unintentionally if the coder is ill informed or does not keep current.

Code Monitoring

Monitoring of CPT codes is done to maximize reimbursement from all third-party payers. First, determine which codes are used most often in the health care organization. Many computer programs can generate a list of codes, ranking them according to frequency of use. If the health care organization does not have a computer, take a sampling of the charge slips to determine the prevalent codes. Once the high-volume codes are known, focus on coding strategies for the best possible reimbursement.

Monitor every remittance advice (RA) and EOB that comes in directly or via patients. Every private insurance, Medicare, Medicaid, and TRICARE payment received should be checked for accuracy to see whether it is consistently the same or if coding changes have occurred. Incorrect payments should be investigated and appealed. Examine all payments made for codes that do not match those submitted. Be sure to appeal every payment that is less than half of what the health care provider bills. An example of a code and payment tracking log to help monitor payments received is shown in Fig. 13.9.

METHODS OF PAYMENT

Most methods of payments are based on individual procedure codes. Private insurance companies, as well as federal and state programs, adopt different methods for establishing payment rates for outpatient services: (1) fee schedules; (2) usual, customary, and reasonable; and (3) relative value scales. Additional reimbursement methods for hospital claims are discussed in Chapter 19.

Fee Schedule

A fee schedule is simply a listing of accepted charges or established allowances for specific medical procedures. A health care organization can have more than one fee schedule unless specific state laws restrict this practice. Charges should be related consistently to the cost of the services and uniformly applied to all patients whether inpatient or outpatient. The following situations can occur:

1. Health care organizations *participating* in the Medicare program typically would be paid by the fee schedule set annually by Medicare. Health care organizations *not participating* in the Medicare program would be paid a limited charge set forth by Medicare and based on the fee schedule set annually be Medicare.

CODE/PAYMENT TRACKING LOG					Date: 1-XX
CPT CODE	Practice fee	Medicare date and amount paid	Medicaid date and amount paid	TRICARE date and amount paid	Blue Shield date and amount paid
99201	$00.00	11-XX $00.00	8-XX $00.00	7-XX $00.00	4-XX $00.00
99202	$00.00	12-XX $00.00	9-XX $00.00	10-XX $00.00	6-XX $00.00
99211	$00.00	12-XX $00.00			11-XX $00.00
99212	$00.00				12-XX $00.00
99221	$00.00				
99231	$00.00				
99232	$00.00				
99241	$00.00				

Fig. 13.9 Example of a code/payment tracking log.

2. Health care providers who treat Medicaid patients cannot bill the patient for any balance after the Medicaid payment is received. These balances must be adjusted off.
3. Health care organizations *participating* with TRICARE would be paid by TRICARE at the TRICARE rate.
4. Health care organizations *not participating* with TRICARE are able to charge 115% of the TRICARE allowed charge. The patient may be billed for the difference between the 115% and the amount TRICARE paid.
5. Health care organizations having a contractual arrangement with in insurance carrier would be paid on the basis of the negotiated contract.
6. Health care organizations rendering services to those who have sustained industrial injuries would be paid based on that state's workers' compensation fee schedule.

Section 1128(b) of the Social Security Act states that a physician may risk exclusion or suspension from the Medicare program if his or her Medicare charges are in excess of its usual charges. To prevent a possible violation of Section 1128(b) of the Social Security Act, the provider should assign one fee for each procedure code when establishing a fee schedule. This fee should be billed to all third-party payers and to self-pay patients. By establishing one fee for each procedure instead of multiple fees for each procedure, the provider helps establish the usual and customary fee for his or her geographic area. It is equally important to monitor third-party payer adjustments to determine how much revenue is lost because of poor contracts and to monitor employee theft.

The fees should be above the maximums paid by the third-party payers to whom the health care organization generally bills. A health care organization may wish to evaluate the fee schedules annually to decide whether fees should be raised for certain procedures or services.

Because mistakes can be costly in terms of lost revenue and possible violations, one fee schedule for all patients, with provisions for financial hardship cases, is usually the safest course for health care providers.

Usual, Customary, and Reasonable

Usual, customary, and reasonable (UCR) is a complex system in which three fees are considered in calculating payment. This is an older payment methodology that was introduced in the Social Security Act of 1965. Although most carriers have stopped using it, it is still a concept that billing specialists should be familiar with. UCR is used mostly in reference to fee-for-service reimbursement. The usual fee is the fee that a health care provider usually charges for a given service to a private patient. A **customary fee** is one that is charged by providers of similar training and experience in a geographic area. A **reasonable fee** is the fee that is, in the opinion of the medical review committee, justifiable considering the special circumstances of the case. Fig. 13.10 illustrates how a surgeon's payment is determined under this method.

Reimbursement is based on the lower of the usual or customary fee and determines the approved or allowed amount. In a UCR system, payment can be extremely low for a rarely performed but highly complex procedure because there may be no history of billed charges from other health care providers on which to base payment. Some private health insurance plans use this method and pay a provider's full charge if it does not exceed UCR charges.

Depending on the policies of each insurance company, the UCR system is periodically updated. UCR is a method chosen by third-party payers and not the provider. If the health care provider has a UCR that is significantly lower than those of other health care organizations in his or her area, document this and ask the third-party payer for a review and possible adjustment. Most plans have discontinued the UCR system and are adopting the Medicare resource-based relative value scale method for physician reimbursement.

Relative Value Studies

In 1956 the California Medical Association Committee on Fees published the first edition of the *California Relative Value Studies* (CRVS). **RVS,** referred to as either **relative value studies** or scale, is a coded listing of procedure codes with unit values that indicate the relative value of the various services performed, taking into account the time, skill, and overhead cost necessary for each service (Example 13.28).

Units in RVS are based on the median charges of all physicians during the period in which the RVS was published. A **conversion factor** is used to translate the abstract units in the scale to dollar fees for each service.

PARTICIPATING SURGEON UCR CALCULATION

Four Example Cases

Surgeon's bill	Usual fee	compared to	Customary fee		Payment
1) $400	$350	→	$350	→ declared reasonable (extenuating circumstances)	$400
2) $400	$350	→	$350	→ declared customary (no unusual circumstances)	$350
3) $375	$350	→	$400	→ declared customary (does not exceed customary level)	$375
4) $350	$350	→	$400	→ declared customary (falls within customary range)	$350

Usual Fee—usual submitted fee for a given service to patient.

Customary Fee—in the range of usual fees charged by providers of similar training and experience in a geographical area (i.e., the history of charges for a given service).

Reasonable Fee—meets the aforementioned criteria or is, in the opinion of the medical review committee, justifiable considering the special circumstances of the case.

Payment—based on the lower of usual and customary fees.

Fig. 13.10 Usual, customary, and reasonable *(UCR)* calculation for four participating surgeons' cases.

EXAMPLE 13.28 Relative Value Scale

Procedure

CODE	Description	Units
10060	Incision & drainage of cyst	0.8

Using a hypothetical figure of $153/unit, this procedure is valued at $122.40.
Math: $153.00 × 0.8 = $122.40

The RVS is a sophisticated system for coding and billing of professional services. After the successful use of the California RVS, many state and medical specialty associations adopted the CRVS method. In 1975 the Federal Trade Commission (FTC) challenged the legality of using the RVS as a fee schedule, stating that it could be interpreted as a form of price fixing in violation of antitrust laws. Since that time, many medical societies and medical specialty associations issued new publications that omitted unit values for the procedures listed but retained the procedure code portion of RVS.

Some states passed legislation mandating the use of RVS codes for procedures and the unit values as the schedule of fees for workers' compensation claims. In these states the conversion factor to be used in applying the units is also stated in the law. The third-party payer pays a specific dollar amount for each unit listed for each procedure in the RVS code book.

An insurer or other third party could devise an RVS on the basis of its own data. This type of RVS would not be created by physicians in an effort to regulate fees and therefore would be acceptable on the basis of FTC guidelines. An example is *Optum's Relative Values for Physicians (RVP)*, which is based on survey data from Relative Value Studies, Inc. Additionally, a national RVS developed under a government contract may be acceptable and would not be in violation of antitrust laws.

Resource-Based Relative Value Scale

The **resource-based relative value scale (RBRVS)** is an RVS developed for CMS by William Hsiao and associates at the Harvard School of Public Health. CMS used it to devise the Medicare fee schedule that was phased in from 1992 through 1996. This approach to fees was developed to redistribute Medicare dollars more equitably among physicians and to control escalating fees that were out of control using the UCR system. This became the basis for physicians' payments nationwide.

This system consists of a fee schedule based on **relative value units (RVUs)**. The formula for obtaining RVUs is somewhat complex and involves a bit of mathematics in computing three components: an RVU for the service, a geographic adjustment factor (GAF), and a monetary conversion factor (CF).

RELATIVE VALUE UNIT FORMULA [(RVU physician work × GCPI physician work) + (RVU practice expense × GPCI practice expense) + (RVU malpractice cost × GCPI malpractice cost)] × CF = Medicare $ for service

CF, Conversion factor; *GPCI,* geographic practice cost index; *RVU,* relative value unit.

RVUs are based on the physician work RVU, the practice expense RVU, and the malpractice insurance RVU. To bring the fees in line for the region where the physician practices and to adjust for regional overhead and malpractice costs, each of the RVUs is adjusted for each Medicare local fiscal agent by geographic practice cost indices (GPCIs).

HCPCS/CPT CODE	WORK RVUs		PRACTICE EXPENSE RVUs		MALPRACTICE RVUs	
91000 RVUs	1.04	+	0.70	+	0.06	
GPCI*	× 1.028		× 1.258		× 1.370	
	1.07		0.88		0.08	= Total adjusted RVUs, 2.03

For 2016, the conversion factor for nonsurgical care is $36.1096 x 2.03 = Allowed amount $73.30

*The geographical practice cost indices (GPCI) for the medical practice whose location in the example is Oakland, California.

Fig. 13.11 Formula used to calculate the fee for a specific procedure using the resource-based relative value scale system. *RVU,* Relative value unit.

A CF is used to convert a geographically adjusted relative value into a payment amount. This CF is updated to a new amount each year. Fig. 13.11 provides an example of calculating payment for one procedure code.

The figures to work out this formula in the chart for each service are published annually in the *Federal Register.*

RVUs help when determining cost accounting because they take into account the practice expense, malpractice expense, work effort, and cost of living. They are also helpful when negotiating the best contract available with managed care plans. A crosswalk is an effective way to see how the practice may be affected by an RBRVS contract (Table 13.6).

Medicare Fee Schedule

Medicare fee schedules are based on RBRVS and are published every year, listing three columns of figures: participating amount, nonparticipating amount, and limiting charge for each procedure code number (Table 13.7). Currently, fee schedules may be accessed online at each local MAC's website.

Developing a Fee Schedule Using Resource-Based Relative Value Scale

Many health care providers and organizations use RBRVS to establish their own fee schedule. Health care fees can be adjusted if they are too high or too low. It is legal to use an RVS guide for setting, realigning, or evaluating fees as long as the physician does not enter into any price-fixing agreements.

TABLE 13.6 Resource-Based Relative Value Scale Crosswalk

A	B	C	D	E	F	G	H
Code	Code Description	RBRVS/RVU	Conversion Factor	FEE	Contract Conversion Factor	Contract FEE	% Contract Payment
99212	Office Visit	0.68	72.06	$49	64.71	$44.00	90%

RBRVS, Resource-based relative value scale; *RVU,* relative value unit.

TABLE 13.7 Mock Medicare Fee Schedule

CPT	Description	Participating	Nonparticipating	Limiting Charge	Global Package
99201	New OV, problem focused	30.43	28.91	33.25	
99202	New OV, expanded problem focused	47.52	45.14	51.91	
99203	New OV, detailed	64.92	61.67	70.92	
99204	New OV, comprehensive, level 4	97.13	92.27	106.11	
99205	New OV, comprehensive, level 5	121.08	115.03	132.28	
99211	Nurse visit	14.70	13.97	16.07	
99212	Est OV, problem focused	26.14	24.83	28.55	
99213	Est OV, expanded prob focused	36.80	34.96	40.20	
99214	Est OV, detailed	56.31	53.79	61.51	
99215	Est OV, comprehensive	88.76	84.32	96.97	
11720	Debridement of nails, 1-5	29.82	28.33	32.58	0
11721	Debridement of nails, 6 or more	29.82	28.33	32.58	0
11750	Exc nail or nail matrix	177.07	168.22	193.45	10
11765	Wedge exc of nail fold	53.04	50.39	57.95	10
19100	Bx breast, needle	88.03	83.63	96.17	0
19101	Bx breast, incisional	257.67	244.79	281.51	10
21330	Nasal fracture, open, complicated	548.71	521.27	599.46	90
27455	Osteotomy, proximal tibia	1142.36	1085.24	1248.03	90
45380	Colonoscopy with biopsy	349.98	332.48	382.35	0

Bx, Biopsy; *CPT, Current Procedural Terminology; est,* established; *exc,* excision; *OV,* office visit.

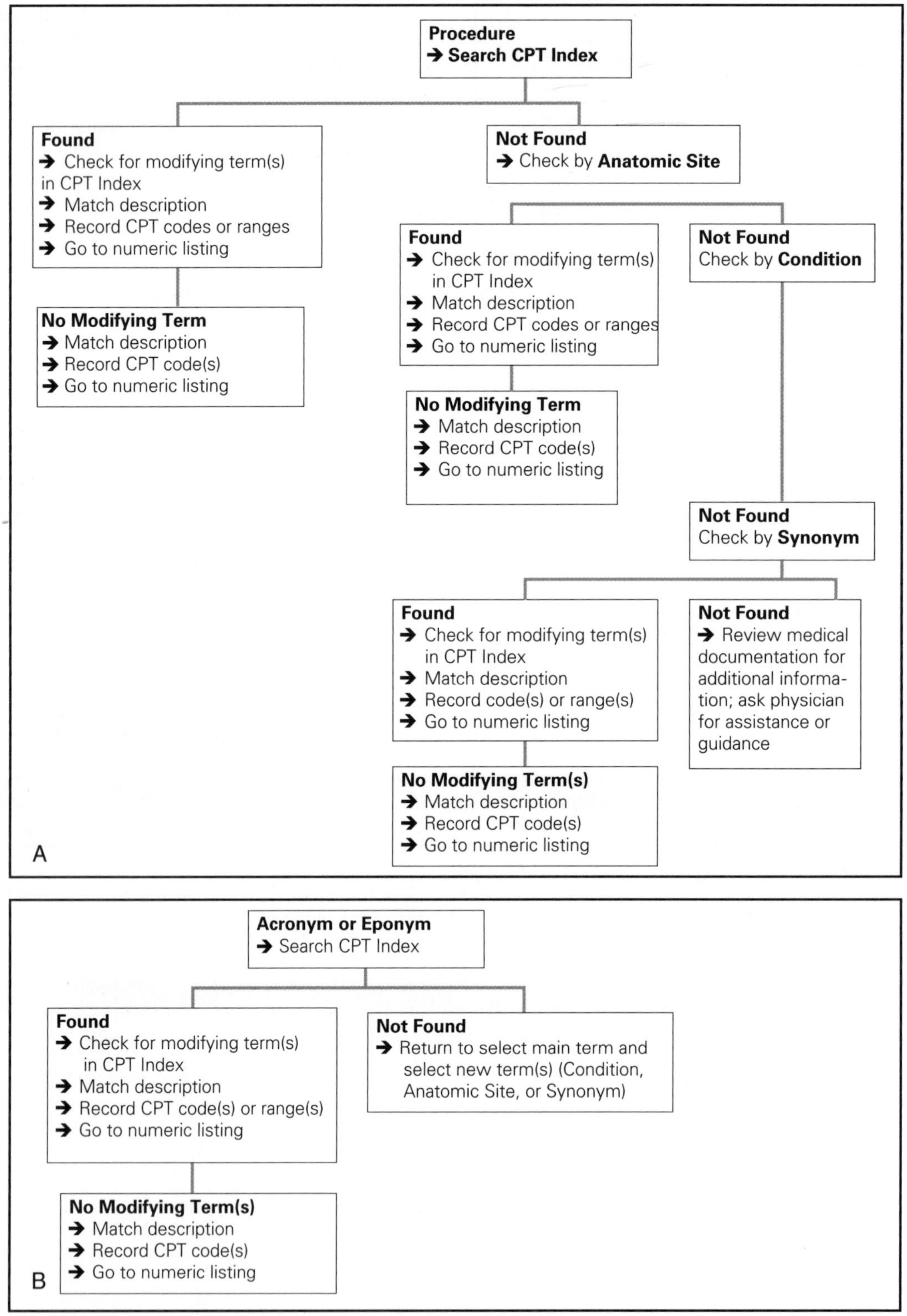

Procedure
➔ **Search CPT Index**

Found
➔ Check for modifying term(s) in CPT Index
➔ Match description
➔ Record CPT codes or ranges
➔ Go to numeric listing

No Modifying Term
➔ Match description
➔ Record CPT code(s)
➔ Go to numeric listing

Not Found
➔ Check by **Anatomic Site**

Found
➔ Check for modifying term(s) in CPT Index
➔ Match description
➔ Record CPT codes or ranges
➔ Go to numeric listing

No Modifying Term
➔ Match description
➔ Record CPT code(s)
➔ Go to numeric listing

Not Found
Check by **Condition**

Not Found
Check by **Synonym**

Found
➔ Check for modifying term(s) in CPT Index
➔ Match description
➔ Record code(s) or range(s)
➔ Go to numeric listing

No Modifying Term(s)
➔ Match description
➔ Record CPT code(s)
➔ Go to numeric listing

Not Found
➔ Review medical documentation for additional information; ask physician for assistance or guidance

A

Acronym or Eponym
➔ Search CPT Index

Found
➔ Check for modifying term(s) in CPT Index
➔ Match description
➔ Record CPT code(s) or range(s)
➔ Go to numeric listing

No Modifying Term(s)
➔ Match description
➔ Record CPT code(s)
➔ Go to numeric listing

Not Found
➔ Return to select main term and select new term(s) (Condition, Anatomic Site, or Synonym)

B

Fig. 13.12 A, Decision tree when coding a medical procedure using the current edition of *Current Procedural Terminology (CPT)* published by the American Medical Association (AMA). **B,** Decision tree when coding a medical procedure using an acronym or eponym and using the current edition of CPT published by the AMA.

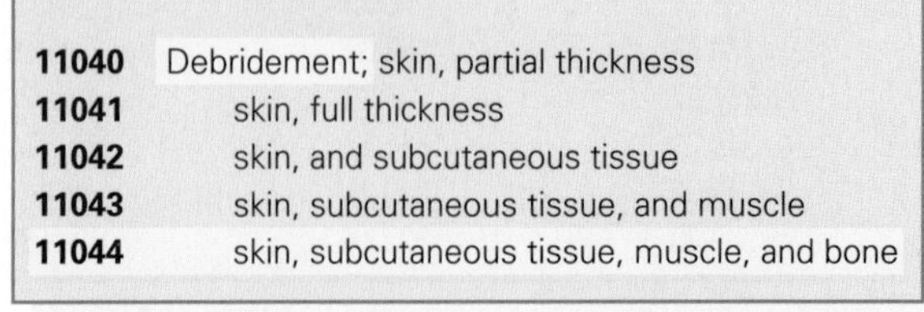

11040	Debridement; skin, partial thickness
11041	skin, full thickness
11042	skin, and subcutaneous tissue
11043	skin, subcutaneous tissue, and muscle
11044	skin, subcutaneous tissue, muscle, and bone

Fig. 13.13 Use of a semicolon.

CODING FOR MULTIPLE LESIONS

Paring or Cutting

11055 Paring or cutting of benign hyperkeratotic lesion (e.g., corn or callus); single lesion

11056 two to four lesions

11057 more than four lesions

A

24. A. DATE(S) OF SERVICE From MM	DD	YY	To MM	DD	YY	B. PLACE OF SERVICE	C. EMG	D. PROCEDURES, SERVICES, OR SUPPLIES (Explain Unusual Circumstances) CPT/HCPCS	MODIFIER	E. DIAGNOSIS POINTER	F. $ CHARGES	G. DAYS OR UNITS	H. EPSDT Family Plan	I. ID. QUAL.	J. RENDERING PROVIDER ID. #
05	11	20XX				11		99203		A	00 00	1		NPI	4627889700
05	11	20XX				11		11057		A	00 00	1		NPI	4627889700
														NPI	
														NPI	
														NPI	
														NPI	

B

Fig. 13.14 A, Procedure codes from the Surgery section of the *Current Procedural Terminology (CPT)* code book. **B,** Blocks 24A through 24J of the revised CMS-1500 (02-12) insurance claim form showing placement of the code on Line 2.

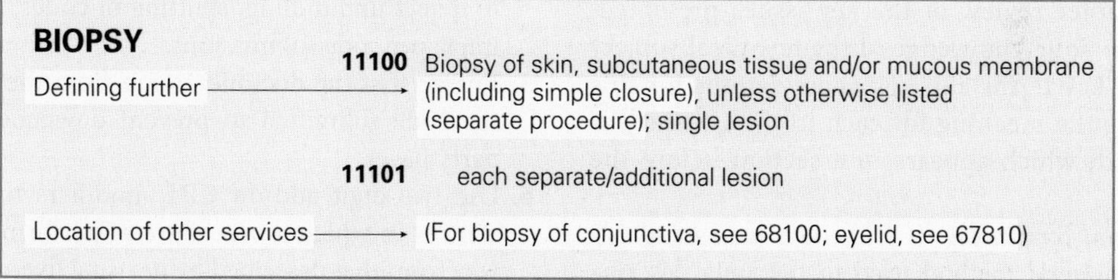

BIOPSY

Defining further → **11100** Biopsy of skin, subcutaneous tissue and/or mucous membrane (including simple closure), unless otherwise listed (separate procedure); single lesion

11101 each separate/additional lesion

Location of other services → (For biopsy of conjunctiva, see 68100; eyelid, see 67810)

Fig. 13.15 Use of parentheses in the Surgery section of the *Current Procedural Terminology* code book.

13150 Repair, complex, eyelids, nose, ears, and/or lips; 1.0 cm or less (See also 40650–40654, 67961–67975)

13151 1.1 cm to 2.5 cm

13152 2.6 cm to 7.5 cm

Fig. 13.16 Metric measurements in the Surgery section of the *Current Procedural Terminology* code book.

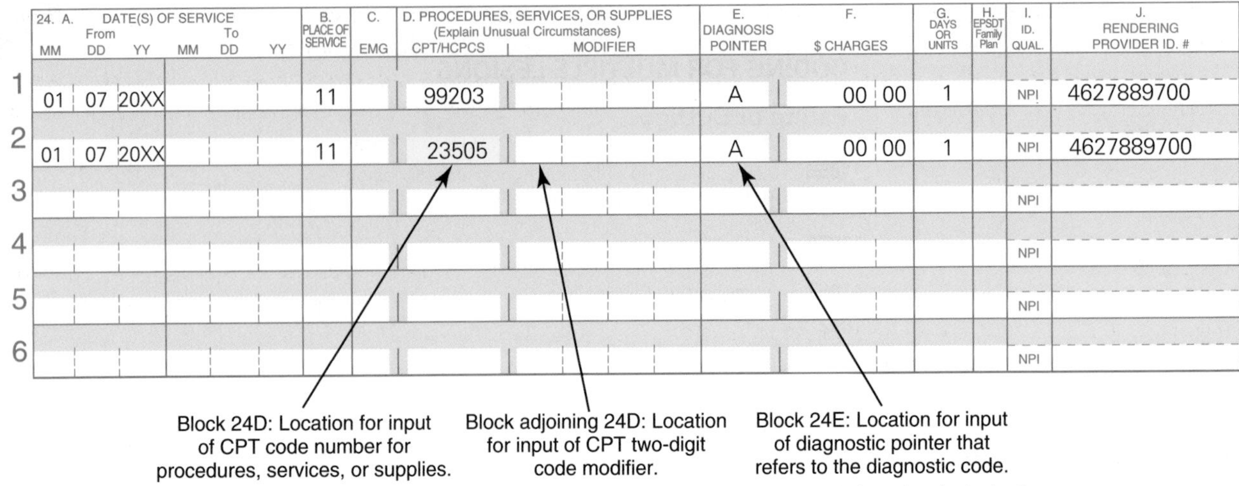

	24. A. DATE(S) OF SERVICE From MM	DD	YY	To MM	DD	YY	B. PLACE OF SERVICE	C. EMG	D. PROCEDURES, SERVICES, OR SUPPLIES (Explain Unusual Circumstances) CPT/HCPCS	MODIFIER	E. DIAGNOSIS POINTER	F. $ CHARGES	G. DAYS OR UNITS	H. EPSDT Family Plan	I. ID. QUAL.	J. RENDERING PROVIDER ID. #
1	01	07	20XX				11		99203		A	00 00	1		NPI	4627889700
2	01	07	20XX				11		23505		A	00 00	1		NPI	4627889700
3															NPI	
4															NPI	
5															NPI	
6															NPI	

Fig. 13.17 The billing portion of a completed claim form for closed manipulation of a clavicular fracture.

EXAMPLE 13.29 Blocks 24A Through 24J of the CMS-1500 Claim Form

Closed Manipulative Treatment of a Clavicular Fracture

Section:	Surgery, Musculoskeletal System
Anatomic subheading:	Shoulder
Condition:	Fracture or Dislocation
Code:	23505

Thus when completing an insurance claim form for closed manipulative treatment, clavicular fracture, the billing portion appears as follows (Fig. 13.17).

KEY POINTS

This is a brief chapter review of the key issues presented. To further enhance your knowledge of the technical subject matter, review the key terms and key abbreviations for this chapter by locating the meaning for each in the Glossary at the end of this text, which appears in a section before the Index.

1. *Current Procedural Terminology* (CPT) codes are a standardized five-digit numeric method used to precisely describe each service and procedure provided by physicians and allied health care professionals.
2. The Healthcare Common Procedure Coding System (HCPCS) has two levels: Level I, the American Medical Association's CPT codes and modifiers, and Level II, Centers for Medicare and Medicaid Services (CMS)–designated codes and alpha modifiers. HCPCS national codes are used to bill for ambulance, medical and surgical supplies, durable medical equipment, drugs administered other than oral method, and so on.
3. Each year when a new CPT code book is published, become familiar with code deletions, new codes, and description changes and observe the symbols and their interpretation in relation to the codes.
4. In CPT coding, *surgical package* is a term used to describe a surgical procedure code that includes the operation; local infiltration, digital block, or topical anesthesia; and normal, uncomplicated postoperative care all included in one fee. Code edits are performed on submitted insurance claims to detect unbundling, splitting of codes, and other types of improper code submissions.
5. Ensure that the documentation from the provider supports the code submitted to prevent downcoding by the third-party payer.
6. Use two-digit add-on CPT modifiers to indicate circumstances in which a procedure as performed differs in some way from that described by its usual five-digit code.
7. A fee schedule is a listing in an insurance policy of procedure code numbers with charges or preestablished allowances for specific medical services and procedures. The Medicare fee schedule is published annually and shows the maximum dollar amounts that Medicare will allow for each service rendered for a beneficiary.
8. The various methods of payment by insurance companies and state and federal programs are (1) fee schedules; (2) usual, customary, and reasonable (UCR); and (3) relative value studies or scale (RVS).
9. In final summary, the seven steps to accurate coding are as follows:
   - **a.** Read the patient's encounter form completely and any notes made by the health care provider.
   - **b.** Highlight words important to the selection of diagnostic and procedural codes.
   - **c.** Ask the provider to clarify any inconsistent or missing information and code only from actual documentation. Do not assume or guess.

d. Code each confirmed diagnosis and accompanying signs or symptoms using the highest level of specificity.
e. Code each medical service, procedure, and treatment provided in the documentation.
f. Verify medical necessity by associating each procedure code to the diagnostic code.
g. Recheck the codes selected by rereading the code descriptions and match them with the provider's notes to confirm the codes assigned.

STUDENT ASSIGNMENT

- Study Chapter 13.
- Answer the fill-in-the-blank, multiple-choice, and true/false review questions in the *Workbook* to reinforce the theory learned in this chapter and help prepare for a future test.
- Complete the assignments in the *Workbook* to assist you in hands-on practical experience in procedural coding and learning medical abbreviations.
- Turn to the Glossary at the end of this text for a further understanding of the key terms and key abbreviations used in this chapter.

UNIT 4

Claims Submission in the Medical Office

14

The Paper Claim CMS-1500

Cheryl Fassett

OBJECTIVES

After reading this chapter, you should be able to:

1. Identify the circumstances in which paper claims continue to be used.
2. Discuss the history of the Health Insurance Claim Form (CMS-1500).
3. Define and discuss the two types of claims submission.
4. Explain the difference between clean, pending, rejected, incomplete, and invalid claims, and discuss specific terms used to describe Medicare claims.
5. List the elements typically abstracted from the health record that are included in a cover letter accompanying an insurance claim.
6. Describe basic guidelines for submitting insurance claims.
7. Explain how the diagnostic fields of the CMS-1500 claim form would be completed.
8. Explain NPI numbers.
9. Discuss claim signatures, the importance of proofreading every paper claim, and supporting documentation for claims.
10. Describe reasons why claims are rejected.
11. Identify claim submission errors and discuss the solutions to correct the errors.
12. Identify techniques required for submission of claims.
13. Demonstrate the ability to complete the CMS-1500 claim form accurately for federal, state, and private payer insurance contracts using current basic guidelines.

KEY TERMS

Administrative Simplification Compliance Act
clean claim
deleted claim
dirty claim
durable medical equipment number
electronic claim
employer identification number
facility provider number
group National Provider Identifier
Health Insurance Claim Form
incomplete claim
intelligent character recognition
invalid claim
National Provider Identifier
National Uniform Claim Committee
optical character recognition
paper claim
pending claim
physically clean claim
rejected claim
Social Security number
state license number
suspended claim
taxonomy code

KEY ABBREVIATIONS

ASCA
CMS-1500
DME
DNA
EIN
EMG
EPSDT
ICR
LMP
MSP
NA, N/A
NPI
NUCC
OCR
SOF
SSN

THE PAPER CLAIM CMS-1500

The Health Insurance Claim Form (CMS-1500) is the standard paper claim form used by health care professionals and suppliers to bill insurance carriers for services provided to patients. The claim form has gone through many transitions throughout the years. The most recent version of the CMS-1500 claim form (02-12) was made mandatory as of April 1, 2014.

Paper claims were once used as our sole method of reporting health insurance claims but most health care organizations now send the majority of their claims to insurance carriers electronically, as a result of the Administrative Simplification Compliance Act (ASCA). ASCA was enacted by Congress to improve administration of the Medicare program by increasing efficiencies gained through electronic claims submission. ASCA required all claims sent to the Medicare program to be submitted electronically starting October 16, 2003. ASCA prohibits payment of services or supplies not submitted to Medicare electronically, with limited exceptions.

The paper claim continues to be an important part of the claims process that the insurance billing specialist must learn as a basic skill set. There are still circumstances under which the paper claim continues to be used, such as the following:

1. ASCA provides an exception to the Medicare electronic claims submission requirements to small health care organizations. ASCA defines a small health care organization or supplier as a provider of services with fewer than 25 full-time equivalent employees or a service provider, health care organization, facility, or supplier (other than a provider of services) with fewer than 10 full-time equivalent employees.
2. ASCA also allows an exemption to any health care organization who may be in an area that has disruptions in electricity and communication connections beyond control and expected to last more than 2 business days. Those health care organizations may report claims to Medicare on paper.
3. ASCA does not preclude health care organizations from submitting paper claims to other health plans. Other payers may allow or require submission of claims on paper.
4. There may be occasions whereby the health care organization's software program experiences technical downtime and the organization is unable to submit claims electronically for a period.
5. Paper claims often are used when reporting special services or require special processing because of unusual circumstances.
6. Paper claims are often used when resubmitting a claim for review after initial denial of the claim.
7. Paper claims can be provided to patients who have coverage with insurance with which the organization does not participate. The patient can then forward the paper claim to the insurance carrier for processing.
8. The paper claim may also be used to report patient encounter data to federal, state, and other public health agencies.

Essentially the paper claim is the basis for electronic claim submission and many software and hardware systems depend on the CMS-1500 claim form. Because of this and because paper claims are still part of the claims process in many circumstances, it is essential for the insurance billing specialist to fully understand the basic guidelines for submitting paper claims and how to properly complete the claim form.

National Uniform Claim Committee

The CMS-1500 claim form was developed by the **National Uniform Claim Committee (NUCC).** NUCC is a voluntary organization co-chaired by the American Medical Association (AMA) and Centers for Medicare and Medicaid Services (CMS). The committee is made up of health care industry stakeholders representing providers, payers, designated standards maintenance organizations, public health organizations, and vendors.

NUCC was formally named in the administrative simplification of the Health Insurance Portability and Accountability Act of 1996 (HIPAA) as the authoritative voice regarding national standard content. The committee is responsible for maintaining the integrity of the data sets and physical layout of the CMS-1500 claim form. It is further charged with the task of standardizing national instructions for completion of the claim form to be used by all payers. This may result in even more changes to the CMS-1500 claim form in the future.

History of the Paper Claim CMS-1500

The paper claim has origins as far back as 1958 when the Health Insurance Association of America (HIAA) and the AMA attempted to standardize the insurance claim form. Over the years, standardization has been the driving force to even further changes (Table 14.1). The current version of the claim form is referred to as the CMS-1500.

TABLE 14.1 History of the Paper Claim CMS-1500

Year	Description
1958	The Health Insurance Association of America (HIAA) and the American Medical Association (AMA) attempted to create a standardized insurance claim form that eventually became known as *COMB-1*, or *Attending Physician's Statement.*
1975	The AMA approved a "universal claim form," called the *Health Insurance Claim Form,* referred to as the *HCFA-1500,* which was an abbreviation for the *Health Care Financing Administration.* The AMA joined forces with the Centers for Medicare and Medicaid Services (CMS) and many other payer organizations, known as the *Uniform Claim Form Task Force,* to standardize and promote the use of their universal health claim form.
1990	The HCFA-1500 (12-90) was revised and printed in red ink, to allow optical scanning of claims. All services for Medicare patients from health care organizations, service providers and suppliers (except for ambulance services) reported after May 1, 1992, had to be billed on the scannable HCFA-1500 (12-90) form.
Mid-1990s	The Uniform Claim Form Task Force was replaced by the National Uniform Claim Committee (NUCC). The committee's goal was to develop the NUCC Data Set (NUCC-DS), a standardized data set for use in an electronic environment but applicable to and consistent with evolving paper claim form standards.
2001	The HCFA-1500 became known as the CMS-1500 when the Health Care Finance Administration was retitled the Centers for Medicare and Medicaid Services (CMS).
2005	It became necessary to change the CMS-1500 (12-90) so that it could accommodate reporting of the National Provider Identifier (NPI) for providers; this form was referred to as the CMS-1500 (08-05).
2009	NUCC began revision of the 1500 Claim Form to accommodate the updated Electronic Claims Submission (Version 5010 837P) changes and implementation of the new diagnosis coding system, ICD-10.
2012	NUCC released the revised version of the 1500 Health Insurance Claim Form (version 02-12), which accommodated changes needed for implementation of ICD-10.
January 6, 2014	Health plans, clearinghouses, and other information support vendors were required to handle and accept the newly revised (02-12) form effective January 6, 2014. Providers were allowed to use either the 08-05 or the revised (02-12) 1500 Claim Form until March 31, 2014.
April 1, 2014	The 1500 Claim Form (08-05) was discontinued and only revised claims (02-12) will be accepted for processing.

Widespread use of the CMS-1500 has saved time and simplified processing of claims for both health care organizations and insurance carriers. It has eliminated the need to complete the many different insurance forms previously brought into the office by patients.

Insurance carriers with various computer programs and equipment may have instructions on completion of the form that vary by locality and program. Local representatives of insurance carriers should always be contacted to find out their specific claim form instructions for completion. Quantities of the CMS-1500 can be purchased from many medical office supply companies or from the AMA by calling toll free to 800-621-8335. Per Medicare guidelines, the red ink versions of the CMS-1500 claim form cannot be duplicated; therefore the claim forms must be originals and not photocopies or they will not be processed.

TYPES OF SUBMITTED CLAIMS

A paper claim is one that is submitted on paper and converted to electronic form by insurance companies. Paper claims may be typed but are typically generated via computer.

In contrast, an electronic claim is one that is submitted to the insurance carrier via dial-up modem, direct data entry, or over the internet by way of digital subscriber line (DSL) or file transfer protocol (FTP). Electronic claims are digital files that are not printed on paper claim forms when submitted to the payer.

! COMPLIANCE ALERT

Compliance and Insurance Claim Forms

The Health Insurance Portability and Accountability Act (HIPAA) federal laws affect insurance claim submission. The provider rendering the service or procedure must be properly identified with the correct provider number. Claims must show only services rendered that have been properly documented and are medically necessary without evidence of fraud or abuse issues. HIPAA mandates use of electronic standards for automated transfer of certain health care data among payers, plans, and health care organizations. The National Provider Identifier (NPI) system for health care providers became effective on May 27, 2007, in connection with the electronic transactions identified in HIPAA.

Claim Status

Paper or electronic claims can be designated as clean, rejected, or pending/suspended.

A **clean claim** is a claim that was submitted within a third party payer's time limit and contains all necessary information so that it can be processed and paid promptly. A **physically clean claim** is one that has no staples or highlighted areas and on which the bar code area has not been deformed.

A **rejected claim** has not been processed or cannot be processed for various reasons. For example, a claim cannot be processed if the patient is not identified in the payer system, the provider is not active in the third-party payer records, or the claim was not submitted in a timely manner. A rejected claim is one that requires investigation, further clarification, and possibly answers to some questions. Such a claim should be resubmitted after proper corrections are made.

A **pending** or **suspended claim** is an insurance claim that is held for review or other reason by the third-party payer. The amount of time a claim is pended varies from carrier to carrier and from claim to claim. Some claims may take only an additional 9 to 10 days to process, whereas others may take more time and may be dependent on additional information requests sent to the health care organization. The insurance billing specialist should handle all additional information requests promptly to eliminate the long-term pending of claims. All pended claims should be monitored and followed up on if they are not promptly cleared for payment or denied.

Medicare Claim Status

In the Medicare program, specific terms are used to describe various claim processing situations. These terms may or may not be used by other insurance programs.

A *clean claim* means the following:

1. The claim has no deficiencies and passes all electronic edits.
2. The carrier does not need to investigate outside of the carrier's operation before paying the claim.
3. The claim is investigated on a postpayment basis, meaning that a claim is not delayed before payment and may be paid. After investigation, payments may be reconsidered and deemed not due. A refund may be requested from the health care organization.
4. The claim is subject to medical review with attached information or forwarded simultaneously with electronic medical claim (EMC) records.

Medicare claims not considered "clean" claims, which require investigation or development on a prepayment basis, are known as *other claims*. Health care organizations that participate in the Medicare program can expect electronic claim submissions to be processed within approximately 14 days of receipt. Health care organizations that are participating in the Medicare program and send paper submissions will not have claims processed until at least 27 days after receipt, and health care organizations that do not participate with the Medicare program will not have claims processed until at least 27 days after receipt.

An **incomplete claim** is any Medicare claim missing required information. It is identified to the health care organization so that it can be resubmitted as a new claim.

An **invalid claim** is any Medicare claim that contains complete, necessary information but is illogical or incorrect. For example, a claim listing an incorrect provider number for a referring physician is invalid. An invalid claim is identified to the health care organization and may be resubmitted.

A **dirty claim** is a claim submitted with errors, one requiring manual processing for resolving problems, or one rejected for payment. Pending or suspended claims are placed in this category because something is holding the claim back from payment.

A **deleted claim** is a claim canceled, deleted, or voided by a Medicare fiscal intermediary for the following reasons:

- CMS-1500 is not used
- Itemized charges are not provided
- More than six line items are submitted on the CMS-1500 claim form

- Patient's address is missing
- Internal clerical error was made
- Certificate of Medical Necessity (CMN) for durable medical equipment was not with the Part B claim or was incomplete or invalid
- Name of the store is not on the receipt that includes the price of the item

The Omnibus Budget Reconciliation Act (OBRA) requires Medicare administrative contractors to pay the prompt payment interest rate on all clean claims not paid in a timely manner. The government updates the interest rate on January 1 and July 1 each year on the United States Treasury Bureau of Fiscal Services page (https://www.fiscal.treasury.gov/fsservices/gov/pmt/promptPayment/rates.htm).

ABSTRACTING FROM MEDICAL RECORDS

The insurance billing specialist must be skilled at abstracting information from medical records. Abstraction of technical and clinical information from patient records may be necessary for claims processing. Insurance carriers often request additional information to process the claim or to support medical necessity before payment of a claim (Fig. 14.1).

Cover Letter Accompanying Insurance Claims

When requesting a review of a denied claim, the insurance billing specialist is required to send a cover letter with the claim. A letter accompanying insurance claims will generally require abstraction of information from the medical record and should include the following:

- Patient's name
- Subscriber's name (if different from that of the patient)
- Subscriber identification number
- Date and type of service
- Total amount of the claim
- A short history
- A clear but concise explanation of the medical necessity, difficulty or complexity, or unusual circumstance (for example, emergency)

The letter and insurance claim should be sent to the attention of the claims supervisor so that it may be directed to the appropriate person for processing.

HEALTH INSURANCE CLAIM FORM (CMS-1500)

Basic Guidelines for Submitting a Claim

The CMS-1500 claim form is accepted by nearly all Medicare, Medicaid, and private third-party payers as well as by TRICARE and workers' compensation. A claim form should be completed and submitted as required by payer rules on behalf of a patient who is covered by third-party insurance. If coverage is in question, the insurance carrier should be contacted about eligibility status. An official rejection from the insurance company is the best answer to present to the patient

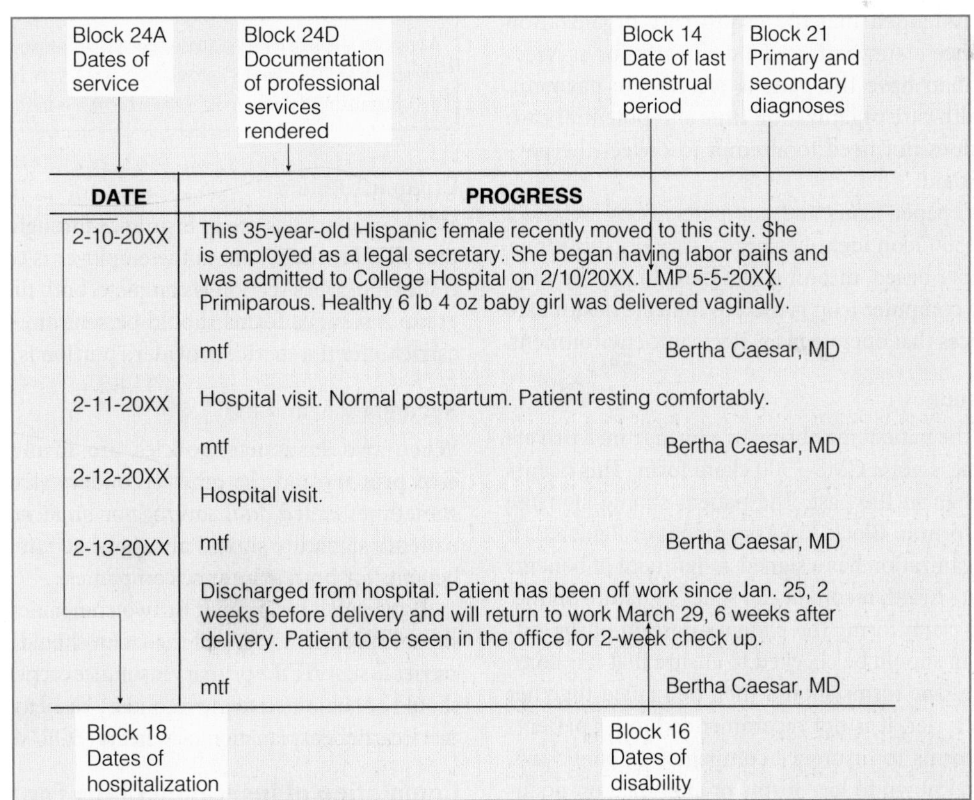

Fig. 14.1 A, Example of a chart note illustrating important information to read through and abstract for insurance claim completion.

14. DATE OF CURRENT: ILLNESS, INJURY, or PREGNANCY(LMP) MM DD YY 05 5 20XX QUAL. 484
15. OTHER DATE QUAL. MM DD YY
16. DATES PATIENT UNABLE TO WORK IN CURRENT OCCUPATION FROM 01 25 20XX TO 03 28 20XX
17. NAME OF REFERRING PROVIDER OR OTHER SOURCE 17a. 17b. NPI
18. HOSPITALIZATION DATES RELATED TO CURRENT SERVICES FROM 02 10 20XX TO 02 13 20XX
19. ADDITIONAL CLAIM INFORMATION (Designated by NUCC)
20. OUTSIDE LAB? YES [X] NO $ CHARGES
21. DIAGNOSIS OR NATURE OF ILLNESS OR INJURY Relate A-L to service line below (24E) ICD Ind. 0
A. O80 B. Z37.0 C. D. E. F. G. H. I. J. K. L.
22. RESUBMISSION CODE ORIGINAL REF. NO.
23. PRIOR AUTHORIZATION NUMBER

	24. A. DATE(S) OF SERVICE From MM DD YY	To MM DD YY	B. PLACE OF SERVICE	C. EMG	D. PROCEDURES, SERVICES, OR SUPPLIES (Explain Unusual Circumstances) CPT/HCPCS MODIFIER	E. DIAGNOSIS POINTER	F. $ CHARGES	G. DAYS OR UNITS	H. EPSDT Family Plan	I. ID. QUAL.	J. RENDERING PROVIDER ID. #
1	02 10 XX		21		59410	A B	1600 00	1		NPI	4305675700
2										NPI	
3										NPI	
4										NPI	
5										NPI	
6										NPI	

25. FEDERAL TAX I.D. NUMBER SSN EIN XX12210XX [X] EIN
26. PATIENT'S ACCOUNT NO.
27. ACCEPT ASSIGNMENT? (For govt. claims, see back) [X] YES NO
28. TOTAL CHARGE $ 1600 00
29. AMOUNT PAID $
30. Rsvd for NUCC Use
31. SIGNATURE OF PHYSICIAN OR SUPPLIER INCLUDING DEGREES OR CREDENTIALS (I certify that the statements on the reverse apply to this bill and are made a part thereof.) Bertha Caesar MD 021520XX SIGNED DATE
32. SERVICE FACILITY LOCATION INFORMATION College Hospital 4500 Broad Avenue Woodland Hills XY 12345-0001 a. X95073106 b.
33. BILLING PROVIDER INFO & PH # (555) 4869002 College Clinic 4567 Broad Avenue Woodland Hills XY 12345-0001 a. 3664021CC b.

ICD-10-CM

O80 Encounter for full-term uncomplicated delivery

Z37.0 Single live birth

CPT

59410 Vaginal delivery only (with or without episiotomy and/or forceps); including postpartum care

B

Fig. 14.1, cont'd B, The location of the abstracted information placed in the blocks on a CMS-1500 insurance claim form in optical character recognition (OCR) format.

in this situation. The patient may be unaware of the status of his or her health care policy coverage and current deductible status. It is recommended that the health care organization submit an insurance claim and get paid directly for services rendered rather than have the patient receive the payment. This saves the health care organization time and potential cash flow issues as it does not need to attempt to collect the payment from the patient.

In this chapter, paper icons and computer icons are used. The paper CMS-1500 icon identifies health care organizations' offices that are paper based, meaning that they do not file electronic claims. The computer icon is used to indicate health care organizations' offices that operate in an electronic environment.

Individual Insurance

In very rare cases the patient may bring in a form from a private insurance plan that is not a CMS-1500 claim form. This occurs less often today than in the past. The patient should sign the CMS-1500 claim form in Block 13 (Assignment of Benefits). If the health care organization has a signed assignment of benefits form in the patient's health record, it can state "signature on file" on the CMS-1500 claim form. The patient's portion of the private insurance form should be checked to ensure that it is complete and accurate. The forms should then be mailed together to the insurance carrier. It is not recommended to let patients direct their own forms to insurance companies or employers. Patients have been known to lose forms or alter data on documents before mailing, forget to send them, or mail them to an incorrect address.

EXAMPLE 14.1 Primary and Secondary Insurance Plans

A husband and wife have insurance through their employers and both have added the spouse to their plans for secondary coverage. If the wife is seen for treatment, the insurance plan to which she is the subscriber is the primary carrier for her.

Group Insurance

When a patient has group insurance through an employer, ensure that all information about the employer is complete and correct. If the employer's section is complete, both the CMS-1500 and the group insurance forms should be sent directly to the insurance carrier after the service provider's portion is completed.

Secondary Insurance

When two insurance policies are involved, one is considered primary and the other secondary (Example 14.1). This is sometimes called *dual coverage* or *duplication of coverage*. The patient's signature should always be acquired for assignment of benefits for both insurance companies.

If the patient is insured by two companies, the primary carrier should be determined and the claim should be submitted to that carrier first. After the primary insurance carrier has paid out, a claim should be submitted to the secondary carrier with a copy of the primary carrier's explanation of benefits (EOB) document attached.

Completion of Insurance Claim Forms

It is recommended that the CMS-1500 claim form be completed following NUCC's Reference Instruction Manual, unless the individual payer has advised otherwise and provided his or her own guidelines for completion of the form. NUCC's guidelines provide block-by-block instructions for completion. Those blocks that are considered to be conditional will be noted in the instructions. If any questions are unanswerable, do not use the abbreviations DNA (does not apply), NA (not applicable), or N/A (not applicable) but leave the space blank.

Diagnosis

In Block 21, the diagnosis field of the CMS-1500 claim form, all accurate diagnostic codes that affect the patient's condition should be inserted, with the primary diagnosis code listed first followed by any secondary or tertiary diagnosis codes. The CMS-1500 claim form has the ability to report 12 diagnostic codes.

A diagnosis should never be submitted without supporting documentation in the medical record. The diagnosis must support the medical necessity of the treatment and services rendered. If there is no formal diagnosis at the conclusion of an encounter, the code(s) for the patient's symptom(s) should be submitted.

It is best to list only one illness or injury and its treatment per form, unless there are concurrent conditions, to avoid confusing services with multiple medical conditions. A concurrent condition is a disorder that coexists with the primary condition, complicating the treatment and management of the primary disorder. It may alter the course of treatment required or lengthen the expected recovery time of the primary condition. It also is referred to as comorbidity.

Service Dates

Dates of service must be entered with no spaces using a 6-digit or 8-digit format; for example, January 2, 20XX, should appear as either 0102XX or 010220XX. The appropriate date of service format to be used is noted in NUCC's instructions section of each Item Number on the CMS-1500 claim form. Do not use ditto marks (") to indicate repetition of dates for services performed on subsequent lines. Charges for services rendered in different years should not be submitted on the same claim form. This type of situation can occur when claims processing is affected by deductible and eligibility factors, thereby delaying reimbursement.

Consecutive Dates

Some carriers allow medical services, hospital services, or office visits to be grouped if each visit is consecutive, occurs in the same month, uses the same procedure code, or results in the same fee. The total fee for the procedures should be listed in Block 24F and the number of times the procedure was performed or service supplied should be listed in Block 24G, as illustrated in the graphic at the bottom of this page (Example: $55.56 × 5 = $277.80). However, some private insurance carriers require a single fee listed in Block 24F rather than the total fee for the procedures. If there is a difference in the procedure code or fee for several visits listed on the claim, each separately coded hospital or office visit must be itemized and each procedure or service code and charge entered on a separate line.

No Charge

Insurance claims should not be submitted for services that have no charge, such as global or surgical package postoperative visit, unless the patient requests that it be sent. These services should only appear documented in the patient's health and financial records.

Physicians' or Service Provider's Identification Numbers

Insurance companies and federal and state programs require certain identification numbers on claim forms to be submitted from health care organizations and service providers. This can be confusing to the beginner, as well as to someone experienced in insurance billing procedures, because there are so many different numbers.

- *State license number.* To practice within a state, each physician or service provider must obtain a state license number. Sometimes this number is requested on forms and is used as a provider number.
- *Employer identification number.* In a health care organization, many service providers may file taxes as a group and thus be under the same employer identification number (EIN) or tax identification number (TIN). This is issued by the Internal Revenue Service for income tax purposes. Some organizations may opt to separate finances and require separate TINs for each provider.

25. FEDERAL TAX I.D. NUMBER	SSN	EIN
74 10640XX	☐	☒

- *Social Security number.* Each service provider has a Social Security number (SSN) for other personal use and use this as an EIN in a solo practice.

A Social Security number is not typically used on the claim form unless the provider does not have an EIN, in which case the Social Security number may be required.

25. FEDERAL TAX I.D. NUMBER	SSN	EIN
082 XX 1707	☒	☐

- *National Provider Identifiers.* The National Provider Identifier (NPI) is a HIPAA administrative simplification standard. Covered health care providers, health care organizations, all health plans, and health care clearinghouses must use the unique 10-digit NPIs in the administrative and financial transactions adopted under HIPAA. Providers began using the NPI on May 23, 2007, except for small health plans whose compliance date was May 23, 2008. The NPI is a lifetime 10-digit number that replaces all other numbers assigned by various health plans. A health care provider is assigned only one NPI, which is retained for a lifetime even if he or she moves to another state. Under HIPAA, providers are required

	24. A. DATE(S) OF SERVICE From MM	DD	YY	To MM	DD	YY	B. PLACE OF SERVICE	C. EMG	D. PROCEDURES, SERVICES, OR SUPPLIES (Explain Unusual Circumstances) CPT/HCPCS	MODIFIER	E. DIAGNOSIS POINTER	F. $ CHARGES	G. DAYS OR UNITS	H. EPSDT Family Plan	I. ID. QUAL.	J. RENDERING PROVIDER ID. #
1	10	04	XX	10	08	XX	21		99232		A	277 80	5		NPI	32783127XX
2															NPI	

to share their NPIs with other providers, organizations, health plans, clearinghouses, and any entity that may need it for their own billing purposes

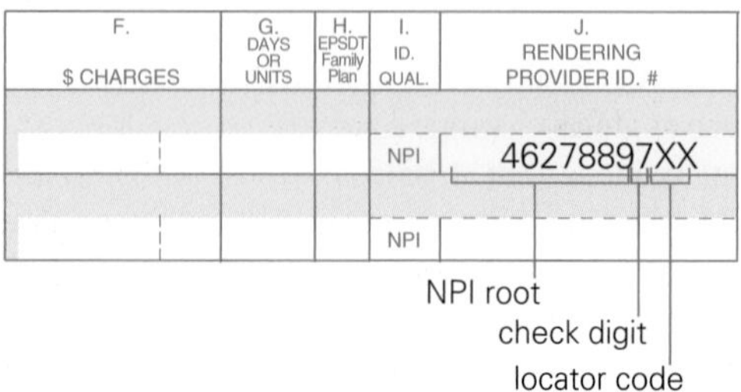

Claims may require several NPI numbers: one for the referring physician, one for the ordering physician, one for the performing physician, and one for the billing entity. It is possible that the ordering physician and performing physician are the same. On rare occasions the number may be the same for all three, but more commonly different numbers are required, depending on the circumstances of the case. For placement of the NPI number on the CMS-1500 claim form, refer to the block-by-block instructions for Blocks 17a, 17b, and 24J. Keep in mind what role the physicians and their numbers represent in relation to the provider listed in Block 33. The following examples of blocks from the CMS-1500 insurance claim form show where these numbers are commonly placed. Insurance billing manuals from major insurers give specific directions.

When a non-physician practitioner (NPP) bills incident-to a physician in the same group but that physician is out of the office on a day the NPP sees the patient, another physician in the same group can provide direct supervision to meet the incident-to requirements. When the ordering and supervising doctors are different individuals, the ordering doctor's name goes in Block 17 and his or her NPI goes in Block 17b. The NPI of the supervising doctor goes in Block 24J and the supervising physician signs the form in Block 31. The group's NPI goes in Block 33a.

To assist with claims completion, a reference list of provider numbers should be compiled for all ordering physicians and physicians who frequently refer patients. For Medicare claims, physicians' provider numbers can be obtained by calling their offices, contacting the Medicare carrier, or searching the NPI Registry on the internet. For license numbers, search the state licensing board on the internet.

Group National Provider Identifier (group NPI). The group NPI is used instead of the individual NPI for the performing provider who is a member of a group practice that submits claims to insurance companies under the group name.

33. BILLING PROVIDER INFO & PH # (555) 4869002
College Clinic
4567 Broad Avenue
Woodland Hills XY 12345-0001
a. 3664021CC b.

- *Durable medical equipment number.* Health care organizations who charge patients a fee for supplies and equipment such as crutches, urinary catheters, ostomy supplies, surgical dressings, and so forth must bill insurance carriers using a **durable medical equipment (DME) number.**

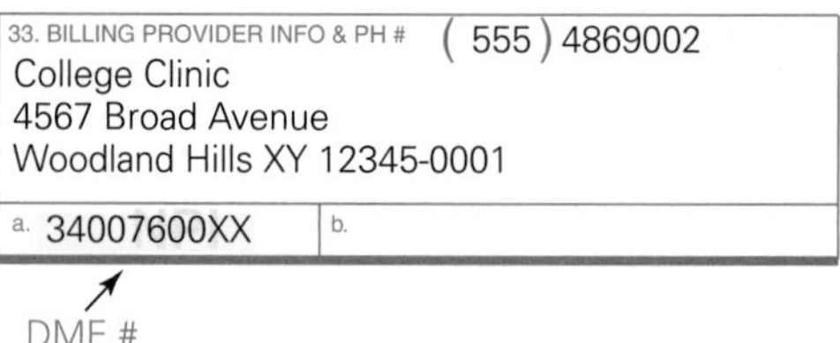
33. BILLING PROVIDER INFO & PH # (555) 4869002
College Clinic
4567 Broad Avenue
Woodland Hills XY 12345-0001
a. 34007600XX b.

- **Facility provider number.** Each facility (for example, hospital, laboratory, radiology office, skilled nursing facility) is issued a facility provider number to be used by the performing physician or service provider to report services done at the location.

32. SERVICE FACILITY LOCATION INFORMATION
College Hospital
4500 Broad Avenue
Woodland Hills XY 12345-0001
a. X9507310XX b.

- **Taxonomy code.** A taxonomy code is assigned to each service provider based on education and training. It is used to define specialty. When applying for an NPI number, a health care provider must select the Health Care Provider Taxonomy code or code description that identifies the health care provider's type, classification, or specialization and report that in its NPI application. Some payers may either assign a provider identifier or prefer that the taxonomy code be inserted on CMS-1500 claim forms. Depending on issues of each case, provider taxonomy codes may or may not be required on the form. When needed, the blocks affected are Blocks 17a, 19, 24I, 24J, 32b, or 33b (Example 14.2).

Physician or Service Provider's Signature

The physician or service provider should sign the insurance claim form above or under their typed or preprinted name. In the computerized office environment, the health care organization's billing system will generate a paper CMS-1500 form.

EXAMPLE 14.2 Service Provider Specialty and Taxonomy Codes

Medicare Specialty Code	Medicare Provider/ Supplier Type Description	Provider Taxonomy Code	Provider Taxonomy Description: Type, Classification, Specialization
33	Physician/ Thoracic Surgery	208G00000X	Allopathic and Osteopathic Physicians/Thoracic Surgery
34	Physician/Urology	208800000X	Allopathic and Osteopathic Physicians/Urology
34	Physician/Urology	2088P0231X	Allopathic and Osteopathic Physicians/Urology, Pediatric Urology

In general, the participating contract with the third-party payer allows the service provider's name to simply be printed in the signature block. This is an acceptable method for the provider's signature.

Insurance Billing Specialist's Initials

If more than one person is assigned to complete insurance paper claims, then the insurance billing specialist should place his or her initials in the bottom left or top right corner of the claim form. Placement of this reference should be consistent. The following are three good reasons to adopt this habit:

- To identify who in the office is responsible for the insurance form
- To decrease errors
- To avoid being accused of someone else's error, especially if another biller submitted a fraudulent claim

Proofread

Ideally every paper claim should be proofread for transposition of numbers (group, policy, physician's ID, procedure, and diagnostic codes), misspelled name, missing date of birth, blanks, and attachments. Larger, more complex claims require special attention because they involve greater sums of money and may be more difficult to complete. Ensure that the bill is for the right patient by checking the address and date of birth to verify the correct individual. Review the encounter form to charge for the correct tests and number of tests so that the patient is not charged more than once for the same service.

Review the bill for the correct number of units when reporting time-based services. For example, a patient seen for 16 minutes should show a billing for one 15-minute session. Check for any overcoding. For example, do not bill for a longer office visit that included paperwork time when only actual face-to-face time should have been charged. Double check to ensure codes are not unbundled. It is fraudulent to bill for charges that should be included in the cost of something else, or codes that are included in another code. Proofreading data prevents subsequent denials and avoids time-consuming responses to questions.

Supporting Documentation

Occasionally claims need supporting documents to further explain services billed and to obtain maximum reimbursement. The following information should be included in case the attachment is separated from the claim during processing.

- The patient's name
- Subscriber's name (if different from that of the patient)
- Date of service
- Insurance identification number

This same information should be placed on each page of the document, front and back if two-sided. If a medication is expensive or experimental, a copy of the invoice received from the supply house or pharmacy should be sent.

When a procedure is complicated, takes additional time to perform, or falls outside of the manner in which the procedure is typically performed, it is reasonable for the health care organization to request additional reimbursement. In those cases, a copy of all pertinent reports (operative, radiology, laboratory, pathology, and discharge summary) should be included with the claim. For a treatment not listed in the procedure code book, a special detailed report should be sent that gives the nature, extent, and need for the services, along with the time, effort, supplies, and equipment required. The correct code number should be used for unlisted services or procedures (Example 14.3).

EXAMPLE 14.3 Unlisted Procedure

951**99**	Unlisted allergy/clinical immunologic service or procedure

Office Pending File

The office copy of the insurance form should be filed in a separate alpha file for insurance claim copies unless the computer system maintains files. This file should be reviewed for follow-up every 30 days. The health care organization's billing system will keep an accurate record of all patients and activity on their accounts.

COMMON REASONS WHY CLAIM FORMS ARE DELAYED OR REJECTED

It is wise to be aware of common billing errors and know how to correct them to reduce the number of appeals and get claims paid faster. This may help to avoid additional administrative burdens, such as telephone calls, resubmission of claims, and appeal letters. Table 14.2 contains some reasons why claims are rejected or delayed and suggested solutions when completing the CMS-1500 insurance claim form blocks.

ADDITIONAL CLAIM SUBMISSION ERRORS

PROBLEM: Carolyn, the insurance billing specialist, telephoned the insurance company and discovered there was no record of the claim at the third-party payer.

SOLUTION: Always keep copies of paper claims. Send claims with large dollar amounts by certified mail with return receipt requested. Another option is to request that the customer service representative search the insurance carrier's imaging file for the period beginning on the date of service and ending on the date you are calling. Sometimes the claim was received and scanned but was never crossed over to the processing unit.

PROBLEM: Claire is in a hurry and submits a claim form that is illegible.

SOLUTION: Never handwrite a claim form. Check printer ink or toner and replace when necessary.

PROBLEM: Untimely or lack of response to claim development letters is discovered.

SOLUTION: Pay close attention to the due date and reply to third-party payer's requests for additional information as soon as possible. Send a copy of the claim with the letter and appropriate medical documentation listing the claim control number, if assigned.

TABLE 14.2 The Paper Claim: Problem Solving

Block Number(s)	Problem	Solution
1	When submitting a paper claim, the wrong block is checked (that is, claim submitted to the secondary insurer instead of the primary insurer).	Obtain data from the patient during the first visit as to which company is the primary insurer, depending on illness, injury, or accident. Submit the claim to the primary carrier and then send in a claim with a copy of the primary carrier's EOB to the secondary carrier.
1–13	Information missing on patient portion of the claim form.	Obtain a complete patient registration form from which information can be extracted. If patients are filling out their portion, educate patients on data requirements at the time of their first visit to the health care organization. Be sure to ask if there have been any changes on subsequent office visits.
1a	Patient's insurance number is incorrect or transposed (especially in Medicare and Medicaid cases).	Proofread numbers carefully from source documents. Always photocopy front and back sides of insurance identification cards.
2	Patient's name and insured's name are entered as the same when the patient is a dependent. A common error is that the patient is listed as the insured when he or she is not the insured (for example, spouse or child). Block 4 is used for listing the insured's name.	Verify the insured party and check for Sr, Jr, and correct birth date.
2	Patient name is missing, illegible, or incorrect.	Patient's name must be entered exactly as it appears on the patient's ID card.
3	Incorrect gender identification, resulting in a diagnosis or procedure code that is inconsistent with patient's gender.	Proofread the claim before mailing and review the patient's medical record to locate gender, especially if the patient's first name could be male or female.
5	Patient address is missing or illegible.	Enter the patient's complete address and telephone number. Do not puncture the address or phone number. When entering a 9-digit zip code, include the hyphen.
9a–9d	Incomplete entry for other insurance coverage.	Accurately abstract data from the patient's registration form and input it to the computer database. Telephone the patient if information is incomplete.
10	Failure to indicate whether patient's condition is related to employment or an "other" type of accident.	Review patient's medical history to find out details of injury or illness and proofread claim before mailing. Telephone the employer to see if permission was given to treat the patient as a workers' compensation case.
14	Date of injury, date of LMP, or dates of onset of illness are omitted. This information is important for determining whether accident benefits apply, patient is eligible for maternity benefits, or there was a preexisting condition.	Do not list unless dates are clearly documented in the patient's medical record. Read the patient's medical history and call the patient to obtain the date of accident or LMP. Compose an addendum to the record if necessary. Always proofread a paper claim before mailing in case data are missing.
17, 17a, 17b	Incorrect or missing name or NPI of referring physician on claim for consultation or other services requiring this information.	Check the patient registration form and the chart note for reference to the referring physician. Develop a list of NPI numbers for all physicians in the area.
19	Attachments (for example, prescription, operative report, manufacturer's invoice) or Medicaid verification (for example, labels, identification numbers) is missing.	Submit all information required for pricing or coverage on an 8.5- × 11-inch paper with the patient's name, subscriber name (if other than patient), and insurance identification number on each attachment (enclosure). Type the word "ATTACHMENT" in Block 19 or 10d. Never staple or clip documentation to a claim.
21	The diagnostic code is missing, incomplete, invalid, or not in standard nomenclature (for example, missing fourth or fifth digit); it includes a written description or does not correspond to the treatment (procedure code) rendered by the physician.	Verify and submit correct diagnostic codes by referring to an updated diagnostic code book and reviewing the patient record. Check with the provider if the diagnosis code listed does not go with the procedure code shown. Do not include decimal point.
24A	Omitted, incorrect, overlapping, or duplicate dates of service.	Verify against the encounter form or medical record that all dates of service are listed and accurate and appear on individual lines on paper claims. Date spans for multiple services must be adequate for the number and types of services provided. Each month should be on a separate line and each year should be on a separate claim.
24B	Missing or incorrect place of service code. If a provider sees a patient in a SNF that is in the same building as a domicile rest home or a hospice, it is possible to incorrectly document the SNF as the site for each patient.	Verify the place of service from the encounter form or medical record and list the correct code for place of service and submitted procedure.

TABLE 14.2 **The Paper Claim: Problem Solving—cont'd**

Block Number(s)	Problem	Solution
24D	Procedure codes are incorrect, invalid, or missing.	Verify the coding system used by the third-party payer and submit correct procedure code(s) by referring to a current procedure code book. For Medicare patients and certain private insurance plans, check the HCPCS manual for CMS national and local procedure codes.
24D	Incorrect or missing modifier(s).	Verify usage of modifiers by referring to a current procedure code book and HCPCS manual. Submit valid modifiers with the correct procedure codes
24E	Diagnosis Pointer is required.	Enter the associated diagnosis by referencing the pointers (A to L) listed in Block 21 that relate to the date of service and the procedures performed. Diagnosis codes must be valid ICD-9 or ICD-10 codes for the date of service.
24F	Omitted or incorrect amount billed.	Be certain that the fee column is filled in. Check the amounts charged with the appropriate fee schedule.
24G	Days/units are required on claim forms.	Enter quantity. Value entered must be greater than zero. (Field allows up to three digits.)
24G	Reasons for multiple visits made in 1 day are not stated on an attachment sheet.	Depending on insurance guidelines, submit documentation explaining reason for multiple visits. Use appropriate modifiers or upcode evaluation and management services to include all visits.
24G	Incorrect quantity billed.	Verify charge amounts. Ensure that the number of units listed is equal to the date span when more than one date of service is billed (for example, hospital visits).
24J	Provider's identification number is missing.	Verify and insert the required provider's number in this block.
24A–24J, Line 6	More than six lines entered on a paper claim.	Insert service date and corresponding procedure on Lines 1 to 6 only. Complete an additional paper claim if more services should be billed.
27	Assignment acceptance must be indicated on the claim.	"Yes" or "No" must be checked.
28	Total amounts do not equal itemized charges.	Total charges for each claim and verify amounts with patient account. If number of units listed in Block 24G is more than one, multiply the units by the fee listed in Block 24F and add to all other charges listed.
31	Physician's signature is missing.	Have the physician or physician's representative sign the claim using a removable indicator "Sign Here" tag to indicate the correct location or key in "SOF" or "signature on file".
32	Information is not centered in block as required when submitting a paper claim.	Enter data centered in block.
33	Provider's address, NPI, or group number is missing.	The billing provider's name and address are required. A physical location must be entered; P.O. boxes are not acceptable. Obtain provider's data from a list that contains all s' professional information.

CMS, Centers for Medicare and Medicaid Services; *EOB*, explanation of benefits; *HCPCS*, Health Care Common Procedure Coding System; *LMP*, last menstrual period; *NPI*, National Provider Identifier; *SNF*, skilled nursing facility.

PROBLEM: Phillip reviews the Medicare remittance advice and discovers a noncovered service that is not considered medically necessary.

SOLUTION: For Medicare claims, check the local coverage determination policies and national coverage determination policies for diagnosis requirements. For private claims, check the insurance policy for the service. Verify that the diagnosis billed indicates necessity for the medical procedure or service.

PROBLEM: Noncovered service occurs because a routine screening procedure is performed in conjunction with a routine examination.

SOLUTION: Determine whether it is a diagnostic or preventive service and if the code is correct. Use the GY modifier when submitting a statutory-excluded service for payment by the secondary insurance carrier.

PROBLEM: Payment is adjusted because the care may be covered by another insurance plan per coordination of benefits.

SOLUTION: Always check all Medicare patients' coverage. Verify eligibility on the Medicare interactive voice recognition system before transmitting the claim.

PROBLEM: Payment is adjusted because the medical service is not paid separately because it is a global surgery or a National Correct Coding Initiative (NCCI) denial.

SOLUTION: Determine the global period for the surgical procedure. Use a modifier to report an unrelated or exception service within a global period. Check the NCCI edits to see if the code selected has been deleted or is a bundled service.

PROBLEM: Irene submits a claim with missing, incomplete, or invalid information regarding where the medical services were performed.

SOLUTION: Include the zip code of where the service was performed.

PROBLEM: In reviewing a Medicare remittance advice (RA) document, Anne notices that it indicates that Mrs. Bentley's medical expenses were incurred before insurance coverage.

SOLUTION: Always verify all Medicare patients' coverage. Review the patient's Medicare card for entitlement and effective dates. Verify eligibility on the Medicare interactive voice recognition system before transmitting the claim. Verify that the claim is submitted with the correct Medicare number, including the alpha suffix.

CLAIM COMPLETION GUIDELINES*

Optical Character Recognition

The majority of paper claims are scanned using **optical character recognition (OCR),** less commonly referred to as **intelligent character recognition (ICR)** or *image copy recognition (ICR)*. This technology has been used across the nation in processing insurance claims to enable greater speed and efficiency. A scanner can transfer printed or typed text and bar codes to the insurance company's computer memory. Scanners read at such a fast speed that they reduce data entry cost and decrease processing time. More control is gained over data input using OCR. It improves accuracy thus reducing coding errors, because the claim is entered exactly as coded by the insurance billing specialist.

Do's and Don'ts for Claim Completion

Basic do's and don'ts for completing claims follow.

Do: Use original claim forms printed in red ink; photocopies and forms generated from ink jet or laser printers cannot be scanned. Laser jet printing is preferable for computer-generated claims.

Do: Computer-generate or type all information in black ink.

Don't: Handwrite information on the document. Handwriting is accepted only for signatures. Handwritten claims require manual processing.

2 nd request

PICA

FECA BLK LUNG (ID#) | OTHER (ID#) | 1a. INSURED'S I.D. NUMBER 111704521 | (For Program in Item 1) A482

Do: Align the printer correctly so that characters appear exactly in the proper fields. Enter all information within designated fields.

PICA

1. MEDICARE (Medicare#) | MEDICAID (Medicaid#) | TRICARE (ID#DoD#) | CHAMPVA (Member ID#) | GROUP HEALTH PLAN (ID#) X | FECA BLK LUNG (ID#) | OTHER (ID#)

2. PATIENT'S NAME (Last Name, First Name, Middle Initial): Forehand, Harry, N

3. PATIENT'S BIRTH DATE MM DD YY: 01 06 1946 SEX M X F

5. PATIENT'S ADDRESS (No., Street): 1456 Main Street

6. PATIENT RELATIONSHIP TO INSURED: Self X Spouse Child Other

CITY: Woodland Hills STATE: XY

8. RESERVED FOR NUCC USE

ZIP CODE: 12345-0000 TELEPHONE (Include Area Code): (555) 4909876

Don't: Allow characters to touch lines

Correct

PICA

FECA BLK LUNG (ID#) | OTHER (ID#) | 1a. INSURED'S I.D. NUMBER 123456789 | (For Program in Item 1)

Incorrect

PICA

FECA BLK LUNG (ID#) | OTHER (ID#) | 1a. INSURED'S I.D. NUMBER 123456789 | (For Program in Item 1)

Don't: Use script, slant, minifont, or italicized fonts or expanded, compressed, or bold print. Use fonts that have the same width for each character.

Do: Keep characters within the borders of each field. Use 10-pitch Pica or Arial or 10-, 11-, or 12-point type.

Don't: Strike over any errors when correcting or crowd preprinted numbers; OCR equipment does not read corrected characters on top of correction tape or correction fluid.

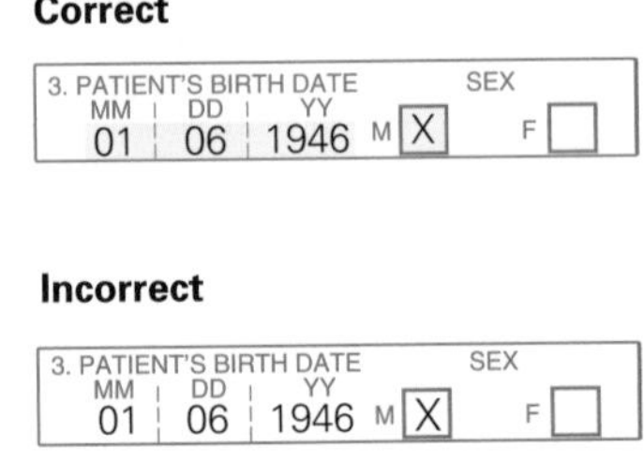
Correct

3. PATIENT'S BIRTH DATE MM DD YY 01 06 1946 SEX M X F

Incorrect

3. PATIENT'S BIRTH DATE MM DD YY 01 06 1946 SEX M X F

Do: Complete a new form for additional services if the case has more than six lines of service.

Correct

6 04 07 XX | 11 | 99214

Correct

24. A. DATE(S) OF SERVICE From MM DD YY To MM DD YY | B. PLACE OF SERVICE | C. EMG | D. PROCEDURES, SERVICES, OR SUPPLIES (Explain Unusual Circumstances) CPT/HCPCS MODIFIER

1 04 10 XX | 21 | 30520

Incorrect

6 040720XX 041020XX | 11 21 | 99214 30520

*Annual update information for CMS-1500 is provided by NUCC in July.

Don't: Use highlighter pens or colored ink on claims.

Don't: Use decimals in Block 21 or dollar signs ($) in the money column.

Correct

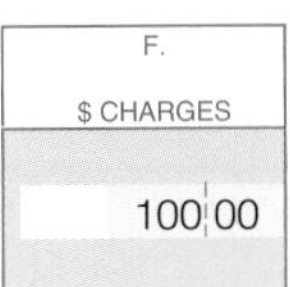

F.
$ CHARGES
100 00

Incorrect

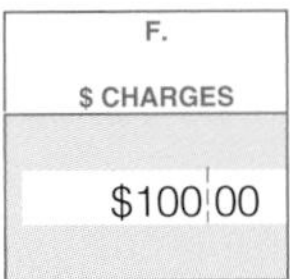

F.
$ CHARGES
$100 00

Don't: Use narrative descriptions of procedures, modifiers, or diagnoses; code numbers are sufficient.

Correct

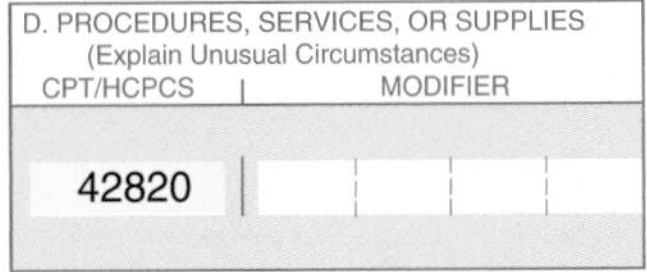

D. PROCEDURES, SERVICES, OR SUPPLIES
(Explain Unusual Circumstances)
CPT/HCPCS | MODIFIER
42820

Incorrect

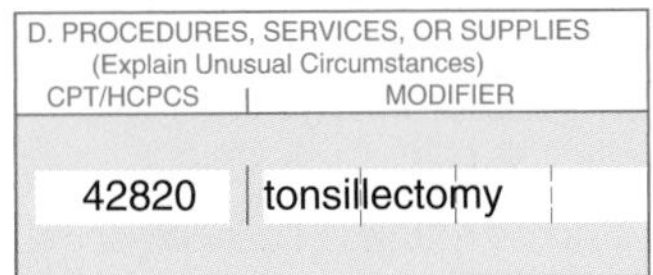

D. PROCEDURES, SERVICES, OR SUPPLIES
(Explain Unusual Circumstances)
CPT/HCPCS | MODIFIER
42820 | tonsillectomy

Don't: Use N/A or DNA when information is not applicable. Leave the space blank.

Correct

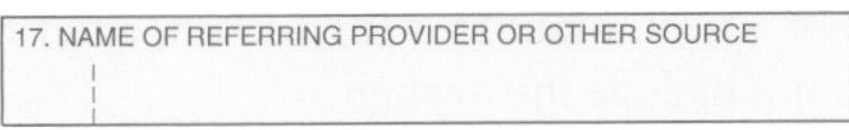

17. NAME OF REFERRING PROVIDER OR OTHER SOURCE

Incorrect

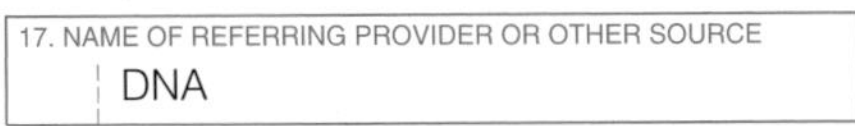

17. NAME OF REFERRING PROVIDER OR OTHER SOURCE
DNA

Don't: Use paper clips, cellophane tape, stickers, rubber stamps, or staples.

Do: Enter 6-digit or 8-digit date formats: 0601XX, 060120XX, or 06-01-20XX, depending on the block instructions.

Correct

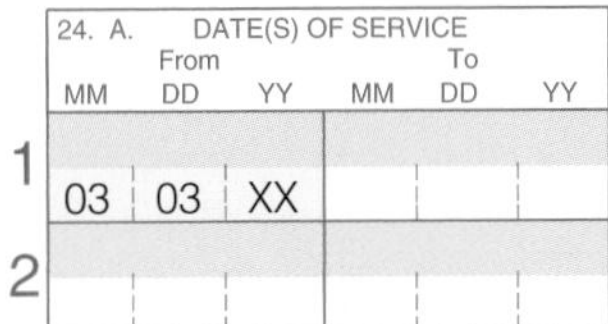

24. A. DATE(S) OF SERVICE	From			To	
	MM	DD	YY	MM	DD	YY
1	03	03	XX			
2						

Correct

24. A. DATE(S) OF SERVICE	From			To		
	MM	DD	YY	MM	DD	YY
1	030320XX					
2						

Do: Keep signature within signature block.

Correct

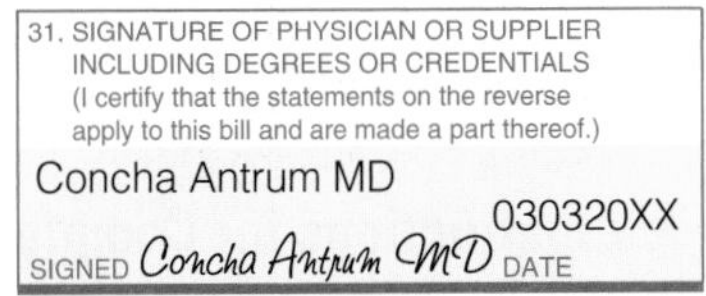

31. SIGNATURE OF PHYSICIAN OR SUPPLIER INCLUDING DEGREES OR CREDENTIALS
(I certify that the statements on the reverse apply to this bill and are made a part thereof.)
Concha Antrum MD
030320XX
SIGNED Concha Antrum MD DATE

Incorrect

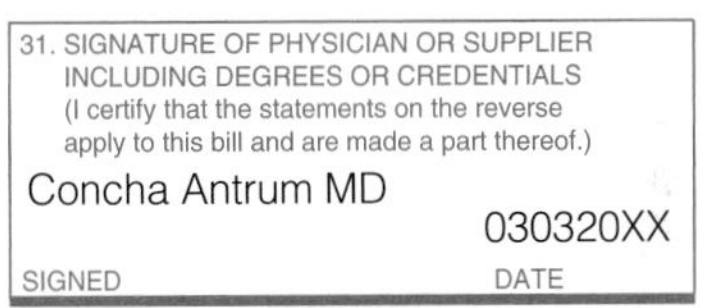

31. SIGNATURE OF PHYSICIAN OR SUPPLIER INCLUDING DEGREES OR CREDENTIALS
(I certify that the statements on the reverse apply to this bill and are made a part thereof.)
Concha Antrum MD
030320XX
SIGNED DATE
Concha Antrum MD

Do: Keep claim form clean and free from stains, tear-off pad glue, notations, circles or scribbles, strike-overs, crossed-out information, or white out.

Don't: Fold or spindle forms when mailing.

Don't: Send claim attachments smaller than 8½ × 11.

INSTRUCTIONS FOR COMPLETING THE HEALTH INSURANCE CLAIM FORM (CMS-1500)

The NUCC has developed a general instruction guide for completing the CMS-1500 claim form, which is referred to as *NUCC's Reference Instruction Manual.** Instructions align with the Health Care Claim Professional 837 and 5010. Updated versions of the instruction manual are released each July.

NUCC's Reference Instruction Manual is not specific to any applicable public or private payer. However, most insurance carriers have adopted the NUCC guidelines for completion of the CMS-1500 claim form. It is recommended that claims be processes using NUCC guidelines unless carriers advise otherwise. NUCC guidelines provide instructions and examples that demonstrate how to enter the data in every field of the CMS-1500 claim form. The instructions on the following pages can be used to complete claims. Blocks should be completed for all carriers as indicated in the "Instructions" unless a more specific guideline for the carrier is indicated.

*Content from the NUCC's 1500 Health Insurance Claim Form Reference Instruction Manual is reprinted by permission of the American Medical Association.

! COMPLIANCE ALERT

HIPAA Transactions and Code Sets Standards

Question

Do the HIPAA transactions and code sets standards apply to paper claims and other nonelectronic transactions?

Answer

No. The HIPAA transactions and code sets standards only apply to electronic transactions conducted by covered entities. Other entities such as employers or casualty insurance plans may decide to use them voluntarily but are not required to do so.

For paper transactions, health plans are free to set their own data requirements. Other federal or state laws may require plans or health care organizations to use specific code sets for certain paper transactions. However, all covered health plans and organizations must be able to use the HIPAA standards for electronic transactions. Health plans may choose to require that paper claims include the same data elements, codes, and identifiers that are required by the HIPAA regulations for electronic transactions.

HIPAA, Health Insurance Portability and Accountability Act.

Block-By-Block Instructions for Completion of the CMS-1500

DRAFT - NOT FOR OFFICIAL USE

HEALTH INSURANCE CLAIM FORM

APPROVED BY NATIONAL UNIFOR MCLAIM COMMITTEE (NUCC) 02/12

PICA | PICA

1. MEDICARE (Medicare#) | MEDICAID (Medicaid#) | TRICARE (ID#DoD#) | CHAMPVA (Member ID#) | GROUP HEALTH PLAN (ID#) [X] | FECA BLK LUNG (ID#) | OTHER (ID#)

1a. INSURED'S I.D. NUMBER (For Program in Item 1): 111704521

2. PATIENT'S NAME (Last Name, First Name, Middle Initial): Forehand, Harry, N

3. PATIENT'S BIRTH DATE MM DD YY: 01 06 1946 SEX M [X] F [ ]

4. INSURED'S NAME (Last Name, First Name, Middle Initial): Forehand, Harry, N

Carrier Block

The carrier block can be found in the upper right corner of the CMS-1500 form. In the upper left corner of the form, a Quick Response (QR) code symbol and the date approved by the NUCC can be located. The payer is the carrier, health plan, third-party administrator, or other payer that will handle the claim. This information directs the claim to the appropriate payer. Note: Some carriers prefer that this area of the claim be left blank because identifying data are printed during the initial insurance claims processing stage.

Instructions: Enter in the white, open carrier area the name and address of the payer to whom the claim is being sent. Information should be entered in the following format:

1st line: Name of insurance carrier

2nd line: First line of address

3rd line: Second line of address (if necessary) (If address only has three lines, leave blank.)

4th line: City, state (two-character state code), and zip code (Examples 14.4 and 14.5)

Do not use punctuation (that is, commas and periods) or other symbols in the address (for example, 123 N Main Street 101 instead of 123 N. Main St, #101). When entering a 9-digit zip code, do not include the hyphen.

PICA | PICA

1. MEDICARE (Medicare#) | MEDICAID (Medicaid#) | TRICARE (ID#DoD#) | CHAMPVA (Member ID#) | GROUP HEALTH PLAN (ID#) [X] | FECA BLK LUNG (ID#) | OTHER (ID#)

1a. INSURED'S I.D. NUMBER (For Program in Item 1): 111704521

2. PATIENT'S NAME (Last Name, First Name, Middle Initial): Forehand, Harry, N

3. PATIENT'S BIRTH DATE MM DD YY: 01 06 1946 SEX M [X] F [ ]

4. INSURED'S NAME (Last Name, First Name, Middle Initial): Forehand, Harry, N

Block 1: Medicare, Medicaid, TRICARE, CHAMPVA, Group Health Plan, FECA, Black Lung, Other

This block is used to identify the insurance type to whom the claim is being submitted and may establish primary liability.

Instructions: Indicate the type of health insurance coverage applicable to this claim by placing an X in the appropriate box. Only one box can be marked. "Other" indicates health insurance, including health maintenance organizations (HMOs), commercial insurance, automobile accident, liability, or workers' compensation. *Note: When completing the* Workbook *assignments for private payer cases or Medicare/Medigap cases, if the insured is employed, assume that the insurance is through the employer and is "group" insurance; otherwise, assume that it is an individual policy and enter "Other."*

EXAMPLE 14.4 **Four-Line Address**

Worldwide Health Insurance Company
Suite 101
123 Main Street
Anytown IL 60605

EXAMPLE 14.5 **Three-Line Address**

Worldwide Health Insurance Company
123 Main Street
Anytown IL 60605

PICA			PICA
1. MEDICARE (Medicare#) ☐ MEDICAID (Medicaid#) ☐ TRICARE (ID#DoD#) ☐ CHAMPVA (Member ID#) ☐ GROUP HEALTH PLAN (ID#) [X] FECA BLK LUNG (ID#) ☐ OTHER (ID#) ☐		1a. INSURED'S I.D. NUMBER (For Program in Item 1) 111704521	
2. PATIENT'S NAME (Last Name, First Name, Middle Initial) Forehand, Harry, N	3. PATIENT'S BIRTH DATE MM DD YY SEX 01 06 1946 M [X] F ☐	4. INSURED'S NAME (Last Name, First Name, Middle Initial) Forehand, Harry, N	

Block 1a: Insured's ID Number The "Insured's ID Number" is the identification number of the insured and identifies the insured to the payer.

Instructions: Enter the "Insured's ID Number" as shown on the insured's ID card for the payer to which the claim is being submitted. If the patient has a unique member identification number assigned by the payer, enter that number in this field.

TRICARE CLAIMS

Enter the sponsor's Department of Defense (DoD) benefits number from the back of the ID card.

CHAMPVA CLAIMS

Enter the sponsor's Social Security number (SSN) or Veterans Affairs (VA) file number.

WORKERS' COMPENSATION CLAIMS

Enter the employee ID or workers' compensation claim number. If none is assigned, enter the employer's policy number.

PROPERTY AND CASUALTY CLAIMS

Enter the federal tax ID or Social Security number (SSN) of the insured person or entity.

PICA			PICA
1. MEDICARE (Medicare#) ☐ MEDICAID (Medicaid#) ☐ TRICARE (ID#DoD#) ☐ CHAMPVA (Member ID#) ☐ GROUP HEALTH PLAN (ID#) [X] FECA BLK LUNG (ID#) ☐ OTHER (ID#) ☐		1a. INSURED'S I.D. NUMBER (For Program in Item 1) 111704521	
2. PATIENT'S NAME (Last Name, First Name, Middle Initial) Forehand, Harry, N	3. PATIENT'S BIRTH DATE MM DD YY SEX 01 06 1946 M [X] F ☐	4. INSURED'S NAME (Last Name, First Name, Middle Initial) Forehand, Harry, N	

Block 2: Patient's Name The "Patient's Name" is the name of the person who received the treatment or supplies.

Instructions: Enter the patient's full last name, first name, and middle initial. If the patient uses a last name suffix (for example, Jr, Sr), enter it after the last name and before the first name. Titles (for example, Sister, Capt, Dr) and professional suffixes (for example, PhD, MD, Esq) should not be included with the name. Use commas to separate the last name, first name, and middle initial. A hyphen can be used for hyphenated names. Do not use periods within the name (Example 14.6). If the patient is the insured, it is not necessary to report the patient's name.

PICA			PICA
1. MEDICARE (Medicare#) ☐ MEDICAID (Medicaid#) ☐ TRICARE (ID#DoD#) ☐ CHAMPVA (Member ID#) ☐ GROUP HEALTH PLAN (ID#) [X] FECA BLK LUNG (ID#) ☐ OTHER (ID#) ☐		1a. INSURED'S I.D. NUMBER (For Program in Item 1) 111704521	
2. PATIENT'S NAME (Last Name, First Name, Middle Initial) Forehand, Harry, N	3. PATIENT'S BIRTH DATE MM DD YY SEX 01 06 1946 M [X] F ☐	4. INSURED'S NAME (Last Name, First Name, Middle Initial) Forehand, Harry, N	

Block 3: Patient's Birth Date, Sex The patient's birth date and gender is information that will identify the patient and it distinguishes persons with similar names.

Instructions: Enter the patient's 8-digit birth date (MM/DD/YYYY). Enter an X in the correct box to indicate sex of the patient. Only one box can be marked. If gender is unknown, leave blank. The patient's age must be as follows to correlate with the diagnosis in Block 21:

- Birth: Newborn diagnosis
- Birth to 17 years: Pediatric diagnosis
- 12 to 55 years: Maternity diagnosis
- 15 to 124 years: Adult diagnosis

EXAMPLE 14.6 Surname Format

Hyphenated name: Smith-White = Smith-White
Prefixed name: MacIverson = MacIverson
Seniority name with numeric suffix: John R. Ellis, III = Ellis III, John, R

PICA							PICA
1. MEDICARE (Medicare#) [ ]	MEDICAID (Medicaid#) [ ]	TRICARE (ID#DoD#) [ ]	CHAMPVA (Member ID#) [ ]	GROUP HEALTH PLAN (ID#) [X]	FECA BLK LUNG (ID#) [ ]	OTHER (ID#) [ ]	1a. INSURED'S I.D. NUMBER (For Program in Item 1) 111704521
2. PATIENT'S NAME (Last Name, First Name, Middle Initial) Forehand, Harry, N			3. PATIENT'S BIRTH DATE MM DD YY 01 06 1946	SEX M [X] F [ ]			4. INSURED'S NAME (Last Name, First Name, Middle Initial) Forehand, Harry, N

Block 4: Insured's Name The "insured's name" identifies the person who holds the policy, which would be the employee for employer-provided health insurance.

Instructions: Enter the insured's full last name, first name, and middle initial. If the insured uses a last name suffix (for example, Jr, Sr), enter it after the last name and before the first name. Titles (for example, Sister, Capt, Dr) and professional suffixes (for example, PhD, MD, Esq) should not be included with the name. Use commas to separate the last name, first name, and middle initial. A hyphen can be used for hyphenated names. Do not use periods within the name.

WORKERS' COMPENSATION CLAIMS

Enter the name of the employer.

PROPERTY AND CASUALTY CLAIMS

Enter the name of the insured person or entity.

5. PATIENT'S ADDRESS (No., Street) 1456 Main Street		6. PATIENT RELATIONSHIP TO INSURED Self [X] Spouse [ ] Child [ ] Other [ ]	7. INSURED'S ADDRESS (No., Street) 1456 Main Street	
CITY Woodland Hills	STATE XY	8. RESERVED FOR NUCC USE	CITY Woodland Hills	STATE XY
ZIP CODE 12345-0000	TELEPHONE (Include Area Code) (555) 4909876		ZIP CODE 12345-0000	TELEPHONE (Include Area Code) (555) 4909876

Block 5: Patient's Address The patient's address is the patient's permanent residence. A temporary address or school address should not be used.

Instructions: Enter the patient's mailing address and telephone number. The first line is for the street address; the second line is for the city and two-character state code; the third line is for the zip code and phone number. If reporting a foreign address, contact payer for specific reporting instructions. If the patient is the insured, it is not necessary to report the patient's address. "Patient's Telephone" does not exist in 5010A1. NUCC recommends that the phone number not be reported.

WORKERS' COMPENSATION CLAIMS

If required by a payer to report a telephone number, do not use a hyphen or space as a separator within the telephone number.

PROPERTY AND CASUALTY CLAIMS

If required by a payer to report a telephone number, do not use a hyphen or space as a separator within the telephone number.

5. PATIENT'S ADDRESS (No., Street)			6. PATIENT RELATIONSHIP TO INSURED	7. INSURED'S ADDRESS (No., Street)		
1456 Main Street			Self [X] Spouse [ ] Child [ ] Other [ ]	1456 Main Street		
CITY Woodland Hills		STATE XY	8. RESERVED FOR NUCC USE	CITY Woodland Hills		STATE XY
ZIP CODE 12345-0000	TELEPHONE (Include Area Code) (555) 4909876			ZIP CODE 12345-0000	TELEPHONE (Include Area Code) (555) 4909876	

Block 6: Patient Relationship to Insured The "Patient Relationship to Insured" indicates how the patient is related to the insured. "Self" would indicate that the insured is the patient. "Spouse" would indicate that the patient is the husband of the wife or qualified partner as defined by the insured's plan. "Child" would indicate that the patient is a minor dependent as defined by the insured's plan. "Other" would indicate that the patient is other than the self, spouse, or child, which may include employee, ward, or dependent as defined by the insured's plan.

Instructions: Enter an X in the correct box to indicate the patient's relationship to the insured when Block 4 is completed. Only one box should be marked.

WORKERS' COMPENSATION CLAIMS

Check "Other."

5. PATIENT'S ADDRESS (No., Street)			6. PATIENT RELATIONSHIP TO INSURED	7. INSURED'S ADDRESS (No., Street)		
1456 Main Street			Self [X] Spouse [ ] Child [ ] Other [ ]	1456 Main Street		
CITY Woodland Hills		STATE XY	8. RESERVED FOR NUCC USE	CITY Woodland Hills		STATE XY
ZIP CODE 12345-0000	TELEPHONE (Include Area Code) (555) 4909876			ZIP CODE 12345-0000	TELEPHONE (Include Area Code) (555) 4909876	

Block 7: Insured's Address The "Insured's Address" is the insured's permanent residence, which may be different from the patient's address in Block 5.

Instructions: Enter the insured's address and telephone number. If Block 4 is completed, this field should be completed. The first line is for the street address; the second line is for the city and state; the third line is for the zip code and phone number. Do not use punctuation or other symbols in the address. For example, use 123 N Main Street 101 instead of 123 N. Main Street, #101. When entering a 9-digit zip code, do not include the hyphen. If reporting a foreign address, contact payer for specific reporting instructions. "Insured's Telephone" does not exist in 5010A1. NUCC recommends that the phone number not be reported.

WORKERS' COMPENSATION CLAIMS

Enter the employer's address. If required by a payer to report a telephone number, do not use a hyphen or space as a separator within the telephone number.

PROPERTY AND CASUALTY CLAIMS

If required by a payer to report a telephone number, do not use a hyphen or space as a separator within the telephone number.

5. PATIENT'S ADDRESS (No., Street)			6. PATIENT RELATIONSHIP TO INSURED	7. INSURED'S ADDRESS (No., Street)		
1456 Main Street			Self [X] Spouse [ ] Child [ ] Other [ ]	1456 Main Street		
CITY Woodland Hills		STATE XY	8. RESERVED FOR NUCC USE	CITY Woodland Hills		STATE XY
ZIP CODE 12345-0000	TELEPHONE (Include Area Code) (555) 4909876			ZIP CODE 12345-0000	TELEPHONE (Include Area Code) (555) 4909876	

Block 8: Reserved for NUCC Use This field is reserved for NUCC use. NUCC will provide instructions for any use of this field.

Instructions: This field was previously used to report "Patient Status." "Patient Status" does not exist in 5010A1, so this field has been eliminated.

9. OTHER INSURED'S NAME (Last Name, First Name, Middle Initial)	10. IS PATIENT'S CONDITION RELATED TO:	11. INSURED'S POLICY GROUP OR FECA NUMBER A482
a. OTHER INSURED'S POLICY OR GROUP NUMBER	a. EMPLOYMENT? (Current or Previous) [ ] YES [X] NO	a. INSURED'S DATE OF BIRTH MM DD YY 01 16 1946 SEX M [X] F [ ]
b. RESERVED FOR NUCC USE	b. AUTO ACCIDENT? PLACE (State) [ ] YES [X] NO	b. OTHER CLAIM ID (Designated by NUCC)
c. RESERVED FOR NUCC USE	c. OTHER ACCIDENT? [ ] YES [X] NO	c. INSURANCE PLAN NAME OR PROGRAM NAME ABC Insurance Company
d. INSURANCE PLAN NAME OR PROGRAM NAME	10d. CLAIM CODES (Designated by NUCC)	d. IS THERE ANOTHER HEALTH BENEFIT PLAN? [ ] YES [X] NO *If yes*, complete items 9, 9a, and 9d.

Block 9: Other Insured's Name The "Other Insured's Name" indicates that there is a holder of another policy that may cover the patient.

Instructions: If Block 11d is marked YES, complete fields 9, 9a, and 9d; otherwise, leave fields 9, 9a, and 9d blank. When additional group health coverage exists, enter other insured's full last name, first name, and middle initial of the enrollee in another health plan if it is different from that shown in Block 2. If the insured uses a last name suffix (for example, Jr, Sr), enter it after the last name and before the first name. Titles (for example, Sister, Capt, Dr) and professional suffixes (for example, PhD, MD, Esq) should not be included with the name. Use commas to separate the last name, first name, and middle initial. A hyphen can be used for hyphenated names. Do not use periods within the name.

9. OTHER INSURED'S NAME (Last Name, First Name, Middle Initial)	10. IS PATIENT'S CONDITION RELATED TO:	11. INSURED'S POLICY GROUP OR FECA NUMBER A482
a. OTHER INSURED'S POLICY OR GROUP NUMBER	a. EMPLOYMENT? (Current or Previous) [ ] YES [X] NO	a. INSURED'S DATE OF BIRTH MM DD YY 01 16 1946 SEX M [X] F [ ]
b. RESERVED FOR NUCC USE	b. AUTO ACCIDENT? PLACE (State) [ ] YES [X] NO	b. OTHER CLAIM ID (Designated by NUCC)
c. RESERVED FOR NUCC USE	c. OTHER ACCIDENT? [ ] YES [X] NO	c. INSURANCE PLAN NAME OR PROGRAM NAME ABC Insurance Company
d. INSURANCE PLAN NAME OR PROGRAM NAME	10d. CLAIM CODES (Designated by NUCC)	d. IS THERE ANOTHER HEALTH BENEFIT PLAN? [ ] YES [X] NO *If yes*, complete items 9, 9a, and 9d.

Block 9a: Other Insured's Policy or Group Number The "Other Insured's Policy or Group Number" identifies the policy or group number for coverage of the insured as indicated in Block 9.

Instructions: Enter the policy or group number of the other or secondary insured. Do not use a hyphen or space as a separator within the policy or group number.

9. OTHER INSURED'S NAME (Last Name, First Name, Middle Initial)	10. IS PATIENT'S CONDITION RELATED TO:	11. INSURED'S POLICY GROUP OR FECA NUMBER A482
a. OTHER INSURED'S POLICY OR GROUP NUMBER	a. EMPLOYMENT? (Current or Previous) [ ] YES [X] NO	a. INSURED'S DATE OF BIRTH MM DD YY 01 16 1946 SEX M [X] F [ ]
b. RESERVED FOR NUCC USE	b. AUTO ACCIDENT? PLACE (State) [ ] YES [X] NO	b. OTHER CLAIM ID (Designated by NUCC)
c. RESERVED FOR NUCC USE	c. OTHER ACCIDENT? [ ] YES [X] NO	c. INSURANCE PLAN NAME OR PROGRAM NAME ABC Insurance Company
d. INSURANCE PLAN NAME OR PROGRAM NAME	10d. CLAIM CODES (Designated by NUCC)	d. IS THERE ANOTHER HEALTH BENEFIT PLAN? [ ] YES [X] NO *If yes*, complete items 9, 9a, and 9d.

Block 9b: Reserved for NUCC Use This field is reserved for NUCC use. NUCC will provide instructions for any use of this field.

Instructions: This field was previously used to report "Other Insured's Date of Birth, Sex." "Other Insured's Date of Birth, Sex" does not exist in 5010A1, so this field has been eliminated.

9. OTHER INSURED'S NAME (Last Name, First Name, Middle Initial)	10. IS PATIENT'S CONDITION RELATED TO:	11. INSURED'S POLICY GROUP OR FECA NUMBER A482
a. OTHER INSURED'S POLICY OR GROUP NUMBER	a. EMPLOYMENT? (Current or Previous) [ ] YES [X] NO	a. INSURED'S DATE OF BIRTH MM DD YY 01 16 1946 SEX M [X] F [ ]
b. RESERVED FOR NUCC USE	b. AUTO ACCIDENT? PLACE (State) [ ] YES [X] NO	b. OTHER CLAIM ID (Designated by NUCC)
c. RESERVED FOR NUCC USE	c. OTHER ACCIDENT? [ ] YES [X] NO	c. INSURANCE PLAN NAME OR PROGRAM NAME ABC Insurance Company
d. INSURANCE PLAN NAME OR PROGRAM NAME	10d. CLAIM CODES (Designated by NUCC)	d. IS THERE ANOTHER HEALTH BENEFIT PLAN? [ ] YES [X] NO *If yes*, complete items 9, 9a, and 9d.

Block 9c: Reserved for NUCC Use This field is reserved for NUCC use. NUCC will provide instructions for any use of this field.

Instructions: This field was previously used to report "Employer's Name or School Name." "Employer's Name or School Name" does not exist in 5010A1, so this field has been eliminated.

9. OTHER INSURED'S NAME (Last Name, First Name, Middle Initial)	10. IS PATIENT'S CONDITION RELATED TO:	11. INSURED'S POLICY GROUP OR FECA NUMBER A482
a. OTHER INSURED'S POLICY OR GROUP NUMBER	a. EMPLOYMENT? (Current or Previous) [ ] YES [X] NO	a. INSURED'S DATE OF BIRTH MM DD YY 01 16 1946 SEX M [X] F [ ]
b. RESERVED FOR NUCC USE	b. AUTO ACCIDENT? PLACE (State) [ ] YES [X] NO	b. OTHER CLAIM ID (Designated by NUCC)
c. RESERVED FOR NUCC USE	c. OTHER ACCIDENT? [ ] YES [X] NO	c. INSURANCE PLAN NAME OR PROGRAM NAME ABC Insurance Company
d. INSURANCE PLAN NAME OR PROGRAM NAME	10d. CLAIM CODES (Designated by NUCC)	d. IS THERE ANOTHER HEALTH BENEFIT PLAN? [ ] YES [X] NO *If yes,* complete items 9, 9a, and 9d.

Block 9d: Insurance Plan Name or Program Name The "Insurance Plan Name or Program Name" identifies the name of the plan or program of the other insured as indicated in Block 9.

Instructions: Enter the other or secondary insured's insurance plan or program name.

MEDICARE/MEDIGAP CLAIMS

To ensure the crossover of Medicare/Medigap claims, complete Blocks 9 through 9d and list the payer identification (PAYRID) number of the MG plan in Block 9d. The PAYRID for Medigap (MG) plans is referred to as Other Carrier Name and Address (OCNA) number and is published in the Medicare newsletter. If automatic crossover capabilities are not offered in one's state, attach the Medicare RA to the claim form and submit to the MG plan separately.

9. OTHER INSURED'S NAME (Last Name, First Name, Middle Initial)	10. IS PATIENT'S CONDITION RELATED TO:	11. INSURED'S POLICY GROUP OR FECA NUMBER A482
a. OTHER INSURED'S POLICY OR GROUP NUMBER	a. EMPLOYMENT? (Current or Previous) [ ] YES [X] NO	a. INSURED'S DATE OF BIRTH MM DD YY 01 16 1946 SEX M [X] F [ ]
b. RESERVED FOR NUCC USE	b. AUTO ACCIDENT? PLACE (State) [ ] YES [X] NO	b. OTHER CLAIM ID (Designated by NUCC)
c. RESERVED FOR NUCC USE	c. OTHER ACCIDENT? [ ] YES [X] NO	c. INSURANCE PLAN NAME OR PROGRAM NAME ABC Insurance Company
d. INSURANCE PLAN NAME OR PROGRAM NAME	10d. CLAIM CODES (Designated by NUCC)	d. IS THERE ANOTHER HEALTH BENEFIT PLAN? [ ] YES [X] NO *If yes,* complete items 9, 9a, and 9d.

Block 10a to 10c: Is Patient's Condition Related To "Is patient's condition related to" indicates whether the patient's illness or injury is related to employment, auto accident, or other accident.

"Employment (current or previous)" indicates that the condition is related to the patient's job or workplace. "Auto accident" indicates that the condition is the result of an automobile accident. "Other accident" indicates that the condition is the result of any other type of accident.

Instructions: When appropriate, enter an X in the correct box to indicate whether one or more of the services described in Block 24 are for a condition or injury that occurred on the job or as a result of an automobile or other accident. Only one box on each line should be marked.

The state postal code where the accident occurred must be reported if "YES" is marked in 10b for "Auto accident." Any item marked "YES" indicates there may be other applicable insurance coverage that would be primary, such as automobile liability insurance. Primary insurance information must then be shown in Block 11.

9. OTHER INSURED'S NAME (Last Name, First Name, Middle Initial)	10. IS PATIENT'S CONDITION RELATED TO:	11. INSURED'S POLICY GROUP OR FECA NUMBER A482
a. OTHER INSURED'S POLICY OR GROUP NUMBER	a. EMPLOYMENT? (Current or Previous) [ ] YES [X] NO	a. INSURED'S DATE OF BIRTH MM DD YY 01 16 1946 SEX M [X] F [ ]
b. RESERVED FOR NUCC USE	b. AUTO ACCIDENT? PLACE (State) [ ] YES [X] NO	b. OTHER CLAIM ID (Designated by NUCC)
c. RESERVED FOR NUCC USE	c. OTHER ACCIDENT? [ ] YES [X] NO	c. INSURANCE PLAN NAME OR PROGRAM NAME ABC Insurance Company
d. INSURANCE PLAN NAME OR PROGRAM NAME	10d. CLAIM CODES (Designated by NUCC)	d. IS THERE ANOTHER HEALTH BENEFIT PLAN? [ ] YES [X] NO *If yes,* complete items 9, 9a, and 9d.

Block 10d: Claim Codes (Designated by NUCC) The "Claim Codes" identify additional information about the patient's condition or the claim.

Instructions: When applicable, use the report "Claim Codes." Applicable claim codes are designated by NUCC. Refer to the most current instructions from the public or private payer regarding the need to report claim codes.

When required by payers to provide the subset of condition codes approved by NUCC, enter the "Condition Code" in this field. The condition codes approved for use on the 1500 Claim Form are available at www.nucc.org, under Code Sets.

Note: When completing the Workbook assignments for Medicaid cases, enter the patient's Medicaid number preceded by "MCD," if Medicaid is the secondary payer. For all other cases, leave blank.

WORKERS' COMPENSATION CLAIMS

A condition code is required when submitting a bill that is a duplicate (W2) or an appeal (W3 = Level 1, W4 = Level 2, W5 = Level 3). The original reference number must be entered in Block 22 for these conditions. *Note:* Do not use condition codes when submitting a revised or corrected bill.

9. OTHER INSURED'S NAME (Last Name, First Name, Middle Initial)	10. IS PATIENT'S CONDITION RELATED TO:	11. INSURED'S POLICY GROUP OR FECA NUMBER A482
a. OTHER INSURED'S POLICY OR GROUP NUMBER	a. EMPLOYMENT? (Current or Previous) ☐ YES ☒ NO	a. INSURED'S DATE OF BIRTH MM DD YY 01 16 1946 SEX M ☒ F ☐
b. RESERVED FOR NUCC USE	b. AUTO ACCIDENT? PLACE (State) ☐ YES ☒ NO	b. OTHER CLAIM ID (Designated by NUCC)
c. RESERVED FOR NUCC USE	c. OTHER ACCIDENT? ☐ YES ☒ NO	c. INSURANCE PLAN NAME OR PROGRAM NAME ABC Insurance Company
d. INSURANCE PLAN NAME OR PROGRAM NAME	10d. CLAIM CODES (Designated by NUCC)	d. IS THERE ANOTHER HEALTH BENEFIT PLAN? ☐ YES ☒ NO *If yes*, complete items 9, 9a, and 9d.

Block 11: Insured's Policy, Group, or FECA Number The "Insured's Policy, Group, or FECA Number" is the alphanumeric identifier for the health, auto, or other insurance plan coverage.

The FECA number is the 9-digit alphanumeric identifier assigned to a patient claiming work-related condition(s) under the Federal Employees' Compensation Act 5 USC 8101.

Instructions: Enter the insured's policy or group number as it appears on the insured's health care identification card. If Block 4 is completed, this field should be completed. Do not use a hyphen or space as a separator within the policy or group number.

9. OTHER INSURED'S NAME (Last Name, First Name, Middle Initial)	10. IS PATIENT'S CONDITION RELATED TO:	11. INSURED'S POLICY GROUP OR FECA NUMBER A482
a. OTHER INSURED'S POLICY OR GROUP NUMBER	a. EMPLOYMENT? (Current or Previous) ☐ YES ☒ NO	a. INSURED'S DATE OF BIRTH MM DD YY 01 16 1946 SEX M ☒ F ☐
b. RESERVED FOR NUCC USE	b. AUTO ACCIDENT? PLACE (State) ☐ YES ☒ NO	b. OTHER CLAIM ID (Designated by NUCC)
c. RESERVED FOR NUCC USE	c. OTHER ACCIDENT? ☐ YES ☒ NO	c. INSURANCE PLAN NAME OR PROGRAM NAME ABC Insurance Company
d. INSURANCE PLAN NAME OR PROGRAM NAME	10d. CLAIM CODES (Designated by NUCC)	d. IS THERE ANOTHER HEALTH BENEFIT PLAN? ☐ YES ☒ NO *If yes*, complete items 9, 9a, and 9d.

Block 11a: Insured's Date of Birth, Sex The "Insured's Date of Birth, Sex" (gender) is the birth date and gender of the insured as indicated in Block 1a.

Instructions: Enter the 8-digit date of birth (MM/DD/YYYY) of the insured and an X to indicate the sex of the insured. Only one box should be marked. If gender is unknown, leave blank.

9. OTHER INSURED'S NAME (Last Name, First Name, Middle Initial)	10. IS PATIENT'S CONDITION RELATED TO:	11. INSURED'S POLICY GROUP OR FECA NUMBER A482
a. OTHER INSURED'S POLICY OR GROUP NUMBER	a. EMPLOYMENT? (Current or Previous) ☐ YES ☒ NO	a. INSURED'S DATE OF BIRTH MM DD YY 01 16 1946 SEX M ☒ F ☐
b. RESERVED FOR NUCC USE	b. AUTO ACCIDENT? PLACE (State) ☐ YES ☒ NO	b. OTHER CLAIM ID (Designated by NUCC)
c. RESERVED FOR NUCC USE	c. OTHER ACCIDENT? ☐ YES ☒ NO	c. INSURANCE PLAN NAME OR PROGRAM NAME ABC Insurance Company
d. INSURANCE PLAN NAME OR PROGRAM NAME	10d. CLAIM CODES (Designated by NUCC)	d. IS THERE ANOTHER HEALTH BENEFIT PLAN? ☐ YES ☒ NO *If yes*, complete items 9, 9a, and 9d.

Block 11b: Other Claim ID (Designated by NUCC) The "Other Claim ID" is another identifier applicable to the claim.

Instructions: Enter the "Other Claim ID." Applicable claim identifiers are designated by the NUCC. The following qualifier and accompanying identifier has been designated for use:

Y4 Agency Claim Number (Property Casualty Claim Number)

Enter the qualifier to the left of the vertical, dotted line. Enter the identifier number to the right of the vertical, dotted line.

WORKERS' COMPENSATION CLAIMS

Claim ID is required if known. Enter the claim number assigned by the payer.

PROPERTY AND CASUALTY CLAIMS

Claim ID is required if known. Enter the claim number assigned by the payer.

9. OTHER INSURED'S NAME (Last Name, First Name, Middle Initial)
a. OTHER INSURED'S POLICY OR GROUP NUMBER
b. RESERVED FOR NUCC USE
c. RESERVED FOR NUCC USE
d. INSURANCE PLAN NAME OR PROGRAM NAME
10. IS PATIENT'S CONDITION RELATED TO:
a. EMPLOYMENT? (Current or Previous) YES [X] NO
b. AUTO ACCIDENT? PLACE (State) YES [X] NO
c. OTHER ACCIDENT? YES [X] NO
10d. CLAIM CODES (Designated by NUCC)
11. INSURED'S POLICY GROUP OR FECA NUMBER A482
a. INSURED'S DATE OF BIRTH MM DD YY 01 16 1946 SEX M [X] F
b. OTHER CLAIM ID (Designated by NUCC)
c. INSURANCE PLAN NAME OR PROGRAM NAME ABC Insurance Company
d. IS THERE ANOTHER HEALTH BENEFIT PLAN? YES [X] NO *If yes*, complete items 9, 9a, and 9d.

Block 11c: Insurance Plan Name or Program Name The "Insurance Plan Name or Program Name" is the name of the plan or program of the insured as indicated in Block 1a.

Instructions: Enter the "Insurance Plan Name or Program Name" of the insured. Some payers require an identification number of the primary insurer rather than the name in this field.

9. OTHER INSURED'S NAME (Last Name, First Name, Middle Initial)
a. OTHER INSURED'S POLICY OR GROUP NUMBER
b. RESERVED FOR NUCC USE
c. RESERVED FOR NUCC USE
d. INSURANCE PLAN NAME OR PROGRAM NAME
10. IS PATIENT'S CONDITION RELATED TO:
a. EMPLOYMENT? (Current or Previous) YES [X] NO
b. AUTO ACCIDENT? PLACE (State) YES [X] NO
c. OTHER ACCIDENT? YES [X] NO
10d. CLAIM CODES (Designated by NUCC)
11. INSURED'S POLICY GROUP OR FECA NUMBER A482
a. INSURED'S DATE OF BIRTH MM DD YY 01 16 1946 SEX M [X] F
b. OTHER CLAIM ID (Designated by NUCC)
c. INSURANCE PLAN NAME OR PROGRAM NAME ABC Insurance Company
d. IS THERE ANOTHER HEALTH BENEFIT PLAN? YES [X] NO *If yes*, complete items 9, 9a, and 9d.

Block 11d: Is There Another Health Benefit Plan? This block indicates that the patient has insurance coverage other than the plan indicated in Block 1.

Instructions: When appropriate, enter an X in the correct box. If marked "YES," complete Blocks 9, 9a, and 9d. Only one box can be marked.

Note: When completing the Workbook assignments for Medicare, leave blank.

READ BACK OF FORM BEFORE COMPLETING & SIGNING THIS FORM.
12. PATIENT'S OR AUTHORIZED PERSON'S SIGNATUREI authorize the release of any medical or other information necessary to process this claim. I also request payment of government benefits either to myself or to the party who accepts assignment below.
SIGNED *Harry N. Forehand* DATE *March 3, 20XX*
13. INSURED'S OR AUTHORIZED PERSON'S SIGNATURE I authorize payment of medical benefits to the undersigned physician or supplier for services described below.
SIGNED *Harry N. Forehand*

A

READ BACK OF FORM BEFORE COMPLETING & SIGNING THIS FORM.
12. PATIENT'S OR AUTHORIZED PERSON'S SIGNATUREI authorize the release of any medical or other information necessary to process this claim. I also request payment of government benefits either to myself or to the party who accepts assignment below.
SIGNED SIGNATURE ON FILE DATE
13. INSURED'S OR AUTHORIZED PERSON'S SIGNATURE I authorize payment of medical benefits to the undersigned physician or supplier for services described below.
SIGNED SIGNATURE ON FILE

B

Block 12: Patient's or Authorized Person's Signature This block indicates that there is an authorization on file for the release of any medical or other information necessary to process and adjudicate the claim. This block should be signed regardless of whether the health care organization participating or nonparticipating. A form created by the health care organization may be used to keep the patient's signature on file in the office. This can be used instead of having a patient sign the CMS-1500. The signed authorization should be kept on file in the patient's health record for an episode of care or for a designated time frame such as one year.

Instructions: Enter "Signature on File," "SOF," or legal signature. When legal signature is entered, enter the date signed in 6-digit (MMDDYY) or 8-digit (MMDDYYYY) format. If there is no signature on file, leave blank or enter "No Signature on File."

SOF situations that may occur in a health care organization are as follows:

Illiterate or physically handicapped. When an illiterate or physically handicapped enrollee signs by mark (X), a witness should sign his or her name and address next to the mark. If the claim is filed for the patient by another person, that person should enter the patient's name and write "By," sign his or her own name and address, indicate relationship to the patient, and state why the patient cannot sign.

Confinement in a facility. Sometimes it is not possible to obtain the signature of a Medicare patient because of confinement in an NF, hospital, or home. In such cases, service provider's should obtain an annual signature authorization from the patient.

Deceased patient. Refer to the section titled "Claims for Deceased Patients" later in this chapter for signature requirements.

Note: When completing the Workbook assignments, enter "Signature on File," not "SOF," in this block.

MEDICARE/MEDIGAP CLAIMS

When transmitting a crossover claim to a Medigap (MG) carrier, obtain an annual signature authorization from the MG patient.

MEDICARE/MEDICAID CLAIMS

Medi-Medi crossover claims do not require a patient's signature.

READ BACK OF FORM BEFORE COMPLETING & SIGNING THIS FORM. 12. PATIENT'S OR AUTHORIZED PERSON'S SIGNATURE I authorize the release of any medical or other information necessary to process this claim. I also request payment of government benefits either to myself or to the party who accepts assignment below.	13. INSURED'S OR AUTHORIZED PERSON'S SIGNATURE I authorize payment of medical benefits to the undersigned physician or supplier for services described below.
SIGNED Harry N. Forehand DATE March 3, 20XX	SIGNED Harry N. Forehand

A

READ BACK OF FORM BEFORE COMPLETING & SIGNING THIS FORM. 12. PATIENT'S OR AUTHORIZED PERSON'S SIGNATURE I authorize the release of any medical or other information necessary to process this claim. I also request payment of government benefits either to myself or to the party who accepts assignment below.	13. INSURED'S OR AUTHORIZED PERSON'S SIGNATURE I authorize payment of medical benefits to the undersigned physician or supplier for services described below.
SIGNED SIGNATURE ON FILE DATE	SIGNED SIGNATURE ON FILE

B

Block 13: Insured's or Authorized Person's Signature This block indicates that there is a signature on file authorizing payment of medical benefits.

Instructions: Enter "Signature on File," "SOF," or legal signature. If there is no signature on file, leave blank or enter "No Signature on File."

Note: When completing the Workbook assignments, enter "Signature on File," not "SOF," in this block.

14. DATE OF CURRENT: ILLNESS, INJURY, or PREGNANCY(LMP) MM DD YY 03 01 20XX QUAL. 431	15. OTHER DATE QUAL. MM DD YY	16. DATES PATIENT UNABLE TO WORK IN CURRENT OCCUPATION MM DD YY FROM MM DD YY TO
17. NAME OF REFERRING PROVIDER OR OTHER SOURCE DN Perry Cardi MD	17a. 17b. NPI 67805027XX	18. HOSPITALIZATION DATES RELATED TO CURRENT SERVICES MM DD YY FROM MM DD YY TO
19. ADDITIONAL CLAIM INFORMATION (Designated by NUCC)		20. OUTSIDE LAB? YES [X] NO $ CHARGES

Block 14: Date of Current Illness, Injury, or Pregnancy (LMP) This block identifies the first date of onset of illness, the actual date of injury, or the last menstrual period (LMP) for pregnancy.

Instructions: Enter the 6-digit (MMDDYY) or 8-digit (MMDDYYYY) date of the first date of the present illness, injury, or pregnancy. For pregnancy, use the date of the LMP as the first date.

Enter the applicable qualifier to identify which date is being reported:

431 Onset of Current Symptoms or Illness

484 Last Menstrual Period

Enter the qualifier to the right of the vertical, dotted line.

14. DATE OF CURRENT: ILLNESS, INJURY, or PREGNANCY(LMP) MM DD YY 03 01 20XX QUAL. 431	15. OTHER DATE QUAL. MM DD YY	16. DATES PATIENT UNABLE TO WORK IN CURRENT OCCUPATION MM DD YY FROM MM DD YY TO
17. NAME OF REFERRING PROVIDER OR OTHER SOURCE DN Perry Cardi MD	17a. 17b. NPI 67805027XX	18. HOSPITALIZATION DATES RELATED TO CURRENT SERVICES MM DD YY FROM MM DD YY TO
19. ADDITIONAL CLAIM INFORMATION (Designated by NUCC)		20. OUTSIDE LAB? YES [X] NO $ CHARGES

Block 15: Other Date The "Other Date" identifies additional date information about the patient's condition or treatment.

Instructions: Enter an "Other Date" related to the patient's condition or treatment. Enter the date in the 6-digit (MMDDYY) or 8-digit (MMDDYYYY) format. Previous pregnancies are not a similar illness. Leave blank if unknown.

Enter the applicable qualifier between the vertical, dotted lines to identify which date is being reported.

454 Initial Treatment

304 Latest Visit or Consultation

453 Acute Manifestation of a Chronic Condition

439 Accident

455 Last X-ray

471 Prescription

090 Report Start (assumed care date)

091 Report End (relinquished care date)

444 First Visit or Consultation

14. DATE OF CURRENT: ILLNESS, INJURY, or PREGNANCY(LMP) MM DD YY 03 01 20XX QUAL. 431	15. OTHER DATE QUAL. MM DD YY	16. DATES PATIENT UNABLE TO WORK IN CURRENT OCCUPATION MM DD YY FROM MM DD YY TO
17. NAME OF REFERRING PROVIDER OR OTHER SOURCE DN Perry Cardi MD	17a. 17b. NPI 67805027XX	18. HOSPITALIZATION DATES RELATED TO CURRENT SERVICES MM DD YY FROM MM DD YY TO
19. ADDITIONAL CLAIM INFORMATION (Designated by NUCC)		20. OUTSIDE LAB? ☐ YES ☒ NO $ CHARGES

Block 16: Dates Patient Unable to Work in Current Occupation Block 16 indicates the time span the patient is or was unable to work.

Instructions: If the patient is employed and is unable to work in current occupation, a 6-digit (MMDDYY) or 8-digit (MMDDYYYY) date must be shown for the "from–to" dates that the patient is unable to work. An entry in this field may indicate employment-related insurance coverage.

Note: When completing the Workbook assignments, enter information when it is documented in the medical record.

o MM DD YY 03 01 20XX QUAL. 431	15. OTHER DATE QUAL. MM DD YY	16. DATES PATIENT UNABLE TO WORK IN CURRENT OCCUPATION MM DD YY FROM MM DD YY TO
17. NAME OF REFERRING PROVIDER OR OTHER SOURCE DN Perry Cardi MD	17a. 17b. NPI 67805027XX	18. HOSPITALIZATION DATES RELATED TO CURRENT SERVICES MM DD YY FROM MM DD YY TO
19. ADDITIONAL CLAIM INFORMATION (Designated by NUCC)		20. OUTSIDE LAB? ☐ YES ☒ NO $ CHARGES

Block 17: Name of Referring Provider or Other Source The name entered is the referring provider, ordering provider, or supervising provider who referred, ordered, or supervised the service(s) or supply(ies) on the claim. The qualifier indicates the role of the provider being reported.

Instructions: Enter the name (first name, middle initial, last name) and credentials of the professional who referred, ordered, or supervised the service(s) or supply(ies) on the claim.

If multiple providers are involved, enter one provider using the following priority order:

1. Referring provider
2. Ordering provider
3. Supervising provider

Do not use periods or commas within the name. A hyphen can be used for hyphenated names.

Enter the applicable qualifier to the left of the vertical, dotted line to identify which provider is being reported.

DN Referring provider
DK Ordering provider
DQ Supervising provider

14. DATE OF CURRENT: ILLNESS, INJURY, or PREGNANCY(LMP) MM DD YY 03 01 20XX QUAL. 431	15. OTHER DATE QUAL. MM DD YY	16. DATES PATIENT UNABLE TO WORK IN CURRENT OCCUPATION MM DD YY FROM MM DD YY TO
17. NAME OF REFERRING PROVIDER OR OTHER SOURCE DN Perry Cardi MD	17a. 17b. NPI 67805027XX	18. HOSPITALIZATION DATES RELATED TO CURRENT SERVICES MM DD YY FROM MM DD YY TO
19. ADDITIONAL CLAIM INFORMATION (Designated by NUCC)		20. OUTSIDE LAB? ☐ YES ☒ NO $ CHARGES

Block 17a: Other ID Number The non-NPI ID number of the referring, ordering, or supervising provider is the unique identifier of the professional or provider designated taxonomy code.

Instructions: The Other ID Number of the referring, ordering, or supervising provider is reported in 17a, the shaded area. The qualifier indicating what the number represents is reported in the qualifier field to the immediate right of 17a.

NUCC defines the following qualifiers used in 5010A1:

0B State License Number
1G Provider UPIN Number
G2 Provider Commercial Number
LU Location Number (This qualifier is used for Supervising Provider only.)

14. DATE OF CURRENT: ILLNESS, INJURY, or PREGNANCY(LMP) MM DD YY 03 01 20XX QUAL. 431	15. OTHER DATE QUAL. MM DD YY	16. DATES PATIENT UNABLE TO WORK IN CURRENT OCCUPATION MM DD YY FROM MM DD YY TO
17. NAME OF REFERRING PROVIDER OR OTHER SOURCE DN Perry Cardi MD	17a. 17b. NPI 67805027XX	18. HOSPITALIZATION DATES RELATED TO CURRENT SERVICES MM DD YY FROM MM DD YY TO
19. ADDITIONAL CLAIM INFORMATION (Designated by NUCC)		20. OUTSIDE LAB? ☐ YES ☒ NO $ CHARGES

Block 17b: NPI The NPI number refers to the HIPAA National Provider Identifier number.

Instructions: Enter the NPI number of the referring, ordering, or supervising provider in Block 17b.

14. DATE OF CURRENT: ILLNESS, INJURY, or PREGNANCY(LMP) MM DD YY 03 01 20XX QUAL. 431	15. OTHER DATE QUAL. MM DD YY	16. DATES PATIENT UNABLE TO WORK IN CURRENT OCCUPATION MM DD YY FROM TO MM DD YY
17. NAME OF REFERRING PROVIDER OR OTHER SOURCE DN Perry Cardi MD	17a. 17b. NPI 67805027XX	18. HOSPITALIZATION DATES RELATED TO CURRENT SERVICES MM DD YY FROM TO MM DD YY
19. ADDITIONAL CLAIM INFORMATION (Designated by NUCC)		20. OUTSIDE LAB? YES [X] NO $ CHARGES

Block 18: Hospitalization Dates Related to Current Services Information in this field refers to an inpatient stay and indicates the admission and discharge dates associated with the service(s) on the claim.

Instructions: Enter the inpatient 6-digit (MMDDYY) or 8-digit (MMDDYYYY) hospital admission date followed by the discharge date (if discharge has occurred). If not discharged, leave discharge date blank. This date is when a medical service is furnished as a result of or subsequent to a related hospitalization.

14. DATE OF CURRENT: ILLNESS, INJURY, or PREGNANCY(LMP) MM DD YY 03 01 20XX QUAL. 431	15. OTHER DATE QUAL. MM DD YY	16. DATES PATIENT UNABLE TO WORK IN CURRENT OCCUPATION MM DD YY FROM TO MM DD YY
17. NAME OF REFERRING PROVIDER OR OTHER SOURCE DN Perry Cardi MD	17a. 17b. NPI 67805027XX	18. HOSPITALIZATION DATES RELATED TO CURRENT SERVICES MM DD YY FROM TO MM DD YY
19. ADDITIONAL CLAIM INFORMATION (Designated by NUCC)		20. OUTSIDE LAB? YES [X] NO $ CHARGES

Block 19: Additional Claim Information (Designated by NUCC) Block 19 identifies additional information about the patient's condition or the claim.

Instructions: Refer to the most current instructions from the public or private payer regarding use of this field. Some payers ask for certain identifiers in this field. For example, when modifier 99 (multiple modifiers) is entered in Block 24D, an explanation of the modifiers might be inserted in Block 19. If identifiers are reported in this field, enter the appropriate qualifiers describing the identifier. Do not enter a space, hyphen, or other separator between the qualifier code and the number.

When reporting a second item of data, enter three blank spaces and then the next qualifier and number/code/information.

NUCC defines the following qualifiers, since they are the same as those used in 5010A1:

0B State License Number
1G Provider UPIN Number
G2 Provider Commercial Number
LU Location Number (This qualifier is used for Supervising Provider only.)
N5 Provider Plan Network Identification Number
SY Social Security Number (The SSN may not be used for Medicare.)
X5 State Industrial Accident Provider Number
ZZ Provider Taxonomy (The qualifier in the 5010A1 for Provider Taxonomy is PXC but ZZ will remain the qualifier for the 1500 Claim Form.)

The list contains both provider identifiers and the provider taxonomy code. The provider identifiers are assigned to the provider either by a specific payer or by a third party in order to uniquely identify the provider. The taxonomy code is designated by the provider in order to identify his or her provider type, classification, and area of specialization. Both provider identifiers and provider taxonomy may be used in this field.

Taxonomy codes reported in this field must not be reportable in other fields, i.e., item numbers 17, 24J, 32 or 33.

When reporting a second item of data, enter three blank spaces and then the next qualifier and number/code/information.

WORKERS' COMPENSATION CLAIMS

Additional claim information is required based on Jurisdictional Workers' Compensation Guidelines.

Supplemental Information - Box 19

For additional claim information, use the qualifier PWK for data followed by the appropriate report type code, the appropriate transmission type code, and then the attachment control number. Do not enter spaces between qualifiers and data. NUCC defines the following qualifiers, since they are the same as those used in 5010A1:

Report Type Code

Code	Description
03	Report Justifying Treatment beyond Utilization
04	Drugs Administered
05	Treatment Diagnosis
06	Initial Assessment
07	Functional Goals
08	Plan of Treatment
09	Progress Report
10	Continued Treatment
11	Chemical Analysis
13	Certified Test Report
15	Justification for Admission
21	Recovery Plan
A3	Allergies/Sensitivities Document
A4	Autopsy Report
AM	Ambulance Certification
AS	Admission Summary
B2	Prescription
B3	Physician Order

B4	Referral Form	OD	Orders and Treatments Document
BR	Benchmark Testing Results	OE	Objective Physical Examination (including vital signs) Document
BS	Baseline	OX	Oxygen Therapy Clarification
BT	Blanket Test Results	OZ	Support Data for Claim
CB	Chiropractic Justification	P4	Pathology Report
CK	Consent Form(s)	P5	Patient Medical History Document
CT	Certification	PE	Parenteral or Enteral Certification
D2	Drug Profile Document	PN	Physical Therapy Notes
DA	Dental Models	PO	Prosthetics or Orthotic Certification
DB	Durable Medical Equipment Prescription	PQ	Paramedical Results
DG	Diagnostic Report	PY	Physician's Report
DJ	Discharge Monitoring Report	PZ	Physical Therapy Certification
DS	Discharge Summary	RB	Radiology Films
EB	Explanation of Benefits (Coordination of Benefits or Medicare Secondary Payer)	RR	Radiology Reports
HC	Health Certificate	RT	Report of Tests and Analysis Report
HR	Health Clinic Records	RX	Renewable Oxygen Content Averaging Report
I5	Immunization Record	SG	Symptoms Document
IR	State School Immunization Records	V5	Death Notification
LA	Laboratory Results	XP	Photographs
M1	Medical Record Attachment		
MT	Models		
NN	Nursing Notes		
OB	Operative Note		
OC	Oxygen Content Averaging Report		

Transmission Type Code

AA	Available on Request at Provider Site
BM	By Mail

Example: PWK03FX12363545465

14. DATE OF CURRENT: ILLNESS, INJURY, or PREGNANCY(LMP) MM DD YY	15. OTHER DATE QUAL. MM DD YY	16. DATES PATIENT UNABLE TO WORK IN CURRENT OCCUPATION MM DD YY FROM TO
03 01 20XX QUAL. 431		
17. NAME OF REFERRING PROVIDER OR OTHER SOURCE	17a. / 17b. NPI	18. HOSPITALIZATION DATES RELATED TO CURRENT SERVICES MM DD YY FROM TO
DN Perry Cardi MD	17b. NPI 67805027XX	
19. ADDITIONAL CLAIM INFORMATION (Designated by NUCC)		20. OUTSIDE LAB? $ CHARGES
		YES [X] NO

Block 20: Outside Lab? $Charges This block indicates that services have been rendered by an independent provider as indicated in Block 32 and the related costs.

Instructions: Complete this field when billing for purchased services by entering an X in "YES." If a "YES" is annotated, enter the purchase price under "$Charges" and complete Block 32. Each purchased service must be reported on a separate claim form because only one charge can be entered.

When entering the charge amount, enter the amount in the field to the left of the vertical line. The entered number should be right justified to the left of the vertical line. Enter 00 for cents if the amount is a whole number. Do not use dollar signs, commas, or a decimal point when reporting amounts. Negative dollar amounts are not allowed. Leave the right field blank.

21. DIAGNOSIS OR NATURE OF ILLNESS OR INJURY Relate A-L to service line below (24E) ICD Ind. 0

A. H66.009 B. C. D.
E. F. G. H.
I. J. K. L.

22. RESUBMISSION CODE ORIGINAL REF. NO.

23. PRIOR AUTHORIZATION NUMBER

24. A. DATE(S) OF SERVICE From MM DD YY	To MM DD YY	B. PLACE OF SERVICE	C. EMG	D. PROCEDURES, SERVICES, OR SUPPLIES (Explain Unusual Circumstances) CPT/HCPCS	MODIFIER	E. DIAGNOSIS POINTER	F. $ CHARGES	G. DAYS OR UNITS	H. EPSDT Family Plan	I. ID. QUAL.	J. RENDERING PROVIDER ID. #
03 03 XX		11		99203		A	70 92	1		NPI	12458977XX

Block 21: Diagnosis or Nature of Illness or Injury The "ICD indicator" identifies the version of the International Classification of Diseases (ICD) code set being reported. The "Diagnosis or Nature of Illness or Injury" is the sign, symptom, complaint, or condition of the patient relating to the service(s) on the.

Instructions: Enter the applicable ICD indicator to identify which version of ICD codes is being reported.

9 ICD-9-CM
0 ICD-10-CM

Enter the indicator between the vertical, dotted lines.

Enter the patient's diagnosis and/or condition codes. List no more than 12 ICD-9-CM or ICD-10-CM diagnosis codes. Relate lines A to L to the lines of service in Block 24E by the letter of the line. Use the highest level of specificity. This block specifically links medical necessity to the billing claim. Do not provide narrative description in this field.

21. DIAGNOSIS OR NATURE OF ILLNESS OR INJURY Relate A-L to service line below (24E) ICD Ind. 0				22. RESUBMISSION CODE	ORIGINAL REF. NO.
A. H66.009	B.	C.	D.	23. PRIOR AUTHORIZATION NUMBER	
E.	F.	G.	H.		
I.	J.	K.	L.		

24. A. DATE(S) OF SERVICE From MM DD YY	To MM DD YY	B. PLACE OF SERVICE	C. EMG	D. PROCEDURES, SERVICES, OR SUPPLIES (Explain Unusual Circumstances) CPT/HCPCS	MODIFIER	E. DIAGNOSIS POINTER	F. $ CHARGES	G. DAYS OR UNITS	H. EPSDT Family Plan	I. ID. QUAL.	J. RENDERING PROVIDER ID. #
03 03 XX		11		99203		A	70 92	1		NPI	12458977XX

Block 22: Resubmission and/or Original Reference Number "Resubmission" means the code and original reference number assigned by the destination payer or receiver to indicate a previously submitted claim or encounter.

Instructions: List the original reference number for resubmitted claims. Refer to the most current instructions from the public or private payer regarding use of this field (that is, code).

When resubmitting a claim, enter the appropriate bill frequency code left justified in the left side of the field.

7 Replacement of prior claim

8 Void/cancel of prior claim

This block is not intended for use of original claim submissions.

21. DIAGNOSIS OR NATURE OF ILLNESS OR INJURY Relate A-L to service line below (24E) ICD Ind. 0				22. RESUBMISSION CODE	ORIGINAL REF. NO.
A. H66.009	B.	C.	D.	23. PRIOR AUTHORIZATION NUMBER	
E.	F.	G.	H.		
I.	J.	K.	L.		

24. A. DATE(S) OF SERVICE From MM DD YY	To MM DD YY	B. PLACE OF SERVICE	C. EMG	D. PROCEDURES, SERVICES, OR SUPPLIES (Explain Unusual Circumstances) CPT/HCPCS	MODIFIER	E. DIAGNOSIS POINTER	F. $ CHARGES	G. DAYS OR UNITS	H. EPSDT Family Plan	I. ID. QUAL.	J. RENDERING PROVIDER ID. #
03 03 XX		11		99203		A	70 92	1		NPI	12458977XX

Block 23: Prior Authorization Number This block identifies the payer assigned number authorizing the service(s).

Instructions: Enter any of the following: prior authorization number, referral number, mammography precertification number, or Clinical Laboratory Improvement Amendments (CLIA) number, as assigned by the payer for the current service.

Do not enter hyphens or spaces within the number.

MEDICARE CLAIMS

When laboratory services are performed in the health care office, the 10-digit CLIA certificate number should be entered in Block 23. Physicians billing patients for outside lab work are not held to CLIA standards but may charge the patient only what the laboratory charges plus any additional services the health care organization provides, such as drawing, shipping, and handling.

Line	24. A. DATE(S) OF SERVICE From MM	DD	YY	To MM	DD	YY	B. PLACE OF SERVICE	C. EMG	D. PROCEDURES, SERVICES, OR SUPPLIES (Explain Unusual Circumstances) CPT/HCPCS	MODIFIER	E. DIAGNOSIS POINTER	F. $ CHARGES	G. DAYS OR UNITS	H. EPSDT Family Plan	I. ID. QUAL.	J. RENDERING PROVIDER ID. #
1	03	03	XX				11		99203		A	70 92	1		NPI	12458977XX
2															NPI	
3															NPI	
4															NPI	
5															NPI	
6															NPI	

25. FEDERAL TAX I.D. NUMBER	SSN	EIN	26. PATIENT'S ACCOUNT NO.	27. ACCEPT ASSIGNMENT? (For govt. claims, see back)	28. TOTAL CHARGE	29. AMOUNT PAID	30. Rsvd for NUCC Use
XX12210XX	☐	☒	010	☒ YES ☐ NO	$ 70 92	$	$

Line	24. A. DATE(S) OF SERVICE From MM	DD	YY	To MM	DD	YY	B. PLACE OF SERVICE	C. EMG	D. PROCEDURES, SERVICES, OR SUPPLIES (Explain Unusual Circumstances) CPT/HCPCS	MODIFIER	E. DIAGNOSIS POINTER	F. $ CHARGES	G. DAYS OR UNITS	H. EPSDT Family Plan	I. ID. QUAL.	J. RENDERING PROVIDER ID. #
1	11	30	XX				21		99231		A	37 74	1		NPI	32783127XX
2	12	01	XX	12	03	XX	21		99231		A	37 74	3		NPI	32783127XX
3															NPI	
4															NPI	
5															NPI	
6															NPI	

25. FEDERAL TAX I.D. NUMBER	SSN	EIN	26. PATIENT'S ACCOUNT NO.	27. ACCEPT ASSIGNMENT? (For govt. claims, see back)	28. TOTAL CHARGE	29. AMOUNT PAID	30. Rsvd for NUCC Use
XX12210XX	☐	☒	102	☒ YES ☐ NO	$ 150 96	$	$

Block 24A: Date(s) of Service (Lines 1 to 6) Block 24A indicates the actual month, day, and year the service(s) was provided. Grouping services refers to a charge for a series of identical services without listing each date of service.

Instructions: Enter date(s) of service, both the "From" and "To" dates. If there is only one date of service, enter that date under "From." Leave "To" blank or re-enter the "From" date. If grouping services, the place of service, procedure code, charges, and individual provider for each line must be identical for that service. Grouping is allowed only for services on consecutive days. The number of days must correspond to the number of units in Block 24G.

When required by payers to provide additional anesthesia services information (for example, begin and end times), narrative description of an unspecified code, National Drug Code (NDC), contract rate, or tooth numbers and areas of the oral cavity, enter the applicable qualifier and number/code/information starting with the first space in the shaded line of this field. Do not enter a space, hyphen, or other separator between the qualifier and the number/code/information. The information may extend to Block 24G.

Line	24. A. DATE(S) OF SERVICE From MM	DD	YY	To MM	DD	YY	B. PLACE OF SERVICE	C. EMG	D. PROCEDURES, SERVICES, OR SUPPLIES (Explain Unusual Circumstances) CPT/HCPCS	MODIFIER	E. DIAGNOSIS POINTER	F. $ CHARGES	G. DAYS OR UNITS	H. EPSDT Family Plan	I. ID. QUAL.	J. RENDERING PROVIDER ID. #
1	03	03	XX				11		99203		A	70 92	1		NPI	12458977XX
2															NPI	
3															NPI	
4															NPI	
5															NPI	
6															NPI	

25. FEDERAL TAX I.D. NUMBER	SSN	EIN	26. PATIENT'S ACCOUNT NO.	27. ACCEPT ASSIGNMENT? (For govt. claims, see back)	28. TOTAL CHARGE	29. AMOUNT PAID	30. Rsvd for NUCC Use
XX12210XX	☐	☒	010	☒ YES ☐ NO	$ 70 92	$	$

Block 24B: Place of Service (Lines 1 to 6) This block identifies the location where the service was rendered.

Instructions: In Block 24B, enter the appropriate two-digit code from the Place of Service Code list for each item used or service performed. The Place of Service Codes can be referenced in Table 14.3 and are available at www.cms.gov/Medicare/Coding/place-of-service-codes/Place_of_Service_Code_set.html.

TABLE 14.3 **Place of Service Codes**

BLOCK 24B	
PLACE OF SERVICE CODES	**PLACE OF SERVICE DESCRIPTION**
01	Pharmacy
02	Telehealth
03	School
04	Homeless shelter
05	Indian health services free-standing facility
06	Indian health services provider-based facility
07	Tribal 638 free-standing facility
08	Tribal 638 provider-based facility
09	Prison/correctional facility
10	Unassigned
11	Doctor's office
12	Patient's home
13	Assisted living facility
14	Group home
15	Mobile unit
16	Temporary lodging
17	Walk-in retail health clinic
18	Place of employment—worksite
19	Off campus—outpatient hospital
20	Urgent care facility
21	Inpatient hospital
22	On campus—outpatient hospital
23	Emergency department—hospital
24	Ambulatory surgical center
25	Birthing center
26	Military treatment facility/uniformed service treatment facility
27–30	Unassigned
31	Skilled nursing facility (swing bed visits)
32	Nursing facility (intermediate/long-term care facilities)
33	Custodial care facility (domiciliary or rest home services)
34	Hospice (domiciliary or rest home services)
35–40	Unassigned
41	Ambulance—land
42	Ambulance—air or water
43–48	Unassigned
49	Independent clinic
50	Federally qualified health center
51	Inpatient psychiatric facility
52	Psychiatric facility—partial hospitalization
53	Community mental health care (outpatient, 24-hours-a-day- services, admission screening, consultation, and educational services
54	Intermediate care facility/mentally retarded
55	Residential substance abuse treatment facility
56	Psychiatric residential treatment facility
57	Non-residential substance abuse treatment facility
58–59	Unassigned
60	Mass immunization center
61	Comprehensive inpatient rehabilitation facility
62	Comprehensive outpatient rehabilitation facility
63–64	Unassigned
65	End-stage renal disease treatment facility
66–70	Unassigned
71	State or local public health clinic
72	Rural health clinic
73–80	Unassigned
81	Independent laboratory
82–90	Unassigned
99	Other place of service not identified above

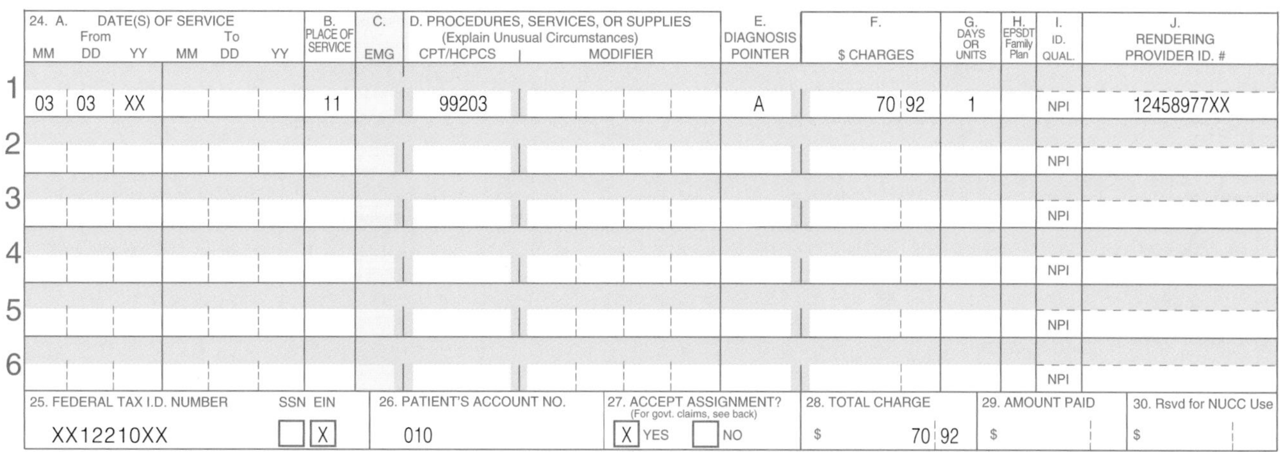

	24. A. DATE(S) OF SERVICE From MM	DD	YY	To MM	DD	YY	B. PLACE OF SERVICE	C. EMG	D. PROCEDURES, SERVICES, OR SUPPLIES (Explain Unusual Circumstances) CPT/HCPCS	MODIFIER	E. DIAGNOSIS POINTER	F. $ CHARGES	G. DAYS OR UNITS	H. EPSDT Family Plan	I. ID. QUAL.	J. RENDERING PROVIDER ID. #
1	03	03	XX				11		99203		A	70 92	1		NPI	12458977XX
2															NPI	
3															NPI	
4															NPI	
5															NPI	
6															NPI	

25. FEDERAL TAX I.D. NUMBER	SSN EIN	26. PATIENT'S ACCOUNT NO.	27. ACCEPT ASSIGNMENT? (For govt. claims, see back)	28. TOTAL CHARGE	29. AMOUNT PAID	30. Rsvd for NUCC Use
XX12210XX	☐ SSN ☒ EIN	010	☒ YES ☐ NO	$ 70 92	$	$

Block 24C: EMG (Lines 1 to 6) "EMG" identifies whether the service was an emergency.

Instructions: Check with the payer to determine whether this element is necessary. If required, enter Y for "YES," or leave blank if "NO," in the bottom, unshaded area of the field. The definition of an emergency would be defined by federal or state regulations or programs or payer contract, or would be as defined in 5010A1.

	24. A. DATE(S) OF SERVICE From MM	DD	YY	To MM	DD	YY	B. PLACE OF SERVICE	C. EMG	D. PROCEDURES, SERVICES, OR SUPPLIES (Explain Unusual Circumstances) CPT/HCPCS	MODIFIER	E. DIAGNOSIS POINTER	F. $ CHARGES	G. DAYS OR UNITS	H. EPSDT Family Plan	I. ID. QUAL.	J. RENDERING PROVIDER ID. #
1	03	03	XX				11		99203		A	70 92	1		NPI	12458977XX
2															NPI	
3															NPI	
4															NPI	
5															NPI	
6															NPI	

25. FEDERAL TAX I.D. NUMBER	SSN EIN	26. PATIENT'S ACCOUNT NO.	27. ACCEPT ASSIGNMENT? (For govt. claims, see back)	28. TOTAL CHARGE	29. AMOUNT PAID	30. Rsvd for NUCC Use
XX12210XX	☐ SSN ☒ EIN	010	☒ YES ☐ NO	$ 70 92	$	$

Block 24D: Procedures, Services, or Supplies (Lines 1 to 6) This block identifies the medical services and procedures provided to the patient.

Instructions: Enter the Current Procedural Terminology (CPT) or Health care Common Procedure Coding System (HCPCS) code(s) and modifier(s) (if applicable) from the appropriate code set in effect on the date of service. This field accommodates the entry of up to four two-digit modifiers. The specific procedure code(s) must be shown without a narrative description.

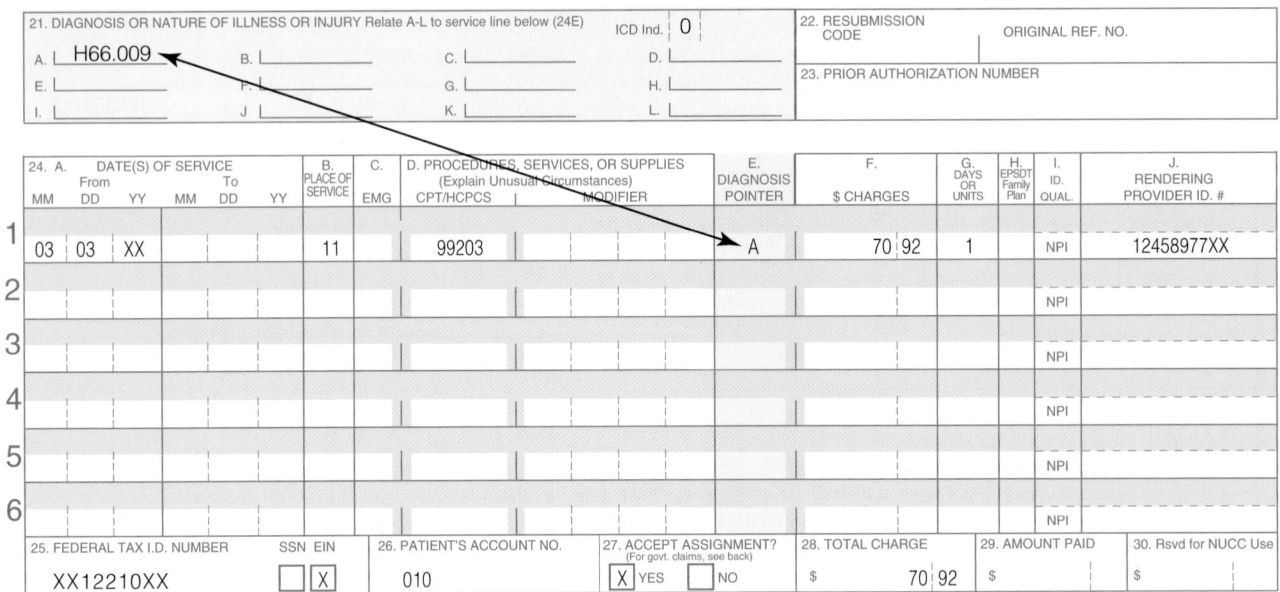

21. DIAGNOSIS OR NATURE OF ILLNESS OR INJURY Relate A-L to service line below (24E) ICD Ind. 0

A. H66.009 B. C. D.
E. F. G. H.
I. J. K. L.

22. RESUBMISSION CODE ORIGINAL REF. NO.

23. PRIOR AUTHORIZATION NUMBER

	24. A. DATE(S) OF SERVICE From MM DD YY	To MM DD YY	B. PLACE OF SERVICE	C. EMG	D. PROCEDURES, SERVICES, OR SUPPLIES (Explain Unusual Circumstances) CPT/HCPCS	MODIFIER	E. DIAGNOSIS POINTER	F. $ CHARGES	G. DAYS OR UNITS	H. EPSDT Family Plan	I. ID. QUAL.	J. RENDERING PROVIDER ID. #
1	03 03 XX		11		99203		A	70 92	1		NPI	12458977XX
2											NPI	
3											NPI	
4											NPI	
5											NPI	
6											NPI	

25. FEDERAL TAX I.D. NUMBER	SSN EIN	26. PATIENT'S ACCOUNT NO.	27. ACCEPT ASSIGNMENT? (For govt. claims, see back)	28. TOTAL CHARGE	29. AMOUNT PAID	30. Rsvd for NUCC Use
XX12210XX	☐ ☒	010	☒ YES ☐ NO	$ 70 92	$	$

Block 24E: Diagnosis Pointer (Lines 1 to 6) The "Diagnosis Pointer" is the line letter from Block 21 that relates to the reason the service(s) was performed.

Instructions: In Block 24E, enter the diagnosis code reference letter (pointer) as shown in Block 21 to relate the date of service and the procedures performed to the primary diagnosis. When multiple services are performed, the primary reference number for each service should be listed first and other applicable services should follow. The reference letter(s) should be A to L or multiple letters as applicable. ICD-9-CM or ICD-10-CM diagnosis codes must be entered in Block 21 only. Do not enter them in Block 24E.

Enter numbers left justified in the field. Do not use commas between the numbers.

	24. A. DATE(S) OF SERVICE From MM DD YY	To MM DD YY	B. PLACE OF SERVICE	C. EMG	D. PROCEDURES, SERVICES, OR SUPPLIES (Explain Unusual Circumstances) CPT/HCPCS	MODIFIER	E. DIAGNOSIS POINTER	F. $ CHARGES	G. DAYS OR UNITS	H. EPSDT Family Plan	I. ID. QUAL.	J. RENDERING PROVIDER ID. #
1	03 03 XX		11		99203		A	70 92	1		NPI	12458977XX
2											NPI	
3											NPI	
4											NPI	
5											NPI	
6											NPI	

25. FEDERAL TAX I.D. NUMBER	SSN EIN	26. PATIENT'S ACCOUNT NO.	27. ACCEPT ASSIGNMENT? (For govt. claims, see back)	28. TOTAL CHARGE	29. AMOUNT PAID	30. Rsvd for NUCC Use
XX12210XX	☐ ☒	010	☒ YES ☐ NO	$ 70 92	$	$

Block 24F: $Charges (Lines 1 to 6) This block indicates the total billed amount for each service line.

Instructions: Enter the charge for each listed service.

Enter numbers right justified in the dollar area of the field. Do not use commas when reporting dollar amounts. Negative dollar amounts are not allowed. Dollar signs should not be entered. Enter 00 in the cents area if the amount is a whole number.

	24. A. DATE(S) OF SERVICE From MM	DD	YY	To MM	DD	YY	B. PLACE OF SERVICE	C. EMG	D. PROCEDURES, SERVICES, OR SUPPLIES (Explain Unusual Circumstances) CPT/HCPCS	MODIFIER	E. DIAGNOSIS POINTER	F. $ CHARGES	G. DAYS OR UNITS	H. EPSDT Family Plan	I. ID. QUAL.	J. RENDERING PROVIDER ID. #
1	03	03	XX				11		99203		A	70 92	1		NPI	12458977XX
2															NPI	
3															NPI	
4															NPI	
5															NPI	
6															NPI	

25. FEDERAL TAX I.D. NUMBER	SSN EIN	26. PATIENT'S ACCOUNT NO.	27. ACCEPT ASSIGNMENT? (For govt. claims, see back)	28. TOTAL CHARGE	29. AMOUNT PAID	30. Rsvd for NUCC Use
XX12210XX	☐ SSN ☒ EIN	010	☒ YES ☐ NO	$ 70 92	$	$

Block 24G: Days or Units (Lines 1 to 6) This block indicates the number of days corresponding to the dates entered in Block 24A or units as defined in CPT or HCPCS coding manual(s).

Instructions: Enter the number of days or units. This block is most commonly used for multiple visits, units of supplies, anesthesia units or minutes, or oxygen volume. If only one service is performed, the numeral 1 must be entered.

Enter numbers left justified in this block. No leading zeros are required. If reporting a fraction of a unit, use the decimal point.

Anesthesia services must be reported as minutes. Units may only be reported for anesthesia services when the codes description includes a time period, such as "daily management."

	24. A. DATE(S) OF SERVICE From MM	DD	YY	To MM	DD	YY	B. PLACE OF SERVICE	C. EMG	D. PROCEDURES, SERVICES, OR SUPPLIES (Explain Unusual Circumstances) CPT/HCPCS	MODIFIER	E. DIAGNOSIS POINTER	F. $ CHARGES	G. DAYS OR UNITS	H. EPSDT Family Plan	I. ID. QUAL.	J. RENDERING PROVIDER ID. #
1	03	03	XX				11		99203		A	70 92	1		NPI	12458977XX
2															NPI	
3															NPI	
4															NPI	
5															NPI	
6															NPI	

25. FEDERAL TAX I.D. NUMBER	SSN EIN	26. PATIENT'S ACCOUNT NO.	27. ACCEPT ASSIGNMENT? (For govt. claims, see back)	28. TOTAL CHARGE	29. AMOUNT PAID	30. Rsvd for NUCC Use
XX12210XX	☐ SSN ☒ EIN	010	☒ YES ☐ NO	$ 70 92	$	$

Block 24H: EPSDT/Family Plan (Lines 1 to 6) The "EPSDT/Family Plan" identifies certain services that may be covered under some state Medicaid plans.

Instructions: For Early and Periodic Screening, Diagnosis, and Treatment (**EPSDT**)–related services, enter the response in the shaded portion of the field as follows.

If there is a requirement to report a reason code for EPDST, enter the appropriate reason code as noted below. (A Y or N response is not entered with the code.) The two-character code is right justified in the shaded area of the field.

The following codes for EPSDT are used in 5010A1:

AV Available—Not Used (Patient refused referral.)

S2 Under Treatment (Patient is currently under treatment for referred diagnostic or corrective treatment or is scheduled for another appointment with screening provider for diagnostic or corrective treatment for at least one health problem identified during an initial or periodic screening service, not including dental referrals.)

ST New Service Requested (Referral to another provider for diagnostic or corrective treatment/scheduled for another appointment with screening provider for diagnostic or corrective treatment for at least one health problem identified during an initial or periodic screening service, not including dental referrals.)

NU Not Used (Used when no EPSDT patient referral was given.)

If the service is Family Planning, enter Y ("YES") or N ("NO") in the bottom, unshaded area of the field.

When there is no requirement to report this is a Family Planning Service, leave the field blank.

	24. A. DATE(S) OF SERVICE From MM	DD	YY	To MM	DD	YY	B. PLACE OF SERVICE	C. EMG	D. PROCEDURES, SERVICES, OR SUPPLIES (Explain Unusual Circumstances) CPT/HCPCS	MODIFIER	E. DIAGNOSIS POINTER	F. $ CHARGES	G. DAYS OR UNITS	H. EPSDT Family Plan	I. ID. QUAL.	J. RENDERING PROVIDER ID. #
1	03	03	XX				11		99203		A	70 92	1		NPI	12458977XX
2															NPI	
3															NPI	
4															NPI	
5															NPI	
6															NPI	

25. FEDERAL TAX I.D. NUMBER	SSN EIN	26. PATIENT'S ACCOUNT NO.	27. ACCEPT ASSIGNMENT? (For govt. claims, see back)	28. TOTAL CHARGE	29. AMOUNT PAID	30. Rsvd for NUCC Use
XX12210XX	☐ SSN ☒ EIN	010	☒ YES ☐ NO	$ 70 92	$	$

Block 24I: ID Qualifier (Lines 1 to 6) If the provider does not have an NPI number, enter the appropriate qualifier and identifying number in the shaded area.

There will always be providers who do not have an NPI and will need to report non-NPI identifiers on their claim forms. The qualifiers will indicate the non-NPI number being reported.

Instructions: Enter in the shaded area of Block 24I the qualifier, identifying if the number is a non-NPI. The Other ID number of the rendering provider should be reported in Block 24J in the shaded area.

NUCC defines the following qualifiers used in 5010A1:

0B State License Number
1G Provider UPIN Number
G2 Provider Commercial Number
LU Location Number
ZZ Provider Taxonomy (The qualifier in the 5010A1 for Provider Taxonomy is PXC but ZZ remains the qualifier for the 1500 Claim Form.)

The list contains both provider identifiers and the provider taxonomy code. The provider identifiers are assigned to the provider either by a specific payer or by a third party in order to uniquely identify the provider. The taxonomy code is designated by the provider in order to identify his or her provider type, classification, and area of specialization. Both provider identifiers and provider taxonomy may be used in this field.

The rendering provider is the person or company (laboratory or other facility) that rendered or supervised the care. In the case where a substitute provider (locum tenens) was used, enter that provider's information here. Report the identification number in Blocks 24I and 24J only when different from data recorded in Blocks 33a and 33b.

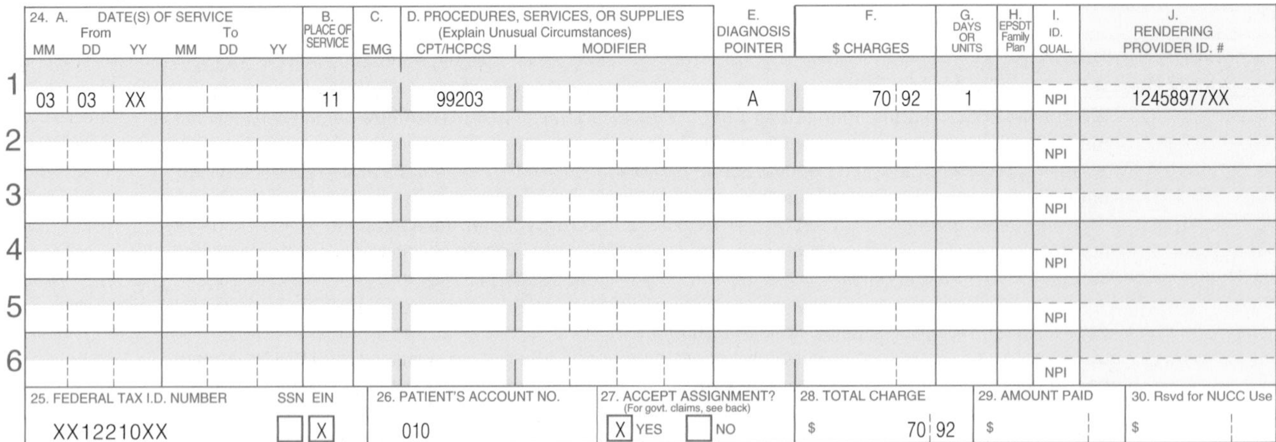

	24. A. DATE(S) OF SERVICE From MM	DD	YY	To MM	DD	YY	B. PLACE OF SERVICE	C. EMG	D. PROCEDURES, SERVICES, OR SUPPLIES (Explain Unusual Circumstances) CPT/HCPCS	MODIFIER	E. DIAGNOSIS POINTER	F. $ CHARGES	G. DAYS OR UNITS	H. EPSDT Family Plan	I. ID. QUAL.	J. RENDERING PROVIDER ID. #
1	03	03	XX				11		99203		A	70 92	1		NPI	12458977XX
2															NPI	
3															NPI	
4															NPI	
5															NPI	
6															NPI	

25. FEDERAL TAX I.D. NUMBER	SSN EIN	26. PATIENT'S ACCOUNT NO.	27. ACCEPT ASSIGNMENT? (For govt. claims, see back)	28. TOTAL CHARGE	29. AMOUNT PAID	30. Rsvd for NUCC Use
XX12210XX	☐ SSN ☒ EIN	010	☒ YES ☐ NO	$ 70 92	$	$

Block 24J: Rendering Provider ID. # (Lines 1 to 6) The individual performing or rendering the service should be reported in Block 24J and the qualifier indicating if the number is a non-NPI goes in Block 24I. The non-NPI ID number of the rendering provider refers to the payer-assigned unique identifier of the professional.

Instructions: The individual rendering the service should be reported in Block 24J. Enter the non-NPI ID number in the shaded area of the field. Enter the NPI number in the unshaded area of the field.

The rendering provider is the person or company (laboratory or other facility) that rendered or supervised the care. In the case where a substitute provider (locum tenens) was used, enter that provider's information here. Report the identification number in Blocks 24I and 24J only when different from data recorded in Blocks 33a and 33b.

Enter numbers left justified in the block.

INSTRUCTIONS AND EXAMPLES OF SUPPLEMENTAL INFORMATION IN BLOCK 24 The following are types of supplemental information that can be entered in the shaded areas of Block 24:

- Narrative descriptions of unspecified codes
- National Drug Codes (NDC) for drugs
- Device Identifier of the Unique Device Identifier for supplies
- Contract rate
- Tooth numbers and areas of the oral cavity

The following qualifiers are to be used when reporting these services:
ZZ Narrative Description of Unspecified Code
N4 National Drug Codes (NDC)
DI Device Identifier of the Unique Device Identifier (UDI)
CTR Contract Rate
JP Universal/National Tooth Designation System
JO ANSI/ADA/ISO Specification No. 3950-1984 Dentistry Designation System for Tooth and Areas of the Oral Cavity

If required to report other supplemental information not listed above, follow payer instructions for the use of a qualifier for the information being reported. When reporting a service that does not have a qualifier, enter two blank spaces before entering the information.

To enter supplemental information, begin at Block 24A by entering the qualifier and then the information. Do not enter a space between the qualifier and the number/code/information. Do not enter hyphens or spaces with the number/code.

More than one supplemental item can be reported in the shaded lines of Block 24. Enter the first qualifier and number/code/information at Block 24A. After the first item, enter three blank spaces and then the next qualifier and number/code/information.

When reporting dollar amounts in the shaded area, always enter the dollar amount, a decimal point, and cents. Use 00 for the cents if the amount is a whole number. Do not use commas. Do not enter dollar signs.

Additional Information for Reporting NDC

When entering supplemental information for NDC, add in the following order: qualifier, NDC code, one space, unit/basis of measurement qualifier, quantity. The number of digits for the quantity is limited to eight digits before the decimal and three digits after the decimal. If entering a whole number, do not use a decimal. Do not use commas.

When a dollar amount is being reported, enter the following after the quantity: one space, dollar amount. Do not enter a dollar sign.

The following qualifiers are to be used when reporting NDC unit/basis of measurement:
F2 International Unit
ME Milligram
ML Milliliter
GR Gram
UN Unit

Additional Information for Reporting Tooth Numbers and Areas of the Oral Cavity

When reporting tooth numbers, add in the following order: qualifier, tooth number (for example, JP16). When reporting an area of the oral cavity, enter in the following order: qualifier, area of oral cavity code (for example, JO10).

When reporting multiple tooth numbers for one procedure, add in the following order: qualifier, tooth number, blank space, tooth number, blank space, tooth number, and so on (for example, JP1 16 17 32).

When reporting multiple tooth numbers for one procedure, the number of units reported in Block 24G is the number of teeth involved in the procedure.

When reporting multiple areas of the oral cavity for one procedure, add in the following order: qualifier, oral cavity code, blank space, oral cavity code, and so on (for example, JO10 20).

When reporting multiple areas of the oral cavity for one procedure, the number of units reported in Block 24G is the number of areas of the oral cavity involved in the procedure.

The following are the codes for tooth numbers, reported with the JP qualifier:
1-32 Permanent dentition
51-82 Permanent supernumerary dentition
A-T Primary dentition
AS-TS Primary supernumerary dentition

The following are the codes for areas of the oral cavity, reported with the JO qualifier:
00 Entire oral cavity
01 Maxillary arch
02 Mandibular arch
10 Upper right quadrant
20 Upper left quadrant
30 Lower left quadrant
40 Lower right quadrant

For further information on these codes, refer to the Current Dental Terminology (CDT) Manual available from the American Dental Association.

25. FEDERAL TAX I.D. NUMBER SSN EIN	26. PATIENT'S ACCOUNT NO.	27. ACCEPT ASSIGNMENT? (For govt. claims, see back)	28. TOTAL CHARGE	29. AMOUNT PAID	30. Rsvd for NUCC Use
XX12210XX ☐ ☒	010	☒ YES ☐ NO	$ 70 92	$	$
31. SIGNATURE OF PHYSICIAN OR SUPPLIER INCLUDING DEGREES OR CREDENTIALS (I certify that the statements on the reverse apply to this bill and are made a part thereof.) Concha Antrum MD 030320XX	32. SERVICE FACILITY LOCATION INFORMATION		33. BILLING PROVIDER INFO & PH # (555) 4869002 College Clinic 4567 Broad Avenue Woodland Hills XY 12345-0001		
SIGNED Concha Antrum MD DATE	a. NPI	b.	a. 3664021CC	b.	

Block 25: Federal Tax ID Number The "Federal Tax ID Number" is the unique identifier assigned by a federal or state agency.

Instructions: Enter the "Federal Tax ID Number" (EIN or SSN) of the billing provider identified in Block 33. This is the tax ID number intended to be used for 1099 reporting purposes. Enter an X in the appropriate box to indicate which number is being reported. Only one box can be marked.

Do not enter hyphens with numbers. Enter numbers left justified in the field.

When completing the Workbook assignments, enter the group's federal tax ID number and check the appropriate box except in Medicare/Medigap cases.

25. FEDERAL TAX I.D. NUMBER SSN EIN	26. PATIENT'S ACCOUNT NO.	27. ACCEPT ASSIGNMENT? (For govt. claims, see back)	28. TOTAL CHARGE	29. AMOUNT PAID	30. Rsvd for NUCC Use
XX12210XX ☐ ☒	010	☒ YES ☐ NO	$ 70 92	$	$
31. SIGNATURE OF PHYSICIAN OR SUPPLIER INCLUDING DEGREES OR CREDENTIALS (I certify that the statements on the reverse apply to this bill and are made a part thereof.) Concha Antrum MD 030320XX SIGNED *Concha Antrum MD* DATE	32. SERVICE FACILITY LOCATION INFORMATION a. NPI b.		33. BILLING PROVIDER INFO & PH # (555) 4869002 College Clinic 4567 Broad Avenue Woodland Hills XY 12345-0001 a. 3664021CC b.		

Block 26: Patient's Account No The "Patient's Account No." is the identifier assigned by the health care organization.

Instructions: Enter the patient's account number assigned by the provider of service's or supplier's accounting system.

Do not enter hyphens with numbers. Enter numbers left justified in the field.

Note: When completing the Workbook *assignments, list the patient account number when provided.*

25. FEDERAL TAX I.D. NUMBER SSN EIN	26. PATIENT'S ACCOUNT NO.	27. ACCEPT ASSIGNMENT? (For govt. claims, see back)	28. TOTAL CHARGE	29. AMOUNT PAID	30. Rsvd for NUCC Use
XX12210XX ☐ ☒	010	☒ YES ☐ NO	$ 70 92	$	$
31. SIGNATURE OF PHYSICIAN OR SUPPLIER INCLUDING DEGREES OR CREDENTIALS (I certify that the statements on the reverse apply to this bill and are made a part thereof.) Concha Antrum MD 030320XX SIGNED *Concha Antrum MD* DATE	32. SERVICE FACILITY LOCATION INFORMATION a. NPI b.		33. BILLING PROVIDER INFO & PH # (555) 4869002 College Clinic 4567 Broad Avenue Woodland Hills XY 12345-0001 a. 3664021CC b.		

Block 27: Accept Assignment? "Accept Assignment?" indicates that the health care organization agrees to accept assignment under the terms of the payer's program.

Instructions: Enter an X in the correct box. Only one box can be marked.

Report "Accept Assignment?" for all payers.

Note: When completing the Workbook assignments, check "Yes" if Medicare or Medicare with other insurance.

MEDICARE/MEDICAID CLAIMS

For Medi-Medi claims, check "Yes" for assignment in Block 27. If the provider does not accept assignment, then payment will go to the patient and Medicaid will not pick up the residual.

25. FEDERAL TAX I.D. NUMBER SSN EIN	26. PATIENT'S ACCOUNT NO.	27. ACCEPT ASSIGNMENT? (For govt. claims, see back)	28. TOTAL CHARGE	29. AMOUNT PAID	30. Rsvd for NUCC Use
XX12210XX ☐ ☒	010	☒ YES ☐ NO	$ 70 92	$	$
31. SIGNATURE OF PHYSICIAN OR SUPPLIER INCLUDING DEGREES OR CREDENTIALS (I certify that the statements on the reverse apply to this bill and are made a part thereof.) Concha Antrum MD 030320XX SIGNED *Concha Antrum MD* DATE	32. SERVICE FACILITY LOCATION INFORMATION a. NPI b.		33. BILLING PROVIDER INFO & PH # (555) 4869002 College Clinic 4567 Broad Avenue Woodland Hills XY 12345-0001 a. 3664021CC b.		

Block 28: Total Charge This block indicates the total billed amount for all services entered in Block 24F (Lines 1 to 6).

Instructions: Enter the total charges for the services (that is, total of all charges in Block 24F).

Enter the amount right justified in the dollar area of the field. Do not use commas. Negative dollar amounts are not allowed. Dollar signs should not be entered. Enter 00 in the cents area if the amount is a whole number.

25. FEDERAL TAX I.D. NUMBER SSN EIN	26. PATIENT'S ACCOUNT NO.	27. ACCEPT ASSIGNMENT? (For govt. claims, see back)	28. TOTAL CHARGE	29. AMOUNT PAID	30. Rsvd for NUCC Use
XX12210XX ☐ ☒	010	☒ YES ☐ NO	$ 70 92	$	$
31. SIGNATURE OF PHYSICIAN OR SUPPLIER INCLUDING DEGREES OR CREDENTIALS (I certify that the statements on the reverse apply to this bill and are made a part thereof.) Concha Antrum MD 030320XX SIGNED *Concha Antrum MD* DATE	32. SERVICE FACILITY LOCATION INFORMATION a. NPI b.		33. BILLING PROVIDER INFO & PH # (555) 4869002 College Clinic 4567 Broad Avenue Woodland Hills XY 12345-0001 a. 3664021CC b.		

Block 29: Amount Paid This block indicates payment received from the patient or other payers.

Instructions: Enter the total amount the patient and/or other payers paid on the covered services only.

Enter the number right justified in the dollar area of the field. Do not use commas when reporting dollar amounts. Negative dollar amounts are not allowed. Dollar signs should not be entered. Enter 00 in the cents area if the amount is a whole number.

25. FEDERAL TAX I.D. NUMBER SSN EIN	26. PATIENT'S ACCOUNT NO.	27. ACCEPT ASSIGNMENT? (For govt. claims, see back)	28. TOTAL CHARGE	29. AMOUNT PAID	30. Rsvd for NUCC Use
XX12210XX ☐ ☒	010	☒ YES ☐ NO	$ 70 92	$	$
31. SIGNATURE OF PHYSICIAN OR SUPPLIER INCLUDING DEGREES OR CREDENTIALS (I certify that the statements on the reverse apply to this bill and are made a part thereof.) Concha Antrum MD 030320XX	32. SERVICE FACILITY LOCATION INFORMATION		33. BILLING PROVIDER INFO & PH # (555) 4869002 College Clinic 4567 Broad Avenue Woodland Hills XY 12345-0001		
SIGNED *Concha Antrum MD* DATE	a. NPI	b.	a. 3664021CC	b.	

Block 30: Reserved for NUCC Use This field is reserved for NUCC use. NUCC will provide instructions for any use of this field.

Instructions: This field was previously used to report "Balance Due." "Balance Due" does not exist in 5010A1, so this field has been eliminated.

25. FEDERAL TAX I.D. NUMBER SSN EIN	26. PATIENT'S ACCOUNT NO.	27. ACCEPT ASSIGNMENT? (For govt. claims, see back)	28. TOTAL CHARGE	29. AMOUNT PAID	30. Rsvd for NUCC Use
XX12210XX ☐ ☒	010	☒ YES ☐ NO	$ 70 92	$	$
31. SIGNATURE OF PHYSICIAN OR SUPPLIER INCLUDING DEGREES OR CREDENTIALS (I certify that the statements on the reverse apply to this bill and are made a part thereof.) Concha Antrum MD 030320XX	32. SERVICE FACILITY LOCATION INFORMATION		33. BILLING PROVIDER INFO & PH # (555) 4869002 College Clinic 4567 Broad Avenue Woodland Hills XY 12345-0001		
SIGNED *Concha Antrum MD* DATE	a. NPI	b.	a. 3664021CC	b.	

Block 31: Signature of Physician or Supplier Including Degrees or Credentials This block refers to the authorized or accountable person and the degree, credentials, or title.

Instructions: Signature of Physician or Supplier Including Degrees or Credentials does not exist in 5010A1.

Enter the legal signature of the practitioner or supplier, signature of the practitioner or supplier representative, "Signature on File," or "SOF." Enter either the 6-digit date (MM/DD/YY), 8-digit date (MM/DD/YYYY), or alphanumeric date (for example, January 1, 2003) on which the form was signed.

25. FEDERAL TAX I.D. NUMBER SSN EIN	26. PATIENT'S ACCOUNT NO.	27. ACCEPT ASSIGNMENT? (For govt. claims, see back)	28. TOTAL CHARGE	29. AMOUNT PAID	30. Rsvd for NUCC Use
XX12210XX ☐ ☒	010	☒ YES ☐ NO	$ 70 92	$	$
31. SIGNATURE OF PHYSICIAN OR SUPPLIER INCLUDING DEGREES OR CREDENTIALS (I certify that the statements on the reverse apply to this bill and are made a part thereof.) Concha Antrum MD 030320XX	32. SERVICE FACILITY LOCATION INFORMATION		33. BILLING PROVIDER INFO & PH # (555) 4869002 College Clinic 4567 Broad Avenue Woodland Hills XY 12345-0001		
SIGNED *Concha Antrum MD* DATE	a. NPI	b.	a. 3664021CC	b.	

Block 32: Service Facility Location Information The name and address of the facility where services were rendered identifies the site where services were provided.

Instructions: Enter the name, address, city, state, and zip code of the location where the services were rendered. Providers of service (name of physician) must identify the supplier's name, address, zip code, and NPI number when billing for purchased diagnostic tests. When more than one supplier is used, a separate 1500 Claim Form should be used to bill for each supplier.

Enter the name and address information in the following format:

1st line: Name
2nd line: Address
3rd line: City, state, and zip code

Do not use punctuation (that is, commas and periods) or other symbols in the address (for example, use 123 N Main Street 101 instead of 123 N. Main Street, #101). Enter a space between the town name and state code; do not include a comma. When reporting a 9-digit zip code, include the hyphen.

If reporting a foreign address, contact payer for specific reporting instructions.

25. FEDERAL TAX I.D. NUMBER SSN EIN	26. PATIENT'S ACCOUNT NO.	27. ACCEPT ASSIGNMENT? (For govt. claims, see back)	28. TOTAL CHARGE	29. AMOUNT PAID	30. Rsvd for NUCC Use
XX12210XX ☐ ☒	010	☒ YES ☐ NO	$ 70 92	$	$
31. SIGNATURE OF PHYSICIAN OR SUPPLIER INCLUDING DEGREES OR CREDENTIALS (I certify that the statements on the reverse apply to this bill and are made a part thereof.) Concha Antrum MD 030320XX	32. SERVICE FACILITY LOCATION INFORMATION		33. BILLING PROVIDER INFO & PH # (555) 4869002 College Clinic 4567 Broad Avenue Woodland Hills XY 12345-0001		
SIGNED *Concha Antrum MD* DATE	a. NPI	b.	a. 3664021CC	b.	

Block 32a: NPI# The NPI number refers to the HIPAA National Provider Identifier number.

Instructions: If a service facility is entered in Block 32, enter the NPI number of the service facility location in Block 32a.

Only report a Service Facility Location NPI when the NPI is different from the Billing Provider NPI.

25. FEDERAL TAX I.D. NUMBER (SSN / EIN)	26. PATIENT'S ACCOUNT NO.	27. ACCEPT ASSIGNMENT? (For govt. claims, see back)	28. TOTAL CHARGE	29. AMOUNT PAID	30. Rsvd for NUCC Use
XX12210XX ☐ SSN ☒ EIN	010	☒ YES ☐ NO	$ 70 92	$	$
31. SIGNATURE OF PHYSICIAN OR SUPPLIER INCLUDING DEGREES OR CREDENTIALS (I certify that the statements on the reverse apply to this bill and are made a part thereof.) Concha Antrum MD 030320XX SIGNED Concha Antrum MD DATE	32. SERVICE FACILITY LOCATION INFORMATION a. NPI b.		33. BILLING PROVIDER INFO & PH # (555) 4869002 College Clinic 4567 Broad Avenue Woodland Hills XY 12345-0001 a. 3664021CC b.		

Block 32b: Other ID# The non-NPI ID number of the service facility is the payer-assigned unique identifier of the facility.

Instructions: Enter the two-digit qualifier identifying the non-NPI number followed by the ID number. Do not enter a space, hyphen, or other separator between the qualifier and number.

NUCC defines the following qualifiers, since they are the same as those used in 5010A1:

0B State License Number
G2 Provider Commercial Number
LU Location Number

25. FEDERAL TAX I.D. NUMBER (SSN / EIN)	26. PATIENT'S ACCOUNT NO.	27. ACCEPT ASSIGNMENT? (For govt. claims, see back)	28. TOTAL CHARGE	29. AMOUNT PAID	30. Rsvd for NUCC Use
XX12210XX ☐ SSN ☒ EIN	010	☒ YES ☐ NO	$ 70 92	$	$
31. SIGNATURE OF PHYSICIAN OR SUPPLIER INCLUDING DEGREES OR CREDENTIALS (I certify that the statements on the reverse apply to this bill and are made a part thereof.) Concha Antrum MD 030320XX SIGNED Concha Antrum MD DATE	32. SERVICE FACILITY LOCATION INFORMATION a. NPI b.		33. BILLING PROVIDER INFO & PH # (555) 4869002 College Clinic 4567 Broad Avenue Woodland Hills XY 12345-0001 a. 3664021CC b.		

Block 33: Billing Provider Info & Ph# The billing provider's or supplier's billing name, address, zip code, and phone number is the billing office location and telephone number of the provider and supplier.

Instructions: Enter the provider's or supplier's billing name, address, zip code, and phone number. The phone number is entered in the area to the right of the field title. Enter the name and address information in the following format:

1st line: Name
2nd line: Address
3rd line: City, state, and zip code

Block 33 identifies the provider that is requesting to be paid for the service rendered and should always be completed. Do not use punctuation (that is, commas and periods) or other symbols in the address (for example, use 123 N Main Street 101 instead of 123 N. Main Street, #101). Enter a space between the town name and two-character state code; do not include a comma. When reporting a 9-digit zip code, include the hyphen. Do not use a hyphen or space as a separator within the telephone number.

If reporting a foreign address, contact the payer for specific reporting instructions.

5010A1 requires the "Billing Provider Address" to be a street address or physical location. NUCC recommends that the same requirements be applied here.

25. FEDERAL TAX I.D. NUMBER (SSN / EIN)	26. PATIENT'S ACCOUNT NO.	27. ACCEPT ASSIGNMENT? (For govt. claims, see back)	28. TOTAL CHARGE	29. AMOUNT PAID	30. Rsvd for NUCC Use
XX12210XX ☐ SSN ☒ EIN	010	☒ YES ☐ NO	$ 70 92	$	$
31. SIGNATURE OF PHYSICIAN OR SUPPLIER INCLUDING DEGREES OR CREDENTIALS (I certify that the statements on the reverse apply to this bill and are made a part thereof.) Concha Antrum MD 030320XX SIGNED Concha Antrum MD DATE	32. SERVICE FACILITY LOCATION INFORMATION a. NPI b.		33. BILLING PROVIDER INFO & PH # (555) 4869002 College Clinic 4567 Broad Avenue Woodland Hills XY 12345-0001 a. 3664021CC b.		

Block 33a: NPI# The NPI number refers to the HIPAA National Provider Identifier number.

Instructions: Enter the NPI number of the billing provider in Block 33a.

25. FEDERAL TAX I.D. NUMBER SSN EIN	26. PATIENT'S ACCOUNT NO.	27. ACCEPT ASSIGNMENT? (For govt. claims, see back)	28. TOTAL CHARGE	29. AMOUNT PAID	30. Rsvd for NUCC Use
XX12210XX ☐ ☒	010	☒ YES ☐ NO	$ 70 92	$	$

31. SIGNATURE OF PHYSICIAN OR SUPPLIER INCLUDING DEGREES OR CREDENTIALS (I certify that the statements on the reverse apply to this bill and are made a part thereof.)	32. SERVICE FACILITY LOCATION INFORMATION		33. BILLING PROVIDER INFO & PH # (555) 489002	
Concha Antrum MD 030320XX			College Clinic 4567 Broad Avenue Woodland Hills XY 12345-0001	
SIGNED *Concha Antrum MD* DATE	a. NPI	b.	a. 3664021CC	b.

Block 33b: Other ID# The non-NPI number of the billing provider refers to the payer-assigned unique identifier of the professional.

Instructions: Enter the two-digit qualifier identifying the non-NPI number followed by the ID number. Do not enter a space, hyphen, or other separator between the qualifier and number.

NUCC defines the following qualifiers used in 5010A1:

0B State License Number

G2 Provider Commercial Number

ZZ Provider Taxonomy (The qualifier in the 5010A1 for provider taxonomy is PXC but ZZ remains the qualifier for the 1500 claim form.)

The list above contains both provider identifiers and the provider taxonomy code. The provider identifiers are assigned to the provider either by a specific payer or by a third party in order to uniquely identify the provider. The taxonomy code is designated by the provider in order to identify his or her provider type, classification, and area of specialization. Both provider identifiers and provider taxonomy may be used in this field.

INSURANCE PROGRAM TEMPLATES The following pages show the completed CMS-1500 insurance claim forms and templates for the most common insurance programs encountered in a health care organization. Add a tab at the page margin for ease in flipping to this reference section when completing the *Workbook* assignments. The following examples illustrate entries for basic cases:

- Fig. 14.2 Private payer.
- Fig. 14.3 Medicaid.
- Fig. 14.4 Medicare.
- Fig. 14.5 Medicaid/Medicare—a crossover claim.
- Fig. 14.6 Medicare/Medigap—a crossover claim.
- Fig. 14.7 MSP—other insurance primary and Medicare secondary.
- Fig. 14.8 TRICARE—standard.
- Fig. 14.9 CHAMPVA.
- Fig. 14.10 Workers' compensation.

PRIVATE PAYER
NO SECONDARY COVERAGE

CARRIER

DRAFT - NOT FOR OFFICIAL USE

HEALTH INSURANCE CLAIM FORM

APPROVED BY NATIONAL UNIFOR MCLAIM COMMITTEE (NUCC) 02/12

PICA PICA

1. MEDICARE (Medicare#) MEDICAID (Medicaid#) TRICARE (ID#DoD#) CHAMPVA (Member ID#) [X] GROUP HEALTH PLAN (ID#) FECA BLK LUNG (ID#) OTHER (ID#)

1a. INSURED'S I.D. NUMBER (For Program in Item 1): 111704521

2. PATIENT'S NAME (Last Name, First Name, Middle Initial): Forehand, Harry, N

3. PATIENT'S BIRTH DATE MM DD YY: 01 06 1946 SEX M [X] F [ ]

4. INSURED'S NAME (Last Name, First Name, Middle Initial): Forehand, Harry, N

5. PATIENT'S ADDRESS (No., Street): 1456 Main Street

6. PATIENT RELATIONSHIP TO INSURED: Self [X] Spouse [ ] Child [ ] Other [ ]

7. INSURED'S ADDRESS (No., Street): 1456 Main Street

CITY: Woodland Hills STATE: XY

8. RESERVED FOR NUCC USE

CITY: Woodland Hills STATE: XY

ZIP CODE: 12345-0000 TELEPHONE (Include Area Code): (555) 4909876

ZIP CODE: 12345-0000 TELEPHONE (Include Area Code): (555) 4909876

9. OTHER INSURED'S NAME (Last Name, First Name, Middle Initial)

10. IS PATIENT'S CONDITION RELATED TO:

11. INSURED'S POLICY GROUP OR FECA NUMBER: A482

a. OTHER INSURED'S POLICY OR GROUP NUMBER

a. EMPLOYMENT? (Current or Previous) [ ] YES [X] NO

a. INSURED'S DATE OF BIRTH MM DD YY: 01 06 1946 SEX M [X] F [ ]

b. RESERVED FOR NUCC USE

b. AUTO ACCIDENT? [ ] YES [X] NO PLACE (State)

b. OTHER CLAIM ID (Designated by NUCC)

c. RESERVED FOR NUCC USE

c. OTHER ACCIDENT? [ ] YES [X] NO

c. INSURANCE PLAN NAME OR PROGRAM NAME: ABC Insurance Company

d. INSURANCE PLAN NAME OR PROGRAM NAME

10d. CLAIM CODES (Designated by NUCC)

d. IS THERE ANOTHER HEALTH BENEFIT PLAN? [ ] YES [X] NO *If yes*, complete items 9, 9a, and 9d.

READ BACK OF FORM BEFORE COMPLETING & SIGNING THIS FORM.

12. PATIENT'S OR AUTHORIZED PERSON'S SIGNATUREI authorize the release of any medical or other information necessary to process this claim. I also request payment of government benefits either to myself or to the party who accepts assignment below.

SIGNED *Harry N. Forehand* DATE *March 3,20XX*

13. INSURED'S OR AUTHORIZED PERSON'S SIGNATURE I authorize payment of medical benefits to the undersigned physician or supplier for services described below.

SIGNED *Harry N. Forehand*

PATIENT AND INSURED INFORMATION

14. DATE OF CURRENT: ILLNESS, INJURY, or PREGNANCY(LMP) MM DD YY: 03 01 20XX QUAL. 431

15. OTHER DATE QUAL. MM DD YY

16. DATES PATIENT UNABLE TO WORK IN CURRENT OCCUPATION MM DD YY FROM TO

17. NAME OF REFERRING PROVIDER OR OTHER SOURCE: DN Perry Cardi MD

17a. 17b. NPI 67805027XX

18. HOSPITALIZATION DATES RELATED TO CURRENT SERVICES MM DD YY FROM TO

19. ADDITIONAL CLAIM INFORMATION (Designated by NUCC)

20. OUTSIDE LAB? [ ] YES [X] NO $ CHARGES

21. DIAGNOSIS OR NATURE OF ILLNESS OR INJURY Relate A-L to service line below (24E) ICD Ind. 0

A. H66.009 B. C. D. E. F. G. H. I. J. K. L.

22. RESUBMISSION CODE ORIGINAL REF. NO.

23. PRIOR AUTHORIZATION NUMBER

	24. A. DATE(S) OF SERVICE From MM DD YY	To MM DD YY	B. PLACE OF SERVICE	C. EMG	D. PROCEDURES, SERVICES, OR SUPPLIES (Explain Unusual Circumstances) CPT/HCPCS MODIFIER	E. DIAGNOSIS POINTER	F. $ CHARGES	G. DAYS OR UNITS	H. EPSDT Family Plan	I. ID. QUAL.	J. RENDERING PROVIDER ID. #
1	03 03 XX		11		99203	A	70 92	1		NPI	1245897700
2										NPI	
3										NPI	
4										NPI	
5										NPI	
6										NPI	

25. FEDERAL TAX I.D. NUMBER SSN EIN: XX12210XX [ ] [X]

26. PATIENT'S ACCOUNT NO.: 010

27. ACCEPT ASSIGNMENT? (For govt. claims, see back) [X] YES [ ] NO

28. TOTAL CHARGE $ 70 92

29. AMOUNT PAID $

30. Rsvd for NUCC Use $

31. SIGNATURE OF PHYSICIAN OR SUPPLIER INCLUDING DEGREES OR CREDENTIALS (I certify that the statements on the reverse apply to this bill and are made a part thereof.)
Concha Antrum MD 030320XX
SIGNED *Concha Antrum MD* DATE

32. SERVICE FACILITY LOCATION INFORMATION
a. NPI b.

33. BILLING PROVIDER INFO & PH # (555) 4869002
College Clinic
4567 Broad Avenue
Woodland Hills XY 12345-0001
a. 3664021CC b.

PHYSICIAN OR SUPPLIER INFORMATION

NUCC Instruction Manual available at: www.nucc.org PLEASE PRINT OR TYPE OMB APPROVAL PENDING

Fig. 14.2 Front side of the scannable Health Insurance Claim Form approved by the American Medical Association's (AMA's) Council on Medical Service. This form is also known as the CMS-1500 and is shown illustrating completion to a private third-party payer with no secondary coverage. Third-party payer, state, and local guidelines vary and may not always follow the visual guide presented here.

MEDICAID
NO SECONDARY COVERAGE

CARRIER

HEALTH INSURANCE CLAIM FORM

APPROVED BY NATIONAL UNIFOR MCLAIM COMMITTEE (NUCC) 02/12

PICA | PICA

1. MEDICARE (Medicare#) [ ] MEDICAID (Medicaid#) [X] TRICARE (ID#DoD#) [ ] CHAMPVA (Member ID#) [ ] GROUP HEALTH PLAN (ID#) [ ] FECA BLK LUNG (ID#) [ ] OTHER (ID#) [ ]

1a. INSURED'S I.D. NUMBER (For Program in Item 1): 276835090

2. PATIENT'S NAME (Last Name, First Name, Middle Initial): Abramson, Adam

3. PATIENT'S BIRTH DATE MM DD YY: 02 12 1995 SEX M [X] F [ ]

4. INSURED'S NAME (Last Name, First Name, Middle Initial): Abramson, Adam

5. PATIENT'S ADDRESS (No., Street): 760 Finch Street

6. PATIENT RELATIONSHIP TO INSURED: Self [X] Spouse [ ] Child [ ] Other [ ]

7. INSURED'S ADDRESS (No., Street): 760 Finch Street

CITY: Woodland Hills STATE: XY

8. RESERVED FOR NUCC USE

CITY: Woodland Hills STATE: XY

ZIP CODE: 12345 TELEPHONE (Include Area Code): (555) 4826789

ZIP CODE: 12345 TELEPHONE (Include Area Code): (555) 4826789

9. OTHER INSURED'S NAME (Last Name, First Name, Middle Initial)

10. IS PATIENT'S CONDITION RELATED TO:

11. INSURED'S POLICY GROUP OR FECA NUMBER

a. OTHER INSURED'S POLICY OR GROUP NUMBER

a. EMPLOYMENT? (Current or Previous) [ ] YES [X] NO

a. INSURED'S DATE OF BIRTH MM DD YY: 02 12 1995 SEX M [X] F [ ]

b. RESERVED FOR NUCC USE

b. AUTO ACCIDENT? [ ] YES [X] NO PLACE (State)

b. OTHER CLAIM ID (Designated by NUCC)

c. RESERVED FOR NUCC USE

c. OTHER ACCIDENT? [X] YES [ ] NO

c. INSURANCE PLAN NAME OR PROGRAM NAME: Medicaid

d. INSURANCE PLAN NAME OR PROGRAM NAME

10d. CLAIM CODES (Designated by NUCC)

d. IS THERE ANOTHER HEALTH BENEFIT PLAN? [ ] YES [X] NO *If yes*, complete items 9, 9a, and 9d.

READ BACK OF FORM BEFORE COMPLETING & SIGNING THIS FORM.

12. PATIENT'S OR AUTHORIZED PERSON'S SIGNATUREI authorize the release of any medical or other information necessary to process this claim. I also request payment of government benefits either to myself or to the party who accepts assignment below.

SIGNED *Adam Abramson* DATE *7/14/XX*

13. INSURED'S OR AUTHORIZED PERSON'S SIGNATURE I authorize payment of medical benefits to the undersigned physician or supplier for services described below.

SIGNED *Adam Abramson*

PATIENT AND INSURED INFORMATION

14. DATE OF CURRENT: ILLNESS, INJURY, or PREGNANCY(LMP) MM DD YY QUAL.

15. OTHER DATE QUAL. MM DD YY

16. DATES PATIENT UNABLE TO WORK IN CURRENT OCCUPATION MM DD YY FROM TO

17. NAME OF REFERRING PROVIDER OR OTHER SOURCE | 17a. | 17b. NPI

18. HOSPITALIZATION DATES RELATED TO CURRENT SERVICES MM DD YY FROM TO

19. ADDITIONAL CLAIM INFORMATION (Designated by NUCC)

20. OUTSIDE LAB? [ ] YES [X] NO $ CHARGES

21. DIAGNOSIS OR NATURE OF ILLNESS OR INJURY Relate A-L to service line below (24E) ICD Ind. 0

A. T16.9xxA B. C. D.
E. F. G. H.
I. J. K. L.

22. RESUBMISSION CODE ORIGINAL REF. NO.

23. PRIOR AUTHORIZATION NUMBER

	24. A. DATE(S) OF SERVICE From MM DD YY	To MM DD YY	B. PLACE OF SERVICE	C. EMG	D. PROCEDURES, SERVICES, OR SUPPLIES (Explain Unusual Circumstances) CPT/HCPCS	MODIFIER	E. DIAGNOSIS POINTER	F. $ CHARGES	G. DAYS OR UNITS	H. EPSDT Family Plan	I. ID. QUAL.	J. RENDERING PROVIDER ID. #
1	07 14 XX		23	Y	99282	25	A	37 00	1		NPI	37640017XX
2	07 14 XX		23	Y	69200		A	49 00	1		NPI	37640017XX
3											NPI	
4											NPI	
5											NPI	
6											NPI	

PHYSICIAN OR SUPPLIER INFORMATION

25. FEDERAL TAX I.D. NUMBER SSN EIN: XX12210XX [X] [ ]

26. PATIENT'S ACCOUNT NO.: 030

27. ACCEPT ASSIGNMENT? (For govt. claims, see back) [X] YES [ ] NO

28. TOTAL CHARGE: $ 86 00

29. AMOUNT PAID: $

30. Rsvd for NUCC Use: $

31. SIGNATURE OF PHYSICIAN OR SUPPLIER INCLUDING DEGREES OR CREDENTIALS (I certify that the statements on the reverse apply to this bill and are made a part thereof.)
Pedro Atrics MD
071420XX
SIGNED *Pedro Atrics MD* DATE

32. SERVICE FACILITY LOCATION INFORMATION
College Hospital
4500 Broad Avenue
Woodland Hills XY 12345-0001
a. X950731067 b.

33. BILLING PROVIDER INFO & PH # (555) 4869002
College Clinic
4567 Broad Avenue
Woodland Hills XY 12345-0001
a. 3664021CC b.

NUCC Instruction Manual available at: www.nucc.org PLEASE PRINT OR TYPE OMB APPROVAL PENDING

Fig. 14.3 A Medicaid case with no secondary coverage, emphasizing basic elements.

MEDICARE
NO SECONDARY COVERAGE

CARRIER

HEALTH INSURANCE CLAIM FORM

APPROVED BY NATIONAL UNIFOR MCLAIM COMMITTEE (NUCC) 02/12

PICA | PICA

1. MEDICARE [X] (Medicare#) | MEDICAID [ ] (Medicaid#) | TRICARE [ ] (ID#DoD#) | CHAMPVA [ ] (Member ID#) | GROUP HEALTH PLAN [ ] (ID#) | FECA BLK LUNG [ ] (ID#) | OTHER [ ] (ID#)

1a. INSURED'S I.D. NUMBER (For Program in Item 1): 123 XX 6789A

2. PATIENT'S NAME (Last Name, First Name, Middle Initial): Hutch, Bill

3. PATIENT'S BIRTH DATE MM DD YY: 05 07 1910 SEX M [X] F [ ]

4. INSURED'S NAME (Last Name, First Name, Middle Initial): Hutch, Bill

5. PATIENT'S ADDRESS (No., Street): 8888 Main Street
CITY: Woodland Hills STATE: XY
ZIP CODE: 12345 TELEPHONE (Include Area Code): (555) 7321544

6. PATIENT RELATIONSHIP TO INSURED: Self [X] Spouse [ ] Child [ ] Other [ ]

7. INSURED'S ADDRESS (No., Street): 8888 Main Street
CITY: Woodland Hills STATE: XY
ZIP CODE: 12345 TELEPHONE (Include Area Code): (555) 7321544

8. RESERVED FOR NUCC USE

9. OTHER INSURED'S NAME (Last Name, First Name, Middle Initial)
a. OTHER INSURED'S POLICY OR GROUP NUMBER
b. RESERVED FOR NUCC USE
c. RESERVED FOR NUCC USE
d. INSURANCE PLAN NAME OR PROGRAM NAME

10. IS PATIENT'S CONDITION RELATED TO:
a. EMPLOYMENT? (Current or Previous) [ ] YES [X] NO
b. AUTO ACCIDENT? [ ] YES [X] NO PLACE (State)
c. OTHER ACCIDENT? [ ] YES [X] NO
10d. CLAIM CODES (Designated by NUCC)

11. INSURED'S POLICY GROUP OR FECA NUMBER
a. INSURED'S DATE OF BIRTH MM DD YY: 05 07 1910 SEX M [X] F [ ]
b. OTHER CLAIM ID (Designated by NUCC)
c. INSURANCE PLAN NAME OR PROGRAM NAME: Medicare
d. IS THERE ANOTHER HEALTH BENEFIT PLAN? [ ] YES [X] NO *If yes*, complete items 9, 9a, and 9d.

READ BACK OF FORM BEFORE COMPLETING & SIGNING THIS FORM.

12. PATIENT'S OR AUTHORIZED PERSON'S SIGNATUREI authorize the release of any medical or other information necessary to process this claim. I also request payment of government benefits either to myself or to the party who accepts assignment below.
SIGNED Signature on file DATE

13. INSURED'S OR AUTHORIZED PERSON'S SIGNATURE I authorize payment of medical benefits to the undersigned physician or supplier for services described below.
SIGNED

PATIENT AND INSURED INFORMATION

14. DATE OF CURRENT: ILLNESS, INJURY, or PREGNANCY(LMP) MM DD YY QUAL.
15. OTHER DATE QUAL. MM DD YY
16. DATES PATIENT UNABLE TO WORK IN CURRENT OCCUPATION FROM MM DD YY TO MM DD YY
17. NAME OF REFERRING PROVIDER OR OTHER SOURCE: DN Gerald Practon MD
17a.
17b. NPI 46278897XX
18. HOSPITALIZATION DATES RELATED TO CURRENT SERVICES FROM MM DD YY TO MM DD YY
19. ADDITIONAL CLAIM INFORMATION (Designated by NUCC)
20. OUTSIDE LAB? [ ] YES [X] NO $ CHARGES
21. DIAGNOSIS OR NATURE OF ILLNESS OR INJURY Relate A-L to service line below (24E) ICD Ind. 0
A. J12.9 B. C. D.
E. F. G. H.
I. J. K. L.
22. RESUBMISSION CODE ORIGINAL REF. NO.
23. PRIOR AUTHORIZATION NUMBER

	24. A. DATE(S) OF SERVICE From MM DD YY	To MM DD YY	B. PLACE OF SERVICE	C. EMG	D. PROCEDURES, SERVICES, OR SUPPLIES (Explain Unusual Circumstances) CPT/HCPCS	MODIFIER	E. DIAGNOSIS POINTER	F. $ CHARGES	G. DAYS OR UNITS	H. EPSDT Family Plan	I. ID. QUAL.	J. RENDERING PROVIDER ID. #
1	03 10 XX		11		99205		A	132 00	1		NPI	64211067XX
2											NPI	
3											NPI	
4											NPI	
5											NPI	
6											NPI	

PHYSICIAN OR SUPPLIER INFORMATION

25. FEDERAL TAX I.D. NUMBER: XX12210XX SSN [X] EIN [ ]
26. PATIENT'S ACCOUNT NO.: 040
27. ACCEPT ASSIGNMENT? (For govt. claims, see back) [X] YES [ ] NO
28. TOTAL CHARGE: $ 132 00
29. AMOUNT PAID: $
30. Rsvd for NUCC Use: $

31. SIGNATURE OF PHYSICIAN OR SUPPLIER INCLUDING DEGREES OR CREDENTIALS (I certify that the statements on the reverse apply to this bill and are made a part thereof.)
Brady Coccidioides
031020XX
SIGNED *Brady Coccidioides MD* DATE

32. SERVICE FACILITY LOCATION INFORMATION
a. NPI b.

33. BILLING PROVIDER INFO & PH #: (555) 4869002
College Clinic
4567 Broad Avenue
Woodland Hills XY 12345-0001
a. 3664021CC b.

NUCC Instruction Manual available at: www.nucc.org | PLEASE PRINT OR TYPE | OMB APPROVAL PENDING

Fig. 14.4 Example of a completed CMS-1500 Health Insurance Claim Form for a basic Medicare case with no other insurance coverage. The provider has accepted assignment. Screened blocks should not be completed for a Medicare case with no other insurance.

MEDICARE/MEDICAID
(primary) (secondary)
CROSSOVER CLAIM

DRAFT - NOT FOR OFFICIAL USE

HEALTH INSURANCE CLAIM FORM

APPROVED BY NATIONAL UNIFORM CLAIM COMMITTEE (NUCC) 02/12

PICA — CARRIER — PICA

1. MEDICARE [X] (Medicare#) MEDICAID [X] (Medicaid#) TRICARE [ ] (ID#DoD#) CHAMPVA [ ] (Member ID#) GROUP HEALTH PLAN [ ] (ID#) FECA BLK LUNG [ ] (ID#) OTHER [ ] (ID#)

1a. INSURED'S I.D. NUMBER (For Program in Item 1): 660 XX 2715A

2. PATIENT'S NAME (Last Name, First Name, Middle Initial): Johnson, Kathryn

3. PATIENT'S BIRTH DATE MM DD YY: 09 07 1937 SEX M [ ] F [X]

4. INSURED'S NAME (Last Name, First Name, Middle Initial): Johnson, Kathryn

5. PATIENT'S ADDRESS (No., Street): 218 Vega Drive

6. PATIENT RELATIONSHIP TO INSURED: Self [X] Spouse [ ] Child [ ] Other [ ]

7. INSURED'S ADDRESS (No., Street): 218 Vega Drive

CITY: Woodland Hills STATE: XY

8. RESERVED FOR NUCC USE

CITY: Woodland Hills STATE: XY

ZIP CODE: 12345-0000 TELEPHONE (Include Area Code): (555) 4829112

ZIP CODE: 12345-0000 TELEPHONE (Include Area Code): (555) 4829112

9. OTHER INSURED'S NAME (Last Name, First Name, Middle Initial): Johnson, Kathryn

10. IS PATIENT'S CONDITION RELATED TO:

11. INSURED'S POLICY GROUP OR FECA NUMBER

a. OTHER INSURED'S POLICY OR GROUP NUMBER: MCD016745289

a. EMPLOYMENT? (Current or Previous) [ ] YES [X] NO

a. INSURED'S DATE OF BIRTH MM DD YY: 09 07 1937 SEX M [ ] F [X]

b. RESERVED FOR NUCC USE

b. AUTO ACCIDENT? [ ] YES [X] NO PLACE (State)

b. OTHER CLAIM ID (Designated by NUCC)

c. RESERVED FOR NUCC USE

c. OTHER ACCIDENT? [ ] YES [X] NO

c. INSURANCE PLAN NAME OR PROGRAM NAME: Medicare

d. INSURANCE PLAN NAME OR PROGRAM NAME: Medicaid

10d. CLAIM CODES (Designated by NUCC)

d. IS THERE ANOTHER HEALTH BENEFIT PLAN? [X] YES [ ] NO *If yes*, complete items 9, 9a, and 9d.

READ BACK OF FORM BEFORE COMPLETING & SIGNING THIS FORM.

12. PATIENT'S OR AUTHORIZED PERSON'S SIGNATURE I authorize the release of any medical or other information necessary to process this claim. I also request payment of government benefits either to myself or to the party who accepts assignment below.

SIGNED *Kathryn Johnson* DATE *10/1/XX*

13. INSURED'S OR AUTHORIZED PERSON'S SIGNATURE I authorize payment of medical benefits to the undersigned physician or supplier for services described below.

SIGNED *Kathryn Johnson*

PATIENT AND INSURED INFORMATION

14. DATE OF CURRENT: ILLNESS, INJURY, or PREGNANCY(LMP) MM DD YY QUAL.

15. OTHER DATE QUAL. MM DD YY

16. DATES PATIENT UNABLE TO WORK IN CURRENT OCCUPATION FROM TO

17. NAME OF REFERRING PROVIDER OR OTHER SOURCE: DN Brady Coccidioides MD

17a.

17b. NPI 64211067XX

18. HOSPITALIZATION DATES RELATED TO CURRENT SERVICES FROM TO

19. ADDITIONAL CLAIM INFORMATION (Designated by NUCC)

20. OUTSIDE LAB? [ ] YES [X] NO $ CHARGES

21. DIAGNOSIS OR NATURE OF ILLNESS OR INJURY Relate A-L to service line below (24E) ICD Ind. 0

A. C43.70 B. C. D.
E. F. G. H.
I. J. K. L.

22. RESUBMISSION CODE ORIGINAL REF. NO.

23. PRIOR AUTHORIZATION NUMBER: 7680560012

	24. A. DATE(S) OF SERVICE From MM DD YY	To MM DD YY	B. PLACE OF SERVICE	C. EMG	D. PROCEDURES, SERVICES, OR SUPPLIES (Explain Unusual Circumstances) CPT/HCPCS	MODIFIER	E. DIAGNOSIS POINTER	F. $ CHARGES	G. DAYS OR UNITS	H. EPSDT Family Plan	I. ID. QUAL.	J. RENDERING PROVIDER ID. #
1	10 01 XX		24		11600		A	195 00	1		NPI	50307117XX
2											NPI	
3											NPI	
4											NPI	
5											NPI	
6											NPI	

PHYSICIAN OR SUPPLIER INFORMATION

25. FEDERAL TAX I.D. NUMBER: XX12210XX SSN [ ] EIN [X]

26. PATIENT'S ACCOUNT NO.: 050

27. ACCEPT ASSIGNMENT? (For govt. claims, see back) [X] YES [ ] NO

28. TOTAL CHARGE: $ 195 00

29. AMOUNT PAID: $

30. Rsvd for NUCC Use: $

31. SIGNATURE OF PHYSICIAN OR SUPPLIER INCLUDING DEGREES OR CREDENTIALS (I certify that the statements on the reverse apply to this bill and are made a part thereof.)
Cosmo Graff MD
100320XX
SIGNED *Cosmo Graff, MD* DATE

32. SERVICE FACILITY LOCATION INFORMATION
Woodland Hills Ambulatory Center
1229 Center Street
Woodland Hills XY 12345-0001
a. X950513700 b.

33. BILLING PROVIDER INFO & PH # (555) 4869002
College Clinic
4567 Broad Avenue
Woodland Hills XY 12345-0001
a. 3664021CC b.

NUCC Instruction Manual available at: www.nucc.org PLEASE PRINT OR TYPE OMB APPROVAL PENDING

Fig. 14.5 Example of a Medicare/Medicaid crossover claim. The CMS-1500 claim form is sent to Medicare (primary payer) and then processed automatically by Medicaid (secondary payer).

MEDICARE/MEDIGAP
(primary) (secondary)
CROSSOVER CLAIM

CARRIER

HEALTH INSURANCE CLAIM FORM

APPROVED BY NATIONAL UNIFOR MCLAIM COMMITTEE (NUCC) 02/12

PICA PICA

PATIENT AND INSURED INFORMATION

1. MEDICARE [X] (Medicare#) MEDICAID [ ] (Medicaid#) TRICARE [ ] (ID#DoD#) CHAMPVA [ ] (Member ID#) GROUP HEALTH PLAN [X] (ID#) FECA BLK LUNG [ ] (ID#) OTHER [ ] (ID#)

1a. INSURED'S I.D. NUMBER (For Program in Item 1): 419 XX 7272A

2. PATIENT'S NAME (Last Name, First Name, Middle Initial): Barnes, Agusta, E

3. PATIENT'S BIRTH DATE MM DD YY: 08 29 1917 SEX M [X] F [ ]

4. INSURED'S NAME (Last Name, First Name, Middle Initial): Barnes, Agusta, E

5. PATIENT'S ADDRESS (No., Street): 356 Encina Avenue

CITY: Woodland Hills STATE: XY

ZIP CODE: 12345-0000 TELEPHONE (Include Area Code): (555) 4672646

6. PATIENT RELATIONSHIP TO INSURED: Self [X] Spouse [ ] Child [ ] Other [ ]

7. INSURED'S ADDRESS (No., Street): 356 Encina Avenue

CITY: Woodland Hills STATE: XY

ZIP CODE: 12345-0000 TELEPHONE (Include Area Code): (555) 4672646

8. RESERVED FOR NUCC USE

9. OTHER INSURED'S NAME (Last Name, First Name, Middle Initial): Barnes, Agusta, E

a. OTHER INSURED'S POLICY OR GROUP NUMBER: MEDIGAP 419167272

b. RESERVED FOR NUCC USE

c. RESERVED FOR NUCC USE

d. INSURANCE PLAN NAME OR PROGRAM NAME: CALFCA002

10. IS PATIENT'S CONDITION RELATED TO:

a. EMPLOYMENT? (Current or Previous) [ ] YES [X] NO

b. AUTO ACCIDENT? [ ] YES [X] NO PLACE (State)

c. OTHER ACCIDENT? [ ] YES [X] NO

10d. CLAIM CODES (Designated by NUCC)

11. INSURED'S POLICY GROUP OR FECA NUMBER: A4612

a. INSURED'S DATE OF BIRTH MM DD YY: 08 29 1917 SEX M [X] F [ ]

b. OTHER CLAIM ID (Designated by NUCC)

c. INSURANCE PLAN NAME OR PROGRAM NAME: ABC Insurance Company

d. IS THERE ANOTHER HEALTH BENEFIT PLAN? [X] YES [ ] NO *If yes*, complete items 9, 9a, and 9d.

READ BACK OF FORM BEFORE COMPLETING & SIGNING THIS FORM.

12. PATIENT'S OR AUTHORIZED PERSON'S SIGNATUREI authorize the release of any medical or other information necessary to process this claim. I also request payment of government benefits either to myself or to the party who accepts assignment below.

SIGNED *Agusta E. Barnes* DATE *11/21/XX*

13. INSURED'S OR AUTHORIZED PERSON'S SIGNATURE I authorize payment of medical benefits to the undersigned physician or supplier for services described below.

SIGNED *Agusta E. Barnes*

PHYSICIAN OR SUPPLIER INFORMATION

14. DATE OF CURRENT: ILLNESS, INJURY, or PREGNANCY(LMP) MM DD YY QUAL.

15. OTHER DATE QUAL. MM DD YY

16. DATES PATIENT UNABLE TO WORK IN CURRENT OCCUPATION MM DD YY FROM TO

17. NAME OF REFERRING PROVIDER OR OTHER SOURCE: DN Gaston Input MD

17a.

17b. NPI 32783127XX

18. HOSPITALIZATION DATES RELATED TO CURRENT SERVICES MM DD YY FROM TO

19. ADDITIONAL CLAIM INFORMATION (Designated by NUCC)

20. OUTSIDE LAB? [ ] YES [X] NO $ CHARGES

21. DIAGNOSIS OR NATURE OF ILLNESS OR INJURY Relate A-L to service line below (24E) ICD Ind. 0

A. R07.89 B. C. D.
E. F. G. H.
I. J. K. L.

22. RESUBMISSION CODE ORIGINAL REF. NO.

23. PRIOR AUTHORIZATION NUMBER

	24. A. DATE(S) OF SERVICE From MM DD YY	To MM DD YY	B. PLACE OF SERVICE	C. EMG	D. PROCEDURES, SERVICES, OR SUPPLIES (Explain Unusual Circumstances) CPT/HCPCS	MODIFIER	E. DIAGNOSIS POINTER	F. $ CHARGES	G. DAYS OR UNITS	H. EPSDT Family Plan	I. ID. QUAL.	J. RENDERING PROVIDER ID. #
1	11 21 XX		11		93350		A	183 00	1		NPI	67805027XX
2	11 21 XX		11		93017		A	68 00	1		NPI	67805027XX
3											NPI	
4											NPI	
5											NPI	
6											NPI	

25. FEDERAL TAX I.D. NUMBER SSN [ ] EIN [ ]

26. PATIENT'S ACCOUNT NO.: 060

27. ACCEPT ASSIGNMENT? (For govt. claims, see back) [X] YES [ ] NO

28. TOTAL CHARGE: $ 251 00

29. AMOUNT PAID: $

30. Rsvd for NUCC Use

31. SIGNATURE OF PHYSICIAN OR SUPPLIER INCLUDING DEGREES OR CREDENTIALS (I certify that the statements on the reverse apply to this bill and are made a part thereof.)
Perry Cardi MD
SIGNED *Perry Cardi, MD* DATE 112220XX

32. SERVICE FACILITY LOCATION INFORMATION
a. NPI b.

33. BILLING PROVIDER INFO & PH # (555) 4869002
College Clinic
4567 Broad Avenue
Woodland Hills XY 12345-0001
a. 3664021CC b.

NUCC Instruction Manual available at: www.nucc.org PLEASE PRINT OR TYPE OMB APPROVAL PENDING

Fig. 14.6 Example of a completed CMS-1500 Health Insurance Claim Form for a Medicare (primary) and Medigap (secondary) crossover claim.

OTHER INSURANCE/MEDICARE-MSP
(primary) (secondary)

DRAFT - NOT FOR OFFICIAL USE

CARRIER

HEALTH INSURANCE CLAIM FORM

APPROVED BY NATIONAL UNIFOR MCLAIM COMMITTEE (NUCC) 02/12

PICA PICA

1. MEDICARE [X] (Medicare#) MEDICAID [ ] (Medicaid#) TRICARE [ ] (ID#DoD#) CHAMPVA [ ] (Member ID#) GROUP HEALTH PLAN [X] (ID#) FECA BLK LUNG [ ] (ID#) OTHER [ ] (ID#)

1a. INSURED'S I.D. NUMBER (For Program in Item 1): 609 XX 5523A

2. PATIENT'S NAME (Last Name, First Name, Middle Initial): Blair, Gwendolyn

3. PATIENT'S BIRTH DATE MM DD YY: 09 01 1931 SEX M [ ] F [X]

4. INSURED'S NAME (Last Name, First Name, Middle Initial): Blair, Gwendolyn

5. PATIENT'S ADDRESS (No., Street): 416 Richmond Street

CITY: Woodland Hills STATE: XY

ZIP CODE: 12345-0000 TELEPHONE (Include Area Code): (555) 4591519

6. PATIENT RELATIONSHIP TO INSURED: Self [X] Spouse [ ] Child [ ] Other [ ]

7. INSURED'S ADDRESS (No., Street): 416 Richmond Street

CITY: Woodland Hills STATE: XY

ZIP CODE: 12345-0000 TELEPHONE (Include Area Code): (555) 4591519

8. RESERVED FOR NUCC USE

9. OTHER INSURED'S NAME (Last Name, First Name, Middle Initial): Blair, Gwendolyn

a. OTHER INSURED'S POLICY OR GROUP NUMBER: 609 XX 5523A

b. RESERVED FOR NUCC USE

c. RESERVED FOR NUCC USE

d. INSURANCE PLAN NAME OR PROGRAM NAME: Medicare

10. IS PATIENT'S CONDITION RELATED TO:

a. EMPLOYMENT? (Current or Previous) [ ] YES [X] NO

b. AUTO ACCIDENT? [ ] YES [X] NO PLACE (State)

c. OTHER ACCIDENT? [ ] YES [X] NO

10d. CLAIM CODES (Designated by NUCC)

11. INSURED'S POLICY GROUP OR FECA NUMBER: 7845931Q

a. INSURED'S DATE OF BIRTH MM DD YY: 09 01 1931 SEX M [ ] F [X]

b. OTHER CLAIM ID (Designated by NUCC)

c. INSURANCE PLAN NAME OR PROGRAM NAME: ABC Insurance Company

d. IS THERE ANOTHER HEALTH BENEFIT PLAN? [X] YES [ ] NO *If yes, complete items 9, 9a, and 9d.*

READ BACK OF FORM BEFORE COMPLETING & SIGNING THIS FORM.

12. PATIENT'S OR AUTHORIZED PERSON'S SIGNATUREI authorize the release of any medical or other information necessary to process this claim. I also request payment of government benefits either to myself or to the party who accepts assignment below.

SIGNED Signature on file DATE

13. INSURED'S OR AUTHORIZED PERSON'S SIGNATURE I authorize payment of medical benefits to the undersigned physician or supplier for services described below.

SIGNED Signature on file

PATIENT AND INSURED INFORMATION

14. DATE OF CURRENT: ILLNESS, INJURY, or PREGNANCY(LMP) MM DD YY QUAL.

15. OTHER DATE QUAL. MM DD YY

16. DATES PATIENT UNABLE TO WORK IN CURRENT OCCUPATION FROM TO

17. NAME OF REFERRING PROVIDER OR OTHER SOURCE: DN Gerald Practon MD

17a.

17b. NPI 46278897XX

18. HOSPITALIZATION DATES RELATED TO CURRENT SERVICES FROM TO

19. ADDITIONAL CLAIM INFORMATION (Designated by NUCC)

20. OUTSIDE LAB? [ ] YES [X] NO $ CHARGES

21. DIAGNOSIS OR NATURE OF ILLNESS OR INJURY Relate A-L to service line below (24E) ICD Ind. 0

A. B35.1 B. C. D.
E. F. G. H.
I. J. K. L.

22. RESUBMISSION CODE ORIGINAL REF. NO.

23. PRIOR AUTHORIZATION NUMBER

	24. A. DATE(S) OF SERVICE From MM DD YY	To MM DD YY	B. PLACE OF SERVICE	C. EMG	D. PROCEDURES, SERVICES, OR SUPPLIES (Explain Unusual Circumstances) CPT/HCPCS	MODIFIER	E. DIAGNOSIS POINTER	F. $ CHARGES	G. DAYS OR UNITS	H. EPSDT Family Plan	I. ID. QUAL.	J. RENDERING PROVIDER ID. #
1	03 15 XX		11		99243	25	A	103 00	1		NPI	54022287XX
2	03 15 XX		11		11750		A	193 00	1		NPI	54022287XX
3											NPI	
4											NPI	
5											NPI	
6											NPI	

25. FEDERAL TAX I.D. NUMBER: XX12210XX SSN [ ] EIN [X]

26. PATIENT'S ACCOUNT NO.: 070

27. ACCEPT ASSIGNMENT? (For govt. claims, see back) [X] YES [ ] NO

28. TOTAL CHARGE: $ 296 00

29. AMOUNT PAID: $ 100 00

30. Rsvd for NUCC Use: $

31. SIGNATURE OF PHYSICIAN OR SUPPLIER INCLUDING DEGREES OR CREDENTIALS (I certify that the statements on the reverse apply to this bill and are made a part thereof.)
Nick Pedro DPM 031620XX
SIGNED *Nick Pedro, DPM* DATE

32. SERVICE FACILITY LOCATION INFORMATION
a. NPI b.

33. BILLING PROVIDER INFO & PH # (555) 4869002
College Clinic
4567 Broad Avenue
Woodland Hills XY 12345-0001
a. 3664021CC b.

PHYSICIAN OR SUPPLIER INFORMATION

NUCC Instruction Manual available at: www.nucc.org PLEASE PRINT OR TYPE OMB APPROVAL PENDING

Fig. 14.7 Template for a case in which another insurance carrier is the primary payer and Medicare is the secondary payer (MSP).

TRICARE
NO SECONDARY COVERAGE

CARRIER

HEALTH INSURANCE CLAIM FORM

APPROVED BY NATIONAL UNIFOR MCLAIM COMMITTEE (NUCC) 02/12

PICA PICA

1. MEDICARE (Medicare#) [ ] MEDICAID (Medicaid#) [ ] TRICARE (ID#DoD#) [X] CHAMPVA (Member ID#) [ ] GROUP HEALTH PLAN (ID#) [ ] FECA BLK LUNG (ID#) [ ] OTHER (ID#) [ ]

1a. INSURED'S I.D. NUMBER (For Program in Item 1): 581147211

2. PATIENT'S NAME (Last Name, First Name, Middle Initial): Smith, Susan, J

3. PATIENT'S BIRTH DATE MM DD YY: 03 16 1976 SEX M [ ] F [X]

4. INSURED'S NAME (Last Name, First Name, Middle Initial): Smith, William D

5. PATIENT'S ADDRESS (No., Street): 420 Maple Street

CITY: Woodland Hills STATE: XY

ZIP CODE: 12345-0000 TELEPHONE (Include Area Code): (555) 7899898

6. PATIENT RELATIONSHIP TO INSURED: Self [ ] Spouse [X] Child [ ] Other [ ]

7. INSURED'S ADDRESS (No., Street): 420 Maple Street

CITY: Woodland Hills STATE: XY

ZIP CODE: 12345-0000 TELEPHONE (Include Area Code): (555) 7899898

8. RESERVED FOR NUCC USE

9. OTHER INSURED'S NAME (Last Name, First Name, Middle Initial)

a. OTHER INSURED'S POLICY OR GROUP NUMBER

b. RESERVED FOR NUCC USE

c. RESERVED FOR NUCC USE

d. INSURANCE PLAN NAME OR PROGRAM NAME

10. IS PATIENT'S CONDITION RELATED TO:

a. EMPLOYMENT? (Current or Previous) [ ] YES [X] NO

b. AUTO ACCIDENT? [ ] YES [X] NO PLACE (State)

c. OTHER ACCIDENT? [ ] YES [X] NO

10d. CLAIM CODES (Designated by NUCC)

11. INSURED'S POLICY GROUP OR FECA NUMBER

a. INSURED'S DATE OF BIRTH MM DD YY: 06 12 1974 SEX M [X] F [ ]

b. OTHER CLAIM ID (Designated by NUCC)

c. INSURANCE PLAN NAME OR PROGRAM NAME: TRICARE

d. IS THERE ANOTHER HEALTH BENEFIT PLAN? [ ] YES [X] NO *If yes,* complete items 9, 9a, and 9d.

PATIENT AND INSURED INFORMATION

READ BACK OF FORM BEFORE COMPLETING & SIGNING THIS FORM.

12. PATIENT'S OR AUTHORIZED PERSON'S SIGNATUREI authorize the release of any medical or other information necessary to process this claim. I also request payment of government benefits either to myself or to the party who accepts assignment below.

SIGNED Signature on file DATE

13. INSURED'S OR AUTHORIZED PERSON'S SIGNATURE I authorize payment of medical benefits to the undersigned physician or supplier for services described below.

SIGNED Signature on file

14. DATE OF CURRENT: ILLNESS, INJURY, or PREGNANCY(LMP) MM DD YY: 10 28 20XX QUAL. 484

15. OTHER DATE QUAL. MM DD YY

16. DATES PATIENT UNABLE TO WORK IN CURRENT OCCUPATION FROM 07 21 20XX TO 09 17 20XX

17. NAME OF REFERRING PROVIDER OR OTHER SOURCE: DN Adam Langerhans MD

17a.

17b. NPI 47680657XX

18. HOSPITALIZATION DATES RELATED TO CURRENT SERVICES FROM 08 06 20XX TO 08 08 20XX

19. ADDITIONAL CLAIM INFORMATION (Designated by NUCC)

20. OUTSIDE LAB? [ ] YES [X] NO $ CHARGES

21. DIAGNOSIS OR NATURE OF ILLNESS OR INJURY Relate A-L to service line below (24E) ICD Ind. 0

A. O80 B. C. D.
E. F. G. H.
I. J. K. L.

22. RESUBMISSION CODE ORIGINAL REF. NO.

23. PRIOR AUTHORIZATION NUMBER

	24. A. DATE(S) OF SERVICE From MM DD YY	To MM DD YY	B. PLACE OF SERVICE	C. EMG	D. PROCEDURES, SERVICES, OR SUPPLIES (Explain Unusual Circumstances) CPT/HCPCS	MODIFIER	E. DIAGNOSIS POINTER	F. $ CHARGES	G. DAYS OR UNITS	H. EPSDT Family Plan	I. ID. QUAL.	J. RENDERING PROVIDER ID. #
1	08 06 XX		21		59400		A	1864 00	1		NPI	43056757XX
2											NPI	
3											NPI	
4											NPI	
5											NPI	
6											NPI	

PHYSICIAN OR SUPPLIER INFORMATION

25. FEDERAL TAX I.D. NUMBER: XX12210XX SSN [ ] EIN [X]

26. PATIENT'S ACCOUNT NO.: 080

27. ACCEPT ASSIGNMENT? (For govt. claims, see back) [X] YES [ ] NO

28. TOTAL CHARGE: $ 1864 00

29. AMOUNT PAID: $

30. Rsvd for NUCC Use: $

31. SIGNATURE OF PHYSICIAN OR SUPPLIER INCLUDING DEGREES OR CREDENTIALS (I certify that the statements on the reverse apply to this bill and are made a part thereof.)
Bertha Caesar MD
SIGNED *Bertha Caesar, MD* DATE 081020XX

32. SERVICE FACILITY LOCATION INFORMATION
College Hospital
4500 Broad Avenue
Woodland Hills XY 12345-0001
a. X950731067 b.

33. BILLING PROVIDER INFO & PH # (555) 4869002
College Clinic
4567 Broad Avenue
Woodland Hills XY 12345-0001
a. 3664021CC b.

NUCC Instruction Manual available at: www.nucc.org PLEASE PRINT OR TYPE OMB APPROVAL PENDING

Fig. 14.8 Example of a completed CMS-1500 claim form used when billing for professional services rendered in a TRICARE standard case.

CHAMPVA
NO SECONDARY COVERAGE

CARRIER

HEALTH INSURANCE CLAIM FORM

APPROVED BY NATIONAL UNIFOR MCLAIM COMMITTEE (NUCC) 02/12

PICA | PICA

1. MEDICARE (Medicare#) [ ] MEDICAID (Medicaid#) [ ] TRICARE (ID#DoD#) [ ] CHAMPVA (Member ID#) [X] GROUP HEALTH PLAN (ID#) [ ] FECA BLK LUNG (ID#) [ ] OTHER (ID#) [ ]

1a. INSURED'S I.D. NUMBER (For Program in Item 1): 560 XX 4444

2. PATIENT'S NAME (Last Name, First Name, Middle Initial): Dexter, Bruce, R

3. PATIENT'S BIRTH DATE MM DD YY: 03 13 1934 SEX M [X] F [ ]

4. INSURED'S NAME (Last Name, First Name, Middle Initial): Dexter, Bruce, R

5. PATIENT'S ADDRESS (No., Street): 226 Irwin Road

CITY: Woodland Hills STATE: XY

ZIP CODE: 12345-0000 TELEPHONE (Include Area Code): (555) 4971338

6. PATIENT RELATIONSHIP TO INSURED: Self [X] Spouse [ ] Child [ ] Other [ ]

7. INSURED'S ADDRESS (No., Street): 226 Irwin Road

CITY: Woodland Hills STATE: XY

ZIP CODE: 12345-0000 TELEPHONE (Include Area Code): (555) 4971338

8. RESERVED FOR NUCC USE

9. OTHER INSURED'S NAME (Last Name, First Name, Middle Initial)

a. OTHER INSURED'S POLICY OR GROUP NUMBER

b. RESERVED FOR NUCC USE

c. RESERVED FOR NUCC USE

d. INSURANCE PLAN NAME OR PROGRAM NAME

10. IS PATIENT'S CONDITION RELATED TO:

a. EMPLOYMENT? (Current or Previous) [X] YES [ ] NO

b. AUTO ACCIDENT? [ ] YES [X] NO PLACE (State)

c. OTHER ACCIDENT? [ ] YES [X] NO

10d. CLAIM CODES (Designated by NUCC)

11. INSURED'S POLICY GROUP OR FECA NUMBER: 023

a. INSURED'S DATE OF BIRTH MM DD YY: 03 13 1934 SEX M [X] F [ ]

b. OTHER CLAIM ID (Designated by NUCC)

c. INSURANCE PLAN NAME OR PROGRAM NAME: CHAMPVA

d. IS THERE ANOTHER HEALTH BENEFIT PLAN? [ ] YES [X] NO *If yes*, complete items 9, 9a, and 9d.

PATIENT AND INSURED INFORMATION

READ BACK OF FORM BEFORE COMPLETING & SIGNING THIS FORM.

12. PATIENT'S OR AUTHORIZED PERSON'S SIGNATUREI authorize the release of any medical or other information necessary to process this claim. I also request payment of government benefits either to myself or to the party who accepts assignment below.

SIGNED Signature on file DATE

13. INSURED'S OR AUTHORIZED PERSON'S SIGNATURE I authorize payment of medical benefits to the undersigned physician or supplier for services described below.

SIGNED Signature on file

14. DATE OF CURRENT: ILLNESS, INJURY, or PREGNANCY(LMP) MM DD YY QUAL.

15. OTHER DATE QUAL. MM DD YY

16. DATES PATIENT UNABLE TO WORK IN CURRENT OCCUPATION FROM MM DD YY TO MM DD YY

17. NAME OF REFERRING PROVIDER OR OTHER SOURCE: DN Gerald Practon MD

17a.

17b. NPI 46278897XX

18. HOSPITALIZATION DATES RELATED TO CURRENT SERVICES FROM 07 29 20XX TO 07 31 20XX

19. ADDITIONAL CLAIM INFORMATION (Designated by NUCC)

20. OUTSIDE LAB? [ ] YES [X] NO $ CHARGES

21. DIAGNOSIS OR NATURE OF ILLNESS OR INJURY Relate A-L to service line below (24E) ICD Ind. 0

A. N40.0 B. C. D.
E. F. G. H.
I. J. K. L.

22. RESUBMISSION CODE ORIGINAL REF. NO.

23. PRIOR AUTHORIZATION NUMBER

	24. A. DATE(S) OF SERVICE From MM DD YY	To MM DD YY	B. PLACE OF SERVICE	C. EMG	D. PROCEDURES, SERVICES, OR SUPPLIES (Explain Unusual Circumstances) CPT/HCPCS	MODIFIER	E. DIAGNOSIS POINTER	F. $ CHARGES	G. DAYS OR UNITS	H. EPSDT Family Plan	I. ID. QUAL.	J. RENDERING PROVIDER ID. #
1	07 29 XX		21		52601		A	1193 00	1		NPI	25678831XX
2											NPI	
3											NPI	
4											NPI	
5											NPI	
6											NPI	

25. FEDERAL TAX I.D. NUMBER: XX12210XX SSN [ ] EIN [X]

26. PATIENT'S ACCOUNT NO.: 090

27. ACCEPT ASSIGNMENT? (For govt. claims, see back) [X] YES [ ] NO

28. TOTAL CHARGE: $ 1193 00

29. AMOUNT PAID: $

30. Rsvd for NUCC Use: $

31. SIGNATURE OF PHYSICIAN OR SUPPLIER INCLUDING DEGREES OR CREDENTIALS (I certify that the statements on the reverse apply to this bill and are made a part thereof.)
Gene Ulibarri MD 073020XX
SIGNED *Gene Ulibarri MD* DATE

32. SERVICE FACILITY LOCATION INFORMATION
College Hospital
4500 Broad Avenue
Woodland Hills XY 12345-0001
a. X950731067 b.

33. BILLING PROVIDER INFO & PH # (555) 4869002
College Clinic
4567 Broad Avenue
Woodland Hills XY 12345-0001
a. 3664021CC b.

PHYSICIAN OR SUPPLIER INFORMATION

NUCC Instruction Manual available at: www.nucc.org PLEASE PRINT OR TYPE OMB APPROVAL PENDING

Fig. 14.9 An example of a completed CMS-1500 Health Insurance Claim Form for a CHAMPVA case with no secondary coverage.

WORKERS' COMPENSATION

DRAFT - NOT FOR OFFICIAL USE

CARRIER

HEALTH INSURANCE CLAIM FORM

APPROVED BY NATIONAL UNIFOR MCLAIM COMMITTEE (NUCC) 02/12

PICA | PICA

1. MEDICARE (Medicare#) | MEDICAID (Medicaid#) | TRICARE (ID#DoD#) | CHAMPVA (Member ID#) | GROUP HEALTH PLAN (ID#) | FECA BLK LUNG (ID#) | OTHER (ID#) [X]

1a. INSURED'S I.D. NUMBER (For Program in Item 1): 667289

2. PATIENT'S NAME (Last Name, First Name, Middle Initial): Barton, Peter, A

3. PATIENT'S BIRTH DATE MM DD YY: 11 14 1976 SEX M [X] F [ ]

4. INSURED'S NAME (Last Name, First Name, Middle Initial): D F Construction

5. PATIENT'S ADDRESS (No., Street): 14890 Daisy Avenue

6. PATIENT RELATIONSHIP TO INSURED: Self [ ] Spouse [ ] Child [ ] Other [X]

7. INSURED'S ADDRESS (No., Street): 1212 Hardrock Place

CITY: Woodland Hills STATE: XY

8. RESERVED FOR NUCC USE

CITY: Woodland Hills STATE: XY

ZIP CODE: 12345-0000 TELEPHONE (Include Area Code): (555) 4277698

ZIP CODE: 12345-0000 TELEPHONE (Include Area Code): (555) 4278200

9. OTHER INSURED'S NAME (Last Name, First Name, Middle Initial)

10. IS PATIENT'S CONDITION RELATED TO:

11. INSURED'S POLICY GROUP OR FECA NUMBER

a. OTHER INSURED'S POLICY OR GROUP NUMBER

a. EMPLOYMENT? (Current or Previous) [X] YES [ ] NO

a. INSURED'S DATE OF BIRTH MM DD YY SEX M [ ] F [ ]

b. RESERVED FOR NUCC USE

b. AUTO ACCIDENT? [ ] YES [X] NO PLACE (State)

b. OTHER CLAIM ID (Designated by NUCC)

c. RESERVED FOR NUCC USE

c. OTHER ACCIDENT? [ ] YES [X] NO

c. INSURANCE PLAN NAME OR PROGRAM NAME

d. INSURANCE PLAN NAME OR PROGRAM NAME

10d. CLAIM CODES (Designated by NUCC)

d. IS THERE ANOTHER HEALTH BENEFIT PLAN? [ ] YES [ ] NO *If yes,* complete items 9, 9a, and 9d.

READ BACK OF FORM BEFORE COMPLETING & SIGNING THIS FORM.

12. PATIENT'S OR AUTHORIZED PERSON'S SIGNATUREI authorize the release of any medical or other information necessary to process this claim. I also request payment of government benefits either to myself or to the party who accepts assignment below.

SIGNED Signature on file DATE

13. INSURED'S OR AUTHORIZED PERSON'S SIGNATURE I authorize payment of medical benefits to the undersigned physician or supplier for services described below.

SIGNED

PATIENT AND INSURED INFORMATION

14. DATE OF CURRENT: ILLNESS, INJURY, or PREGNANCY(LMP) MM DD YY: 01 04 20XX QUAL. 431

15. OTHER DATE QUAL. MM DD YY

16. DATES PATIENT UNABLE TO WORK IN CURRENT OCCUPATION FROM 01 04 20XX TO 03 27 20XX

17. NAME OF REFERRING PROVIDER OR OTHER SOURCE 17a. 17b. NPI

18. HOSPITALIZATION DATES RELATED TO CURRENT SERVICES FROM TO

19. ADDITIONAL CLAIM INFORMATION (Designated by NUCC)

20. OUTSIDE LAB? [ ] YES [ ] NO $ CHARGES

21. DIAGNOSIS OR NATURE OF ILLNESS OR INJURY Relate A-L to service line below (24E) ICD Ind. 0

A. M24.419 B. C. D. E. F. G. H. I. J. K. L.

22. RESUBMISSION CODE ORIGINAL REF. NO.

23. PRIOR AUTHORIZATION NUMBER

	24. A. DATE(S) OF SERVICE From MM DD YY	To MM DD YY	B. PLACE OF SERVICE	C. EMG	D. PROCEDURES, SERVICES, OR SUPPLIES (Explain Unusual Circumstances) CPT/HCPCS	MODIFIER	E. DIAGNOSIS POINTER	F. $ CHARGES	G. DAYS OR UNITS	H. EPSDT Family Plan	I. ID. QUAL.	J. RENDERING PROVIDER ID. #
1	02 27 XX		11		29055		A	150 00	1		NPI	12678547XX
2											NPI	
3											NPI	
4											NPI	
5											NPI	
6											NPI	

25. FEDERAL TAX I.D. NUMBER: XX12210XX SSN [ ] EIN [X]

26. PATIENT'S ACCOUNT NO.: 100

27. ACCEPT ASSIGNMENT? (For govt. claims, see back) [ ] YES [ ] NO

28. TOTAL CHARGE: $ 150 00

29. AMOUNT PAID: $

30. Rsvd for NUCC Use: $

31. SIGNATURE OF PHYSICIAN OR SUPPLIER INCLUDING DEGREES OR CREDENTIALS (I certify that the statements on the reverse apply to this bill and are made a part thereof.)

Raymond Skelton MD

SIGNED *Raymond Skelton, MD* DATE 022820XX

32. SERVICE FACILITY LOCATION INFORMATION a. NPI b.

33. BILLING PROVIDER INFO & PH # (555) 4869002

College Clinic
4567 Broad Avenue
Woodland Hills XY 12345-0001

a. 3664021CC b.

PHYSICIAN OR SUPPLIER INFORMATION

NUCC Instruction Manual available at: www.nucc.org | PLEASE PRINT OR TYPE | OMB APPROVAL PENDING

Fig. 14.10 An example of a completed CMS-1500 Health Insurance Claim Form for a workers' compensation case.

KEY POINTS

This is a brief chapter review of the key issues presented. To further enhance your knowledge of the technical subject matter, review the key terms and key abbreviations for this chapter by locating the meaning for each in the Glossary at the end of this book, which appears in a section before the Index.

1. There are two types of claims submitted to insurance companies for payment: *paper claims* and *electronic claims.*
2. A *clean claim* is one that was submitted to the third-party payer within the time limit, had the necessary information for processing, and was paid promptly. Under the Medicare program, a clean claim is one that has passed all electronic edits and is routed for payment.
3. Other types of claims are called *dirty* when a claim is submitted with errors; *incomplete* when missing required information; *invalid* when illogical or incorrect; *pending* when held in suspense for review; *rejected* when the claim needs investigation and answers to some questions; or *deleted* when the Medicare fiscal intermediary cancels, deletes, or voids a claim.
4. When two insurance policies are involved *(dual coverage* or *duplication of coverage),* one is considered primary and the other secondary. First, an insurance claim is submitted to the primary plan; after payment, the secondary carrier is billed with a copy of the explanation of benefits (EOB) from the primary carrier.
5. A diagnosis should never be submitted on an insurance claim without supporting documentation in the medical record.
6. Every insurance claim should be proofread for completeness and accuracy of content before it is submitted to the insurance carrier.
7. Be aware of common billing errors and learn how to correct them for quicker claim settlements and to reduce the number of appeals.
8. HIPAA transactions and code sets standards only apply to electronic transactions conducted by covered entities.
9. Copies of submitted insurance claim forms should be filed in a tickler file and reviewed for follow-up every 30 days unless the computer system maintains the files.
10. Ensure that the correct NPI is shown on the claim for the health care provider rendering the medical service to the patient.

STUDENT ASSIGNMENT

- Study Chapter 14.
- Answer the fill-in-the-blank, multiple-choice, and true/false questions in the *Workbook* to reinforce the theories learned in this chapter and to help prepare you for a future test.
- Complete the assignments in the *Workbook* to give you hands-on experience in abstracting information from case histories and financial accounting record cards as well as in completing insurance claim forms.
- Study the claim sample in the *Workbook* and try to locate as many errors as possible on the basis of the instructions you have been given in this chapter.
- Turn to the Glossary at the end of this text for a further understanding of the key terms and key abbreviations used in this chapter.

15

The Electronic Claim

Cheryl Fassett

OBJECTIVES

After reading this chapter, you should be able to:

1. Define and discuss electronic data interchange.
2. Summarize the advantages of electronic claim submission.
3. Describe the clearinghouse process that follows after a claim is electronically received.
4. Identify the transactions and code sets to use for insurance claims transmission.
5. State which insurance claim data elements are required or situational for the 837P standard transaction format.
6. Define a claim attachment and discuss claim attachments standards.
7. Compare and contrast standard unique provider identifiers, health plan identifiers, and patient identifiers.
8. Describe necessary components when adopting a practice management system.
9. Describe the use of patient encounter forms and scannable encounter forms in electronic claim submission.
10. Name and discuss some methods of interactive computer transactions for transmitting insurance claims.
11. Discuss interactive transactions and relate the electronic funds transfer process and mandated requirements under the Affordable Care Act (ACA).
12. Define an electronic remittance advice and identify the ASC X12 Health Care Claim Payment/Advice (835).
13. List the six basic procedures for transmission of an electronic claim and discuss methods for sending claims.
14. Explain the difference between carrier-direct and clearinghouse electronically transmitted insurance claims.
15. List computer transmission problems that can occur.

KEY TERMS

Accredited Standards Committee X12 Version 5010
Administrative Simplification Enforcement Tool
American National Standards Institute
application service provider
ASC X12 Version 5010
audit trail
batch
business associate agreement
cable modem
carrier-direct system
claim attachments
clearinghouse
code sets
covered entity
data elements
digital subscriber line
direct data entry
electronic data interchange
electronic funds transfer
electronic remittance advice
encoder
encryption
HIPAA Transaction and Code Sets rule
National Standard Format
real time
standard transactions
T-1
taxonomy codes
trading partner
trading partner agreement

KEY ABBREVIATIONS

ANSI
ASC X12
ASET
ASP
ATM
DDE
DHHS
DSL
EDI
EFT
EHR
EMC
EOMB
ERA
HPID
IRS
MAC
NDC
NSF
PMS
TCS rule

ELECTRONIC DATA INTERCHANGE

Electronic data interchange (EDI) is the exchange of data through computer systems. For example, health insurance claims are exchanged between health care organizations and insurance carriers. This is a process by which understandable data are sent back and forth in a standardized format via computer linkages between entities, or trading partners, that function alternately as sender and receiver. Technology and the use of EDI have made processing of transactions more efficient and have reduced administrative overhead costs in health care and many other industries.

For security purposes, electronic transmissions are sent encrypted so that they cannot be opened and read if received by the wrong individual. Encryption is used to assign a "secret code" to represent data, which makes data unintelligible to unauthorized parties. In encrypted versions, the data look like gibberish to unauthorized users and must be decoded to use or read.

In electronically secure environments, the sending computer system encrypts or encodes the data being sent and the receiving computer decodes the data to make them understandable. Therefore both computers must speak the same "language." Standardizing transaction and code sets is required to use EDI effectively. To achieve this, the Health Insurance Portability and Accountability Act (HIPAA) implemented standard formats, procedures, and data content.

ELECTRONIC CLAIMS

An electronic claim, like a paper claim, is constructed from data that are used in the reimbursement process. However, the method for submitting an electronic claim is EDI rather than the US Postal Service or paper fax transmission.

Since the 1960s and early 1970s, claims processing has transitioned from paper claims to electronic claims submission. The federal government has taken steps through the Administrative Simplification Compliance Act (ASCA) that require providers to submit claims electronically unless they have a waiver on file with their Medicare Administrative Contractor (MAC). Third-party payers have followed this lead, offering and encouraging electronic claims submission. Today most health care providers submit electronic claims for reimbursement.

ADVANTAGES OF ELECTRONIC CLAIM SUBMISSION

Electronic claim submission offers many advantages to health care organizations. Unlike paper claims, electronic transactions require no signature or stamp, no search for a third-party payer's address, no postage fees or trips to the post office, and no storage of claim forms in a file cabinet. Electronic transactions build an audit trail, which is a chronologic record of submitted data that can be traced to the source to determine the place of origin. Generally, cash flow is improved and less time is spent processing claims, thereby freeing staff for other duties. Information goes from one computer to another, which reduces overhead by decreasing labor costs and human error. After electronic submission of claims, payment can be received in 2 weeks or less. In comparison, when claims are completed manually and sent by mail, payment may take 4 to 6 weeks on average. With EDI, the audit trail offers proof of receipt and is generated by the carrier, thus eliminating the potential for insurance payers to make the excuse that the claim was never received and therefore not processed.

Another important advantage of electronic claims submission is the online error-edit process that may be incorporated in the software in the health care organization's office, clearinghouse, or insurance company. This feature alerts the person processing the claim to any errors immediately so that a correction can be made before transmission of the claim. Information about problem claims can be telecommunicated immediately, allowing quicker submission of corrected or additional data.

Both paper and electronic claims begin with gathering data before, during, and after the service is rendered. You have learned that the information you need to obtain is crucial when submitting a paper claim for payment. Accurate information is key to successful electronic claim submission as well.

CLEARINGHOUSES

A clearinghouse is an entity that receives the EDI from the health care organization's office and translates it to a standard format prescribed in HIPAA regulations. Claims are sent to clearinghouse in batches, or groups of claims for different patients sent at the same time from one health care organization. Once the clearinghouse receives a batch, it separates the claims by carrier, performs software edits on each claim to check for errors, and transmits claims electronically to the correct insurance payer (Fig. 15.1).

After receiving the claims transmission, a typical clearinghouse process is as follows:

- Claims are checked electronically (scrubbed) for missing or incorrect information using an elaborate editing process. Claims that do not meet all required data for further processing are rejected and not forwarded to the payer.
- Claims that are rejected during the editing process are sent back to the health care organization electronically along with a report that lists the needed corrections.
- Batches of claims that pass all edits are then sent to each separate insurance payer. Several claims can be submitted to various insurance payers in a single-batch electronic transmission.

Using a clearinghouse offers the following advantages:

- Translation of various formats to the HIPAA-compliant standard format
- Reduction in time of claims preparation
- Cost-effective method through loss prevention
- Fewer claim rejections
- Fewer delays in processing and quicker response time
- More accurate coding with claims edits
- Consistent reimbursement

Some health care organizations choose not to use the services of a clearinghouse and have carrier-direct links to the insurance companies. For example, the Centers for Medicare

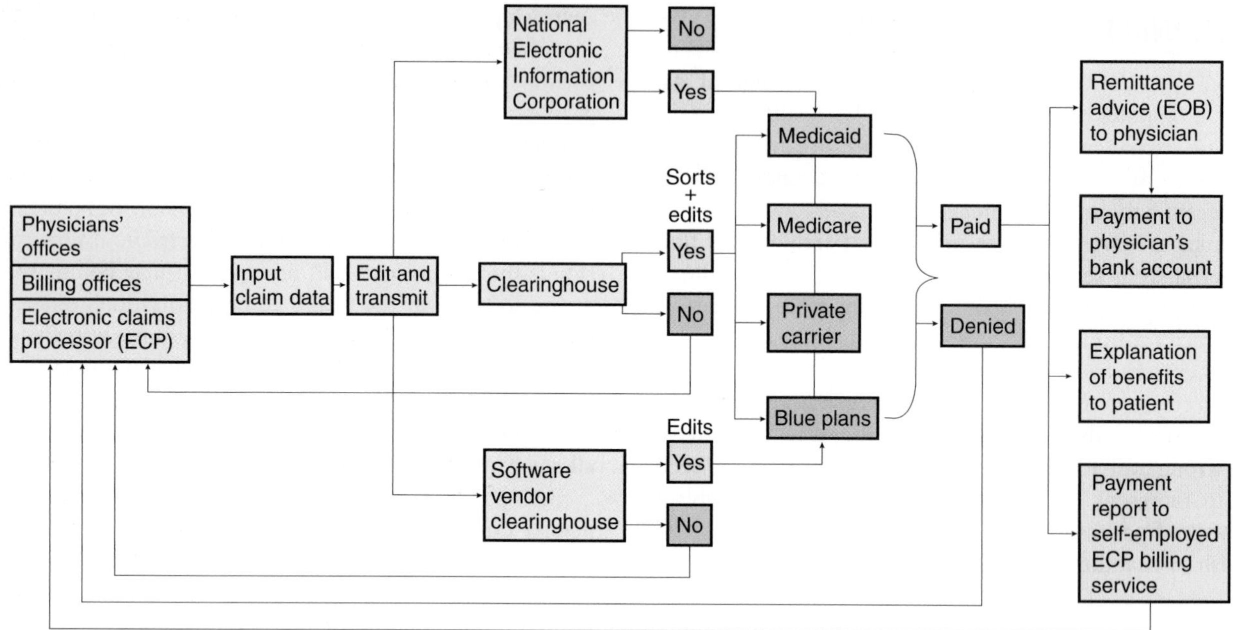

Fig. 15.1 Flow sheet of electronic transmission systems showing path for claim payment via the National Electronic Information Corporation (NEIC), clearinghouse, and independent software vendor. This system also indicates when a payment is made to the health care organization and depicts where claims may not pass an edit or are denied. *EOB,* Explanation of benefits.

and Medicaid Services (CMS) allows health care organizations to submit claims electronically to a MAC if they are using a computer with software that meets electronic filing requirements as established under HIPAA claim standards. Institutional claims can be submitted to CMS MACs via direct data entry screens. The system called *electronic medical claims (*EMCs*)* is used for nearly all Medicare transactions, including claims submission, payment, direct deposit, online eligibility verification, coordination of benefits, and claims status.

TRANSACTION AND CODE SETS REGULATIONS: STREAMLINING ELECTRONIC DATA INTERCHANGE

Under HIPAA Title II Administrative Simplification, the Secretary of the US Department of Health and Human Services (DHHS) is required to adopt standards to support the electronic exchange of health care transactions between health care providers and plans. The purposes and objectives of this component of HIPAA were to achieve a higher quality of care and reduce administrative costs by streamlining the processing of routine administrative and financial transactions. As a result, the HIPAA Transaction and Code Sets (TCS) rule was developed to introduce efficiencies in the health care system. The DHHS estimated that by implementing TCS almost $30 billion over 10 years would be saved.

The intent of TCS requirements is to achieve a single standard. A code set is any set of codes with their descriptions used to encode data elements, such as a table of terms, medical concepts, medical diagnostic codes, or medical procedure codes. Before HIPAA, there were more than 400 versions of a National Standard Format (NSF) that existed to submit a claim for payment. The TCS regulation, which took effect October 16, 2003, required the implementation of specific standards for transactions and code sets so health care organizations could submit to all carriers in the same format.

HIPAA standardization actions are similar to using a bank's automatic teller machine (ATM) or the grocery store's self-checkout. A magnetic strip on a bank card or the bar code on a grocery item can be swiped across a scanning device, allowing customers to process a transaction more quickly than with traditional methods. As these methods are adapted, there are benefits to both the end user and the business providing the technology (Table 15.1). Health care organizations benefit from less paperwork and standardizing data results in more accurate information and a more efficient organization.

As discussed earlier, HIPAA governs how a covered entity may handle health information. Whether a provider transmits health information in electronic form in connection with a transaction covered by HIPAA will determine whether a provider is considered a covered entity (Fig. 15.2). Under HIPAA, the following circumstances would likely make the provider a covered entity:

- If the provider submits electronic transactions to any payer, the provider is considered a covered entity.
- If the provider submits paper claims to Medicare and has 10 or more employees, the provider was required to convert to electronic transactions no later than October 16, 2003. Therefore HIPAA compliance is required.

A provider is *not* considered a covered entity under HIPAA in the following circumstances:

- If the provider has fewer than 10 employees and submits claims only on paper to Medicare. The provider may continue to submit on paper and therefore is not required to comply with HIPAA guidelines.

TABLE 15.1 Recognized Benefits of Transaction and Code Sets and Electronic Data Interchange

Benefit	Result
More reliable and timely processing—quicker reimbursement from payer	Fast eligibility evaluation; reduced time in claim life cycle; industry averages for claim turnarounds are 9–15 days for electronic versus 30–45 days for paper claims, improving cash flow
Improved accuracy of data	Decreases processing time, increases data quality, and leads to better reporting
Easier and more efficient access to information	Improves patient support
Better tracking of transactions	Assists tracking of transactions (that is, when sent and received), allowing for monitoring (for example, prompt payments)
Reduction of data entry/manual labor	Electronic transactions assist automated processes (for example, automatic payment posting)
Reduction in office expenses	Lowers office supplies, postage, and telephone expenses

Data from HIPAAdocs Corporation, Columbia, MD.

- If the provider submitted only paper claims until and after April 14, 2003, and does not send claims to Medicare, the provider is not required to comply with sending electronic claims.

! COMPLIANCE ALERT

Providers Who Must Submit Claims Electronically

According to the Centers for Medicare and Medicaid Services, "Providers who are not small providers (institutional organizations with fewer than 25 full-time employees or providers with fewer than 10 full-time employees) must send all claims electronically in the HIPAA format."

Transaction and Code Sets Standards

TCS standards have been adopted for health care transactions. HIPAA **standard transactions** are the specific electronic file formats in which medical data are compiled to be used throughout the health care industry.

In general, code sets are the allowable sets of codes used to enter information into a specific field on a form. All health care organizations using electronic transactions have to use and accept the code sets systems required under HIPAA that document specific health care data elements. These data elements include medical diagnoses and procedures, drugs, physician services, and medical suppliers. These codes have already been in common use throughout the industry and should have helped ease the transition to the new transaction requirements. What was a standard in the health care industry and recognized by most payers has now been *mandated* under HIPAA.

HIPAA standard codes are used in conjunction with the standard electronic transactions. This standardization eliminates uncertainty when processing transactions. In turn, it improves the quality of data submitted for processing and improves the reimbursement cycle. *Medical code sets* are data elements used uniformly to document why patients are seen (that is, diagnosis, *International Classification of Diseases, Tenth Revision, Clinical Modification* [ICD-10-CM]) and what is done to them during their encounter (that is, procedure, *Current Procedural Terminology, Fourth Edition* [CPT-4], and *Healthcare Common Procedure Coding System* [HCPCS]). Each covered entity organization is responsible for implementing the updated codes in a timely manner and deleting old or obsolete ones (Table 15.2). Because of this, health care organizations may opt to subscribe to coding software or data files that have frequent updates and include new, updated, and deleted codes. Deleted codes become obsolete but are not removed because they have been used when billing past accounts.

Data Requirements

Your role as an insurance billing specialist will require you to understand which data elements are required to construct a HIPAA standard transaction compared with those essential for a paper CMS-1500 form or an electronic claim.

The health care organization's billing software system produces the required HIPAA standard electronic formats. If the software is not capable of producing such formats, the use of clearinghouses translates data to the HIPAA standard format.

! COMPLIANCE ALERT

Standard Transaction

When a patient comes to your office and is treated, his or her confidential health information is collected and put in the computerized billing system. The services rendered are assigned a standard code from the HIPAA-required *code sets* (for example, CPT) and the diagnosis is selected from another code set (for example, ICD-10-CM). When claims are generated for electronic submission, all data collected are compiled and constructed into a HIPAA *standard transaction.* This electronic data interchange (EDI) is recognized across the health care sector in computers maintained by health care organizations, clearinghouses, and insurance payers. The harmony among the covered entities results in a more efficient claim life cycle.

Required and Situational

In addition to the major code sets (ICD-10 and CPT/HCPCS), several *supporting code sets* encompass both medical and nonmedical data. When constructing a claim, the supporting code sets are made up of "required" and "situational" data elements, similar to those on the CMS-1500 paper form. These supporting code sets are embedded in the data elements identified by the HIPAA standard electronic formats. You do not need to know all of these specific codes, but it is helpful to know that they do exist, especially if you are active in the claims processing procedures. When reviewing reports from the clearinghouse or the insurance payer, you may have to correct claims that were rejected for not having correct data elements.

Required refers to data elements that must be used to be in compliance with a HIPAA standard transaction. Conversely, *situational* means that the item depends on the data content or context (Examples 15.1 and 15.2). For the required and situational status of data elements when electronically transmitting HIPAA-compliant electronic claim files (837P claims), refer to the extreme right column of Table 15.5, which appears later in this chapter.

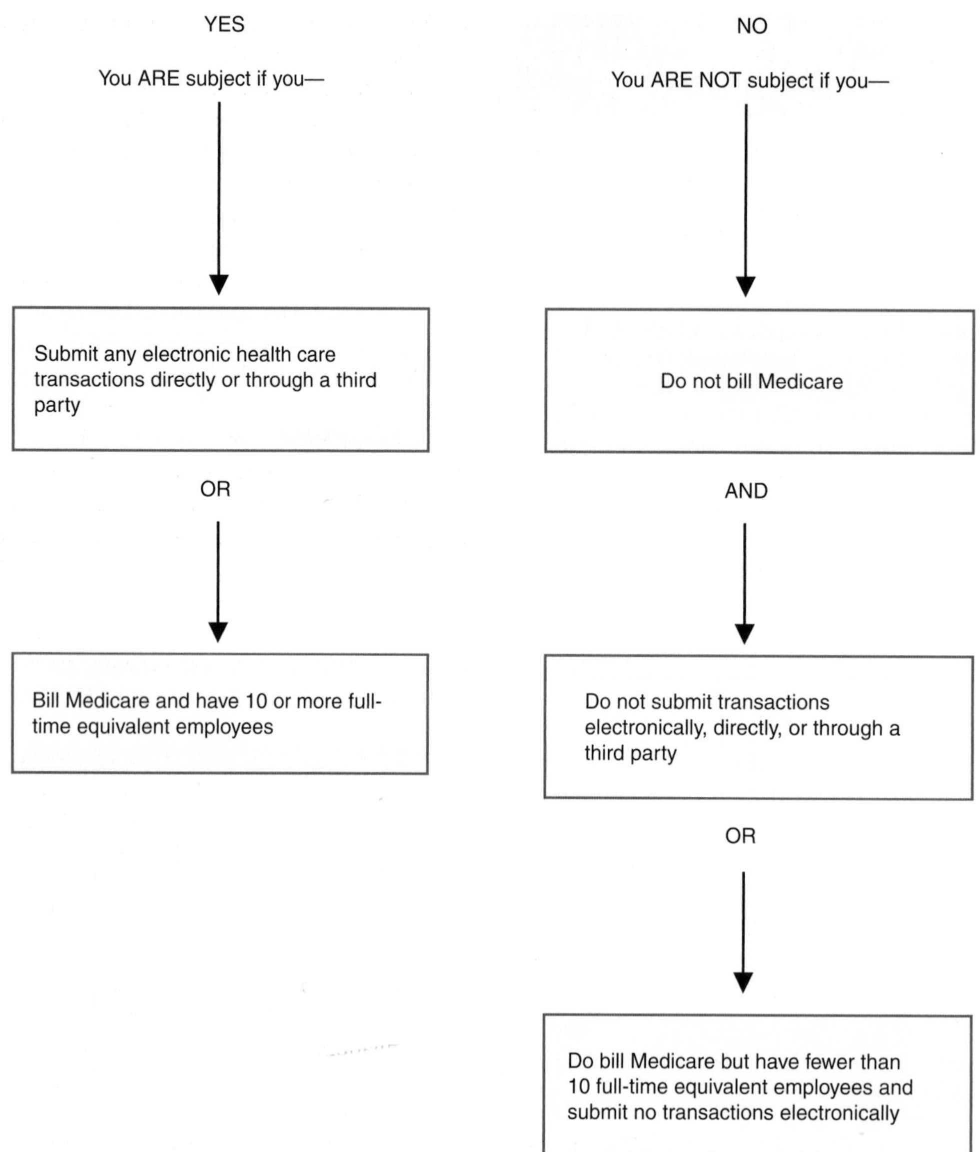

Fig. 15.2 Decision flow chart of who is subject to the HIPAA Transaction and Code Sets rule.

EXAMPLE 15.1 Required Data

Patient's birth date.
Patient's gender.

EXAMPLE 15.2 Situational Data

Baby's birth weight when an infant is delivered.
Last menstrual period (LMP) when a woman is pregnant.

Determining the required and situational data elements not currently collected for the CMS-1500 claim or NSF electronic format can be complex; you will learn this process when you are in the office performing claims processing duties. As an insurance billing specialist, you are directly involved in the claims processing procedures and need to know the most important items to look for related to required and situational data to successfully construct a compliant and payable insurance claim.

In addition to other data elements required under HIPAA TCS standards, examples include the following:

Taxonomy Codes: Taxonomy is defined as the science of classification; thus these are numeric and alpha provider specialty codes (10 characters in length) that classify each health care provider. The taxonomy codes are self-selected by the provider, organized based on education and training, and used to define specialty, not specific services that are rendered. Common **taxonomy codes** include "general practice 208D0000X," "family practice 207Q00000X," and "nurse practitioner 363L00000X." Beginning January 2, 2007, CMS required providers submitting claims to include a taxonomy code. Taxonomy codes are necessary because some institutional providers may choose not to apply for a unique national provider number for each of its subparts (for example, psychiatric unit or rehabilitation unit). Taxonomy codes are maintained by the National Uniform Claim Committee (NUCC).

Patient Account Number: To be assigned to every claim.

TABLE 15.2 HIPAA Medical Code Sets and Elements

Standard Code Sets	Medical Data Elements
Healthcare Common Procedure Coding System (HCPCS)	Items and supplies and nonphysician services not covered by the American Medical Association's (AMA's) CPT-4 codes
Current Procedure Terminology (CPT) codes	Medical procedures and physicians services
International Classification of Diseases, Tenth Revision, Clinical Modification (ICD-10-CM)	Diseases, injuries, impairments, and other health-related problems and their manifestations
International Classification of Diseases, Tenth Revision, Procedural Coding System (ICD-10-PCS)	Procedures or other actions taken for diseases, injuries, and impairments on hospital inpatients reported by hospitals, including prevention, diagnosis, treatment, and management
National Drug Code (NDC)	Pharmaceuticals and biologics
Code on Dental Procedures and Nomenclature, *Current Dental Terminology* (CDT)	Dental services
Place of service (POS) codes	Indicates the setting in which services are provided

Relationship to Patient: Expanded to 25 different relationships, including indicators such as "grandson," "adopted child," "mother, and "life partner."

Facility Code Value: Facility-related element that identifies the place of service with at least 29 locations to choose from, including "office," "ambulance air or water," and "end-stage renal disease treatment facility."

ELECTRONIC STANDARD HIPAA 837P

The American National Standards Institute (ANSI) formed the Accredited Standards Committee X12 (ASC X12), which developed the US standards body for the cross-industry development, maintenance, and publication of electronic data exchange standards. In the health care industry, processing administrative functions can be costly and involve many paper forms and communications via telephone, fax, and postal services. Also, the security and privacy of an individual's health information may be jeopardized. To address the burden of these high overhead costs, the uniform adoption of HIPAA standards has brought forth electronic formats to complete the following health care–related transactions:

- Obtain authorization to refer to a specialist
- Submit a claim for reimbursement
- Request and respond to additional information needed to process a claim
- Record health care claims or equivalent encounter information
- Provide health care payment and remittance advice
- Provide coordination of benefits
- Determine health care claim status
- Enroll and disenroll in a health plan
- Determine eligibility for a health insurance plan
- Make health plan premium payments
- Provide referral certification and authorization
- Make first report of injury
- Add health claims attachments
- Other transactions that DHHS may prescribe by regulation

Each of these standard transactions is identified by a three-digit number preceded by "ASC X12N" (Table 15.3). However, the transactions are referred to in the office simply by the three-digit number (for example, 837 or 837P [Professional]). The 837P replaces the paper CMS-1500 form and more than 400 versions of the electronic NSF.

Levels of Information for 837P Standard Transaction Format

Because the 837P is an electronic claims transmittal format, data collected to construct and submit a claim are grouped by levels. It is important for claims processing staff to know the language when following up on claims. You do not need to know exactly how these are grouped. However, if the clearinghouse or payer states that you have an invalid item at the "high level," you need to understand that it could be incomplete or erroneous information pertaining to the provider, subscriber, or payer (Table 15.4).

An easier way to understand this new stream-of-data format is to show a crosswalk between the legacy CMS-1500 paper claim and the 837P (Table 15.5). Note that dates on HIPAA transactions will be in the 8-digit YYYYMMDD (for example, 20090806) electronic claim format.

Accredited Standards Committee X12 Version 5010

The programs for transmission of insurance claims data must be upgraded periodically due to the continual changes to policies and regulations for payment of claims. Implementation of ICD-10-CM/PCS in 2015 resulted in the need to upgrade to HIPAA transaction standard ASC X12 Version 5010 for electronic claim submission. Providers, payers, and clearinghouses were required to implement and start using this standard on January 1, 2012. Version 5010 allows providers and payers to transmit either ICD-9 or ICD-10 data. Version 5010 also requires health insurers to specify when they received the claim from a health care organization, which allows organizations to calculate interest due on untimely payments. There are many additional system improvements, such as returning claims that need corrections to the provider sooner, assignment of claim numbers closer to the time received by the payer, and more consistency of claims editing and error handling. A newer electronic transaction standard, the Version 6020, was tabled in 2015, and Version 7030 is under development.

CLAIM ATTACHMENTS STANDARDS

Claim attachments are supplemental documents providing additional medical information to the claims processor that cannot be accommodated within the claim format. Common attachments are Certificates of Medical Necessity (CMNs), discharge summaries, and operative reports. Practice management and claims software include a data field that allows you to indicate that a paper claims attachment is included with the claim.

TABLE 15.3 HIPAA Transaction Functions and Formats

Standard Transaction Function	Industry Format Name
Official Title: Health Care Eligibility Benefit Inquiry and Response **Purpose:** Eligibility verification/response • When obtaining issues regarding benefits and coverage, this standard is used from a health care provider to a health plan or between two health plans. • The 270 is the "inquiry for eligibility verification." • The 271 is the "response."	ASC X12N 270/271
Official Title: Health Care Claim Status Request and Response **Purpose:** Health claim status inquiry/response • The 276 is the "inquiry" to determine the status of a claim. • The 277 is the "response."	ASC X12N 276/277
Official Title: Health Care Services Review—Request for Review and Response **Purpose:** Referral certification and authorization for patient health care services	ASC X12N 278
Official Title: Payroll Deducted and Other Group Premium Payment for Insurance Products **Purpose:** Health plan premium payments, including payroll deductions	ASC X12N 820
Official Title: Benefit Enrollment and Maintenance **Purpose:** Transmission of subscriber enrollment information to a health plan to establish coverage or terminate the policy	ASC X12N 834
Official Title: Payment and Remittance Advice **Purpose:** Transmission indicating the explanation of benefits or remittance advice from a health plan payer to the health care provider • This also may be data sent from a health plan directly to the provider's financial institution (bank) and may include payment and information about the processing of the claim.	ASC X12N 835
Official Title: Health Care Claim or Equivalent Encounter **Purpose:** To obtain payment for the transmitted health services encounter information • The 837P (Professional) replaces the paper CMS-1500 form and the electronic National Standard Format (NSF). • The 837I (Institutional) replaces the paper UB-04 often used in hospitals. • The 837D (Dental) is used for dentistry. • Additionally, the coordination of benefits (COB) for claims and payment will be transmitted through the 837 format.	ASC X12N 837 includes: A. 837P—Health Care Claim, Professional B. 837I—Health Care Claim, Institutional C. 837D—Health Care Claim, Dental
Proposed Official Title: First Report of Illness, Injury, or Incident **Potential Purpose:** This standard will be used to report information on a claim pertaining to factors such as date of onset of illness or date of accident.	PROPOSED ASC X12N 148
Proposed Official Title: Health Claims Attachment **Potential Purpose:** Transmit additional information to claim 1. This means no more photocopied attachments stapled to paper claims or additional information mailed after the claim is initially received.	PROPOSED ASC X12 275 and HL7

TABLE 15.4 Data Grouping in 837P Standard Transaction Format

Level	Information
High-level information: Applies to the entire claim and reflects data pertaining to the billing provider, subscriber, and patient	• Billing/pay to provider information • Subscriber/patient information • Payer information
Claim-level information: Applies to the entire claim and all service lines and is applicable to most claims	Claim information
Specialty claim–level information: Applies to specific claim types	Specialty
Service line–level information: Applies to specific procedure or service that is rendered and is applicable to most claims	Service line information
Specialty service line–level information: Applies to specific claim types; required data are required only for the specific claim type	Specialty service line information
Other information	• Coordination of benefits • Repriced claim/line • Credit/debit information • Clearinghouse/value added network tracking

HIPAA identified a health claim attachment as one of the transactions for which electronic standards were to be adopted. However, the final rule was never adopted. The Affordable Care Act (ACA) mandatory compliance date of January 1, 2016 has come and gone. Despite this, various organizations have continued to research and develop the electronic attachment issue. It is hoped that it will be addressed in the upcoming Version 7030 standard for electronic claims submission.

STANDARD UNIQUE IDENTIFIERS

Standard Unique Identifiers are used to identify the specific entities associated with the electronic claims process.

Standard Unique Employer Identifier

The employer identification number (EIN) is assigned by the Internal Revenue Service (IRS) and used to identify employers

TABLE 15.5 Comparison of CMS-1500 and 837P v5010*

1500 FORM LOCATOR		ANSI 837P VERSION 5010		
Item Number	**Title**	**Loop ID**	**Segment/Data Element**	**Notes**
N/A	Carrier Block	2010BB	NM103 N301 N302 N401 N402 N403	
1	Medicare, Medicaid, TRICARE, CHAMPUS, CHAMPVA, Group Health Plan, FECA, Black Lung, Other	2000B	SBR09	Required: **Claim filing indicator code.** Must = MB for Medicare Part B claims.
1a	Insured's ID Number	2010BA	NM109	Required: **Subscriber Primary Identifier.** Enter the patient's Health Insurance Claim Number.
2	Patient's Name	2010BA	NM103 NM104 NM105 NM107	Required: **Subscriber last, first and middle name.** Enter the patient's name as shown on their insurance card.
3	Patient's Birth Date, Sex	2010BA	DMG02 DMG03	Required: **Subscriber birth date and gender code.** Enter the patient's birth date and sex.
4	Insured's Name	2330A	NM103 NM104 NM105 NM107	Situational: **Other insured last name, first name, middle name.** If there is insurance primary to Medicare, either through the patient's or spouse's employment or any other source, list the name of the insurance here. Required: If any other payers are known to potentially be involved in paying the claim.
5	Patient's Address	2010BA	N302 N401 N402 N403	Required: **Subscriber address, city, state and zip code.** Enter the patient's mailing address.
6	Patient Relationship to Insured	2000B 2320	SBR02 PAT01	Situational: **Individual relationship code.** Required when subscriber is the same as the patient. Individual relationship code is required if any other payers are known to potentially be involved in paying this claim.
7	Insured's Address	2330A	N301 N302 N401 N402 N403	Situational: **Other subscriber address, city, state, zip code.** Enter the mailing address of the insured. Required if any other payers are known to potentially be involved in paying this claim and the information is available.
8	Reserved for NUCC use.	Leave blank.	N/A	
9	Other Insured's Name	2330A	NM103 NM104 NM105 NM107	Situational: **Other insured last name, first name and middle name.** Enter the last name, first name and middle name of the insured. Required if other payers are known to potentially be involved in paying this claim.
9a	Other Insured's Policy or Group Number	2320 2320A	SBR03	Situational: **Other insured identifier and insured group or policy number.** Enter the policy number of the insured. Required if other payers are known to potentially be involved in paying this claim. Enter the insured's group or plan number.
9b	Reserved for NUCC use.	Leave blank.	N/A	
9c	Reserved for NUCC use.	2330B	N/A	Situational: **Other payer city name, state code, zip code.** Enter the city, state and zip code of the insurer. Required if any other payers are known to potentially be involved in paying this claim.
9d	Insurance Plan Name or Program Name	2330B	SBR04	Situational: **Other payer primary identifier, other payer organization name.** Enter the insurer's unique identifier. Enter the name of the insured's other insurance.

Continued

TABLE 15.5 Comparison of CMS-1500 and 837P v5010*—cont'd

1500 FORM LOCATOR		ANSI 837P VERSION 5010		
Item Number	**Title**	**Loop ID**	**Segment/Data Element**	**Notes**
10a 10b 10c	Is Patient's Condition Related to: Employment? Auto accident? Other accident?	2300	CLM11	Situational: **Employment-related indicator, auto accident indictor, other accident indicator.** Required if date of accident (DTP01 = 439) is used and the service is employment related or the result of an accident. Situational: **Auto Accident State or Province Code.** Identify state where automobile accident occurred if auto accident.
10d	Reserved for local use	2300	K3	This is specific for reporting workers' compensation condition codes
11	Insured's Policy, Group, or FECA Number	2000B	SBR03	Situational: **Insured group or policy number.** If there is insurance primary to Medicare, enter the insured's policy or group number. Required if other payers are known to potentially be involved in paying this claim.
11a	Insured's Date of Birth, Sex	2010BA	DMG02 DMG03	
11b	Other Claim ID (Designated by NUCC)	Leave blank.	N/A	
11c	Insurance Plan Name or Program Name	2000B	SBR04	Situational: **Other insured group name, other payer organization name, other payer primary identifier.** Enter the complete insurance plan or program name. Enter the payer ID of the other insurer.
11d	Is there another Health Benefit Plan?	2320		
12	Patient's or Authorized Person's Signature	2300	CLM09	Required: **Release of information code.** This item authorizes release of medical information necessary to process the claim. It also authorizes payment of benefits to the provider of service or supplier when assignment is accepted on the claim.
13	Insured's or Authorized Person's Signature	2300	CLM08	Required: **Benefits assignment certification.** This item authorizes payment of medical benefits to the service provider or supplier.
14	Date of Current Illness, Injury, Pregnancy	2300	DTP03	Situational: **Accident date, onset of current illness or injury, initial treatment date.** Required if CLM 11-1 or 2 = (AA) or (OA) and on all claims involving spinal manipulations.
15	Other Date	Leave blank.	N/A	
16	Dates Patient Unable to Work in Current Occupation	2300	DTP03	Situational: **Initial disability period start and end.** If the patient is employed and is unable to work in his/her current occupation, enter the date(s) when patient is unable to work.
17	Name of Referring Provider or Other Source	2310A (referring) 2310D (supervising)	NM103 NM104 NM105 NM107	Situational: **Referring provider, ordering provider and/or supervising provider last name, first name and middle name.** Enter the name of the referring or ordering physician if the service or item was ordered or referred by a physician. All service providers who order service or refer Medicare beneficiaries must report this data. This is also used if Medicare policy requires you to report a supervising physician. When a claim involves multiple referring and/or ordering physicians, a separate claim should be submitted for each.
17a	Other ID#	2310A (referring) 2310D (supervising)	REF02	
17b	NPI#	2310A (referring) 2310D (supervising)	NM109	Situational: **Referring provider ID, Ordering provider ID and/or supervising provider ID.** Enter "XX" in the NM108 data element to indicate an NPI is present in NM109. Enter the NPI of the referring, ordering, or supervising physician or nonphysician practitioner listed in Item 17.
18	Hospitalization Dates Related to Current Services	2300	DTP03	Situational: **Related Hospitalization Admission and Discharge Dates.** Enter the date when a medical service is furnished as a result of, or subsequent to, a related hospitalization.

TABLE 15.5 **Comparison of CMS-1500 and 837P v5010*—cont'd**

1500 FORM LOCATOR		ANSI 837P VERSION 5010		
Item Number	**Title**	**Loop ID**	**Segment/Data Element**	**Notes**
19	Reserved for local use	2300	NTE PWK	Situational: **Last seen date.** Enter the date patient was last seen and the NPI of his/her attending physician when a physician providing routine foot care submits claim. Situational: **Supervising provider ID.** Enter "XX" in the NM108 data element to indicate an NPI is present in NM 109. Enter the NPI of his/her attending physician when a physician providing routine foot care submits claim. Situational: **Test Results.** Enter R1 or R2 in the MEA02 to qualify the Hemoglobin or Hematocrit test results. Enter the test results in the MEA03. Situational: **Code Category, Certification Condition Indicator, Homebound Indicator.** Required when an independent lab renders an EKG tracing or obtains a specimen from a homebound or institutionalized patient. Situational: **Extra narrative data.** Enter all applicable modifiers when modifier -99 is entered on the service line. Enter the statement, "Testing for hearing aid" when billing services involving the testing of a hearing aid is used to obtain intentional denials when other payers are involved. When dental examinations are billed, enter the specific surgery for which the exam is performed. Situational: **Description.** Enter the drug's name and dosage when submitting a claim for Not Otherwise Classified drugs. Enter a concise description of an unlisted procedure code or a Not Otherwise Classified drug. Enter the specific name and dosage amount when low osmolar contract material is billed, but only if HCPCS codes do not cover them. Situational: **Demonstration Project Identifier.** Required on claim where a demonstration project is being billed. Situational: **Assumed and Relinquished care dates.** Enter the date for a global surgery claim when providers share post-operative care. Situational: **Purchases Service Provider Identifier.** Enter "XX" in the NM108 data element to indicate an NPI is present in NM109. Enter the NPI of the service provider who is performing the technical or professional component of a diagnostic test that is subject to the anti-markup payment limitation. Subjective: **Last X-ray.** Enter the x-ray date for chiropractic services (if an x-ray, rather than a physical exam was the method used to demonstrate subluxation). Situational: **Benefits Assignment Certification Indicator.** When a patient refuses to assign benefits to the provider, enter code "W".
20	Outside Lab Charges	2400	PS102	Situational: **Purchases service provider identifier, charge amount and service provider.** Required when billing for diagnostic tests subject to the anti-markup payment limitations. Loop 2420B is required when a 2400/PS1 segment is present. When submitting a PS1 segment, you must also submit the facility information in either loop 2310C or 2420C.
21	Diagnosis or Nature of Illness or Injury	2300	HI01-2 HI02-2 HI03-2 HI04-2	Required: **Principal diagnosis code.** Required on all claims. Do not transmit the decimal points in the diagnosis codes. The decimal point is assumed. Enter the patient's diagnosis/condition. All physician and nonphysician specialties use diagnosis codes to the highest level of specificity for the date of service. Enter the diagnoses in priority order. Situational: **Secondary and tertiary diagnosis codes.**
22	Resubmission and/or Original Reference Number	2300 2300	CLM05-3 REF02	Titled Claim Frequency Code in the 837P. Titled Payer Claim Control Number in the 837P.

Continued

TABLE 15.5 **Comparison of CMS-1500 and 837P v5010*—cont'd**

1500 FORM LOCATOR		ANSI 837P VERSION 5010		
Item Number	**Title**	**Loop ID**	**Segment/Data Element**	**Notes**
23	Prior Authorization Number	2300	REF02	Titled Prior Authorization Number in the 837P.
		2300	REF02	Titled Referral Number in the 837P.
		2300	REF02	Titled Clinical Laboratory Improvement Amendment Number in the 837P.
		2300	REF02	Titled Mammography Certification Number in the 837P.
24A	Date(s) of Service	2400	DTP03	Required: **Service date.** Enter the service date for each procedure or supply.
24B	Place of Service	2300	CLM05-1	Titled Facility Code Value in the 837P.
		2400	SV105	Required: **Place of Service Code.** Enter the appropriate place of service code. Identify the setting, using a place of service code, for each item used or service performed.
24C	EMG	2400	SV109	Titled Emergency Indicator in the 837P.
24D	Procedures, Services, or Supplies	2400	SV101-2 SV101-3 SV101-4 SV101-5 SV101-6	Required: **Procedure code.** In product's Service ID Qualifier (SV101-1) enter (HC) for HCPCS codes. Enter the procedures, services or supplies using the HCPCS coding system. Situational: **Procedure modifier.** When applicable, show the HCPCS modifiers with the HCPCS codes.
24E	Diagnosis Pointer	2400	SV107-1 SV107-2 SV107-3 SV107-4	Required: **Diagnosis code pointer.** A submitter must point to the primary diagnosis for each service line. Use remaining diagnosis pointers in declining level of importance to service line.
24F	$Charges	2400	SV102	Required: **Line item charge amount.** Enter the charge amount for each service.
24G	Days or Units	2400	SV104	Required: **Service unit count.** Enter the number of days or units. For anesthesia, show the elapsed time. Convert hours into minutes and enter the total minutes required for the procedure.
24H	EPSDT/Family Plan	2400	SV111 SV112	Titled EPSDT Indicator and Family Planning Indicator in the 837P.
24I Shaded Line	ID Qualifier	2310B 2420A	PRV02 REF01 PRV02 REF01	Titled Reference Identification Qualifier in the 837P. Titled Reference Identification Qualifier in the 837P.
24J Shaded line	Rendering Provider ID#	2310B 2420A	PRV03 REF02	Titled Provider Taxonomy Code and Rendering Provider Secondary Identifier in the 837P.
24J	Rendering Provider ID#	2310B 2420A	NM109	Situational: **Rendering provider identifier.** Enter "XX" in the NM 108 data element to indicate an NPI is present in NM109. Enter the rendering provider's NPI number. This is required when the information is different than that in 2010AA billing provider.
25	Federal Tax ID Number	2010AA	REF01 REF02	Required: **Billing Provider Tax Identification Number/Social Security Number.** Enter the provider of services or supplier Federal Tax ID number or Social Security number.
26	Patient's Account No.	2300	CLM01	Required: **Patient control number.** Enter the patient's account number assigned by the provider of service's or supplier's accounting system.
27	Accept Assignment?	2300	CLM07	Required: **Assignment or Plan Participation Code.** A=Assigned B=Assignment accepted on Clinical Lab services only C=Not assigned
28	Total Charge	2300	CLM02	Required: **Total claim charge amount.** Enter the total charges for the services.
29	Amount Paid	2300 2320	AMT02	Situational: **Patient amount paid.** Required if patient has paid any amount toward the claim for covered services only.
30	Reserved for NUCC Use.	Leave blank.	N/A	
31	Signature of Physician or Supplier Including Degrees or Credentials	2300	CLM06	Required: **Provider or supplier signature indicator.** A "Y" value indicates the provider signature is on file, an "N" value indicates the provider signature is not on file.

TABLE 15.5 Comparison of CMS-1500 and 837P v5010*—cont'd

1500 FORM LOCATOR		ANSI 837P VERSION 5010		
Item Number	**Title**	**Loop ID**	**Segment/Data Element**	**Notes**
32	Service Facility Location Information	2310C	NM103 N301 N401 N402 N403	Situational: **Laboratory or Facility Name, Address, City/State/Zip.** Required when the location of service is different than that carried in Loop ID-2010AA. If a modifier is billed indicating the service was rendered in a Health Professional Shortage Area or Physician Scarcity Area, the physical location where the service was rendered shall be entered. If an independent laboratory is billing, enter the place where the test was performed outside a health care organization's office. Providers of service shall identify the supplier's name, address, and NPI when billing for anti-markup tests. Situational: **Ambulance Pick-up and Drop-off Location, address, city, state and zip.** Required when billing for ambulance or nonemergency transportation services. Situational: **Mammography certification.** If the supplier is a certified mammography screening center, enter the FDA-approved certification number.
32a		2310C	NM109	Situational: **Laboratory/Facility Primary Identifier.** Enter "XX" in the NM108 data element to indicate an NPI is present in NM109. Enter the NPI of the service facility.
32b	Other ID#	2310C	REF01 REF02	Titled Reference Identification Qualifier and Laboratory or Facility Secondary Identifier in the 837P.
33	Billing Provider Info & Ph #	2010AA	NM103 NM104 NM105 NM107 N301 N401 N402 N403 PER04	Required: **Provider last or organization name, provider first name, middle initial, address, city, state, zip code, phone number.** Enter the provider of service/supplier's billing name, address, zip code and telephone number.
33a	NPI#	2010AA	NM109	Required: **Billing provider Identifier.** Enter "XX" in the NM108 data element to indicate an NPI is present in NM109. Enter the NPI of the billing provider or group.
33b	Other ID#	2000A 2010AA	PRV03 REF01 REF02	Titled Provider Taxonomy Code in the 837P. Titled Reference Identification Qualifier and Billing Provider Additional Identifier in the 837P.

*This crosswalk relates to the CMS-1500 (08-05) claim form.

CHAMPUS, Civilian Health and Medical Program of the Uniformed Services; *CHAMPVA,* Civilian Health and Medical Program of the Department of Veterans Affairs; *CLIA,* Clinical Laboratory Improvement Amendments; *EKG,* electrocardiogram; *EMG,* emergency; *EPSDT,* Early Periodic Screening, Diagnosis, and Treatment; *FDA,* Food and Drug Administration; *FECA,* Federal Employees' Compensation Act; *HCPCS,* Healthcare Common Procedure Coding System; *ID,* identification; *NPI,* National Provider Identifier; *NUCC,* National Uniform Claim Committee.

for tax purposes. HIPAA requires that the EIN be used to identify employers rather than inputting the name of the company when submitting claims. Employers use their EINs to identify themselves in transactions involving premium payments to health plans on behalf of their employees or to identify themselves or other employers as the source or receiver of information about eligibility. Employers also will use EINs to identify themselves in transactions when enrolling or disenrolling employees in a health plan.

Standard Unique Health Care Provider Identifier

In the past, health insurance plans have assigned an identifying number to each provider with whom they conduct business. This resulted in providers having many different identifier numbers when submitting claims to several different payers.

Under HIPAA, all providers were required to obtain a National Provider Identifier (NPI) that is assigned to each provider for use in transactions with all health plans. The NPI is all numeric and 10 characters in length and became a requirement on all claims effective May 23, 2007.

According to CMS, NPI is a lasting identifier. It will not change with changes to a health care provider's name, address, ownership, membership in health plans, or Healthcare Provider Taxonomy classification.

Standard Unique Health Plan Identifier

Previously health plans were identified in electronic transactions with multiple identifiers that differed in length, format, and meaning. The current versions of the adopted standards

(ASC X12N) allow health plans to use these various identifiers in standard transactions that result in inconsistent use of identifiers for health plans.

The ACA required implementation of standard unique health plan identifiers (**HPIDs**). The standard unique HPID rule assigned a standard identifier to identify health plans that process and pay certain electronic health care transactions. On October 4, 2012, a corrected and final rule was posted in the *Federal Register,* which stated that health plans (with the exception of small health plans) were required to obtain an HPID by November 5, 2014. Small health plans had to obtain an HPID by November 5, 2015. Covered entities were required to use HPIDs in the standard transactions on or after November 7, 2016.

The adoption of the HPID increased standardization within HIPAA standard transactions and provided a platform for other regulatory initiatives. The use of HPIDs brought a higher level of automation to health care organizations as they process billing and perform other insurance-related tasks, such as verification of patient eligibility and processing of remittance advices.

Standard Unique Patient Identifier

In addition to standardization of a unique provider identifier and a unique HPID, both HIPAA and the ACA support the creation of a unique patient identifier system. However, privacy and security concerns have stalled the efforts to implement the proposal. The intention to create a standard for a uniform patient identifier has also prompted protest among public interest groups who consider a universal identifier to be a civil liberties threat. Therefore the issue of a universal patient identifier is "on hold."

PRACTICE MANAGEMENT SYSTEM

The most important function of a practice management system (**PMS**) or billing system is accounts receivable. Many offices use features such as scheduling, electronic health record (**EHR**), and word processing to run an efficient office. However, maximum value can only be attained if the PMS is also able to prepare, send, receive, and process HIPAA standard electronic transactions. For older PMS versions, a clearinghouse converts old formats to HIPAA standard transactions. Keep in mind that HIPAA does not apply to the format of stored data within the PMS databases. Computer systems are free to use any data format when storing data because HIPAA standards apply only to the format in which data are transmitted.

If your health care organization is in the market for a new PMS, it is important to find a vendor that understands HIPAA thoroughly—including the Privacy and Security Rules. A PMS can help with administrative burdens, such as tracking the receipt of the Notice of Privacy Practices (NPP), noting a patient's treatment consent or authorization, and mapping disclosures. A HIPAA-ready PMS should do the following:

- Set security access to patient files in the software
- Indicate date of receipt and signature of NPP
- Insert date of patient's authorization
- Maintain files of the health care organization's authorization and notification forms
- Track requests for amendments, requests for restrictions on use and disclosure of protected health information (PHI), and indications of whether the service provider agreed to or denied the request
- Track expiration dates

When assessing the PMS's functionality in accounts receivable management, consider the ability to perform the following:

- Set up all of the organization's providers as individuals to bill using correct and appropriate identifiers for each and every health care provider
- Key in all patient demographics and insurance information
- Perform electronic claim batch submission, either direct to payer or through a clearinghouse

Note that some PMS vendors sell an "add-on" module to go directly to some carriers, such as Medicare, Medicaid, and Blue Cross Blue Shield.

BUILDING THE CLAIM

Encounter or Multipurpose Billing Forms

As mentioned earlier, an *encounter form* is a document used to record information about the service rendered to a patient. The style and format of the billing form varies because it is customized to meet the needs of each health care office, based on the health care organization's specialty. For easy reference, many billing forms include preprinted procedural and diagnostic codes. The provider circles the codes and the insurance billing specialist takes that information and enters it in the computer system.

Some encounter forms are designed so that they may be scanned to input charges and diagnoses in the patient's computerized account. Time is saved and fewer errors occur because no keystrokes are involved (Fig. 15.3).

Keying Insurance Data for Claim Transmission

When entering patient data into a software program, a prompt appears on the screen and the data are keyed in reply to the prompt (Fig. 15.4). Reusable data are entered initially in a file and identified by a number. Each treating physician, referring physician, patient, and third-party payer has an assigned computer code number. Notice in Figs. 15.4 to 15.6 that a patient, Charles Weber, is input as account number WEBCH000; Star Insurance is STA00; and the provider is keyed as DIW, the initials of the provider. This information is stored in the database and is the same as that necessary for completing a claim manually. It is automatically retrieved by the system when a computer code number is keyed in and used to generate a computerized claim or electronic claim. Because there are computer code numbers and prompts for each item, there is less chance of error or omitting mandatory information. The program checks that data are complete and in proper format. It is important to understand how your particular management system works.

Some general do's and don'ts for keying in data and billing electronic claims follow.

Do: Use the patient account numbers to differentiate between patients with similar names.

CFR

PAT 4140.0	**DOCTOR: 2 FRANK CHI, M.D.**	**APPT DATE:**	**05/27/XX**
	ROOM:	APPT TIME:	2:30 PM
	APPTLOC:	APPT LEN:	10 min.
( ) 985-6575 01/22/1936 F63	APPTCD:	DEPT/LOC:	0, n/a
PRI: (Y) BLUE SHIELD ENVOY	REASON: OX, F/U visit	DSET/PRT:	1, 12
201-XX-9969	LAST DX: 000.0 No diagnosis applicable	ACCT BAL:	75.00
SEC:	SSN/STA: 201-XX-9969, 1 Active	PAT DUE:	0.00
	OVERLAY: 1 INTERNAL MEDICINE	VOUCHER:	7887

①②③④P/L **NEW PT OFFICE VISITS**
①②③④P/L 99203 NP LEVEL THREE
①②③④P/L 99204 NP LEVEL FOUR
①②③④P/L 99205 NP LEVEL FIVE
①②③④P/L **EST PT OFFICE VISIT**
①②③④P/L 99211 EST PT LEVEL ONE
①②③④P/L 99212 EST PT LEVEL TWO
①②③④P/L 99213 EST PT LEVEL THREE
①②③④P/L 99214 EST PT LEVEL FOUR
①②③④P/L 99215 EST PT LEVEL FIVE
①②③④P/L 00003 GLOBAL VISIT

OTHER PROCEDURES
①②③④P/L 99000 COLL & PREP/PAP TEST
①②③④P/L 93000 EKG WITH INTERPRETATION
①②③④P/L 82270 HEMOCCULT
①②③④P/L 81000 URINALYSIS

INJECTIONS
①②③④P/L ~FLU, FLU INJ/ADMIN/MCR
①②③④P/L ~9065 FLU INJ/NON MCR
①②③④P/L ~PNEU PNEUMO/ADMIN/MCR
①②③④P/L ~9073 PNEUMO INJ NON MCR

UNLISTED PROCEDURES

____

STOP FOR VERIFICATION

BREASTS
①②③④P/L N60.29 FIBROADENOSIS, BREAST
①②③④P/L N63 LUMP OR MASS IN BREAST

CARDIOVASCULAR
①②③④P/L I71.4 ABDOM AORTIC ANEURYSM
①②③④P/L I20.9 ANGINA
①②③④P/L I74.11 AORTIC VALVE DISORDER
①②③④P/L I48.91 ATRIAL FIBRILLATION
①②③④P/L I48.92 ATRIAL FLUTTER
①②③④P/L I49.1 ATRIAL PREMATURE BEATS
①②③④P/L I44.0 ATRIOVENT BLOCK-1ST DE
①②③④P/L R01.1 CARDIAC MURMURS NEC
①②③④P/L I51.7 CARDIOMEGALY
①②③④P/L I50.9 CONGESTIVE HEART FAILU
①②③④P/L I42.1 HYPERTR OBSTR CARDIOMY
①②③④P/L I25.10 ISCHEMIC CHR HEART DIS
①②③④P/L R00.2 PALPITATIONS
①②③④P/L I47.1 PAROX ATRIAL TACHYCARD
①②③④P/L I47.2 PAROX VENTRIC TACHYCAR

CHEST
①②③④P/L J20.9 BRONCHITIS, ACUTE
①②③④P/L J41.0 BRONCHITIS, CHRONIC
①②③④P/L J44.9 CH OB ASTH W/O STAT AS
①②③④P/L J45.20 EXT ASTHMA W/O STAT AS

①②③④P/L J44.1 OBS CHR BRNC W ACT EXA
①②③④P/L J44.9 OBS CHR BRNC W/O ACT E

ENDOCRINE
①②③④P/L E10.40 DMI NEURO CMP CONTROLL
①②③④P/L E10.9 DMI WO CMP CONTROLLED
①②③④P/L E10.65 DMI UNCONTROLLED
①②③④P/L E11.40 DMII NEURO CMP CONTROL
①②③④P/L E11.9 DMII WO CMP CONTROLLED
①②③④P/L E11.65 DMII UNCONTROLLED
①②③④P/L E78.0 HYPERCHOLESTEROLEMIA
①②③④P/L E78.1 HYPERGLYCERIDEMIA
①②③④P/L E03.9 HYPOTHYROIDISM
①②③④P/L E66.01 MORBID OBESITY
①②③④P/L E04.1 THYROID NODULE

EXTREMITIES
①②③④P/L E60.9 EDEMA
①②③④P/L I74.3 LOWER EXT EMBOLISM
①②③④P/L I80.0- PHLEBITIS-LEG
①②③④P/L I70.219 PVD W/CLAUDICATION
①②③④P/L I83.90 VARICOSE VEIN OF LEG

GI
①②③④P/L R10.13 ABDMNAL PAIN EPIGASTRI
①②③④P/L R10.12 ABDMNAL PAIN LFT UP QU
①②③④P/L R10.32 ABDMNAL PAIN LT LWR QU
①②③④P/L R10.33 ABDMNAL PAIN PERIUMBIL
①②③④P/L R10.31 ABDMNAL PAIN RT LWR QU
①②③④P/L R10.11 ABDMNAL PAIN RT UPR QU
①②③④P/L K92.1 BLOOD IN STOOL
①②③④P/L K81.2 CHOLECYSTITIS, ACUTE
①②③④P/L K59.00 CONSTIPATION
①②③④P/L R19.7 DIARRHEA
①②③④P/L K57.32 DIVERTICULITIS
①②③④P/L K57.30 DIVERTICULOSIS
①②③④P/L K580.20 GALLSTONE(S), CHRONIC
①②③④P/L K29.00 GASTRITIS
①②③④P/L K51.9 GERD
①②③④P/L K64.4 HEMORRHOID, EXT W/O COM
①②③④P/L K64.8 HEMORRHOID, INT W/O COM
①②③④P/L K58.9 IRRITABLE COLON
①②③④P/L R11.2 NAUSEA WITH VOMITING
①②③④P/L K62.5 RECTAL & ANAL HEMORRHA
①②③④P/L K21.0 REFLUX ESOPHAGITIS
①②③④P/L Z12.12 SCREEN COLORECTAL

GU
①②③④P/L N41.0 ACUTE PROSTATITIS
①②③④P/L N40.0 BPH
①②③④P/L N20.0 CALCULUS OF KIDNEY
①②③④P/L N20.1 CALCULUS OF URETER
①②③④P/L N30.00 CYSTITIS, ACUTE
①②③④P/L N30.10 CYSTITIS, CHRONIC
①②③④P/L R31.9 HEMATURIA
①②③④P/L N52.9 IMPOTENCE, ORGANIC ORI
①②③④P/L R80.9 PROTEINURIA

HEENT
①②③④P/L H61.23 CERUMEN, IMPACTED
①②③④P/L H10.019 CONJUNCTIVITIS
①②③④P/L R04.0 EPISTAXIS
①②③④P/L R51 HEADACHE
①②③④P/L J04.0 LARYNGITIS/TRACHEITI
①②③④P/L J06.0 LARYNGOPHARYNGITIS, A
①②③④P/L R42 LIGHT-HEADEDNESS
①②③④P/L G43.109 MIGRAINE
①②③④P/L J00 NASOPHARYNGITIS, ACUT
①②③④P/L H65.00 OTITIS MEDIA
①②③④P/L J02.9 PHARYNGITIS, ACUTE
①②③④P/L J30.1 RHINITIS ALLERGIC
①②③④P/L J01.00 SINUSITIS, ACUTE
①②③④P/L R55 SYNCOPE/VERTIGO

HEMATOLOGIC
①②③④P/L D50.0 CHR BLOOD LOSS ANEMI
①②③④P/L D50.8 IRON DEF ANEMIA DIET
①②③④P/L D51.0 PERNICIOUS ANEMIA

HYPERTENSION
①②③④P/L I13.11 BEN HY HT/REN/CHF
①②③④P/L I12.9 BEN HTN REN W/O REN
①②③④P/L I12.0 BEN HYP WITH REN FAI
①②③④P/L I10 BENIGN HYPERTENSION
①②③④P/L I10 MALIGNANT HYPERTENSI
①②③④P/L I95.1 ORTHOSTATIC HYPOTENS

NEURO
①②③④P/L G40.309 GEN CNV EPIL W/O INT
①②③④P/L I82.3 TIA
①②③④P/L I65.29 CAROTID STENOSIS
①②③④P/L I67.2 CEREBRAL ATHEREOSCLER

OB GYN
①②③④P/L B37.3 CANDIDAL VULVOVAGINI
①②③④P/L N95.1 MENOPAUSAL SYMPTOMS
①②③④P/L Z12.4 SCREEN MAL NEOP-CERV

RHEUMATOLOGIC
①②③④P/L M54.2 CERVICAL PAIN
①②③④P/L M10.00 GOUT
①②③④P/L M54.5 LUMBAGO/BACK PAIN
①②③④P/L M79.609 PAIN IN LIMB
①②③④P/L M54.6 PAIN IN THORACIC SPI
①②③④P/L M06.9 RHEUMATOID ARTHRITIS
①②③④P/L M54.30 SCIATICA
①②③④P/L M32.10 SYST LUPUS ERYTHEMAT

MISC
①②③④P/L R50.9 FEVER UNKN ORGIN
①②③④P/L B00.9 HERPES SIMPLEX NOS
①②③④P/L R06.02 SHORTNESS OF BREATH

UNLISTED DIAGNOSIS
①②③④P/L STOP FOR VERIFICATION

①②③④P/L **REFERRALS**	①②③④P/L **LOCATIONS**	①②③④P/L **DOCTORS**	①②③④P/L **NEXT VISIT**
①②③④P/L	①②③④P/L	①②③④P/L	①②③④P/L ____ DAYS
①②③④P/L	①②③④P/L	①②③④P/L F. CHI, MD	①②③④P/L _1_ WEEKS
①②③④P/L	①②③④P/L	①②③④P/L A. SWERD, MD	①②③④P/L ____ MONTHS
①②③④P/L	①②③④P/L	①②③④P/L J. STEVEN, MD	①②③④P/L

Fig. 15.3 Scannable encounter form. Primary service or procedure is marked (with a no. 2 pencil) in the number 1 location and linked to the primary diagnosis, which also is marked in the number 1 location. The secondary procedures are marked in the number 2 location, as is the secondary diagnosis. The primary linkage for all services and procedures is connected to the service provider and the location in which it took place. Because there are five levels for both new and established patient office visits, an encounter form should include all levels. If information is missing, as shown in this example, an audit could be triggered because it appears to construe that this health care organization never bills any service lower than a Level 3, indicating fraud to an auditor. (Form template from Pearson NCS, Inc., Bloomington, Minn. Form data are fictitious and not a part of the template.)

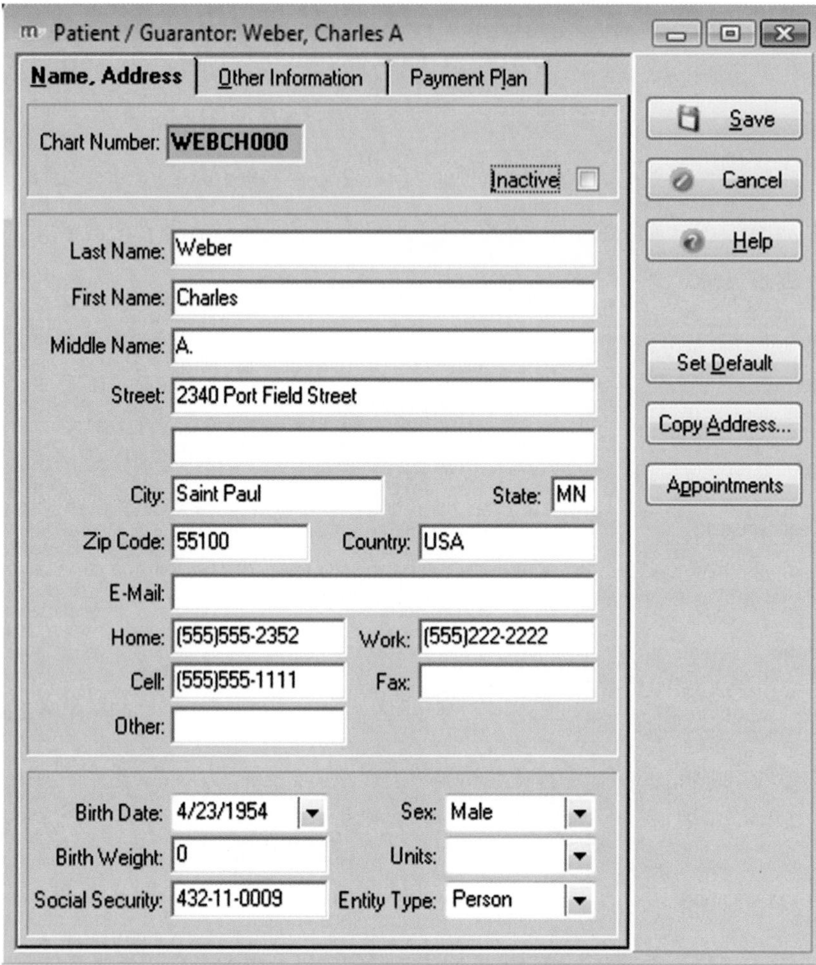

Fig. 15.4 Patient entry screen using practice management software. (Screenshot used by permission of MCKESSON Corporation. All rights reserved. ©MCKESSON Corporation 2012.)

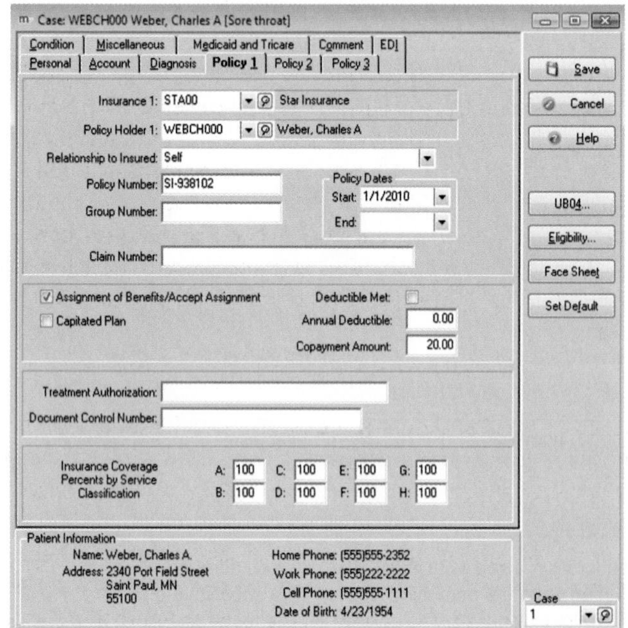

Fig. 15.5 Insurance information using practice management software. Notice that the code for the payer is "STA00." (Screenshot used by permission of MCKESSON Corporation. All rights reserved. ©MCKESSON Corporation 2012.)

Do: Use correct numeric locations of service code and current valid CPT, or HCPCS procedure codes.

Do: Print an insurance billing worksheet or perform a front-end edit (online error checking) to look for and correct all errors before the claim is transmitted to the third-party payer.

Do: Request electronic error reports from the third-party payer to make corrections to the system.

Do: Obtain and cross-check the electronic status report against all claims transmitted.

Don't: Bill codes using modifier -22 electronically unless the carrier receives documents (called *attachments*) to justify more payment.

After input is complete, the information is stored in memory and a claim may be transmitted individually or in batches. Batched claims can be divided according to insurance type or date(s) of service and are ideally sent during low-volume times.

Because the health care provider is responsible for submitting an accurate bill, the insurance billing specialist must accurately input the codes. Medicare and other third-party payer's claims examiners are forbidden to recode a claim. During the edit and error process, software code editors identify invalid codes, age conflicts, gender conflicts, procedural and diagnostic code conflicts, and other data before issuing payment. If certain information, such as a patient's name or

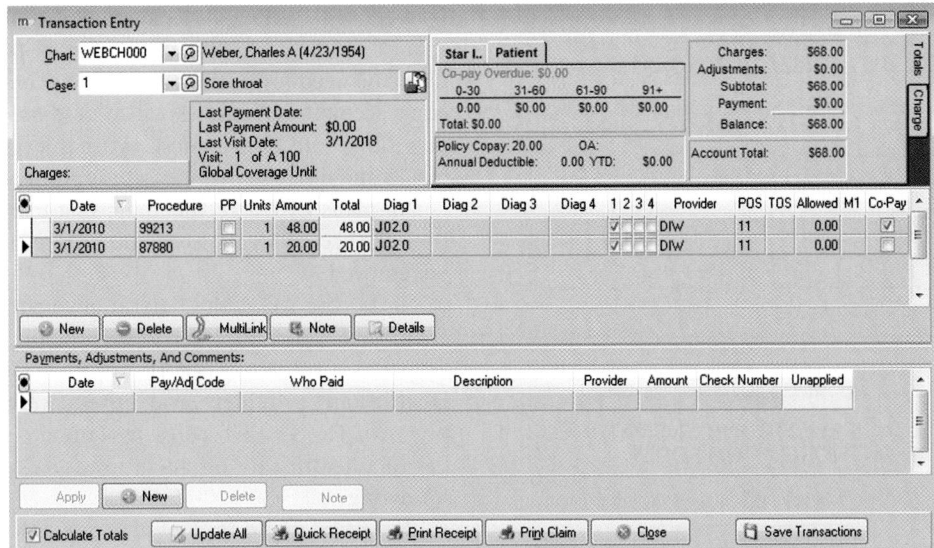

Fig. 15.6 Entering patient information in an electronic encounter form. Notice that the provider's initials are DIW. (Screenshot used by permission of MCKESSON Corporation. All rights reserved. ©MCKESSON Corporation 2012.)

insurance identification number, is submitted incorrectly, the claim is rejected and must be resubmitted with correct data. Incorrect coding may be keying errors or it may be a deliberate attempt to obtain fraudulent payment. The edit check allows immediate feedback about the status of an electronically transmitted claim. The service provider may revise coding on the health record and on the claim to reflect the services more accurately until the time at which the claim is transmitted for payment.

Encoder

An **encoder** is add-on software to a PMS that can greatly reduce the time it takes to build or review a claim before batching and can improve overall coding accuracy. The insurance billing specialist is prompted with a series of questions or choices leading to or affecting a specific code assignment by displaying code-specific edits. Using an encoder can enhance a health care organization's compliance program when it comes to accuracy in its billing procedures. Used as an audit tool, the encoder can also be helpful in performance improvement by identifying problem areas in the billing process.

However, there are instances when an encoder does not accurately assign codes; therefore one must never be completely dependent on code-assist software. For example, if a patient has three thorns incised and extracted (removed), the CPT code 10120 "incision and removal of foreign body, subcutaneous tissue; simple (integumentary system)" might be generated by the encoder. However, if internally audited, the case may warrant CPT code 27372 "removal of foreign body, deep, thigh region in knee area (musculoskeletal system)." Thus one learns that not all procedures involving the skin are found in the integumentary system and, if deeper skin layers are affected, a code may be found in another system.

The final considerations in building a claim are the signature requirements for both the patient and the service provider.

Signature Requirements

Service Provider

The service provider's signature on the agreement or contract with the third-party payer is a substitute for his or her signature on the claim form.

Patient

For assignment of benefits, each patient's signature must be obtained and retained in the office records because there are no handwritten signatures on electronic claims (Fig. 15.7). A clause on the patient registration form or an authorization and assignment release document may be designed specifically to obtain signatures for transmitting electronic claims and acceptance of financial responsibility by the patient. The CMS-1500 Health Insurance Claim Form also may be used for this purpose and the patient should sign in Block 12 or 13 for a specific date of service. Most PMSs ask whether the patient's signature is on file and require a "yes" or "no" answer to complete the required field when the claim is submitted. When a service provider sees a patient in the hospital who has never been to the office, the authorizations obtained by the hospital apply to that provider's filing of a claim.

Clean Electronic Claims Submission

Because a denied claim can delay payment for 30 to 100 days or more, clean claims are the key to a healthy revenue cycle. By ensuring that clean claims are submitted initially, your chances of getting paid promptly are increased. According to industry experts, 90% of claim denials are preventable. The following is a review of some methods used to ensure clean electronic claims:

- Incorporate claim scrubber software (prebill/edit processing) to identify errors and correct them on initial submission.
- Verify, file, and keep all transmission reports.
- Track clearinghouse claims to ensure successful transmission.

PATIENT'S MEDICARE ELECTRONIC SIGNATURE MONTHLY AUTHORIZATION FORM

I authorize any holder of medical or other information about me to release to the Social Security Administration and Centers for Medicare and Medicaid Services or its intermediaries or carriers any information needed for this or a related Medicare claim. I permit a copy of this authorization to be used in place of the original, and request payment of medical insurance benefits either to myself or to the party who accepts assignment.

Signature of Patient ____________ Date ____________

A

PATIENT'S MEDICARE ELECTRONIC SIGNATURE ONE-TIME AUTHORIZATION FORM

I request that payment of authorized Medicare benefits be made either to me or on my behalf to ____________ for services furnished me by that physician or supplier. I permit a copy of this authorization to be used in place of the original and authorize any holder of medical information about me to release to the Centers for Medicare and Medicaid Services or its agents any information needed to determine these benefits or the benefits payable for related services.

Signature of Patient ____________ Date ____________

B

Fig. 15.7 Examples of patients' Medicare electronic signature authorization forms. **A,** Monthly form. **B,** One-time form.

- Ensure that your computer software is consistent with the claims rules.
- Verify that your software correctly prints the CMS-1500 claim form.
- Use encoder software.
- Use an electronic clearinghouse.
- Perform single and batch claims review.

PUTTING HIPAA STANDARD TRANSACTIONS TO WORK

Interactive Transactions

Interactive transactions involve back-and-forth communication between two computer systems. One requests information and the other provides information during what is referred to as *online real time.* **Real time** allows for instant information. An inquiry is made and an answer received within seconds. It can involve eligibility verification, deductible status, claim inquiries, status of claims, and other insurance claim data. Other information, such as fee schedules, allowables, procedure codes, and postoperative days for specific procedures, also may be accessed. Many insurance companies, provide access to information on assigned pending and paid claims. Additional information that may be determined includes whether the individual has other coverage and which third-party payer should be billed as primary.

Electronic Funds Transfer

Many third-party payers deposit payments in the health care organization's bank account automatically via **electronic funds transfer (EFT).** EFT is a paperless computerized system that enables funds to be debited, credited, or transferred and eliminates the need for personal handling of checks. A deposit-only bank account, sometimes called *zero-balance account (ZBA),* provides protection against cyber-thieves. This account has blocks and filters so that it accepts only deposits. However, if the health plan's EFT agreement allows it to recoup overpayments from the provider's bank account, this restriction would have to be removed.

Under the ACA, the federal government has established a uniform procedure for electronically transferring funds as part of HIPAA Title II Administrative Simplification. Health care providers and others were required to comply with CMS's EFT rules by January 1, 2014. The benefits to a health care organization for using EFT include the following:

- Reduction in the amount of paper in the office
- Time savings for staff
- Avoiding the hassles associated with depositing checks at the bank
- Elimination of the risk of paper checks being lost or stolen in the mail
- Faster access to funds
- Easier reconciliation of payments with bank statements

Electronic Remittance Advice

An **electronic remittance advice (ERA)** is a notice of payments and adjustments sent to providers, billers, and suppliers. After a claim has been received and processed, the insurance carrier produces the ERA, which may serve as a companion to a claim payment or as an explanation when there is no payment. The ERA explains reimbursement decisions, including the reasons for payments and adjustments of processed claims. The ERA is similar to the remittance advice (RA) for paper claims, except that the ERA offers additional information and administrative efficiencies.

If the health care organization elects to set the software system to automatically post the information to patients' accounts, then data entry is not required. The computer tests the claims computer data against various guidelines or parameters known as *screens.* If the services billed on the claim exceed the screens, the claim is denied, returned to the service provider for more information, or sent for review. If a claim is denied or rejected, the insurance billing specialist receives a printout stating the reason. The missing, miscoded, or incomplete information should be added or corrected and the claim resubmitted. This process is more efficient than remaining on a telephone, on hold, or resubmitting a claim via standard mail.

A Medicare ERA, formerly known as *explanation of Medicare benefits* (EOMB or *EOB*), is based on the ANSI ASC X12 Health Care Claim Payment/Advice (835), or ANSI 835. The use of ANSI 835 Version 5010 generates an electronic Medicare RA similar to the Standard Paper Remittance Advice (SPR) (Fig. 15.8). To improve cash flow, ANSI 835 also allows EFT of Medicare payments to the health care organization's bank account, which is called *direct deposit.*

No. 1 ABC INSURANCE COMPANY	5780 MAIN STREET				WOODLAND HILLS		XY	12345	TEL # 5557639836	
No. 2 Prov #	No. 3 Prov Name			No. 4 Part B			No. 5 Paid Date:		No. 6 Remit #	Page:
PATIENT NAME	PATIENT CNTRL NUMBER			RC	REM	DRG #	DRG OUT AMT	COINSURANCE	PAT REFUND	CONTRACT ADJ
No. 7	No. 12			No. 20	No. 21	No. 22	No. 27	No. 30	No. 34	No. 38
HIC NUMBER	ICN NUMBER			RC	REM	OUTCD CAPCD		COVD CHGS	ESRD NET ADJ	PER DIEM RTE
No. 8	No. 13			No. 20	No. 21	Nos. 23 24		No. 31	No. 35	No. 39
FROM DT–THRU DT	NACHG	HICHG	TOB	RC	REM	PROF COMP	MSP PAYMT	NCOVD CHGS	INTEREST	PROC CD AMT
Nos. 9 10	Nos. 14	15	16	No. 20	No. 21	No. 25	No. 28	No. 32	No. 36	No. 40
CLM STATUS	COST	COVDY	NCOVDY	RC	REM	DRG AMT	DEDUCTIBLES	DENIED CHGS	PRE PAY ADJ	NET REIMB
No. 11	Nos. 17	18	19	No. 20	No. 21	No. 26	No. 29	No. 33	No. 37	No. 41
SUBTOTAL FISCAL YEAR							No. 27	No. 30	No. 34	No. 38
								No. 31	No. 35	No. 39
						No. 25	No. 28	No. 32	No. 36	No. 40
	Nos. 17	18	19			No. 26	No. 29	No. 33	No. 37	No. 41
SUBTOTAL PART B							No. 27	No. 30	No. 34	No. 38
								No. 31	No. 35	No. 39
						No. 25	No. 28	No. 32	No. 36	No. 40
	Nos. 17	18	19			No. 26	No. 29	No. 33	No. 37	No. 41

A

Medicare Standard Remittence Advice

Claim Adjustment Reason Codes (CARCs) provide financial information about claim decisions. CARCs communicate an adjustment, or why a claim (or service line) was paid differently than it was billed.

1	Deductible amount
2	Coinsurance amount
3	Copayment amount
4	The procedure code is inconsistent with the modifier used or a required modifier is missing.
5	The procedure code/bill type is inconsistent with the place of service.
6	The procedure/revenue code is inconsistent with the patient's age.

Remittance Advice Remark Codes (RARCs) are used in conjunction with CARCs on the Medicare remittance advice to further explain an adjustment or to indicate if and what appeal rights apply. RARCs are maintained by CMS, but may be used by any health care payer when appropriate.

M2	Not paid separately when the patient is an inpatient.
M19	Missing oxygen certification/recertification
M20	Missing/invalid HCPCS code

B

Fig. 15.8 A, Example of a computer-generated Medicare Part B remittance advice (RA) document received by a provider from the payer or fiscal intermediary. **B,** Medicare standard remittance advice.

METHODS OF SENDING CLAIMS

The methods for getting claims submitted to either the payer or the clearinghouse vary according to the office system in place. Methods can include the following:

1. Data transmission via **cable modem, digital subscriber line (DSL)**, or **T-1**
   a. *Cable modem.* A modem used to connect a computer to a cable television system that offers online services.
   b. *DSL.* A high-speed connection through a telephone line jack and usually a means of accessing the internet.
   c. *T-1.* A T-carrier channel that can transmit voice or data channels quickly.

2. Data directly keyed into payer system: Direct data entry (DDE) via dial-up modem or internet
   a. *DDE.* Keying claim information directly into the payer system by accessing it over modem dial-up or DSL. This is a technology used to directly enter the information into the payer system via the access, whether it is dial-up or DSL.
3. *PMS.* An in-house shared system or application service provider (ASP)
   a. *ASP.* "Renting" a PMS available over the internet. All data are housed on the server of the ASP but the accounts are managed by the health care provider's staff. Claims are batched and submitted as though the software is stored on the desktop at the provider's office.

COMPUTER CLAIMS SYSTEMS

Carrier-Direct

There are different types of claims submission systems. Fiscal agents for Medicaid, Medicare, TRICARE, and many private third-party payers use the carrier-direct system. With this system, the data are transmitted electronically directly to the payer's system. This eliminates the need for a clearinghouse. It is necessary to have a signed agreement with each carrier with whom the service provider or health care organization wishes to submit electronic claims.

Once enrollment is complete, a submitter number may be assigned. Submitters must send a test file to the insurance carrier to ensure accurate file format, completeness, and validity. Any problems discovered during the test period must be corrected and a new test submitted for review before final approval. Test submissions may be a cross-section of claim type data from previously adjudicated claims. The test file must consist of a minimum number of claims, dependent on the requirements of the insurance carrier, for each claim type to be billed. The test procedure must be completed for each claim type. A new test must be submitted when software is upgraded or the submission method changes. Test claims are not processed for payment. It is only after receiving written notification from the insurance carrier that claims may be transmitted electronically.

Clearinghouses

Clearinghouses may charge a flat fee per claim or a monthly fee. Some clearinghouses offer to file claims free of charge to the provider but they recoup the expense from the payer. Most often, a vendor agreement of sorts will be in place between the clearinghouse and the provider submitting the claims. These contracts may be a business associate agreement, a trading partner agreement, or other contract.

TRANSMISSION REPORTS

Whether claims are submitted carrier-direct or through a clearinghouse, reports are generated to track each function of the claims process. Examples are as follows:

- **Send and Receive File Reports:** Shows that a file is received by the clearinghouse and/or payer and notifies the billing specialist when a file has been sent to the service provider's account for review (Fig. 15.9).
- **Batch Claim Report Billed Summary:** Lists each patient's name, total charges for medical services, batch number, billing number, name of insurance company billed, and chronologic date on which the claim was transmitted (Fig. 15.10).
- **Scrubber Report:** Indicates the total number of claims, the charges, and the dollar amounts that were received by the clearinghouse and scrubbed for claims submitted to Massachusetts Insurance Plan (Fig. 15.11). The insurance billing specialist reviews the scrubber report for each insurance payer when claims have been transmitted through the clearinghouse.
- **Transaction Transmission Summary:** Shows how many claims were originally received by the clearinghouse and/or payer and how many claims were rejected automatically (Fig. 15.12).
- **Rejection Analysis Report:** Identifies the most common reasons that claims are rejected and indicates what claims were not included for processing (Fig. 15.13). Corrections must be made by the insurance billing specialist and the claims need to be refiled.
- **Electronic Inquiry or Claims Status Review:** Lists files received from the provider's office and indicates the progress of the claim. For example, if a claim is sent to a clearinghouse and forwarded to a payer, the clearinghouse can indicate that the status is confirmed received by the payer.

Electronic Processing Problems

Some problems can occur in electronic claims submission. Usually a status report of claims is received electronically from the third-party payer. It consists of an acknowledgment report and indicates assigned and unassigned claims, crossed over and not crossed over claims, claims accepted with errors, and rejected claims (see Fig. 15.13). Data transmission problems arise periodically because of hardware or software problems.

Changes to the standard electronic claims submission process can also result in errors. The upgrade to HIPAA transaction standard ASC X12 Version 5010 resulted in these common errors:

Billing Provider Address: The 5010 guidelines require providers to enter the physical address; post office boxes or lock box addresses cannot be used as a health care organization's address.

Zip Code: The 5010 guidelines require a nine-digit zip code when reporting billing provider and service facility locations.

Anesthesia Minutes: The 5010 guidelines require that anesthesia services be reported in actual minutes rather than units.

Primary Identification Code Qualifiers: The 5010 guidelines allow only an NPI as a primary identifier. EINs or Social Security numbers cannot be used as a primary identifier.

Billing Provider NPI Number: The 5010 guidelines require that a consistent NPI number be reported with all payers.

National Drug Code (NDC): The 5010 guidelines require that a drug quantity and unit of measure be reported on the claim form when an NDC is used.

A

```
Raw 837
=========

Electronic Technologies, Inc.
=========================

ISA*00* *00*
*ZZ*1234*ZZ*VB6786786*041110*0310*U*00401*123456789*0*P*:~GS*HC*12
34*VB6786786*20041110*0310*123456789*X*004010X098A1~ST*837*0001~B
HT*0019*00*1*20041110*0310*CH~REF*87*004010X098A1~NM1*41*2*GERI
ATRIC ASSOCIATES LLC*****46*1234~PER*IC*JIM
JONES*TE*8005551212~NM1*40*2*MASSACHUSETTS INS
PLAN*****46*XYZ1~HL*1**20*1~NM1*85*2*ALABAMA MEDICAL
ASSOC*****24*54-5555555~N3*PO BOX
123456~N4*BOSTON*MA*12345~REF*1D*123456789~HL*2*1*22*0~SBR*P*1
8*******MC~NM1*IL*1*JONES*DEBRA*K***MI*123456789123~N3*11
JEFFERS POND
ROAD~N4*BOSTON*MA*12345~DMG*D8*19640812*F~NM1*PR*2*VMAP
FHSC FA*****PI*DMAS~N3*PO BOX
123~N4*BOSTON*MA*12345~CLM*123456*150***11::1*Y*A*Y*Y*B~REF*X
4*1242522DD~HI*BK:6110~NM1*DN*1*JACKSON*DONALD~REF*1D*12345
6789~NM1*82*1*ROWLAND*DAVID****24*54-
5555555~PRV*PE*ZZ*207ZP0102X~REF*1D*123456789~NM1*77*2*NORTH
OFFICE*****24*54-5555555~N3*123 LIPPLE
AVENUE~N4*BOSTON*MA*12345~LX*1~SV1*HC:88305:26*150*UN*1***1~
DTP*472*D8*20041028~REF*6R*11265594~
.
.
.
.
.
SE*160*0001~GE*1*123456789~IEA*1*123456789~
```

B

```
Human-Readable 837
==================
Electronic Technologies, Inc.
=========================

================================================================
INTERCHANGE HEADER - Production File
================================================================
Authorization: none                     Password: none
SubmitterID: 1234                       ReceiverID: VB6786786
Date: 11.10.2004                        Time: 0310
Run #: 003                              Control #: 123456789
Request Acknowledgement: No Sub-element Separator: :

FUNCTIONAL GROUP HEADER - HC
================================================================
Submitter ID: 1234                      ReceiverID: VB6786786
Date: 11.10.2004                        Time: 0310 Control #: 123456789
ANSI X10 Version: 004010X098A1

TRANSACTION SET HEADER- 837
================================================================
Control #: 0001
Structure Code: 0019                    Purpose Code: 00
Reference ID: 1                         Type: CH
Date: 11.10.2004                        Time: 0310
Functional Category: 004010X098A1

Submitter - Non-Person
---------
GERIATRIC ASSOCIATES LLC (Electronic Transmitter ID #,1234)
Contact: JIM JONES
Phone Number: 800.555.1212

Receiver - Non-Person
--------
MASSACHUSETTS INS PLAN (Electronic Transmitter ID #,XYZ1)

BATCH #1
================================================================

Billing Provider - Non-Person
----------------
ALABAMA MEDICAL ASSOC (Employer ID Number,54-5555555)
PO BOX 123456
BOSTON, MA 12345
Provider Number: 123456789

PATIENT #1
================================================================
Primary Insurance
-----------------
Patient Relationship: Self

Subscriber - Person
----------
JONES, DEBRA K (Member ID Number,123456789123)
11 JEFFERS POND ROAD
BOSTON, MA  12345

Date of Birth: 19640812 Gender Code: F

Payer - Non-Person
-----
VMAP FHSC FA (Payer ID Number,DMAS)
PO BOX 123
BOSTON, MA 12345

Account Number:                         123456
Claim Amount:                           $150
Facility:                               Office
This Claim is                           ORIGINAL
Provider Signature:                     On File Assignment Code: Assigned
Assignment of Benefits Indicator:       Y
Release of Information:                 Yes, Provider Has a Signed Statement
Permitting Release of Medical Billing
Data Related to a Claim
CLIA Number:                            1242522DD
Principal Diagnosis Code:               6110

Referring Prov. - Person
---------------
JACKSON, DONALD
MA Provider Number: 123456789

Rendering Prov. - Person
---------------
ROWLAND, DAVID  (Employer ID Number,54-5555555)
Provider Taxonomy Code: 207ZP0102X
MA Provider Number: 123456789

Service Location - Non-Person
----------------
NORTH OFFICE (Employer ID Number,54-5555555)
123 LIPPLE AVENUE
BOSTON, MA 12345

Service Line # 1
----------------
Service Code:                           88305
Modifier:                               26
Amount:                                 $150 Measurement: Unit Quantity: 1
Diagnosis Pointer:                      1
Date of Service:                        20041028
Prov. Control #:                        11265594

PATIENT #2
================================================================
.
.
.
.
.
.
TRANSACTION SET TRAILER
================================================================
Included Segments: 160
Control #: 0001

FUNCTIONAL GROUP TRAILER
================================================================
Transaction Sets Included: 1
Group Control #: 123456789

INTERCHANGE TRAILER
================================================================
Included Functional Groups: 1
Control #: 123456789
```

Fig. 15.9 A, Raw 837 clearinghouse transmission report. If you print the 837 electronic claims transmission file, it looks similar to this; however, the report becomes readable after it comes back from the clearinghouse showing the patients' claims that were submitted. **B,** Readable 837 clearinghouse transmission report. (Reports supplied by Electronic Technologies, Inc., Delmar, NY.)

BATCH CLAIM REPORT Billed Summary

Patient code	Total charges	Batch #	Billing #	Insurance co. billed	Date sent
BORTOLUSSI	465.00	2	1005	ABCI000001	05/25/2005
BLACKWOOD	16.07	3	1006	TRICARE	05/25/2005
HELMS	33.25	4	1007	MDCR	05/25/2005
JAMESON	41.07	5	1008	ROYAL	05/25/2005
KELSEY	66.23	8	1010	XYZI000001	06/09/2005
	621.62				

Fig. 15.10 Batch Claim Report Billed Summary by chronologic date.

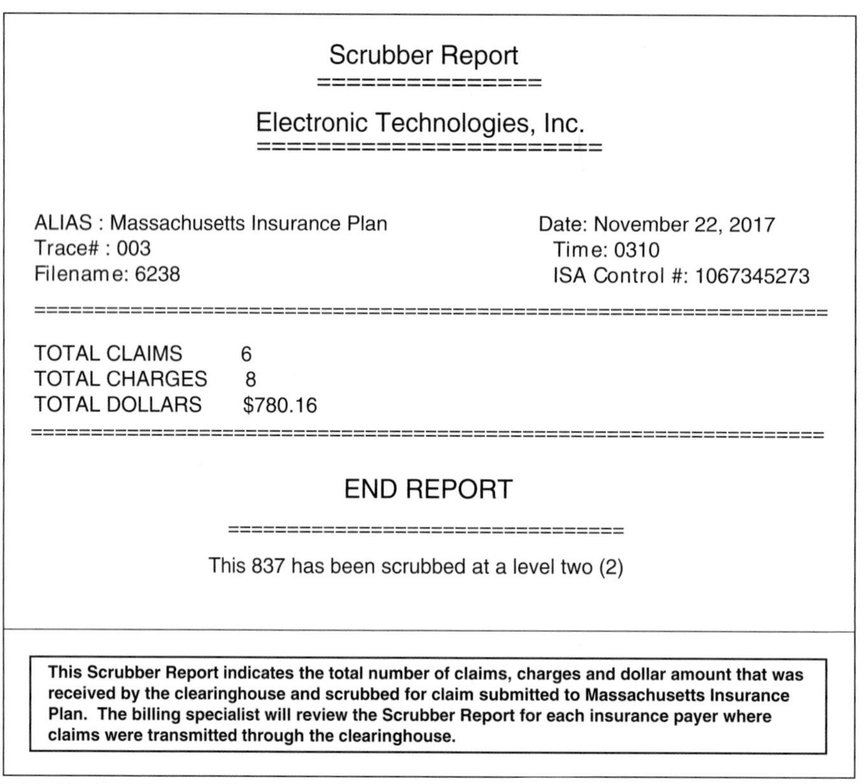

Scrubber Report

Electronic Technologies, Inc.

ALIAS : Massachusetts Insurance Plan
Trace# : 003
Filename: 6238

Date: November 22, 2017
Time: 0310
ISA Control #: 1067345273

TOTAL CLAIMS 6
TOTAL CHARGES 8
TOTAL DOLLARS $780.16

END REPORT

This 837 has been scrubbed at a level two (2)

This Scrubber Report indicates the total number of claims, charges and dollar amount that was received by the clearinghouse and scrubbed for claim submitted to Massachusetts Insurance Plan. The billing specialist will review the Scrubber Report for each insurance payer where claims were transmitted through the clearinghouse.

Fig. 15.11 Clearinghouse scrubber report. (Report supplied by Electronic Technologies, Inc., Delmar, NY.)

Most billing software bundles claims into a batch and then the claims are transmitted together. If one claim in the batch contains an error, such as, missing a patient name or missing a diagnosis code, the third-party payer may reject the entire batch and return all claims to the provider.

Some batches contain errors that occur in every transaction in the batch. These are called *syntax errors*. Syntax errors are inaccuracies that violate the HIPAA standard transaction format, such as incorrect sequence of patient information or incorrect batch header. Such errors make it difficult for the third-party payer's software to read the transactions in a batch.

There are other errors in which only one transaction in the batch has a syntax error or one of the batch's transactions has a data content error. In these instances, it would be inappropriate for a third-party payer to reject the entire batch. Usually the payer returns any noncompliant claims and processes the remaining claims in the batch. To avoid these types of rejections, it is important to use software that will separate out noncompliant transactions so that those can be removed from the batch and fixed before submission.

Solutions to Electronic Processing Problems

1. Review claims filed electronically by validating that you received confirmation that the claims were processed by the clearinghouse and received by the insurance carrier. Check for error messages from the clearinghouse and payer. Immediately respond to rejected claims.
2. Produce monthly aging of accounts and check the large amounts not paid in the 60-day aging column. Look at service dates of claims and the amounts. If there are many outstanding claims with the same service dates, it is possible that these claims did not reach the payer. Immediately confirm with the payer whether the claims were received and refile if appropriate.

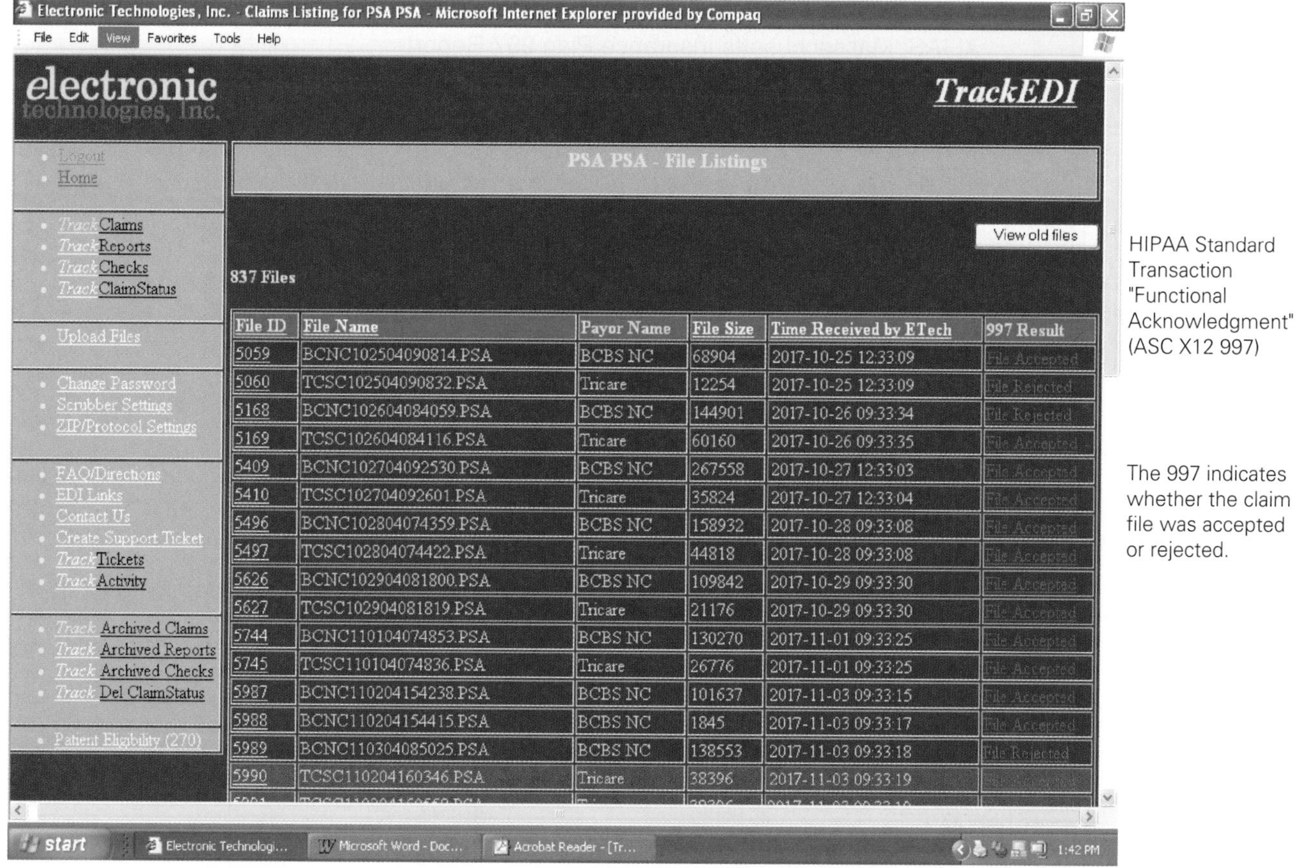
Electronic Technologies, Inc. - Claims Listing for PSA PSA - Microsoft Internet Explorer provided by Compaq
File Edit View Favorites Tools Help
electronic technologies, Inc.
TrackEDI
Logout
Home
Track Claims
Track Reports
Track Checks
Track ClaimStatus
Upload Files
Change Password
Scrubber Settings
ZIP/Protocol Settings
FAQ/Directions
EDI Links
Contact Us
Create Support Ticket
Track Tickets
Track Activity
Track Archived Claims
Track Archived Reports
Track Archived Checks
Track Del ClaimStatus
Patient Eligibility (270)
PSA PSA - File Listings
View old files
837 Files
File ID | File Name | Payor Name | File Size | Time Received by ETech | 997 Result
5059 | BCNC102504090814.PSA | BCBS NC | 68904 | 2017-10-25 12:33:09 | File Accepted
5060 | TCSC102504090832.PSA | Tricare | 12254 | 2017-10-25 12:33:09 | File Rejected
5168 | BCNC102604084059.PSA | BCBS NC | 144901 | 2017-10-26 09:33:34 | File Rejected
5169 | TCSC102604084116.PSA | Tricare | 60160 | 2017-10-26 09:33:35 | File Accepted
5409 | BCNC102704092530.PSA | BCBS NC | 267558 | 2017-10-27 12:33:03 | File Accepted
5410 | TCSC102704092601.PSA | Tricare | 35824 | 2017-10-27 12:33:04 | File Accepted
5496 | BCNC102804074359.PSA | BCBS NC | 158932 | 2017-10-28 09:33:08 | File Accepted
5497 | TCSC102804074422.PSA | Tricare | 44818 | 2017-10-28 09:33:08 | File Accepted
5626 | BCNC102904081800.PSA | BCBS NC | 109842 | 2017-10-29 09:33:30 | File Accepted
5627 | TCSC102904081819.PSA | Tricare | 21176 | 2017-10-29 09:33:30 | File Accepted
5744 | BCNC110104074853.PSA | BCBS NC | 130270 | 2017-11-01 09:33:25 | File Accepted
5745 | TCSC110104074836.PSA | Tricare | 26776 | 2017-11-01 09:33:25 | File Accepted
5987 | BCNC110204154238.PSA | BCBS NC | 101637 | 2017-11-03 09:33:15 | File Accepted
5988 | BCNC110204154415.PSA | BCBS NC | 1845 | 2017-11-03 09:33:17 | File Accepted
5989 | BCNC110304085025.PSA | BCBS NC | 138553 | 2017-11-03 09:33:18 | File Rejected
5990 | TCSC110204160346.PSA | Tricare | 38396 | 2017-11-03 09:33:19 |
start
Electronic Technologi...
Microsoft Word - Doc...
Acrobat Reader - [Tr...
1:42 PM
HIPAA Standard Transaction "Functional Acknowledgment" (ASC X12 997)
The 997 indicates whether the claim file was accepted or rejected.

Fig. 15.12 Clearinghouse 997 report that shows which 837 claim files were accepted and rejected. (Report supplied by Electronic Technologies, Inc., Delmar, NY.)

3. File claims within the time limits because many payers have a 90-day filing deadline. Payers will not reimburse a time delinquent claim unless you can prove that the payer received the claim. Electronic confirmation that a claim reached the clearinghouse is not sufficient.
4. Double check that the correct code for place of service is shown, especially if your service provider does procedures in different locations. The payment amount may be more or less, depending on the location.
5. Be accurate in linking the correct diagnosis codes to the procedure codes. Usually payers use the first diagnosis codes to process claims. Additional diagnostic codes may be used only for informational purposes or not considered at all.

Billing and Account Management Schedule

Maintaining a schedule will help with EDI transmissions, which will enable better cash flow. Table 15.6 suggests guidelines and procedures that can be tailored to the needs of your billing office.

Administrative Simplification Enforcement Tool

To address issues of noncompliance with the HIPAA TCS rule, the federal government has implemented the use of an web-based tool to assist health care providers, payers, clearinghouses, and others to submit complaints. This online tool, the Administrative Simplification Enforcement Tool (ASET), enables individuals or organizations to file a complaint online against a covered entity "that fails to adopt and follow the HIPAA rules for transactions and code sets". Failure to implement these standards can result in civil monetary penalties.

ALIAS: Massachusetts Insurance Plan 997 Report
==
CLAIMS 997 ACKNOWLEDGMENT FILE

Trace#: 941 | ID: 114120941
SUBMISSION DATE: 11.22.2004 | 997 DATE: 11.23.2017
TIME SUBMITTED: 0112 | 997 TIME: 111346
=============== ==

ERROR CODE	PATIENT ACCT #	LINE# / CHARGE#
251:NM1:9	628263478	2893

DESCRIPTION: Payer Name
Segment Has Data Element Errors
DETAIL: Subscriber Identifier - (Mandatory data element missing)
SUBMITTED:

ERROR CODE	PATIENT ACCT #	LINE# / CHARGE#
251:NM1:10	123456	5454545

DESCRIPTION: Payer Name
Segment Has Data Element Errors
DETAIL: (Invalid character in data element)
SUBMITTED:

ERROR CODE	PATIENT ACCT #	LINE# / CHARGE#
251:NM1:8	4515485	3157654

DESCRIPTION: Payer Name
Segment Has Data Element Errors
DETAIL: Identification Qualifier (Conditional required data element missing)
SUBMITTED:

This transaction was :	Rejected
Rejection Reason :	One or More Segments in Error
This Functional Group was :	Rejected
Transaction Sets Included :	1
Transaction Sets Received :	1
Transaction Sets Accepted :	0

Fig. 15.13 Clearinghouse 997 report showing the claims acknowledgment file. This report shows error codes and details the types of errors made. It also shows patient account numbers and names of the payers. (Report supplied by Electronic Technologies, Inc., Delmar, NY.)

TABLE 15.6 Daily, Weekly, and End-of-Month Guidelines and Protocols

Daily	Weekly	End of Month
Post charges in practice management system. Post payments in practice management system.	Batch, scrub, edit, and transmit claims (daily or weekly). Analyze previous week's rejected and resubmitted claims.	Run month-end aging reports. Review all claim rejection reports (clearinghouse and payer), ensuring all problems are resolved and claims accepted.
Batch, scrub, edit, and transmit claims (daily or weekly); retrieve transmission reports.	Note any problematic claims and resolve outstanding files.	Update practice management system with payer information, such as EIN and NPI.
Run daysheet.	Research unpaid claims.	Run patient statements in office or through clearinghouse.
Review clearinghouse/payer transmission confirmation reports.	Make follow-up calls to resolve reasons for rejections, such as incorrect NPI, missing patient ID, incomplete data elements, and wrong format.	
Audit claims batched and transmitted with confirmation reports. Correct rejections and resubmit claims.		

EIN, Employer identification number; *ID*, identification; *NPI*, National Provider Identifier.

KEY POINTS

This is a brief chapter review of the key issues presented. To further enhance your knowledge of the technical subject matter, review the key terms and key abbreviations for this chapter by locating the meaning for each in the Glossary at the end of this book, which appears in a section before the Index.

1. The American National Standards Institute (ANSI) formed the Accredited Standards Committee X12 (ASC X12), which developed the US standards body for the cross-industry development, maintenance, and publication of electronic data exchange standards.
2. Through HIPAA regulations, standardized transaction and code sets have been implemented to use electronic data interchange effectively.
3. A clearinghouse receives the electronic transmission of claims from the health care provider's office and translates it to a standard format prescribed in HIPAA regulations.
4. Under HIPAA rules, a provider who sends Medicare claims is considered a covered entity that has 10 or more employees and must transmit claims electronically. Health care organizations with fewer than 10 employees are not considered covered entities and are not required to submit Medicare claims electronically.
5. Practice management software (PMS) is used to input data, which helps generate a variety of documents including the 837P (Professional) in electronic National Standard Format (NSF), formerly the CMS-1500 paper form.
6. When constructing an insurance claim, the supporting code sets are made up of "required" and "situational" data elements identified by the HIPAA standard electronic formats.
7. Ten-character, alphanumeric provider-specialty taxonomy codes are assigned and classify each health care provider. These codes are used when transmitting electronic insurance claims.
8. Employers use their employer identification numbers (EINs) to identify themselves in transactions involving premium payments to health plans on behalf of their employees or to identify themselves to other employers as the source or receiver of information about eligibility. Employers use EINs to identify themselves in transactions when enrolling or disenrolling employees in health plans.
9. HIPAA requires that a National Provider Identifier (NPI), a 10-character numeric identifier, be assigned to each provider to be used in transactions with all health plans.
10. An encoder is helpful because it can reduce the time it takes to build or review a claim and help to improve coding accuracy before batching and transmitting to a third-party payer.
11. An electronic remittance advice (ERA) is the equivalent of a paper summarized statement called an *explanation of benefits (EOB)*, which gives the status of insurance claims with payment details for one or more beneficiaries. It is referred to as *ANSI 835* or *Health Care Claim Payment/Advice (835)*.
12. Several methods are available for submitting claims to either the payer or a clearinghouse, such as cable modem, digital subscriber line (DSL), T-1, direct data entry (DDE), and application service provider (ASP).

STUDENT ASSIGNMENT

- Study Chapter 15.
- Answer the fill-in-the-blank, multiple-choice, and true/false review questions in the *Workbook* to reinforce the theories learned in this chapter and to help prepare for a future test.
- Complete the assignments in the *Workbook* to edit and correct insurance claims that have been transmitted and rejected with errors.
- Turn to the Glossary at the end of this text for a further understanding of the key terms and key abbreviations used in this chapter.

UNIT 5

The Claim Follow-Up and Payment Process

16

Receiving Payments and Insurance Problem Solving

Linda M. Smith

OBJECTIVES

After reading this chapter, you should be able to:

1. Identify and discuss three health insurance payment policy guidelines.
2. Assess reimbursement payment time frames for all submitted claims.
3. Identify the components of an explanation of benefits document and interpret and post an explanation of benefits document to a patient's account.
4. Discuss secondary insurance and guidelines to billing secondary insurance.
5. List and describe three health insurance claim management techniques.
6. Explain reasons for claim inquiries and identify strategies to discover why payments are delayed.
7. Define terminology pertinent to problem claims filing, and discuss types of problems as well as find solutions.
8. Identify specific reasons for rebilling a claim.
9. Describe situations for filing appeals and discuss the review and appeals process.
10. Review Medicare's five levels in the redetermination (appeal) process and determine which forms to use for each level.
11. Review and discuss the TRICARE review and appeal process, including expedited and nonexpedited appeals, as well as reconsideration.
12. List four objectives of state insurance commissioners.
13. Mention seven problems to submit to insurance commissioners.
14. Discuss the type of information necessary to include in an insurance commission request.
15. Explain the importance of claim denial management.

KEY TERMS

administrative law judge hearing
aging report
appeal
claim denial management
delinquent claim
denied claim
explanation of benefits
inquiry
insurance payment poster
insurance payment posting
lost claim
medical necessity
overpayment
peer review
Qualified Independent Contractor
reassess
rebill (resubmit)
reimbursement
rejected claim
remittance advice
revenue cycle management
review
state insurance commissioner
suspended claim
suspense
tracer

KEY ABBREVIATIONS

ALJ
CMS
DAB
EOB
HIPAA
NPI
QIC
RA
RCM

REVENUE CYCLE MANAGEMENT

Revenue cycle management (RCM) is the process that health care organizations use to track services provided and patient care episodes from registration and appointment scheduling to the final payment of the associated fees. As discussed in Chapter 1, an insurance billing specialist's primary goal is to assist in management of the revenue cycle. The insurance billing specialist will help to obtain maximum insurance benefits for services provided and ensure cash flow to the health care organization they are employed by. Revenue is the total income produced by a health care organization and the cycle is the regularly repeating set of events for producing it.

Everything that you have learned in the preceding chapters has led up to submission of the claim to the insurance carrier. Now that the claim has been successfully submitted to the insurance carrier, the next step in the revenue cycle is to track the claim until a response is received from the responsible party and the service has been paid in full.

RESPONSE FROM A SUBMITTED CLAIM

An insurance company can accept responsibility to pay the claim and reimburse the health care organization, they can suspend the claim to investigate the details of the claim further, or they can deny the claim for a variety of reasons. Delay in reimbursements, or payments to the health care organization, can also occur when health insurance companies state that they did not receive the claim at all. At times, the insurance company may reimburse claims lower than expected, after which an appeal can be filed. An appeal is a documented request to the insurance company to review (reassess) a claim and reconsider for payment.

This chapter begins with the provisions for payment in the insurance contract and explains how this affects the timeliness for payment. Then the text demonstrates how to interpret the document that accompanies payment and how to manage and organize financial records. To improve cash flow, numerous problems that can occur are presented and some solutions are offered. Finally, the review and appeal processes for various programs are discussed.

The management of the reimbursement process and insurance company denials is often referred to as claim follow-up. By developing proficient skills and experience in following up on claims, an insurance billing specialist can become a valuable asset to his or her employer and bring in revenue that might otherwise be lost to the health care organization.

CLAIM POLICY GUIDELINES

A patient who seeks medical care with a health insurance card is presenting the contract that he or she has with the insurance company. In other words, the insurance company issued the card to the patient as evidence that it takes responsibility to pay the health care organization for the services the patient receives. In order for the health care organization to get paid for these services, insurance companies require them to submit a claim form. The insurance company dictates the guidelines for claims submission, such as which services are covered, the reimbursement rates, and the time limits for claim submission and payment.

Insured

A patient's insurance card does not specify the detailed benefits and coverages. However, before rendering services to the patient, it is in the health care providers' best interest to be aware of their patients' insurance benefits and coverages. For example, maternity care is an optional benefit; therefore a health care provider should be aware that by providing maternity care to a patient with no coverage, the provider risks not being reimbursed. Another example is that there may be a provision that the claimant has an obligation to notify the insurance company of a loss (injury, illness, or accident) within a certain period or the insurer has the right to deny benefits for that loss.

In some policies, if the insured disagrees with the insurer for settlement of a claim, a suit must begin within 3 years after the claim is submitted. Another provision might state that an insured person cannot bring legal action against an insurance company until 60 days after a claim is submitted.

Contracts and Fee Schedules

A fee schedule is included when a health care organization or physician signs a contract with an insurance company or group to become a participating with the insurance plan. The participating health care organization/physician agrees to the fee schedule, which is typically less than the provider's standard fee for service, and agrees not to charge the patient for the difference. In certain circumstances, health care organizations will agree to a contract capitation in which they agree to provide services by accepting the patient's copayment and the monthly stipend paid per patient.

Reimbursement Time Frames

All health insurance companies are obligated to reimburse health care organizations for services rendered promptly. However, time limits vary in this provision from one third-party payer to another. Specific time limits will be stated in either the insurance contract or the payer's manual. It is reasonable to expect payment within 4 to 12 weeks if claims are submitted on paper or in as little as 7 days when they are transmitted electronically.

Many states have implemented prompt payment laws to set standards for the prompt, fair, and equitable settlements of patient claims and provider services. For example, New York requires insurers to pay claims and bills within 45 days of receipt. Furthermore, the law requires the insurance carrier to make an interest payment on any claim that is not paid within the 45-day period. It is important that the insurance billing specialist research to see if there are prompt pay laws in the state they are filing claims in.

If a payment delay occurs and the insurance company is slow or ignores, denies, or exceeds time limits to pay a claim, then it is prudent to contact the insurance company. In the letter the contracted time limit should be stated and the reason the claim has not been paid should be sought, and a copy should be retained for the office files.

EXPLANATION OF BENEFITS

An explanation of benefits (EOBs) is a document issued to both the health care provider filing the claim and the patient that explains the allowable amount, the paid amount, the amount that must be written off, and any financial responsibility of the patient. The EOB also provides details about claims that are denied and provides the reasons why. A denied claim is the refusal of an insurance carrier to honor a request to pay for health care services. Sometimes EOBs will provide details on specific claims that need to be refunded and the reasons why. Finally, if a payment is explained in the EOB, a check will be attached or evidence of an electronic transfer of funds will be evident. Medicare and other payers may refer to the EOB as a remittance advice (RA). The elements within the RA document are the same as an EOB document. A suspended claim is one that is processed by a third-party payer but is held in an indeterminate (pending) state. The claim is usually suspended because of an error or the need for additional information from the provider of service or the patient. The EOB also states the allowed amount for the service provided based on the contracted fee schedule by the third-party payer, as shown in Fig. 16.1. The allowed amount is the maximum dollar value that the insurance company assigns to each medical service. If the health care provider is contracted with the health insurance company, the provider will receive a copy of the EOB along with payment. If the provider is not participating with the insurance company, payment can be sent to the patient, in which case the patient should be billed.

Components of an Explanation of Benefits

Unfortunately, there is no standard format for EOB forms from one carrier to the next but the information contained in each one is usually the same. At first glance, the EOB may seem difficult to understand; however, if one line at a time is read, the description and calculations for each patient may be understood easily. The EOB breaks down how payment was determined and contains the following information in categories or columns:

1. Insurance company's name and address
2. Provider of services
3. Dates of services
4. Service or procedure (*Current Procedural Terminology* [CPT]) code
5. Amounts billed by the health care provider
6. Reduction or denial codes: comment codes (reasons, remarks, or notes) indicating reasons that payments were denied or reduced, asking for more information to determine coverage and benefits, or stating amounts of adjustment because of payments by other insurance companies (coordination of benefits)
7. Claim control number
8. Subscriber's and patient's name and policy numbers
9. Analysis of patient's total payment responsibility (allowed amount, copayment amount, deductible, coinsurance, other insurance payment, and patient's total responsibility)
10. Copayment amount(s) due from the patient
11. Deductible amounts subtracted from billed amounts
12. Total amount paid by the insurance carrier

Interpreting an Explanation of Benefits

Reading and interpreting an EOB may be overwhelming initially, so take time to read the document carefully. If several patients' claims are submitted to a third-party payer, the EOB may reflect the status of all of those claims and one check voucher may be issued. The EOB shown in Fig. 16.1 should be read line by line to interpret the meanings under each category or column and the numbered explanations should be referred to when necessary. A helpful way to separate patients and their corresponding payments is to use a highlighter or ruler to underline the entire row across the EOB. This helps reduce errors when posting payments.

Posting an Explanation of Benefits

Insurance payment posting is the process of applying payments to the patient account while writing off all adjustments. Posting of insurance payments is done by line item. In Fig. 16.1 each line item, or coded service, is explained separately. The insurance payment poster, the individual responsible for posting payments in patient accounts, must be careful to review lines that are posted and lines that are denied. Denials should be presented to the insurance billing specialist's attention as soon as possible; many denials or pending claims have a window of time in which additional information can be forwarded to process the claim.

If there are any remaining balances after posting of the payment, the insurance billing specialist must determine the appropriate course of action. If the patient has secondary insurance, the secondary insurance should be billed at this time. If there is a remaining balance and the patient has no secondary insurance, the patient should be billed for the balance. It is during the posting process that payments are evaluated for correctness according to the insurance company contracted requirements. Refer to Chapter 4 and see Fig. 4.14, which illustrates a patient's financial accounting record that shows posting of professional service descriptions, fees, payments, adjustments, and running balance due.

If services are reimbursed but the EOB is difficult to understand, a phone call to the payer usually clarifies and resolves the problem so that posting can be completed. Most private insurance companies offer secure internet portal access that provides quick reference to the patient's EOB, contracted fee schedule, pending claims, and denied claims.

Claims paid with no errors are designated closed. The best method to store EOBs that have been posted is to create a scanned e-file cabinet in which the patient account in the software system contains a link to the EOB.

Secondary Insurance

In some cases, patients carry secondary insurance to cover the coinsurance for which the patient is responsible. There are some guidelines to billing secondary insurance:

1. The secondary insurance cannot be billed until the primary insurance has paid.

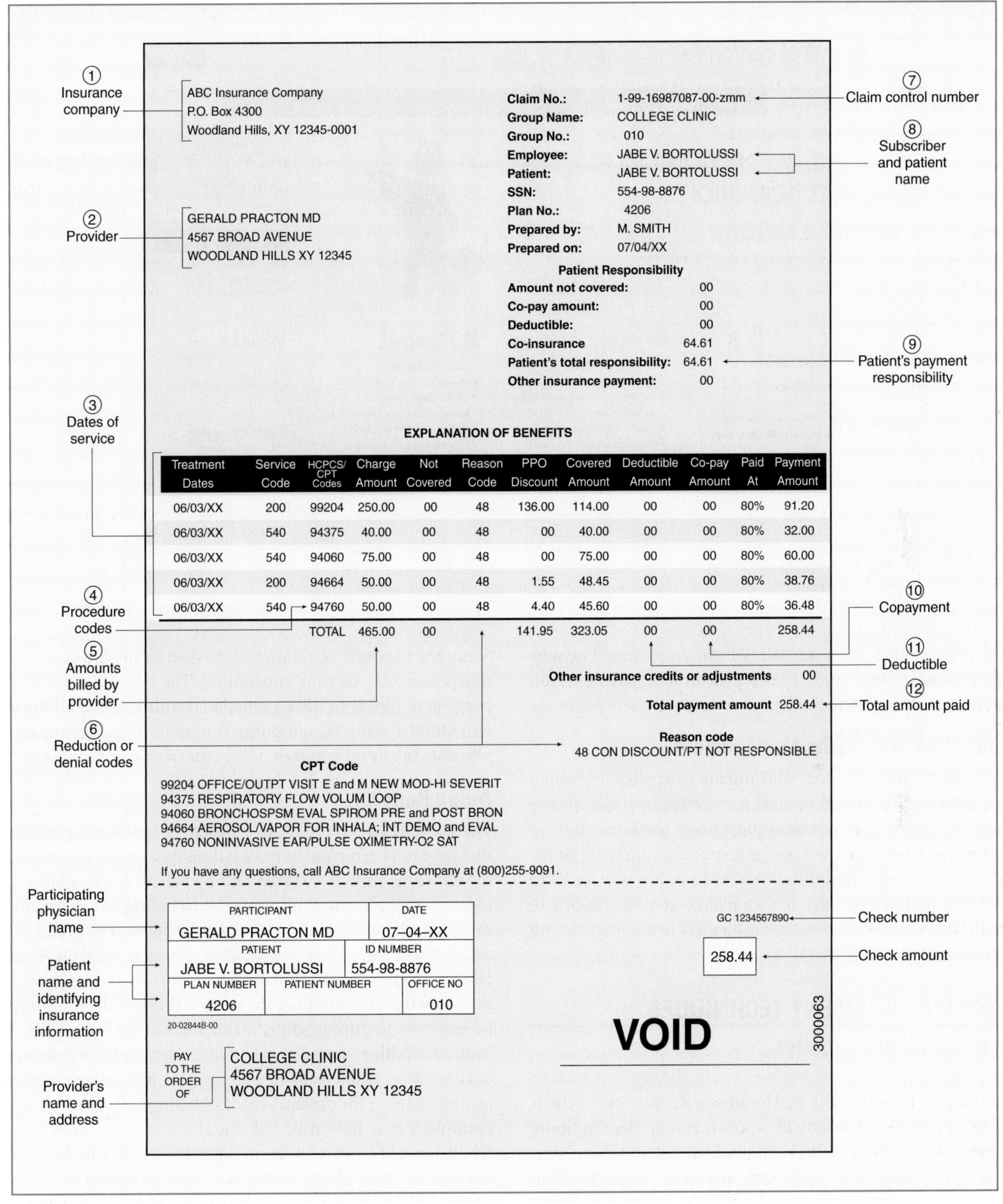

ABC Insurance Company
P.O. Box 4300
Woodland Hills, XY 12345-0001

GERALD PRACTON MD
4567 BROAD AVENUE
WOODLAND HILLS XY 12345

Claim No.: 1-99-16987087-00-zmm
Group Name: COLLEGE CLINIC
Group No.: 010
Employee: JABE V. BORTOLUSSI
Patient: JABE V. BORTOLUSSI
SSN: 554-98-8876
Plan No.: 4206
Prepared by: M. SMITH
Prepared on: 07/04/XX

Patient Responsibility

Amount not covered: 00
Co-pay amount: 00
Deductible: 00
Co-insurance 64.61
Patient's total responsibility: 64.61
Other insurance payment: 00

EXPLANATION OF BENEFITS

Treatment Dates	Service Code	HCPCS/CPT Codes	Charge Amount	Not Covered	Reason Code	PPO Discount	Covered Amount	Deductible Amount	Co-pay Amount	Paid At	Payment Amount
06/03/XX	200	99204	250.00	00	48	136.00	114.00	00	00	80%	91.20
06/03/XX	540	94375	40.00	00	48	00	40.00	00	00	80%	32.00
06/03/XX	540	94060	75.00	00	48	00	75.00	00	00	80%	60.00
06/03/XX	200	94664	50.00	00	48	1.55	48.45	00	00	80%	38.76
06/03/XX	540	94760	50.00	00	48	4.40	45.60	00	00	80%	36.48
		TOTAL	465.00	00		141.95	323.05	00	00		258.44

Other insurance credits or adjustments 00

Total payment amount 258.44

Reason code
48 CON DISCOUNT/PT NOT RESPONSIBLE

CPT Code
99204 OFFICE/OUTPT VISIT E and M NEW MOD-HI SEVERIT
94375 RESPIRATORY FLOW VOLUM LOOP
94060 BRONCHOSPSM EVAL SPIROM PRE and POST BRON
94664 AEROSOL/VAPOR FOR INHALA; INT DEMO and EVAL
94760 NONINVASIVE EAR/PULSE OXIMETRY-O2 SAT

If you have any questions, call ABC Insurance Company at (800)255-9091.

PARTICIPANT		DATE
GERALD PRACTON MD		07–04–XX
PATIENT		ID NUMBER
JABE V. BORTOLUSSI		554-98-8876
PLAN NUMBER	PATIENT NUMBER	OFFICE NO
4206		010

20-02844B-00

GC 1234567890

258.44

VOID

3000063

PAY TO THE ORDER OF
COLLEGE CLINIC
4567 BROAD AVENUE
WOODLAND HILLS XY 12345

Fig. 16.1 An example of an explanation of benefits (RA) document with accompanying check that the provider received from a private third-party payer. These payment voucher documents vary among insurance companies.

2. Blocks 9a–d of the CMS-1500 form should include information about the primary insurance that paid the first part of the claim.
3. Block 30 of the CMS-1500 form should reflect the balance after the claim was paid and the amount exceeding the allowable is written off.
4. Depending on the Medicare Administrative Contractor, Medicare will automatically forward the claim it paid on to the secondary insurance. If the claim was forwarded to the secondary insurance, the EOB will state to which insurance company the EOB was forwarded. When this happens, there is no need to bill secondary insurance.

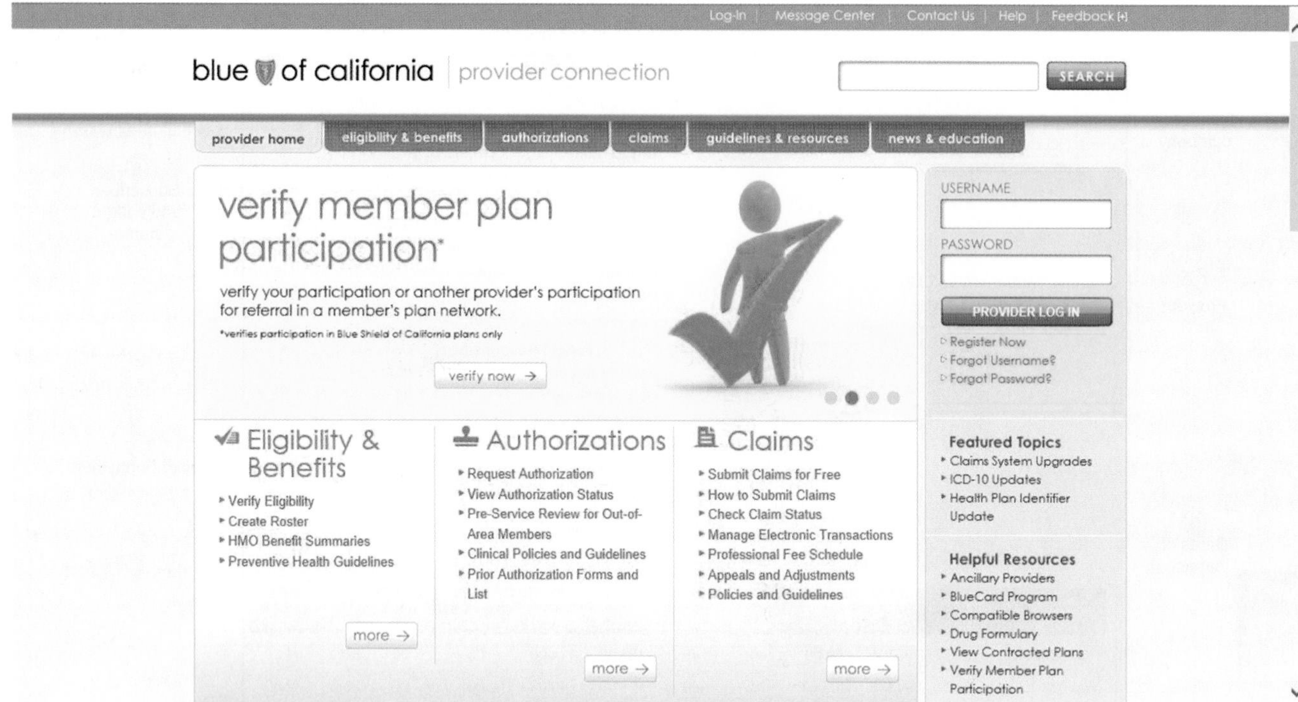

Fig. 16.2 Online health insurance provider portals provide quick and easy access to patient eligibility, authorization for services, insurance claim status, and remittance advice documents.

5. Reimbursements from secondary insurances should be designated separately from primary insurance payments on patient account statements.

Explanation of Benefits Management

After posting payments and adjustments to applicable patient accounts, the EOB should be filed in a designated area clearly marked in a folder. Some offices may group these remittances by payer, by month received, or by some other method. Some health care organizations billing systems allow for EOB forms to be scanned into the software and some do automatic posting of payment by downloading electronic files that work in sync with the format of the remittances.

CLAIM MANAGEMENT TECHNIQUES

Insurance Claims Register

Because most claims are submitted electronically, it is vital to check Batch Claim Reports and Scrubber Reports on a scheduled basis. An acknowledgment report from the clearinghouse will list each insurance claim submitted per patient; this report should be followed up on each week to ensure that every claim is processed to prevent **delinquent claims**, or claims that are not paid within 30 to 45 days of the service date. Once the insurance company confirms receipt of the claim, insurance billing specialists can view and confirm patient claim status using secure internet portals (Fig. 16.2).

Purging Paid Files

When claims are paid off and have a zero balance, they are purged, or removed in bulk, from the insurance claim file. Some medical offices remove files when EOBs are posted, but this process can be time consuming. The most effective way to purge paid files is to have a scheduled time that the billing system automatically runs a purge program. Many organizations schedule the purge program to be run weekly or monthly.

Aging Reports

The account **aging report** is a listing of outstanding accounts that have not been paid. In most billing systems the report can be separated by insurance carrier and by patient responsibility. The report lists the amount of money outstanding and is organized by the amount of time the money has been owed (Fig. 16.3). The aging report categorizes outstanding claims as current, 30 days, 60 days, 90 days, and 120 days. The report should be generated each month. After running the report, proper follow-up should be made by inquiring why a claim has not yet been paid. The insurance billing specialist can write notes on the aging report documenting phone calls to the payer or adjustments made or include notes in the patient's medical billing software profile. For example, a note indicating that the claim is to be corrected and rebilled would be helpful; many software systems allow the user to create alerts for when the status of the claim should be reviewed again. The key to getting the most reimbursements is prompt action with clear and regular documentation of the action taken.

Because time is of the essence, it is wise to be aggressive on claims that are outstanding for more than 30 to 45 days, especially when there are issues concerning timely filing.

Using the health care organization's medical billing software, monthly reports can be generated and are useful when tracking the payment history of insurance companies. This is an easy method to discover which companies pay slowly or pay

AETNA									
				Aging Analysis					
Patient Name	Acct #	Primary Insurance	Secondary Insurance	0-30	31-60	61-90	91-120	over 120	Total Balance
Bassett, Eleanor	75846	AETNA		$145.00	$0.00	$0.00	$0.00	$0.00	$145.00
Herron, John	83029	AETNA		$0.00	$42.41	$0.00	$0.00	$0.00	$42.41
Holt, Maxine	64739	AETNA	BLUE SHIELD	$145.00	$0.00	$0.00	$0.00	$0.00	$145.00
Kellog, Keenan	24537	AETNA		$0.00	$0.00	$145.00	$0.00	$0.00	$145.00
Lincoln, Frank	85940	AETNA		$0.00	$15.00	$0.00	$0.00	$0.00	$15.00
Markham, Melanie	14263	AETNA	MEDICARE	$0.00	$0.00	$0.00	$260.00	$0.00	$260.00
McDonald, Lydia	56374	AETNA		$260.00	$0.00	$0.00	$0.00	$0.00	$260.00
McLean, Mary	24395	AETNA		$0.00	$0.00	$0.00	$0.00	$260.00	$260.00
Aetna Aging Total :				**$550.00**	**$57.41**	**$145.00**	**$260.00**	**$260.00**	**$1,272.41**

Fig. 16.3 The aging report shows patient account balances according to the number of days after the date of service.

less on certain services. Billing and accounts receivable reports are helpful to understand trends in the financial operations of the health care office and to prepare for negotiations of future insurance contracts.

An insurance company payment history system can help to avoid potential problems and pinpoint requirements that must be met to secure additional payment on a reduced or denied claim.

CLAIM INQUIRIES

When reviewing an aging report, unpaid claims that are more than 30 to 45 days old require that an **inquiry** on claim status be made to the health insurance company. These claims could be delayed because they may not have been received by the insurance company or for other reasons relating to the member's health plan. Different types of claim inquiries can focus on denial codes on the EOB or can be related to patient coinsurance or deductible responsibilities. To reduce the number of phone calls to the insurance companies, many private insurance organizations have set up online web portals that allow insurance billing specialists to review patient claim status and benefit information. If more information about the claim is needed beyond the scope of the online portal, insurance benefit specialists can be reached by calling the member services number on the back of the patient's ID card. The following are reasons for making inquiries:

- There was no response to a submitted claim within 30 to 45 days.
- Payment was not received within the time limit for the plan or program.
- Payment was received but the amount is incorrect.
- Payment was received but the amount allowed and the patient's responsibility was not defined.
- A duplicate payment or overpayment was made.
- Payment received was for a patient not seen by the provider. It is possible to receive a payment check made out to a payee's name that is different from the patient's name. Making a call may quickly clarify for whom the payment is being made.

In addition to nonpayment or reduced payment, there are other reasons for inquiries to an insurance company, including the following:

- EOB shows that a professional or diagnostic code was changed from what was submitted.
- EOB shows that the service was disallowed when it was a benefit.
- EOB shows that additional information was needed and it was sent in a timely manner but payment has not been sent.
- The claim should be revised and resubmitted. Check to see whether the procedure codes were correct and that the services listed were described fully enough to justify the maximum allowable benefits.
- There is an error on the EOB.
- The check received was issued to the wrong health care provider.

Inquire about the claim if any of these situations occurs. Although there are many online web portals for private insurance claims inquiry, sometimes government health plans do not offer the same online tools. For this reason, government health plans have their own inquiry or **tracer** forms available online that needs to be submitted in writing along with a copy of the claim. If a claim must be reviewed after payment has been rendered, send the letter as shown in Fig. 16.4. Remember that effective follow-up centers around effective documentation, so document the name of the person spoken to, the date and time of call, the department or extension of the person, and an outline of the conversation, and save these notes in the patient account.

PROBLEM CLAIMS

Problems in claims filing will delay the reimbursement process. Determining the most appropriate amount of time to follow up on a claim after it has been submitted will vary from insurance carrier to insurance carrier. Many types of problem claims (for example, delinquent, in **suspense** [pending], lost, rejected, denied, downcoded, partial payment, payment lost in the mail, payment made to patient, and overpayment) exist. Table 16.1 contains a complete list of the types of problems and their descriptions.

To keep accounting accurate and up to date, these problems require some type of follow-up action. The claim status may be indicated on an EOB; however, sometimes a claim is submitted and no status is reported. As mentioned, visiting the insurance carrier's online web portal is the most efficient way to view claim status. If the insurance carrier does not have a web portal, calling to confirm claim status is the most efficient step.

COLLEGE CLINIC
4567 Broad Avenue
Woodland Hills, XY
12345-0001
Telephone 555/486-9002
Fax (555) 487-8976

Committee on Physician's Services

Re: Underpayment
Identification No.: M18876782
Patient: Peaches Melba
Type of Service: Plastic & Reconstructive Surgery
Date of Service: 1 - 3 - XX
Amount Paid: $ 75.00
My Fees: $ 180.00

Dear Sirs:

Herewith a request for a committee review of the above-named case, since I consider the allowance paid very low having in mind the location, the extent, the type, and the necessary surgical procedure performed: The skin graft, one inch in diameter, included the lateral third of eyebrow and was full thickness to preserve hair follicles.

Operative report for the surgery has been sent to you with the claim.

Considering these points I hope that you will authorize additional payment in order to bring the total fee to within reasonable and customary charges.

Sincerely,

Cosmo Graff, M.D.

Cosmo Graff, M.D.

mf
enclosure

Fig. 16.4 A letter signed by the physician appealing a fee reduction. This letter lists information specific to the patient claim in question and is sent to the third-party payer after payment has been received and the physician feels that the reimbursement should be higher.

The individual working at the front desk must collect insurance information accurately and update patient demographic information (for example, insurance identification number and address) at every office visit or medical encounter. The person posting to accounts must be certain to post to the correct patient account and ensure that secondary insurances are billed after the primary insurance company has paid. Identified errors should be brought to the attention of the responsible individuals to improve the accuracy of outgoing claims and to avoid future problems.

There is a significant difference in the way problem claims are handled when filed by paper or filed electronically. Because most health insurance claims should be submitted electronically, the problems and solutions listed will focus mainly on electronic submission.

Types of Problems

The following are specific claim problems and practical solutions.

Delinquent, Pending, or Suspense

PROBLEM: Delinquent claims are typically beyond 30 to 45 days overdue on the aging report. The nonpayer can be an insurance company, managed care plan, or intermediary for the Medicaid, Medicare, or TRICARE programs. Sometimes nonpayment is caused by a claim in review or in suspense because of an error or the need for additional information. The carrier may be investigating a claim because of preexisting conditions or possibly because the patient may have a work-related injury. If a service is not covered, sometimes there is no response; however, a follow-up should be initiated to further investigate.

SOLUTION: Use claim management techniques to keep on top of delinquent claims so that follow-up can be accomplished in a timely manner. If the office handles a large volume of claims, divide the unpaid claims into four groups, one for each of the three largest insurers and the fourth for all others. Work on one group each week so that the work is spread out over the 4 weeks in each month. Routinely visit the online web portals to check for claims status and look for evidence of the claim being submitted while reconciling the electronic data interchange (EDI) clearinghouse acknowledgement report for up-to-date information. If the claim was submitted and confirmed received, it is wise to look at how the claim was billed (for example, accurate coding). If this information is correct and the dates on the claim

TABLE 16.1 Insurance Claim Processing Problems

Type	Description
Delinquent claims	• Payment overdue from nonpayer
Denied claims	• Lack of insurance coverage (canceled, service provided before effective insurance, or lapsed beyond renewal date) • Selected diagnoses not covered • Frequency limitations or restrictions per benefit period • Procedure performed by ineligible specialty provider (e.g., podiatrist would not be paid for neurosurgery) • Bundled with other services • Payable only in certain locations (e.g., outpatient only) • Prior approval needed and not obtained • Service or procedure not justified by diagnosis • Missing or incorrect POS code • Missing physician signature • Missing necessary and/or requested medical documentation • Insurance policy issue (preexisting condition or preauthorization required under plan) • Experimental procedure not reimbursable • Incorrect code for service rendered • Code selected from incorrect system (CPT code instead of HCPCS Level II national code) • Unbundled codes when one code should have been submitted • Unspecified diagnostic code reported
Downcoded claims	• Computer software selects procedure code at lower level than medical service requires
Lost claims	• Claim not received by third-party payer
Overpayment	• Third-party payer pays more than the bill or the allowed amount • Third-party payer pays more than one's fee or contract rate • Third-party payer sends provider payment intended for patient • Provider receives duplicate payments from two or more insurance companies or from the patient and one or more third-party payers • Provider receives payment for someone who is not the provider's patient
Payment errors	• Third-party payer sends provider payment intended for patient • Patient paid by third-party payer when provider should have been paid
Pending (suspense) claims	• Claim has an error • Additional information required • Claim review needed by third-party payer (complex procedure, high reimbursement, utilization management)
Rejected (soft denial) claims	• Claim contains technical error (missing or incorrect information, numbers transposed, invalid diagnostic or procedural code numbers, duplicate charges, duplicate dates of service, etc.) • Third-party payer instructions not followed
Underpayment	• Third-party payment at less than negotiated contract rate

CPT, Current Procedural Terminology; HCPCS, Healthcare Common Procedure Coding System; *POS,* place of service.

are correct, contact the payer to find out what information is holding up the claim or why the claim was denied. If the claim was not successful in being received by the clearinghouse and there is no apparent reason on reports or on investigating the claim data showing exactly what information was amiss, then perhaps there was a problem with the format. To have more insight as to why the claim was not successfully received or was rejected, contact the clearinghouse. The insurance billing specialist can contact the payer immediately after finding out that the claim is delinquent, or the payer can be contacted after initial steps of investigation take place, such as in-house editing and contacting the clearinghouse.

Lost Claims

PROBLEM: Lost claims are insurance claims that cannot be located after sending to an insurance carrier. Lost claims are more common with paper claim submission; sometimes managing large volumes of claims leads to some getting lost from time to time. Paper claims can get lost in the mail, be sent to the incorrect address, or be mismanaged through the health insurance mail management system. It is important to track all claims, as some insurance contracts may have deadlines to file claims 30 days after the date of service.

SOLUTION: The insurance company should be contacted if there has been no response to a claim that has aged 30 to 45 days. The first step is to check the claim status with the private insurance company online through the online provider web portal or to call the local government agency office. If there is no record of the claim, all lost claims should be resubmitted. If a claim is determined to be lost, submit a copy of the original claim referencing it as "copy of the original claim submitted on (date)"; on rare occasions, insurance companies may accept the resubmission of a claim in the form of a fax if the fax references the original submission date. Before sending it, verify the correct mailing address (for example, post office box number and zip code).

Ask if there is a backlog of claims to resolve the situation. This indicates that the claim probably has not been logged into the system. Always verify that the patient is insured by the insurance company and is covered for the basic benefits claimed.

Always retain the electronic response or confirmation from the carrier saying that it received the specific claim. Keep all clearinghouse reports that confirm received transmissions and relay information regarding claim status. Medical billing software programs display the date of every claim submitted. Tamper-proof data recorded by the computer may be used as a legal form of proof that the claim was submitted to the third-party payer. Unfortunately, this does not "prove" that the payer received the claim, so some payers do not always accept this. Send a printed copy of the electronic proof of timely filing to the third-party payer, along with a copy of the claim and a copy of the denial you may have received for exceeding the timely filing limit.

Rejected Claims

A rejected claim is a submitted claim that does not follow specific third-party payer instructions or contains a technical error.

Such claims may be disapproved or discarded by the system and returned to the biller. Technical errors consist of missing or incorrect information and are found through computer edits, screening processes for benefit provisions, and proofreading. Common reasons why health insurance claims are rejected can be found in Box 16.1.

PROBLEM: Paper or electronic claim rejections may occur as a result of one or more of the following:

- Transposed numbers
- Missing required Health Insurance Portability and Accountability Act (HIPAA) transaction code sets
- Missing subscriber date of birth
- Missing, invalid, or incorrect procedure codes and modifiers
- Missing or invalid place of service (POS)
- Mismatch of POS to type of service
- Missing referring physician when billing tests
- Missing or invalid provider number when the patient was referred
- Incorrect, invalid, nonspecific, or missing diagnostic code numbers
- Incorrect dates of service
- Incorrect year of service
- Incorrect number of days in the month (for example, February)
- Code description that does not match services rendered
- Duplicate dates of service
- Duplicate charges

SOLUTION: It is likely that an electronic claim will not make it into a batch to be transmitted to the payer if a series of computer edits have been performed before batching (that is, grouping claims together). The system will flag this particular claim as needing edits and will not batch it with the rest. If the claim does go through to the payer and is reported as being rejected, review the rejection reason code and correct the field. Then resubmit the claim. Never send a corrected claim for review or appeal because this type of claim should always be resubmitted.

BOX 16.1 Common Reasons Why Health Insurance Claims Are Rejected

Code description does not match services rendered
Duplicate charges
Duplicate dates of service
Incorrect dates of service
Incorrect electronic submission code
Incorrect number of days in the month (e.g., February)
Incorrect year of service
Incorrect, invalid, nonspecific, or missing diagnostic code numbers
Mismatch of POS to type of service
Missing NPI number for the provider and/or facility
Missing or invalid POS
Missing or invalid provider number when the patient was referred
Missing referring physician when billing tests
Missing required HIPAA transaction code sets
Missing subscriber date of birth
Missing, invalid, or incorrect procedure codes and modifiers
Missing physician signature
Transposed numbers

HIPAA, Health Insurance Portability and Accountability Act; *NPI,* National Provider Identifier; *POS,* place of service.

PROBLEM: A claim is submitted for several services. One line item is rejected for incomplete information, but the other services are paid.

SOLUTION: Generate a new claim for the rejected services online and note in Block 19 of the CMS-1500 claim form that it is a resubmission.

PROBLEM: A third-party payer requests further information or information about another insurance carrier.

SOLUTION: A common mistake during the patient registration process is not obtaining the insurance subscriber's name, employer, and date of birth. It is important to verify insurance information with the patient (including confirmation of the patient's primary, and possibly secondary, insurance information), obtain a signed patient release of information form that follows HIPAA guidelines, and call or mail the information to the insurance company. Identify the subscriber, subscriber ID number, and date of service on all correspondence.

PROBLEM: A resubmitted claim is returned a second time.

PAPER CLAIM SOLUTION: Review the EOB statement to determine whether there is a denial code or narrative explanation. Examine the claim for missing, incomplete, or incorrect information, and if found, correct it. Evaluate the claim to determine whether it is a candidate for the appeal process. Determine whether a specific appeal form must be submitted. Submit chart notes, a detailed summary, or a copy of the operative or pathology report, as applicable, to clearly identify the procedure or service. Enclose a cover letter with the resubmitted data. The letter must specifically state what course of action is being requested (that is, review) and it must have the name and signature of the person requesting the review.

A common claim denial reason is lack of medical necessity. *Medical necessity* refers to health care services that a health care provider, exercising his or her best clinical judgment, would provide to a patient for evaluating, diagnosing or treating an illness, injury, disease or its symptoms. Services are considered medically necessary if they are:

- in accordance with the generally accepted standards of medical practice;
- clinically appropriate, in terms of type, frequency, extent, site and duration, and considered effective for the patient's illness, injury or disease;
- not primarily for the convenience of the patient or health care provider; and
- not costlier than an alternative service or sequence of services at least as likely to produce equivalent therapeutic or diagnostic results as to the diagnosis or treatment of that patient's illness, injury or disease.

Claims that do not support medical necessity guidelines are denied. These types of denials are sometimes caused by diagnosis and procedure code not matching. An example of this would be a denial for hammertoe surgery with a broken wrist diagnosis. Because these denials can be related to lack of supporting documentation or errors in coding, they should be returned to the original coder to be corrected and resubmitted.

Denied Claims

Claims are often denied because they do not meet the criteria in a coverage policy. For example, a patient may have acupuncture services; however, those services are listed as a noncovered service in the patient's insurance contract.

When a claim is denied, and the responsible party is indicated on the EOB to be the patient, transfer the entire balance to the patient's account. State laws require insurance companies to notify the insured of a denial and state why the claim was denied. However, if the insurance company has not contacted the patient, notify the patient by phone or mail as soon as possible to keep him or her informed. Always retain the correspondence from the insurance company so that it can be retrieved quickly in case a patient inquires and has additional questions.

When a claim is denied, simply changing information on the claim and resubmitting it will not resolve the problem. If it is determined that the claim was denied incorrectly, and the service meets the benefits requirements, the recourse is to challenge the insurance carrier's decision and file an appeal.

It stands to reason that insurance companies save money when a claim is denied, and only a small percentage of individuals pursue appeals. The appeals process for denied claims varies among third-party payers.

Common reasons why insurance claims are not paid because of denial include the following:

- Selected diagnoses not covered
- Frequency limitations or restrictions per benefit period
- Procedure performed by ineligible specialty provider (for example, a podiatrist would not be paid for neurosurgery)
- Bundled with other services
- Payable only in certain locations (for example, outpatient only)
- Prior approval needed and not obtained
- Service or procedure not justified by diagnosis
- Missing or incorrect POS code

Additional examples with suggested solutions are as follows:

PROBLEM: The medical service provided was not covered for the patient (for example, routine physical examination, routine tests, routine foot care, routine dental care, cosmetic surgery, custodial care, eye or hearing examinations for glasses or hearing aids, and some immunizations). Plastic surgery and maternity care can be considered a general exclusion in many insurance policies.

SOLUTION: Send the patient a statement with a notation of the response from the insurance company. Before providing services, always verify coverage for routine physical examinations or tests and services by calling or checking the online provider web portal regarding whether the health insurance will accept financial responsibility. Discuss this with the patient before service is provided and advise of the likelihood of the claim being denied; in these instances, it may be appropriate to request payment at the time of service.

PROBLEM: Insurance coverage is canceled or temporarily lapsed before the date of service.

SOLUTION: It is a good practice to verify insurance coverage for each patient before his or her appointment for services by visiting the online web portal or by calling to verify coverage. If the claim is then denied after services were rendered, send the patient a statement with notation of the insurance determination on the bill.

PROBLEM: The health insurance company indicates that the provided service was not medically necessary. "Medical necessity" has become the encompassing denial reason that indicates that the insurance company does not agree with the services provided to the patient because they were not necessary. This makes clearing the medical necessity denial reason most challenging to overturn. The following are a few reasons why insurance companies deny medical necessity:

- The diagnosis code and the procedure code do not match
- The procedure code and the place or type of service do not match
- The procedure is performed by a physician of a different specialty
- The frequency of the same procedure rendered is more than authorized
- The procedure is experimental and has not yet been approved for reimbursement by the insurance company
- Supporting documentation is unclear or limited

SOLUTION: Determine under what circumstances the third-party payer considers the service to be medically necessary. It is vital that the service provider's documentation be specific enough to support the necessity of the services provided. If the service provider believes that the patient's condition supported the medical necessity for the service, send an appeal for review to the insurance company, explaining in detail the reasons why the service was necessary. Keep a list of codes that have been denied for medical necessity and what further determinations were made in the insurance company payment history. Check the insurance contract to determine whether the patient may be billed. Consider asking patients to sign an Advance Beneficiary Notice or Waiver of Liability form before treatment. Do not have every patient sign such documents because then these documents would be considered a blanket waiver if the claim is denied.

PROBLEM: Service was for an injury that is approved and covered under workers' compensation.

SOLUTION: Create a workers' compensation information sheet asking the employee and employer to fill out separate sections with space for the following: explanation of the injury, insurance information, claim adjuster's name and telephone number, and claim or case number. Because most workers' compensation insurance companies typically accept paper claims, all correspondence should be made directly with the claims adjuster via phone or mail. Locate the carrier for the industrial injury, request permission to treat, and send the carrier a report of the case with a bill. Notify the patient's health insurance carrier monthly about the status of the case.

PROBLEM: A service was not preauthorized for a surgery, hospitalization, or diagnostic procedure.

SOLUTION: Contact the insurance company or check the online web portal to determine whether preauthorization was necessary for the service or if any sanctions were imposed. The office may want to institute a standard procedure that all surgical procedures and durable medical equipment and supplies be confirmed with insurance companies before rendering services. Document the contact name, date, and time of the call, or if using the online provider portal, print out the preauthorization information for the patient's chart. If there were problems or difficulties with the case leading to the reason that precertification was not obtained, write a letter of appeal noting the history. Insurance payers can change their policies on certain procedure codes throughout the year.

PROBLEM: The deductible was not met.

SOLUTION: Before rendering services to the patient, confirm with the insurance company the patient's current deductible and the amount for which the patient will be financially responsible for medical services. Inform the patient at the prescreening appointment that the deductible must be collected at that appointment or the procedure should be rescheduled.

PROBLEM: Elective surgery or procedures were billed that are not typically covered by health insurance.

SOLUTION: Inform the patient before scheduling the appointment that he or she is responsible to pay for services upfront, before the procedure.

PROBLEM: The claim is incomplete and denied because essential elements are missing and/or inaccurate.

SOLUTION: Prevention measures to avoid denied claims are as follows:

1. Be proactive and verify insurance coverage before the first visit; this saves time and prevents surprises for everyone. Ensure that the demographic information is current at each visit.
2. Include progress notes and orders for tests for extended hospital services.
3. Submit a letter from the prescribing physician documenting necessity when ambulance transportation is used.
4. Clarify the type of service (for example, primary surgical services versus assist-at-surgery services).
5. Use modifiers to further describe and identify the exact service rendered.
6. Keep abreast of the latest policies for all contracted payers as well as for the federal programs by going to the Centers for Medicare and Medicaid Services (CMS) website to read currently posted Medicare Transmittals. For example, know the Medicare local coverage determinations (LCDs) and national coverage determinations (NCDs) that state which conditions and services are covered and the limitations on coverage. Read news releases from the Blue Plans, Medicaid, TRICARE, workers' compensation insurance companies, and managed care plans.
7. Obtain current provider manuals for all contracted payers as well as the Blue Plans, Medicaid, Medicare, and TRICARE for quick reference. When bulletins or pages are received from these programs during the year, keep the manuals up to date by inserting the current material.
8. Become familiar with the modifier descriptions and their appropriate use and verify that the payer recognizes them.

Downcoding

PROBLEM: The insurance carrier has downcoded the claim, thereby reducing reimbursement. The procedure or diagnosis code submitted on the claim was general and unspecified.

SOLUTION: Be sure to read through all procedure notes and provider orders to determine the most specific diagnosis code related to the patient's condition. If the patient experiences complications, these should be added to the code. If the service provider's notes are not specific enough to determine a more specific diagnosis, emphasize to the provider the importance of specificity, especially regarding diagnosis.

Payment Made to Patient

PROBLEM: An insurance payment sent to the patient instead of the provider can occur for two reasons: Either the provider is considered out of network from the patient's health plan or the assignment of benefits was not signed by the patient.

SOLUTION: Call the insurance company or visit the online web portal to verify whether the payment was made, to whom, for which dates of service, the amount, the check number, and the date of issue. If the provider has a participating agreement, the insurance company is obligated to pay the provider and must proceed by correcting the error. The following are two different courses of action to take after this has been verified:

1. Call the patient, explain that the insurance company sent payment to the patient in error, and ask when full payment can be expected. Document the commitment in the patient's financial record. If the patient cannot be reached by telephone, send a letter by certified mail to the patient. Document each effort that was made toward collection of the payment from the patient and the patient's responses.
2. Send a letter to the insurance company, including a copy of the claim with EOB indicating that payment was made to the patient and a copy of the assignment of benefits. Demand payment from the insurance company, stating the need to honor the assignment and the signed participation agreement. The insurance company must recover the payment from the patient. If the insurance company admits that there is an assignment of benefits and that it inadvertently paid the patient, the insurance company must pay the service provider within 2 to 3 weeks and honor the assignment even before it recovers its money from the patient. The insurance company then files for payment from the patient.

Underpayment

It is important that the insurance billing specialist perform random checks and monitor large claim payments made during the first 3 months of a new contract to ensure that the third-party payer's system has the contracted payment fee schedule correctly loaded into the software. Track the charge, allowable, deductible, and paid amount to determine whether the amounts are correct (Fig. 16.5).

PROBLEM: Claims are underpaid.

SOLUTION: Print the incorrectly paid claims and send them by mail to the third-party payer's contract negotiator to be resolved. Ask them to re-adjudicate the claims based on the agreed-upon contracted amount; include a letter with the claims clearly stating that they are not duplicate claims but do need to be reviewed for appropriate payment. Use codes or notations on the claims to indicate that they are updated.

Method for Calculating Over- and Underpayments

Third-party payer: ______________

Patient name	Procedure/ service	Claims paid date	Provider charge	Allowed amount	Amount paid	Overpayment (+) Underpayment (−)
May Ito	Colonoscopy	5/2/20XX	$1500	$900	$2000	$1100+

Fig. 16.5 Audit method used for calculating overpayments and underpayments. Subtract the allowed amount, which is the insurance contract's fee schedule amount minus any patient copayment or deductible from the amount paid. Any positive (+) number is an overpayment and any negative (−) number is an underpayment.

Overpayment

An overpayment is a sum of money paid by the insurance company or patient to the provider of service that is more than the account balance or more than the allowed amount. Overpayments can happen for a variety of reasons, and handling them can be challenging. Overpayments can happen for any one of the following reasons:

- A payment was made twice for the same date of service. This usually happens when a claim is rebilled before receiving confirmation of the health insurance receipt.
- A payment was made that was greater than the contracted allowable amount.
- A payment was made for a patient and date of service that do not exist.
- A payment was made for a service that was not performed for the specific patient.

The insurance payment poster usually discovers overpayments when payments are posted in patient accounts. The Office of the Inspector General (OIG) strongly advises providers to return overpayments promptly. Not doing so can lead to severe fines and implicate fraudulent activity.

Some states have laws or court decisions restricting insurance carriers from recovering payments made in error from health care providers. It is essential to research the law pertaining to the handling of overpayments in the state that the health care organization is located. First, determine whether an overpayment exists by reviewing the available financial documents on the case in question. Second, decide how to handle the overpayment. Be sure to get advice from the health care organization's attorney on the extent to which the demand for repayment can be challenged based on state law or court decisions.

It is wise to develop an overpayment policy and a procedure for each type of insurer, program, or managed care plan and for every type of overpayment situation that may occur.

PROBLEM: Overpayment scenarios that may occur are:

- Receiving more than one's fee from a third-party payer
- Receiving more than the contract rate from a managed care plan
- Receiving payments that should have been paid to the patient
- Receiving duplicate payments from two or more insurance companies or from the patient and one or more third-party payers
- Receiving payment made for someone who is not the provider's patient

SOLUTION: When an overpayment occurs, post the activity to the appropriate patient account with an additional notation that it was received in error and a refund was made. Creating an account specifically for overpayments is advisable to track all funds in this category. In any type of overpayment situation, cash the third-party payer's check and make out a refund check payable to the originator of the overpayment. Keep a copy of the third-party payer's check before it is deposited. The refund check should always be sent to the attention of a specific person at the insurance company. In case of an audit, this establishes documentation showing that the problem has been resolved. Usually insurance companies process a credit of the overpayment amount to the next check voucher.

Refund checks should be given top priority and written as soon as reasonably possible. Ensure that the office policy is clearly stated and adhered to in all cases. If the patient pays and a third-party pays and the overpayment must be refunded to the patient, always write a check—never refund in cash. Send the patient a letter with a check to explain the overpayment. If the patient pays by credit card, wait until the charges have cleared to draft a check or preferably process a credit card refund to the credit card company.

If the patient cannot be located to return the money, send a check by registered mail to the patient's last known address. When it comes back marked "undeliverable," retain the document as legal proof that an honest effort was made to return the overpayment. The money should be listed as taxable income and put in the bank.

REBILLING

If a claim has not been paid within a reasonable amount of time, do not automatically rebill (resubmit) the third-party payer without researching the reason why it is still outstanding. Simply rebilling claims can be considered duplicate claims and the insurance company may audit the health care organization for trying to collect duplicate payment. Instead, follow up on the claim as indicated in the previous section. If it is discovered that an error has been made in completing the insurance claim form, make the changes and resubmit the form, indicating that the new claim is corrected.

Patient accounts with a balance should be billed monthly, even when an insurance payment is expected, so that patients understand what has been submitted and what is pending.

The statement should clearly identify the claim that has been submitted and what action is expected from the patient. If collection becomes a problem, action can be referenced to the date of service if the patient has been billed consistently.

In December 2004, the CMS implemented a process that allows providers to resubmit corrected Medicare claims that have been rejected for minor errors or omissions rather than appealing those claims. For example, claims with missing or incorrect provider numbers, claims with incorrect modifiers, or claims with keying errors (incorrect date or POS) can be rebilled. These claims can be corrected through the clearinghouse and resubmitted electronically. Other insurance carriers may have similar resubmission processes.

REVIEW AND APPEAL PROCESS

An appeal is a request for review and reconsideration of a claim that has been underpaid, incorrectly paid, or denied by an insurance company. Some insurance carriers may refer to appeals as redeterminations. Before starting the appeals process, examine the insurance carrier's policy to determine whether there is a time limit for making an appeal. Most carriers have rather stringent time limits for filing an appeal after the original claim determination.

The first step in the appeals process is to carefully review the RA sent to the service provider. If the claim was paid, the insurance billing specialist should carefully check the reimbursement amount against the appropriate fee schedule for that insurance carrier. It is important to confirm that the insurance carrier has paid correctly. If payment was not made in accordance with the fee schedule, the reimbursement amount will need to be appealed.

If the claim was denied, the RA should be carefully reviewed to determine the reason the claim was denied. The decision to appeal a claim should be based on several factors. The health care provider should determine that there is sufficient information to back up the claim and the amount of money in question should be sufficient in the provider's opinion. Ultimately, the decision to appeal rests in the provider's hands, not the insurance billing specialist's. An appeal is filed in the following circumstances:

- Payment is denied and the reason for denial is not known.
- Service was denied as a noncovered service.
- Payment is received but the amount is incorrect. Verify that initially the correct amount was billed. Perhaps there was an excessive reduction in the allowed payment.
- The service provider disagrees with the decision by the third-party payer about a preexisting condition.
- Unusual circumstances warranted medical treatments that are not reflected in the payment.
- Precertification was not obtained within contract provisions because of extenuating circumstances and the claim was denied.
- Service was considered inclusive in a more comprehensive service performed on the same date of service.
- Service was considered inclusive in a global surgical period.
- Inadequate payment was received for a complicated procedure.
- "Not medically necessary" is stated as the reason for denial and the service provider disagrees.

FILING AN APPEAL

Appeals can be time consuming and costly. The insurance billing specialist should be well prepared for the appeals process and well-versed in the basic guidelines for filing an appeal.

The process for filing appeals varies from insurance carrier to insurance carrier. Some will require that the appeal be written, whereas others may allow telephone or online appeals. Some insurance carriers will require completion of a specific form of appeals, whereas others will request a written letter of appeals.

Most payers have a specific structure for appeals that move through various stages starting at the lowest level of appeals and moving to the highest level of the appeals process. The first step might simply consist of a simple request for reconsideration, whereas the highest level of appeals may involve a **peer review** or a medical director. A peer review is an evaluation done by a group of unbiased practicing physicians or other health care professionals to judge the effectiveness and efficiency of professional care rendered. This group determines the medical necessity and subsequent payment for the case in question.

When performing a telephone appeal, the insurance billing specialist should follow these basic guidelines:

- Assemble all documents needed (for example, patient's health record, copy of the insurance claim form, and EOB).
- Always remain courteous.
- Obtain the name and extension number of the insurance claims representative or adjuster and keep this with the telephone records. After developing a rapport, you may wish to call on him or her in the future for help. Ask for any toll-free numbers that the company may have and keep these for future reference.
- Listen carefully. Jot down the date and take notes of how to solve the problem. This may be of help if another problem of the same type occurs.

When performing written appeals, always send a copy of the original claim, EOB, and any other documents to justify the appeal. Refer to Procedure 16.1 at the end of this chapter for the procedure to follow when composing a letter of appeal (Fig. 16.6).

It is important to keep track of the status after inquiry or appeal until payment for the case is resolved. Use the insurance claims register or a separate active file labeled "Appeals Pending."

If the appeal is won but copies of the same documents must be submitted each time this issue arises, ask the third-party payer how future claims with the same issue may be handled. Keep track of this information in a file.

If an appeal is denied, the service provider may want to proceed to the next step of the insurance carrier's appeal process.

Medicare Review and Redetermination Process

CMS has its own appeals process. A service provider or beneficiary has the right to appeal a claim after Medicare payment or denial. The Medicare program has five levels of redetermination and special guidelines to follow:

- Level 1: Redetermination Medicare Administrative Contractor (MAC) that processed the original claim.

PHYSICIAN'S LETTERHEAD

January 2, 20XX

Committee on Physician's Services
Medicare
Street address of fiscal intermediary
City, State, ZIP Code

Dear Madam or Sir:

Re: Underpayment

Identification No.:	1910-2192283-101
Patient:	Mrs. Sarah C. Nile
Type of Service:	Exploratory laparotomy
Date of Service:	December 1, 20XX
Amount Paid:	$000.00
My Fees:	$0000.00

Herewith a request for a committee review of the above-named case, since I consider the allowance paid very low having in mind the patient's condition prior to surgery, the location, the extent, the type, and the necessary surgical procedure performed.

Enclosed are photocopies of the history and physical showing the grave status of the patient prior to surgery, operative report, pathology report, and discharge summary. The Medicare Remittance Advice and the Medicare CMS-1500 claim originally submitted are also enclosed.

Considering these points, I hope that you will authorize additional payment in order to bring the total fee to a more reasonable amount.

Sincerely,

Hugh R. Aged, MD
Hugh R. Aged, MD
NPI# 73542109XX

mf

Fig. 16.6 A cover letter signed by the physician appealing a claim.

TABLE 16.2 Medicare Part B Redetermination Process

Level		Time Limit for Request	Amount in Controversy	Jurisdiction	Form
1	Redetermination (telephone, letter, or CMS-20027 form)	120 days from initial claim determination	None	Medicare carrier/MAC	CMS-20027 form CMS-1500 (02-12) corrected claim resubmitted
2	Reconsideration (QIC)	180 days from receipt of MRN	None	Carrier/QIC	CMS-20033
3	ALJ hearing	60 days from receipt of the Hearing Officer's (HO's) determination	$160 or more (2018)	Carrier/Social Security Bureau of Hearings and Appeals	OMHA-101
4	Medicare Appeals Council	60 days from receipt of hearing decision	None	Federal district court	DAB-101
5	US district court	60 days from receipt of the Departmental Appeals Board's (**DAB**'s) decision	At least $1600 (2018) increased annually		

ALJ, Administrative law judge; *CMS,* Centers for Medicare and Medicaid Services; *MAC,* Medicare administrative contractor; *MRN,* Medicare Redetermination Notice; *QIC,* Qualified Independent Contractor.

- Level 2: Reconsideration by a Qualified Independent Contractor
- Level 3: Administrative law judge hearing
- Level 4: Medicare Appeals Council review
- Level 5: Judicial review by a federal district court

Table 16.2 illustrates the Medicare Part B appeals process. Because Medicare guidelines change frequently, refer to their website at www.cms.gov.

Redetermination (Level 1)

Redetermination is the first step to resolve a denied claim. Information about the denied claim is found on the Medicare RA. The insurance billing specialist should fill out a Redetermination Request Form and send it to the MAC. A written request for redetermination must include the following information:

- Beneficiary name
- Medicare Health Insurance Claim (HIC) number
- Specific service and/or item(s) for which a redetermination is being requested
- Specific date(s) of service
- Name and signature of the party or the representative of the party

If the claim was denied because of a simple error made by the insurance billing specialist, such as omission of the National Provider Identifier (NPI) of the referring physician or failure to code a diagnosis, then complete a Medicare Redetermination Request form and resubmit a corrected claim (Fig. 16.7). Include only the denied services and indicate in Block 19 "resubmission, corrected claim." The MAC must respond within 60 days of receipt of a request for redetermination from a beneficiary or provider. It must include reasons for the decision, a summary of clinical or scientific evidence used in making the redetermination, a description of how to obtain additional information, a notification of the right to appeal, and instructions on how to appeal the decision to the next level. If requested, the Medicare intermediary must provide information about the policy, manual, or regulation used in making the redetermination decision. The decision must be written in language that the beneficiary can understand.

Reconsideration (Level 2)

The next step in the appeals process is a reconsideration request. A Qualified Independent Contractor (QIC) will conduct the reconsideration. QICs are independent contractors that did not take part in the level 1 appeals decision. When making reconsideration decisions, QICs are expected to give weight to local and national coverage policies and conduct a panel review of denials when necessary. The request must be made within 180 days from the date the Medicare redetermination notice was received. The CMS-2033 form can be used to request reconsideration of a claim (Fig. 16.8).

The request for reconsideration should clearly explain why you disagree with the redetermination. Attach the following with the reconsideration request:

1. Copy of the original insurance claim
2. Copy of the RA showing the denial
3. Photocopy of other documents, such as operative or pathology report or detailed summary about the procedure, with appropriate words highlighted to help the reviewer
4. The reconsideration form with explanation of the procedure indicating justification for the services and the reason that the provider should receive more reimbursement

Mail the documents by certified mail with return receipt requested and retain copies of all documents sent to the carrier in the provider's pending file.

Generally, the QIC will send its decision to all parties within 60 days of receipt of the request for reconsideration. If the provider is not satisfied with the results of the review, move to the next level of appeals.

If a claim is unassigned, the beneficiary (patient) can pursue the review or appoint the service provider as an authorized representative. The patient completes form SSA-1696 (Rec 06/12) (Fig. 16.9) and obtains the service provider's acceptance signature. Decisions on unassigned claims are sent to the patient.

Administrative Law Judge Hearing (Level 3)

The third level of appeals is an administrative law judge (ALJ) hearing. If the service provider disagrees with the reconsideration decision, an ALJ hearing may be requested. The level of appeals can be done via telephone, video teleconference, or occasionally in person. The hearing provides an opportunity to explain your position to an ALJ.

To request a hearing by the ALJ, the amount remaining in controversy must meet the minimum threshold of $160 (for calendar year 2018). Claims may be combined to meet the minimum threshold. The request must be made within 60 days of receiving the reconsideration officer's decision (Fig. 16.10). Because of the number of appeal requests, it may take up to 18 months to receive an ALJ assignment.

Proof that the claim represents an unusual case and warrants special consideration may lead to a successful conclusion. However, the decision might be reversed, it might allow partial adjustment of the carrier's payment, or payment might be denied. If the final judgment is not satisfactory, proceed to the next level.

Medicare Appeals Council (Level 4)

If the service provider is dissatisfied with the ALJ's decision, the provider may request the fourth level of appeals, a review by the Medicare Appeals Council. The Medicare Appeals Council is part of the Office of Hearings and Appeals of the Social Security Administration. There are no requirements regarding the amount of money in controversy. A request must be made within 60 days of the ALJ decision; if there is a question that the final judgment was not made in accordance with the law, the council by its own election may review the ALJ decision. If the council denies a review, the provider may file a civil action for a federal district court hearing.

Federal District Court (Level 5)

To pursue the highest level of appeals, a judicial review in federal district court, the amount of the case must meet a minimum dollar amount. For 2018 the minimum dollar amount is $1600. It is acceptable to combine claims to meet this dollar amount. The hearing must be requested within 60 days from receipt of the level 4 appeals. An attorney must be hired to represent the provider and manage the case. The case may be filed where the health care organization is located. Contact the local medical society for suggestions of names of attorneys experienced at this level of the appeals process.

DEPARTMENT OF HEALTH AND HUMAN SERVICES
CENTERS FOR MEDICARE & MEDICAID SERVICES

MEDICARE REDETERMINATION REQUEST FORM – 1ST LEVEL OF APPEAL

1. Beneficiary's name: Carolyn N. Harvey
2. Medicare number: 072-XX-1461
3. Item or service you wish to appeal: Office Visit (99215)
4. Date the service or item was received: 07-24-20XX
5. Date of the initial determination notice (please include a copy of the notice with this request):
(If you received your initial determination notice more than 120 days ago, include your reason for the late filing.)
09-02-20XX

5a. Name of the Medicare contractor that made the determination (not required):
Palmetto GBA

5b. Does this appeal involve an overpayment? ☐ Yes ☒ No
(for providers and suppliers only)

6. I do not agree with the determination decision on my claim because:
Established patient is 60 years old and has diabetic nephropathy with increasing edema and dyspnea.
7. Additional information Medicare should consider:
Comprehensive history and comprehensive examination was performed because patient had not been seen for a year. Her case had to be discussed with a cardiologist because of possibility of congestive heart failure condition.
8. ☒ I have evidence to submit. Please attach the evidence to this form or attach a statement explaining what you intend to submit and when you intend to submit it. You may also submit additional evidence at a later time, but all evidence must be received prior to the issuance of the redetermination.

☐ I do not have evidence to submit.

9. Person appealing: ☐ Beneficiary ☒ Provider/Supplier ☐ Representative
10. Name, address, and telephone number of person appealing: Gerald Practon, MD
4567 Broad Avenue, Woodland Hills, XY 12345 555-486-9002
11. Signature of person appealing: Gerald Practon, MD
12. Date signed: 10-04-20XX

PRIVACY ACT STATEMENT: The legal authority for the collection of information on this form is authorized by section 1869 (a)(3) of the Social Security Act. The information provided will be used to further document your appeal. Submission of the information requested on this form is voluntary, but failure to provide all or any part of the requested information may affect the determination of your appeal. Information you furnish on this form may be disclosed by the Centers for Medicare and Medicaid Services to another person or government agency only with respect to the Medicare Program and to comply with Federal laws requiring or permitting the disclosure of information or the exchange of information between the Department of Health and Human Services and other agencies. Additional information about these disclosures can be found in the system of records notice for system no. 09-70-0566, as amended, available at 71 Fed. Reg. 54489 (2006) or at http://www.cms.gov/PrivacyActSystemofRecords/downloads/0566.pdf

Form CMS-20027 (12/10)

Fig. 16.7 Medicare Redetermination Request Form—1st Level of Appeal, CMS-20027, which can be used by the Medicare beneficiary or physician when requesting a redetermination of a submitted claim.

Centers for Medicare and Medicaid Services Regional Offices

One final suggestion (and this can be done with steps for a hearing or a review) is to write or telephone the medical director at one of the CMS regional offices. Sometimes a regional officer intercedes or takes steps to correct problems or inequities. CMS regional offices may be located by accessing the Medicare website.

Medigap

Insurance companies that sell Medigap (MG) policies must be certified by the state insurance commissioner before being

DEPARTMENT OF HEALTH AND HUMAN SERVICES
CENTERS FOR MEDICARE & MEDICAID SERVICES

MEDICARE RECONSIDERATION REQUEST – 2ND LEVEL OF APPEAL

1. Beneficiary's name: Jose F. Perez
2. Medicare number: 032-XX-6619
3. Item or service you wish to appeal: Electrocadiographic Monitoring, 24 hrs (93224)
4. Date the service or item was received: 01-21-20XX
5. Date of the redetermination notice (please include a copy of the notice with this request):
(If you received your redetermination notice more than 180 days ago, include your reason for the late filing.)
03-24-20XX

5a. Name of the Medicare contractor that made the redetermination (not required if copy of notice attached):
Palmetto GBA

5b. Does this appeal involve an overpayment? ☐ Yes ☒ No
(for providers and suppliers only)

6. I do not agree with the redetermination decision on my claim because:
Patient had heart palpitations, tachycardia, and lightheadedness (near syncopal episode). Although patient had a previous Holter monitor within the 60 months time limitation, it did not provide any clinical evidence of disease. Patient underwent recent monitoring after experiencing additional symptoms that were more severe then the inital.
7. Additional information Medicare should consider:

8. ☒ I have evidence to submit. Please attach the evidence to this form or attach a statement explaining what you intend to submit and when you intend to submit it. You may also submit additional evidence at a later time, but all evidence must be received prior to the issuance of the reconsideration.

☐ I do not have evidence to submit.

9. Person appealing: ☐ Beneficiary ☒ Provider/Supplier ☐ Representative
10. Name, address, and telephone number of person appealing: Gerald Practon, MD
4567 Broad Avenue, Woodland Hills, XY 12345 555-486-9002
11. Signature of person appealing: Gerald Practon, MD
12. Date signed: 06-05-20XX

PRIVACY ACT STATEMENT: The legal authority for the collection of information on this form is authorized by section 1869 (a)(3) of the Social Security Act. The information provided will be used to further document your appeal. Submission of the information requested on this form is voluntary, but failure to provide all or any part of the requested information may affect the determination of your appeal. Information you furnish on this form may be disclosed by the Centers for Medicare and Medicaid Services to another person or government agency only with respect to the Medicare Program and to comply with Federal laws requiring or permitting the disclosure of information or the exchange of information between the Department of Health and Human Services and other agencies. Additional information about these disclosures can be found in the system of records notice for system no. 09-70-0566, as amended, available at 71 Fed. Reg. 54489 (2006) or at http://www.cms.gov/PrivacyActSystemofRecords/downloads/0566.pdf

Form CMS-20033 (12/10)

Fig. 16.8 Medicare Reconsideration Request Form—2nd Level of Appeal, CMS-20033, which can be used when requesting a reconsideration of Medicare Part B claims.

allowed to sell in each state. The certification can be lifted from any insurer that does not honor its contract agreements. If payment is slow in coming or is not received from an MG insurer, first try the paper or electronic claim solutions for delinquent claims mentioned previously in this chapter. As a last resort, tell the insurer, "If I do not receive payment, I will have no alternative but to contact the state insurance commissioner."

TRICARE Review and Appeal Process

Denials made by a TRICARE contractor can be appealed by the beneficiary or a participating provider. A provider who treats a TRICARE patient but is out of network is not able to obtain information from TRICARE. Contact the patient for his or her assistance. Also, out-of-network providers who wish to treat an obstetric case may need a nonavailability request form

DEPARTMENT OF HEALTH AND HUMAN SERVICES
CENTERS FOR MEDICARE & MEDICAID SERVICES

Form Approved
OMB No. 0938-0950

APPOINTMENT OF REPRESENTATIVE

Name of Party	Medicare Number (beneficiary as party) or National Provider Identifier Number (provider as party)

Section 1: Appointment of Representative

To be completed by the party seeking representation (i.e., the Medicare beneficiary, the provider or the supplier):

I appoint this individual, ______________________________ to act as my representative in connection with my claim or asserted right under Title XVIII of the Social Security Act (the "Act") and related provisions of Title XI of the Act. I authorize this individual to make any request; to present or to elicit evidence; to obtain appeals information; and to receive any notice in connection with my appeal, wholly in my stead. I understand that personal medical information related to my appeal may be disclosed to the representative indicated below.

Signature of Party Seeking Representation		Date
Street Address		Phone Number (with Area Code)
City	State	Zip Code

Section 2: Acceptance of Appointment

To be completed by the representative:

I, ______________________________, hereby accept the above appointment. I certify that I have not been disqualified, suspended, or prohibited from practice before the Department of Health and Human Services (DHHS); that I am not, as a current or former employee of the United States, disqualified from acting as the party's representative; and that I recognize that any fee may be subject to review and approval by the Secretary.

I am a / an ______________________________
(Professional status or relationship to the party, e.g. attorney, relative, etc.)

Signature of Representative		Date
Street Address		Phone Number (with Area Code)
City	State	Zip Code

Section 3: Waiver of Fee for Representation

Instructions: This section must be completed if the representative is required to, or chooses to waive their fee for representation. (Note that providers or suppliers that are representing a beneficiary and furnished the items or services may not charge a fee for representation and **must** complete this section.)

I waive my right to charge and collect a fee for representing ______________________________ before the Secretary of DHHS.

Signature	Date

Section 4: Waiver of Payment for Items or Services at Issue

Instructions: Providers or suppliers serving as a representative for a beneficiary to whom they provided items or services must complete this section if the appeal involves a question of liability under section 1879(a)(2) of the Act.(Section 1879(a)(2) generally addresses whether a provider/supplier or beneficiary did not know, or could not reasonably be expected to know, that the items or services at issue would not be covered by Medicare.)

I waive my right to collect payment from the beneficiary for the items or services at issue in this appeal if a determination of liability under §1879(a)(2) of the Act is at issue.

Signature	Date

Form CMS-1696 (11/15) 1

Fig. 16.9 Form CMS-1696 (Rev 06/12) completed by a Medicare patient appointing the physician as his or her authorized representative. (From Department of Health and Human Services, Washington, DC, March 2017.)

Charging of Fees for Representing Beneficiaries before the Secretary of DHHS

An attorney, or other representative for a beneficiary, who wishes to charge a fee for services rendered in connection with an appeal before the Secretary of DHHS (i.e., an Administrative Law Judge (ALJ) hearing, Medicare Appeals Council review, or a proceeding before an ALJ or the Medicare Appeals Council as a result of a remand from federal district court) is required to obtain approval of the fee in accordance with 42 CFR 405.910(f).

The form, "Petition to Obtain Representative Fee" elicits the information required for a fee petition. It should be completed by the representative and filed with the request for ALJ hearing or request for Medicare Appeals Council review. Approval of a representative's fee is not required if: (1) the appellant being represented is a provider or supplier; (2) the fee is for services rendered in an official capacity such as that of legal guardian, committee, or similar court appointed representative and the court has approved the fee in question; (3) the fee is for representation of a beneficiary in a proceeding in federal district court; or (4) the fee is for representation of a beneficiary in a redetermination or reconsideration. If the representative wishes to waive a fee, he or she may do so. Section III on the front of this form can be used for that purpose. In some instances, as indicated on the form, the fee must be waived for representation.

Approval of Fee

The requirement for the approval of fees ensures that a representative will receive fair value for the services performed before DHHS on behalf of a beneficiary, and provides the beneficiary with a measure of security that the fees are determined to be reasonable. In approving a requested fee, the ALJ or Medicare Appeals Council will consider the nature and type of services rendered, the complexity of the case, the level of skill and competence required in rendition of the services, the amount of time spent on the case, the results achieved, the level of administrative review to which the representative carried the appeal and the amount of the fee requested by the representative.

Conflict of Interest

Sections 203, 205 and 207 of Title XVIII of the United States Code make it a criminal offense for certain officers, employees and former officers and employees of the United States to render certain services in matters affecting the Government or to aid or assist in the prosecution of claims against the United States. Individuals with a conflict of interest are excluded from being representatives of beneficiaries before DHHS.

Where to Send This Form

Send this form to the same location where you are sending (or have already sent) your: appeal if you are filing an appeal, grievance if you are filing a grievance, initial determination or decision if you are requesting an initial determination or decision. If additional help is needed, contact your Medicare plan or 1-800-MEDICARE (1-800-633-4227). TTY users please call 1-877-486-2048.

CMS does not discriminate in its programs and activities. To request this publication in an alternative format, please call: 1-800-MEDICARE or email: **AltFormatRequest@cms.hhs.gov**

According to the Paperwork Reduction Act of 1995, no persons are required to respond to a collection of information unless it displays a valid OMB control number. The valid OMB control number for this information collection is 0938-0950. The time required to prepare and distribute this collection is 15 minutes per notice, including the time to select the preprinted form, complete it and deliver it to the beneficiary. If you have comments concerning the accuracy of the time estimates or suggestions for improving this form, please write to CMS, PRA Clearance Officer, 7500 Security Boulevard, Baltimore, Maryland 21244-1850.

Form CMS-1696 (11/15) 2

Fig. 16.9, cont'd.

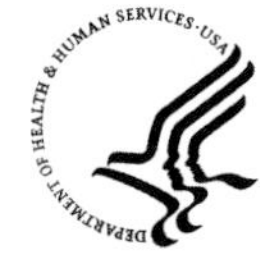

DEPARTMENT OF HEALTH AND HUMAN SERVICES
Office of Medicare Hearings and Appeals
REQUEST FOR ADMINISTRATIVE LAW JUDGE (ALJ) HEARING OR REVIEW OF DISMISSAL

Section 1: Which Medicare Part are you appealing (if known)? (*Check one*)

☐ Part A ☐ Part B ☐ Part C (*Medicare Advantage*) or Medicare Cost Plan ☐ Part D (*Prescription Drug Plan*)

Section 2: Which party are you, or which party are you representing? (*Check one*)

☐ The Medicare beneficiary or enrollee, or a successor (such as an estate), who received or requested the items or services being appealed, or is appealing a Medicare Secondary Payer issue.

☐ The provider or supplier that furnished the items or services to the Medicare beneficiary or enrollee, a Medicaid State agency, or an applicable plan appealing a Medicare Secondary Payer issue.

☐ Other. *Please explain*:

Section 3: What is your (the appealing party's) information? (*Representative information in next section*)

Name (*First, Middle Initial, Last*)		Firm or Organization (*if applicable*)	
Address where appeals correspondence should be sent	City	State	ZIP Code
Telephone Number	Fax Number	E-Mail	

Section 4: What is the representative's information? (*Skip if you do not have a representative*)

Name		Firm or Organization (*if applicable*)	
Mailing Address	City	State	ZIP Code
Telephone Number	Fax Number	E-Mail	

Did you file an appointment of representation (form CMS-1696) or other documents authorizing your representation at a prior level of appeal?

☐ No. *Please file the document(s) with this request.*
☐ Yes

Section 5: What is being appealed? *Submit a separate request for each Reconsideration or Dismissal that you wish to appeal. If the appeal involves multiple beneficiaries or enrollees, use the multiple claim attachment (OMHA-100A).*

Name of entity that issued the Reconsideration or Dismissal (*or attach a copy of the Reconsideration or Dismissal*)		Reconsideration (Medicare Appeal or Case) Number (*or attach a copy of the Reconsideration or Dismissal*)	
Beneficiary or Enrollee Name		Health Insurance Claim Number	
Beneficiary or Enrollee Mailing Address	City	State	ZIP Code
What item(s) or service(s) are you appealing? (*N/A if appealing a Dismissal*)		Date(s) of service being appealed (*if applicable*)	
Supplier or Provider Name (*N/A for Part D appeals*)		Supplier or Provider Telephone Number (*N/A for Part D appeals*)	
Supplier or Provider Mailing Address (*N/A for Part D appeals*)	City	State	ZIP Code

Section 6: For appeals of prescription drugs ONLY (*Skip for all other appeals*)

Part D Prescription Drug Plan Name	What drug(s) are you appealing?

Are you requesting an expedited hearing?
(*An expedited hearing is only available if your appeal is not solely related to payment (for example, you do not have the drug) and applying the standard time frame for a decision (90 days) may jeopardize your health, life, or ability to regain maximum function*)

☐ No. ☐ Yes. *On a separate sheet, please explain or have your prescriber explain why applying the standard time frame for a decision (90 days) may jeopardize your health, life, or ability to regain maximum function.*

OMHA-100 (03/17) **PAGE 1 OF 2** PSC Publishing Services (301) 443-6740. EF

Fig. 16.10 Request for Medicare hearing by an administrative law judge, form OMHA-100. (From Department of Health and Human Services, Centers or Medicare & Medicaid Service, Washington, DC, November 2015.)

Section 7: Why do you disagree with the Reconsideration or Dismissal being appealed? *(Attach a continuation sheet if necessary)*

Section 8: Are you submitting evidence with this request, or do you plan to submit evidence?

☐ I am not planning to submit evidence at this time. *(Skip to Section 9, below)*

☐ I am submitting evidence with this request.

☐ I plan to submit evidence. Indicate what you plan to submit and when you plan to submit it:

Was the evidence already submitted for the matter that you are appealing?	☐ No. *Part A and Part B appeals only. If you are a provider or supplier, or a provider or supplier that is representing a beneficiary, you must include a statement explaining why the evidence is being submitted for the first time and was not submitted previously.* ☐ Yes.

Section 9: Is there other information about your appeal that we should know?

Are you aggregating claims to meet the amount in controversy requirement? *(If yes, attach your aggregation request. See 42 C.F.R. § 405.1006(e) and (f), and 423.1979(c) for request requirements.)*	☐ No	☐ Yes
Are you waiving the oral hearing before an ALJ and requesting a decision based on the record? *(If yes, attach a completed form OMHA-104 or other explanation. N/A if requesting review of a dismissal.)*	☐ No	☐ Yes
Does the request involve claims that were part of a statistical sample? *(If yes, please explain the status of any appeals for claims in the sample that are not included in this request.)*	☐ No	☐ Yes

Section 10: Certification of copies sent to other parties *(Part A and Part B appeals only)*

If another party to the claim or issue that you are appealing was sent a copy of the Reconsideration or Dismissal, you must send a copy of your request for an ALJ hearing or review of dismissal to that party.

Indicate the party (or their representative) to whom and address where you are sending a copy of the request, and when the copy will be sent *(attach a continuation sheet if there are multiple parties).*

Name of Recipient		
Mailing Address		
City	State	ZIP Code
Date of Mailing		

☐ Check here if no other parties were sent a copy of the Reconsideration or Dismissal.

Section 11: Filing instructions

Your appealed claim must meet the current amount in controversy requirement to file an appeal. See the Reconsideration or Dismissal or visit www.hhs.gov/omha for information on the current amount in controversy. Send this request form to the entity in the appeal instructions that came with your reconsideration (for example, requests for hearing following a Part C reconsideration are generally sent to the entity that conducted the reconsideration). If instructed to send to OMHA, use the addresses below.

Beneficiaries and enrollees, send your request to:	**For expedited Part D appeals, send your request to:**	**All other appellants, send your request to:**
OMHA Centralized Docketing Attn: Beneficiary Mail Stop 200 Public Square, Suite 1260 Cleveland, Ohio 44114-2316	OMHA Centralized Docketing Attn: Expedited Part D Mail Stop 200 Public Square, Suite 1260 Cleveland, Ohio 44114-2316	OMHA Centralized Docketing 200 Public Square, Suite 1260 Cleveland, Ohio 44114-2316

We must receive this request within 60 calendar days after you received the Reconsideration or Dismissal that you are appealing. We will assume that you received the Reconsideration or Dismissal 5 calendar days after the date of the Reconsideration or Dismissal, unless you provide evidence to the contrary. *If you are filing this request late, attach a completed form OMHA-103 or other explanation for the late filing.*

PRIVACY ACT STATEMENT

The legal authority for the collection of information on this form is authorized by the Social Security Act (section 1155 of Title XI and sections 1852(g)(5), 1860D-4(h)(1), 1869(b)(1), and 1876 of Title XVIII). The information provided will be used to further document your appeal. Submission of the information requested on this form is voluntary, but failure to provide all or any part of the requested information may affect the determination of your appeal. Information you furnish on this form may be disclosed by the Office of Medicare Hearings and Appeals to another person or governmental agency only with respect to the Medicare Program and to comply with Federal laws requiring the disclosure of information or the exchange of information between the Department of Health and Human Services and other agencies.

If you need large print or assistance, please call 1-855-556-8475

OMHA-100 (03/17) **PAGE 2 OF 2**

Fig. 16.10, cont'd.

completed and processed before a patient can receive care. There must be a reason the patient cannot go to a providing facility, and TRICARE determines whether it will approve the request. Otherwise, claims will be denied.

All TRICARE inquiries are done through the online portal or the automated phone system. TRICARE managed care contracts have been adopted throughout the United States, and the appeals procedures that TRICARE contractors use in these areas may vary. For information on how to file reviews and appeals for those contracts, ask the contracting insurance company for instructions and forms.

There are two types of TRICARE appeals, expedited and nonexpedited. Expedited appeals must be filed within 3 days of the receipt of the initial denial. These appeals should include an expedited review of a prior authorization denial. This process varies slightly depending on the regional contractor, so research the appeals process with the local TRICARE contractor.

Nonexpedited appeals must be filed no more than 90 days after the receipt of the initial denial. The steps to file a nonexpedited appeal follow:

1. Send a letter to the regional TRICARE contractor at the address specified in the notice to appeal. The appeal letter must be submitted no more than 90 days after the date of the RA. Include in the appeal the RA stating the denial, along with a claim form and all medical documentation relating to the claim. If for some reason essential paperwork for the insurance claim is not available to be sent, include this reason in the appeal letter. Keep copies of all paperwork for future reference and follow-up.
2. The TRICARE contractor will review the case and make a decision. If the decision is not favorable, the next level of appeal is TRICARE Quality Monitoring Contractor (TQMC).
3. Send a letter to TQMC including all the documentation from the original appeal and the decision received from the regional TRICARE contractor. The letter must be received by TRICARE no more than 90 days after the date of the appeal decision. Again, if all documentation is not available to be sent along with the appeal, include the reasons why in the appeal letter. Keep all paperwork for future reference and follow-up.
4. The TQMC issues a second reconsideration decision. If the claim is for less than $300, the TQMC decision is final. If there is still a dispute about a claim that is more than $300, an independent hearing may be requested with the TRICARE Management Activity (TMA).

Reconsideration

Participating providers may appeal certain decisions made by TRICARE and request reconsideration. Providers who do not participate may not appeal but TRICARE patients and parents or guardians of patients younger than 18 years of age who seek care from nonparticipating providers may file appeals. Providers who do not participate may not receive any information about a claim without the signed authorization of the patient or the patient's parent or guardian.

Matters that can be appealed include the following:

1. Medical necessity disagreements (inappropriate care, level of care, investigational procedures)
2. Factual determinations (hospice care, foreign claims, provider sanction cases)
   a. Denials or partial denials of requests for preauthorization for certain services or supplies
   b. Coverage issues—notification that TRICARE will not pay for services before or after a certain date

Matters that cannot be appealed include the following:

1. Denial of services received from a provider not authorized to provide care under TRICARE
2. A specific exclusion of law or regulation
3. Allowable charges for particular services
4. Issues relating to the establishment and application of diagnosis-related groups
5. Decisions by the claims processor to ask for additional information on a case
6. A determination of a person's eligibility as a TRICARE beneficiary

The TRICARE department that handles appeals also collects and organizes all information necessary to review the case effectively. Usually a determination decision is made within 60 days from receipt of the appeal. Disagreements about the amount allowed for a claim may be reviewed by the claims processor to determine whether it was calculated correctly. However, an individual cannot appeal the amount that the TRICARE contractor determines to be the allowable charge for a certain medical service.

Requests must be sent to the claims processor of the state in which services were provided and must be postmarked within 90 days of the date the provider receives the Summary Payment Voucher (formerly referred to as an RA). Include photocopies of the claim, the Summary Payment Voucher, and other supporting documents with the request form or letter. The claim identification number assigned by the claims processor should be included in any inquiry concerning payment of the claim. If TRICARE denies the initial request, the other two levels of review—formal review and hearing—may be pursued.

STATE INSURANCE COMMISSIONER

Commission Objectives

There is no federal regulatory agency that oversees insurance companies. Instead, insurance companies are regulated primarily by the individual states. Insurance regulations vary widely from state to state. If a complaint arises about an insurance policy, medical claim, or insurance agent or broker, the insurance department of the state of residence or the state in which the insurance company's corporate office is headquartered should be contacted. This department is generally referred to as the **state insurance commissioner.** State insurance commissioners are public officials who regulate the insurance industry in their state.

State insurance departments usually have various objectives, including the following:

- To register insurance companies
- To establish standards and best practices
- To make certain that the financial strength of insurance companies is not unduly diminished

- To monitor the activities of insurance companies to ensure that the interests of the policyholders are protected
- To verify that all contracts are carried out in good faith
- To ensure that all organizations authorized to transact insurance, including agents and brokers, are in compliance with the insurance laws of that state
- To release information on how many complaints have been filed against a specific insurance company in a year
- To help explain correspondence related to insurance company bankruptcies and other financial difficulties
- To assist if a company funds its own insurance plan
- To help resolve insurance conflicts

The insurance commissioner can hold a hearing to determine whether licensed insurers, agents, or brokers are in compliance with the insurance laws of the state, but the commissioner does not have the authority vested in a court of law to order an insurance company to make payment on a specific claim.

The insurance commissioner reviews the policy to determine whether the denial of a claim by the insurance company was based on legal provisions of the insurance contract and advises the patient if there is an infraction of the law. If there is an infraction, the patient should consult an attorney to determine whether the claim should be submitted to a court of law.

Types of Problems

Problems that should be submitted to the insurance commissioner are as follows:

1. Improper denial of a claim or settlement for an amount less than that indicated by the policy after proper appeal has been made
2. Delay in settlement of a claim after proper appeal has been made
3. Illegal cancellation or termination of an insurance policy
4. Misrepresentation by an insurance agent or broker
5. Misappropriation of premiums paid to an insurance agent or broker
6. Problems about insurance premium rates
7. Two companies that cannot determine which is primary

Commission Inquiries

An insurance billing specialist may not be in a position to know the particulars about a case and should never assume or accuse unless he or she is certain or has concrete evidence. Remember, "Jump to conclusions, suffer contusions."

Requests to the insurance commissioner must be submitted online. In some states the insurance commissioner requires that the complaint come from the patient even if an assignment of benefits form has been signed. In such a case a letter or form should be prepared for the patient to sign and then submit. Depending on the circumstances of the case, one may wish to send copies to the state medical association or an attorney. Mail may be sent certified, return receipt requested. The request should contain the following information:

1. The inquiring person's (patient) or policyholder's name—the commissioner's responsibility is to the patient (the consumer), not the health care organization
2. The policyholder's address
3. The policyholder's telephone number
4. The insured's name
5. Name, address, and title of the insurance agent or official of the insurance company
6. A statement of the complaint including, if possible, a copy of the policy, medical bills, unpaid medical insurance claim, canceled checks, and any correspondence from the company pertaining to the claim
7. The patient's signature
8. The name and address of the insurance company, agent, or broker, or the name and address of the finance company if the premium was financed
9. The policy or claim number
10. The date of loss
11. The date on which the patient signed the complaint form

If an insurance company is continually a slow payer, one method to speed up payments is to include a note to the carrier that reads, "Unless this claim is paid or denied within 30 to 45 days, a formal written complaint will be filed with the state insurance commissioner."

Another method is to send a letter to the insurance commissioner with a copy notation inserted at the end to the insurance company. It might read, "The attached claim has been submitted to the XYZ Insurance Company. It has not been paid or denied. Please accept this letter as a formal written complaint against the XYZ Insurance Company."

Insurance companies are rated according to the number of complaints received about them, so they do not want the insurance commissioner to be alerted to any problems. Some states have information available to the public on how many claims have been submitted against a company if this information is necessary.

CLAIM DENIAL MANAGEMENT

Every health care organization will experience claim denials. Denied claims represent unpaid services, and failure to promptly work denials from insurance carriers results in lost revenue for the health care organization. Denials also present a significant burden on the health care organization from the perspective of staff time spent managing and working denials. In fact, some organizations are unable to devote the needed manpower to the denied claim effort and eventually the denials are written off as bad debt. Health care organizations leave millions of dollars on the table because of inefficient claim denial management processes. **Claim denial management** represents a significant opportunity for revenue cycle cash flow improvement and has become a critical component of any health care organization's strategic effort toward this goal.

Identification. Effective claim denial management starts with identifying the reason for denials. The insurance billing specialist will need to review RAs carefully to determine the specific reason for denial. The reason for the denial is usually identified on the RA with a reason code that translates to a specific denial description. If the denial description is unclear, it may be necessary for the insurance billing specialist to call the insurance carrier for additional information.

Review and appeal. The health care organization should have a process in place to ensure that the denial will be reviewed and appealed within a week from receipt of the RA. Techniques for appealing the claim are outlined previously in this chapter. Creating a strong workflow for claim denied claims is key to the denial management process. To do this, a workflow must be established that will track the claims as they enter and leave the organization's billing system. Keep in mind that many insurance carriers have time limits associated with how quickly a denial can be appealed.

Categorize. In addition to working denials and appealing claims, the denials must be categorized by reason, source and other pertinent factors. As the reasons for denials are identified, processes can be modified to reduce the number of denials. Examples of reasons for denial include:

- Registration errors such as incorrect payer, incorrect insurance identification number, and so on
- Charge entry errors
- Referral and preauthorization errors
- Duplicate claims incorrectly submitted
- Medical necessity
- Documentation
- Coding errors
- Bundled/noncovered services
- Incorrect/invalid modifier usage
- Credentialing issues

Measure. Using medical billing software, the health care organization can track, report, and measure claim denials. The organization should compute denials as a percentage of all claims submitted to understand what the volume and reasons for denials reveal about the organization's revenue cycle. Gathering this type of data will provide important content to analyze your health care organization's processes and overall performance. It may be helpful to continue to drill down through the denial, based on even greater specificity. For example:

Step 1: The organization calculates a high percentage of denials for medical necessity.

Step 2: The next step would be to measure the amount of medical necessity denials per provider. In doing this, one provider is identified who has a higher percentage of medical necessity denials than other providers.

Step 3: The final step in this situation would be to measure the amount of medical necessity denials for this provider by procedure code. In doing this it is identified that excision of benign lesions has the highest medical necessity denial rate of all procedures performed by this provider.

By doing this type of analysis, the organization is able to pinpoint the specific reason for the high percentage of denials and can now strategize at how to correct the problem.

Strategize. As denial categories are analyzed and measured, the organization will develop strategies to change processes that will prevent future denials. Strategies might include adjusting workflows, retraining staff, assisting providers with documentation issues, reviewing medical necessity policies, implementing system alerts and notifications, researching coding issues, clarifying carrier guidelines and policies, implementing internal audit processes, and providing incentives for improving collection of patient information.

Denial management is a roadmap for change. Every time a denial is reduced, the health care organization will get paid correctly and will have eliminated all the rework required when a claim is denied. Denial management is key to improving any organization's cash flow.

PROCEDURE 16.1 File an Appeal

Objective

To compose, format, key, proofread, and print a letter of appeal and attach photocopies of information to substantiate reimbursement requested

Equipment/Supplies

Typewriter or computer, printer, letterhead paper, envelope, attachments (if necessary), thesaurus, English dictionary, medical dictionary, and pen or pencil

Directions

Follow these basic step-by-step procedures, which include rationales, to learn this skill and practice it by completing the *Workbook* assignment.

1. Refer to CMS 16-10 at the end of Chapter 4 and follow the procedure to compose, format, key, proofread, and print a letter.
2. Include the beneficiary's name, health insurance claim number, date of initial determination, dates of service in question, items or services in question, name and address of the provider, and signature of appellant.
3. Compose a letter with an introduction that stresses the service provider's qualifications, the provider's commitment to complying with regulations and providing appropriate services, and the importance of the health care organization to the payer's panel of health care professionals.
4. Provide a detailed account of the necessity of the treatment given and its relationship to the patient's problems and chief complaint. You might cross-reference the health record and emphasize parts of it that the reviewer may have missed.
5. Explain the reason why the provider does not agree with the claim denial listed on the explanation of benefits or remittance advice.
6. Abstract excerpts from the coding resource book and attach a photocopy of the article or pertinent information showing the name of the article, coding resource, and date of publication.
7. Send copies of similar cases with increased reimbursement from the same insurance company if available from the insurance company payment history file.
8. Call the insurance company and speak to the individual responsible for appeals; explain what the resubmission is trying to accomplish. Direct the correspondence to this person.
9. Retain copies of all data sent for the health care organization's files.
10. Use a method that confirms the payer received the letter, such as a certified return receipt or signature using Federal Express or Airborne Express services.

KEY POINTS

This is a brief chapter review, or summary, of the key issues presented. To further enhance your knowledge of the technical subject matter, review the key terms and key abbreviations for this chapter by locating the meaning for each in the Glossary at the end of this book, which appears in a section before the Index.

1. Payment from a third-party payer after submission of a paper claim should occur within 4 to 12 weeks and of an electronic claim should occur within 7 days. When a payment problem develops, and the insurance company is slow, ignores, denies, or exceeds time limits, contact the third-party payer.
2. An explanation of benefits (EOB) or electronic Medicare remittance advice (RA) should be read and interpreted line by line and checked to establish whether the amount paid is correct. Amounts should then be posted to each patient's financial account.
3. Routine periodic checks of the insurance claims electronic tracking report or insurance paper claims register (log) should be done to follow up on delinquent claims.
4. The individual handling the front desk must collect insurance information accurately and update patient demographic information routinely to avoid future collection problems.
5. To avoid denied claims and to assist in solving claim problems, keep abreast of the latest policies for all contracted payers as well as for the federal programs.
6. A decision to appeal a claim should be based on whether there is ample information to back up the claim and if a substantial amount of money is in question.
7. The levels of a Medicare appeal are (1) redetermination by telephone, letter, or form; (2) reconsideration by a hearing officer; (3) hearing by an administrative law judge; (4) review by the Medicare Appeals Council; and (5) judicial review in the federal district court.
8. The types of a TRICARE appeal are expedited and nonexpedited.
9. To complain about a problem with an insurance contract or claim involving a private third-party payer or a Medigap (MG) supplemental plan, the state insurance commission must be contacted.
10. Always file the appropriate form or write a letter to begin the appeal process for resolving an insurance problem or complaint.
11. Denial management is critical to improving any organization's cash flow.

STUDENT ASSIGNMENT

- Study Chapter 16.
- Answer the fill-in-the-blank, multiple-choice, and true/false review questions in the *Workbook* to reinforce the theory learned in this chapter and to help prepare you for a future test.
- Complete the assignments in the *Workbook* to fill in a form for tracing a delinquent claim, to locate errors on a returned claim, and to complete a form to appeal a Medicare case.
- Turn to the Glossary at the end of this text for a further understanding of the key terms and key abbreviations used in this chapter.

17

Collection Strategies

Linda M. Smith

OBJECTIVES

After reading this chapter, you should be able to:

1. Explain the cash flow cycle in a health care organization.
2. Define *accounts receivable* and explain how it is handled.
3. Describe procedures for collecting complete and accurate patient information.
4. State policies for managing patient accounts and collection in a health care organization
5. Describe guidelines for missed appointments.
6. Recite and discuss types of fee adjustments available to patients.
7. Discuss fees with patients.
8. Name and describe payment options available to patients.
9. Define how to use the aging account receivable report effectively in collections.
10. Discuss dun messages, electronic media, and manual and computer billing, as well as state the role of a billing service in the collection process.
11. List the names of the federal credit laws applicable to the health care setting.
12. Explain statutes of limitations of three kinds of financial accounts.
13. Perform oral and written communication collection techniques.
14. Describe insurance collection from the patient and from third-party payers.
15. State and discuss the role of a collection agency in the collection process.
16. Explain the purpose of small claims court in the collection process.
17. Name and discuss basic actions in tracing a debtor who has moved and left no forwarding address.
18. Identify and describe special collection issues.

KEY TERMS

accounts receivable
age analysis
automatic stay
balance
bankruptcy
bonding
cash flow
collateral
collection ratio
credit
credit card
creditor
cycle billing
debit card
debt
debtor
discount
dun messages
embezzlement
estate administrator
estate executor
fee schedule
financial accounting record
garnishment
itemized statement
lien
netback
no charge
nonexempt assets
professional courtesy
secured debt
skip
statute of limitations
unsecured debt
write-off

KEY ABBREVIATIONS

A/R
ATM
e-check
ERISA
FACT
FCBA
FCRA
FDCPA
FEHBA
FTC
N/A
NC
NSF
TILA
W2

COLLECTION STRATEGIES

As discussed in earlier chapters, the insurance billing specialist's primary goal is to assist in management of the revenue cycle. *Revenue cycle management* refers to the processes a health care organization uses to collect unpaid bills, and it determines the organization's profitability. The insurance billing specialist strives to obtain maximum reimbursement for services provided and ensure a strong cash flow to the health care organization he or she is employed by. Collections of unpaid bills from patients is another component of revenue cycle management.

The practice of medicine in the United States is both a profession and a business. Although the service provider decides what type of health care services he or she will provide, it is often the health care organization's administrator who takes over the responsibilities for the business portion of the organization. It is extremely important for the health care administrator, service providers, and insurance billing specialist to work together to provide all patients with the best possible medical care and ensure that the services rendered are paid fairly.

Today this process has become increasingly complex. Billing practices for health care organizations have evolved from the barter system of days past. Since the Great Depression, the availability of **credit** and **credit cards** has become a common feature of the financial marketplace. The word *credit* comes from the Latin word *credere,* which means "to believe" or "to trust." This trust is in an individual's business integrity and his or her financial ability to meet obligations when they become due. For many, the idea of credit has changed and may simply mean to put off paying today what one can pay tomorrow.

A large percentage of reimbursement to health care organizations is generated from third-party payers (private insurance, government plans, managed care contracts, and workers' compensation). However, patients continue to take on more financial responsibility for their health care as a result of high-dollar-deductible health plans and rising copays and coinsurance. Financial responsibility by patients has steadily increased, and their responsibility can range from approximately 10.5% (inpatients) to 27.0% (outpatients) of the health care services.

It is essential for health care organizations to place more emphasis on the collection of unpaid balances. In today's environment, revenue cycle management requires focusing on patient collection strategies to maximize cash collections as well as provide a positive patient experience.

Fig. 17.1 shows a flow chart and overview of a health care organization's billing procedures that illustrates the sequence from beginning to end.

ACCOUNTS RECEIVABLE

Accounts receivable (A/R) is the total amount of unpaid **balances** that are due to a health care organization from patients and third-party payers for services that have been rendered. A/R management is vital to a health care organization's financial stability, and each organization will have a policy about handling A/R.The effectiveness of this policy and its enforcement are reflected in the organization's cash flow. The **cash flow** is the ongoing availability of actual cash in the organization. The primary goal in management of an account receivable is to reduce the amount of time an account is outstanding and to ensure payment of all services. When payment is collected at the time of service , the days in A/R is zero. In an ideal situation, all outstanding balances are paid within 60 days; however, this is not possible for the following reasons:

1. Health care expenses have increased and exceed the expenses the patient pays for everyday living.
2. Laws have been enacted and health care organizations have instituted policies to ensure that all patients, regardless of their financial situations, receive the best possible health care. In many situations, care of the indigent becomes an unreimbursable expense in the health care organization.
3. Legal proceedings often delay the payment of medical expenses.
4. Third-party payers do not always pay claims in a timely manner, resulting in further delays in the collection of patient copayments.
5. Managed care plans seek discounted rates for their members obtaining medical services.

By monitoring A/R, the insurance billing specialist can evaluate the effectiveness of the collection process. Later in this chapter, A/R ratio formulas are presented in the section titled Accounts Receivable and Age Analysis by Aging Report.

The best way to keep A/R down is to verify insurance benefits before providing care to the patient (if possible), collect copayments and deductibles at the time of service, obtain authorizations when required, and monitor A/R weekly. Set up automatic alerts when patients with a balance in their account want to schedule an appointment. This reminds the receptionist to ask for a copayment, deductible, or noncovered fee. Electronic claims that have not been paid within 30 days of submission may have problems that can range from the carrier asking for additional information from the patient to the patient not being one of the carrier's insured.

The **collection ratio** is the relationship of the amount of money owed to a health care organization and the amount of money collected on the A/R. A collection rate of 100% is obviously desirable, although unrealistic, and should always be sought as a goal for the person managing collections in the health care office. To calculate the collection ratio for a 1-month period, divide the amount of monies collected during the current month by the total amount of A/R.

PATIENT EDUCATION

Most Americans do not fully understand how health insurance works, so the burden of educating them falls on the health care organization's staff. Front office medical staff should strive to educate the patient in the following aspects of health care:

- Benefits, including how many appointments are allowed per year, copays, and deductibles
- The approximate out-of-pocket expense for patients after insurance has paid
- The cost of medications, medical equipment, and ambulatory services

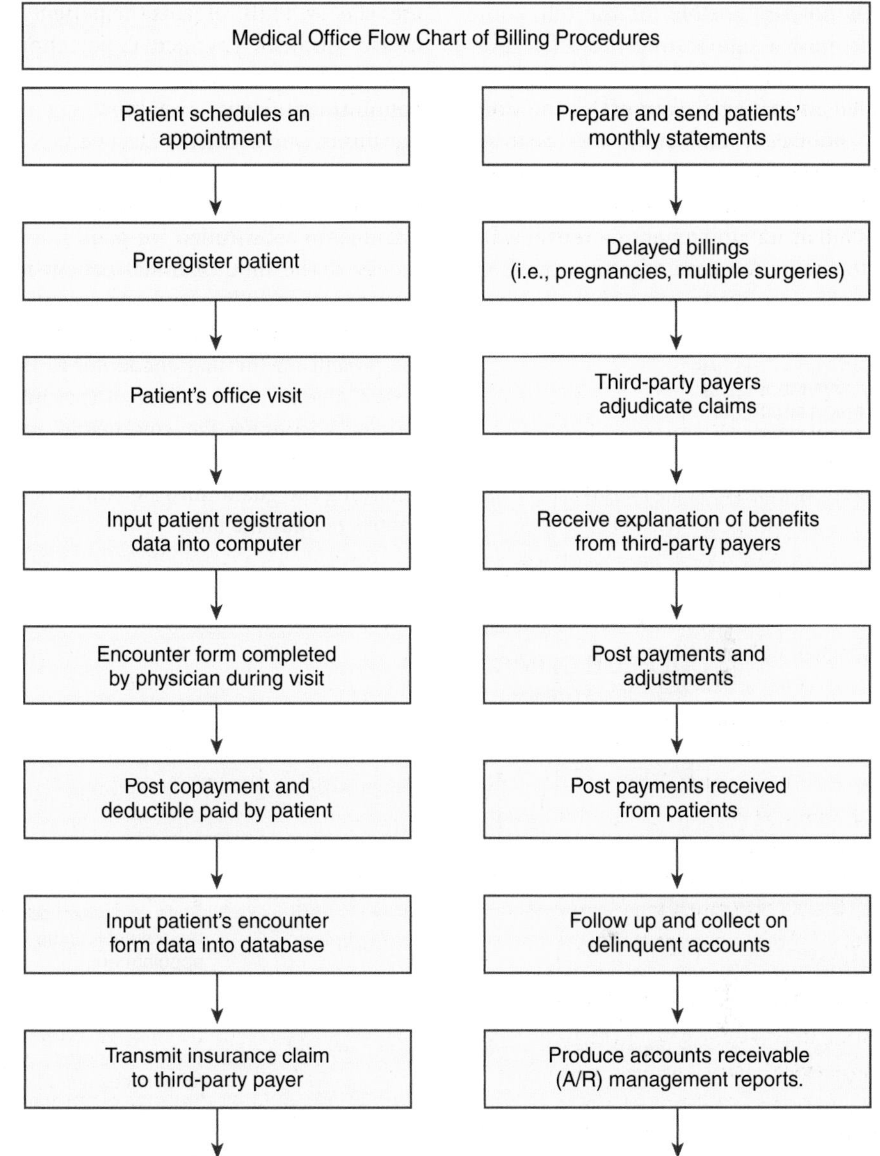

Fig. 17.1 Flow chart showing a health care organization's billing procedures from scheduling the patient's appointment to producing accounts receivable management reports.

- The difference between emergency and urgent care and the costs involved

The Affordable Care Act of 2013 was enacted to allow more Americans access to quality health care. Some of the provisions include free preventive care, elimination of preexisting conditions, expanded Medicaid coverage, and discount medications for seniors (Fig. 17.2).

The Affordable Care Act also provides subsidized health insurance for lower-income individuals and allows young adults up to age 26 to remain on their parent's health care plan. This Act does not affect how health care organization are reimbursed; probably the biggest change that the medical office has experienced is that the number of self-pay patients has decreased.

A new patient information packet should be provided to the patient on the initial encounter to the health care organization that contains information about payment policies. This decreases the number of billing statements sent and increases collections. Never allow a patient to

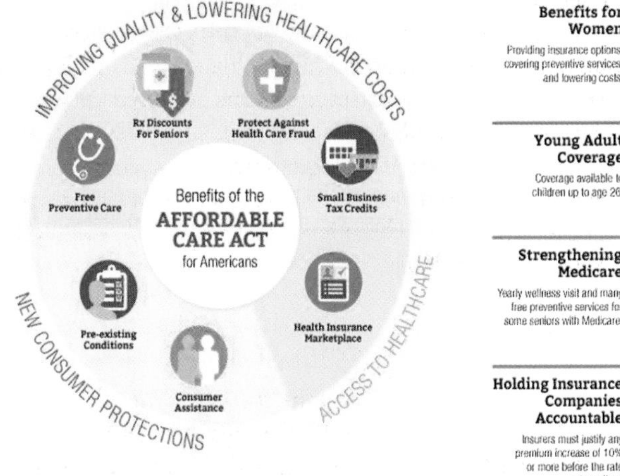
IMPROVING QUALITY & LOWERING HEALTHCARE COSTS
Rx Discounts For Seniors
Protect Against Health Care Fraud
Free Preventive Care
Small Business Tax Credits
Benefits of the
AFFORDABLE CARE ACT
for Americans
Pre-existing Conditions
Health Insurance Marketplace
Consumer Assistance
NEW CONSUMER PROTECTIONS
ACCESS TO HEALTHCARE
Benefits for Women
Providing insurance options, covering preventive services, and lowering costs.
Young Adult Coverage
Coverage available to children up to age 26.
Strengthening Medicare
Yearly wellness visit and many free preventive services for some seniors with Medicare.
Holding Insurance Companies Accountable
Insurers must justify any premium increase of 10% or more before the rate takes effect.

Fig. 17.2 The Affordable Care Act is focused on improving quality of patient care, reducing costs of health care, protecting patients' right to access care, and other consumer protections.

believe that he or she is not responsible for the bill; some medical offices prefer to post a sign stating the office policy (Fig. 17.3). Discuss copayment requirements with patients who are enrolled in managed care plans and convey the organization's policy of collecting this amount when registering the patient for services. A new-patient information pamphlet or brochure and confirmation letter (Fig. 17.4) may be e-mailed as an attachment or sent to welcome the new patient to the health care organization. This

YOUR CO-PAY IS
EXPECTED AT THE TIME
OF SERVICE, UNLESS
PRIOR FINANCIAL
ARRANGEMENTS
HAVE BEEN MADE.

Fig. 17.3 Signs for payment like this are commonly found in the health care organization.

message or letter informs the patient about the organization, clearly outlines payment expectations, provides collection policies and procedures in printed form, includes a missed appointment clause, establishes a contact person, invites questions, and confirms all specific details discussed.

Patient Registration Form

There is no substitution for good information-gathering techniques at the time of initial patient registration because this assists later in billing and collection. Always obtain complete and accurate demographic and identifying information from the patient on the first encounter to the health care organization. Confirm the accuracy of that information on each subsequent encounter. For commercial insurance plans, have the guarantor agree in writing to pay for all medical treatment. By obtaining the guarantor's signature, he or she is then bound by contract to pay the bill.

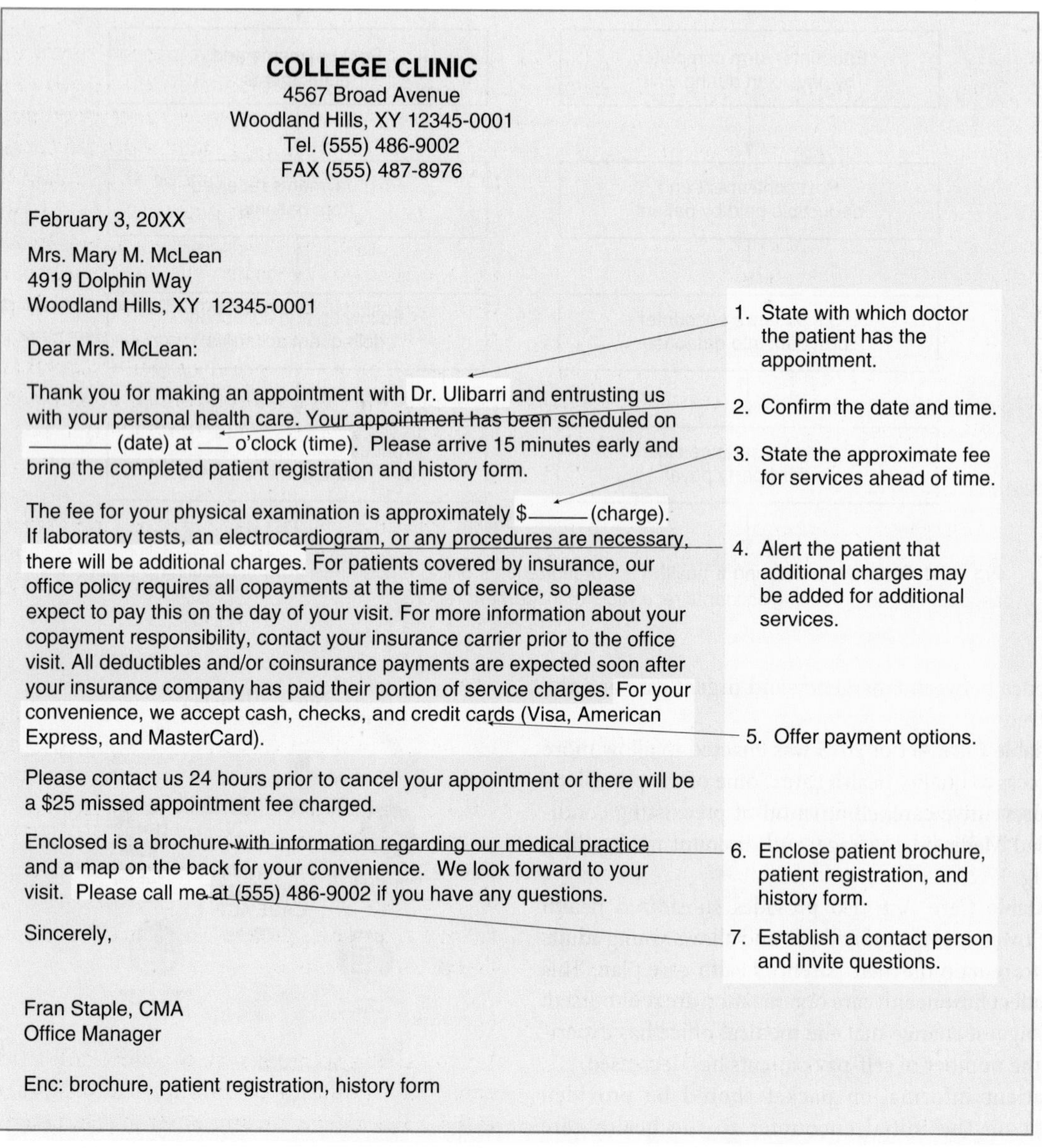

COLLEGE CLINIC
4567 Broad Avenue
Woodland Hills, XY 12345-0001
Tel. (555) 486-9002
FAX (555) 487-8976

February 3, 20XX

Mrs. Mary M. McLean
4919 Dolphin Way
Woodland Hills, XY 12345-0001

Dear Mrs. McLean:

Thank you for making an appointment with Dr. Ulibarri and entrusting us with your personal health care. Your appointment has been scheduled on ______ (date) at ___ o'clock (time). Please arrive 15 minutes early and bring the completed patient registration and history form.

The fee for your physical examination is approximately $______ (charge). If laboratory tests, an electrocardiogram, or any procedures are necessary, there will be additional charges. For patients covered by insurance, our office policy requires all copayments at the time of service, so please expect to pay this on the day of your visit. For more information about your copayment responsibility, contact your insurance carrier prior to the office visit. All deductibles and/or coinsurance payments are expected soon after your insurance company has paid their portion of service charges. For your convenience, we accept cash, checks, and credit cards (Visa, American Express, and MasterCard).

Please contact us 24 hours prior to cancel your appointment or there will be a $25 missed appointment fee charged.

Enclosed is a brochure with information regarding our medical practice and a map on the back for your convenience. We look forward to your visit. Please call me at (555) 486-9002 if you have any questions.

Sincerely,

Fran Staple, CMA
Office Manager

Enc: brochure, patient registration, history form

Fig. 17.4 New patient confirmation letter emphasizing information to incorporate when writing to a new patient.

Learn as much as possible about the patient before any services are provided. This is when the patient is likely to be the most cooperative. Information provided on the patient information sheet will prove critical to any billing and collection efforts. The patient should be instructed to answer all questions and indicate any spaces on the form that do not apply by marking N/A (not applicable). A helpful tip is to assist the patient to focus on vital information needed by using a yellow highlighter and blocking all necessary information. One field often overlooked is the subscriber information and date of birth, even though dependents may have insurance cards issued in their name. Reviewing the completed patient information sheet ensures that all blanks have been addressed and accurate information has been collected. It also alerts office staff of an account that may be a future problem. Items often overlooked are the street address, when a post office box is given; an apartment or mobile home park number; a cellphone number; and a business telephone number with department and extension. These help the insurance billing specialist to trace a patient who has moved. If a patient refuses to divulge any information, invoking privacy laws, it should be policy to require payment for services at the time that care is rendered. A potential nonpaying patient may be recognized at this time. Some indications to look for include the following:

- Incomplete information on the registration form
- Multiple changes of residence
- Questionable employment record
- No telephone numbers (business, cell, or home)
- Post office box listed with no street address
- A motel address
- Incomplete insurance information or no insurance coverage
- No referral information or authorization from a primary care physician (PCP) for patients enrolled in a managed care plan

Employers are changing health plans with increasing frequency and patients are more transient than ever, so update this form each time the patient is seen. This can be done by printing out a data sheet or having the patient review a copy of their registration form. The patient should sign or initial any changes or corrections.

FEES

Fee Schedule

Most health care organizations operate with a set of fees that must be applied uniformly to all patients receiving services. Health care organizations set their own fees, and they are generally based on the Medicare fee schedule. As discussed in previous chapters, a fee schedule is a listing of accepted charges or established allowances for specific medical procedures. Always quote fees and state policies about the collection of fees to the patient at the initial encounter. Under federal regulations, a list of the most common services the health care organization offers, including procedure code numbers with a description of each service and its price, must be available to all patients.

Missed Appointments

Missed appointments are expensive for health care organizations, so patients should be informed of the importance of keeping appointments. The medical staff should inform patients from the very first encounter about the missed appointment fee, which is typically $35 to $50. Regardless of the type of insurance the patient carries, he or she should be held responsible for the fee if the appointment is missed without calling in. Missed appointment charges should not be billed to the insurance company; the patient is responsible for these fees regardless of the insurance he or she carries. To avoid possible discrimination or civil rights violations, ensure that the missed appointment fee is applied to all patients within the health care organization.

Some health care organizations hold a specific 24- to 48-hour appointment cancellation policy. As a professional courtesy to patients, staff should call or contact patients to remind them of the date and time of the appointment just before this cancellation period. The staff should also inform the patient of the cancellation fee if the patient was to miss the appointment.

Fee Adjustments

Discounted Fees

A health care organization may choose to discount its fees, but this practice is ill-advised and may be illegal in some circumstances. A discount is a reduction of the normal fee based on a specific amount of money or a percentage of the charge. When a health care organization offers a discount, it must apply to the total bill, not just the portion that is paid by the patient (copayment or coinsurance amount). By following this rule, the health care provider is giving a discount to both the patient and the insurance company. The same discount must be given to each member of the insurance plan. This practice could reduce the health care organization's payment schedule with the insurance company and trigger a reduction in the organization's allowable reimbursement schedule. Consequently, the health care organization should weigh the long-term outcome of discounting fees. All discounts must be electronically posted to the patient's financial accounting record (ledger) and any financial reasons or special circumstances should be documented in the patient's health record. This ensures complete record keeping and safeguards any questions that may be asked during a financial audit.

Cash Discounts

Cash discounts may be offered to patients who pay the entire fee, in cash, at the time of service (Fig. 17.5). If a cash discount system is offered, this policy should be posted in the medical office and every active patient sent notification. Research your state laws because some states do not allow cash discounts; check the health care organization's insurance contracts to determine whether they are affected. Also, refer to the health care organization's compliance protocol to ensure that any such discounts do not implicate fraud.

Financial Hardship

Financial hardship cases are the most difficult for the health care organization to determine. The insurance billing specialist should never assume anything about a patient's financial status, nor judge a patient's ability to pay based on his or her appearance. The Department of Health and Human

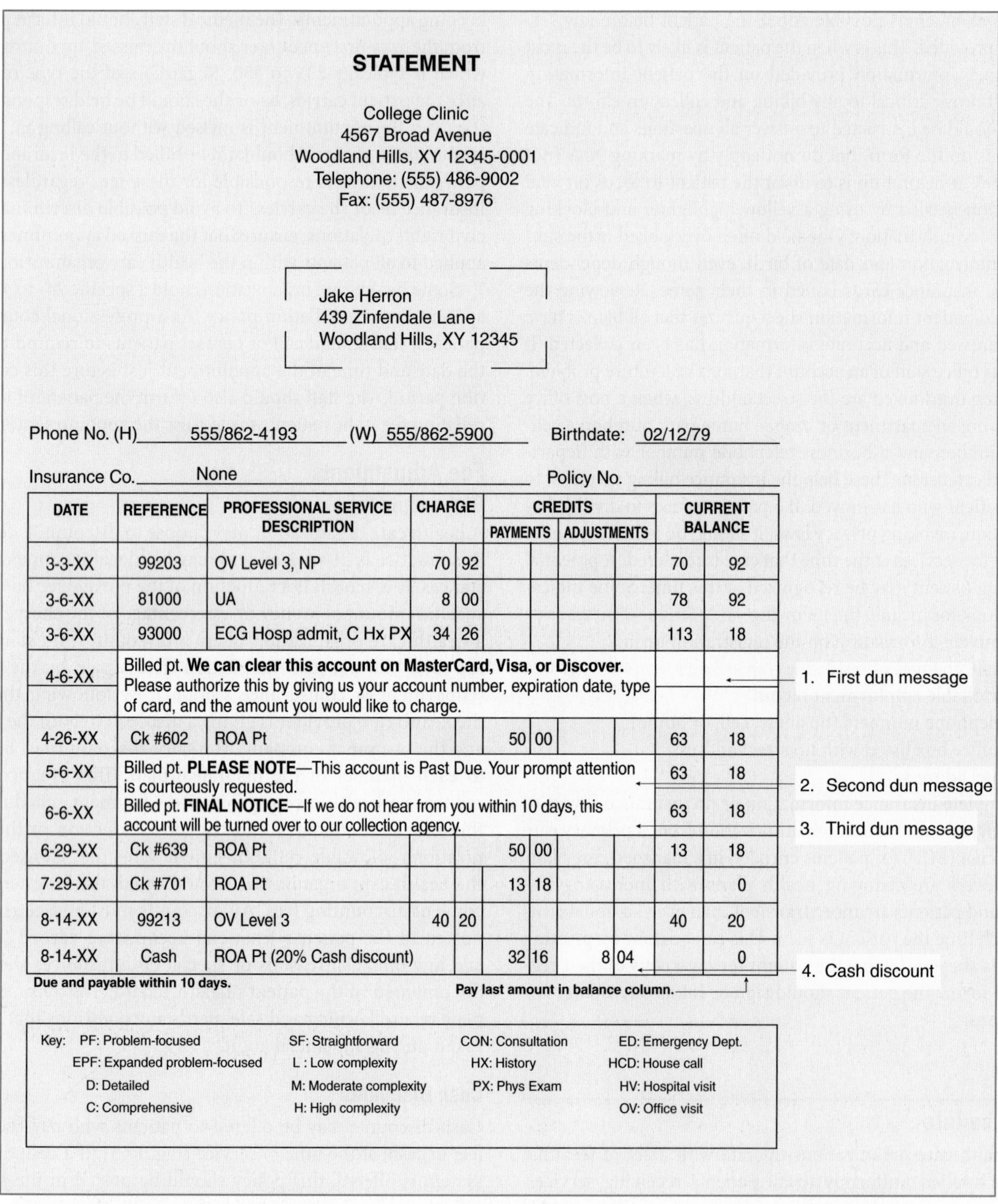

STATEMENT

College Clinic
4567 Broad Avenue
Woodland Hills, XY 12345-0001
Telephone: (555) 486-9002
Fax: (555) 487-8976

Jake Herron
439 Zinfendale Lane
Woodland Hills, XY 12345

Phone No. (H) 555/862-4193 (W) 555/862-5900 Birthdate: 02/12/79

Insurance Co. None Policy No.

DATE	REFERENCE	PROFESSIONAL SERVICE DESCRIPTION	CHARGE		CREDITS PAYMENTS		CREDITS ADJUSTMENTS		CURRENT BALANCE	
3-3-XX	99203	OV Level 3, NP	70	92					70	92
3-6-XX	81000	UA	8	00					78	92
3-6-XX	93000	ECG Hosp admit, C Hx PX	34	26					113	18
4-6-XX	Billed pt. **We can clear this account on MasterCard, Visa, or Discover.** Please authorize this by giving us your account number, expiration date, type of card, and the amount you would like to charge.									
4-26-XX	Ck #602	ROA Pt			50	00			63	18
5-6-XX	Billed pt. **PLEASE NOTE**—This account is Past Due. Your prompt attention is courteously requested.								63	18
6-6-XX	Billed pt. **FINAL NOTICE**—If we do not hear from you within 10 days, this account will be turned over to our collection agency.								63	18
6-29-XX	Ck #639	ROA Pt			50	00			13	18
7-29-XX	Ck #701	ROA Pt			13	18				0
8-14-XX	99213	OV Level 3	40	20					40	20
8-14-XX	Cash	ROA Pt (20% Cash discount)			32	16	8	04		0

Due and payable within 10 days.

Pay last amount in balance column.

Key: PF: Problem-focused; EPF: Expanded problem-focused; D: Detailed; C: Comprehensive; SF: Straightforward; L: Low complexity; M: Moderate complexity; H: High complexity; CON: Consultation; HX: History; PX: Phys Exam; ED: Emergency Dept.; HCD: House call; HV: Hospital visit; OV: Office visit

Fig. 17.5 Electronic hard copy of a patient's financial accounting record showing dun messages, posted payments, and cash discount.

Services (DHHS) annually publishes a guideline on poverty income (Fig. 17.6), which is used to determine eligibility for uncompensated services under the Hill-Burton, Community Services Block Grant, and Head Start programs. Health care organizations may choose to follow these guidelines to direct patients to government-sponsored programs, obtain public assistance, and determine who is eligible for a hardship waiver. A hardship waiver can vary from 25% to 100% of the bill. Various financial forms are available to obtain this information; a copy of the patient's wage and tax statement (W2) or income tax return should be examined to make a reliable decision. The patient also should sign a written explanation to verify true financial hardship. This helps in the collection process and allows the health care organization to accept the insurance as payment in full, in certain circumstances, without being suspected of insurance fraud. The reason for a fee reduction must be documented in the patient's health record. Very large medical organizations or

HHS POVERTY GUIDELINES FOR 2017

The 2017 poverty guidelines are in effect as of January 26, 2017.See also the Federal Register notice of the 2017 poverty guidelines, published January 31, 2017

2017 POVERTY GUIDELINES FOR THE 48 CONTIGUOUS STATES AND THE DISTRICT OF COLUMBIA	
PERSONS IN FAMILY/HOUSEHOLD	POVERTY GUIDELINE
For families/households with more than 8 persons, add $4,180 for each additional person.	
1	$12,060
2	$16,240
3	$20,420
4	$24,600
5	$28,780
6	$32,960
7	$37,140
8	$41,320

2017 POVERTY GUIDELINES FOR ALASKA	
PERSONS IN FAMILY/HOUSEHOLD	POVERTY GUIDELINE
For families/households with more than 8 persons, add $5,230 for each additional person.	

2017 POVERTY GUIDELINES FOR ALASKA	
PERSONS IN FAMILY/HOUSEHOLD	POVERTY GUIDELINE
1	$15,060
2	$20,290
3	$25,520
4	$30,750
5	$35,980
6	$41,210
7	$46,440
8	$51,670

2017 POVERTY GUIDELINES FOR HAWAII	
PERSONS IN FAMILY/HOUSEHOLD	POVERTY GUIDELINE
For families/households with morethan 8 persons, add $4,810 for each additional person.	
1	$13,860
2	$18,670
3	$23,480

Fig. 17.6 Department of Health and Human Services (DHHS) 2017 guidelines on poverty income. (From Office of the Assistant Secretary for Planning and Evaluation. HHS poverty guidelines for 2017. Available at http://aspe.hhs.gov.)

medical offices whose services may not be covered by insurance can create and use a sliding scale fee schedule based on federal poverty levels, and patients pay according to their financial situation.

Be careful about giving a discount because it can be construed as discriminatory if not given to other patients consistently. To avoid problems, develop a written policy about what qualifies a patient for a financial hardship discount.

Write-Off or Courtesy Adjustment

A write-off, or *courtesy adjustment,* is a debt that has been determined to be uncollectable and is taken off (subtracted/credited) the accounting books. It is considered lost income but may not be claimed as a loss for tax purposes. The insurance billing specialist should obtain financial information on all patients who request a write-off. Office policies about adjustments and all discounts should be in writing, and all staff members should be informed. Write-off policies should clearly state who must approve all discounts, adjustments, and special payment arrangements before patient contract signature.

! COMPLIANCE ALERT

Compliance Guidelines for Deviations From Standard Collection Procedures

The Office of the Inspector General issued guidance to health care organizations that they are free to use whatever policy they want on charity care, discounts, write-offs, and collections, as long as it is done consistently and the reasons for granting these are documented in the organization's compliance manual. Ensure that these deviations from standard collection procedures are not tied to or conditional on referrals or use of the provider's services. The policy must also state the minimum effort in collection of debts, such as one or more letters or telephone calls. The health care organization that uses minimum collection efforts can waive the obligations of patients in financial need in accordance with office policy and try to collect more aggressively from other patients who are not financially needy.

The health care organization must appoint a designated individual to approve the portion of the charge to be credited to the financial record before the debt is forgiven. A write-off is possible in three circumstances. The first is as stated in the preceding discussion, when the patient has proved a financial hardship.

2017 POVERTY GUIDELINES FOR HAWAII	
PERSONS IN FAMILY/HOUSEHOLD	POVERTY GUIDELINE
4	$28,290
5	$33,100
6	$37,910
7	$42,720
8	$47,530

The separate poverty guidelines for Alaska and Hawaii reflect Office of Economic Opportunity administrative practice beginning in the 1966-1970 period. Note that the poverty thresholds — the original version of the poverty measure — have never had separate figures for Alaska and Hawaii. The poverty guidelines are not defined for Puerto Rico, the U.S. Virgin Islands, American Samoa, Guam, the Republic of the Marshall Islands, the Federated States of Micronesia, the Commonwealth of the Northern Mariana Islands, and Palau. In cases in which a Federal program using the poverty guidelines serves any of those jurisdictions, the Federal office which administers the program is responsible for deciding whether to use the contiguous-states-and-D.C. guidelines for those jurisdictions or to follow some other procedure.

The poverty guidelines apply to both aged and non-aged units. The guidelines have never had an aged/non-aged distinction; only the Census Bureau (statistical) poverty thresholds have separate figures for aged and non-aged one-person and two-person units.

Programs using the guidelines (or percentage multiples of the guidelines — for instance, 125 percent or 185 percent of the guidelines) in determining eligibility include Head Start, the Supplemental Nutition Assistance Program (SNAP), the National School Lunch Program, the Low-Income Home Energy Assistance Program, and the Children's Health Insurance Program. Note that in general, cash public assistance programs (Temporary Assistance for Needy Families and Supplemental Security Income) do NOT use the poverty guidelines in determining eligibility. The Earned Income Tax Credit program also does NOT use the poverty guidelines to determine eligibility. For a more detailed list of programs that do and don't use the guidelines, see the Frequently Asked Questions (FAQs).

The poverty guidelines (unlike the poverty thresholds) are designated by the year in which they are issued. For instance, the guidelines issued in January 2016 are designated the 2016 poverty guidelines. However, the 2016 HHS poverty guidelines only reflect price changes through calendar year 2015; accordingly, they are approximately equal to the Census Bureau poverty thresholds for calendar year 2015. (The 2015 thresholds are expected to be issued in final form in September 2016; a preliminary version of the 2015 thresholds is now available from the Census Bureau.)

The poverty guidelines may be formally referenced as "the poverty guidelines updated periodically in the Federal Register by the U.S.Department of Health and Human Services under the authority of 42 U.S.C. 9902(2)."

Fig. 17.6, cont'd.

The second is when it will cost more to bill the balance than what is owed. For example, the balance may be $1.05. It will cost the health care organization more than this amount to collect the balance. This type of write-off is known as a *small balance write-off.* The third situation is when the health care organization has made a good faith effort to collect the balance with no success. In this case the balance is written off and the account may or may not be sent to a professional collection agency depending on whether the agency accepts balances less than, for example, $35 for collection.

Professional Courtesy

Professional courtesy is a concept attributed to Hippocrates, but the foundations are derived from Thomas Percival's *Code of Medical Ethics,* written in 1803. The *American Medical Association (AMA) Code of Ethics,* formulated and adopted in 1847, closely mirrored Percival's code. The practice of professional courtesy served to build bonds between health care providers and reduce the incentive for providers to treat their own families. Most health care providers agree that one of the greatest honors and privileges in the practice of medicine is to be asked to care for another health care provider or a provider's family members. The practice of professional courtesy often was extended to others in the health care profession and members of the clergy. Now most health care providers have insurance coverage for medical expenses. Consequently, most hospitals and health care organizations have given up the practice of free care through professional courtesy.

Professional courtesy means either a discount or an exemption from charges that may be given to certain people at the discretion of the provider rendering the service.

An interim rule from the Centers for Medicare and Medicaid Services (CMS), effective September 5, 2007, identifies proper ways to offer professional courtesy.

1. The professional courtesy is offered to all health care providers on the entity's bona fide medical staff or in the entity's local community or service area without regard to volume or value of referrals or other business generated between the parties.
2. The health care items and services provided are of a type routinely provided by the entity.
3. The entity's professional courtesy policy is written and approved in advance by the entity's governing body.
4. The professional courtesy is not offered to a health care provider (or immediate family member) who is a federal health care program beneficiary unless there has been a good faith showing of financial need.
5. If the professional courtesy involves any whole or partial reduction of any coinsurance obligation, the insurer is informed in writing of the reduction.
6. The arrangement does not violate the Anti-Kickback statute (section 1128B[b] of the Act) or any federal or state law or regulation governing billing or claims submission.

Health care organizations must examine their policies on professional courtesy to ensure that they do not violate the contractual terms in private, managed care, or government-sponsored insurance policies. If the treating provider does not bill the health care provider–patient for services rendered, the third-party payer is relieved of its contractual obligation. If the treating provider waives the deductible and copayment, he or she may be accused of not treating others with the same insurance coverage in an equal manner. Although there may be some situations in which it is defensible to not charge for services to health care professionals, the health care organization should ensure that this professional courtesy is not linked to patients who have been referred. Laws prohibit any inducement or kickbacks from health care organizations or physicians that could influence the decision of a service provider to refer patients or that may affect a patient's decision to seek care.

! COMPLIANCE ALERT

Professional Courtesy Guidelines

Professional courtesy may violate fraud and abuse laws depending on how the recipients of the professional courtesy are selected and how the courtesy is extended. If selection depends on referral of individuals, it may implicate the Anti-Kickback statute. An insurance claim submitted as a result of such a professional courtesy may also be affected by the False Claims Act.

Copayment Waiver

Waiving copayments is another way that health care organizations have reduced the cost of medical care for patients in the past. In doing so, the organization accepts the insurance payment only. In most situations, both private insurers and the federal government ban waiving the copayment, so it is not recommended. Waiving copayments could violate the contract between the patient and third-party payer. If the health care organization has contracted with a third-party payer, waiving the copayment may be a violation of the insurance contract. Some insurance companies look at this as a means of recouping its losses by undergoing litigation against the health care organization or demanding the return of all payments made to the service provider.

No Charge

No charge (NC) means waiving the entire fee for professional care. This is permitted as long as it is not part of a fraudulent scheme and is offered to all patients. All NC services must be fully documented in the clinical portion of the patient's health record.

No charge situations may occur on a patient's account when follow-up visits are posted after a patient undergoes surgery considered under a surgical package or Medicare global fee structure. When posting such charges in a medical billing system, *Current Procedural Terminology* (CPT) code 99024 (postoperative follow-up visit included in global fee) may be used.

Reduced Fee

Precautions should be taken before reducing the fee of a patient who dies. The health care organization's sympathy in this case could be misinterpreted and result in a malpractice suit. A fee reduction should never be based on a poor result in the treatment of a patient.

If a patient disputes a fee and the health care organization agrees to settle for a reduced fee, the agreement should be in writing in the patient account file.

! COMPLIANCE ALERT

Discussion of Financial Matters With Patients

Because the patient's financial history is personal, conversations about fees must be private so that other individuals cannot overhear. The patient should be made to feel comfortable so that he or she feels free to discuss any financial problems. Be firm. Use tact. Always use a courteous but businesslike approach when discussing financial matters.

Discussing Fees

People have a difficult time asking each other for money and talking about financial obligations. Financial arrangements should be discussed up front and in great detail before any services are provided. Many health care organizations create their own collection problems by not being clear about how and when they expect to be paid. If patients are not told that payment is due at the time of service, most assume they can pay at a later time. Patients are unaware of additional absorbed services given to patients during an encounter. Fig. 17.7 presents a detailed description of some of those tasks that may be pointed out to patients so that they have a better understanding of the time expended by the health care provider and staff. The following are some guidelines to help communicate effectively about money.

1. Be courteous at all times but express a firm, businesslike approach that will not offend the patient.
2. Never badger or intimidate a patient into paying; merely state the payment policy and educate the patient.

ABSORBED MEDICAL SERVICES

- ✔ Create and maintain patient's permanent medical records.
- ✔ Order, review/interpret, document/file, and telephone laboratory test results to the patient.
- ✔ Order x-rays, review/interpret, compare with previous studies if abnormal, consult with radiologist, document/file, and telephone results to the patient.
- ✔ Write and send consultation reports/letters to referring or consulting physicians and other providers.
- ✔ Telephone consultations with physicians.
- ✔ Complete family medical leave forms, disability forms, waivers for handicapped plates, waivers of insurance premiums, automotive forms, life insurance premium forms, travel insurance forms, and school, camp, or athletic participation forms.
- ✔ E-mail responses to patients.
- ✔ Write letters of referral to specialists.
- ✔ Create patient education materials.
- ✔ Conduct medical research pertinent to the patient's case.
- ✔ Write prescriptions and communicate with pharmacies about patients' prescriptions.
- ✔ Transmit (or complete) patients' insurance claim forms and complete insurance application forms.
- ✔ Conduct utilization review negotiations with hospitals and insurance companies.
- ✔ Review and maintain documentation for patients' hospital medical records.
- ✔ Write medical orders for hospitalized patients and orders for those in nursing facilities.
- ✔ Write letters to obtain medical services, instruments, or equipment for patients.
- ✔ Arrange for hospital admissions and follow-up consultations with nurses and other physicians.

Fig. 17.7 Details of additional absorbed medical services the health care organization and staff give to patients during an encounter, depending on the complexity of a medical problem.

3. Inform patients of their full financial responsibility and balance due in a clear manner.
4. Verify the patient's copayment listed on his or her insurance card and collect this amount before the patient's encounter for services.
5. Make it easier for patients to pay rather than leave without making payment.
6. Do not give patients an option by asking if they would like to pay now or have a bill sent.
7. Motivate patients to pay by appealing to their honesty, integrity, and pride.

The following are examples of communicating in a positive manner and letting the patient know exactly what is expected:

- "Today's services are $62, Mrs. Smith. Would you like to pay by cash, check, credit card, or debit card?"
- "Your copayment for today's service is $20, Mr. Jones, and you can pay by cash, check, credit card, or debit card."
- "Your insurance policy shows a $100 deductible that is your responsibility and currently has not been met, Miss Rodriguez. You must pay the full fee today, which is $100."
- "Mrs. Merryweather, I must collect $4.77 today for your vitamin B_{12} injection. The injection is not covered by your insurance policy."
- "We look forward to seeing you on Tuesday, March 3, at 10 AM, Mr. Gillespie. The consultation fee will be approximately $150 and payment is expected at the time of service. We accept cash, check, credit cards, or debit cards for your convenience."

Collecting Fees

Payment at the Time of Service

Collecting applicable copayments and other amounts due from the patient at each health care encounter is strongly recommended. To avoid difficulties in collecting at a future date, ask for fixed copayments before the patient is seen by the provider. This will alleviate billing for small amounts. The importance of collecting outstanding bills, coinsurance amounts, and money from cash-paying patients up front should be communicated to office staff. One-on-one communication is the best way to motivate a debtor. Each patient's account balance (amount due) should

PROCEDURE 17.1 Create a Financial Agreement With a Patient

Objective

To assist the patient in making credit arrangements by completing and signing a Truth in Lending form

Equipment/Supplies

Patient's financial accounting record (ledger), calendar, Truth in Lending form, typewriter or computer, calculator, and quiet private room

Directions

Follow the step-by-step procedures, which include rationales, to learn this job skill. An assignment is presented in the *Workbook* to practice this skill.

1. Explain the patient's balance due and answer questions about credit.
2. Inform the patient of the health care organization's office policy about extending credit payments.
3. Discuss an installment plan concerning the amount of the total debt, the down payment, the amount and date of each installment, and the date of final payment.
4. Subtract the down payment from the total debt. Divide the remaining amount by the number of months the debt is being carried to determine the monthly installment amounts and the date of final payment.
5. Complete a Truth in Lending form after mutually agreeing on the terms if the payments require more than four installments. This procedure complies with Regulation Z.
6. Review the completed Truth in Lending form with the patient.
7. Ask the patient to sign the Truth in Lending form.
8. Make a photocopy of the Truth in Lending form for the patient to retain.
9. File the original Truth in Lending form in the patient's financial file in the office.

be reviewed before his or her appointment. If the appointment schedule is on a computer system, print the account balance by each patient's name. If an appointment book is used, make a copy of the page showing the day's schedule. Write overdue balances by the patient's name after obtaining overdue amounts from each patient's financial accounting record. This information also should be recorded on the transaction slip for that day's encounter and may be "flagged" when the transaction slips are printed or written. Treat this information confidentially, and keep it out of view of other patients. When a patient arrives whose name is flagged, alert the patient accounts manager.

To do effective preappointment collection counseling, the patient should be taken to a quiet area away from the general activity of the office. Sit down with the patient and discuss the situation. Use an understanding attitude and helpful nature while verbalizing phrases such as "I understand" and "I can help." Ask direct questions to learn exactly what problems the patient is facing. Answers to questions such as "When do you expect your next paycheck?" and "How much are you able to pay today?" help to determine the strategy. The goal should be to collect the full amount. If that is not possible, try to collect a portion of the balance. Get a promise to pay for the remaining balance by a specific date. If the patient is unable to comply, set up a payment plan. The chances of reaching a mutually satisfactory resolution are greatly improved when the two parties are face to face. Refer to Procedure 17.1 to create a financial agreement with the patient.

A face-to-face interview is better than a telephone interview because a financial agreement can be signed when the debtor is present (Fig. 17.8), resulting in a better follow-up response. Let the patient know that the health care organization is willing to help and that the debtor should inform the insurance billing specialist if he or she runs into further problems making the payment. This personal contact helps if a renegotiation of the agreement is necessary. A health care organization cannot refuse to let an established patient see the doctor because of a debt, but the office staff has every right to ask for payment while the patient is in the office.

Encounter Forms

Multipurpose billing forms are known by many names, including *encounter form*. These forms are helpful when collecting fees at the time of service. Encounter forms can be given to patients to bill their insurance companies, used to inform patients of current charges and outstanding balances, and used as receipts for payment (Fig. 17.9).

Patient Excuses for Nonpayments

Nonpayers tend to dismiss financial arrangements with curt remarks. Look directly at the patient, confidently expecting payment. Demonstrate to the patient the right to request payment. Be ready if excuses are offered. Table 17.1 shows examples of patients' excuses and possible responses.

When a patient chatters nervously, it may be a way of setting up reasons to rationalize not paying. Do not let this be distracting. Pause after asking for payment and do not say another word until the patient responds. Many people feel uncomfortable with silence, but pauses may be advantageous and help to complete a transaction. The cash flow and collection ratio are increased by taking this approach, while billing chores and collection costs are decreased. The quick identification of nonpayers may be obtained and the person responsible for collections notified.

Credit and Debit Cards

The current economic trend is heading toward the use of credit and debit cards. Patients find these easier to use and tend to always have them on hand. Accepting credit cards can improve a health care organization's financial management in many ways:

- Lower risk of embezzlement by current employees
- Fewer trips to the banks for deposit; funds are electronically transferred to the health care organization's account
- Fewer concerns about check fraud
- Convenient for patients

Credit card payment is an option that provides patients with an alternative to clear their account balances. Credit cards are issued by organizations that entitle the cardholder to credit at their establishments. This method of payment may be most useful as a down payment on uninsured or elective procedures. According to a survey by American Express, 33% of patients said they would use a credit card to pay for health care–related expenses if the option were given. Credit cards can help to manage A/R by improving cash flow, reducing billing costs, lowering overhead, and reducing the risk of bad debts. If a health

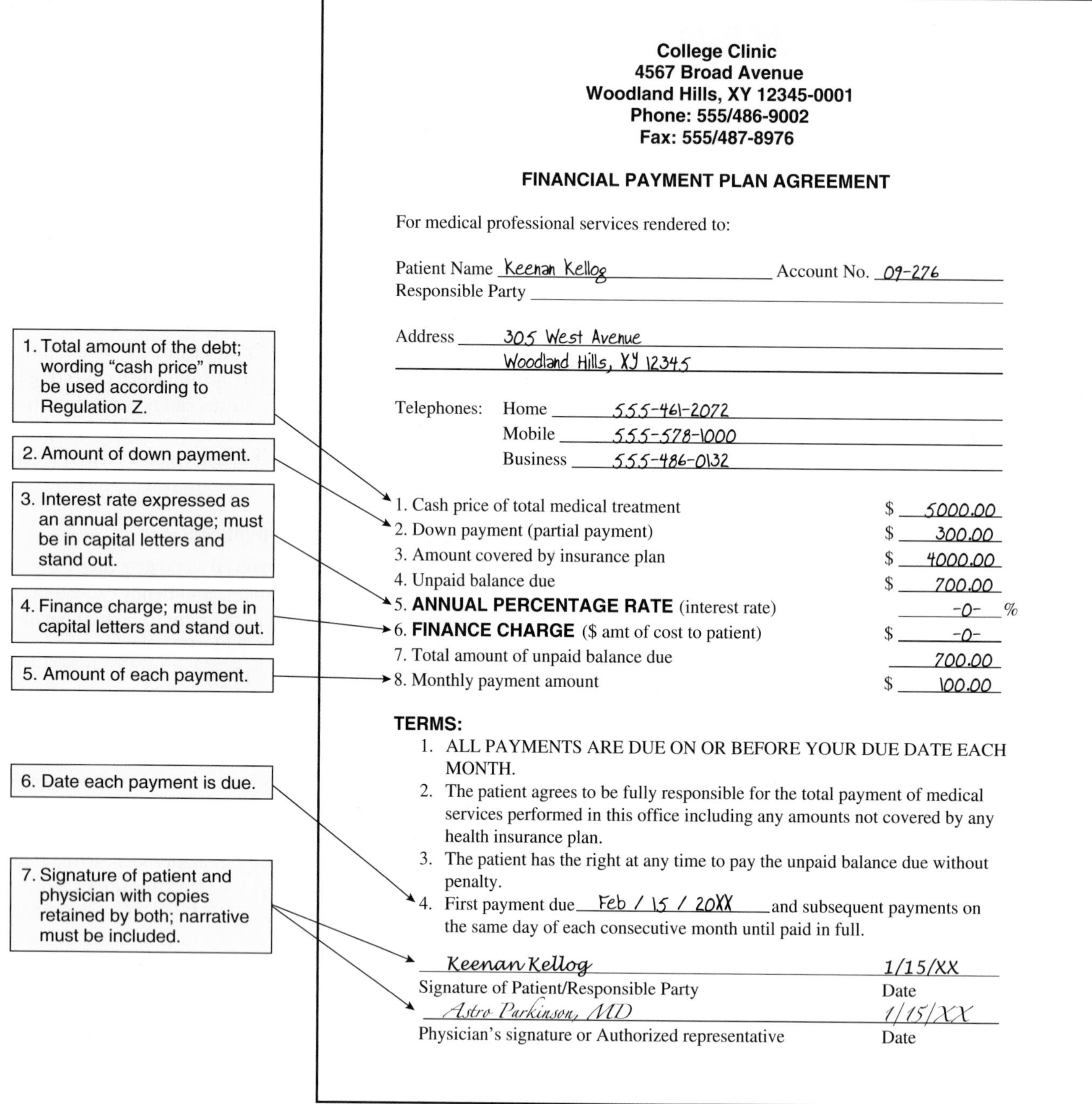
College Clinic
4567 Broad Avenue
Woodland Hills, XY 12345-0001
Phone: 555/486-9002
Fax: 555/487-8976

FINANCIAL PAYMENT PLAN AGREEMENT

For medical professional services rendered to:

Patient Name Keenan Kellog Account No. 09-276
Responsible Party

Address 305 West Avenue
Woodland Hills, XY 12345

Telephones: Home 555-461-2072
Mobile 555-578-1000
Business 555-486-0132

1. Cash price of total medical treatment $ 5000.00
2. Down payment (partial payment) $ 300.00
3. Amount covered by insurance plan $ 4000.00
4. Unpaid balance due $ 700.00
5. **ANNUAL PERCENTAGE RATE** (interest rate) -0- %
6. **FINANCE CHARGE** ($ amt of cost to patient) $ -0-
7. Total amount of unpaid balance due 700.00
8. Monthly payment amount $ 100.00

TERMS:
1. ALL PAYMENTS ARE DUE ON OR BEFORE YOUR DUE DATE EACH MONTH.
2. The patient agrees to be fully responsible for the total payment of medical services performed in this office including any amounts not covered by any health insurance plan.
3. The patient has the right at any time to pay the unpaid balance due without penalty.
4. First payment due Feb / 15 / 20XX and subsequent payments on the same day of each consecutive month until paid in full.

Keenan Kellog 1/15/XX
Signature of Patient/Responsible Party Date
Astro Parkinson, MD 1/15/XX
Physician's signature or Authorized representative Date

Fig. 17.8 Financial payment plan agreement that provides full disclosure of all information by the Truth in Lending Act, Regulation Z.

care organization accepts credit cards, advise all patients in the following ways:

- Display a credit card acceptance sign.
- Include an insignia or message on the patient account statement.
- Include the credit card policy in the new patient brochure or new patient welcome letter.
- Have staff members verbalize to patients that this option is available.

Patients may prefer to clear a debt immediately and make monthly payments to the credit card company instead of owing money to their service provider.

Verifying Credit Cards

The insurance billing specialist should check credit card warning bulletins to ensure that the card has not been canceled or stolen. Large health care organizations may have an electronic credit card machine that allows the insurance billing specialist to swipe the card through the machine, which is linked to the credit card company. Transactions are then approved, processed, and deposited in a bank account, usually in 2 working days. A receipt is generated for the patient.

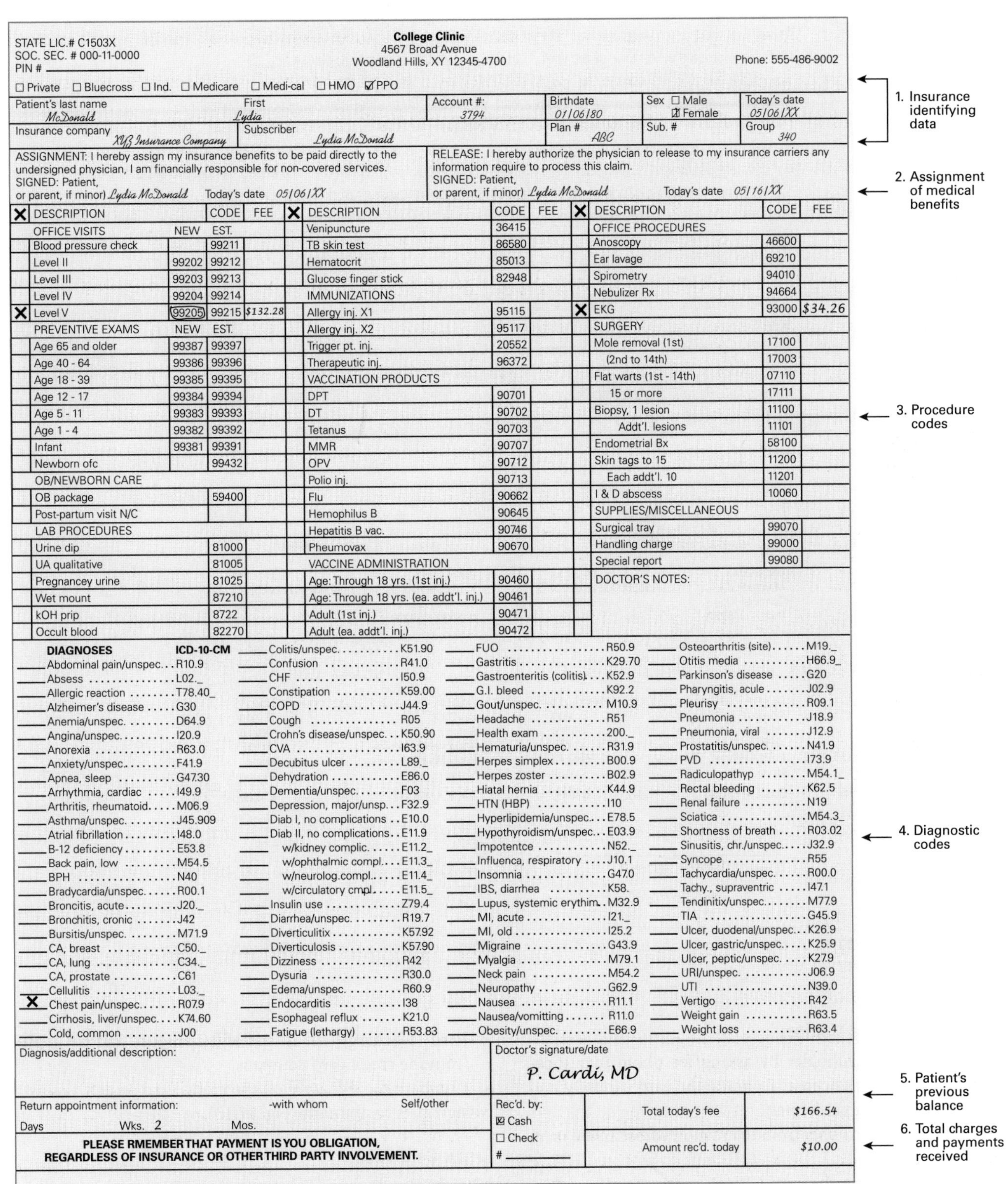

STATE LIC.# C1503X
SOC. SEC. # 000-11-0000
PIN # ______

College Clinic
4567 Broad Avenue
Woodland Hills, XY 12345-4700

Phone: 555-486-9002

☐ Private ☐ Bluecross ☐ Ind. ☐ Medicare ☐ Medi-cal ☐ HMO ☑ PPO

Patient's last name	First	Account #:	Birthdate	Sex	Today's date
McDonald	*Lydia*	*3794*	*01/06/80*	☐ Male ☒ Female	*05/06/XX*

Insurance company	Subscriber	Plan #	Sub. #	Group
XYZ Insurance Company	*Lydia McDonald*	*ABC*		*340*

ASSIGNMENT: I hereby assign my insurance benefits to be paid directly to the undersigned physician, I am financially responsible for non-covered services. SIGNED: Patient, or parent, if minor) *Lydia McDonald* Today's date *05/06/XX*

RELEASE: I hereby authorize the physician to release to my insurance carriers any information require to process this claim. SIGNED: Patient, or parent, if minor) *Lydia McDonald* Today's date *05/16/XX*

X	DESCRIPTION		CODE	FEE
	OFFICE VISITS	NEW	EST.	
	Blood pressure check		99211	
	Level II	99202	99212	
	Level III	99203	99213	
	Level IV	99204	99214	
X	Level V	(99205)	99215	*$132.28*
	PREVENTIVE EXAMS	NEW	EST.	
	Age 65 and older	99387	99397	
	Age 40 - 64	99386	99396	
	Age 18 - 39	99385	99395	
	Age 12 - 17	99384	99394	
	Age 5 - 11	99383	99393	
	Age 1 - 4	99382	99392	
	Infant	99381	99391	
	Newborn ofc		99432	
	OB/NEWBORN CARE			
	OB package		59400	
	Post-partum visit N/C			
	LAB PROCEDURES			
	Urine dip		81000	
	UA qualitative		81005	
	Pregnancey urine		81025	
	Wet mount		87210	
	kOH prip		8722	
	Occult blood		82270	

X	DESCRIPTION	CODE	FEE
	Venipuncture	36415	
	TB skin test	86580	
	Hematocrit	85013	
	Glucose finger stick	82948	
	IMMUNIZATIONS		
	Allergy inj. X1	95115	
	Allergy inj. X2	95117	
	Trigger pt. inj.	20552	
	Therapeutic inj.	96372	
	VACCINATION PRODUCTS		
	DPT	90701	
	DT	90702	
	Tetanus	90703	
	MMR	90707	
	OPV	90712	
	Polio inj.	90713	
	Flu	90662	
	Hemophilus B	90645	
	Hepatitis B vac.	90746	
	Pneumovax	90670	
	VACCINE ADMINISTRATION		
	Age: Through 18 yrs. (1st inj.)	90460	
	Age: Through 18 yrs. (ea. addt'l. inj.)	90461	
	Adult (1st inj.)	90471	
	Adult (ea. addt'l. inj.)	90472	

X	DESCRIPTION	CODE	FEE
	OFFICE PROCEDURES		
	Anoscopy	46600	
	Ear lavage	69210	
	Spirometry	94010	
	Nebulizer Rx	94664	
X	EKG	93000	*$34.26*
	SURGERY		
	Mole removal (1st)	17100	
	(2nd to 14th)	17003	
	Flat warts (1st - 14th)	07110	
	15 or more	17111	
	Biopsy, 1 lesion	11100	
	Addt'l. lesions	11101	
	Endometrial Bx	58100	
	Skin tags to 15	11200	
	Each addt'l. 10	11201	
	I & D abscess	10060	
	SUPPLIES/MISCELLANEOUS		
	Surgical tray	99070	
	Handling charge	99000	
	Special report	99080	

DOCTOR'S NOTES:

	DIAGNOSES	ICD-10-CM
	Abdominal pain/unspec.	R10.9
	Absess	L02._
	Allergic reaction	T78.40_
	Alzheimer's disease	G30
	Anemia/unspec.	D64.9
	Angina/unspec.	I20.9
	Anorexia	R63.0
	Anxiety/unspec.	F41.9
	Apnea, sleep	G47.30
	Arrhythmia, cardiac	I49.9
	Arthritis, rheumatoid	M06.9
	Asthma/unspec.	J45.909
	Atrial fibrillation	I48.0
	B-12 deficiency	E53.8
	Back pain, low	M54.5
	BPH	N40
	Bradycardia/unspec.	R00.1
	Broncitis, acute	J20._
	Bronchitis, cronic	J42
	Bursitis/unspec.	M71.9
	CA, breast	C50._
	CA, lung	C34._
	CA, prostate	C61
	Cellulitis	L03._
X	Chest pain/unspec.	R07.9
	Cirrhosis, liver/unspec.	K74.60
	Cold, common	J00
	Colitis/unspec.	K51.90
	Confusion	R41.0
	CHF	I50.9
	Constipation	K59.00
	COPD	J44.9
	Cough	R05
	Crohn's disease/unspec.	K50.90
	CVA	I63.9
	Decubitus ulcer	L89._
	Dehydration	E86.0
	Dementia/unspec.	F03
	Depression, major/unsp.	F32.9
	Diab I, no complications	E10.0
	Diab II, no complications	E11.9
	w/kidney complic.	E11.2_
	w/ophthalmic compl.	E11.3_
	w/neurolog.compl.	E11.4_
	w/circulatory cmpl.	E11.5_
	Insulin use	Z79.4
	Diarrhea/unspec.	R19.7
	Diverticulitix	K57.92
	Diverticulosis	K57.90
	Dizziness	R42
	Dysuria	R30.0
	Edema/unspec.	R60.9
	Endocarditis	I38
	Esophageal reflux	K21.0
	Fatigue (lethargy)	R53.83
	FUO	R50.9
	Gastritis	K29.70
	Gastroenteritis (colitis)	K52.9
	G.I. bleed	K92.2
	Gout/unspec.	M10.9
	Headache	R51
	Health exam	200._
	Hematuria/unspec.	R31.9
	Herpes simplex	B00.9
	Herpes zoster	B02.9
	Hiatal hernia	K44.9
	HTN (HBP)	I10
	Hyperlipidemia/unspec.	E78.5
	Hypothyroidism/unspec.	E03.9
	Impotentce	N52._
	Influenca, respiratory	J10.1
	Insomnia	G47.0
	IBS, diarrhea	K58.
	Lupus, systemic erythim.	M32.9
	MI, acute	I21._
	MI, old	I25.2
	Migraine	G43.9
	Myalgia	M79.1
	Neck pain	M54.2
	Neuropathy	G62.9
	Nausea	R11.1
	Nausea/vomitting	R11.0
	Obesity/unspec.	E66.9
	Osteoarthritis (site)	M19._
	Otitis media	H66.9_
	Parkinson's disease	G20
	Pharyngitis, acule	J02.9
	Pleurisy	R09.1
	Pneumonia	J18.9
	Pneumonia, viral	J12.9
	Prostatitis/unspec.	N41.9
	PVD	I73.9
	Radiculopathyp	M54.1_
	Rectal bleeding	K62.5
	Renal failure	N19
	Sciatica	M54.3_
	Shortness of breath	R03.02
	Sinusitis, chr./unspec.	J32.9
	Syncope	R55
	Tachycardia/unspec.	R00.0
	Tachy., supraventric	I47.1
	Tendinitix/unspec.	M77.9
	TIA	G45.9
	Ulcer, duodenal/unspec.	K26.9
	Ulcer, gastric/unspec.	K25.9
	Ulcer, peptic/unspec.	K27.9
	URI/unspec.	J06.9
	UTI	N39.0
	Vertigo	R42
	Weight gain	R63.5
	Weight loss	R63.4

Diagnosis/additional description:

Doctor's signature/date *P. Cardi, MD*

Return appointment information: -with whom Self/other
Days ____ Wks. *2* Mos. ____

PLEASE RMEMBER THAT PAYMENT IS YOU OBLIGATION, REGARDLESS OF INSURANCE OR OTHER THIRD PARTY INVOLVEMENT.

Rec'd. by: ☒ Cash ☐ Check # ______

Total today's fee	*$166.54*
Amount rec'd. today	*$10.00*

Fig. 17.9 Encounter form; diagnostic codes from *International Classification of Diseases, Tenth Revision, Clinical Modification* (ICD-10-CM) and procedural codes for professional services from *Current Procedural Terminology* (CPT). (Courtesy Bibbero Systems, Inc., Petaluma, Calif.; telephone: 800-242-2376; fax: 800-242-9330; www.bibbero.com.)

TABLE 17.1 Possible Responses to Patients' Excuses for Avoiding Payment

Excuse	Response
"Just bill me."	"As we explained when we made your appointment, Mr. Barkley, our practice bills for charges more than $50. Amounts less than $50 are to be paid at the time of the visit. That will be $25 for today's visit, please."
"I have insurance to cover this."	"We will be billing your insurance for you, Miss Butler, but your policy shows a deductible in the amount of $300 that still must be met. We must collect the full fee for today's visit, which is $150 to meet that deductible responsibility."
"I get paid on Friday; you know how it is."	"I understand. Why don't you write the check today and postdate it for Saturday? We will hold the check and deposit it on the next business day." (Depending on office policy.)
"If I pay for this, I won't be able to pay for the prescription."	"Our payment policy is very much like the pharmacy's: We expect payment at the time of service. Let me check and see if the doctor can dispense some medication samples to last until you can get your prescription filled."
"I don't have that much with me."	"How much can you pay, Mrs. Fish? I can accept $10 now and give you an envelope to send us the balance within the week or I can put it on your credit or debit card." (Get a commitment and write the balance due under the sealing flap of the envelope. Also write the date on a tickler calendar or the patient's financial accounting record while the patient is watching.)
"I'll take care of it."	"I know you will, Mr. Stone; I just need to know when that will be so that I can document your intentions for our bookkeeper." (Get a commitment and input the date in the patient's financial accounting record while the patient is watching. Hand him an envelope with the amount due written under the sealing flap.)
"I forgot my checkbook."	"We take Visa, MasterCard, and American Express, Mr. Storz." (If the patient still does not pay, provide him with a self-addressed envelope and write the patient's name, account number, date of service, amount due, and expected payment date under the sealing flap. Restate the expected payment date as you hand the patient the envelope. Input the date in the patient's financial accounting record while the patient is watching.)

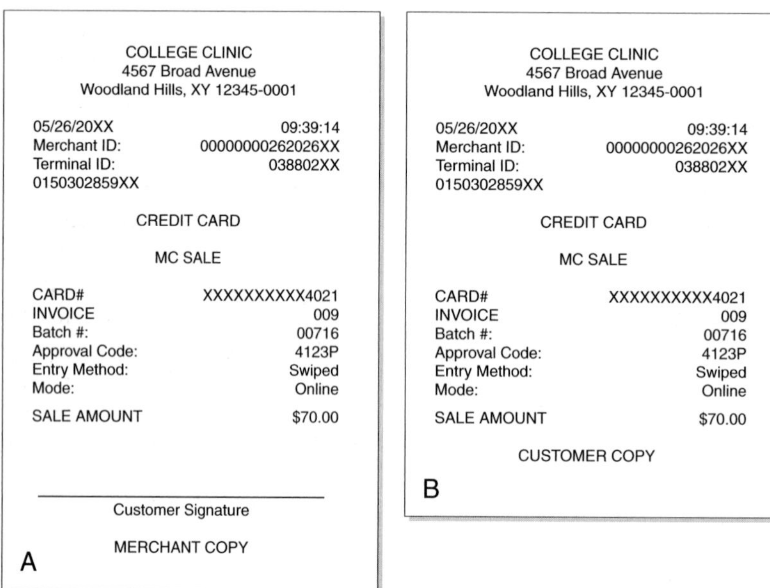

COLLEGE CLINIC
4567 Broad Avenue
Woodland Hills, XY 12345-0001

05/26/20XX	09:39:14
Merchant ID:	00000000262026XX
Terminal ID:	038802XX
0150302859XX	

CREDIT CARD

MC SALE

CARD#	XXXXXXXXXX4021
INVOICE	009
Batch #:	00716
Approval Code:	4123P
Entry Method:	Swiped
Mode:	Online
SALE AMOUNT	$70.00

Customer Signature

MERCHANT COPY

A

COLLEGE CLINIC
4567 Broad Avenue
Woodland Hills, XY 12345-0001

05/26/20XX	09:39:14
Merchant ID:	00000000262026XX
Terminal ID:	038802XX
0150302859XX	

CREDIT CARD

MC SALE

CARD#	XXXXXXXXXX4021
INVOICE	009
Batch #:	00716
Approval Code:	4123P
Entry Method:	Swiped
Mode:	Online
SALE AMOUNT	$70.00

CUSTOMER COPY

B

Fig. 17.10 A, Merchant copy of a credit card receipt showing the patient's signature. **B,** Customer copy of a credit card receipt.

Verifying Credit Card Holders

Always verify the cardholder by asking for photo identification, such as a driver's license. Examine the card carefully and observe the following guidelines:

- Accept a credit card only from the person whose name is on the card.
- Match the name on the card with the patient's other identification and ensure that the expiration date has not passed.
- Look on the back of the card for the word *void.* This is an alert that the card has been heated, which is a method used to forge a signature.
- Check the "hot list" for problem cards.
- Verify all charges regardless of the amount and get approval from the credit card company.
- Compare the signature on the credit card receipt against the signature on the card (Fig. 17.10).

Credit Card Fees

Most banks directly deposit the amount on the credit card receipt and subtract the monthly fees from the health care organization's bank account. A statement from the bank indicates how much has been credited to the account. The fees can be negotiated on the basis of volume but usually range from 2% to 10% on each transaction. Some health care organizations charge patients a service fee for using credit cards. Do not issue cash or

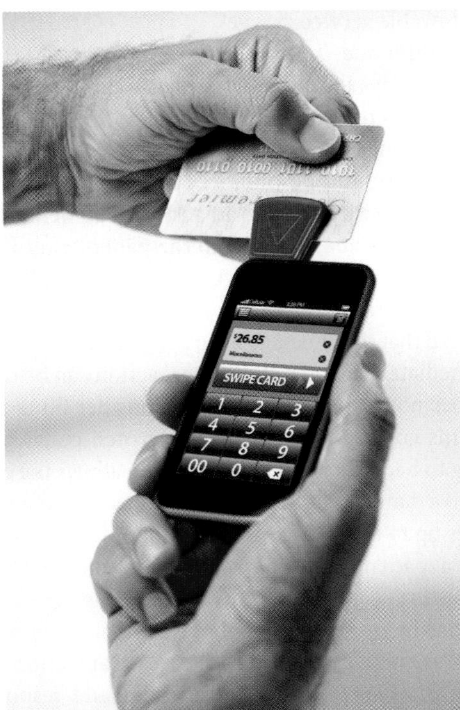

Fig. 17.11 Square device used with a tablet to collect credit card payments. (Photo copyright iStock.com.)

check refunds for any payments made by credit card. Patients who want to make payments may have their credit cards charged for each scheduled payment. Some health care organizations choose to impose a nominal fee (50 cents) for all credit and debit card transactions to recoup the fee charged by the credit card company. Simple credit card reader terminal devices attached to a smartphone or tablet are available (Fig. 17.11).

Credit Card Options

Online bill payment or e-payment, such as PayPal, is another way patients can pay their health care bills. It is done through the health care organization's secure website. Payment can be verified immediately and deposited directly into the organization's bank account.

Other cards are used for credit in a health care office. Automated teller machine (ATM) cards are sometimes accepted for medical care if the health care organization has a credit card scanner. An ATM card is a magnetically encoded bankcard used to make deposits and withdraw cash from checking or savings accounts. Private-label cards are credit vehicles that can be used only to pay for health care. Some large health care organizations offer their own private-label health cards. Smart cards also are used in some locations. They are small credit or debit cards that contain a computer chip that can store money in the form of electronic data. Special-use smart cards for telephone calls, gas stations, and fast food are now in use, as are common cards having multiple uses. These cards may also contain patient health care data.

Visa offers a credit card service unique to the health care market. It has a preauthorized health care form that allows patients to authorize the health care organization to bill their account directly for copayments and the balance not covered by insurance. Patients who need a series of treatments, such as allergy injections or chemotherapy, can fill out one form designating these services, which authorizes the staff to charge the patient's account directly.

Debit Cards

A debit card is a card that permits bank customers to withdraw cash at any hour from any affiliated ATM in the country. The holder may make cashless purchases from funds on deposit without incurring revolving finance charges for credit. Health care organizations that offer credit card payment may use the same electronic credit card machine to swipe the debit card for verification and approval. Separate debit card machines are also available for businesses that do not accept credit cards. Debit cards take the place of check writing; however, once the debit card is approved for a certain amount, the bank that issued the debit card is responsible for paying the funds that were approved. There are no returned checks for nonsufficient funds (NSF) with this method of payment.

Payment by Check

E-Checks

Another payment option that is becoming popular is payment by e-check. With an e-check, the patient gives their checking account information, such as account number and bank routing number. A signature to confirm the electronic transaction is required and the check is deposited immediately.

Paper Check Verification

Check verification requires the insurance billing specialist to become familiar with the appearance of a good check. A personal check is the most common method of payment in most medical offices, but it is not a personal guarantee of payment. A driver's license and one other form of identification always should be required. Check these against existing records. Call the bank to verify all out-of-state and suspicious checks. A verification service (which is a private company with resources to identify patient information quickly over the telephone) or a check authorization system may be worthy of consideration for clinics and larger health care organizations.

Check Forgery

Forgery is false writing or alteration of a document to injure another person or with intent to deceive. An example of forgery is signing another person's name on a check to obtain money or pay off a debt without permission. To guard against forgery, always check that the endorsement on the back of the check matches the name on the front. Be suspicious if the beneficiary or provider states that he or she did not receive the check but the third-party payer shows it as being cashed, or if the payee of the check claims that the signature is not theirs.

Payment Disputes

Problem checks appear in many forms. One is the check for partial payment when the debtor (the patient) writes "payment in full" on the check. If the creditor (the health care organization) cashes the check, it may be argued that the debt is paid in full. A legal theory called *accord and satisfaction* may apply to this situation if the debt is truly disputed by the debtor. If the check is cashed by the health care organization, it can be considered "accord and satisfaction" and the organization cannot procure the balance from the patient. The operative words are *truly disputed*. If there is a legitimate, genuine dispute over the amount of the bill and an amount less than the full amount of the bill is accepted, the health care organization could be precluded from seeking the balance. However, acceptance of payment does not necessarily mean acceptance of the "paid in full" remark. Even if a check marked "paid in full" is accidentally cashed, 90 days may be available to rectify the situation by returning the funds to the patient and informing him or her that the accord and satisfaction is not acceptable. A patient who is paying less may be dissatisfied with the health care organization in some way. This may help to defuse any lurking issues and to address the patient's underlying problem.

Postdated Checks

Checks dated to be payable 3 to 6 months in the future are not honored by the bank. Always read the date on every check. Federal collection law states that if a check dated more than 5 days in advance is accepted, the patient must be notified no more than 10 days and no less than 3 days before the check is deposited. State laws vary but some states have regulations in addition to federal laws.

Unsigned Checks

Another problem is unsigned checks. Ask the patient to come to the office and sign the check or send a new one. If the insurance billing specialist is unable to reach the patient or if there is a transportation or time limitation problem, they should write the word "over" or "see reverse" on the signature line on the front of the check. On the back of the check, where the n endorsement should appear, write "lack of signature, guaranteed," the health care organization's name, and one's own name and title. This endorsement in effect is a guarantee that the health care organization will absorb the loss if the patient's bank or the patient does not honor the check.

Returned Checks

When the health care organization receives notice that a check was not honored, the reason should be stated on the back of the check. The most common reason is NSF. Call the bank to find out if there are adequate funds in the account to cover the check and take the NSF check to the bank immediately. The insurance billing specialist might telephone the patient to see if he or she suggests redepositing it. Check the state laws about NSF checks. There is a time limit for making the check good, and there are additional charges (up to 10% of the value of the check) that the patient must make to restore the check. If the patient does not respond, the matter may be turned over to a regional district attorney or satisfaction may be obtained through small claims court. An NSF demand letter (Fig. 17.12) should be sent by certified mail with return receipt requested and include the following:

1. Check date
2. Check number
3. Name of the bank where the check is drawn
4. Name of person the check was payable to
5. Check amount
6. Any allowable service charges
7. Total amount due
8. Number of days the check writer has to take action

Future payments should be in the form of cash, money order, or a cashier's check. If the patient wants the check to be returned, it should be photocopied and kept in the financial record because it serves as an acknowledgment of the debt. The bad check may be returned to the patient after it has been replaced with a valid payment. A notation should be placed on the patient's record to this effect.

If notified that the checking account is closed, send a demand letter immediately. In most states, legal action can be taken if the patient does not respond in 30 days. Consider filing a claim in small claims court. Most states have written codes or statutes pertaining to bad checks. Often legislation allows the creditor to add punitive damages to the amount of the debt being collected, sometimes up to three times the amount of the check.

When a patient stops payment on a check, it is usually done to resolve a good faith dispute. In this case the patient believes that he or she has legal entitlement to withhold payment. Representatives of the health care organization may want to contact a lawyer to discuss legal rights and responsibilities before sending a demand letter and trying to collect.

Itemized Patient Statements

Every patient receives an **itemized statement** (Fig. 17.13) of his or her account showing the dates of service, a list of detailed charges, copayments and deductibles paid, the date the insurance claim was filed, applicable adjustments, and the account balance. These items also are listed on the patient's account or financial accounting record card (see Fig. 17.5). Timeliness, accuracy, and consistency have a significant effect on the cash flow and collection process when sending itemized statements. A credit card option should be printed on the statement to encourage easier and faster payment.

Professional bills are a reflection of the health care organization. The billing statement should be patient oriented and easy to read and understand. Avoid technical terms and abbreviations that might lead to misunderstandings and confusion. Enclose a return envelope with the address payments should be mailed to or that have a window that displays the health care organization's mailing address. Addressed envelopes should contain the statement "forwarding service requested" so that the postal service can forward the mail and provide the health care organization with a notice of the patient's new address. When this notice is received by the health care organization, it should be circulated to all necessary departments to record the new information.

Patients can be oriented to the billing process by having the insurance billing specialist electronically generate a printed statement as the patient leaves the service provider's office that explains pertinent information, such as account number, dates of service, payments, procedures, interest fees, copayments, and deductibles. Patients may choose to receive their statements electronically, so ask software providers for this component. If using standard mail, patient information pamphlets about common health concerns (such as blood pressure, cholesterol, or back pain) can be sent with the bill to convey a caring attitude.

COLLEGE CLINIC
4567 Broad Avenue
Woodland Hills, XY 12345-0001
Tel. (555) 486-9002
FAX (555) 487-8976

August 15, 20XX

Mrs. Maxine Holt
444 Labina Lane
Woodland Hills, XY 12345-0001

Dear Mrs. Holt:

The following check has been dishonored by the bank and returned without payment:

Date:	08/04/20XX
Check No.:	755
Amount:	$106.11
Payable to:	Perry Cardi, MD
Bank:	Woodland Hills National Bank
Reason:	Nonsufficient funds

This is a formal notice demanding payment in the amount of $106.11 within 15 days from today's date or your account will be considered for legal action.

Please make payment immediately by cash, cashier's check, or money order at the above address. Your immediate attention will be appreciated.

Sincerely,

Delores Yee, CMA-A

Patient Accounts Manager
for Perry Cardi, MD

Fig. 17.12 Demand letter for returned check. This letter serves as a formal notice to collect payment and notifies a patient of impending legal action.

The health care organization is likely to experience an increase in telephone calls from inquiring patients when statements go out in the mail. A patient account representative or department should handle all billing questions, ensuring a consistent response.

Accounts Receivable and Age Analysis by Aging Report

Age analysis is a term used for the procedure of systematically arranging the A/R by age from the date of service. Accounts are usually aged in periods of 30, 60, 90, and 120 days and older. An aging report can be generated by the organization's medical billing system. This helps collection follow up by providing easy recognition of overdue accounts and allows the insurance billing specialist to determine which accounts need action in addition to a regular statement.

The formula for determining the A/R ratio is to divide the month-end A/R balance by the monthly average charges for the prior 12-month period. An average total A/R (all monies not collected at the time of service) should be one and a half to two times the charges for 1 month of services (Examples 17.1 and 17.2).

Accounts that are 90 days or older should not exceed 15% to 18% of the total A/R. To calculate this figure, divide the total amount of A/R by the amount of accounts that are 90 days old and older (Example 17.3). The medical billing system should calculate this automatically when an aging report is required.

A decision tree showing time frames for sending statements and making telephone calls is presented in Fig. 17.14.

Dun Messages

Dun messages are phrases printed on statements to inform or remind a patient about a delinquent account and to promote payment (see Fig. 17.5). The best and most effective collection statements include a handwritten note; however, this is seldom possible. Dun messages also can be printed by the computer system or applied with brightly colored labels. Examples of dun messages follow:

- "If there is a problem with your account, please call me at (555) 486-0000—Maralyn."
- "This bill is now 30 days past due. Please remit payment."
- "This bill is now 60 days past due. Please send payment immediately."
- "Your account is 90 days past due. Please remit payment now to avoid collection action."

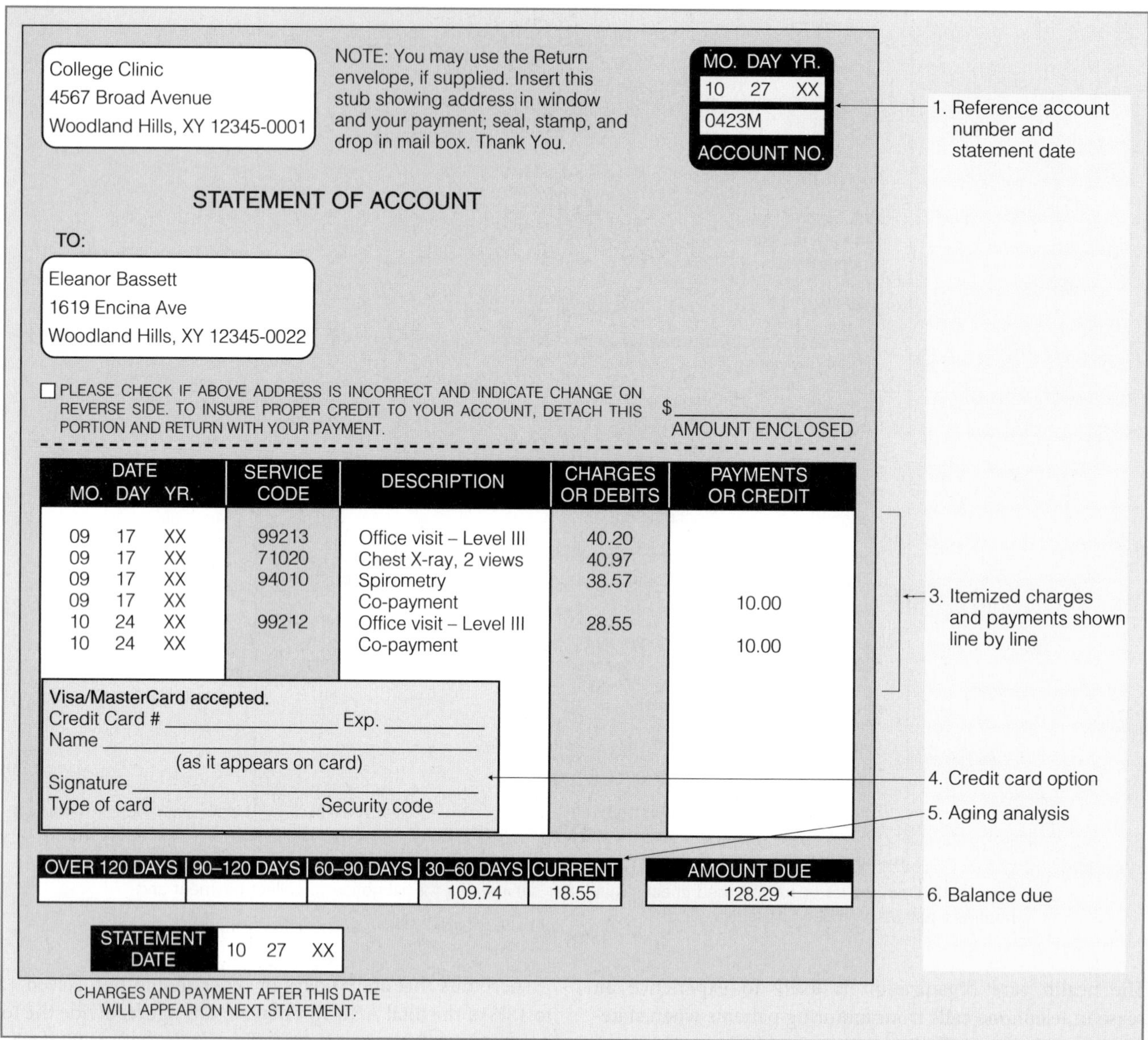
College Clinic
4567 Broad Avenue
Woodland Hills, XY 12345-0001

NOTE: You may use the Return envelope, if supplied. Insert this stub showing address in window and your payment; seal, stamp, and drop in mail box. Thank You.

MO. DAY YR.
10 27 XX
0423M
ACCOUNT NO.

STATEMENT OF ACCOUNT

TO:

Eleanor Bassett
1619 Encina Ave
Woodland Hills, XY 12345-0022

☐ PLEASE CHECK IF ABOVE ADDRESS IS INCORRECT AND INDICATE CHANGE ON REVERSE SIDE. TO INSURE PROPER CREDIT TO YOUR ACCOUNT, DETACH THIS PORTION AND RETURN WITH YOUR PAYMENT.

$________ AMOUNT ENCLOSED

DATE MO. DAY YR.	SERVICE CODE	DESCRIPTION	CHARGES OR DEBITS	PAYMENTS OR CREDIT
09 17 XX	99213	Office visit – Level III	40.20	
09 17 XX	71020	Chest X-ray, 2 views	40.97	
09 17 XX	94010	Spirometry	38.57	
09 17 XX		Co-payment		10.00
10 24 XX	99212	Office visit – Level III	28.55	
10 24 XX		Co-payment		10.00

Visa/MasterCard accepted.
Credit Card # ____________ Exp. ________
Name ______________________
(as it appears on card)
Signature ______________________
Type of card ____________ Security code _____

OVER 120 DAYS	90–120 DAYS	60–90 DAYS	30–60 DAYS	CURRENT	AMOUNT DUE
			109.74	18.55	128.29

STATEMENT DATE 10 27 XX

CHARGES AND PAYMENT AFTER THIS DATE WILL APPEAR ON NEXT STATEMENT.

Fig. 17.13 Patient account statement. A credit card option should be printed near the bottom of the statement to encourage payment. (Form adapted courtesy Bibbero Systems, Inc., Petaluma, Calif.; telephone: 800-242-2376; fax: 800-242-9330; www.bibbero.com.)

EXAMPLE 17.1 Formula

Health care organization's charges monthly total	$50,000 × 1.5 = $75,000 Or $50,000 × 2.0 = $100,000	Total outstanding accounts receivable

Total outstanding accounts receivable should range from $75,000 to $100,000.

EXAMPLE 17.2 Calculation of Accounts Receivable Ratio

Annual gross charges	$150,000
Average monthly gross charges (150,000 ÷ 12 months)	$12,500
Current accounts receivable balance	$20,000
Accounts receivable ratio: 20,000 ÷ 12,500 = 1.60 months	

EXAMPLE 17.3 Formula for Determining Percentage of Accounts over 90 Days

Amount of A/R over 90 days	A/R total	Percentage of A/R over 90 days
$12,000 ÷	$75,000	= 16%

A/R, Accounts receivable.

- "FINAL NOTICE: If we do not hear from you within 10 days, this account will be turned over to our collection agency."

Do not send intimidating, impatient, or threatening statements. These serve only to antagonize patients. Dun messages should be printed in different languages and sent to patients who speak English as a second language. Examples are as follows:

- "No payment yet; your payment by return mail will be appreciated."

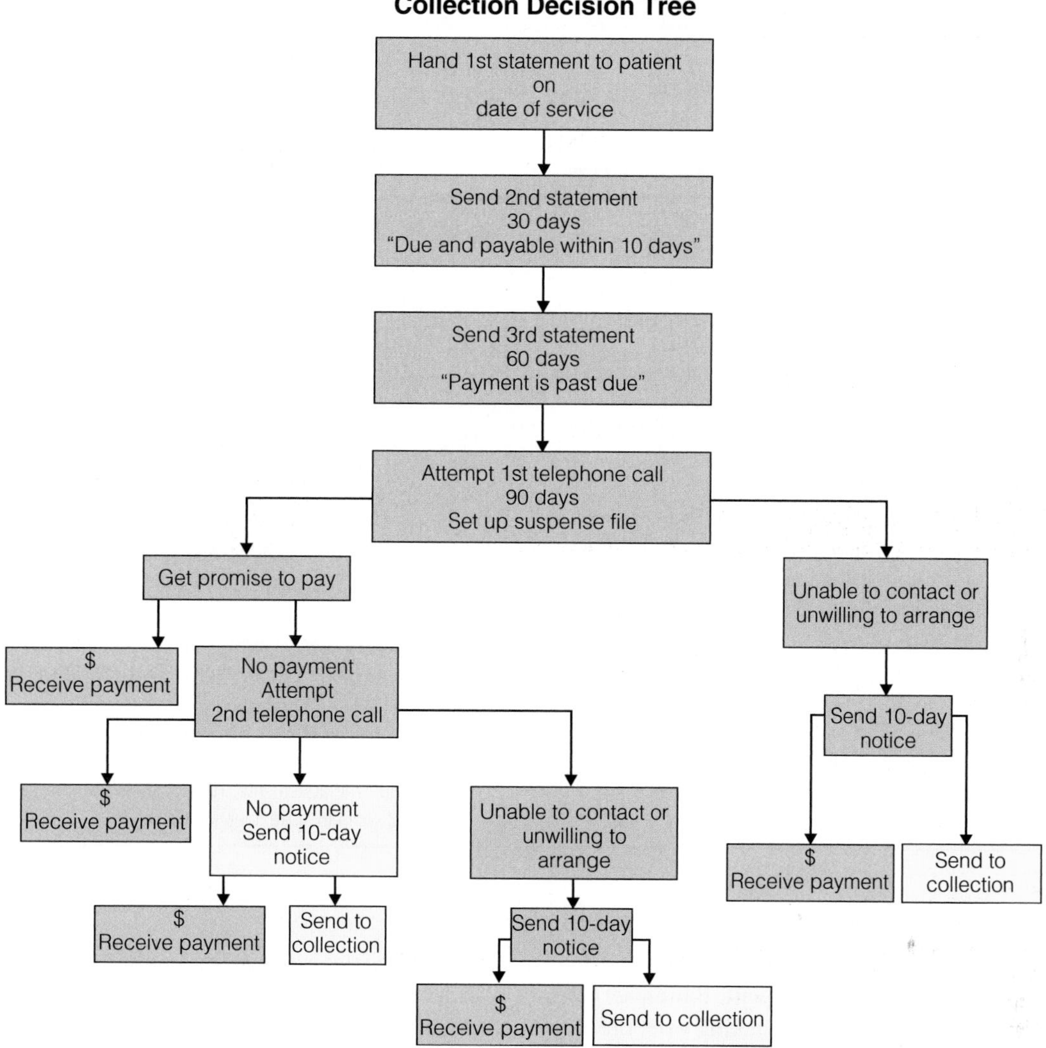

Fig. 17.14 Collection decision tree. This is a quick reference used to help determine when to send statements, make telephone calls, and send accounts to a collection agency.

- "No hemos recibido pago. Agracieramos remita por correo."
- "Payment needed now. No further credit will be extended."
- "Se requiere pago hoy. No se le estendera mas credito."

Electronic Media

Health care organizations may receive e-mail messages about their bills, but it is advisable that a response not be given to patients via e-mail because of privacy concerns. An e-mail consent form must be signed and dated by the patient, and e-mail is then limited to appointment requests, prescription refills, requests for information, nonurgent health care questions, updates to information, or exchange of noncritical information, such as changes in office hours, holiday schedules, recalls or infectious diseases, immunizations, insurance changes, financial eligibility information, and so on. Some organizations use their websites for live chat with patients because it is secure and similar to a telephone call. It is especially suitable for hearing impaired patients. It is acceptable to receive online payments from patients via the health care organization's website. It is not advisable to send debt communications through social media, such as Twitter and Facebook, because a written notice is required that must be received by the debtor and no other person. Too many people have access to social media over the internet.

Computer Billing

Because most health care organizations use the computer to generate billing statements, the manual system is not discussed in this edition. Computerized patient statements are generated by the organization's medical billing system. All charges, payments, and adjustments are reflected on hard copy and made readily available to mail to the patient (see Fig. 17.5) The computer program usually offers choices of billing types, including patient billing, insurance balance billing, billing according to types of adjustments, and no bill. The insurance billing specialist can instruct the computer to print all bills of a specific type. The computer also can be instructed to print bills according to specific accounts, dates, and insurance types. Accounts are automatically aged and standard messages can be printed on the statements for each of the aged dates (that is, 30, 60, 90, or 120 days). Some systems allow personalized messages to be inserted that override the standard messages.

PROCEDURE 17.2 Seven-Step Billing and Collection Guidelines

Objective

To properly bill and collect payments for medical services rendered to patients

Equipment/Supplies

Patients' financial accounting statements, envelopes, calendar, and telephone

Directions

Follow these step-by-step procedures and guidelines, which include rationales, to learn this job skill.

1. Present the first statement at the time of service. This can be a formal statement or an encounter form (multipurpose billing form).
2. Mail the second itemized statement within 30 days of treatment. The phrase "due and payable within 10 days" should be printed on each statement. Local paycheck issuing patterns should be considered before selecting a date for statements to be mailed. Choose which billing routine the office will use.
   a. Monthly billing. Using the monthly billing system, all statements are mailed at the same time during the month. Choose a mail-out day at the beginning of the month so that the patient will receive the bill near the fifteenth or send statements near the end of the month so that the patient receives the bill on the first.
   b. Cycle billing. **Cycle billing** is a system of billing accounts at spaced intervals during the month based on a breakdown of accounts by alphabet, account number, insurance type, or date of first service. This relieves the pressure of having to get all statements out at one time and allows collection at a faster, more organized rate than accounts collected at random. It also allows continuous cash flow throughout the month and distributes the influx of incoming calls from patients about problem accounts. The number of cycles may be determined by how the collector wishes to divide the workload. Using two cycles per month, statements would be sent on the twenty-fifth to arrive by the first and on the tenth to arrive by the fifteenth of the month. Using four cycles per month, statements should be sent every Tuesday or Wednesday to arrive at the end of the week. If a cycle that was established by the first date of service is used and the patient was first seen on the eleventh of the month, then he or she should receive a bill every month on the eleventh.
3. Send the third statement 30 days after the second statement was sent. Indicate that the payment is past due.
4. If there is no response to the third statement, place the first telephone call to the patient depending on office policy (7 – 14 days). Ask if there is a problem. Ask for a payment commitment and set up a suspense file. Accounts are put in a suspense file for active follow-up. Action must be taken within the time frame mentioned, after the patient has been so advised.
5. Check for payment as promised. Allow 1 day for mail delay. Place the second telephone call to the patient and ask for payment. Set up a new payment date. Allow 5 days.
6. Check for payment as promised. Send a 10-day notice advising the patient that unless payment is received in 10 days, the account will be turned over for legal action.
7. Check for payment. Promptly surrender the account for collection or legal action. Fig. 17.15 shows a collection decision tree to be used when determining when to send statements, 10-day notices, and accounts to a collection agency and when to make telephone calls.

Billing Services

Health care organizations can contract with billing services to reduce administrative paperwork by taking over the task of preparing, submitting, and following up for third-party health insurance companies and patients. They may provide data entry of patients' demographic and billing information, charges, receipts, and adjustments; tracking of payments from patients and third-party payers; production of management reports; purging of inactive accounts; and collection of accounts.

Some advantages of billing services are advanced technology, professional and understandable bills, experts answering all billing-related telephone inquiries, and no downtime caused by vacations or medical or personal leave. This service allows the health care organization to have fewer disruptions and freedom from worry about financial matters when trying to provide medical care.

The health care organization sends billing and receipt information to the billing service daily. This may be done in writing or through a computer system. The billing service then prepares the bills, mails them, and may also receive payments. Regular reports, whether weekly or monthly, are sent to the health care organization summarizing the transactions. Billing services may offer full account management services and in many cases, customize a service that meets the needs of the health care organization. Most medical billing services charge a percentage of every claim collected, typically 5% to 10%. Using a billing service company is most commonly referred to as *outsourcing*. When choosing a billing service, make a list of important questions and visit the facility. Also ask for references to obtain valuable feedback from other health care offices that have used the same billing service.

! COMPLIANCE ALERT

Guidelines When Contracting With a Billing Service

Have a written directive in place that gives the billing company permission to communicate directly with the insurance company and a Medicare administrative contractor (MAC) about denied or problem claims. When changing billing services, be sure to revoke such authorizations with each carrier and MAC.

Billing Guidelines

Billing procedures are determined by the size of the health care organization, the number of accounts, and the number of staff members assigned to the collection process. Adopt a specific method of handling accounts and decide which billing routine best fits the organization. Check insurance contracts carefully to determine which circumstances allow for patients to be billed. Be sure to conform to federal guidelines if there is a need to bill patients. See Procedure 17.2 at the end of this chapter for the procedure for seven-step billing and collection guidelines.

PAYMENT PLAN SCHEDULE

Balance due amount	Minimum monthly payment	Time frame for full payment
$0 - $200	$35	6 months
$201 - $500	$50	1 year
$501 - $1000	$100	1 year
$1001 - $3000	$125	2 years
$3001 - $5000	$150	2 years
>$5001*	$200	5 years

*Accounts over $5000 must complete a credit card application to certify the minimum required payment and are subject to approval by the office manager.

Fig. 17.15 Payment plan schedule used in the health care organization to negotiate monthly payments shows balance due amounts, minimum monthly payment, and payment time frames.

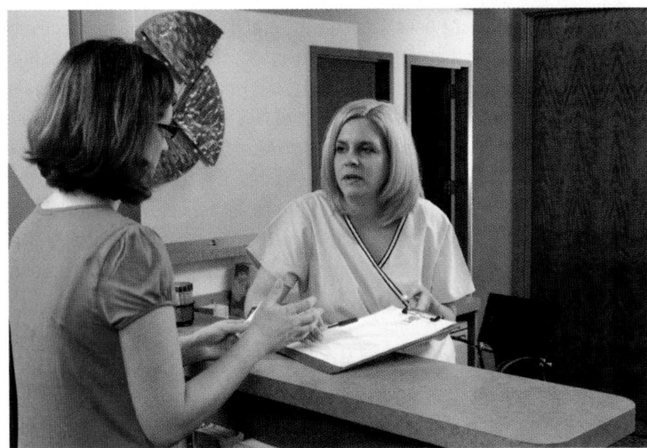

Fig. 17.16 Insurance billing specialist setting up a payment plan with a patient.

Payment Plans

Payment plans offer the patient a way of paying off an account by spreading out the amount due over time. Caution should be taken when offering patients a payment plan. The Truth in Lending Consumer Credit Cost Disclosure law (see the following section, Credit and Collection Laws), also referred to as *Regulation Z,* requires full written disclosure about the finance charges for large payment plans involving four or more installments, excluding a down payment. However, this regulation does not apply if the patient agrees to pay in one sum or in fewer than four payments and then decides independently to make drawn-out partial payments. Patients often think that if they make any amount of payment, the health care organization is required to accept that payment and not take any additional action. This is incorrect. The health care organization can take action, including sending the account to a collection agency. Have a written payment plan schedule when working with accounts in which payment plans may be offered. Fig. 17.15 illustrates sample guidelines that may be used or revised according to the specific needs of a health care organization (Fig. 17.16).

When patients seek care from the health care organization but are honest about their financial status, it is necessary to develop a financial payment plan agreement. This agreement (see Fig. 17.8) provides the patient with a clear understanding of all fees, the agreed-upon monthly payment amount, and the monthly due date. It may be wise to set up an automatic monthly withdrawal from the patient's bank account or credit card to ensure receipt of the patient's payment. A statement that provides the account balance should be sent to the patient every month after a payment is made.

EXAMPLE 17.4 Sample Appeal Letter Citing State Prompt Payment Law

Date

To Whom It May Concern:

Thank you for the opportunity to submit this denied claim for reconsideration of payment. We are contacting you about the medical services rendered to [patient's name, date of service, and medical services].

We request immediate payment of the above-referenced claim. According to our records, this claim was filed on [date of filing] but payment has not been received.

Failure to release payment may be a violation of [name of state and code number]. [Insert wording of the state's code.] Please adjudicate this claim immediately based on this state's mandate.

Thank you for your reconsideration.

Sincerely, [your name], Account Representative

CREDIT AND COLLECTION LAWS

The following laws are important because they provide the legal framework within which the insurance billing specialist must execute the health care organization's collection policy. In addition, each state may have specific collection laws that must be researched and obeyed. Most states have *prompt payment laws* designed to govern actions of insurers and third-party payers to pay insurance claims in a timely manner. See Example 17.4 for wording an appeal letter citing prompt payment law of the state in which the health care organization is located. Box 17.1 includes names and descriptions of the federal credit and collection laws that affect health care organizations.

! COMPLIANCE ALERT

Red Flags Rule

The Red Flags Rule is a set of Federal Trade Commission (**FTC**) requirements for businesses that have more than 20 employees and issue credit to their clients. This rule aims to prevent fraud and identity theft of a person's personal data for illegal use. A health care organization must create a plan to help recognize warning signs (or "red flags") associated with fraud and identity theft, or face civil penalties for violation. A health care organization must notify patients if their data have been stolen.

Statute of Limitations

A formal regulation or law setting time limits on legal action is known as a **statute of limitations.** Regarding collections, the statute of limitations is the maximum time during which a legal collection suit may be rendered against a debtor. However, for a lawsuit to be successful, a concerted effort should be made to collect on an account from the time services are rendered. The patient should receive regular statements indicating that if the insurer does not pay, the patient will be held responsible.

BOX 17.1 Federal Credit and Collection Laws

Equal Credit Opportunity Act (ECOA)

Prohibits discrimination in all areas of granting credit. Detailed credit information should be obtained before performing services to prevent accusations of impartiality. New patients should be informed that payment is due at the time of service and that they should arrive 20 minutes early to fill out a credit application if they wish to establish credit for treatment. Data, such as the patient's address, previous addresses, length of residence, employment history, and approximate wage, can be verified with a credit bureau. The report will also contain the patient's name changes, the patient's bill-paying history, and any history of bankruptcy. If the patient has a poor credit rating, credit may be denied, and the patient then has 60 days to request the reason in writing. The law prohibits discrimination against any applicant for credit for the following reasons:

- Age, color, marital status, national origin, race, religion, or sex
- Receiving income from alimony or any public assistance program

Fair Credit Reporting Act (FCRA)

Regulates agencies that either issue or use reports on consumers (patients) in connection with the approval of credit. Credit reporting agencies can provide reports only when the following occurs:

- A court order is issued.
- The report is requested by the consumer (patient) or instructions are given by the patient to provide the report.
- There is a legitimate business need for the information.

If credit is refused, the health care organization must provide the patient with a reason credit was denied and the name and address of the agency from which the report came. Specific information about what the report contains is not necessary and should not be given. The patient must have an opportunity to correct any inaccuracies if they occur.

Fair and Accurate Credit Transactions (FACT) Act (Public Law 108-159)

Establishes (as of December 4, 2003) medical privacy provisions as part of consumer credit law. The bill amends the FCRA to include improved medical privacy protections and protections against identity theft. Credit bureaus and creditors must comply with many medical privacy restrictions that ban the sharing of medical information. Title IV of the FACT Act limits the use and sharing of medical information in the financial system and provides an expanded definition of medical information. For military personnel, it provides an active-duty alert that can be placed on the credit file for a year at the three major credit bureaus. This means that a creditor cannot issue new credit or a card without first contacting the active-duty individual whose name is on the card.

Fair Credit Billing Act (FCBA)

Applies to "open end" credit accounts, such as credit cards and revolving charge accounts for department store accounts. It does not cover installment contracts, such as loans or extensions of credit repaid on a fixed schedule. Consumers often buy cars, furniture, and major appliances on an installment basis and they repay personal loans in installments as well. The FCBA settlement procedures apply only to disputes about "billing errors," such as unauthorized charges. Federal law limits the consumer's responsibility for unauthorized charges to $50; charges that list the wrong date or amount; charges for goods and services that the consumer did not accept or were not delivered as agreed; math errors; failure to post payments and other credits, such as returns; failure to send bills to the current address, provided the creditor receives the change of address, in writing, at least 20 days before the billing period ends; and charges for which an explanation or written proof of purchase along with a claimed error or request for clarification are requested. The consumer must write to the creditor at the address given for "billing inquiries," not the address for sending payments, and include one's name, address, account number, and a description of the billing error. Send the letter so that it reaches the creditor within 60 days after the first bill was mailed that contained the error. Send the letter by certified mail, return receipt requested, for proof of what the creditor received. Include copies (not originals) of sales slips or other documents that support the position. Keep a copy of the dispute letter. The creditor must acknowledge the complaint in writing within 30 days after receiving it, unless the problem has been resolved. The creditor must resolve the dispute within two billing cycles (but not more than 90 days) after receiving the letter. Payment may be withheld on the disputed amount (and related charges) during the investigation. Any part of the bill not in question must be paid, including finance charges on the undisputed amount.

The creditor may not take any legal or other action to collect the disputed amount and related charges (including finance charges) during the investigation. Although the account cannot be closed or restricted, the disputed amount may be applied against the credit limit. If the creditor's investigation determines that the bill is correct, one must be told promptly and in writing how much is owed and why. Copies of relevant documents may be requested. At this point the disputed amount is owed plus any finance charges that accumulated while the amount was in dispute. The minimum amount that was missed because of the dispute may have to be paid. If the results of the investigation are disputed, the creditor may be written to within 10 days after receiving the explanation and the disputed amount may be refused. At this point the creditor may begin collection procedures. Any creditor who fails to follow the settlement procedure may not collect the amount in dispute, or any related finance charges, up to $50, even if the bill turns out to be correct. For example, if a creditor acknowledges the complaint in 45 days—15 days too late—or takes more than two billing cycles to resolve a dispute, the penalty applies. The penalty also applies if a creditor threatens to report, or improperly reports, one's failure to pay to anyone during the dispute period.

Electronic Fund Transfer Act (EFTA)

Limits consumers' liability if there has been an unauthorized use of an ATM card, debit card, or other electronic banking device.

Truth in Lending Act (TILA)

Applies to anyone who charges interest or agrees to payment of a bill in more than four installments, excluding a down payment. When a specific agreement is reached between patient and health care organization, Regulation Z of this consumer protection act requires that a written disclosure of all pertinent information be made, regardless of the existence of a finance charge (see Fig. 17.8). This full disclosure must be discussed at the time the agreement is first reached between patient and health care organization and credit is extended. According to the Federal Trade Commission (FTC), the Truth in Lending provision is not applicable and no disclosures are necessary if a patient decides on his or her own to pay in installments or whenever convenient.

It is essential to include the following items:

1. Total amount of the debt
2. Amount of down payment
3. Finance charge
4. Interest rate expressed as an annual percentage
5. Amount of each payment
6. Date each payment is due
7. Date final payment is due
8. Signature of patient and service provider with copies retained by both
9. Account balance with total interest and total amount paid by the patient at the end of the contract

Health care organizations that implement late payment charges that meet the criteria defined in the TILA as a finance charge must comply with a host of requirements that revolve around proper disclosure to patients.

Charges must meet the following criteria to qualify as late payment charges:

1. The account balance must be paid in full at the time of initial billing.
2. The account is treated as delinquent when unpaid.

BOX 17.1 Federal Credit and Collection Laws—cont'd

3. The charge is assessed to a patient's account only because of their failure to make timely payments.
4. Installments are limited to no more than three.
5. The creditor (health care organization's insurance billing specialist) makes a "commercially reasonable" effort to collect these accounts.

When a health care organization continues to treat a patient with an overdue account, the courts have viewed this as continuation of care and an extension of credit. Patients who fall into this delinquent status should be referred elsewhere. After the patient has paid the overdue amount, the patient can be taken back and treated on a cash-only basis.

Truth in Lending Consumer Credit Cost Disclosure

Requires businesses to disclose all direct and indirect costs and conditions related to the granting of credit. All interest charges, late charges, collection fees, finance charges, and so forth must be explained up front, before the time of service. Include the following on all statements to charge interest and bill the patient monthly:

- Amount of each payment
- Due date
- Unpaid balance at the beginning of the billing period
- Finance charges
- Date balance is due

Fair Debt Collection Practices Act (FDCPA)

Addresses the collection practices of third-party debt collectors and attorneys who regularly collect debts for others. Although this Act does not apply directly to health care organizations collecting for themselves, a professional health care collector must avoid the actions that are prohibited for collection agencies. The main intent of the Act is to protect consumers from unfair, harassing, or deceptive collection practices. Refer to the guidelines in Box 17.2, which are taken from the FDCPA, to help avoid illegalities, enhance collections, and maintain positive patient relations. For more information about collection laws in your state, contact your state attorney general's office. The stricter law prevails if there is a conflict between state and federal laws.

Statutes vary according to the following three kinds of accounts:

1. *Open book accounts* (also called *open accounts*) are open to charges made from time to time. Payment is expected within a specific period but credit has been extended without a formal written contract. Patient accounts are usually open book accounts.
2. *Written contract accounts* have a formal written agreement in which a patient signs to pay their bill in more than four installments (see the Truth in Lending Act section in Box 17.1).
3. *Single-entry accounts* have only one entry or charge, usually for a small amount.

THE COLLECTION PROCESS

For collections to be handled effectively, staff members should be trained in collection techniques. Most insurance billing specialists can be trained to be efficient collectors when given the correct tools. New collectors need time to gain confidence, which is an important aspect of being a good collector.

Telephone Collection Procedures

Telephone collections are made easier if the insurance billing specialist is convinced that he or she can collect before trying to convince the patient to pay. Two important factors to consider are the insurance billing specialist's ability to contact the patient and the patient's ability to pay the bill. The following are helpful suggestions for using the telephone to address a collection problem:

- Contact the patient in a timely manner at the first sign of payment delay. Prepare before making a telephone collection call by reviewing the account and noting anything unusual. Locate information as to where the patient is employed (or if unemployed) by reviewing the patient registration form.
- Decide what amount will be settled for if payment cannot be made in full. Make the first call count. Act in a calm, businesslike manner and combine empathy with diligence. Be positive and persuasive. Listen to what patients have to say, even if they get angry and raise their voice. Lower the volume of your own voice and respond in a composed manner. Try to pick up clues from what the patient is saying; the patient may be giving the real reason for nonpayment.
- Ask questions, show interest, and let the patient know that they are being listened to.
- Respond in a respectful manner and carefully word the reply; when patients are distressed, they do not always make sense. The goal is to encourage the patient to pay, not agitate the patient.
- Use all resources and learn to negotiate.

Office Policy

The most organized approach to making collection calls is to print out the aging report and target accounts in the 60- to 90-day categories. The most effective results come from this group. Before making each call, review the patient's financial account in the medical billing system for notes on previous patient encounters. Start with the largest amount owed and work the accounts in decreasing amounts owed. After this category has been completed, move on to the 90- to 120-day accounts. Finally, go after accounts that are more than 120 days old.

Most state collection laws allow telephone calls to the debtor between 8 AM and 9 PM. Never call between 9 PM and 8 AM because to do so may be considered harassment. According to collection experts, the best time to telephone is between 5:30 PM and 8:30 PM on Tuesdays and Thursdays, and between 9 AM and 1 PM on Saturdays. Regardless of when the call is made, track the times when the most patients are contacted and adjust the calling schedule accordingly. Perhaps the insurance billing specialist's hours should be increased to include one evening a week or Saturday mornings to make collection calls. Another option is the use of flex time, in which the employee can choose their own working hours from within a broad range of hours approved by management. Use a private telephone away from the busy operations of the office to eliminate interruptions. Patients may be embarrassed about not being able to pay their bills and patient confidentiality must be maintained. Follow the guidelines stated in the Fair Debt Collection Practices Act (Box 17.2).

BOX 17.2 Fair Debt Collection Practices Act Guidelines

1. Contact debtors only once a day; in some states, repeated calls in 1 day or the same week could be considered harassment.
2. Place calls after 8 AM and before 9 PM.
3. Do not contact debtors on Sunday or any other day that the debtor recognizes as a Sabbath.
4. Identify yourself and the health care organization represented; do not mislead the patient.
5. Contact the debtor at work only if unable to contact the debtor elsewhere; no contact should be made if the employer or debtor disapproves.
6. Contact the attorney if an attorney represents the debtor; contact the debtor only if the attorney does not respond.
7. Do not threaten or use obscene language.
8. Do not send postcards for collection purposes; keep all correspondence strictly private.
9. Do not call collect or cause additional expense to the patient.
10. Do not leave a message on an answering machine indicating that you are calling about a bill.
11. Do not contact a third party more than once unless requested to do so by the party, or the response was erroneous or incomplete.
12. Do not convey to a third party that the call is about a debt.
13. Do not contact the debtor when notified in writing that a debtor refuses to pay and would like contact to stop, except to notify the debtor in writing that there will be no further contact or that there will be legal action.
14. Stick to the facts; do not use false statements.
15. Do not prepare a list of "bad debtors" or "credit risks" to share with other health care providers.
16. Take action immediately when stating that a certain action will be taken (for example, filing a claim in small claims court or sending the patient's case to a collection agency).
17. Send the patient written verification of the name of the creditor and the amount of debt within 5 days of the initial contact.

Some health care organizations have found success in reaching patients by text messaging. The health care organization must receive permission to text the patient during the initial patient encounter before using this tool. There are many online companies that will text patients with appointment reminders. Be careful not to include any information that will violate the privacy of the patient, so keep the messages general, such as "The Mountain Valley Physical Therapy Associates has a message for you about your account; please call (888) 873-9472."

Be alert for new ideas or approaches to collection by watching how banks and other retailers implement sophisticated collection skills. Decide whether any of these could be used to the health care organization's advantage and present the techniques to the office manager. Keep abreast of improvements made to collection software that improve collection results and allow more collectors to work from their homes. Other advances (for example, call block, which is an expanded telephone service) have made it more difficult to make collection calls. This service was originally intended to screen out unwanted telemarketing calls by intercepting blocked, unlisted, or unknown numbers. Standard numbers are usually allowed to go through. The key to averting a block is to ensure that the number the call is being placed from is listed and within the patient's area.

For a step-by-step procedure on making telephone collection calls, see Procedure 17.3 at the end of this chapter.

Telephone "Don'ts"

Communication is important, especially when trying to work with a patient on difficulties in making payments. Remain professional at all times and treat the patient with respect. The following is a list of *don'ts* for telephone collections:

- Do not raise your voice and antagonize the patient.
- Do not accuse the patient of dishonesty or lying.
- Do not act like a "tough guy" or threaten a patient.
- Do not consent to partial payments until payment in full has been asked for and do not agree to a long string of small partial payments.
- Do not engage in a debate.
- Do not report a disputed account to a collection agency or bureau until the patient's dispute is disclosed as part of the record.

Telephone collection calls are effective on the day before patients are due for their appointments. State the date and time of the appointment and then remind the patient of the balance owed and ask whether they could please bring payment to the appointment.

Telephone Collection Scenarios

The most difficult part of one-on-one collections is preparing for the many situations that may be encountered and the various responses the patient may make. Table 17.2 lists some statements that patients make about not paying an account and examples of responses that the insurance billing specialist can make.

Collection Letters

Collection letters are another method of reaching patients and reminding them of their debt. Knowledge of the patient base and of individual patients may help to determine the effectiveness of collection letters. Every health care organization is unique, and the type of service provided, the number of accounts, the geographic spread of patients, the staff size, and the amount of time collectors have to spend on individual accounts helps determine which collection method best suits the organization.

The positive aspect of collection letters is that they can reach many patients rapidly and the cost is relatively low, especially if form letters are used (Fig. 17.17).

Collection letters have some negative aspects, such as the following:

- Letters usually take 2 or 3 days to reach the patient and may lie unopened for a week or more.
- Letters are one-way communication and thus lack the ability to provide the reason for nonpayment.
- Response and recovery through letters are relatively poor.
- Manual preparation takes time (especially if a decision must be made before sending each letter).
- The costs of postage and supplies are increasing.

PROCEDURE 17.3 Telephone Collection Plan

Objective

To obtain payment of a delinquent account balance due by making the first collection telephone call

Equipment/Supplies

Telephone, pen or pencil, patient's financial accounting record, computerized account, or collection telephone log

Directions

Follow these step-by-step procedures and guidelines, which include rationales, to learn this job skill.

1. Set the mood of the call by the manner of speech and tone of voice. The first 30 seconds of the call sets the scene for the relationship with the patient. Follow the Fair Debt Collection Practices Act when making a telephone call.
2. State the name of the caller and the health care organization represented and identify the patient. Be certain the debtor is being spoken to before revealing the nature of the call.
3. Identify oneself and the health care organization.
4. Verify the debtor's address and any telephone numbers.
5. State the reason for the call by asking for full payment and stating the total amount owed. Ask for payment courteously but firmly.
6. Take control of the conversation and establish urgency by asking for full payment now. Speak slowly in a low voice; staying calm and polite prevents quarreling.
7. Ask when payment will be made, how it will be made, and if it will be sent by mail or in person.
8. Pause for effect. This turns the conversation back to the patient to respond to the demand or explain why payment has not been made. Never assume that if a patient does not respond, it means "no."
9. Find out if the patient needs clarification of the bill.
10. Inquire if the patient has a problem. Ask if the health care organization can be of assistance, especially when the patient is unable to give a reason for nonpayment.
11. If the patient is reluctant to agree to an amount, question him or her by asking one of the following: "How much are you willing to pay?" "Do you have a regular paycheck?" "Will payment be made through a checking account?"
12. Obtain a promise to pay with an agreeable amount and a due date; be clear how and when payment is expected but give the patient a choice of action. Set immediate deadlines for payment.
13. Ask for half of the amount if full payment is not possible.
14. Discuss a payment plan if the patient is not able to pay half of the balance owed. Be realistic and reasonable. It is self-defeating to set up payment arrangements the patient cannot afford. Advise the patient that the entire balance will become due and payable if the payment is even 1 day late. Ask the patient to please call before the due date with an explanation if any problems arise to prevent payment.
15. Restate the importance of the agreement.
16. Tell the patient to write down the amount and due date.
17. Document the agreement on the patient's financial accounting record by inserting the date of the call and abbreviated notations, in the computer system, or in a collection telephone log. Note the time the patient was spoken to.
18. Send confirmation of the agreement (Fig. 17.21) as a follow-up to the telephone call.
19. Check the account the day after the payment was due; allow 1 day for mail delay. If the patient fails to make payment as promised, make another telephone call and ask the patient if there is still a problem. Get a new commitment to pay and confirm again. If the patient continues to avoid payment, advise the patient that the account will be turned over to a collection agency and follow through as stated.

TABLE 17.2 Telephone Collection Scenarios

Statement	Response
"I can't pay anything now."	"Are you employed? Are you receiving unemployment compensation, welfare, or Social Security benefits?" You are determining the patient's ability to pay.
"I can't pay the whole bill now."	"How long will it take you to pay this bill?" Ask this question instead of "How much can you pay?"
"I can pay but not until next month."	"When do you get paid?" Ask for payment the day after payday. "Do you have a checking account?" Ask for a postdated check.
"I have other bills."	"This is also one of your bills that should be paid now. Let's talk about exactly how you plan payment."
"How about $10 a month (on a $300 bill)?"	"I'd like to accept that but our accountant does not allow us to stretch out payments beyond 90 days, which would be $100 a month." This adheres to (Truth in Lending law) regulations for collecting payment in installments without a written agreement. If the patient tries to cooperate, then compromise. If not, turn the account over to a collection agency.
"I sent in the payment."	"When was the payment sent? To what address was it sent? Was it a check? On what bank was it drawn and for what amount? What is the canceled check number?" Investigate to determine whether the check was posted to a wrong account. If not, call the patient back and ask if he or she would call their bank to see if it cleared; if it has not cleared, the patient should stop payment. Ask the patient to call back and verify the status of the check. If the patient is not being truthful, he or she will not follow through. Ask for a new check and tell the patient that a refund will be made if the other one shows up.
"I cannot make a payment this month."	"The collection agency picks up all of our delinquent accounts next Monday. I don't want to include yours, but I need a check today."
"The check is in the mail."	"May I have the check number and date it was mailed?" Call back in 3 days if not received.
"I'm not going to pay the bill because the doctor didn't spend any time with me."	"May I confirm the doctor you saw, the date, and time? For what reason did you see the doctor? Do you still have the problem for which you saw the doctor?" Get as much information as possible and research the office schedule on the day the patient was seen. Let the doctor know about the patient's complaint and inquire how he or she would like to handle the complaint.
"I thought the insurance company was paying this."	"Your insurance paid most of the bill; now the balance is your responsibility. Please send your check before Friday to keep your account current." Explain why (deductible, copayment benefit) the service is not covered under the insurance plan.

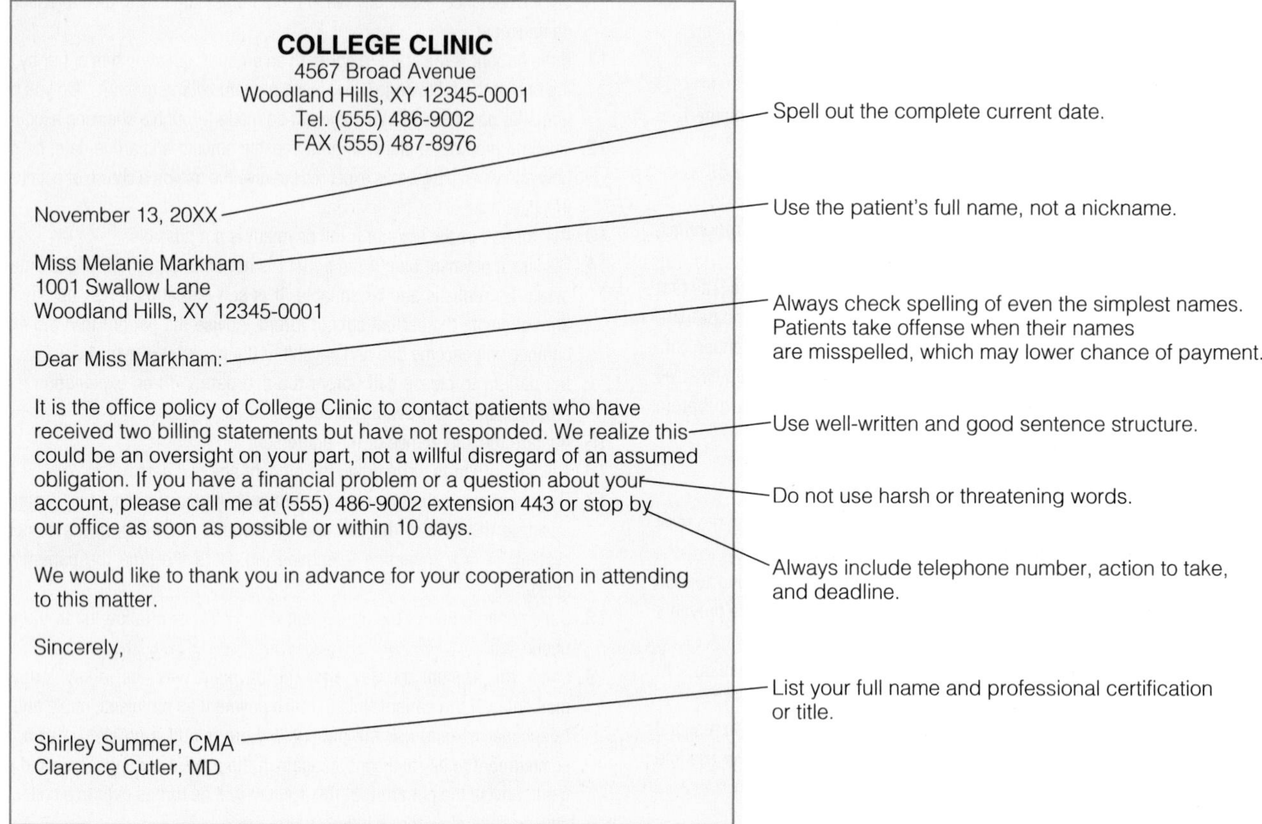

COLLEGE CLINIC
4567 Broad Avenue
Woodland Hills, XY 12345-0001
Tel. (555) 486-9002
FAX (555) 487-8976

November 13, 20XX

Miss Melanie Markham
1001 Swallow Lane
Woodland Hills, XY 12345-0001

Dear Miss Markham:

It is the office policy of College Clinic to contact patients who have received two billing statements but have not responded. We realize this could be an oversight on your part, not a willful disregard of an assumed obligation. If you have a financial problem or a question about your account, please call me at (555) 486-9002 extension 443 or stop by our office as soon as possible or within 10 days.

We would like to thank you in advance for your cooperation in attending to this matter.

Sincerely,

Shirley Summer, CMA
Clarence Cutler, MD

Fig. 17.17 Collection form letter sent to all patients who have not responded after two billing cycles.

The insurance billing specialist is often the one who composes collection letters and devises a plan for collection follow-up. A series of collection letters may be written using varying degrees of forcefulness, starting with a gentle reminder. When a collection letter is written, use a friendly tone and ask why payment has not been made. Imply that the patient has good intentions to pay. This may be done by suggesting that the patient has overlooked a previous statement. Communicate the health care organization's sincere interest in the patient. Always invite the patient to explain the reason for nonpayment in a letter, telephone call, or service encounter. It should sound as though the patient is eager to clear the debt.

When collection letters are sent toward the end of the year, include a statement letting the patient know that if the account is paid in full by the end of the year, the medical expense may be used as an income tax deduction. Another tactic is to send a notice advising the patient that he or she may skip December's payment because of increased expenses during the holidays. This tactic may be used as an opportunity to build patient relationships, but the collector must be firm and clear when offering such leeway. Collection letters sent after the first of the year can suggest that the patient clear the debt by using an income tax refund check.

Types of Collection Letters

A form letter saves time and can go out automatically at specific times during the billing cycle (Fig. 17.18).

Collection letters should contain the following information:

- Full amount owed
- Services performed
- What action the patient should take
- Time frame in which the patient should respond
- How the patient should take care of the bill
- Why the patient should take care of the bill
- Address to which the patient should send payment
- Telephone number to contact the office
- Contact person's name
- Signature, which can be listed as "Financial Secretary," "Insurance Billing Specialist," or one's name and title with the health care organization's name below it

When pursuing collection, the insurance billing specialist should stay within the authorization of the health care organization. All letters should be noted on the back of the financial accounting record, in the collection log, or in the computer comment area. Abbreviations can be used to indicate which letter was sent (Table 17.3) as well as the date on which the letter was mailed. Letters can be sent in brightly colored envelopes to attract attention. The envelope should include "address service requested" or "forwarding service requested" on the outside to ensure that the letter is forwarded if the patient has moved so that the office will be notified of the patient's new address. Always include a self-addressed stamped envelope.

Collection Abbreviations

Collection abbreviations can be used to save time and space while documenting efforts to collect and patients' responses. A few of the most common abbreviations are listed in Table 17.3. Always use standard abbreviations so that anyone working on the account will know exactly what attempts have been made to collect and what action has been taken.

COLLEGE CLINIC
4567 Broad Avenue
Woodland Hills, XY 12345-0001
Tel. (555) 486-9002
FAX (555) 487-8976

March 16, 20XX

Mr. Frank Lincoln
3397 Westminster Avenue
Woodland Hills, XY 12345-0001

Account No. 593287
Amount Due: $ ______________

Dear Mr. Lincoln:

The care of our patients is more important than writing letters about overdue accounts. Yet, as you must realize, the expense of furnishing care can only be met by payments from appreciative patients.

Your account is seriously past due and has been removed from our current files because of its delinquent status. Our office policy indicates that your account should be placed with a collection agency.However, we would prefer to hear from you regarding your preference in this matter.

Enclosed is a current statement of your account. Please indicate your payment choice.

- ☐ I would prefer to settle this account immediately. Please find payment in full enclosed.
- ☐ I would prefer to make monthly payments (up to six months). To exercise this option, please call and make arrangements to come into our office to sign a financial agreement.
- ☐ Please charge the full amount to my credit card. (We accept American Express, MasterCard, and Visa). To exercise this option, please telephone our office or fill in the enclosed form and return it with the envelope provided.

____
Signature Date

Please select one of the three options above, sign the form, and return this notice within 10 days from the date indicated in the letter. A postmarked return envelope is provided. Failure to respond will result in an automatic referral to our collection agency. Please do not hesitate to call if you have any questions regarding this matter.

Sincerely,

Gil Steinberg
Office Manager

Enc. Envelope, Credit Card Agreement Form

Fig. 17.18 Multipurpose collection letter with checklist. This advises the patient of a seriously past due account, offers the patient three payment options, and warns the patient that failure to respond will result in a referral to a collection agency.

TABLE 17.3 **Collection Abbreviations**

Abbreviation	Description	Abbreviation	Description
Atty	Attorney	NSN	No such number
B	Bankrupt	OFC	Office
Bal	Balance	OOT	Out of town
Bk*	Bank	OOW	Out of work
BLG	Belligerent	PA	Payment arrangement
BTTR	Best time to reach	PH or PH'D	Phoned
CB	Call back	Ph/Dsc*	Phone disconnected
CLM	Claim	PIF	Payment in full
DA*	Directory assistance	PIM	Payment in mail
DFB	Demand for balance	PMT	Payment
DNK	Did not know	POE	Place of employment
DSC	Disconnected	POW	Payment on way
EMP	Employed	PP	Promise to pay or partial payment
EOM	End of month	PT	Patient
EOW	End of week	RCD	Received
FA	Further action	R/D*	Reverse directory
FN	Final notice	RE	About
H	He (or husband)	RES	Residence
HHCO	Have husband call office	S	She (or wife)
HSB	Husband	SEP	Separated
HTO	He phoned office	SK*	Skip or skipped
HU	Hung up	SOS	Same old story
INS	Insurance	SP/DEL*	Special delivery
L1, L2	Letter one, letter two (sent)	STO	She phoned office
LB	Line busy	TB	Phoned business
LD	Long distance	TR	Phoned residence
LM	Left message	TXT	Texted
LMCO	Left message, call office	TT	Talked to
LMVM	Left message, voice mail	TTA	Turned to agency
LTR	Letter	UE or U/Emp	Unemployed
MR	Mail return	UTC	Unable to contact
N1, N2	Note one, note two (sent)	VFD	Verified
NA	No answer	Vfd/E	Verified employment
NFA*	No forwarding address	Vfd/I	Verified insurance
NHD*	Never heard of debtor	W/	Will
NI	Not in	WCO	Will call office
NLE	No longer employed	WCIO	Will come in office
NPL	No phone listed	W/I	Walk-in
NPN	Nonpublished number	WVO	Will visit office
NR	No record	X	By
NSF	Nonsufficient funds		

*Used in skip tracing.

Insurance Collection

Most patients carry some form of insurance; however, filing an insurance claim is only the first step in collecting fees owed. As discussed in previous chapters, good follow-up techniques are necessary to ensure payment from the third-party payer and copayment or coinsurance payment from the patient.

First, affirm that a clean insurance claim was submitted electronically with all necessary preauthorization and documentation for services. Next, follow up in a timely manner with electronic submission reports from the clearinghouse. Track all denials to learn what services are being denied and which insurance companies are denying payment.

History of Accounts

If the third-party payer seems to be ignoring all efforts to trace the claim, an exact history of the account may be the best weapon with which to proceed. A history of the account is a chronologic record of all events that have occurred. Keep all communications received from the third-party payer, note all telephone calls, and keep copies of all documents sent. Send a copy of the history of the account directly to the third-party payer and demand a reply. This may also be done in the case of an insurance company dispute or a refusal to pay.

Coinsurance Payments

Use a letter or statement to collect from patients who have insurance coverage. Clearly indicate to the patient that the insurance billing specialist has submitted an insurance claim and advise the patient what action is expected. The status of the insurance claim should be noted on all statements. Notify patients promptly when insurance payment has been received. Ask patients to get involved in the insurance process or to pay the bill within 10 days if a problem exists. The following are examples of notations on statements for patients with insurance coverage:

- "We have received payment from your insurance company. The balance of $_____ is now your responsibility."
- "Your insurance company has paid its share of your bill. This statement is for the amount payable directly by you."
- "Your insurance company has paid $_____ for the above services. The remaining portion of $_____ is now your responsibility."
- "The balance of this account is your share of the cost. Please remit today. For questions, call 486-9002."
- "Your insurance company has not responded. The account is due and payable. Please contact your insurance company about payment. Thank you for your assistance."

Insurance Checks Sent to Patients

Send a letter immediately to notify patients who receive insurance checks. Advise such patients that they have received payment from their insurance company and that their account is due and payable within 10 days. Do not send continuous monthly bills; instead, speed up the collection process. If the patient refuses to pay and the health care organization does not want the patient to return, send a 10-day notification advising the patient that the account will go to a collection agency. If there is no response, refer to the health care organization's policy for discharging a patient and proceed accordingly.

MANAGED CARE

Managed Care Organizations

When a health care organization deals with numerous insurance carriers, trying to remember all of the contract information can be confusing. A managed care desk reference can help staff members to find information quickly. "Promised payment date" along with all the other information on the desk reference grid or matrix can be easily referred to by the insurance billing specialist when trying to collect from managed care organizations. Ensure that all referral authorizations are in place before the patient is to be seen. If a patient shows up without a referral, offer to reschedule or inform the patient that the visit must be paid for in cash before leaving the office. If the patient has no money, a promissory note may be executed, but this action is not preferred and should be carried out as a last option. When dealing with managed care contracts, do not sign any contract that holds a third party "harmless." The "hold harmless" clause is a way for one party to shift financial responsibilities to another party. Such "hold harmless" clauses often include phrases that state that the third party is "held harmless" to pay claims, liabilities, costs, expenses, judgments, or damages awarded by any court to all patients who bring any legal action against the health care organization. If the third party goes out of business or goes bankrupt before the contract is honored, the health care organization cannot collect any money from the patient that the third party was to have paid. To avoid such possibilities, ensure that payments from all managed care organizations are current. Check to see that all third-party payers are insured by a federal agency. Such insurance would pay the health care organization in the event that the managed care organization could not.

MEDICARE

Health care organizations must make genuine efforts to collect the unpaid deductible and coinsurance amounts from all Medicare patients. Reasonable efforts must include subsequent billings, telephone calls, and in-person collection efforts done in the same manner as with all patients. Accounts may not be written off until sequential statements (spaced 15 to 30 days apart) have been sent, with an increasing intensity in the collection message. A telephone call should be placed to the debtor asking for payment; a request for payment should be made when the patient is seen in person as well.

MEDICARE

Medigap Insurance

When a patient has Medigap (MG) insurance, ensure that the patient's signature appears in Block 13 of the CMS-1500 insurance claim form. Do not routinely enter "signature on file" unless the insured has signed an insurance-specific statement authorizing assignment of benefits to the service provider named on the claim form. A signed statement allowing the health care organization to bill and receive payment for MG-covered services until the beneficiary revokes authorization is preferred. A Medicare "signature on file" is not sufficient.

WORKERS' COMPENSATION

Verify the validity of work-related injury and illness through the patient's employer and obtain accurate billing information, including the date of injury. Send timely bills and reports using the correct coding system and fee schedule. Always keep the adjuster assigned to the case informed of ongoing treatment. The patient and employer should both be notified if a problem exists. Document all correspondence, including telephone authorizations for treatment and any tracing efforts. Any disputed or unresolved workers' compensation cases may be revised to self-pay or referred to a financial service representative or the proper state-level authority. The service provider may file for mediation on behalf of the patient if proper authorization was obtained and a claim form sent at the time of the patient's treatment. A claim may also be filed with the state labor board, naming the patient's employer and workers' compensation carrier, whenever there is difficulty getting full payment. The industrial board has the employer pressure the carrier to resolve the matter. If an insurance company has not paid or has sent a written notice of nonpayment, the service provider may file a request for default judgment from the state authority. If the judgment is in the provider's favor, the payer is ordered to pay in full.

Suing a Third-Party Payer

As stated in the Statute of Limitations section, there are periods during which an insured person may sue the insurance company to collect the amount that the claimant believes is owed. An insured person may not initiate a legal action against the insurer until 60 days after the initial claim has been submitted. A lawsuit against the insurer must be filed within 3 years of the date on which the initial claim was submitted for payment.

When the insurance company does not respond to reason or negotiation after the health care organization's office has tried to collect from an insurance plan, the only alternatives are surrender or litigation. A lawsuit may be worthwhile if a high-dollar claim is in question. Third-party payers may be sued for payment under two circumstances: claim for plan benefits or breach of contract and claim for damages.

Claims for plan benefits are used when the claim is governed by the Employee Retirement Income Security Act (ERISA), and Federal Employee Health Benefit Act (FEHBA). ERISA governs health insurance that is provided as a benefit of employment. FEHBA governs all health insurance provided as a benefit to federal employees. An insured person is entitled to appeal a denied claim under these two federal laws. A timely request must be filed to sue for payment. The time limit for ERISA is within 60 days of denial; the time limit for FEHBA is within 6 months. Federal laws apply across the country and overrule all state laws. Suits based on claims for plan benefits may be made when denial is based on the following:

- Medical necessity
- Preexisting condition
- Usual and customary rate issues
- Health care organizations or providers that are not covered
- Services that fall within an exclusion to coverage
- Failure to offer Consolidated Omnibus Budget Reconciliation Act (COBRA) coverage by a plan administrator

When the claim falls outside the scope of these federal laws, it is possible to sue if the conduct of the payer constitutes a violation of state laws relating to unfair insurance practices.

Suing based on claim for damages falls entirely under state law in the state where the health care organization is located. This is most likely to occur if the patient has no plan benefit but the patient or service provider's office is led to believe so by the insurer or plan administrator. Examples include the following:

- Insurer misquoting benefits during a verification of those benefits
- Denial of payment because of lack of medical necessity when preauthorization of treatment was obtained

Collection Agencies

Delinquent accounts should be turned over to a collection agency only after all reasonable attempts have been made to collect by the health care organization. Knowing when to turn accounts over helps determine the success of the collection agency. The longer the balance is unpaid, the less chance the agency has to collect the account, so the determination that an account is uncollectable should be made quickly. Following are some situations in which a health care organization should consider turning an account over to a collection agency:

- When a patient states that they will not pay or there is a denial of responsibility
- When a patient breaks a promise to pay
- When a patient makes partial payments and 60 days have lapsed without payment
- When a patient fails to respond to the health care organization's letters or telephone calls
- When payment terms fail for no valid reason
- When a check is returned by the bank because of NSF and the patient does not make an effort to rectify the situation within 1 week of notification
- When delinquency coexists with marital problems, divorce proceedings, or child support agreements
- When a patient is paid by the insurance company and does not forward the payment to the health care organization (This constitutes fraud and may be pursued with legal action.)
- When a patient gives false information
- When a patient moves, and the office has used all resources to locate the patient

Not all accounts should go to a collection agency. Such accounts include those of personal friends, elderly widows or widowers living on pensions, and accounts with balances less than $25. Many health care organizations prefer to adjust small bad debts off the books rather than increase administrative costs. All disputed accounts should be reviewed and approved by the individual designated by administration before they are sent to collection; to expedite the collection process, it is important for the health care organization and the office manager to establish a standard policy for deciding which accounts are sent to collections. There should be a systematized approach for turning accounts over to a collection agency that still allows room for exceptions.

Choosing an Agency

The collection agency is a reflection of the health care organization, so it is important to choose one wisely. Choose a reputable agency that is considerate and efficient, with a high standard of ethics. The agency should specialize in health care accounts and have an attitude toward debtors with which the organization agrees. Find out how long the agency has been in business and request a list of at least 10 references and statistics on their collection effectiveness. The average collection rate varies greatly but falls between 20% and 60% on assigned accounts. Ensure that the reported rate includes all accounts more than 1 year old and does not exclude accounts with small balances.

An agency's performance can be evaluated by the amount collected, less the agency's fees, which is called the **netback**. For instance, if a collector recovered 25% of $5000 ($1250) and takes a 50% commission, the health care organization's netback is $625. If a different collector recovered 25% of the $5000 ($1250) and charged a 30% commission, the netback is $375. Although the second agency collected the same amount, its lower commission afforded the health care organization more money.

When choosing a collection agency, make sure (1) to set up a separate post office box or lock box for the collection project; (2) to set up a separate bank account for the collection project; (3) that the contract stipulates that all correspondence be sent to the post office box (no correspondence is sent to the collection agency's physical or payment address); (4) that all e-checks and credit card receipts are deposited into the health care organization's bank account; and (5) that under no circumstance is the collection agency to receive any payments.

If collected funds go directly to the collection agency (whether insured, bonded, registered, or licensed), there is nothing to stop the agency from stealing the health care organization's money. The collection agency also could have a hidden lawsuit against it or an income tax lien and the organization may lose all its money if the money goes to the agency's bank account. Do not put "hold harmless" clauses in contracts. Hold the collection agency responsible for its actions. Many states do not regulate collection agencies and simply require that these agencies be registered. In addition to checking references, check with the state's Department of Corporations to determine whose name is on the collection agency's registration, if the tax identification number is correct and current, and if the address listed is different from the one the agency gave. Contact the circuit court to determine whether there are any lawsuits or judgments against the collection agency. Find out how many of the collection agency's employees will be assigned to the account, then monitor them once the contract is signed. They may have the best credentials and references and belong to all the correct organizations, but if they acquire an increasing number of accounts and the amount of recoupment remains constant each month or is less than the national average, they may be picking and choosing the accounts. This is especially true when they are overanxious to receive a new file. If this happens, consider looking for another collection agency. Ensure that an account can be recalled without a penalty. The patient may have coverage with an insurance carrier that the health care organization has a contract with, so find out if the collection agency has the ability to resend a claim or if the billing company or office staff handles this. If so, does the contract have provisions for this and does the collection agency receive recoupment for obtaining insurance information?

The biggest key to the agency's effectiveness is the health care organization's own credit and collection policy. A comprehensive patient registration form, along with verifying employment, turning accounts over quickly when they qualify, and giving the agency all available information, helps the agency to pick up the paper trail and secure payment. A good collection agency has membership in a national collection society and the approval of the local medical society. Review the agency's financial statement and ensure that the agency is licensed, bonded, and carries "hold harmless clause" insurance. If a patient should sue because of harassment, this insurance will protect the health care organization from being sued as well. The local bar association and state licensing bureaus can be contacted to determine whether any complaints have been lodged against the agency or law firm. Find out if the agency reports uncollectable debtors ("deadbeats") to a credit bureau and investigate which one is used.

Types of Agencies

There are local, regional, and national agencies. National agencies and those that use the internet may have better results when tracing **skips** (patients who owe balances on their accounts and move without leaving a forwarding address). Local agencies are more aware of the socioeconomic status of patients. Some agencies pay their staff commissions and bonuses for high productivity and others are low key and more customer oriented. Find out the experience level of the staff and ensure that the agency values the health care organization's business.

Another option is to use a collection service, such as CollectNet, which gives small and midsized facilities with limited budgets the collection capabilities of large collection systems by connecting to databases. The health care organization is able to make calling lists, print collection letters, search for telephone numbers and addresses, access patient credit reports, write and format reports, monitor collection progress, and set automatic callback reminders. Optional features include BankruptcyNet, SkipNet, LetterNet, and BureauNet. Collection agencies use this service, but it is also available to large groups and clinics.

Agency Operating Techniques

Collection agencies must follow all the laws stated in the Fair Debt Collection Practices Act. They may not "harass" the debtor or make false threats and they may not use letters that appear to be legal documents. A provision should be included for the agency to seek permission from the health care organization's office before suing a debtor in municipal court and charging a percentage of the judgment. A progress report should be provided to the health care organization on a regular basis at least monthly. The agency also should return any uncollectable accounts within a reasonable time and not charge for these accounts. All procedures used to make collections should be shown to the health care organization, including collection letters and telephone scripts. The health care organization should be aware if the agency uses a personalized or standard approach. A personal visit to the premises of the collection agency can provide a firsthand view of its operating techniques.

Agency Charges

Agencies may be paid a flat rate on all accounts according to volume. Some agencies may leave the accounts in the control of the health care organization, where the staff speaks with the patient and posts all delinquent incoming monies. Other agencies charge a commission based on a percentage of an account and the health care organization refers all calls to the agency once the account is turned over to it. A standard rate needed for most agencies to break even is one third of all monies collected and an average rate charged is 50%. Make sure the commission is based on how much is collected on the overdue accounts and not the total amount of overdue accounts turned over to the agency.

Agency Assigned Accounts

Patients' accounts turned over to a collection agency should have a letter of withdrawal sent by certified mail. Place a note on all financial accounting records indicating the date on which the account was assigned. Once an account has been given to a collection agency, it is illegal to send the patient a monthly statement. Financial management consultants usually recommend that the patient's balances be written off the A/R at the time the account is assigned. A portion of the account balance can be written back on if and when the agency collects on the debt. Accounts also should be listed in a separate journal to help track the effectiveness of the agency. Allow enough columns to show the future date, amount, and percentage of an account collected by the agency as well as the total account balance.

PROCEDURE 17.4 File a Claim in Small Claims Court

Objective

To file a claim to obtain payment for a delinquent or uncollectable financial account in small claims court

Equipment/Supplies

Small claims court filing form, photocopy of the patient's financial accounting record, computer or typewriter, pen or pencil, envelope, and check for filing fee

Directions

Follow these step-by-step procedures and guidelines, which include rationales, to learn this job skill.

1. Obtain a Claim of Plaintiff or Plaintiff's Original Petition form to notify the patient that action is being filed. This can be obtained from the clerk's office located at the municipal or justice court. Obtain booklets and material to help guide the claimant through the process.
2. Complete and file the papers with the small claims court; make sure to have the patient's correct name and street address.
3. Make a photocopy of the small claims court form for the office files.
4. Pay the clerk the small filing fee. Filing fees vary by state, by county within some states, and by the amount of the claim.
5. Make arrangements to serve the defendant. The summons or citation can be served on the patient by a sheriff or court-appointed officer by paying a small fee plus mileage for the constable who serves it. The person serving the defendant must fill out a proof of service form.
6. After being served, a patient has one of four options.
   a. Pay the claim to the court clerk. This will be forwarded to the health care organization, but the filing fee or service charge will not be refunded.
   b. Ignore the claim. The health care organization will win by default. In some states, a judgment may be requested in writing, but in other states, the health care organization or its representative must appear on a specified date. If the patient does not appear, the judgment is granted in the health care organization's favor and usually court costs are included in the judgment.
   c. Request a small claims hearing. The court clerk will let both parties know when to appear. The patient may file a counterclaim against the health care organization at this time.
   d. Demand a jury trial. The case will be taken out of small claims court. The health care organization will be notified by the court clerk to file a formal complaint in a higher court and an attorney must represent the health care organization.
7. Appear in court (service provider or health care organization representative) on the specified date; otherwise, the claim will be dismissed and cannot be refiled.
8. Basic information required by the court follows:
   a. Health care organization and service provider's name, address, and telephone number
   b. Patient's name and address
   c. Delinquent amount
   d. Summary of the claim, including the date the health care organization's bill was due, date of the last encounter, date of the last payment, unpaid amount, and all records of telephone contacts and letters sent
9. Determine what the judge needs to hear to decide a favorable case. Good preparation for the trial can make the difference between success and failure.
10. Organize all exhibits in a notebook, in chronologic order. A timeline showing the sequence of events can be useful.
11. Take a businesslike professional approach at the hearing by giving concise and accurate answers to the judge's questions, speaking slowly and clearly. The service provider or the health care organization's representative must bring any witnesses, statements, receipts, contracts, notes, dishonored checks, or other evidence to court. The judge will question the service provider or the health care organization's representative and the patient, review the evidence, and then make a ruling.
12. Put a lien on the debtor's wages, automobile, bank or personal assets, or real property if the judgment, which is usually effective for many years, is in the service provider's favor. This is the service provider's legal right. The small claims office will show the service provider or the health care organization's representative how to execute a judgment.
13. Pay a small fee if the health care organization decides to execute against the patient's assets. It is recoverable from the patient.

Each patient account that has been sent to collection should have an alert pop up every time the file is opened in the medical billing system. This will alert all medical staff of the situation if the patient calls on short notice or walks in to be seen. If the patient sends payment to the health care organization after the account has been turned over to an agency, notify the collection agency immediately. Any calls about accounts that have gone to collection should be referred to the agency.

Small Claims Court

Small claims court is a part of our legal system that allows laypeople access to a court system without the use of an attorney. Some advantages are a modest filing fee, minimal paperwork, exclusion of costly lawyers, and a short time frame from filing the action to trial date.

Most states have small claims courts (also called *conciliation courts, common pleas, general sessions, justice courts,* or *people's courts*). Each state has monetary limits on the amount that can be handled in small claims court and accounts should be reviewed for eligibility. The dollar amount varies from state to state and sometimes from one county to another. The national median small claims jurisdiction is $5300. Several legislative bills being considered by the US Senate and House committees address raising the dollar limit. Several states have already had such bills signed into law. The new limits in these states vary from $3000 to $25,000. There also may be limits on the number of claims filed per year that are for more than a specific dollar amount.

When filing a claim, the health care organization filing the petition is referred to as the *plaintiff* and the party being brought to suit (the patient) is called the *defendant.* It is generally recommended that the plaintiff send a written demand to the defendant before filing a lawsuit to give the defendant a final opportunity to resolve the claim.

For a step-by-step procedure on filing a claim in small claims court, see Procedure 17.4 at the end of this chapter.

After filing a claim, a trial date will be set and both plaintiff and defendant will be ordered to appear before the judge. Often a postcard is sent notifying the plaintiff when the defendant has been served. If the amount of delinquent debt is more than the monetary limit for small claims court, consider "cutting the claim to fit" the limit. For example, if the amount of debt is $2757 and the state limit is $2500, consider waiving (giving up) the $257 (difference) to bring the amount down to the limit. The claim cannot be divided into two different suits of $1378.50 and suing twice on the same claim is not allowed.

Claim Resolutions

The defendant has the following four options after he or she is served:

1. **Pay the claim.** The court clerk will receive the money and forward it to the health care organization, but the filing fee or service charges will not be refunded.
2. **Ignore the claim.** The judge may ask the health care organization's attorney or representative to state its case. The judgment will be awarded in the health care organization's favor, usually including court costs.
3. **Answer the petition.** A contested court hearing will be held. The health care organization has the burden of proving its claim to the court. A counterclaim may be filed by the patient at this time.
4. **Demand a jury trial.** The case will be taken out of small claims court and the health care organization will be notified by the county clerk to file a formal complaint in a higher court. An attorney must represent the health care organization if this occurs.

Trial Preparation

The plaintiff and defendant must both appear on the trial date or the claim will be dismissed and cannot be refiled. Instead of attending the trial in person, the health care organization may send a representative. If the claim is settled before trial, a dismissal form should be dated, signed, and filed with the clerk.

Preparation for the trial is essential and can mean the difference between success and failure. Decide what the judge should hear to conclude in the health care organization's favor. Although being represented in court by a lawyer is not allowed, a lawyer can be asked for advice before going to court. Recommendations to help prepare for trial are as follows:

1. Be on time; otherwise, the court may give a judgment in the defendant's favor.
2. Be ready to submit the basic data required by the court: the health care organization and service provider's name, address, and telephone number; the patient's name and address; the delinquent amount being claimed; and a brief summary of the claim.
3. Show all dates of service and amounts owed, the date on which the bill was due (if a series of treatments is involved), the last date service was provided, the date of the last payment (if any payment was made), and the amount still unpaid.
4. Include all attempts to collect the debt and organize all exhibits in chronologic order. Include documentation, such as copies of statements, letters, notes, receipts, contracts, dishonored checks, telephone calls, other discussions with the patient, and other evidence to present to the court. A timeline showing the sequence of events may be useful.
5. Speak slowly and clearly, present the case in a concise manner, and use a businesslike approach. Answer all questions accurately but briefly.
6. Present a witness if live testimony is relevant. A notarized statement from a witness is admissible but not as effective.
7. Try to anticipate the opposing party's evidence and arguments so that a rebuttal may be prepared. Keep in mind that a third party will be making the decision.

The judge will question the health care organization's representative and the patient, review the evidence, and then make a ruling. Winning the case gives the health care organization the right to attach a debtor's bank assets, salary, car, personal assets, or real property. The small claims office can advise on how to execute a judgment. Judgments are usually effective for many years. There is a small charge if the health care organization decides to execute against the patient's assets but this charge is recoverable from the defendant.

A losing defendant may appeal and request a new trial in superior court. The defendant may ask the judge to make small installment payments, but not all judges order this alternative. If the defendant fails to pay, a writ of execution may be obtained from the clerk's office to enforce judgment. This writ of execution permits the marshal to obtain funds from a losing party's bank account or take items of the losing party's property to satisfy the judgment.

Federal Wage Garnishment Laws

Garnishment is a court order attaching a debtor's property or wages to pay off a debt. Federal wage garnishment laws provide a limit on the amount of employee earnings withheld in a work week or pay period when a debtor's future wage is seized to pay off a debt. They also protect the employee from being dismissed if their pay is garnished for only one debt, regardless of the number of levies that must be made to collect. This law is enforced by the compliance officers of the Wage and Hour Office of the US Department of Labor. The laws do not apply to federal government employees, court-ordered support of any person, court orders in personal bankruptcy cases, or state or federal tax levies. The patient's employer becomes involved as the "trustee" because the employer owes money to the debtor for wages earned.

Once a garnishment has been ordered by the court, an employer must honor it by satisfying the terms of garnishment before wages can be paid to the debtor. Only a percentage of the wage (usually 25%) is garnished and paid to the creditor. This amount is determined from the employee's disposable earnings. Disposable earnings are the amount left after Social Security and federal, state, and local taxes are deducted. The statute resulting in the smaller garnishment applies when state garnishment laws conflict with federal laws. This method of collection should be considered a last resort for a health care organization and used only with large bills.

Tracing a Skip

A patient who owes a balance on their account and moves but leaves no forwarding address is called a *skip*. In these cases, an unopened envelope is returned to the office marked

BOX 17.3 Search Techniques Used to Trace a Debtor

1. Cross-check the address on the returned envelope with the patient registration form and account to ensure that it was mailed correctly.
2. Check the zip code directory to determine whether the zip code corresponds with the patient's street address or post office box.
3. File a request with the local post office to obtain a new or corrected address.
4. Call the primary care physician for updated information when investigating for a health care organization.
5. Determine whether the patient has been seen at the hospital; if so, speak to someone in the accounts department.
6. Inquire at the patient's place of employment. If the patient is no longer employed, ask to speak to the personnel department in an effort to locate the patient. Do not divulge the reason for the call.
7. Contact persons listed on the patient registration form, including personal referrals.
8. Request information from the Department of Motor Vehicles if a driver's license number is available.
9. Request information from utility companies.
10. Inquire at the patient's bank to determine whether he or she is still a customer.
11. Obtain the services of a local credit bureau to check reports and receive notification if the patient's Social Security number shows up under a different name or at a new address.
12. Check public records, such as tax records, voter registration, court records, death and probate records, hunting and fishing licenses, and marriage licenses.

"returned to sender, addressee unknown." Place the words "forwarding service requested" below the health care organization's return address on the envelope and the post office will make a search and forward the mail to the new address. The health care organization will be informed of this new address for a nominal fee. Complete a Freedom of Information Act form at the post office if the address is a rural delivery box number and the US Postal Service will provide the physical location of a person's residence. When patients send payments by mail, precautions must be taken to avoid discarding envelopes with a change of address. Always match the address on the envelope, along with the check, against the patient's account. One staff person should be responsible for updating all patients' addresses in all locations to prevent this problem.

Skip Tracing Techniques

Once it is determined that a patient is a skip, tracing should begin immediately. Office policies should be established stating how the skip will be traced and at what point the account will be sent to a collection agency. Some offices choose to make only one attempt, whereas others prefer to do most of the detective work themselves. Box 17.3 lists techniques that can be used to initiate the search for the debtor.

Never state one's business with the patient when trying to make any of these contacts. Keep all information confidential. A good skip tracer should have patience and the ability to pursue all necessary steps with tenacity and tact. A good imagination, a detective's instincts, and the ability to get along with people help in this tedious job.

Skip Tracing Services

There are several outside services from which to choose. Some agencies offer customized service with several levels of skip tracing available. Each level is more extensive and costly. The health care organization decides at which level it would like the search conducted. The first level usually involves verifying the patient's information and checking for typographic errors. The highest level uses every resource available to find the patient. The age of the account, the account balance, and the cost of the level of skip tracing service are all considerations when deciding which level to choose. A collection agency or credit bureau (as mentioned) may offer the services of skip tracing as well.

Search via Computer

Another method of skip tracing is to use electronic databases or online services. "Information wholesalers" also exist. They cater to bill collectors and similar interested parties. There are a number of bills pending in Congress aimed at restricting the flow of personal data in cyberspace. Perhaps in the future this information will not be so easy to obtain; however, conducting a successful electronic search is relatively easy at present. The following are several methods used to search electronic databases to locate a debtor's address and home telephone number:

- *Surname scan* can be done locally, regionally, or nationally using data banks that have been compiled from public source documents.
- *Address search* provides property search and any change of address from all suppliers of data to the database, including the US Postal Service. Names of other adults in the household who may have the debtor's telephone number listed under their name may be included.
- *Credit holder search* is used to establish occupation.
- *Phone number search* permits access to the names of other adults within the same household who have a telephone number.
- *Neighbor search* displays the names, addresses, and telephone numbers of the debtor's former neighbors.
- *Zip code search* provides the names, addresses, and telephone numbers of everyone within that zip code who has the same last name as the debtor.
- *City search* locates everyone with the same last and first name within a given city as well as all people who live in that city.
- *State search* finds all people with the same last name or same last and first name within the state and lists their addresses and telephone numbers.
- *National search* operates the same way as the state search. It is recommended for people with unusual last names.
- *Business search* lists all the names of the businesses in the neighborhood of the patient's last known residence. This search may help find where the patient has relocated or verify the patient's place of employment.

Explore several directories to cross-check results because data change frequently. Information is not secure when using the internet. The patient's right to privacy must never be violated.

Special Collection Issues

Bankruptcy

Bankruptcy is a condition under which a person or corporation is declared unable to pay debts. Bankruptcy laws are federal laws applicable in all states that ensure equal distribution of the assets of an individual among the individual's creditors. There are two kinds of bankruptcy petitions: voluntary and involuntary. A voluntary petition is one filed by a person asking for relief under the Bankruptcy Reform Act (the Code). An involuntary petition is one filed against a person by their creditors requesting that a person obtain relief under the Code.

When a patient files for bankruptcy, he or she becomes a ward of the court and has its protection. The patient is granted an **automatic stay** against creditors, which means that the health care organization may contact the patient only for the name, address, and telephone number of their attorney. The insurance billing specialist should no longer send statements, make telephone calls, or attempt to collect the account. A creditor can be fined for contempt of court if it continues to proceed against the debtor. If a collection agency has the account and has been notified of the bankruptcy, the situation is the same as if the health care organization has been notified. If the health care organization is notified first, the collection agency should be called and informed of the bankruptcy. Notification of bankruptcy does not have to be in writing; verbal communication is valid (for example, if a patient contacts the health care organization to inform it of the bankruptcy). Bankruptcy remains part of the debtor's permanent credit record for 10 years.

After a patient informs the health care organization of the bankruptcy, determine what type of bankruptcy the debtor has filed. Refer to Box 17.4 for a listing of the five types of bankruptcy cases.

BOX 17.4 Types of Bankruptcy Cases

Chapter 7 Case

Chapter 7 bankruptcy is sometimes called a *straight petition in bankruptcy* or *absolute bankruptcy*. In Chapter 7 bankruptcy, the court considers the individual's property as a possible means for paying back creditors. Once the individual files bankruptcy, all their property becomes part of the bankruptcy estate. Certain property is exempt from being sold to repay creditors, while other property is not exempt. The property that is not exempt is called **nonexempt assets**. In this case, all of the nonexempt assets of the bankrupt person are liquidated and distributed according to the law to the creditors. Secured creditors are first in line for payment of all **secured debt**.

Unsecured creditors are last. A person declares those to whom he or she owes money and is not required to make payment, thus eliminating all the debtor's outstanding legal obligations for **unsecured debt**. Most medical bills are considered unsecured debt because they are not backed by any form of **collateral**. Collateral would be valuables or possessions such as automobiles, furniture, stocks, or bonds that secure or guarantee the discharge of an obligation. The only debt that is discharged in Chapter 7 bankruptcy is the debt that had been incurred up to the point of filing for protection under Chapter 7. So, if a patient files before services are rendered, the bankruptcy laws do not apply for the treatment provided. A Chapter 7 bankruptcy does not necessarily result in the discharge of all debts. If the patient lies about their financial status, the debt may not be dischargeable. If the debt incurred was for a luxury service (for example, facelift), immediately preceding the filing, it is possible that it may not be discharged. Consult the health care organization's attorney before adjusting the debt off the books in such a situation. All creditors are notified by the Administrator in Bankruptcy as to the proceedings and may choose either to attend the proceedings or to make a claim against whatever assets remain.

Chapter 9 Case

This case is used for reorganization proceedings when a city or town is insolvent or unable to meet its debts. A plan is put into effect to adjust such debts.

Chapter 11 Case

This case is used for reorganization of a business enterprise when the company is unable to meet its debts but would like to continue business and would be unable to do so if creditors took away its assets. A plan of arrangement is confirmed by the court and each class of creditor must accept the plan or receive at least that which it would receive on liquidation of the company.

Chapter 12 Case

This case is used for reorganization when farmers are unable to meet their debts.

Chapter 13 Case

This is sometimes called a *wage earner's bankruptcy*. It is designed to protect the wage earner from creditors while allowing the wage earner to make arrangements to repay a portion of his or her bills (about 70%) over a 3- or 5-year period. The debtor pays a fixed amount agreed on by the court to the trustee in bankruptcy. A claim needs to be filed as directed by the debtor's attorney.

Bankruptcy Rules

Under the bankruptcy rules effective October 17, 2005, debtors must meet an income test and must have insufficient assets to be eligible for filing a Chapter 7 bankruptcy. Otherwise they are forced into Chapter 13 bankruptcy, in which a debt repayment plan is ordered.

When filing a claim, the proper form may be obtained from a stationery store or by writing to the presiding judge of the bankruptcy court. If a creditor fails to file a claim, the creditor will lose the right to any proceeds from the bankruptcy. A plan for payment will be approved by the court. The trustee may be contacted from time to time to check the status of the claim and the payments that should be expected. Once a patient has obtained credit counseling and petitioned for bankruptcy, there must be a time lapse of 6 years before he or she can file again. The only exception to this is Chapter 13 bankruptcy.

Terminally Ill Patients

Although it may be difficult to collect from patients who are terminally ill, it is usually harder to collect from the estates after they have died. When a patient is too sick or scared to communicate necessary information, consult the health care provider about whether to obtain the patient's permission to speak to family members and stress the need for help. Usually, terminally ill patients want to do the right thing. Call the patient before he or she comes in to receive service. Ensure that the patient is aware of the existing balance and try to work with the patient

PROCEDURE 17.5 File an Estate Claim

Objective

To file a claim on an estate for a deceased patient who has an outstanding balance on his or her financial accounting record

Equipment/Supplies

Statement of Claim form, computer or typewriter, pen or pencil, photocopy machine, patient's financial accounting record, US Postal Service certified mail forms, and envelope

Directions

Follow these step-by-step procedures and guidelines, which include rationales, to learn this job skill.

1. Confirm the date and place of death with the hospital, nursing home, or funeral home.
2. Pursue payment from all third-party payers first.
3. Contact the Register of Wills office in the county where the patient lived or the probate department of the superior court, County Recorder's Office. Request a Statement of Claim form or the county's proper document to formally register a claim against an estate.
4. File the claim according to the instructions received with the claim form. When probate is filed, a notification will be sent advising the court of probate, the attorney representing the estate, and the **estate executor** or **estate administrator**. Perhaps a small fee should be included for court costs.
5. Send a photocopy of the patient's financial accounting record (itemized statement) by certified mail, return receipt, to the attorney and copies to the executor and the court. If the health care organization treated the deceased patient's last illness, that fact should be clearly indicated on the statement.
6. Allow the legal system to take its course. A call to the executor can be made periodically to check on the status of the estate.

to eliminate at least a portion of the balance before the next appointment. Estimate costs and prepare a plan that is agreeable to both the health care organization and the patient.

Estate Claims

Great care and sensitivity should be taken when trying to collect on a deceased patient's account. When the health care organization discovers that a patient has died, first pursue insurance coverage. The entire probate system was set up to help protect families from painful involvement in estate settlements. Do not offend the deceased's family by making contact during the time of bereavement. However, file a claim after the first or second week so that the health care organization's name can be added to the list of creditors.

Refer to Procedure 17.5 at the end of this chapter for filing an estate claim.

After filing, the claim is denied or accepted. If accepted, an acknowledgment of the debt is sent to the health care organization. Many delays arise because of the legal complications of settling an estate but the debts are paid according to a priority system when the estate is settled. Usually funeral expenses are paid first; following in order are estate administration expenses, claims due for the deceased person's last illness, and taxes and other debts. Any amounts left are divided among family members. A lien or lawsuit may be filed against the estate in the rare case of a rejection of the claim.

Various state time limits and statutes govern the filing of a claim against an estate. Check with the county court in your state to obtain filing deadlines. Deadlines may range from 2 months to 3 years but must be adhered to for successful collection from an estate.

Litigation

A difficult question arises when the health care organization is advised that a patient is involved in a pending litigation related to the services provided to the patient. It may not be necessary to wait until the litigation is resolved to pursue payment. Assess whether the patient has the ability to pay before possibly receiving a settlement in a lawsuit. Before withholding collection activity, the health care organization should get a guarantee that it will be paid in full before the patient (debtor) receives money from a settlement. The agreement must be guaranteed by the lawyer representing the patient. If the patient is working, regular payments should be required pending the settlement of the patient's litigation. It is always advisable to contact a malpractice attorney in such cases.

Liens

A **lien** is a claim on the property of another as security for a debt. This may include a claim on a future settlement of a lawsuit. The health care organization may be asked to accept a lien by a patient or the patient's attorney when the patient has been involved in an automobile accident and is awaiting a settlement (Fig. 17.19). In litigation cases, a lien is a legal promise to satisfy a debt owed by the patient to the health care organization out of any proceeds received on the case.

Patient Complaints

It is generally in the health care organization's best interest to resolve patient complaints and billing disputes quickly, accurately, and amicably. Always address collection complaints seriously. Listen to the patient with an open mind. Note specifically what the patient is saying and what the patient wants to do. Look beyond the complaint to determine what caused the problem. The source of the problem, not just the symptom of the problem, should be resolved. A patient complaint form may be adapted to prompt staff to pay close attention to positive customer relations. This form may help to screen poor collection techniques by staff members, pinpoint billing department problems, and identify policies and procedures that need improvement.

The patient may refuse to pay the health care organization if the patient's complaint is not addressed. Some guidelines to follow when a patient calls or writes a letter complaining about medical care are:

1. Listen carefully (or read the letter carefully) and establish exactly what the patient complaint is and what the patient wants done about it.
2. Thank the person for calling (or writing); demonstrate appreciation of his or her input on the situation.
3. Apologize, regardless of whether the patient is right or wrong.
4. Answer the complaint. Explain what happened, if applicable, and state what is being done about it.

REQUEST FOR ALLOWANCE OF LIEN ASSIGNMENT AND AUTHORIZATION

WHEREAS, I have a right or cause of action out of personal injury, to wit:

I, ________________hereby authorize________________________ ,
patient's name physician's name

to furnish upon request, to my attorney,______________________________ , any and all medical records, or reports of examination, diagnosis, treatment, or prognosis but not necessarily limited to those items as set forth herein, in addition to an itemized statement of accounts for services rendered therefore or in connection therewith, which my attorney may from time to time request in connection with the injuries described above and sustained by me on the___________day of________________, 20XX.

I hereby irrevocably authorize and direct my said attorney set forth herein to pay to _____________________all charges for attendance in court,
patient's name

if required as an expert witness whether he testifies or not; reports or other data supplied by him; depositions given by said doctor; medical services rendered or drugs supplied; and any other responsible and customary charges incurred by my attorney as submitted by_______________and in
physician's name

connection with said injury. Said payment or payments are to be made from any money or monies received by my attorney whether by judgment, decree, or settlement of this case, prior to disbursement to me and payment of the amount as herein directed shall be the same as if paid by me. This authorization to pay the aforementioned doctor shall constitute and be deemed as assignment of so much of my recovery I receive. It is agreed that nothing herein relieves me of the primary responsibility and obligation of paying my doctor for services rendered, and I shall at all times remain personally liable for such indebtedness unless released by the aforementioned doctor or by payment disbursed by my attorney. I accept the above assignment:

Dated:________________Patient:____________________

As the attorney of record for the above-named, I hereby agree to observe the terms of this agreement, and to withhold from any award in this case such sums as are required for the adequate protection of Dr.___________________,

Date:________________Attorney:____________________

Fig. 17.19 A patient's authorization to release information to an attorney and grant lien to the health care organization against proceeds of settlement in connection with accident, industrial, or third-party litigation cases.

5. Use a professional and sincere approach. If the patient is wrong, state that the complaint is unjustified but first explain your interpretation of the situation and its resolution. Otherwise, the patient is likely to become quite upset. Do not be sarcastic, condescending, or insulting.
6. Take all complaints seriously. Do not respond in a lighthearted manner or use humor; it will only serve to upset the patient.
7. Respond in letter form. Whether the complaint has been received by telephone or by letter, take the time to write to answer the complaint. This indicates that the matter is not being taken lightly.
8. Be cordial and sincere. Express to the patient the hope of continuing a friendly relationship but that payment is necessary. Treat the patient with respect, good will, and sincere appreciation. Often, kindness can turn a negative into a positive. The complaint can be turned into a payment.
9. Follow-up after the complaint has been resolved by looking at the root of the problem and taking the necessary time to communicate this to administration. This follow-up allows creation of a plan of action that can help to prevent the same type of problem from recurring.

Bonding

Insurance billing specialists, claims assistance professionals, or anyone who handles checks or cash should be bonded or insured. When a health care organization carries a fidelity or honesty bond, it means that an insurance company will prosecute any employees found guilty of stealing. **Bonding** is an insurance contract by which a bonding agency guarantees

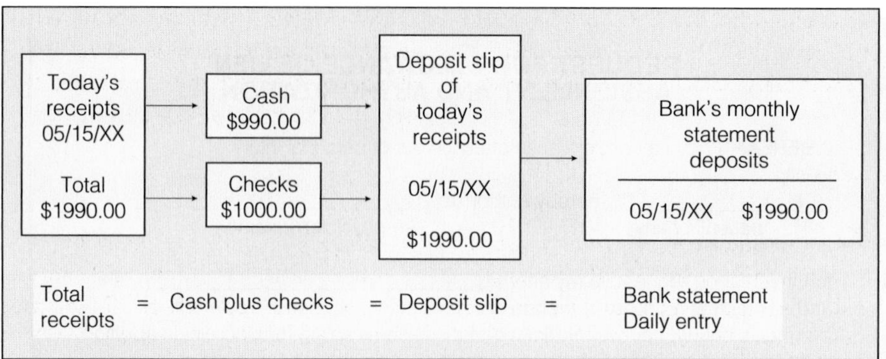

Fig. 17.20 Auditing the daily collection in the medical office to reconcile with the bank deposit.

payment of a certain sum to a health care organization in case of a financial loss caused by an employee or some contingency over which the payee has no control. Bonding methods for an organization with three or more office employees are:

- *Position-schedule bond* covers a designated job, such as a bookkeeper or nurse, rather than a named individual. If one employee in a category leaves, the replacement is automatically covered.
- *Blanket-position bond* provides coverage for all employees regardless of job title.
- *Personal bond* provides coverage for those who handle large sums of money. A thorough background investigation is required.

Such bonding contracts may be obtained from a casualty insurance agent or broker. Bond coverage should be reviewed periodically with the insurance agent to ensure that coverage is keeping pace with the expansion of the business.

Collection Controls

Embezzlement. Embezzlement is stealing money that has been entrusted in one's care. In many cases of insurance claims embezzlement, the health care organization is held as the guilty party and must pay huge sums of money to the third-party payer when false claims are submitted by an employee. If an undiscovered embezzler leaves the organization, the employee who is hired to replace that person could be accused some months later of doing something that he or she did not do. Take precautions as an employee and to protect the health care organization.

Precautions for financial protection. To prevent the temptation to steal from a health care organization, the following policies should be routinely practiced. The organization must have a process by which management must approve all entries posted about adjustments, discounts, and write-offs. If a patient owes money that is uncollectable and adjusted off, seek management approval and confirm that the balance due has been brought to zero. Implement a process whereby an auditor or an outside consultant is occasionally brought in to check an entire day's records (the patient sign-in log and appointment schedule) with the daysheet, patients' financial accounting records, encounter forms, and cash receipt slips. A daily trail of the balance of A/R, including daily deposit of checks and cash, can assist in reviewing monthly income and aid in discovering

COLLEGE CLINIC
4567 Broad Avenue
Woodland Hills, XY 12345-0001
Tel. (555) 486-9002
FAX (555) 487-8976

October 2, 20XX

Mr. Leonard Blabalot
981 McCort Circle
Woodland Hills, XY 12345-0001

Dear Mr. Blabalot:

I am glad we had an opportunity to discuss your outstanding balance with our practice during our phone conversation on October 1, 20XX. This will confirm and remind you that you agreed to pay $100 on your account on or before October 15, 20XX.

A return envelope is enclosed for your convenience.

Sincerely,

Charlotte Rose Routingham
Business Office

Enc. envelope

Fig. 17.21 Letter confirming telephone payment discussion sent to remind the patient of the payment terms agreed upon.

embezzlement. Audit the daily collection and reconcile with the bank deposit (Fig. 17.20). If poor bookkeeping and record keeping are noticed, bring this to the management's attention immediately.

All insurance payment checks should be immediately stamped within the endorsement area on the back "For Deposit Only," called a *restrictive endorsement.* The bank should be given instructions never to cash a check made payable to the health care organization.

Encounter forms, transaction slips, and cash receipts should be prenumbered. If a mistake is made when completing one, void it and keep the slip as part of the financial records. It is imperative to have prenumbered insurance forms to eliminate the filing of fictitious insurance claims.

As a precautionary measure, insurance billing specialists should always type their initials at the bottom left or top right corner of the insurance claim forms that they submit. This will indicate to office personnel who did the work. Always retain the explanation of benefits (EOB) or remittance advice (RA) documents that accompany checks from insurance companies.

Only a few of the many precautions for protection are mentioned here; embezzlement can occur in A/R, accounts payable, with petty cash, with the use of computers, and in various other aspects of a health care organization.

KEY POINTS

This is a brief chapter review, or summary, of the key issues presented. To further enhance your knowledge of the technical subject matter, review the key terms and key abbreviations for this chapter by locating the meaning for each in the Glossary at the end of this book, which appears in a section before the Index.

1. The health care organization, administrators responsible for financial affairs, service providers, the insurance billing specialist, and the patient must understand insurance contracts, which list payment provisions, medical services not covered, the portion of the bill for which the patient is responsible, and the process for reimbursing the office.
2. The insurance billing specialist must monitor the accounts receivable (A/R) weekly to determine the effectiveness of collection. An average A/R should be one and a half to two times the charges for 1 month of services.
3. Collect copayments and deductibles from patients at the time service is rendered. The health care organization can charge a missed appointment fee regardless of the health insurance the patient carries; the patient is responsible for paying the missed appointment fee.
4. Under the Health Insurance Portability and Accountability Act (HIPAA), health care organizations are free to use whatever policies they want on charity care, discounts, write-offs, and collections, but this must be done consistently and the reasons must be documented. Professional courtesy should be kept to a minimum.
5. When payments are made by check, require two forms of verification. Always take immediate action when the bank returns a check for nonsufficient funds (NSF). When payments are made by credit card, require picture ID verification.
6. Online services such as Square can be used to accept credit cards at any time. Fees vary depending on the amount of transactions for the health care organization. It is customary for the health care organization to impose a nominal fee on the patient for credit transactions.
7. Review overdue accounts to determine when to send dun messages on statements, make telephone calls, or send to a collection agency.
8. Use alternative payment methods to help cash flow and reduce collection costs such as credit card payments, debit cards, e-checks, and payment plans.
9. Follow all federal and state laws that affect collection of delinquent accounts.
10. Contact the patient in a timely manner by telephone at the first sign of payment delay and then send a collection letter as a reminder.
11. Delinquent accounts should be turned over to a collection agency only after all reasonable attempts have been made to collect.
12. Learn and use all techniques in skip tracing a debtor.
13. It is in the health care organization's best interest to resolve patient complaints and billing disputes quickly, accurately, and amicably.

STUDENT ASSIGNMENT

- Study Chapter 17.
- Answer the fill-in-the blank, multiple-choice, and true/false review questions in the *Workbook* to reinforce the theory learned in this chapter and to help prepare you for a future test.
- Complete the assignment in the *Workbook* to give you hands-on experience in selecting a dun message, posting a courtesy adjustment and insurance or patient payment, composing a collection letter, and accepting three methods of credit card payments.
- Turn to the Glossary at the end of this text for a further understanding of the key terms and key abbreviations used in the chapter.

UNIT 6

Healthcare Facility Billing

18

Ambulatory Surgery Center

Rachael D'Andrea

OBJECTIVES

After reading this chapter, you should be able to:

1. Explain the revenue cycle of reimbursement systems for ambulatory surgical center claims.
2. Understand the ambulatory surgery center billing process used by ambulatory surgical centers.
3. Discuss the importance of medical coder and biller roles in reimbursement.
4. Describe the components of the outpatient prospective payment and ambulatory surgical payment systems.
5. Recognize the features of the relative value unit and factors of the resource-based relative value scale payment system with the emphasis on the ambulatory surgery center (ASC) rate.
6. Explain the role of the *International Classification of Diseases,* Tenth Revision, Clinical Modification, Coding System (ICD-10-CM).
7. Explain the role of *Current Procedural Terminology* Fourth Revision, Procedure Coding System (CPT-4) in ambulatory surgical billing.
8. Identify the role of Healthcare Common Procedural Coding System (HCPCS).
9. Describe the significance of assigning modifiers.
10. Define payment status indicators and their use in the Medicare ASC reimbursement process.
11. Understand the impact of local coverage determinations and national coverage determinations in the ASC reimbursement cycle.
12. Recognize and assess the reimbursement methods used when determining various payers for ambulatory surgical services.
13. Identify the Ambulatory Quality Reporting (ASCQR) measures and the effect on the ASC payment rates.

KEY TERMS

Accreditation Association for Ambulatory Health Care
ambulatory care
ambulatory payment classifications
ambulatory surgery center
Ambulatory Surgery Center Quality Reporting
ASC payment system
CMS-1500
Current Procedural Terminology
conversion factor
discounted fee-for-service
discounting
first-listed diagnosis
geographic practice cost index
Healthcare Common Procedure Coding System
***International Classification of Diseases,* Tenth Revision, Clinical Modification (ICD-10-CM)**
local coverage determination
medical necessity
Medicare Part B
Medicare Physician Fee Schedule
modifiers
national coverage determinations
National Correct Coding Initiative
national unadjusted payment
outpatient prospective payment system
packaged
pass throughs
preadmission
preauthorization
prospective payment system
relative value units
resource-based relative value scale
revenue code
revenue cycle
revenue cycle management
status (payment) indicator
Uniform Bill 04

KEY ABBREVIATIONS

AAAHC
APC
ASC
ASCQR
ASU
CF
CMS
CPT
ECS
EMR
HCPCS
ICD-10-CM
LCD
MPFS
NCDs
NCCI
OPPS
PPS
RBRVS
RCM
RVU
UB-04

This chapter builds on concepts that have already been covered in other chapters of this text. These concepts include the basics of health insurance, privacy, compliance, and revenue cycle management. The focus of this chapter is concepts that are unique to ambulatory surgical centers.

Outpatient hospital care is often called ambulatory care and covers various types of services that do not require an overnight hospital stay. Ambulatory surgery centers, known as ASCs, are health care facilities specifically focused on providing same-day surgical care, including diagnostic and preventive procedures and services. ASCs allow patients greater access to care, a higher level of convenience, and more focused and cost-effective care when undergoing surgical procedures.

HISTORY OF AMBULATORY SURGERY CENTERS

For the past four decades, ambulatory surgery centers have increased their health care presence by providing procedures and services in the outpatient setting. Reasons for their significant growth include reduced health care costs for patients, providers, and payers; expansion of types of surgeries and services performed; and the national technologic advancement of health care ambulatory surgery facilities.

In the past, almost all surgery was performed in hospitals. Surgery was scheduled in advance, with preoperative tests, such as bloodwork and x-ray examinations, done during the initial inpatient stay. Surgery was done on the second inpatient day, and recovery added to the length of stay.

Technologic advancements created a movement of specific types of high-volume surgeries, such as for cataracts and biopsies, to the outpatient setting, initiating an upsurge in the outpatient services for hospitals.

The first freestanding ASC facility was launched in 1970 in Phoenix, Arizona, by two physicians who wanted to provide timely, convenient, and comfortable surgical services to patients in their community. Since that time, the number of ASCs has increased nationally. It is estimated that there are approximately 5500 Medicare-certified ASCs in the United States (MedPAC 2017). Fig. 18.1 displays the number of Medicare-certified ASCs by state. Common ASC specialties include Ophthalmology, Gastroenterology, Pain Management, Orthopedics and Dermatology.

Fig. 18.2 identifies the specialties served in ASCs Ambulatory Surgery Center Association (ACSA).

TYPES OF AMBULATORY SURGERY CENTERS

According to the Medicare Claims Processing Manual Chapter 14, section 10.1, "An ASC for Medicare purposes is a distinct entity that operates exclusively for the purpose of furnishing outpatient surgical services to patients."

There are two types of ASCs:

1. Independent ASCs are typically freestanding and they are usually privately owned. They are not integrated as part of a hospital, they are not directly associated with a hospital, and they are not included in a hospital's cost report.

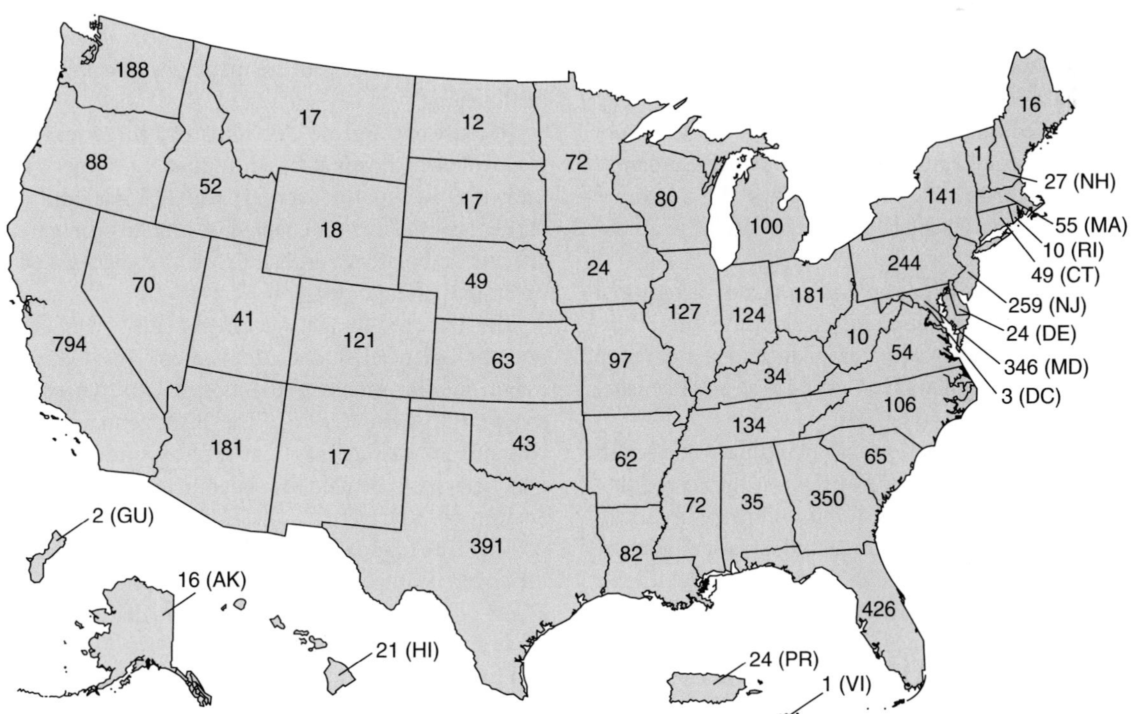

Based on data provided by the Centers for Medicare & Services (CMS), June 2018

Fig. 18.1 Medicare-certified ambulatory surgery centers by state. (Copyright Ambulatory Surgery Center and ASCA Foundation. All rights reserved. https://www.ascassociation.org/advancingsurgicalcare/asc/numberofascsperstate, June 2018.)

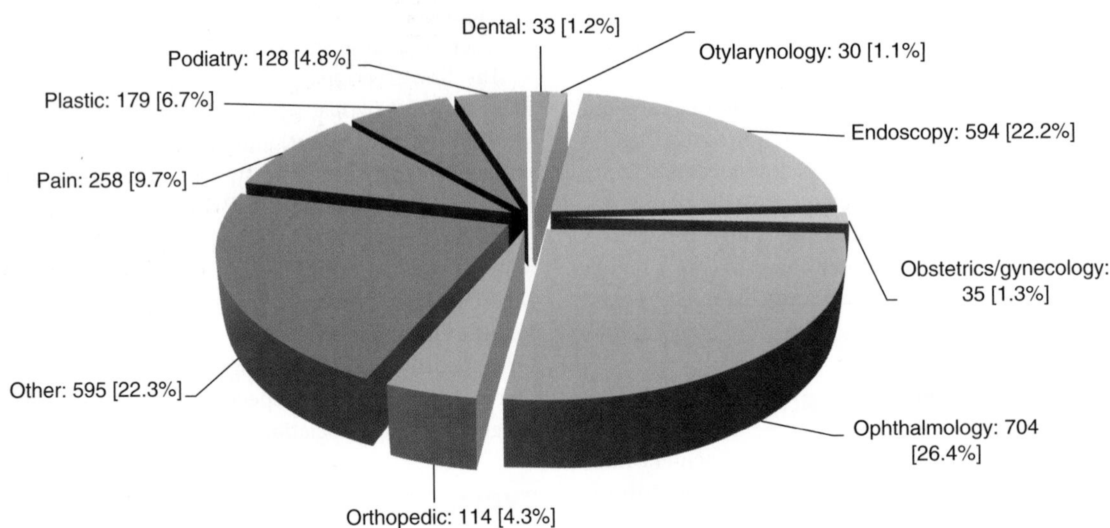

Fig. 18.2 Specialties served in ambulatory surgery centers (ASCs). (Copyright Ambulatory Surgery Center and ASCA Foundation. All rights reserved. https://www.ascassociation.org/advancingsurgicalcare/asc/whatisanasc, June 2017.)

2. Hospital-based ASCs are affiliated with or owned by a hospital. They can be freestanding (but hospital based) or located within a hospital.

It is important for the medical billing specialist to understand the difference between a hospital-based ASC and an independent ASC because different billing and coding rules apply and reimbursement is based on different payment systems.

Chapter 14 of the Medicare Claims Processing Manual includes the ambulatory surgery Medicare payment rules. Refer to the Center for Medicare and Medicaid (CMS) services website, https://www.cms.gov/Regulations-and-Guidance/Guidance/Manuals/downloads/clm104c14.pdf. It displays the Medicare Claims Processing Manual Chapter 14, which is specific to ambulatory surgery centers.

To provide services and bill as an ASC, a facility is required to be certified, and most states also require licensure. Initial certification will involve a survey with compliance to standards to meet Medicare and state regulations. Certification and licensure must be maintained on an ongoing basis.

The **Accreditation Association for Ambulatory Health Care (AAAHC)** has been designated by CMS as the accrediting body for ambulatory surgery centers. This voluntary organization was founded in 1979 to encourage and assist ambulatory health care organizations to provide the highest achievable level of care for recipients in the most efficient and economically sound manner. The organization provides ongoing consultative and education survey processes to ambulatory care facilities as they strive to set the highest of standards and to continuously advance patient care.

Legislative Background

Launched by Congress in 1965, the Medicare program was composed of both inpatient and outpatient services and based on hospital-specific, reasonable costs. As a result of the upsurge in demand for health care services, the fast-emerging presence of new technology, and the increased economic factors, national health care costs grew exponentially. This escalation prompted the Social Security Amendments of 1983 (Public Law 98-21, Section 1886 [d]), and the enactment of the **prospective payment system (PPS)** for inpatient services in 1983. Implementation of this payment system for inpatient services proved to be successful in managing the increasing costs of health care.

Because of the growth of outpatient surgeries that were being performed in hospital-based outpatient surgery departments, known as **ambulatory surgery units (ASUs)** and ASCs, federal legislation was further enacted in 1986 to segregate and pay for specific ambulatory surgical procedures performed at hospitals on an outpatient basis.

The Balanced Budget Act of 1997 (BBA) (Public Law 105-33) and the Balanced Budget Refinement Act of 1999 established major modifications to the hospital **outpatient prospective payment system (OPPS)**. The BBA demanded that the outpatient PPS include inpatient services under Part B for certain beneficiaries to be paid via separate fee schedules, as defined in Section 1833(t)(1)(B).

The BBA mandated that the outpatient classification system for covered outpatient services be developed using the calculation of relative payment weight, median hospital costs, and labor and geographic-adjusted costs. The OPPS was developed and implemented in August 2000 by CMS to pay for outpatient services provided in hospitals. The payment system is for services such as x-rays examinations, emergency department visits, and partial hospitalization services in hospital outpatient departments (HOPDs). The system is based on **ambulatory payment classifications (APCs)**, which reimburse the facility a fixed fee based on the procedure performed and the resources required to provide the service.

CMS did not implement APCs in the ASC system because the ASC claims processing system will not allow or track the type of packaging of ancillaries necessary for creating APCs. For example, CMS packages surgical recovery services into the payment for the surgery, although the hospital will bill the services separately on the claim.

Payment for ASC services is also based on rates set under Medicare Part B and is referred to as the **ASC payment system.** It required Medicare to pay the same rates to hospitals and ASC facilities for all outpatient procedures approved for ASC coverage.

Medicare Certification for Ambulatory Surgery Centers—42 CFR Part 416

In 2008, CMS, under the Medicare Prescription Drug, Improvement and Modernization Act (MMA) of 2003, revised the ambulatory surgery center payment system, based on the hospital OPPS. A 4-year transition, which ended in 2011, led to the fully implemented ASC payment groups that exist currently.

In 2009, 42 CFR Part 416 defined Medicare-certified ASCs with the following criteria (https://www.cms.gov/Medicare/Provider-Enrollment-and-Certification/SurveyCertificationGenInfo/Accreditation-of-Medicare-Certified-Providers-and-Suppliers.html):

- An ASC must be certified and approved to enter into a written agreement with CMS. Participation as an ASC is limited to any distinct entity that operates exclusively for the purpose of providing surgical services to patients not requiring hospitalization and in which the expected duration of services would not exceed 24 hours after an admission. An unanticipated medical circumstance may arise that would require an ASC patient to stay in the ASC longer than 24 hours but such situations should be rare.
- The regulatory definition of an ASC does not allow the ASC and another entity, such as an adjacent physician's office, to mix functions and operations in a common space during concurrent or overlapping hours of operations.
- ASCs are not permitted to share space with a critical access hospital (CAH) outpatient surgery department or with a Medicare participating independent diagnostic testing facility (IDTF). Specific radiology services that are reasonable, necessary, and integral to covered surgical procedures may be provided by an ACS.

It is expected that CMS will continue to look at ASC payment reform, specifically site neutrality and efficiency of care (MedPAC 2017).

AMBULATORY SURGERY CENTER PAYMENT SYSTEM

The federal government offers Medicare coverage to individuals who are 65 years or older, have certain disabilities, or suffer from end-stage renal disease or amyotrophic lateral sclerosis (ALS).

Medicare Part B covers outpatient and physician-based ambulatory services. Providers furnishing the services primarily receive Medicare reimbursement via the hospital Outpatient Prospective Payment System (HOPPS) or the **Medicare Physician Fee Schedule (MPFS).**

Medicare publishes a booklet titled "Ambulatory Surgical Center Payment System." This is a useful and supportive resource and can be found online at the CMS website (https://www.cms.gov/Outreach-and-Education/Medicare-Learning-Network-MLN/MLNProducts/Downloads/AmbSurgCtrFeepymtfctsht508-09.pdf).

For Medicare patients, payment for ASC services is based on rates set under Medicare Part B. This ASC payment system is used when paying for covered surgical procedures and the ASC facility services that are furnished in connection with the covered surgical procedure. CMS updates the OPPS/ASC regulations together in one rule annually, with public comment periods before implementation of the final rule.

CMS pays hospitals where Medicare Part B beneficiaries receive outpatient care under the OPPS. The federal agency sets OPPS reimbursement rates using the APCs, a package of similar services based on clinical factors and costs. The federal agency identifies the services using **Healthcare Common Procedure Coding System (HCPCS)** codes.

Medicare makes facility payments to ASCs only for the specific ASC covered surgical procedures on the ASC list of covered surgical procedures. Medicare makes separate payment to ASCs for certain covered ancillary services that are provided integral to a covered ASC surgical procedure.

All other non-ASC services, such as physician services and prosthetic devices, may be covered and separately billable under other provisions of Medicare Part B. The Medicare definition of covered ASC facility services for a covered surgical procedure includes services that would be covered if furnished on an inpatient or outpatient basis in connection with a covered surgical procedure. This includes operating and recovery rooms, patient preparation areas, waiting rooms, and other areas used by the patient or offered for use to patients needing surgical procedures. It includes all services and procedures provided in connection with covered surgical procedures furnished by nurses, technical personnel, and others involved in patient care.

These do not include physician services or medical and other health services for which payment may be made under other Medicare provisions (e.g., services of an independent laboratory located on the same site as the ASC, anesthetist professional services, or nonimplantable durable medical equipment [DME]).

ASCs must accept Medicare's payment as payment in full for services with respect to those services defined as ASC services. The physician and anesthesiologist may bill and be paid for the professional component of the service also.

The unit of payment in the ASC payment system is the surgical procedure. Each of the approximately 3500 procedures approved for payment in an ASC is classified into an APC group on the basis of clinical and cost similarity. There are several hundred APCs. All services within an APC have the same payment rate. The ASC system uses the same APCs as the OPPS.

Each APC receives a scaled relative payment weight that represents the average health care costs for the services included in the package. Then the weight is multiplied by a conversion factor (CF) to create a **national unadjusted payment** rate. CMS also adjusts OPPS rates by the hospital wage index to offset geographic variations in health care costs.

Within each APC, CMS packages ancillary items and services with the service performed. CMS pays separately for certain ancillary items and services when they are integral to surgical procedures. For example, CMS pays separately for corneal tissue acquisition, brachytherapy sources, certain radiology services, and many drugs.

In addition, ASCs can receive separate payments for implantable devices that are eligible for **pass-through** payments under the OPPS. Pass-through payments are for specific, new technology items that are used in the delivery of services Facilities using the pass-through drugs and devices receive extra payments for these products. Congress established the pass-through provision in the Medicare law to encourage the distribution of new technologies.

Medicare maintains and updates the covered procedure list, defined by ***Current Procedural Terminology* (CPT)**/HCPCS codes, of all services offered in an ASC.

PAYMENT FOR AMBULATORY SURGERY CENTER SERVICES

Facility Payment

The ASC List of Covered Surgical Procedures are Category I CPT codes within the surgical range of CPT codes, 10000 through 69999. Included within that code range are Level II HCPCS and Category III CPT codes that crosswalk, or are clinically similar, to Category I CPT codes.

Medicare and other payers may consider a procedure a noncovered service when performed in an ASC for several reasons. It may be considered cosmetic, or it may appear on the list of procedures not payable by Medicare or the payer contract for an ASC.

Some surgical procedures are covered by Medicare but not on the list of ASC covered surgical procedures. For those not covered in ASCs, the related professional services may be billed by the rendering provider as Part B services. However, the beneficiary is liable for the facility charges that are not covered by Medicare.

For a procedure or service to be considered medically necessary, the following criteria must be met:

- The procedure or service matches the diagnosis.
- The procedure or service is not experimental or investigational.
- The procedure or service is necessary.
- The procedure or service is provided at the most appropriate level that is safe and effective.
- The procedure or service is not elective.

For example, a blepharoplasty procedure may be either cosmetic or functional. When it is a cosmetic procedure, it is considered an elective procedure, so the patient will pay both the physician's fee and the facility fee.

Payments made to ASCs from private insurers are based on the contract the facility has with the payer. Insurance carriers use fee schedules that are contracted and maintained on an annual basis with the ASC.

Medicare's ASC reimbursement is twofold:

1. Services performed by the facility. These services are covered under Part B and must be identified on Medicare's covered ASC list. This includes the following:
   - Surgical supplies, nursing services and equipment;
   - Use of the operating and recovery rooms, patient preparation areas, waiting room, and other areas used by the patient or offered for use by the patient's relatives, attendants, companions, or other person(s) accompanying the injured worker in connection with surgical services;
   - Drugs, biologicals, intravenous fluids and tubing, surgical dressings, splints, casts, surgical supplies, and equipment required for both the patient and the ASC personnel (for example, fiber-optic scopes and their associated supplies);
   - Gowns, masks, drapes, case packs and their contents, and operating and recovery room equipment routinely furnished by the ASC in connection with the surgical procedure;
   - Simple diagnostic and preoperative testing performed by an ASC on the date of surgery, such as urinalysis, blood hemoglobin or hematocrit, blood glucose, or venipuncture to obtain specimens that are included in the ASC facility charges; and
   - Materials for conscious sedation and general anesthesia, including the anesthesia pharmaceuticals and any materials, whether disposable or reusable, necessary for its administration.

   In addition, ASCs receive a separate payment for radiology services that are integral to the covered surgical procedure if separate payment is made for the radiology service in the OPPS; brachytherapy sources implanted during a surgical procedure; pass-through and non–pass-through drugs that are paid for separately under the OPPS when provided as part of a covered surgical procedure; and devices with pass-through status under the OPPS.
2. The cost of the physician's professional services for performing the procedure is the other cost. The payment system for physicians and other health professionals is known as the Medicare Physician Fee Schedule.

Non-ASC facility services that are separately reimbursable include the physician's professional services; sale, lease, or rental of DME for ASC patients to use at home; services performed by an independent laboratory; and hospital-based ambulance services.

As previously stated, ASCs must accept Medicare's payment as payment in full for services with respect to those services defined as ASC services. The physician and anesthesiologist will bill and be paid for separately for the professional component of the service.

ASCs must include charges for packaged services into the charges reported for the separately payable services with which they are provided.

Inpatient Only List

The Inpatient Only List is updated annually by CMS. The list of approximately 1700 procedures affects patient selection criteria to identify and consider those appropriate outpatient procedures for patients who are in excellent health,

TABLE 18.1 Addendum for ASC List of Covered Procedures

CPT Code	Short Description	Subject to Multiple Procedure Discounting	2018 Payment Indicator	2018 Payment Weight	2018 Payment Rate
27060	Removal of ischial bursa	Yes	A2	28.084	$1,279.91
27062	Remove femur lesion/bursa	Yes	A2	28.084	$1,279.91
27065	Remove hip bone les super	Yes	A2	28.084	$1,279.91
27066	Remove hip bone les deep	Yes	A2	28.084	$1,279.91
27067	Remove/graft hip bone lesion	Yes	A2	59.712	$2,721.37
27080	Removal of tail bone	Yes	A2	28.084	$1,279.91
27086	Remove hip foreign body	Yes	A2	11.912	$542.88

CPT, Current Procedural Terminology.
From CMS October 2018 ASC Approved HCPCs Codes and Payment Rates—Updated 9/28/18. Retrieved from https://www.cms.gov/Medicare/Medicare-Fee-for-Service Payment/ASCPayment/11_Addenda_Updates.html.

who have limited or no comorbidities, and who will have appropriate caregiver support after discharge.

For example, a change noted in 2018 states that knee replacements may be performed on either an inpatient or an outpatient basis.

Addendum for ASC List of Covered Procedures

The ASC list of covered surgical procedures lists those procedures that CMS determines do not pose a significant safety risk and are not expected to require an overnight stay after the surgical procedure.

Addendum AA is the Final ASC Covered Surgical Procedures for CY 2018 including Surgical Procedures for which the payment is packaged. This spreadsheet lists the following formatted information:

- Column A: HCPCS Short Descriptor
- Column B: CPT Code
- Column C: Subject to Multiple Procedure Discounting
- Column D: Final CY 2018 Comment Indicator
- Column E: Final 2018 Payment Indicator
- Column F: Final 2018 Payment Weight
- Column G: Final 2018 Payment Rate

See Table 18.1 for the list of addenda files.

ASC Exclusion List

Medicare will not pay for surgical procedures in an ASC if the procedure meets any of the following criteria for exclusion:

- Is on the inpatient only list
- Poses a significant safety risk to the beneficiary
- Typically requires active medical monitoring and care past midnight
- Directly involves major blood vessels
- Requires major or prolonged invasion of body cavities
- Generally results in extensive blood loss
- Is emergent in nature
- Is life-threatening in nature
- Commonly requires systemic thrombolytic therapy
- Can only be reported using an unlisted surgical procedures code

Addendum EE identifies the surgical procedures excluded from payment in ASCs. Column A displays the HCPCS code and column B is the code's short description.

Table 18.2 details Addendum EE.

TABLE 18.2 Surgical Procedures Excluded From Payment in the ASC

CPT Code	Short Description
22857	Lumbar artif discectomy
22861	Revise cerv artific disc
22862	Revise lumbar artif disc
22864	Remove cerv artif disc
22865	Remove lumb artif disc
22899	Spine surgery procedure
22999	Abdomen surgery procedure
23200	Resect clavicle tumor
23210	Resect scapula tumor
23220	Resect prox humerus tumor
23335	Shoulder prosthesis removal
23470	Reconstruct shoulder joint

CPT, Current Procedural Terminology.
From CMS' List of Surgical Procedures to be Excluded from Payment in ASCs—Updated October 2018 (Addendum EE) Resource. Retrieved from https://www.cms.gov/Medicare/Medicare-Fee-for-Service-Payment/ASCPayment/11_Addenda_Updates.html.

Physician Payment

Medicare Part B covers outpatient and physician-based ambulatory services. Providers furnishing the services primarily receive Medicare reimbursement via the HOPPS or the MPFS.

Physicians who furnish services in ASCs bill for and receive separate payment under Part B. Physicians' services include the services of anesthesiologists administering or supervising the administration of anesthesia to beneficiaries in ASCs and the beneficiaries' recovery from the anesthesia. The services include routine pre- or postoperative services, such as office visits, consultations, diagnostic tests, removal of stitches, changing of dressings, and other services.

Medicare payment for physician services is based on the MPFS, a list of payment rates for services as described by HCPCS codes.

Unlike in the OPPS and ASC payment systems, payments for services are not packaged together in the physician payment system. Providers generally receive a separate payment for each service provided.

Medicare Physician Fee Schedule

Payment for most physicians' services are determined by the standard system for pricing called the resource-based relative value scale (RBRVS). Under RBRVS, CMS assigns relative value units (RVUs) to each surgical procedure using three factors that affect physicians' costs: the amount of physician work involved, practice expenses, and malpractice/professional liability insurance. The work RVU, practice expense RVU, and malpractice RVU are each multiplied by separate geographic practice cost indexes (GPCI). The adjusted RVUs are added together and multiplied by the physician fee schedule CF to calculate the total payment rate.

In an ASC the practice expense RVU is generally lower because the ASC facility incurred part of the expenses, so the physician will receive an additional payment from Medicare.

Payment modifiers affect specific payments. For example, many diagnostic procedures have the professional component, which covers physician interpretation of test results, and the technical component that covers the expenses of providing the diagnostic service. For example, if the provider bills for the service "globally," he or she is reimbursed for interpretation of the results as well as for the use of space, equipment, supplies, and technical staff support used in actually performing the procedure.

For example, an ASC service will generate both a payment to the physician and a payment to the ASC.

PAYMENT RATES

Payment for ASC services is based on rates set under Medicare Part B. This system for payment is called the ASC Payment System and is used when paying for covered surgical procedures, including ASC facility services that are furnished in connection with the covered surgical procedure. CMS updates the HOPPS/ASC regulations together in one rule annually, with comment periods open before implementation of the final rule. CMS uses the Consumer Price Index for urban customers (CPI-U) to update the ASC payments.

MEDICARE SETTING COMPONENT WITHIN BASE RATE

The payment rate for each service is calculated by multiplying the relative weight for the applicable APC by the ASC conversion factor (CF), which is updated annually. Fig. 18.3 is an example of an ASC payment. Although the relative weights of the ASC payment system are linked to the OPPS relative weights, the CF used to convert the relative weights into payment amounts are different. The ASC CF is lower than the OPPS conversion factor, resulting in lower ASC payment rates for the same service.

The MedPAC Payment Basics 2018 chart displayed in Fig. 18.4 describes the algorithm used for the ASC payment system.

The complete list of the ASC-covered surgical procedures and ASC-covered ancillary services, payment indicators, payment rates for each covered surgical procedure and ancillary service before adjustment for regional wage variations, wage-adjusted payment rates, and wage indices are available on the CMS website.

Medicare pays ASCs 80% of the lesser of the actual charge or the ASC facility payment rate for the covered services performed. The beneficiary is responsible for 20% of the lesser of the submitted charge or the ASC facility payment rate for the covered services performed.

Exceptions include the screening flexible sigmoidoscopy and screening colonoscopy; with these services, Medicare pays 75% and the beneficiary is responsible for 25%.

A single payment is made to an ASC for facility services furnished by the ASC in connection with a covered surgical procedure. Payments to ASCs are "packaged," which means related services are bundled together and paid in one lump sum. Additional payments may be made to the ASC for covered ancillary services, specifically brachytherapy sources, certain implantable devices with pass-through status under the OPPS, corneal tissue acquisition, drugs and biologicals for which separate payment is allowed under the OPPS, radiology services for which separate payment is allowed under the OPPS, and certain other integral services not included in the primary procedure payment.

2016 APC CF	Wage index adjusted CF	Service/RW	Adjusted CF x RW	Total Payment
$74.17	(74.17 x .60 x .9444) + (74.17 x .40) 42.02 + 29.67 = 71.69	99282/1.5206	$71.69 x 1.5206	$109.01

Fig. 18.3 Example of ambulatory surgery center payment with relative weights (RW). *APC,* Ambulatory payment center; *CF,* conversion factor. (From Centers for Medicare and Medicaid Services, https://www.cms.gov/Medicare/Medicare-Fee-for-Service-Payment/HospitalOutpatientPPS/Addendum-A-and-Addendum-B-Updates.html.)

Covered ancillary services, for which separate payment is made, must be provided integral to covered surgical procedures, specifically just before, during, or immediately after the covered surgical procedure.

The ASC facility services include intraocular lens (IOL) and new technology intraocular lens (NTIOL), approved by the Food and Drug Administration (FDA) for insertion during or subsequent to cataract surgery.

SEPARATELY PAYABLE SERVICES

Some items and services covered under Medicare may be furnished in an ASC that are not considered ASC services and that payment for ASC services does not include.

These non-ASC services are covered and paid for under other applicable provisions of Part B.

For example, the ASC may be part of a medical complex that includes other entities, such as an independent laboratory, supplier of durable medical equipment, or a physician's office and covered as separate entities under Part B.

If the ASC furnishes an implantable DME to a patient, the ASC bills and receives a single payment from the local contractor for the covered surgical procedure and the implantable device, as long as the implantable device does not have pass-through status under the OPPS.

In general, an item or service provided in a separate part of the medical complex is not considered an ASC service.

When the ASC performs multiple surgical procedures in the same operative session that are subject to the multiple procedure discount, contractors pay 100% of the highest paying surgical procedure on the claim, plus 50% of the applicable payment rate(s) for the other ASC covered surgical procedures subject to the multiple procedure discount that are furnished in the same session. Fig. 18.5 displays an example of two surgical procedures performed on the same day with sequencing and discounting.

In determining the ranking of procedures for the assignment of the multiple procedure reduction, payment is based on the lower of the billed charge or the ASC payment amount.

For example, a procedure performed bilaterally in one operative session is reported as two procedures, either as a single unit on two separate lines or with "2" in the units field on one line. Depending on whether the claim includes other services to which the multiple procedure discount applies, the payer will assign the multiple procedure reduction of 50% to the payment for at least one of the CPT code payment rates.

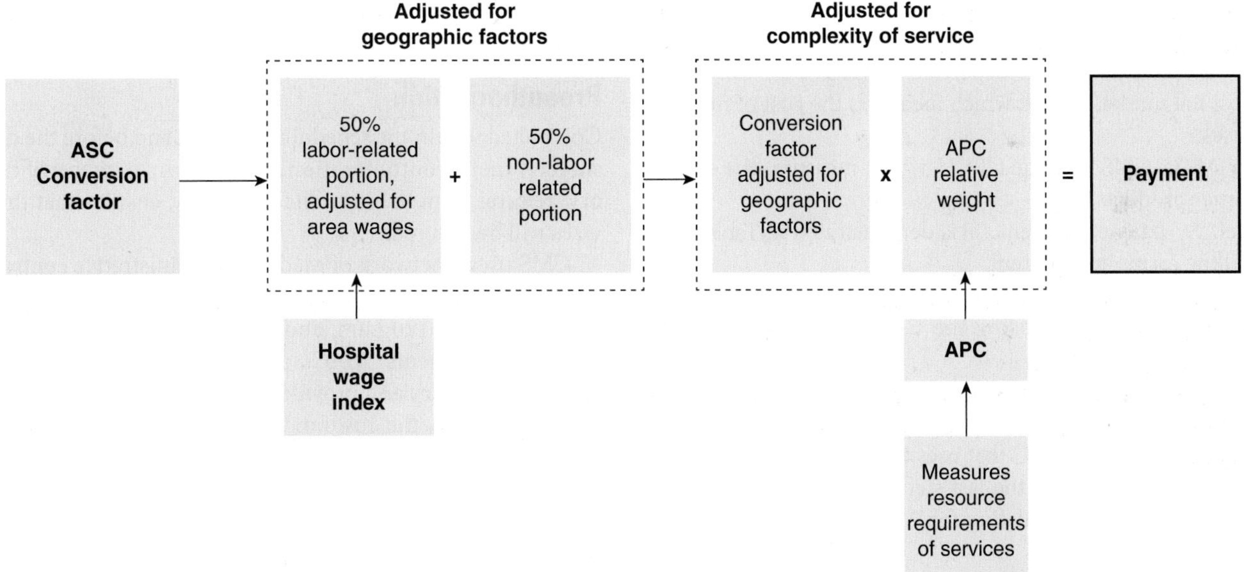

Fig. 18.4 MedPAC payment basics, 2018. *APC,* Ambulatory payment center; *ASC,* ambulatory surgery center. (From MedPAC, medpac.gov, Washington, DC.)

Service Sequence	CPT Code	Description	Fee	%
1st Service	13132	Repair, complex, 2.6 cm – 7.5 cm	$486.62	Higher code at 100%
2nd Service	15120	Split thickness autograft	$212.59	Lesser code at 50%
			Total	$699.21

Fig. 18.5 Example of surgical procedures performed together on the same day with discount. *CPT,* Current Procedural Terminology. (From Department of Health and Human Services, Office of Inspector General, https://oig.hhs.gov/oas/reports/region7/70302666.pdf.)

HOSPITAL OUTPATIENT PROSPECTIVE PAYMENT

For Medicare, an ASC in a hospital setting groups services using HCPCS codes into APCs. Services within the same APC are organized with similar cost and clinical characteristics and are paid the same amount. In addition, CMS packages integral services and items with the primary service into each APC.

There are hospital outpatient services that do not fit into an APC, such as some diagnostic and nonsurgical therapeutic procedures, blood and blood products, clinic and emergency department visits, certain preventative services, and some drugs.

The comprehensive APC (C-APC) payment model is being developed to simplify reporting and payment provision for high cost, complex outpatient procedures by accounting for all costs and component services typically involved in the provision of the complete primary procedure.

DIFFERENCES BETWEEN ASC AND HOSPITAL OUTPATIENT DEPARTMENT REIMBURSEMENT MODELS

CMS determines reimbursement rates for hospital outpatient departments and ASCs using two different measures of inflation, resulting in important cost differentials.

For hospital outpatient departments (HOPDs), CMS uses the hospital market basket, which measures the cost of medical expenses.

For ASCs, CMS uses the CPI-U, which measures the cost of consumer products.

The ASC payment system CF is demonstrated in Table 18.1. The billing forms are different.

Ambulatory surgical center claims are submitted to Medicare and Medicaid using the CMS-1500 claim form or the 837P.

HOPD claims to the payers are filed using the Uniform Bill 04 (UB-04) or the 837I (Fig. 18.6).

In a hospital-based ASC that uses the UB-04 and electronic medical records (EMRs), the last step to coding the Medicare ambulatory record is calculating the APC. This is accomplished with APC software.

In the hospital-based ASC, the integrated outpatient code editor (I/OCE) program processes claims for outpatient institutional providers, including hospitals that are subject to the OPPS as well as hospitals that are not (non-OPPS). Claims are identified as OPPS or non-OPPS.

The OCE targets individual errors and indicates what actions should be taken and the reasons why these actions are necessary.

The modifiers published in the CPT appendix titled "Modifiers Approved for Ambulatory Surgery Center (ASC) Hospital Outpatient Use" may be used in facility surgical coding. This differs from those just labeled "Modifiers," which are used for physician surgical coding.

REVENUE CYCLE MANAGEMENT

The Revenue Cycle

Revenue cycle management (RCM) is an important process that supports the financial strength of the ambulatory surgery center. The revenue cycle encompasses many interrelated and mutually dependent processes.

The revenue cycle starts with patient registration and scheduling and includes medical coding, claims management, managed care contracting, and collections.

Most ASCs use electronic billing software with automated tools for payer contract maintenance and claims scrubber that integrate with the clearinghouse for insurance verification, claim submission, and electronic remittance processing. The clearinghouse prescreens the claims for errors and aggregates and transfers the electronic claims to the payer securely, using Health Insurance Portability and Accountability Act (HIPAA) standards.

Most ASCs employ billing contractors for the claims adjudication.

Preadmission

When a new patient is registered at the ASC, he or she will complete the patient information form in the preadmission process. The patient's and guarantor's demographic and insurance information will be used for the verification of eligibility of insurance benefits.

Preauthorization

Completed within the scheduling process and before the date of surgery, the preauthorization, also known as precertification, or a referral from the insurance company, ensures that the services will be covered.

CMS uses a network of Medicare administrative contractors (MACs) to process Medicare claims, enroll health care providers in the Medicare program, and educate providers on Medicare billing requirements. MACs also handle claims appeals and answer beneficiary and provider inquiries.

Contact with the insurance carrier, with whom the ASC has contracted, can be accomplished electronically, by fax, or by phone call. The insurance carrier will require the patient's demographic and insurance information, including the policy's effective dates, the date of the planned surgery, and reason(s) for the procedure or services. Medical necessity, the use of services and/or supplies as determined by the insurance corporation's medical director or his or her designee, is essential for the determination of the patient's coverage and verification of benefits (VOB). For a service to be considered medically necessary, it must be reasonable and necessary to treat the patient's medical condition or diagnosis.

Each insurance provider will have special requirements for the information provided on the claim form and the effective due dates for submission. Examine the insurance provider's claim manual for the details before transmitting the claim to the insurance provider or clearinghouse via electronic claims submission (ECS).

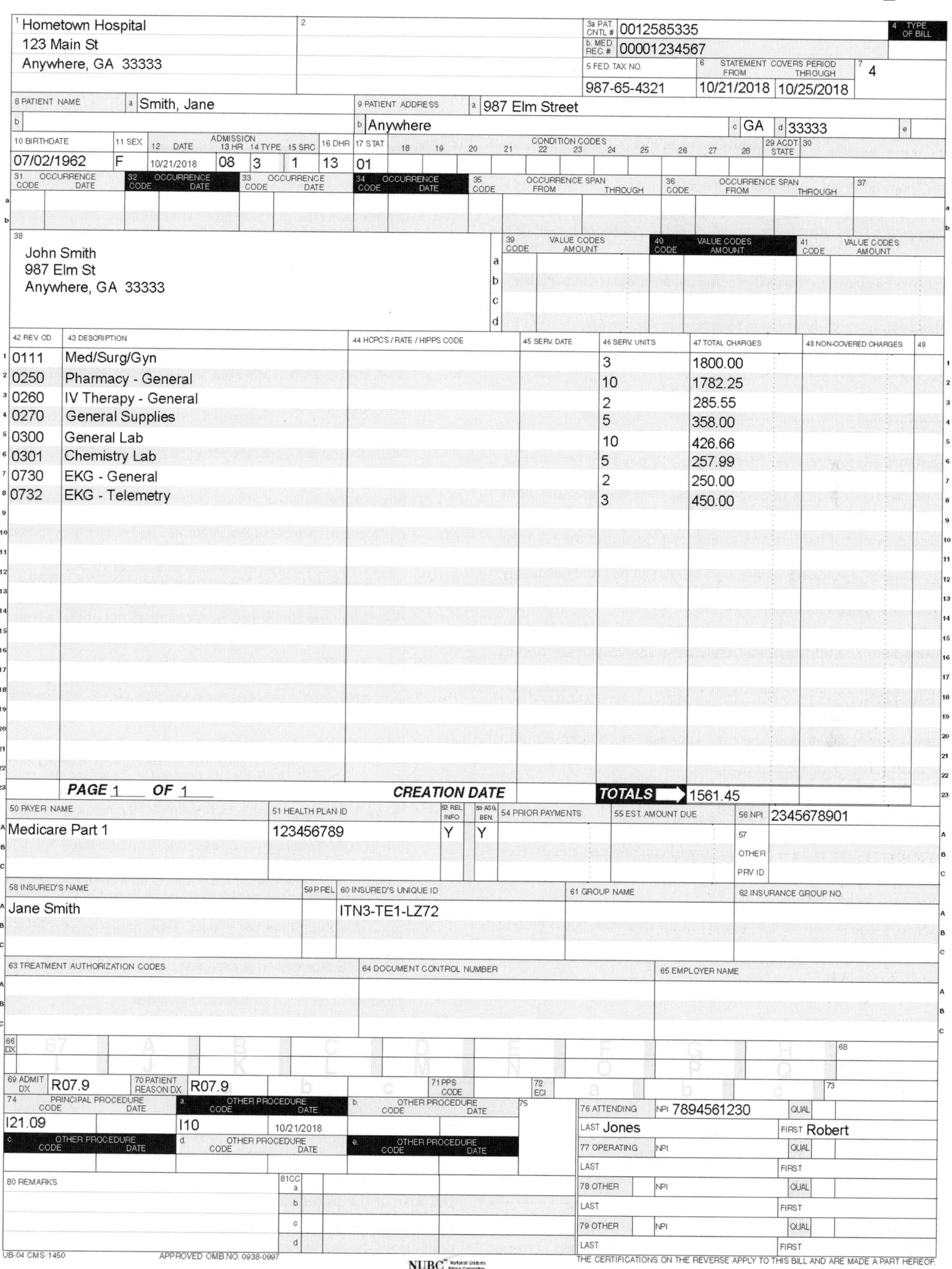

1 Hometown Hospital
123 Main St
Anywhere, GA 33333

3a PAT. CNTL # 0012585335
b. MED. REC. # 00001234567
4 TYPE OF BILL
5 FED. TAX NO. 987-65-4321
6 STATEMENT COVERS PERIOD FROM 10/21/2018 THROUGH 10/25/2018
7 4

8 PATIENT NAME a Smith, Jane
9 PATIENT ADDRESS a 987 Elm Street
b Anywhere c GA d 33333

10 BIRTHDATE	11 SEX	12 ADMISSION DATE	13 HR	14 TYPE	15 SRC	16 DHR	17 STAT
07/02/1962	F	10/21/2018	08	3	1	13	01

38
John Smith
987 Elm St
Anywhere, GA 33333

42 REV. CD.	43 DESCRIPTION	44 HCPCS / RATE / HIPPS CODE	45 SERV. DATE	46 SERV. UNITS	47 TOTAL CHARGES	48 NON-COVERED CHARGES	49
0111	Med/Surg/Gyn			3	1800.00		
0250	Pharmacy - General			10	1782.25		
0260	IV Therapy - General			2	285.55		
0270	General Supplies			5	358.00		
0300	General Lab			10	426.66		
0301	Chemistry Lab			5	257.99		
0730	EKG - General			2	250.00		
0732	EKG - Telemetry			3	450.00		
	PAGE 1 OF 1	CREATION DATE		TOTALS	1561.45		

50 PAYER NAME	51 HEALTH PLAN ID	52 REL. INFO	53 ASG. BEN.	54 PRIOR PAYMENTS	55 EST. AMOUNT DUE	56 NPI
Medicare Part 1	123456789	Y	Y			2345678901

58 INSURED'S NAME	59 P. REL	60 INSURED'S UNIQUE ID	61 GROUP NAME	62 INSURANCE GROUP NO.
Jane Smith		ITN3-TE1-LZ72		

63 TREATMENT AUTHORIZATION CODES
64 DOCUMENT CONTROL NUMBER
65 EMPLOYER NAME

69 ADMIT DX R07.9
70 PATIENT REASON DX R07.9

74 PRINCIPAL PROCEDURE CODE 121.09
a. OTHER PROCEDURE CODE I10 DATE 10/21/2018

76 ATTENDING NPI 7894561230
LAST Jones FIRST Robert
77 OPERATING NPI
78 OTHER NPI
79 OTHER NPI

80 REMARKS

UB-04 CMS-1450 APPROVED OMB NO. 0938-0997
NUBC National Uniform Billing Committee
THE CERTIFICATIONS ON THE REVERSE APPLY TO THIS BILL AND ARE MADE A PART HEREOF.

Fig. 18.6 Uniform Bill 04 (UB-04) or the 837I. (From the National Uniform Billing Committee, American Hospital Association, Chicago, Illinois.)

UB-04 NOTICE: THE SUBMITTER OF THIS FORM UNDERSTANDS THAT MISREPRESENTATION OR FALSIFICATION OF ESSENTIAL INFORMATION AS REQUESTED BY THIS FORM, MAY SERVE AS THE BASIS FOR CIVIL MONETARTY PENALTIES AND ASSESSMENTS AND MAY UPON CONVICTION INCLUDE FINES AND/OR IMPRISONMENT UNDER FEDERAL AND/OR STATE LAW(S).

Submission of this claim constitutes certification that the billing information as shown on the face hereof is true, accurate and complete. That the submitter did not knowingly or recklessly disregard or misrepresent or conceal material facts. The following certifications or verifications apply where pertinent to this Bill:

1. If third party benefits are indicated, the appropriate assignments by the insured /beneficiary and signature of the patient or parent or a legal guardian covering authorization to release information are on file. Determinations as to the release of medical and financial information should be guided by the patient or the patient's legal representative.
2. If patient occupied a private room or required private nursing for medical necessity, any required certifications are on file.
3. Physician's certifications and re-certifications, if required by contract or Federal regulations, are on file.
4. For Religious Non-Medical facilities, verifications and if necessary re-certifications of the patient's need for services are on file.
5. Signature of patient or his representative on certifications, authorization to release information, and payment request, as required by Federal Law and Regulations (42 USC 1935f, 42 CFR 424.36, 10 USC 1071 through 1086, 32 CFR 199) and any other applicable contract regulations, is on file.
6. The provider of care submitter acknowledges that the bill is in conformance with the Civil Rights Act of 1964 as amended. Records adequately describing services will be maintained and necessary information will be furnished to such governmental agencies as required by applicable law.
7. For Medicare Purposes: If the patient has indicated that other health insurance or a state medical assistance agency will pay part of his/her medical expenses and he/she wants information about his/her claim released to them upon request, necessary authorization is on file. The patient's signature on the provider's request to bill Medicare medical and non-medical information, including employment status, and whether the person has employer group health insurance which is responsible to pay for the services for which this Medicare claim is made.
8. For Medicaid purposes: The submitter understands that because payment and satisfaction of this claim will be from Federal and State funds, any false statements, documents, or concealment of a material fact are subject to prosecution under applicable Federal or State Laws.
9. For TRICARE Purposes:
   (a) The information on the face of this claim is true, accurate and complete to the best of the submitter's knowledge and belief, and services were medically necessary and appropriate for the health of the patient;
   (b) The patient has represented that by a reported residential address outside a military medical treatment facility catchment area he or she does not live within the catchment area of a U.S. military medical treatment facility, or if the patient resides within a catchment area of such a facility, a copy of Non-Availability Statement (DD Form 1251) is on file, or the physician has certified to a medical emergency in any instance where a copy of a Non-Availability Statement is not on file;
   (c) The patient or the patient's parent or guardian has responded directly to the provider's request to identify all health insurance coverage, and that all such coverage is identified on the face of the claim except that coverage which is exclusively supplemental payments to TRICARE-determined benefits;
   (d) The amount billed to TRICARE has been billed after all such coverage have been billed and paid excluding Medicaid, and the amount billed to TRICARE is that remaining claimed against TRICARE benefits;
   (e) The beneficiary's cost share has not been waived by consent or failure to exercise generally accepted billing and collection efforts; and,
   (f) Any hospital-based physician under contract, the cost of whose services are allocated in the charges included in this bill, is not an employee or member of the Uniformed Services. For purposes of this certification, an employee of the Uniformed Services is an employee, appointed in civil service (refer to 5 USC 2105), including part-time or intermittent employees, but excluding contract surgeons or other personal service contracts. Similarly, member of the Uniformed Services does not apply to reserve members of the Uniformed Services not on active duty.
   (g) Based on 42 United States Code 1395cc(a)(1)(j) all providers participating in Medicare must also participate in TRICARE for inpatient hospital services provided pursuant to admissions to hospitals occurring on or after January 1, 1987; and
   (h) If TRICARE benefits are to be paid in a participating status, the submitter of this claim agrees to submit this claim to the appropriate TRICARE claims processor. The provider of care submitter also agrees to accept the TRICARE determined reasonable charge as the total charge for the medical services or supplies listed on the claim form. The provider of care will accept the TRICARE-determined reasonable charge even if it is less than the billed amount, and also agrees to accept the amount paid by TRICARE combined with the cost-share amount and deductible amount, if any, paid by or on behalf of the patient as full payment for the listed medical services or supplies. The provider of care submitter will not attempt to collect from the patient (or his or her parent or guardian) amounts over the TRICARE determined reasonable charge. TRICARE will make any benefits payable directly to the provider of care, if the provider of care is a participating provider.

SEE http://www.nubc.org/ FOR MORE INFORMATION ON UB-04 DATA ELEMENT AND PRINTING SPECIFICATIONS

Fig. 18.6, cont'd.

REIMBURSEMENT PROCESS

After payment is received by the insurance provider, review the remittance advice (RA) to make sure that the correct amount was paid. Contact the insurance provider immediately with any discrepancies.

Collections

Because of the potential for added staff costs and legal complications, many ASCs hire billing contractors for the billing and collections tasks. By arranging the payment early in the ASC registration and scheduling process, the billing contractor can follow up in adjudicating the claim.

Appeals

Insurers are required to report why they denied the claim or reimbursed a lower-than-expected charge, and they must state how and when their decisions can be disputed in an appeal process. Deadlines in which appeals can be submitted vary among insurers. Contact the insurance provider immediately to resolve the issue.

Often the billing and collections contractor will manage this process.

OTHER TYPES OF REIMBURSEMENT

Self-Pay

As health care costs continue to rise, patients are taking on larger self-pay responsibilities, so ASCs are observing that the growing portion of their revenue comes from direct payments by patients. Collecting self-pay is a process that can require significant work and cost.

The ASC's self-pay policy, including the fee and payment schedule, should be provided to the patient before his or her visit. This will enable best practice for communication with the patient, moving forward through the encounters, including preoperative, postoperative, and follow-up for collections by the billing company.

Capitation

Capitation payments are used by insurance carriers to control health care costs. Capitation payments control use of health care resources by putting the physician at financial risk for services provided to patients. At the same time, to ensure that patients do not receive suboptimal care through underutilization of health care services, managed care organizations measure rates of resource utilization in physician practices. These reports are made available to the public as a measure of health care quality and can be linked to financial rewards, such as bonuses.

Capitation is a fixed amount of money per patient per unit of time paid in advance to the ASC for the delivery of health care services. The amount paid is determined by the ranges of services provided, the number of patients involved with the ASC, and the period during which the services are provided. Capitation rates are developed using local costs and average utilization of services and can vary nationally.

When the health care provider signs a capitation agreement, a list of specific services that must be provided to patients is included in the contract. The amount of the capitation will be determined in part by the number of services provided and will vary from health plan to health plan.

This can include contractually agreed-on fee schedules that are discounted compared with the local usual and customary fees.

Fee-for-Service

The most common health care payment model in the United States, fee-for-service (FFS) prompts patients to pay for individual services after they are received.

FFS is health care's most traditional payment model, in which physicians and health care providers are reimbursed by insurance companies and government agencies (third-party payers) based on the number of services they provide or the number of procedures they order. Payments are unbundled and paid for separately each time patients have a procedure in the ASC.

With the **discounted fee-for-service**, the provider agrees to provide services on a fee-for-service basis but with the fees discounted by a certain percentage from the usual charges.

Box 18.1 is an example of the ASC calculation for Blue Cross/Blue Shield (BC/BS).

BOX 18.1 Ambulatory Surgery Center Fee Schedule Allowance Calculation Examples

Amounts are displayed for illustrative purposes only. These examples demonstrate allowed amount calculations, not the Florida Blue payment because member deductible, coinsurance, and/or copayment liability have not been applied.

For the below examples, the following sample contracted percentage is used:

Fee Schedule (FS) Surgery

The allowance is determined by:

Fee Schedule Allowance × Fee Schedule Percent = Allowance

24515 $591 × 100% (1.0) = $591

Multiple Fee Schedule Surgery

The allowance is determined by:

Surgical procedure with the highest fee schedule will have an allowance of 100% (1.0)

Fee Schedule Allowance × Fee Schedule Percent = Allowance

24515 $591 × 100% (1.0) = $591

Additional procedures will have an allowance of 50% (.50) of the applicable fee schedule.

23650 $312 × 50% (.50) = $156

12005 $419 × 50% (.50) = $209.50

Total Allowance $956.50

From Florida Blue, Manual for Physicians and Provider, 2018. Retrieved from https://www.floridablue.com/providers/tools-resources/provider-manual.

MEDICAID OVERVIEW

Medicaid is an assistance-based federal and state-sponsored program for low-income individuals that pays for their health care costs. Each state defines who is eligible for Medicaid coverage, but the program generally covers individuals who have limited income.

The difference between Medicare and Medicaid is evident in that each state controls its own Medicaid program. Consequently, every Medicaid program differs based on the state regulations.

CPT Code	Procedure Description	Allowed Amount
27060	Removal of ischial bursa	$181.20
27062	Remoe femur lesion/bursa	$181.20
27065	Remoe hip bone les super	$168.00
27066	Remoe hip bone les deep	$252.00
27067	Remoe/graft hip bone lesion	$545.10
27080	Removal of tail bone	$210.00
27086	Removal hip foreign body	$25.20

Physicians performing surgeries in an ASC will report the surgical code for their professional services and will be reimbursed under a Medicaid Physician Fee Schedule (PFS). This is an example of a Medicaid PFS from 2018; State of Rhode Island Medicaid Program.

Fig. 18.7 Medicaid physician fee schedule. *ASC,* Ambulatory surgery center. (From Executive Office of Health & Human Services, Cranston, Rhode Island, http://www.eohhs.ri.gov/Portals/0/Uploads/Documents/Fee%20Schedules/Medicaid%20Fee%20Schedule.pdf.)

TABLE 18.3 Example of ASC Fee Schedule

CPT Code	Short Description	Payment Group Legend	Reimbursement Based on ASC Fee Schedule Legend	Comment	Translation of Comment Based on ASC Fee Schedule Legend
23040	Exploratory shoulder surgery	3	$366.60		
23044	Exploratory shoulder surgery	4	$415.35		
23066	Biopsy shoulder tissues	2	$339.40		
23071	Exc shoulder les sc>3cm	3	$366.60		
23073	Exc shoulder tum deep >5 cm	3	$366.60		
23075	Exc shoulder les sc<3 cm	2	$339.40		
23076	Removal of shoulder lesion	2	$339.40		
23077	Removal tumor of shoulder	3	$366.60		
23078	Resect should tum >5cm	3	$366.60		
23100	Biopsy of shoulder joint	2	$339.40	(CPA Age 21+)/(No PA Age <21)	Contractor requires prior authorization for patients age 21+; No prior authorization required for patients less than 21.
23101	Shoulder joint surgery	7	$$563.90	(CPA Age 21+)/(No PA Age <21)	Contractor requires prior authorization for patients age 21+; no prior authorization required for patients less than 21.

Medicaid Fee Schedule from Washington State Health Care Authority's Medicaid ASC Fee Schedule; Updated May 2, 2018. Retrieve from https://www.hca.wa.gov/billers-providers-partners/prior-authorization-claims-and-billing/provider-billing-guides-and-fee-schedules#billing-guides-fee-schedules.

Some Medicaid reimbursement models use fee-for-service, managed care, or a combination of both to pay providers. Fig. 18.7 displays an example of BC/BS Medicaid physician fee schedule. Table 18.3 presents an example of a Medicaid ASC fee schedule.

MEDICAL RECORDS FOR REIMBURSEMENT

A complete patient chart will include the patient's medical record, payment and benefit plan agreements, and insurance identification, verification, and authorization. The medical coder will review the entire medical record for the clinical documentation to assign the appropriate CPT/HCPCS codes, **International Classification of Diseases, Tenth Revision, Clinical Modification (ICD-10-CM)** diagnosis codes, modifiers, and status (that is, payment) indicators.

Audits of coding compliance require the knowledge of ASC coding in accordance with ICD and HCPCS coding rules as well as proper billing procedures from both Medicare and private payers. Audits are on the increase and will continue to be a factor in coding and billing compliance (AHIMA 2017).

An ASC claim for payment for terminated surgery must include an operative report kept on file by the ASC.

MEDICAL CODING AND BILLING GUIDANCE

Diagnosis Coding

The admission diagnosis, the condition assigned to the patient on admission to the ASC, must be coded according to the ICD-10-CM guidelines. This initial diagnosis is documented by the patient's surgeon who determined that the surgery was necessary. This is also known as the preoperative diagnosis.

The **first-listed diagnosis,** the condition treated or investigated during the episode of care, is coded also according to ICD-10-CM. This diagnosis is documented by the surgeon and located on the operative report upon completion of the surgery. Often this is called the postoperative diagnosis.

Secondary, or additional, diagnoses, coded with ICD-10-CM, are the conditions that coexist during the episode of care and affect the treatment provided to the patient. These can include comorbidities, complications, and other diagnoses that are documented by the surgeon.

Procedure Coding

The first-listed procedure, coded with CPT/HCPCS, can be either therapeutic or diagnostic, and is documented by the surgeon on completion of the surgery. The CPT codes should be entered on the claim in descending order of reimbursement. The highest paying procedure will be entered as the first-listed procedure, with a logical clinical connection between the first-listed diagnosis and the first-listed procedure.

The secondary procedures are also assigned in CPT/HCPCS. During ambulatory surgery, secondary procedures are often performed that are considered integral to the first-listed procedure. When a separate and distinct procedure is performed, modifier -59 can be appended to the code.

The provider must document the diagnoses for all services performed. "Linking" the diagnosis to the procedure or service performed on the claim form is an essential action to substantiate medical necessity.

Billing

The Medicare global period for the procedure is important to consider in this step. The global components include the preoperative, interoperative, and postoperative services rendered to the patient for the specific service. Separate billing is not allowed for visits or other services that are included in the global package (CMS 2016).

A free source of information about the number of global surgical days assigned to a code is the Medicare Fee Schedule Lookup Tool.

Scrutiny of coding compliance, which requires knowledge of ASC coding in accordance with ICD and HCPCS coding rules as well as proper billing procedures from both Medicare and private payers, has been on the increase recent years and will continue to be a factor in coding and billing compliance audits in the future.

In an ASC, the ambulatory surgery fee schedule provides the contracted charges for the surgery. The insurance carrier, including Medicare, Medicaid, and other payers, will list the fee schedule.

Generally the list will be organized numerically by HCPCS/CPT code along with any applicable discounting and payment.

CLAIMS MANAGEMENT AND HEALTH CARE CLAIM SUBMISSION

Billing Forms

The Administrative Simplification Act (ASCA) requires that all initial claims reimbursed by Medicare be submitted electronically, with limited exceptions.

ASC claims are different from hospital claims. The appropriate billing form depends on the type of facility. ASC claims will be reported to Medicare, Medicare Advantage Plans, and Medicaid using the CMS-1500 or 837P form. Professional charges are also filed on the CMS-1500.

Hospital outpatient surgery claims will be reported with the UB-04 or 837I form. The UB-04 is often used to file medical claims to the other payers.

CMS-1500

The following CMS-1500 837P claim form instructions relate to ambulatory surgery centers.

Field 23 Prior Authorization Number: Enter the authorization number.

Field 24B Place of Service: Enter 24, Ambulatory Surgery Center.

Field 24D ASC Modifier: Enter F for Specialty 49.

Notes: Field 21, diagnosis or nature of illness or injury, must relate, or link, to Field 24E, the diagnosis pointer.

The Place of Service Codes Set is required for use in the implementation guide adopted as the national standard for electronic transmission of professional health care claims under the provisions of HIPAA.

Uniform Bill 04

Box 4, the bill type for submitting claims on the UB-04, is 83X. The first digit denotes the type of facility: 8—Special Facility, Hospital ASC Surgery.

The second digit denotes the bill classification: 3—Outpatient. The third digit signifies the frequency, which is represented by the variable X:

1—Admit through Discharge Claim
7—Replacement of Prior Claim or Corrected Claim
8—Void or Cancel of the Prior Claim

Most often, the third digit is 1.

The **revenue code** used to report ASC care is 490 in Box 42.

See Fig. 18.6 for an example of the UB-04 form using modifier 50 to identify a bilateral procedure that requires additional significant time.

Some insurers require revenue codes, which identify specific categories for payment purposes, for eligible supplies, durable medical equipment, prosthetic devices, and implants. The CPT or HCPCS code will be entered in locator 44 of the UB-04 claim form and the revenue code in locator 42. For example, enter HCPCS code L1885 prosthetic device in locator 44 and associated revenue code 274.

MODIFIERS

CPT codes can be customized to the procedure or service performed. Procedures and services are often complex, so the modifiers provide additional information about the procedure. The CPT modifier can describe whether multiple procedures were performed, why that procedure was necessary, where the procedure was performed on the body, how many surgeons worked on the patient, and other information that may be critical to a claim's status with the insurance payer.

CPT **modifiers** are two characters and may be numeric or alphanumeric, as you remember. Modifiers are added to the end of a CPT code. In the case of more than one modifier, sequencing is important. Assign the "functional" modifier, and then "informational" modifier, listing the "functional" modifier that most directly affects the reimbursement process first. Different payers require the use of different modifiers.

CMS-1500, the form that is used for ASC and physician billing, and UB-04, the form used for facility billing, provide space for four modifiers. Some payers will not examine the modifiers after the first two, so it is always a good practice to assign the most significant modifier first, as stated previously.

Many CPT modifiers necessitate supplemental reports to the health insurance payer for payment. For example, the payer could question the reason why a procedure was discontinued. The supplementary report would state the reason.

Note that there may be some overlap or contradiction with the set of HCPCS modifiers because HCPCS has its own set of modifiers. The Level II modifiers consist of two alpha or alphanumeric characters in the sequence AA to VP.

Medicare Modifiers

Medicare ASC coding requires the following modifiers when assigning specific CPT procedure codes on the ASC claims.

Modifier RT: Right side

Modifier LT: Left side

Modifier TC: Technical component

Modifier 52: This modifier has a special use in Medicare ASC coding that differs from what is published in CPT. It is used for coding reduced services for discontinued radiology procedures and other procedures not requiring anesthesia that are partially reduced or discontinued at the physician's discretion. In this usage the payment is 50% of the allowed amount.

Modifier 59: Distinct separate procedure

Modifier 73: Procedure discontinued after preparation for surgery. For example, this modifier can be used before anesthesia administration but not when there is an elective cancellation of the procedure. The surgical or diagnostic procedure may be canceled subsequent to surgical preparation but before the administration of anesthesia. Payment is at 50% of the allowable amount for the procedure.

Modifier 74: Procedure discontinued after anesthesia administered. An example is after the procedure has commenced or after the anesthesia was administrated. Payment is at 100% of the allowable amount for the procedure.

Modifier FB: Device furnished at no cost/full credit

Modifier FC: Device furnished at partial credit

Modifier PA: Wrong body part

Modifier PB: Surgery wrong patient

Modifier PC: Wrong surgery on patient

Modifier PT: Colorectal screening converted to diagnostic or therapeutic procedure/surgery

Modifier GW: Surgery not related to hospice patient's terminal condition

Medicaid Modifiers

Medicaid requires the use of modifier SG, which identifies the claim as an ASC claim.

Other Insurer Modifiers

Billing guidelines will vary by insurer and by state. For example, BC/BS generally requires the use of modifier 50, which identifies the procedure as bilateral and two units of service. However, Medicare requires modifier RT or modifier LT on separate lines with one unit of service.

Unlisted codes end in "99." An example is "66999 Unlisted code anterior segment." Unlisted codes should not be used for facility coding because they will not be reimbursed. Medicare contractors are unable to evaluate these codes or assign a payment value.

Anatomic modifiers: E1-E4, FA, F1-F9, TA, T1-T9, LT, RT, LC, LD, RC, LM, RI

Global surgery modifiers: 24, 25, 57, 58, 78, 79

Other modifiers: 27, 59, 91, XE, XP, XS, XU

STATUS (PAYMENT) INDICATORS

In the OPPS, every CPT/HCPCS code has a **status indicator.** The status indicator provides information about the procedure including whether or not it is covered under the OPPS, if it is subject to discounting, and if it is an inpatient procedure only. For example, status indictors G and H identify pass-through drugs and devices.

Discounting is when the reimbursement to the ASC is reduced. For example, when two or more surgical procedures are performed in the same operative session, the first surgical procedure is paid at 100%, and the subsequent procedure is paid at 50%. The status indicator T for the CPT codes associated with the major procedures will identify that they are subject to the discounting.

Addendum DD1 is the file that provides clarification of the status (payment) indicators.

NATIONAL CORRECT CODING INITIATIVE EDITS

The CMS developed the **National Correct Coding Initiative (NCCI)** to promote national correct coding and to control improper coding leading to wrong payment in Part B claims.

NCCI bundling instructions apply to processing claims from ASC facilities services. In general, if an ASC bills a CPT code that is considered to be part of another more comprehensive code that is also billed for the same beneficiary on the same date of service, only the more comprehensive code is covered, provided that code is on the list of ASC approved codes.

Because an ASC bills to Part B of Medicare, the physician NCCI edits are the ones that apply. The list of edits is updated quarterly, and coding personnel need to keep up-to-date on these updates.

The NCCI contains one table of Procedure-to-procedure (PTP) edits for physicians/practitioners and one table of PTP edits for outpatient hospital services. The Column One/Column Two Correct Coding Edits table and the Mutually Exclusive Edits table have been combined into one table and include PTP code pairs that should not be reported together for a number of reasons, which are explained in the Coding Policy Manual.

These code pair edits are applied to claims submitted by physicians, non-physician practitioners, and ASCs, provided the code is listed as one of the Medicare-approved ASC procedures.

Accurate coding and reporting of services are critical aspects of proper billing. Service that is denied based on PTP code pair edits or medically unlikely edits may not be billed to Medicare beneficiaries. The NCCI tools located on the CMS website (including the National Correct Coding Initiative Policy Manual for Medicare Services) help providers avoid coding and billing errors and subsequent payment denials (CMS 2018 n.).

OTHER PAYERS

Although some payers may follow the NCCI process, most pay a case rate for the service according to their respective contract. It is recommended that the biller review the specific contract to see if the NCCI ruling is applicable or if the payer uses their own.

LOCAL COVERAGE DETERMINATIONS AND NATIONAL COVERAGE DETERMINATIONS

National Coverage Determinations

National coverage determinations (NCDs) are developed by CMS to describe the circumstances for Medicare coverage nationwide for a specific medical service procedure or device and define the conditions for which a service is considered to be covered or not covered.

Published as a CMS program instruction, an NCD is required on all Medicare carriers/DME regional carriers (DMERC), also called durable medical equipment Medicare administrative contractors (DME MACs); fiscal intermediaries (FIs); quality improvement organizations (QIOs, formerly known as peer review organizations or PROs); and program safeguard contractors (PSCs); and for Medicare+Choice organizations (such as Medicare Advantage).

In the absence of a national coverage policy, an item or service may be covered at the discretion of the Medicare contractors based on a **local coverage determination (LCD)**.

The contractor will apply the NCDs when reviewing claims for items or services addressed by NCDs.

The Medicare Coverage Database's website is: https://www.cms.gov/medicare-coverage-database/overview-and-quick-search.aspx

The list of NDCs is available at: https://www.cms.gov/medicare-coverage-database/indexes/ncd-alphabetical-index.aspx

Local Coverage Determinations

An LCD is a decision by a MAC regarding whether to cover a particular item or service on a MAC-wide basis in accordance with Section 1862(a)(1)(A) of the Social Security Act (that is, a determination as to whether the item or service is reasonable and necessary).

Contractors develop and publish LCDs when there is no NCD or when there is a need to further define an NCD.

In rare instances, if there is contradicting information in the NCD and LCD, the NCD overrides the LCD.

Contractors review claims on either a prepayment or postpayment basis regardless of whether an NCD, coverage provision in an interpretive manual, or LCD exists for that item or service.

Denials are made when clear policy or certain other conditions exist within the claim in the automated process. When making individual claim determinations, the contractor will determine whether the item or service in question is covered based on an LCD or the clinical judgment of the medical reviewer. An item or service may be covered by a contractor if it meets all the conditions.

AMBULATORY SURGERY CENTER QUALITY REPORTING (ASCQR)

The Affordable Care Act required the Secretary of Health and Human Services to develop a plan to implement a value-based purchasing (VBP) program for payments under the Medicare program for ASCs.

The **Ambulatory Surgery Center Quality Reporting Program (ASCQR)**, sponsored by CMS, began in 2014. The pay-for-reporting, quality data program requires ASCs to report their quality of care data for standardized measures to receive the full ASC payment rate.

The ASC quality measures are focused on the goals for quality improvement and accurate decision making. Also, efficiency and patient satisfaction are evaluated. High-impact events, such as surgery performed on the wrong site, and safety issues, such as patient falls, are examples of the quality measures. Data sources for the information include chart abstraction from the health record entered into the Web-based ASCQR program and the assignment of data quality codes (QDCs) on the claim form (CMS-1500).

The ASC measures are updated annually. For 2019 the measures for payment determination include the following:

ASC-1 Patient Burn
ASC-2 Patient Fall
ASC-3 Wrong Site, Wrong Side, Wrong Patient, Wrong Procedure, Wrong Implant

ASC-4 All-Cause Hospital Transfer/Admission
ASC-8 Influenza Vaccination Coverage among Healthcare Personnel
ASC-9 Endoscopy/Polyp Surveillance: Appropriate Follow-Up Interval for Normal Colonoscopy in Average Risk Patients
ASC-10 Endoscopy/Polyp Surveillance: Colonoscopy Interval for Patients with a History of Adenomatous Polyps—Avoidance of Inappropriate Use
ASC-11 Cataracts: Improvement in Patient's Visual Function within 90 Days Following Cataract Surgery
ASC-12 Facility 7-Day Risk-Standardized Hospital Visit Rate after Outpatient Colonoscopy

ASCs that do not meet the reporting requirements will experience a 2% reduction to their payment.

CMS provides excellent resources that detail the complexities of the ASCQR program. See the Quality Net website for further information: http://www.qualitynet.org.

CMS has planned to look at intraoperative and postoperative measures in the future.

CONSUMER ASSESSMENT OF HEALTH CARE PROVIDERS AND SYSTEMS OUTPATIENT AND AMBULATORY SURGERY SURVEY

CMS has developed the Consumer Assessment of Health Care Providers and Systems Outpatient and Ambulatory Surgery Survey (OAS CAHPS) standardized survey to measure and assess the experience of care for patients who have a surgery or procedure performed in an HOPD or ASC.

The survey measures patients' experiences on topics such as:

- communication and care provided by health care providers and office staff;
- preparation for the surgery or procedure;
- postoperative care coordination; and
- patient-reported outcomes.

Participating HOPDs and ASCs can compare their patient responses against their state and the national averages.

The program is currently voluntary.

STUDENT ASSIGNMENT

- Study Chapter 18.
- Answer the fill-in-the-blank, multiple-choice, and true/false review questions in the *Workbook* to reinforce the theory learned in this chapter and to help you prepare for a future test.
- Complete the assignments in the *Workbook*.
- Turn to the Glossary at the end of this text for a further understanding of the key terms and key abbreviations used in this chapter.

19

Hospital Outpatient and Inpatient Billing

Nanette Sayles

OBJECTIVES

After reading this chapter, you should be able to:

1. Explain the revenue cycle of hospital claims.
2. Manage the Discharge Not Final Billed report.
3. Discuss the 72-hour rule.
4. Explain utilization management and its role in the hospital reimbursement system.
5. Explain the chargemaster.
6. Explain the *International Classification of Diseases, Tenth Revision, Procedure Coding System* (ICD-10-PCS).
7. Explain the role of the ICD-10-PCS in hospital billing.
8. Explain the role of *Current Procedural Terminology* in hospital billing.
9. Explain the role of *Healthcare Common Procedural Coding System.*
10. Assign the present on admission indicator.
11. Explain the reimbursement methods used when receiving reimbursement for Medicare hospital services.

KEY TERMS

72-hour rule
admission
admission review
against medical advice
ambulatory payment classifications
capitation
case mix groups
chargemaster
concurrent review
complication
comorbidity
continued stay review
cost outlier
covered entity
diagnosis-related groups
discharge disposition
Discharge Not Final Billed
discounting
downcoding
DRG creep
Emergency Medical Treatment and Labor Act
gatekeeper
grouper
Health Insurance Portability and Accountability Act
hospital-acquired condition
inpatient
Inpatient Prospective Payment System
Inpatient Psychiatric Facility Prospective Payment System
Inpatient Rehabilitation Facility Patient Assessment Instrument
Inpatient Rehabilitation Facility Prospective Payment System
inpatient only
International Classification of Diseases, Tenth Revision, Clinical Modification
International Classification of Diseases, Tenth Revision, Procedure Coding System
Long-Term Care Hospital Prospective Payment System
major complication/comorbidity
major diagnostic categories
Medicare administrative contractor
Medicare Severity Diagnosis-Related Group
National Uniform Billing Committee
observation
Outpatient Prospective Payment System
per diem
physician advisor
preadmission
preadmission testing
preauthorization
present on admission
principal diagnosis
prospective payment system
prospective utilization reviews
quality improvement organization
Reason for encounter
relative weight
Resource-Based Relative Value Scale
retrospective review
revenue code
revenue cycle
rehabilitation impairment category
self-pay
status indicator
swing bed
Tax Equity and Fiscal Responsibility Act of 1982
Transaction and Code Set Rule
transaction set
Uniform Bill 04
upcoding
utilization management

KEY ABBREVIATIONS

ABN	DNFB	IRF PAI	PAT
AMA	DRG	IRF PPS	POA
ANSI	EMTALA	LTCH	PPS
APC	HAC	LTCH PPS	QIO
ASC	HIPAA	MAC	RBRVS
CC	ICD-10-CM	MCC	RICs
CE	ICD-10-PCS	MDC	TEFRA
CMG	IPO	MS-DRG	UB-04
CMS	IPF PPS	OPPS	UM
CPT	IPPS	PA	

This chapter builds on concepts that have already been covered in other chapters of this text. These concepts include the basics of health insurance, privacy, compliance, and revenue cycle management. The focus of this chapter is concepts that are unique to hospitals.

REVENUE CYCLE

The revenue cycle of a hospital is a complex process. The **revenue cycle** is "the process of how patient financial and health information moves into, through, and out of the health care facility, culminating with the facility receiving reimbursement for services provided" (AHIMA 2017, 208). The revenue cycle process begins with the scheduling of an appointment for services in the case of scheduled services or when the patient arrives at the hospital for emergency services. The revenue cycle includes preadmission, preauthorization, admission, capture of charges, submission of claim, and receipt of reimbursement among others. This process can be divided into three periods: preadmission, patient care, and posthospitalization. Fig. 19.1 shows the key steps in the process.

Preadmission

The steps discussed in this period occur before the patient's arrival. For nonemergency hospital services, inpatient and outpatient, the patient goes through a preadmission process. **Preadmission** is the process of preparing for the patient's care by collecting demographic information and insurance information. An **inpatient** is a patient who receives nursing and other care around the clock. To be an inpatient, there must be a physician order admitting the patient to the hospital.

Medicare has a **72-hour rule.** This rule states that if a patient receives any treatment related to the inpatient admission, such as diagnostic laboratory tests, x-ray examinations, medical equipment, or emergency services, or any outpatient services within 72 hours of admission to the same hospital, then all these services are bundled with the inpatient service claim. If the service is unrelated to the hospitalization, the rule does not apply. For example, routine preadmission blood work would be submitted to Medicare for payment as an outpatient service if it is completed within 72 hours of admission and if it is related to the reason for admission. If the patient was scheduled to be admitted to have a hysterectomy as an inpatient and the patient comes to the hospital

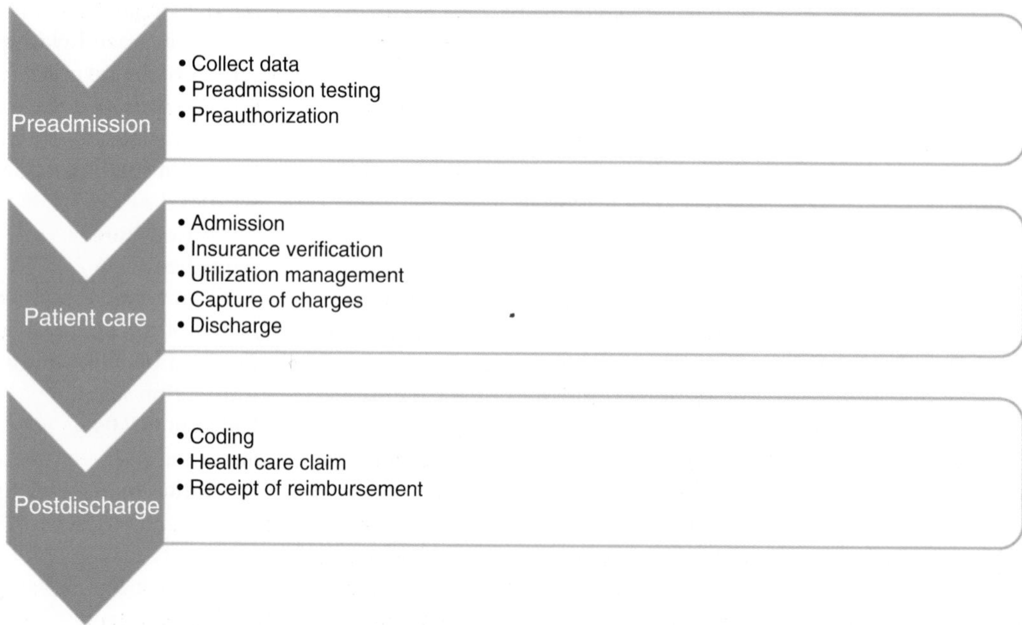

Fig. 19.1 Revenue cycle process.

to have routine blood work for a medication that was prescribed by her dermatologist for her acne, the outpatient claim can be submitted to Medicare. There are exceptions to the 72-hour rule:

- Services provided by home health facilities, hospices, nursing facilities, and ambulance services
- Physician's professional portion of a diagnostic service (the technical portion of a diagnostic service must be included in the inpatient bill)
- Preadmission laboratory testing when the laboratory is not contracted with the hospital

This rule does not apply to non-Medicare insurers.

To obtain necessary diagnostic information and speed up patient care, a patient is often sent to the hospital for preadmission testing (PAT) a day or two before being admitted for surgery. These preadmission tests can include diagnostic studies, such as routine blood and urine tests, radiology imaging, and electrocardiogram. These tests generally fall within the 72-hour rule and therefore are billed as part of the inpatient claim.

Preauthorization

Some services require prior approval from the insurer before they can be performed. This is known as preauthorization. Common examples of services that require preauthorization are magnetic resonance imaging, colonoscopies, and inpatient hospitalizations. The services vary by insurer. The hospital may appeal the need for preauthorization if the procedure/hospitalization is performed in a medical emergency. The authorization number received from the insurer is entered on the health care claim. Local care determinations and national care determinations should be consulted to determine whether Medicare will pay for the services to be provided.

Inpatient Only List

Some insurers, including Medicare, have created a list of procedures that they will reimburse hospitals for only if the procedure is performed on an inpatient basis. The procedures on this inpatient only list (IPO) are considered to be too risky to be performed on an outpatient basis. Examples include open heart procedures and amputations.

Patient Care

This period of the revenue cycle are the stages that occur while the patient is receiving treatment at the hospital. This may be as an inpatient, outpatient, or observation patient. The physician order must identify which patient type the patient should be. Inpatients are said to be admitted to the hospital. An admission is when the patient is formally accepted into the hospital for care. Observation is when outpatients stay overnight in the hospital to determine what is wrong with the patient and if inpatient services are needed. These observation patients generally stay a day or two. Observation patients may be admitted as an inpatient or sent home depending on what is found.

During this admission process, additional information is collected and consent and other forms are signed. Either during preadmission or admission, the patient's insurance is verified, meaning that the insurer is contacted to ensure that the patient's insurance is in effect and to determine what the insurance covers, what the patient will pay, and if preauthorization is needed. A copy or scan of the insurance card is made and maintained by patient accounts department. If the patient is an inpatient or observation patient, the patient is assigned a room. The location depends on the physician order. Locations include regular nursing units, intensive care units, and more.

Utilization Management

Utilization management (UM) is "a collection of systems and processes to ensure that facilities and resources, both human and nonhuman, are used maximally and are consistent with patient care needs" (AHIMA 2017, 239). UM is performed to control costs and to ensure the patient's care is medically necessary. There are two types of reviews: admission and continuing stay.

An admission review is an evaluation for appropriateness and necessity of admission. The health record is reviewed and compared with utilization review criteria. This criterion is established by the insurer to identify when patients should be admitted to the hospital. This criterion generally evaluates the patient's "severity of illness" and "intensity of service"—in other words, how sick they are and what is being done for them. A continued stay review examines patients' health records to determine whether or not patients should stay in the hospital. If the documentation does not meet the criteria for admission or continued stay, the admission is referred to a physician advisor (PA). A PA is a physician who works for the hospital, either part time or full time to conduct a medical review to determine whether the patient's hospitalization is appropriate. The PA reviews the health record and talks to the attending physician. The PA then makes a medical judgment on the appropriateness of the patient's hospitalization. Insurers may also call and talk to utilization review coordinators to gain an understanding of the patient's current condition to make their medical evaluation. If either the PA or the insurer determines that the patient's hospitalization is not justified, an advanced beneficiary notice (ABN) should be awarded if the patient is not discharged. For additional information on the ABN, refer to Chapter 6.

UM can be performed prospectively or retrospectively. Prospective utilization reviews are used to determine the medical necessity and appropriate setting for service before the service. *Appropriate setting* refers to whether the service should be performed as an outpatient or inpatient of the hospital or some other settings. A concurrent review is an evaluation of health care services to determine medical necessity and appropriateness of the care provided during the time services are being provided. A retrospective review is performed after the service is performed. An example of when a retrospective review occurs is when the patient is admitted and discharged before the review being performed, such as over a weekend or holiday.

Posting Charges

Charges for services rendered are posted, or entered, into the patient accounting system. These charges include supplies, procedures, room and board, equipment, medications, and much more. Many items have a barcode stamped on them to facilitate data entry and to improve data quality. The charges for all these items are recorded in the chargemaster.

Chargemaster

The chargemaster, also called charge description master, is a list or database of all of the services, supplies, equipment, and so forth provided by the hospital and the charges that are associated with them. Other data elements in the chargemaster include a unique identifier for each item, the department providing the service, a revenue code, and the procedure codes (discussed later in this section). Services that are provided by multiple departments have an entry for each department. A revenue code is a four-digit code used to group similar charges together, such as clinical laboratory services or room and board. See Table 19.1 for examples of revenue codes.

When a charge is posted in the patient's account, the appropriate code is hardcoded, meaning that it is already coded based on the charge. The chargemaster is used for laboratory, radiology, and other routine services. This prevents the coders from having to manually assign the code for these routine services.

This chargemaster should be constantly monitored and updated as codes change, services are added or discontinued, and charges change. A chargemaster coordinator normally controls the day-to-day management of the chargemaster under the direction of the chargemaster committee. This chargemaster committee is responsible for the design and contents of the chargemaster. This committee should be made up of billers, coders, clinical staff, and others involved in the revenue cycle process.

Charges may include a professional charge and a technical charge. The hospital will charge a technical charge for its services such as a chest radiograph and pathologic testing. This technical charge would cover, for example, the costs of the x-ray examination itself, the radiology technician performing the procedure, supplies, and any other costs. The professional charge is for the physician services. In the case of the radiology example, the professional charge for physician services would reimburse the radiologist for reading and interpreting the radiology report. A professional charge would not be added for medications, supplies, room charges, and so forth. This professional charge will be billed by the hospital only if the physician or other health care professional is an employee of the hospital; otherwise, the professional charge is made by the health care professional's practice.

Discharge

A discharge occurs when the physician writes an order releasing the patient from the hospital. This order should include where the patient should go. Possible locations include home, home with home health, another acute care hospital, rehabilitation, and more. There are times when a patient wants to leave the hospital and the physician believes the patient needs continued hospitalization. If the patient insists, the patient leaves against medical advice (AMA). This should be documented in the health record. The location where the patient is being discharged to is known as the discharge disposition. This discharge disposition is entered in the hospital information system at the time of discharge for inclusion on the health care claim.

TABLE 19.1 Sample Revenue Codes

Revenue Code	Description
0270	Medical/Surgical Supplies
0305	Laboratory—Clinical Diagnostic: Hematology
0619	Magnetic Resonance Tech. (MRT): Other MRT
0720	Labor Room

Adapted from Centers for Medicare and Medicaid Services (2018A).

Postdischarge

The postdischarge phase includes all the steps that occur after the patient's discharge: coding, health care claim, receipt of reimbursement, hospital-acquired conditions, and the Discharge Not Final Billed report. This section will also cover many of the types of reimbursement used in hospitals.

Coding

Diagnosis and procedure codes are assigned to each inpatient and outpatient health record. These codes are included on the health care claim. Diagnosis codes are assigned for all patient types using the *International Classification of Disease, Tenth Edition, Clinical Modification (ICD-10-CM).* The coding system used for procedures depends on if the patient is an outpatient or inpatient. Outpatient procedures, which include outpatient surgery, emergency room, observation, and other outpatient services, use Healthcare Common Procedural Coding System (HCPCS). HCPCS is made up of two tiers. Tier I is the American Medical Association's *Current Procedural Terminology* (CPT). Because CPT does not include codes for medications, durable medical equipment, and other procedures, tier II was developed by the Centers for Medicare and Medicaid Services (CMS) to address these gaps. Inpatient procedures are coded using the *International Classification of Disease, Tenth Edition, Procedure Coding System (ICD-10-PCS).* See Chapter 13 for more on CPT and HCPCS.

International Classification of Disease, Tenth Edition, Clinical Modification. ICD-10-CM is divided into two volumes. Volume 1 is an alphabetic list of the diagnoses. Volume 2 is a tabular list where the diagnoses are listed in order by the code. Diagnosis codes are made up of three to seven alphanumeric characters depending on the level of detail required for the diagnosis. ICD-10-CM codes always begin with an alphabetic character, and there is always a three-character category code. Codes may have one to four additional characters, which may be numeric or alphabetic. Examples of codes are I10, K46.0, and S55.019A. One of the key concepts in coding inpatient services is the definition of the principal diagnosis. It is the reason, after study, for admission to the hospital. This code is listed first on the health care claim. Two examples of how this definition is applied are as follows:

- A patient may come to the hospital with chest pain. After running tests, the physician determines that the chest pain is caused by an acute myocardial infarction. The acute myocardial infarction is the principal diagnosis, not the chest pain.
- A patient is admitted to the hospital for gastroenteritis. While in the hospital, the patient falls and fractures her arm. Surgery is required for the fracture. The principal diagnosis remains the gastroenteritis.

The term used for the first code on the outpatient claim is *reason for encounter.* Additional diagnosis codes are added to both inpatient and outpatient claims based on coding guidelines and health care facility policy. For example, codes for diabetes and chronic obstructive pulmonary disease would be coded when the patient comes into the hospital for appendicitis, but acne would not be coded in this situation.

International Classification of Disease, Tenth Edition, Procedure Coding System. The ICD-10-PCS is structured in a table format. To know what table to refer to, an alphabetic index is used. The coding system is based on the intent of the procedures. The term *root operation* is used to identify the intent. Examples of the root operation are resection, extraction, control, and release. Rather than looking up a cholecystectomy in the alphabetic index, the coder would locate the term *resection* because this is the root operation for the removal of the entire body part. All ICD-10-PCS codes contain seven alphanumeric characters. Each of these characters has a specific meaning, such as root operation and body part, but the values for each character vary by body system. See Table 19.2 for an example of how an ICD-10-PCS code is structured. Table 19.3 is a list of all of the Medical and Surgical section root operations.

The section character identifies the specialty areas of the procedure. The majority of the codes in ICD-10-PCS fall into the Medical and Surgical section; however, there are a number of other specialty sections such as Radiation Therapy and Obstetrics. The body section character identifies the body system on which the procedure is being performed, such as the cardiovascular or respiratory system. The operation character identifies the root operation or intent of the procedure as discussed earlier. It identifies whether the procedure removes the entire body part, a piece of the body part, restricts a body part, removes foreign body, or other procedure. The body part character identifies the specific body part, which may or may not be the entire part. It may also be a region such as the trunk. For example, body parts can include right lower leg, gallbladder, or left lobe of the liver. The ICD-10-PCS does include laterality of the procedure as shown in the example in Table 19.2. The approach identifies how the surgery was performed. Some of the options are open (where the procedure is performed directly through an incision), laparoscopically (through small incisions using a camera), and endoscopically (through a natural or artificial opening). A device is an item left in place after surgery such as an artificial hip or pacemaker. Most procedures do not have a device; however, a character identifying this is still part of the code. The seventh character is a qualifier. This is used to provide additional information, such as origin of tissue for transplant and whether the removal of tissue was for diagnostic purposes. A placeholder character must be present even when there is no additional information provided.

The principal procedure is the procedure code that is listed first on the health care claim. The principal procedure should be associated with the principal procedure. For example, an appendectomy would be a surgical treatment associated with the principal diagnosis of appendicitis. Additional significant procedure codes are added. Significant procedure codes have risk, require special training, and include both surgical (such as appendectomy) and diagnostic procedures (such as cardiac catheterization). What is coded is determined by coding guidelines and the health care facility's policy.

The principal diagnosis only applies to inpatient hospitalizations and is sequenced first on the health care claim. The first listed code identifies why the patient sought health care services. It is only used for outpatient services.

ICD-10-PCS is maintained by CMS. The coding guidelines and codes are update each October 1.

Health Care Claim

After the patient's discharge, the hospital claim is dropped, meaning that the claim is submitted to the insurer. There is generally a period between the patient's discharge and the bill

TABLE 19.2 ICD-10-PCS Structure Total Abdominal Cholecystectomy

Character	Name of Character	Total Abdominal Cholecystectomy
1	Section	0: Medical and Surgical
2	Body System	F: Hepatobiliary System and Pancreas
3	Operation	T: Resection
4	Body Part	4: Gallbladder
5	Approach	0: Open
6	Device	Z: No Device
7	Qualifier	Z: No qualifier
Entire Code		0FT40ZZ

ICD-10-PCS, International Classification of Disease, Tenth Edition, Procedure Coding System.
Adapted from Centers for Medicare and Medicaid Services. (2018b). *ICD-10 Procedure Coding System (ICD-10-PCS) 2018 Tables and Index.* Retrieved from https://www.cms.gov/Medicare/Coding/ICD10/Downloads/2018-ICD-10-PCS-Tables-And-Index.zip.

TABLE 19.3 Medical and Surgical Root Operations

Alteration	Inspection
Bypass	Map
Change	Occlusion
Control	Reattachment
Creation	Release
Destruction	Removal
Detachment	Repair
Dilation	Replacement
Division	Reposition
Drainage	Resection
Excision	Restriction
Extirpation	Revision
Extraction	Supplement
Fragmentation	Transfer
Fusion	Transplantation
Insertion	

dropping. The purpose of the period is to allow time for any late charges to be entered.

An important part of the billing process is the content and formatting requirements for the health care claim. Much of this was defined by the Health Insurance Portability and Accountability Act of 1996. The **Health Insurance Portability and Accountability Act of 1996 (HIPAA)** had a major impact on the submission of health care claims. HIPAA is a federal law that mandated a number of requirements, including the privacy and security of protected health information, as discussed in Chapter 2. It also established standards for the sharing of data for administrative purposes. The focus of this section is the **Transactions and Code Set Rule.** To be subject to the HIPAA, an organization must meet the definition of a **covered entity (CE).** A CE is a health care provider, a health plan (insurer), or a health care clearinghouse that performs one or more of the identified transactions electronically.

The code set portion of the rule mandated the use of ICD-10-CM, ICD-10-PCS, HCPCS Level II, CPT, and other code sets for use on health care claims.

It also established transaction standards for the following (CMS, 2017a):

- "Health claims
- Eligibility and benefit verification
- Prior authorization and referrals
- Claim status inquiry and response
- Claim payment
- Electronic remittance advice
- Coordination of benefits
- Referral certification
- Retail pharmacy subrogation
- Enrollment/disenrollment in a health plan
- Premium payment/explanation"

A **transaction set** "is the collection of data that is exchanged to convey meaning between the parties engaged in electronic data interchange" (X12 2017). All the transactions listed with the exception of selected pharmacy transactions use the American National Standards Institute (**ANSI**) Accredited Standards Committee (**ASC**) X12N standards. These standards must be used to perform any of the listed activities. These standards provide the format and other directions on how to submit the claims or other activity.

The **Uniform Bill 04 (UB-04),** also known as the CMS-1450, is the claims form used to submit paper claims for institutional health care facilities such as hospitals (acute care and specialty) and skilled nursing facilities. The electronic version is known as ASC X12N 837. The UB-04 is maintained by the **National Uniform Billing Committee** to create a national standard for the health care claim. Both the UB-04 and the ASC X12N 837 contain the same data and use the same format. The UB-04 does not list every item for which the patient was charged; rather it is a summary of the charges. Another document, known as an itemized bill, lists each individual item used in the patient's care, such as medications, laboratory tests, radiology tests, gauze, syringes, room charges, and so forth. Auditors often require access to both the UB-04 and the itemized bill to conduct an audit of the claim.

On the UB-04, there are 81 form locators, or fields. These form locators are divided into five sections. These sections are as follows:

- Provider information (form locators 1 to 7): These form locators provide information on the health care facility, such as name, address, account number, dates of service that the claim covers, and the federal tax identifier.
- Patient information (form locators 8 to 38): These form locators provide identification about the patient, such as patient name, address, date of birth, and gender. This section also contains admission date, type of admission (emergency, urgent, and elective), and admission time.
- Billing information (form locators 39 to 49): The billing information section includes revenue codes, description of services, HCPCS codes, service units, and charges. The service units provide the number of items/units—for example, four units of a medical/surgical room when the patient is an inpatient in the hospital for 4 days.
- Payer information (form locators 50 to 65): The payer information section includes insurer, health plan identifier, insured's name, and other insurance information.
- Diagnostic information (form locators 66 to 81): Diagnostic information includes diagnosis and procedure codes, date of procedures, and admitting diagnosis.

A sample of a completed CMS-1450 form for inpatient services is found in Fig. 19.2. A sample of a completed CMS-1450 form for outpatient services is found in Fig. 19.3.

Receipt of Reimbursement

When the primary insurer pays a claim, the insurer notifies the hospital via remittance advice. The amount is documented in the patient's account and any adjustments are made. If there is a secondary insurer, that insurer is billed and any payment is posted. The patient is billed for any remaining balance as appropriate.

Hospital Acquired Conditions

CMS identified a number of conditions that indicated a quality issue if the patient developed these conditions while an inpatient at an acute care hospital. These conditions are collectively known as **hospital-acquired conditions (HACs).** Some of these conditions include administration of wrong blood type, foreign body left in patient during surgery, trauma due to fall, and air embolism. For a full list, refer to Table 19.4. Documentation in the health record is key to the HAC program as the documentation has to indicate whether or not these conditions are **present on admission (POA)** or not. Table 19.5 shows the indicators that are assigned to each diagnosis on inpatient claims.

To identify whether or not the condition was POA or not, acute care hospitals are mandated to report a POA indicator for each diagnosis included on a Medicare inpatient claim. These indicators are Y for yes, N for no, U for documentation does not indicate when the condition occurred, and W for when the physician cannot determine when the condition occurred (CMS, 2017b). Although mandated only for Medicare patients, hospitals collect this information for all inpatient discharges. If a patient developed one of the

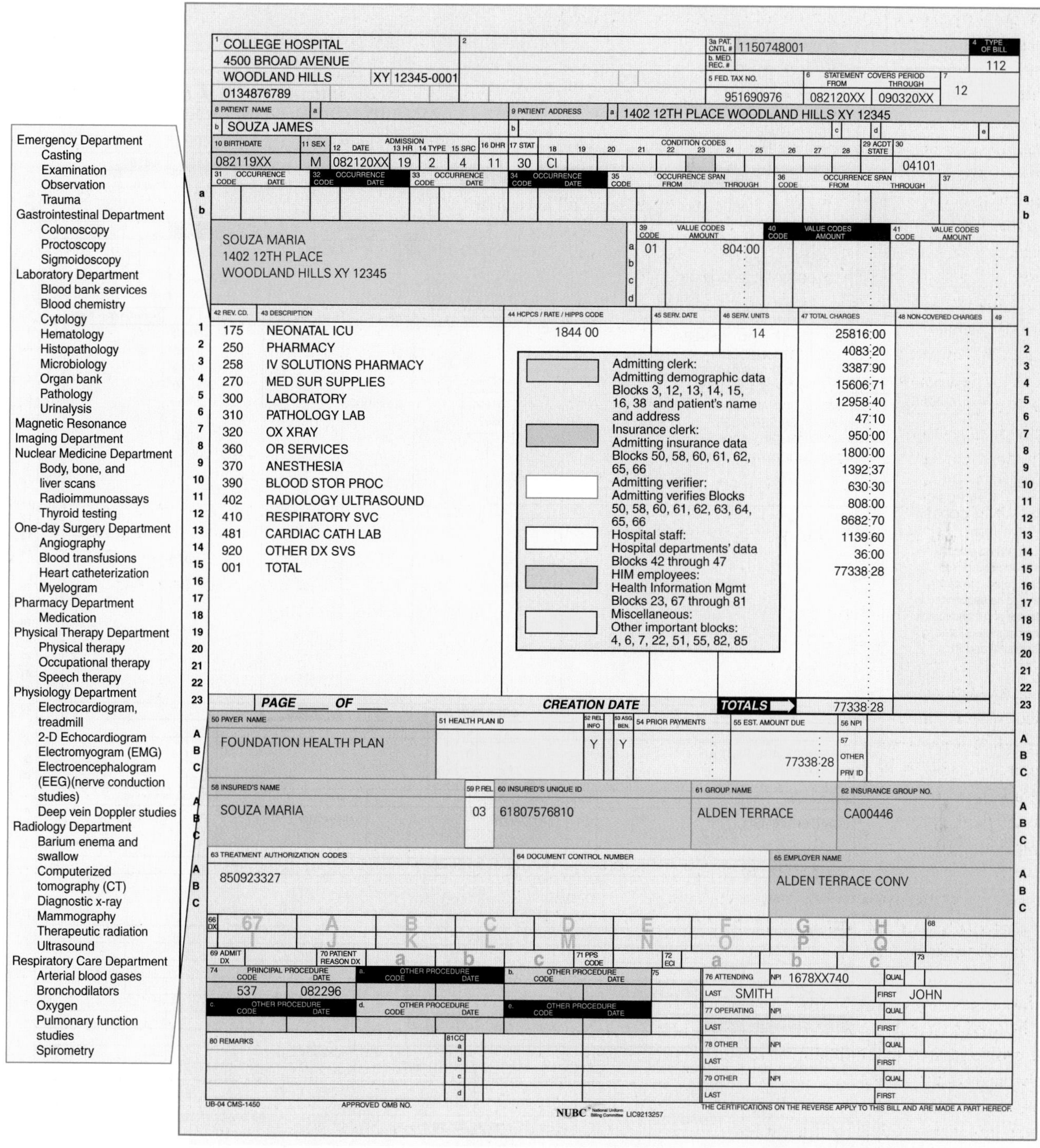

Emergency Department
Casting
Examination
Observation
Trauma
Gastrointestinal Department
Colonoscopy
Proctoscopy
Sigmoidoscopy
Laboratory Department
Blood bank services
Blood chemistry
Cytology
Hematology
Histopathology
Microbiology
Organ bank
Pathology
Urinalysis
Magnetic Resonance Imaging Department
Nuclear Medicine Department
Body, bone, and liver scans
Radioimmunoassays
Thyroid testing
One-day Surgery Department
Angiography
Blood transfusions
Heart catheterization
Myelogram
Pharmacy Department
Medication
Physical Therapy Department
Physical therapy
Occupational therapy
Speech therapy
Physiology Department
Electrocardiogram, treadmill
2-D Echocardiogram
Electromyogram (EMG)
Electroencephalogram (EEG)(nerve conduction studies)
Deep vein Doppler studies
Radiology Department
Barium enema and swallow
Computerized tomography (CT)
Diagnostic x-ray
Mammography
Therapeutic radiation
Ultrasound
Respiratory Care Department
Arterial blood gases
Bronchodilators
Oxygen
Pulmonary function studies
Spirometry

1 COLLEGE HOSPITAL
4500 BROAD AVENUE
WOODLAND HILLS XY 12345-0001
0134876789

3a PAT. CNTL # 1150748001
b. MED. REC. #
4 TYPE OF BILL 112
5 FED. TAX NO. 951690976
6 STATEMENT COVERS PERIOD FROM 082120XX THROUGH 090320XX
7 12

8 PATIENT NAME b SOUZA JAMES
9 PATIENT ADDRESS a 1402 12TH PLACE WOODLAND HILLS XY 12345

10 BIRTHDATE 082119XX
11 SEX M
ADMISSION 12 DATE 082120XX 13 HR 19 14 TYPE 2 15 SRC 4
16 DHR 11
17 STAT 30
CONDITION CODES 18 CI
29 ACDT STATE
30 04101

31–36 OCCURRENCE CODE / DATE; OCCURRENCE SPAN CODE / FROM / THROUGH; 37

38 SOUZA MARIA
1402 12TH PLACE
WOODLAND HILLS XY 12345

39 VALUE CODES CODE AMOUNT: a 01 804:00
40 VALUE CODES CODE AMOUNT
41 VALUE CODES CODE AMOUNT

42 REV. CD.	43 DESCRIPTION	44 HCPCS / RATE / HIPPS CODE	45 SERV. DATE	46 SERV. UNITS	47 TOTAL CHARGES	48 NON-COVERED CHARGES
175	NEONATAL ICU	1844 00		14	25816:00	
250	PHARMACY				4083:20	
258	IV SOLUTIONS PHARMACY				3387:90	
270	MED SUR SUPPLIES				15606:71	
300	LABORATORY				12958:40	
310	PATHOLOGY LAB				47:10	
320	OX XRAY				950:00	
360	OR SERVICES				1800:00	
370	ANESTHESIA				1392:37	
390	BLOOD STOR PROC				630:30	
402	RADIOLOGY ULTRASOUND				808:00	
410	RESPIRATORY SVC				8682:70	
481	CARDIAC CATH LAB				1139:60	
920	OTHER DX SVS				36:00	
001	TOTAL				77338:28	

PAGE ___ OF ___ CREATION DATE TOTALS 77338:28

Admitting clerk: Admitting demographic data Blocks 3, 12, 13, 14, 15, 16, 38 and patient's name and address
Insurance clerk: Admitting insurance data Blocks 50, 58, 60, 61, 62, 65, 66
Admitting verifier: Admitting verifies Blocks 50, 58, 60, 61, 62, 63, 64, 65, 66
Hospital staff: Hospital departments' data Blocks 42 through 47
HIM employees: Health Information Mgmt Blocks 23, 67 through 81
Miscellaneous: Other important blocks: 4, 6, 7, 22, 51, 55, 82, 85

50 PAYER NAME: FOUNDATION HEALTH PLAN
51 HEALTH PLAN ID
52 REL. INFO Y
53 ASG. BEN. Y
54 PRIOR PAYMENTS
55 EST. AMOUNT DUE 77338:28
56 NPI
57 OTHER PRV ID

58 INSURED'S NAME: SOUZA MARIA
59 P. REL 03
60 INSURED'S UNIQUE ID 61807576810
61 GROUP NAME ALDEN TERRACE
62 INSURANCE GROUP NO. CA00446

63 TREATMENT AUTHORIZATION CODES 850923327
64 DOCUMENT CONTROL NUMBER
65 EMPLOYER NAME ALDEN TERRACE CONV

66 DX 67 A B C D E F G H I J K L M N O P Q 68
69 ADMIT DX 70 PATIENT REASON DX a b c 71 PPS CODE 72 ECI a b c 73
74 PRINCIPAL PROCEDURE CODE 537 DATE 082296
a. OTHER PROCEDURE CODE DATE b. OTHER PROCEDURE CODE DATE
c. OTHER PROCEDURE CODE DATE d. OTHER PROCEDURE CODE DATE e. OTHER PROCEDURE CODE DATE
75
76 ATTENDING NPI 1678XX740 QUAL
LAST SMITH FIRST JOHN
77 OPERATING NPI QUAL LAST FIRST
78 OTHER NPI QUAL LAST FIRST
79 OTHER NPI QUAL LAST FIRST
80 REMARKS
81CC a b c d

UB-04 CMS-1450 APPROVED OMB NO. NUBC National Uniform Billing Committee LIC9213257
THE CERTIFICATIONS ON THE REVERSE APPLY TO THIS BILL AND ARE MADE A PART HEREOF.

Fig. 19.2 Scannable Uniform Bill (CMS-1450 [UB-04]) insurance paper claim form completed for an inpatient showing hospital department that input data for hospital services. Colored blocks indicate data obtained by various hospital personnel. Job titles and the exact data each person obtains may vary from facility to facility. Form locator guidelines vary and may not always follow the visual guide presented here.

conditions while in the hospital, the hospital is not reimbursed by Medicare a higher weighted Medicare-severity diagnosis-related group (discussed later in this chapter) that the HAC causes. If the condition was POA, then the hospital is reimbursed. Although the conditions affected are limited, not receiving reimbursement would have a serious impact on the hospital's reimbursement.

Discharge Not Final Billed Report

The Discharge Not Final Billed (DNFB) report is a list of all hospital (inpatient and outpatient) claims that have not been submitted to the insurer. The claim may be on the DNFB for a number of reasons such as: not coded, missing data, still in window of time waiting for late charges, missing discharge disposition, and more. The DNFB is monitored to identify

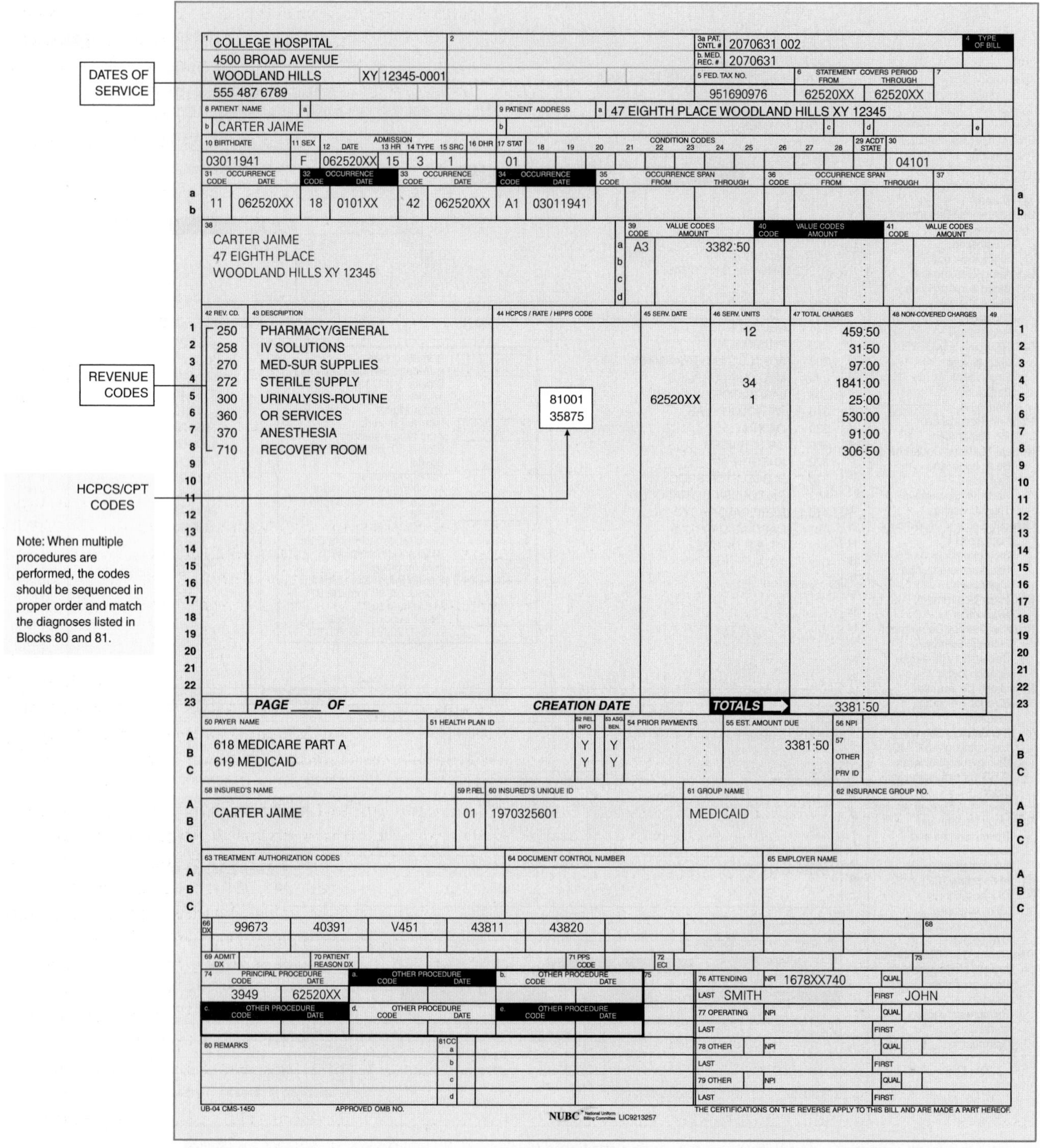

DATES OF SERVICE

REVENUE CODES

HCPCS/CPT CODES

Note: When multiple procedures are performed, the codes should be sequenced in proper order and match the diagnoses listed in Blocks 80 and 81.

1 COLLEGE HOSPITAL
4500 BROAD AVENUE
WOODLAND HILLS XY 12345-0001
555 487 6789

2

3a PAT. CNTL # 2070631 002
b. MED. REC. # 2070631

4 TYPE OF BILL

5 FED. TAX NO. 951690976

6 STATEMENT COVERS PERIOD FROM 62520XX THROUGH 62520XX

7

8 PATIENT NAME a
b CARTER JAIME

9 PATIENT ADDRESS a 47 EIGHTH PLACE WOODLAND HILLS XY 12345

10 BIRTHDATE	11 SEX	12 ADMISSION DATE	13 HR	14 TYPE	15 SRC	16 DHR	17 STAT	18–28 CONDITION CODES	29 ACDT STATE	30
03011941	F	062520XX	15	3	1		01			04101

31 OCCURRENCE CODE	DATE	32 OCCURRENCE CODE	DATE	33 OCCURRENCE CODE	DATE	34 OCCURRENCE CODE	DATE	35 OCCURRENCE SPAN CODE	FROM	THROUGH	36 OCCURRENCE SPAN CODE	FROM	THROUGH	37
11	062520XX	18	0101XX	42	062520XX	A1	03011941							

38 CARTER JAIME
47 EIGHTH PLACE
WOODLAND HILLS XY 12345

39 VALUE CODES CODE	AMOUNT	40 VALUE CODES CODE	AMOUNT	41 VALUE CODES CODE	AMOUNT
a A3	3382:50				

	42 REV. CD.	43 DESCRIPTION	44 HCPCS / RATE / HIPPS CODE	45 SERV. DATE	46 SERV. UNITS	47 TOTAL CHARGES	48 NON-COVERED CHARGES	49
1	250	PHARMACY/GENERAL			12	459:50		
2	258	IV SOLUTIONS				31:50		
3	270	MED-SUR SUPPLIES				97:00		
4	272	STERILE SUPPLY			34	1841:00		
5	300	URINALYSIS-ROUTINE	81001	62520XX	1	25:00		
6	360	OR SERVICES	35875			530:00		
7	370	ANESTHESIA				91:00		
8	710	RECOVERY ROOM				306:50		
23		PAGE ___ OF ___	CREATION DATE		TOTALS	3381:50		

50 PAYER NAME	51 HEALTH PLAN ID	52 REL. INFO	53 ASG. BEN.	54 PRIOR PAYMENTS	55 EST. AMOUNT DUE	56 NPI
618 MEDICARE PART A		Y	Y		3381:50	57 OTHER PRV ID
619 MEDICAID		Y	Y			

58 INSURED'S NAME	59 P. REL.	60 INSURED'S UNIQUE ID	61 GROUP NAME	62 INSURANCE GROUP NO.
CARTER JAIME	01	1970325601	MEDICAID	

63 TREATMENT AUTHORIZATION CODES | 64 DOCUMENT CONTROL NUMBER | 65 EMPLOYER NAME

66 DX 99673 40391 V451 43811 43820 | 68

69 ADMIT DX | 70 PATIENT REASON DX | 71 PPS CODE | 72 ECI | 73

74 PRINCIPAL PROCEDURE CODE 3949 DATE 62520XX | a. OTHER PROCEDURE CODE DATE | b. OTHER PROCEDURE CODE DATE | 75
c. OTHER PROCEDURE CODE DATE | d. OTHER PROCEDURE CODE DATE | e. OTHER PROCEDURE CODE DATE

76 ATTENDING NPI 1678XX740 QUAL
LAST SMITH FIRST JOHN
77 OPERATING NPI QUAL
LAST FIRST
78 OTHER NPI QUAL
LAST FIRST
79 OTHER NPI QUAL
LAST FIRST

80 REMARKS | 81CC a b c d

UB-04 CMS-1450 APPROVED OMB NO. NUBC National Uniform Billing Committee LIC9213257

THE CERTIFICATIONS ON THE REVERSE APPLY TO THIS BILL AND ARE MADE A PART HEREOF.

Fig. 19.3 Scannable Uniform Bill (CMS-1450 [UB-04]) insurance paper claim form showing placement of ambulatory payment classification (APC) data for an outpatient for submission to an insurance company.

the claims that have issues preventing the claim from dropping. One of the most common reasons that the claim remains on the DNFB is that the diagnosis and procedure codes have not been entered. The missing codes may be due to missing a health record in the paper environment, waiting on a physician for documentation, backlogs in coding, and other reasons. Administration typically monitors this report and may have a dollar threshold that they want the report to stay below. This threshold varies widely depending on the size of the hospital and other factors. For example, the threshold of a 60-bed community hospital may be $300,000, whereas a 900-bed tertiary hospital that provides transplants and trauma services, has a burn unit, and offers other advanced services may have a threshold of $2,000,000.

TABLE 19.4 Hospital-Acquired Conditions
Air embolism
Blood incompatibility
Catheter-associated urinary tract infection
Deep vein thrombosis and pulmonary embolism following specific orthopedic procedures
Falls and trauma
Foreign object left in patient after surgery
Iatrogenic pneumothorax with venous catheterization
Symptoms of poor glycemic control
Pressure ulcers (stages III and IV)
Surgical site infection following bariatric surgery for obesity
Surgical site infection following insertion of cardiac implantable electronic device
Surgical site infection following specified orthopedic procedures
Surgical site infection, mediastinitis, following a coronary artery bypass graft
Vascular catheter-associated infection

Adapted from Centers for Medicare and Medicaid Services. (n.d.). *FY 2013, FY 2014, and FY 2015 Final HAC List (no changes have been made)*. Retrieved from https://www.cms.gov/Medicare/Medicare-Fee-for-Service-Payment/HospitalAcqCond/Downloads/FY_2013_Final_HACsCodeList.pdf.

TABLE 19.5 Present on Admission
Y: Diagnosis was present at time of admission.
N: Diagnosis was not present at time of admission.
U: Documentation in the health record is insufficient to determine whether the condition was POA.
W: The physician is unable to clinically determine whether the condition was POA.
1: The diagnosis is exempt from POA reporting.

POA, Present on admission.

TYPES OF REIMBURSEMENT METHODOLOGIES

Many different reimbursement methodologies are used to reimburse for health care services. These reimbursement methodologies include the following:

- Self-pay: **Self-pay** is when the patient pays out of pocket for the health care services. This method may be used because the patient does not have insurance, because the service is not covered by insurance, or for other reasons. For example, a patient may not want an HIV test to be submitted to the insurer or may not want his spouse to know he had health care services.
- Prospective payment system: In a **prospective payment system (PPS),** the health care provider knows the amount of reimbursement that will be received before the service being provided. One method of a PPS is **diagnosis-related groups (DRGs).** There are many different DRG systems, including the Medicare Severity Diagnosis-Related Groups discussed later in this chapter.
- Capitation: Capitation is often used in managed care. In **capitation,** a health care provider is given a set amount of money each month to provide all the care for a patient for a period. The amount remains the same regardless of whether the patient does not come to the hospital or is in the hospital for the entire month. In a capitated environment, a gatekeeper is often used. A **gatekeeper** is a primary care physician (family practice, internist, pediatrician) who provides the care for the patient. For the patient to go to a specialist (cardiologist, dermatologist, and so forth), the gatekeeper must refer the patient.
- Fee-for-service: In the fee-for-service reimbursement, the health care provider is paid for each service provided.

MEDICARE

Medicare is an important insurer to understand in hospital reimbursement. For general information regarding Medicare, refer to Chapter 6. This section will address the reimbursement methods, the role of the Medicare administrative contractor, and quality improvement organizations.

Medicare Administrative Contractor

A **Medicare administrative contractor (MAC)** is an organization that contracts with Medicare to process the Medicare claims and to perform other activities. MACs also create the local coverage determinations that were discussed in Chapter 6. They work with appeals and so much more.

Quality Improvement Organizations

Quality improvement organizations (QIOs) are hired by the CMS to improve patient care, ensure the medical necessity of care provided, review the appropriateness of the setting (inpatient vs. outpatient), and address beneficiary complaints (CMS, 2016a).

Some of the reviews performed by QIOs in hospitals include the following (Quality Improvement Organizations nd):

- Higher weighted DRG: The higher weighted DRG reviews evaluate whether or not the higher reimbursement Medicare severity DRG is justified by the health record. Medicare severity DRGs are discussed later in this chapter.
- Readmission: Readmission reviews are conducted when the patient is readmitted to the hospital for the same condition. The purpose of the review is to determine whether or not the patient was discharged from the hospital too soon.
- Emergency Medical Treatment and Labor Act: The **Emergency Medical Treatment and Labor Act (EMTALA)** is a federal law that prohibits patients from being transferred to another hospital if they are medically unstable or are in active labor. These reviews determine if patients were transferred appropriately. The health record must support the need for transfer and that the patient is medically stable. This law was established because patients without insurance were being transferred to other hospitals while in critical conditions or in active labor. There were times when patients gave birth on the way to the other hospital or died en route.

Whenever a problem is identified during a review, such as the patient's admission was not medically necessary, the QIO sends a denial letter to the hospital. The reimbursement that the hospital received for that hospitalization is returned to Medicare. To have the reimbursement returned, the hospital would need to appeal the decision. In this example, the hospital would need to work with the physician to get him or her to write the letter justifying the need for hospitalization. For additional information on denial management and QIOs, refer to Chapter 6.

Medicare Reimbursement Methodologies

The Tax Equity and Fiscal Responsibility Act of 1982 (TEFRA) mandated the use of prospective payment systems for Medicare. TEFRA mandated the use of the PPS for acute care hospital's inpatient discharges. Today a number of PPS systems are in use for Medicare reimbursement of hospital services, including the following:

- Acute Inpatient Prospective Payment System
- Outpatient Prospective Payment System
- Resource-Based Relative Value Scale
- Long-Term Care Hospital Prospective Payment System
- Inpatient Rehabilitation Facility Prospective Payment System
- Psychiatric Prospective Payment System
- Ambulance Fee Schedule

Changes to these reimbursement systems go into effect each October 1. These reimbursement systems apply to the traditional Medicare program but not Medicare Part C. Each of these reimbursement systems is discussed in the following sections.

Acute Inpatient Prospective Payment System

The Acute Inpatient Prospective Payment System (IPPS) is the prospective reimbursement system used for Medicare inpatient claims. Reimbursement is made based on Medicare Severity Diagnosis-Related Groups (MS-DRGs). The MS-DRG system groups similar conditions that consume similar resources (costs are similar) together. The hospital receives one MS-DRG for each admission. The MS-DRG is assigned by a software application known as a grouper. The grouper uses the principal diagnosis, procedures, discharge disposition, complications, comorbidities, major complications and comorbidities, and patient age to assign the MS-DRG. The MS-DRG system has a three-tiered DRG system based on the severity of the patient's condition. Each MS-DRG is assigned a relative weight, geometric mean length of stay, and arithmetic mean length of stay. Many, but not all, of the MS-DRGs have a structure in which the diagnosis and sometimes the diagnosis and procedure is linked to the following three-tiered structure:

- No complication or comorbidity
- A complication or comorbidity
- A major complication or comorbidity

An example of this three-tiered approach is as follows:

- MS-DRG 037 Extracranial procedures with MCC
- MS-DRG 038 Extracranial procedures with CC
- MS-DRG 039 Extracranial without CC/MCC (2018c)

A complication is a diagnosis or condition that arises during the patient's hospitalization that increases the patient's length of stay in 75% of the cases. A comorbidity is a condition that the patient has on admission that increases the patient's length of stay in 75% of the cases. Together these are known as complication/comorbidities (CCs). Medicare has identified some conditions as major complications/comorbidities (MCCs). These complications and comorbidities have a significant impact on the patient's care and therefore result in additional compensation for the acute care hospital.

The MS-DRGs are grouped into major diagnostic categories (MDCs). Many of the MDCs are based on the body system, but others are based on factors such as injuries.

The hospital receives one MS-DRG payment as reimbursement. If the MS-DRG payment is more than the costs of providing care, the hospital has a profit; however, if the MS-DRG payment is less than the costs, the hospital has a loss unless the loss is significant enough to qualify as a cost outlier. A cost outlier is additional reimbursement for patient care when the costs of the hospitalization are excessively large. Each MS-DRG is assigned a threshold for the amount necessary for the admission to qualify for the cost outlier.

The amount of reimbursement for the assigned MS-DRG is based on the relative weight. The relative weight is assigned to each MS-DRG by CMS. The "average" relative weight is 1.0000 (all relative weights go four digits past the decimal point). Each hospital is assigned a base rate that covers salary and nonsalary costs. This base rate varies based on the cost of living in that area. The MS-DRG relative weight is multiplied by the base rate. If the hospital qualifies for an add-on, then that amount is added to the amount. There are four types of add-ons: teaching medical residents, disproportionate number of indigent patients, use of approved technologies, and cost outliers (CMS, 2016b). There may also be adjustments to the IPPS in special circumstances. Fig. 19.4 shows an example of how a basic MS-DRG works.

Under four circumstances, the MS-DRG payment is reduced. These circumstances are as follows (CMS, 2016b):

- Length of stay is 1 or more days shorter than the geometric mean length of stay for the MS-DRG.
- Patient is transferred to another acute care hospital subject to the IPPS or in certain circumstances to a postacute setting. Postacute settings include rehabilitation hospitals and skilled nursing facilities, long-term care hospitals, and more.
- The patient is transferred to an acute care hospital not subject to the IPPS.
- Patient is transferred to a critical access hospital. A critical access hospital is one that meets specific criteria, including a rural location. These hospitals are in locations that do not have other hospitals in the surrounding area.

MS-DRG 192

Base rate $4,567.00X Relative weight 0.7234 = MS-DRG Amount $3,303.77

MS-DRG Amount $3,303.77 + Add-on $765.00 = Reimbursement received $4068.77

Fig. 19.4 Calculating the basic Medicare Severity Diagnosis-Related Group *(MS-DRG)* reimbursement.

Upcoding is assigning codes to increase reimbursement when the health record does not support the diagnosis and procedure codes. DRG creep is the result of upcoding. DRG creep results in increased reimbursement to a level that is not deserved by the hospital. Another term to know is downcoding. Downcoding is coding a lower level of care when the health record would support a higher level. Some facilities practice this to not be accused of fraudulent claims. Downcoding results in poor data quality from the inappropriate codes as well as a smaller reimbursement amount.

Hospital Outpatient Prospective Payment System

The Outpatient Prospective Payment System (OPPS) is used for hospital outpatient services, including surgical procedures; radiology, laboratory, and emergency services; observation; and more. Acute care hospitals are paid based on ambulatory payment classifications (APCs). APCs group similar services with similar costs together. A hospital can receive multiple APCs for services rendered. For example, if a patient came to the hospital to have a routine mammogram, a urinalysis and a chest radiograph, the hospital would receive three APCS, one for each service.

APCs use packaging, which means that all supplies, medications, and other components of a service are included in the APC. Because of this, the hospital would not bill for these components separately. For example, if a patient has a cholecystectomy performed on an outpatient basis, the APC would include the surgery, anesthesia, postoperative observation, medications, supplies, and more.

In the OPPS, every HCPCS code (including CPT), discussed earlier, is given a status indicator. The status indicator provides information about the procedure, including whether or not it is covered under the OPPS, if it is subject to discounting, if it is an inpatient-only procedure, and more. Another component of the OPPS is the use of discounting. Discounting is when the APC reimbursement to the hospital is reduced. Discounting occurs in the following circumstances:

- The patient is prepared for surgery and is taken to the operating or procedure room before the surgery is cancelled. The anesthesia may or may not have been administered.
- Two or more surgical procedures are performed at the same operative session. When this occurs, the first surgical procedure is paid at 100% and the subsequent procedures are paid at 50% of the APC amount. The logic behind this is that there is only one administration of anesthesia, one recovery, and so forth. The status indicator for the HCPCS codes associated with these procedures must indicate that they are subject to the discounting. This is indicated with a status indicator of T. A full list of status indicators and their definitions is published in Addendum D1 of the OPPS/ASC proposed and final rules each year. The status indicator for each HCPCS code is shown in OPPS Addendum B. The link to Addendum B is: https://www.cms.gov/Medicare/Medicare-Fee-for-Service-Payment/HospitalOutpatientPPS/Addendum-A-and-Addendum-B-Updates.html

To determine reimbursement, each APC is assigned a relative weight, which is multiplied by a national number known as the conversion factor. That figure is then adjusted for the geographic location, including both labor and nonlabor costs. There may be other adjustments depending on the circumstances, including a cost outlier.

Resource-Based Relative Value Scale

The Resource-Based Relative Value Scale (RBRVS) is the prospective payment system used for physician reimbursement. This would only be used by hospitals if the physician is an employee of the hospital. For more on RBRVS, refer to Chapters 6 and 13.

Long-Term Care Hospital Prospective Payment System

Long-Term Care Hospital Prospective Payment System (LTCH PPS) is the prospective reimbursement system used by long-term care hospitals. To qualify as a long-term care hospital, the average length of stay must be at least 25 days. These hospitals provide services to patient who no longer need acute care but whose level of care needed is still significant. The LTCH PPS includes a subset of the same MS-DRGs used in the IPPS program. The MS-DRGs used are the ones that might require extended hospitalization, such as those where the patient is on mechanical ventilation. The relative weight of the LTCH DRGs is higher to accommodate the longer average length of stay.

The LTCH DRG can be reduced in certain circumstances; some of these are as follows (CMS, 2016c):

- Short stay outlier: When a patient is discharged before staying 5/6 of the length of stay given to each LTCH DRG, reimbursement is reduced.
- High cost outlier: As discussed under the IPPS.

APC	Status Indicator	Reimbursed at
1	T	This APC example is subject to discounting so the hospital would receive either 100% or 50% depending on whether APC 1 or APC 4 is reimbursed at a higher rate. The higher APC rate is reimbursed at 100% and the lower reimbursement APC is reimbursed at 50%.
2	S	100% as S payment indicators are not subject to discounting
3	J1	100% as J1 payment indicators are not subject to discounting
4	T	This APC example is subject to discounting so the hospital would receive either 100% or 50% depending on whether APC 1 or APC 4 is reimbursed at a higher rate. The higher APC rate is reimbursed at 100% and the lower reimbursement APC is reimbursed at 50%.

Fig. 19.5 Example of discounting. Discounting is applied when the patient goes to surgery and has three procedures performed at the same time. *APC,* Ambulatory payment classification.

- Interrupted stay: This occurs if a patient leaves the LTCH and is then readmitted. This may be for continued care not provided by the LTCH or to go home. If the interruption is 3 days or less and the patient received care elsewhere, the LTCH is responsible for reimbursement of the other health care provider. If the interruption is more than 3 days and the patient was discharged to an acute care hospital, rehabilitation hospital, or skilled nursing facility and returns to the same LTCH, the LTCH hospitalization may be considered one hospitalization. This is based on fixed-day periods. The acute care hospital, rehabilitation hospital, and skilled nursing facility, including swing beds, are each assigned a range of days, known as fixed-day periods, that qualifies the LTCH for the greater than 3-day interruption. For example, if a patient is admitted to the acute care hospital between 4 and 9 days and then returns to the original LTCH during that period, it is considered to be the original LTCH hospitalization. A **swing bed** is a bed in an acute care hospital that can be used for acute care or for a skilled nursing facility.

Inpatient Rehabilitation Facility Prospective Payment System

The **Inpatient Rehabilitation Facility Prospective Payment System (IRF PPS)** is the reimbursement system used for rehabilitation hospitals. To qualify for this reimbursement system, 60% of the hospital's inpatients must be treated for one of 13 conditions. These conditions are (CMS, 2017c, 3-4):

- Stroke
- Spinal cord injury
- Congenital anomaly
- Amputation of limb
- Multiple trauma
- Fracture of femur
- Injury to the brain
- Specified neurologic disorders (for example, Parkinson disease)
- Burns
- Specific arthropathies causing difficulty with activities of daily living
- Systemic vasculitides with inflammation of the joints causing difficulty with activities of daily living
- Osteoarthritis (severe)
- Knee and/or hip replacement (procedure must be bilateral, patient obese, or patient 85 years of age or older)

The discharge is grouped into a **rehabilitation impairment category (RIC)** based on the patient's primary diagnosis or condition. Under each RIC are **case mix groups (CMGs).** The discharge will be assigned to one of these CMGs. CMGs are based on the patient's functional motor and cognitive (mental) scores as well as their age and comorbidities. These functional motor and cognitive skills are evaluated by the **Inpatient Rehabilitation Facility Patient Assessment Instrument (IRF PAI).** The CMGs is broken into four tiers based on the patient's comorbidities. The higher the tier, the higher the reimbursement (CMS, 2017c).

The CMG payment may be adjusted because of interrupted stays, short stays (defined as less than 3 days), transfer to another facility, and cost outliers. CMG payments are also affected by characteristics of the inpatient rehabilitation facilities: wage index, rural/urban, proportion of indigent patients, and teaching hospitals (CMS, 2017c).

Each year, Medicare sets a national base rate. This base rate is adjusted for local wages and nonlabor expenses. This rate is multiplied by the CMG weight. There may be adjustments as a result of location, number of indigent patients, and whether or not the facility is a teaching facility (CMS, 2017c).

Psychiatric Prospective Payment System

The **Inpatient Psychiatric Facility Prospective Payment System** (IPF PPS) is the reimbursement system used for psychiatric hospitals and acute care hospitals' psychiatric units, which are exempt from the MS-DRG system. The physician must certify that the patient's condition justifies the need for inpatient hospitalization. A recertification of the patient's need for hospitalization is performed at day 12 and at least every 30 days thereafter. If the patient's condition changes significantly between recertifications, a recertification would be needed when that significant change occurs. The IPF PPS is based on a **per diem** rate. *Per diem* means that they are paid a specific rate for each day that the patient is hospitalized. This base rate, a dollar amount, is established each year by CMS. There are other factors that influence reimbursement, including the following (CMS, 2017d):

- DRG
- Age
- Length of stay
- Emergency department
- Number of electroconvulsive shock treatments

In addition to these factors, the payment is adjusted based on the wage index for the area of the hospital, whether or not the facility is a teaching hospital, and additional funds if the facility is a rural hospital. For an illustration of the structure of the IPF PPS payment, refer to Fig. 19.6.

Ambulance Fee Schedule

The **Ambulance Fee Schedule** is the reimbursement system used by Medicare to reimburse for ambulance services. Not all ambulances are owned by hospitals, but some are. To pay for ambulance transport, the services must meet the following criteria (CMS, 2017e):

- Medically necessary
- Local destination
- Patient covered by Medicare
- Appropriate health care facility

The payment is a base rate plus mileage to the closest appropriate facility. This fee schedule includes both ground ambulance transport and air ambulance. Air ambulance is only covered in critical circumstances such as multiple trauma or when the patient requires specialized services not provided at all hospitals (CMS, 2017e).

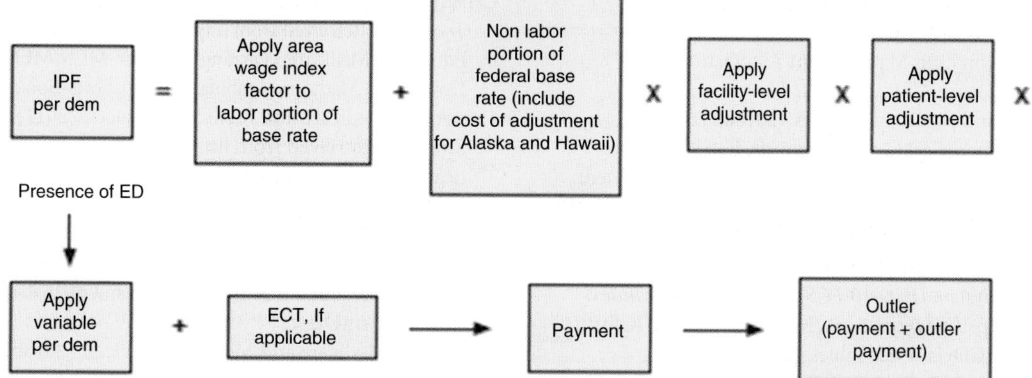

Fig. 19.6 Payment rates under the Inpatient Psychiatric Facility Prospective Payment System (IPF PPS). *ECT,* electroconvulsive therapy; *ED,* emergency department. (From Centers for Medicare and Medicaid Services. (2016d). *Inpatient Psychiatric Facility Prospective Payment System: Payment System Series.* Retrieved from https://www.cms.gov/Outreach-and-Education/Medicare-Learning-Network-MLN/MLNProducts/Downloads/Inpatient-Psychiatric-Facility-Prospective-Payment-System.pdf.)

KEY POINTS

This is a brief chapter review, or summary, of the key issues presented. To further enhance your knowledge of the technical subject matter, review the key terms and key abbreviations for this chapter by locating the meaning for each in the Glossary at the end of this book, which appears in a section before the index.

1. Medicare reimbursement systems are paid based on prospective payment systems.
2. The Discharge Not Final Billed is used to monitor unbilled claims.
3. Utilization managements ensure the medical necessity and appropriateness of service.
4. The Acute Inpatient Prospective Payment System is the prospective payment system used for reimbursement of Medicare inpatient services based on the Medicare Severity Diagnosis-Related Group.
5. The Outpatient Prospective Payment System is the Medicare reimbursement system used for hospital outpatient services.
6. The Long-Term Care Hospital Prospective Payment System is the Medicare reimbursement system used for long-term acute care hospital services.
7. The Inpatient Rehabilitation Facility Prospective Payment System is the reimbursement system used for inpatient services at a rehabilitation hospital.
8. The Psychiatric Prospective Payment System is the reimbursement system used for inpatient services at a psychiatric hospital.
9. The Ambulance Fee Schedule is the reimbursement system used for both ground and air ambulances.

STUDENT ASSIGNMENT

- Study Chapter 19.
- Answer the fill-in-the-blank, multiple-choice, and true/false review questions in the *Workbook* to reinforce the theory learned in this chapter and to help you prepare for a future test.
- Complete the assignments in the *Workbook.*
- Turn to the Glossary at the end of this text for a further understanding of the key terms and key abbreviations used in this chapter.

REFERENCES

American Health Information Management Association. (2017). *AHIMA Pocket Glossary*. Chicago: AHIMA Press.

Centers for Medicare and Medicaid Services. (2018a). *2018 NPRM OPPS Revenue Code-to-Cost Center Crosswalk*. Retrieved from https://www.cms.gov/apps/ama/license.asp?file=/Medicare/Medicare-Fee-for-Service-Payment/HospitalOutpatientPPS/Downloads/CMS-1678-P-OPPS-Revenue-Code-to-Cost-Center-Crosswalk.zip.

Centers for Medicare and Medicaid Services. (2018b). *ICD-10 Procedure Coding System (ICD-10-PCS) 2018 Tables and Index*. Retrieved from https://www.cms.gov/Medicare/Coding/ICD10/Downloads/2018-ICD-10-PCS-Tables-And-Index.zip.

Centers for Medicare and Medicaid Services. (2018c). *Care Severity Diagnosis-Related Groups (MS-DRGs), Relative Weighting, Metric and Arithmetic Mean Length of State—FY 2018 Correction Notice. Retrieved from* https://www.cms.gov/Medicare/Medicare-Fee-for-Service-Payment/AcuteInpatientPPS/Downloads/FY2018-CMS-1677-FR-Table-5.zip.

Centers for Medicare and Medicaid Services. (2017a). *Transactions Overview.* Retrieved from. https://www.cms.gov/Regulations-and-Guidance/Administrative-Simplification/Transactions/Transactions Overview.html.

Centers for Medicare and Medicaid Services. (2017b). *Hospital-Acquired Conditions and Present on Admission Indicator Reporting Provision.*

Centers for Medicare and Medicaid Services. (2017c). *Inpatient Rehabilitation Facility Prospective Payment System: Payment System Series.* Retrieved from https://www.cms.gov/Outreach-and-Education/Medicare-Learning-Network-MLN/MLNProducts/Downloads/wPOA-Fact-Sheet.pdf.

Centers for Medicare and Medicaid Services. (2017d). *Inpatient Psychiatric Facility Prospective Payment System PC PRICER.* Retrieved from https://www.cms.gov/Medicare/Medicare-Fee-for-Service-Payment/PCPricer/inppsy.html.

Centers for Medicare and Medicaid Services. (2017e). *Medicare Ambulance Transports.* Retrieved from https://www.cms.gov/Outreach-and-Education/Medicare-Learning-Network-MLN/MLNProducts/Downloads/Medicare-Ambulance-Transports-Booklet-ICN903194.pdf.

Centers for Medicare and Medicaid Services. (2017). *Ambulance Fee Schedule.* Retrieved from https://www.cms.gov/Outreach-and-Education/Medicare-Learning-Network-MLN/MLNProducts/Downloads/AmbulanceFeeSched_508.pdf.

Centers for Medicare and Medicaid Services. (2016a). *Quality Improvement Organizations.* Retrieved from. https://www.cms.gov/Medicare/Quality-Initiatives-Patient-Assessment-Instruments/Quality-ImprovementOrgs/.

Centers for Medicare and Medicaid Services. (2016b). *Acute Care Hospital Inpatient Prospective Payment System.* Retrieved from https://www.cms.gov/Outreach-and-Education/Medicare-Learning-Network-MLN/MLNProducts/downloads/AcutePaymtSysfctsht.pdf.

Centers for Medicare and Medicaid Services. (2016c). *Long Term Care Hospital Prospective Payment System.* Retrieved from https://www.cms.gov/Outreach-and-Education/Medicare-Learning-Network-MLN/MLNProducts/Downloads/Long-Term-Care-Hospital-PPS-Fact-Sheet-ICN006956.pdf.

Centers for Medicare and Medicaid Services. (2016d). *Inpatient Psychiatric Facility Prospective Payment System: Payment System Series.* Retrieved from. https://www.cms.gov/Outreach-and-Education/Medicare-Learning-Network-MLN/MLNProducts/Downloads/Inpatient-Psychiatric-Facility-Prospective-Payment-System.pdf.

Centers for Medicare and Medicaid Services. (n.d.). *FY 2013, FY 2014, and FY 2015 Final HAC List (no changes have been made).* Retrieved from https://www.cms.gov/Medicare/Medicare-Fee-for-Service-Payment/HospitalAcqCond/Downloads/FY_2013_Final_HACsCodeList.pdf.

Quality Improvement Organizations. (n.d.). *10th to 11th Scope of Work (SoW): The New QIO Program.* Retrieved from http://qioprogram.org/sites/default/files/ProviderCallSlides_FINAL_7-25-14.pdf.

UNIT 7

Employment

20

Seeking a Job and Attaining Professional Advancement

Linda M. Smith

OBJECTIVES

After reading this chapter, you should be able to:

1. Prepare to find a position as an insurance billing specialist, claims assistance professional, or electronic claims processor.
2. State types of certifications available to insurance billers and coders.
3. State and discuss various actions to take to search for a job.
4. Search online for employment opportunities and discuss job fairs.
5. List guidelines for completing job application form.
6. Compose a letter of introduction to accompany the résumé.
7. Analyze education and experience to prepare a traditional or electronic résumé.
8. Prepare responses to common interview questions.
9. Identify illegal interview questions.
10. Name the items to assemble for a job portfolio and discuss follow-up letters.
11. Explore the business aspects of self-employment.

KEY TERMS

application form
auditor
blind mailing
business associate agreement
certification
Certified Coding Specialist
Certified Coding Specialist–Physician
Certified Medical Assistant
Certified Medical Billing Specialist
Certified Professional Coder
chargemaster coordinator
chronologic résumé
clinical documentation improvement specialist
coding specialist
combination résumé
compliance specialist
continuing education
cover letter
employment agencies
functional résumé
interview
mentor
National Certified Insurance and Coding Specialist
networking
portfolio
Registered Medical Assistant
Registered Medical Coder
résumé
Revenue Cycle Manager
self-employment
service contract

KEY ABBREVIATIONS

AAPC
AHIMA
CAP
CCAP
CCS
CCS-P
CECP
CMA
CMBS
CMRS
CPC
CPC-A
CPC-H
ECP
EEOC
FCS
HRS
NCICS
PAHCOM
RMA
RMC
USCIS

EMPLOYMENT OPPORTUNITIES

Insurance Billing Specialist

Employment opportunities are available throughout the United States for insurance billing specialists who attain coding skills, knowledge of insurance programs, and expertise in completing insurance claims accurately.

Because of the complexities of billing for health care services, there is a corresponding increase in the need for insurance billing specialists. Health care organizations are looking for individuals who have knowledge of state and federal laws associated with the billing process, a solid understanding of Health Insurance Portability and Accountability Act (HIPAA) laws, and a solid foundation in fraud and abuse controls. They are also looking for individuals who have knowledge of the primary insurances that are routinely billed by health care organizations, such as Medicare, Medicaid, workers' compensation, and third-party payers. They are looking for insurance billing specialists who understand coding, the claims submission process, the reimbursement process, and revenue cycle management (Fig. 20.1).

The complexities of billing for health care services has also resulted in a wide range of career titles the individual may see advertised as positions available. Some of these job titles will be broad and cover the entire billing process, whereas others may be very specific and focused on a narrow set of job skills. Some of the job titles may be listed as follows:

- Electronic claims processor (ECP)
- Medicare or Medicaid billing specialist
- Workers' compensation specialist
- Reimbursement specialist
- Collection specialist
- Claims examiner
- Claims assistance professional (CAP)

Advanced Job Opportunities

As the insurance billing specialist gains experience and additional knowledge, there may be employment opportunities in more advanced roles. More advanced job opportunities might include the following positions.

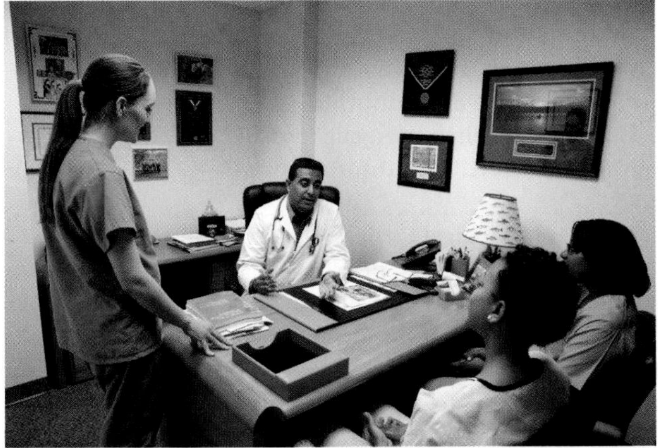

Fig. 20.1 Staff conference discussing applicants for potential interviews.

Coding specialist. Coding specialists are responsible for assigning the diagnosis and procedure codes that are included on the insurance claim. To assign the code, the medical coder must understand the health record, anatomy, diseases and conditions, procedures, pharmacology, medical terminology, and more. The coder must be able to identify key information in the health record and assign the code based on the official coding guidelines and other resources.

The coder has a tremendous amount of responsibility because the health care organization's reimbursement is usually based on the diagnosis and procedure codes. Coding errors can cost the health care organization hundreds if not thousands of dollars and possibly result in accusations of fraud and abuse. As a result, coders are expected to code with a 95% to 98% accuracy rate. Because of the importance of coding, coders are constantly learning about changes in the coding system, changes in procedures, and more.

Coders typically must earn a certificate in coding or an associate degree in health information management. Prospective students seeking a certificate in medical coding should look for a coding program that has been recognized as a Professional Certificate Approval Program. The two most widely known associations that award these certifications are the American Health Information Management Association (AHIMA) and the American Academy of Professional Coders (AAPC).

Clinical documentation improvement (CDI) specialist. The clinical documentation improvement specialist works with physicians and other health care professionals to ensure that the documentation in the health record is complete and granular (at the appropriate level of detail). The clinical documentation improvement (CDI) specialist must understand medical coding health care documentation, diseases, coding systems, and so forth just as the coders do. Clinical documentation improvement is the process an organization undertakes to improve clinical specificity and documentation that will allow coding professionals to assign more concise disease classification codes.

Some of the ways that the CDI specialist improves clinical documentation include offering educational programs to physicians and other health care providers, writing articles for newsletters, and writing queries. The intent of CDI programs is to improve the quality of documentation available to the coders. For example, the physician may write that the patient has pneumonia but does not provide the organism causing the pneumonia. In this case the coder must assign the generic pneumonia code when a more specific diagnosis code could be used if the organism was specified. Another example is a fracture of the tibia. This diagnostic statement does not provide the coder with information regarding which portion of the tibia is fractured, nor does it document laterality (right or left). Without detailed information, the specific code cannot be assigned, so a nonspecific code must be used. Coding quality issues that result from incomplete documentation may result in poor decisions because the data being used are not specific. Both AHIMA and the AAPC offer certifications related to clinical documentation improvement.

Chargemaster coordinator. The chargemaster coordinator oversees managing the contents of the chargemaster, including updating codes, adding new services, deleted services no longer provided, and updating charges. The chargemaster lists all the services provided by the health care facility and the amount charged for the service. It also includes the codes. The chargemaster coordinator must work with the clinical services, billers, financial department, and others to ensure the entries in the chargemaster meets their needs. Failure to maintain the chargemaster will result in overpayments for services, underpayments for services, submitting claims with invalid codes, and many other problems. This position in critical to the revenue cycle as data in the chargemaster is used in the creation of health care claims.

Revenue cycle manager. Revenue cycle managers are responsible for overseeing billing accounts and helping departments resolve their revenue cycle problems. They oversee the billing teams that manage accounts, communication with insurance companies, collections, contract analysis, cash posting, billing transactions with clients, and report creation. Revenue cycle managers help ensure that these areas run smoothly, and they must detect problems in the billing systems and correct them accordingly.

A revenue cycle manager must be an innovative person because new solutions and automation in various billing areas must be created by a revenue cycle manager. The revenue cycle manager usually implements a system to ensure that billing communication to and from the customer reaches the billing system smoothly. When there are problems with billing related to patients or insurance, a revenue cycle manager must develop a solution. The revenue cycle manager may work in a medical facility or office setting but also may move around the facility to communicate with various departments.

Auditor. Auditors monitor revenue cycle activities. The title varies according to what they are monitoring. Examples include diagnosis-related group (DRG) auditor and revenue cycle auditor. Auditors may be responsible for ongoing auditing of health care claims, documentation, and other components of the revenue cycle. The auditor must have an overall understanding of the functions of the revenue cycle so that issues can be found. This includes understanding coding, documentation, revenue cycle, auditing, statistical analysis, federal and state laws, and more. The purpose of the audits is to identify and correct issues in the revenue cycle process before the Center for Medicare and Medicaid Services investigate the health care organization for fraud and abuse practices. Auditors ensure that policies and procedures are being followed. They also monitor the quality of billing, coding, and other revenue cycle steps to ensure the steps are being performed accurately. The auditor generates statistical reports that are then shared with management. These reports show number of audits, error rates, types of errors, who is making the errors, and more.

Compliance specialist. Compliance specialists are responsible for the development and management of the health care organization's compliance program. These individuals assist in development of policies and procedures, audit programs, ensure programs are being followed, and identify issues and the corrective actions to be taken. The individual in this role must understand the compliance program, federal and state laws, data analysis, management of people, problem resolution, and much more.

PROFESSIONAL ORGANIZATIONS

Membership in professional organizations is a networking opportunity that will surround you with others in your field and will help you in keeping up to date with current trends. They offer continuing education opportunities through various types of publications, webinars, and conferences (local, regional, and national). Professional organizations can also assist with problem solving, provide reliable resources, and may direct you to employment opportunities. Most of these associations have student, as well as active and associate, membership categories. In general, there are local chapters or state organizations affiliated with the national association. In addition to the professional organizations listed in Table 20.1, the Medical Association of Billers (MAB), the Healthcare Billing and Management Association (HMBA), AHIMA, and AAPC are some of the most popular professional organizations that insurance billing specialists affiliate with.

Certification

An additional benefit to belonging to a professional organization is the opportunity to become certified. Certification is a process of earning a credential through a combination of advanced education and experience. Upon satisfactory completion of the requirements of the board or association, they will issue a certification statement verifying that a person meets the professional standards of that organization (see Table 20.1). Professional certifications identify the experts in the field and can contribute to career advancement. Some of the certifications that the insurance billing specialist may want to explore include the following:

- Certified Medical Billing Specialist (CMBS)
- Certified Medical Reimbursement Specialist (CMRS)
- Certified Professional Coder (CPC)
- Certified Professional Coder–Apprentice (CPC-A)
- Certified Professional Coder–Hospital (CPC-H)
- Certified Coding Specialist (CCS)
- Certified Coding Specialist–Physician (CCS-P)
- Certified Electronic Claims Processor (CECP)
- Certified Claims Assistance Professional (CCAP)
- Facility Coding Specialist (FCS)
- Health Care Reimbursement Specialist (HRS)
- National Certified Insurance and Coding Specialist (NCICS)
- Registered Medical Coder (RMC)

Becoming certified is an essential goal if one seeks career advancement. Credentials validate individuals' knowledge and expertise in the field and show their commitment in following the standards and code of ethics set by the professional organization they belong to. Credentials help insurance billing specialists to advance their career, help health care organizations to effectively manage their revenue cycle, ensure compliance, and prepare for the future changes in health care.

TABLE 20.1 Certifications

Certification Title (Abbreviation)	Description to Obtain Certification or Registration	Professional Association Mailing Address	Telephone Number	Website	E-Mail Address
• Advanced Coding Specialist (ACS) • Specialty Coding Professional (SCP) • Certified Compliance Professional–Physician (CCP-P)	2 to 3 years of experience and working knowledge of coding in the specialty	Board of Medical Specialty Coding 9737 Washington Blvd. Suite 200 Gaithersburg, MD 20878	(800) 897-4509	www.medicalspecialtycoding.com	info@medicalspecialtycoding.com
• Certified Billing and Coding Specialist (CBCS) • Certified Electronic Health Records Specialist (CEHRS)	Graduate of health care training program or 1 or more year(s) of full-time job experience; exam or home study certification program	National Healthcare Association 11161 Overbrook Rd. Leawood, KS 66211	(800) 499-9092	www.nhanow.com	info@nhanow.com
• Certified Bookkeeper (CB)	Self-study program and employment experience; pass three tests	American Institute of Professional Bookkeepers 6001 Montrose Rd. Suite 500 Rockville, MD 20852	(800) 622-0121	www.aipb.org	info@aipb.org
• Certified Coding Associate (CCA) • Certified Coding Specialist (CCS) • Certified Coding Specialist–Physician (CCS-P) • Certified in Healthcare Privacy and Security (CHPS)	Self-study program; pass certification examination	American Health Information Management Association (AHIMA) 233 N. Michigan Ave. 21st Floor Chicago, IL 60601-5809	(800) 335-5535	www.ahima.org	info@ahima.org
• Certified Cardiology Coding Specialist (CCCS) • Certified ENT Coding Specialist (CENTCS) • Certified Family Practice Coding Specialist (CFPCS) • Certified Gastroenterology Coding Specialist (CGCS) • Certified General Surgery Coding Specialist (CGSCS) • Certified Internal Medicine Coding Specialist (CIMCS) • Certified Nephrology Coding Specialist (CNCS) • Certified OB/GYN Coding Specialist (COBGCS) • Certified Orthopedics Coding Specialist (COCS) • Certified Pediatrics Coding Specialist (CPEDCS) • Certified Podiatry Coding Specialist (CPODCS) • Certified Pulmonary Medicine Coding Specialist (CPMCS) • Certified Urology Coding Specialist (CUCS) • Certified Multi-Specialty Coding Specialist (CMSCS)	Active member of Professional Association of Healthcare Coding Specialists, employed as a coder with 2 years' experience, 6 college credit course hours in coding	Professional Association of Healthcare Coding Specialists (PAHCS) 218 E. Bearss Ave. #354 Tampa, FL 33613	(888) 708-4707	www.pahcs.org	info@pahcs.org
• Certified Specialist Accounting and Finance (CSAF)	2 or more years in health care	Healthcare Financial Management Association (HFMA) 3 Westbrook Corporate Center Suite 600 Westchester, IL 60154-5700	(800) 252-4362	www.hfma.org	webmaster@Financial-Professionalhfma.com

Continued

TABLE 20.1 Certifications—cont'd

Certification Title (Abbreviation)	Description to Obtain Certification or Registration	Professional Association Mailing Address	Telephone Number	Website	E-Mail Address
Claims assistant professional (CAP)	No formal certification process	Alliance of Claims Assistance Professionals (ACAP) 9600 Escarpment Suite 745-65 Austin, TX 78749	(888) 394-5163	www.claims.org	capinfo@claims.org
Certified Healthcare Billing and Management Executive (CHBME)	Complete comprehensive program; pass proficiency test	Healthcare Billing and Management Association (HMBA) 2025 M St. NW Suite 800 Washington, D.C. 20036	(877) 640-4262	www.hbma.com	info@hbma.com
Certified in Healthcare Compliance (CHC)	Have work experience and continuing education credits and pass examination	Health Care Compliance Association 6500 Barrie Rd. Suite 250 Minneapolis, MN 55435	(888) 580-8373 (952) 405-7900	www.hcca-info.org	info@hcca-info.org
Certified Health Data Analyst (CHDA)	Eligibility requirements and pass examination; pass CHPS examinations	American Health Information Management Association (AHIMA) 233 N. Michigan Ave. 21st Floor Chicago, IL 60601-5809	(800) 335-5535	www.ahima.org	info@ahima.com
• Certified Information Systems Security Professional (CISSP) • Systems Security Certified Practitioner (SSCP)	Pass examination and submit endorsement form	International Information Systems America 1625 Prince St. Suite 230 Alexandria, VA 22314	(866) 462-4777	www.isc2.org	isc2@asestores.com
Certified Medical Assistant (CMA)	Graduate from accredited medical assisting program; apply to take national certifying examination	American Association of Medical Assistants (AAMA) 20 North Wacker Dr. Suite 1575 Chicago, IL 60606	(800) 228-2262	www.aama-ntl.org	Visit website
Certified Medical Billing Specialist (CMBS)	Complete 6 courses and provide evaluation of billing performance by supervisor	Medical Association of Billers (MAB) 2620 Regatta Dr. Suite 102 Las Vegas, NV 89128	(702) 240-8519	www.physician-swebsites.com	medassocb@aol.com
Certified Medical Manager (CMM)	Examination for supervisors or managers of small-group and solo practices	Professional Association of Health Care Office Management (**PAHCOM**) 1576 Bella Cruz Dr. Suite 360 Lady Lake, FL 32159	(800) 451-9311	www.pahcom.com	pahcom@pahcom.com

• Certified Medical Practice Executive (CMPE) • Nominee first level • Certification second level • Fellow third level	• First level—Eligible group managers join; membership/nominee • Second level—Complete 6- to 7-hour examination • Third level—Mentoring project of thesis	Medical Group Management Association (MGMA), American College of Medical Practice Executives (affiliate) 104 Inverness Terrace East Englewood, CO 80112-5306	(877) 275-6462	www.mgma.com	acmpe@mgma.com
• Certified Medical Coder (CMC) • Certified Medical Insurance Specialist (CMIS) • Certified Medical Compliance Officer (CMCO)	Self-study program and successfully pass exam	Practice Management Institute 8242 Vicar Dr. San Antonio, TX 78218	(800) 259-5562	www.pmimd.com	info@pmimd.com
Certified Medical Reimbursement Specialist (CMRS)	Self-study program; successfully pass 18 sections of examination	American Medical Billing Association (AMBA) 2465 E. Main Davis, OK 73030	(580) 369-2700	www.ambanet.net/cmrs.htm	larry@brightok.net
Registered Healthcare Documentation Specialist (RHDS) Certified Healthcare Documentation Specialist (CHDS)	Self-study program and successfully pass written and practical examinations offered by Medical Transcription Certification Commission (MTCC)	Association for Healthcare Documentation Integrity (AHDI) 4120 Dale Rd. Suite J8-233 Modesto, CA 95356	(800) 982-2182	www.ahdionline.org	ahdi@ahdionline.org
• Certified Revenue Cycle Executive (CRCE) • Certified Revenue Cycle Professional (CCRCP) • Certified Revenue Integrity Professional (CRIP) • Certified Revenue Cycle Specialist (CRCS) • Certified Compliance Technician (CCT)	Complete self-study course; pass standard examination administered twice yearly	American Association of Healthcare Administrative Management (AAHAM) National Certification Examination Program 11240 Waples Mill Rd. Suite 200 Fairfax, VA 22030	(703) 281-4043	www.aaham.org	moayad@aaham.org
• Certified Professional Coder (CPC) • Certified Outpatient Coder • Certified Inpatient Coder • Certified Professional Biller	Independent study program; pass examination approximately 5 hours (CPC) and 8 hours (CPC-H) in length	American Academy of Professional Coders (AAPC) 2233 South Presidents Dr. Suite F Salt Lake City, UT 84120	(800) 626-2633	www.aapc.com	info@aapc.com

Continued

TABLE 20.1 Certifications—cont'd

Certification Title (Abbreviation)	Description to Obtain Certification or Registration	Professional Association Mailing Address	Telephone Number	Website	E-Mail Address
Certified Healthcare Reimbursement Specialist (CHRS) Certified HIPAA Information Specialist (CHIS)	Successfully complete open-book examination	National Electronic Billers Alliance (NEBA) 2226-A Westborough Blvd. #504 South San Francisco, CA 94080	(650) 359-4419	www.nebazone.com	mmedical@aol.com
National Certified Insurance and Coding Specialist (NCICS)	Graduate from an insurance program; sit for certification examination given by independent testing agency at many school sites across the nation	National Center for Competency Testing 7007 College Blvd. Suite 385 Overland Park, KS 66211	(800) 875-4404	www.ncctinc.com	staff@ncctinc.com
Registered Medical Assistant (RMA)	Sit for certification exam	American Medical Technologists (AMT) 10700 West Higgins Rd. Suite 150 Rosemont, IL 60018	(800) 275-1268	www.americanmedtech.org	amtmail@aol.com
Utilization Review Accreditation Commission (URAC) Accredited Consultant	Application	Utilization Review Accreditation Commission (URAC) 1220 L St. NW Suite 400 Washington, DC 20005	(202) 216-9010	www.urac.org	ita@urac.org
Compliance Certification Board (CCB)	Examination, work experience, and continuing education	Health Care Compliance Association 6500 Barrie Rd. Suite 250 Minneapolis, MN 55435	(888) 580-8373	www.hcca-info.org	info@hcca-info.org
	Pass examination and submit endorsement form	ISC Americas 311 Park Place Blvd. Suite 400 Clearwater, FL 33759	(866) 462-4777	www.isc2.org	isc2@asestores.com

Certified members to professional organizations must keep up-to-date by continuing to take educational sessions and earning **continuing education** credits to maintain their certification credential. Continuing education is intended to improve or maintain professional competence.

JOB SEARCH

In addition to the skills necessary for performance on the job, ask yourself the following questions to determine whether you need to sharpen your job-seeking techniques:

- Are you motivated and interested in finding a job?
- Can you communicate effectively in an interview?
- Do you enjoy good health?
- Are you mature?
- Do you have good grooming and manners?

You can seek employment in several ways. You may wish to be employed by a physician, hospital, medical facility, insurance company, or managed care organization (MCO). You may choose to be self-employed if you have had a number of years of experience, or you may even choose some type of combination situation. The following lists suggested actions to take to search for a job:

1. Explore the internet using a smartphone, tablet, or computer. Visit websites of professional billing and coding organizations. Make it easy to be found, such as being on LinkedIn, ExecuNet, or other professional networking sites. Upload your résumé to as many databases as possible. Search names of professional offices and hospitals near your location to contact.
2. Join a professional organization, to network with others in the same career field and to hear about job openings (Fig. 20.2). Put a notice about your availability in the chapter newsletter.
3. Attend meetings and workshops in this career field to keep up to date and network with others.
4. Contact the school placement personnel, complete the necessary paperwork, and leave a résumé on file if you have just completed a course at a community college or trade school.
5. Spread the word to those who work in medical settings and those who might hear of openings in medical facilities, such as classmates, instructors, school counselors, relatives, and friends. If you are introducing yourself to a hiring manager identified via a professional colleague, type the colleague's name in the e-mail subject line (for example, "John Doe referred me") so that the manager is less likely to delete your e-mail.
6. Contact pharmaceutical representatives who visit physicians' offices and hospitals for employment information or leads.
7. Visit public and private **employment agencies,** including temporary and temporary-to-permanent agencies. Before signing with an agency, ask whether the employer or applicant pays the agency fee.
8. Inquire at state and federal government offices and their employment agencies.

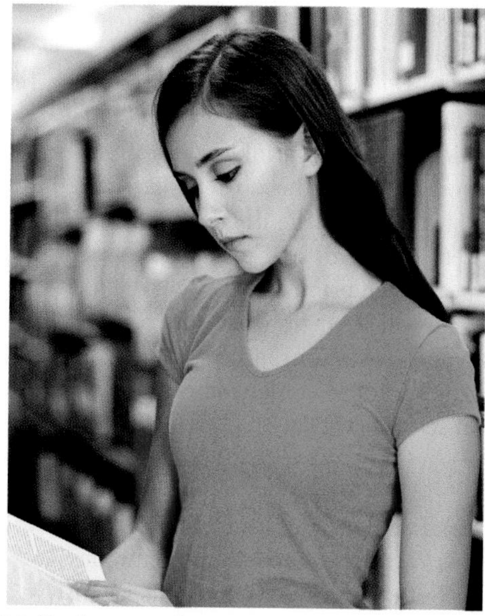

Fig. 20.2 Student scanning a professional journal for job leads.

9. Look for part-time employment that might lead to a permanent full-time position.
10. Check bulletin boards in personnel offices of hospitals and clinics frequently for posted job offerings.
11. Go to your local medical society to determine whether it has a provision for supplying job leads.
12. Send a blind mailing of the résumé, including a cover letter, to possible prospects. A **blind mailing** means to send information to employers whom you do not know personally and who have not advertised for a job opening.
13. Visit your city's chamber of commerce and ask for some of their publications that contain membership directories and names of major professional employers in specific areas.
14. Subscribe to an online principal newspaper of the city where employment is desired. Read help wanted advertisements in the classified section, especially in the Sunday newspaper. Do not be discouraged by specific requirements in an advertisement; apply anyway. Send or transmit an e-mail with your résumé and a cover letter the next day. Some employers give priority to candidates who respond within the first 3 or 4 days after a job announcement because they believe it is an indication that someone is truly interested in the position.
15. E-mail or telephone job hotlines of large medical clinics in your area.
16. Visit job locations unannounced (referred to as "cold calling").

Online Job Search

Because of the internet, newspaper and magazine classified advertisements may become resources of the past. An individual with internet access through a mobile device, tablet, or computer can locate potential employers who are offering jobs to health care workers at their websites. In general, you can find detailed descriptions of positions that are available, and you can respond to a specific job of interest by completing an online application or delivering an online résumé. Employers may use automated résumé scanning to sort e-mailed résumés for key words. Use standard typefaces and font sizes between 10 to 14 points. Keep text lines under 65 characters and use boldface for section headings. You must have a 95% to 100% key word match for the position; therefore sprinkle your résumé and cover letter with the verbiage used in the job advertisement. Key words can be entered at the end of the document. To make them unnoticeable, select the words and make the font color white; they will not appear when printed or viewed on the monitor, but the electronic scan will see them when sorting.

If you do not have internet access, your school may allow you to use the campus internet Many libraries have computers with free internet service (Fig. 20.3).

Internet

Helpful websites are www.jobsearch.about.com and www.indeed.com.com/jobs, which feature résumé templates and examples. Check out websites such as www.ziprecruiter.com, www.glassdoor.com, www.careerbuilder.com, and www.monster.com, which list job postings that you can browse according to field, location, and career type. Many of these sites also allow job seekers to post their résumés at no cost.

Job Fairs

Annual community events feature job fairs at community colleges and technical trade schools. Some job fairs are sponsored by professional associations. Job recruiters set up booths with information about their companies and available positions; however, they do not have much time to spend with each job seeker. Thus it is wise to go prepared and practice a 30-second introduction before attending. This introduction should consist of a quick overview of your career goals, experience, skills, training, education, and personal strengths. Be sure to explain what you can offer the employer. These are usually daylong events, and you may want to investigate several participating employers' booths.

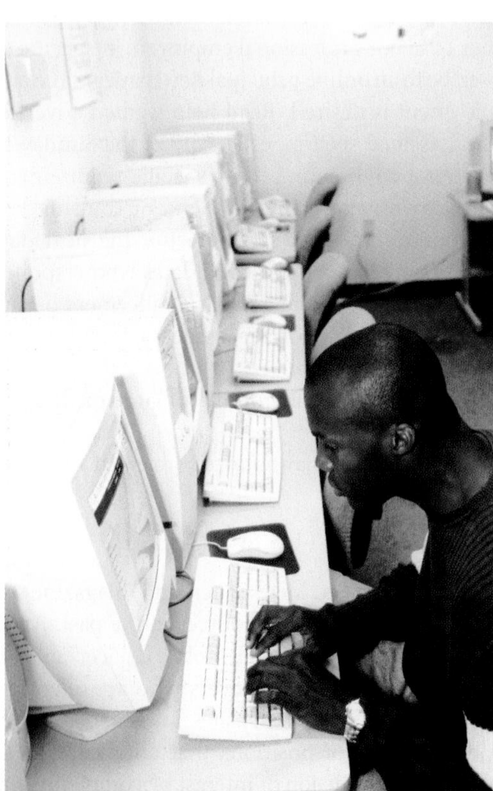

Fig. 20.3 Student doing an online job search.

Go prepared by dressing professionally and carrying a binder or folder with plenty of copies of your résumé to give to the company representatives you meet. Résumés should be neat, clean, and not folded, wrinkled, or coffee stained. Take a pen, pencil, and notepad to obtain information. Research the employers attending so that you know which ones you will visit. Keep a positive attitude and approach each employer with confidence and enthusiasm. Show the job recruiter that you are interested and knowledgeable.

Take home the business card and brochure of anyone you talk to who genuinely interests you. After the fair, send that person a follow-up letter or e-mail message to reaffirm your interest.

Application

When visiting a potential employer, ask for an **application form** to complete and inquire whether the facility keeps potential job applicants on file and for how long (Fig. 20.4). Study each question on the application form carefully before answering and follow instructions. Furnish as much information as possible; if a question does not apply or cannot be answered, insert "no," "none," "NA" (not applicable), or "DNA" (does not apply). Some application forms may request information that could be considered discriminatory. If this situation occurs, use your best judgment on whether to insert or omit an answer.

Follow these guidelines when completing an application form:

1. Read the whole application before completing; some instructions may appear on the last page or last line.
2. Read the fine print and instructions: "Please print," "Put last name first," or "Complete in your own handwriting." This indicates an ability to follow instructions.
3. Print if your handwriting is poor and abbreviate only when there is lack of space.
4. Complete the application in black ink unless pencil is specified.
5. Refer to data from a portfolio, sample application form, or résumé that has been checked for accuracy; use this information to copy onto each new application form. Be neat.
6. List correct dates of previous employment so they will be accurate if the employer seeks verification. If a question is presented asking the reason for leaving a position, insert "to be discussed during the interview."
7. Name specific skills such as procedural coding, diagnostic coding, knowledge of insurance programs, ability to complete and/or transmit the CMS-1500 (02-12) claim form, keyboarding (number of words per minute), fluency in a second language, knowledge of medical terminology, and knowledge and use of computer software.
8. When a question is asked about salary amount, write in "negotiable" or "flexible" and then discuss this during the interview.
9. Sign the application after completion.

APPLICATION FOR POSITION / Medical or Dental Office
AN EQUAL OPPORTUNITY EMPLOYER

(In answering questions, use extra blank sheet if necessary)

No employee, applicant, or candidate for promotion, training or other advantage shall be discriminated against (or given preference) because of race, color, religion, sex, age, physical handicap, veteran status, or national origin.

Date of application 7-2-20XX

PLEASE READ CAREFULLY AND WRITE OR PRINT ANSWERS TO ALL QUESTIONS. DO NOT TYPE.

A. PERSONAL INFORMATION

Name - Last: Valasquez First: Jennifer Middle: M
Home Tel. (555) 439-4800 E-mail (optional) valasquezj@gmail.com
Bus. Tel. ( ) Cell Phone (optional) 555-301-2612
Present address: Street 1234 Martin Street (Apt.#) City Woodland Hills State XY Zip 12345
Person to notify in case of emergency or accident - name: Elena Sanchez
Address: 20 South M Street Woodland Hills, XY 12345 Telephone: 555-261-0707

B. EMPLOYMENT INFORMATION

Position desired: insurance biller X Full-time Part-time Either Date available for employment: 7-6-20XX Wage/salary expectations: negotiable
List hrs./days you prefer to work: M-F 8-5 PM List any hrs./days you are not available: (Except for times required for religious practices or observances) Can you work overtime, if necessary? X Yes No
Are you employed now?: Yes X No If so, may we inquire of your present employer? No Yes, if yes: Name of employer: Phone number: ( )
Have you applied for a position with this office before? X No Yes If Yes, when?: Month and year ________ Location ________
Are you able to perform the essential functions of the job for which you are applying? .... X Yes No
If no, describe the functions that cannot be performed. ________
Have you ever been convicted of a criminal offense (felony or serious misdemeanor)? *(Convictions for marijuana-related offenses that are more than two years old need not be listed.)* Yes No
If yes, state nature of the crime(s), when and where convicted and disposition of the case. ________

(Note: We comply with the ADA and consider reasonable accommodation measures that may be necessary for eligible applicants/employees to perform essential functions. Hire may be subject to passing a medical examination, and to skill and agility tests.)

(Note: No applicant will be denied employment solely on the grounds of conviction of a criminal offense. The nature of the offense, the date of the offense, the surrounding circumstances and the relevance of the offense to the position(s) applied for may, however, be considered.)

Referred by/or where did you learn of this job? Read advertisement in newspaper
Can you, upon employment, submit verification of your legal right to work in the United States? X Yes No
Submit proof that you meet legal age requirement for employment? X Yes No
Language(s) applicant speaks or writes (if use of a language other than English is relevant to the job for which the applicant is applying: Spanish

C. EDUCATION HISTORY

	Name and address of schools attended (include current)	Number of months/ years attended	Highest grade/ level completed	Diploma/degree(s) obtained/areas of study
High school	ABC High School, Woodland Hills, XY	2000-2004	12	Diploma
College	Vocational-Tech School, Woodland Hills, XY	2005		Degree/major Certificate
Post graduate	Montana State Univ., Woodland Hills, XY	2005-2007		Degree/major 24 credits
Business/trade/technical				Course/diploma/license/ certificate
Other				Course/diploma/license/ certificate

Specific training, skills, education, or experiences which will assist you in the job for which you have applied See resume
Membership/professional or civic organizations (excluding those that disclose race, color, religion or national origin) Amer. Acad. of Professional Coders
Future educational plans Continuing education—preparing for certification in coding
Military - did you serve in the armed forces? X No Yes, if yes, branch? ________
Training relevant to position for which you are applying:

D. SPECIAL SKILLS (Check below the kinds of work you have done)

Front Office		Back Office	
X Accounts receivable	X Filing	Blood counts	Phlebotomy
Bookkeeping	X Medical terminology	Dental assistant	Urinalysis
X Collections	Medical transcription	Dental hygienist	X-ray
X Data entry	Receptionist	Injections	Other:
X Electronic/medical billing	Other:	Nursing/assisting	Other:

Other kinds of tasks performed or skills that may be applicable to position:
Office equipment/machines used: computer, calculator, printer
Keyboarding/typing speed 65 wpm
Computer programs used: Word, Excel

ORDER # 72-110 • © 1976 BIBBERO SYSTEMS, INC. • PETALUMA, CA. • (Rev. 3/03)
TO REORDER CALL TOLL FREE: (800) BIBBERO (800-242-2376) OR FAX (800) 242-9330 MFG IN U.S.A.
(PLEASE COMPLETE OTHER SIDE)

Fig. 20.4 Application for Position/Medical or Dental Office form. (Courtesy Bibiru Systems, Inc., Petaluma, Calif. Telephone: [800] 242-2376; fax: [800] 242-9330; website: www.bibbero.com.)

E. EMPLOYMENT RECORD ☐ INFORMATION SUPPLIED ON ATTACHED RÉSUMÉ

LIST MOST RECENT EMPLOYMENT FIRST (Full or Part-Time) **May we contact your previous employer(s) for a reference?** ☒Yes ☐No

1) Employer/Company name: St. John's Outpatient Clinic	Type of business: Hospital outpatient medical clinic
Address Street City State Zip code: 24 Center St. Woodland Hills, XY 12345	Worked performed. Be specific:
Phone number: (555) 782-0155	
Your position: Insurance billing specialist — Dates From Mo. 6 Yr. 07 To Mo. 6 Yr. 09	
Supervisor's name: Candice Johnson — Hourly rate/salary Starting $12/hr Final $15/hr	
Reason for leaving: Professional advancement	
2) Employer/Company name: Eastern Airlines	Type of business: Airline transportation
Address Street City State Zip code: Orlando FL	Worked performed. Be specific:
Phone number: (555) 350-7000	
Your position: Receptionist — Dates From Mo. 1 Yr. 99 To Mo. 1 Yr. 2000	
Supervisor's name: Gary Stevens — Hourly rate/salary Starting $9/hr Final $11.50/hr	
Reason for leaving: Career change	
3) Employer/Company name	Type of business:
Address Street City State Zip code	Worked performed. Be specific:
Phone number ( )	
Your position — Dates Mo. Yr. Mo. Yr. From To	
Supervisor's name — Hourly rate/salary Starting Final	
Reason for leaving	

F. REFERENCES – *List below two persons NOT related to you who have knowledge of your work performance within the last three years.*

(1) Furnished upon request
Name Address Telephone number (☐Work ☐Home) Occupation Years acquainted

(2)
Name Address Telephone number (☐Work ☐Home) Occupation Years acquainted

Please feel free to add any information which you feel will help us consider you for employment

DO NOT ANSWER ANY QUESTIONS IN THIS SECTION UNLESS THE BOXES ARE CHECKED - If the employer has checked the box next to the question, the information requested is needed for a legally permissible reason, including, without limitation, national security considerations, a legitimate occupational qualification or business necessity. The Civil Rights Act of 1964 prohibits discrimination in employment because of race, color, religion, sex or national origin. Federal law also prohibits discrimination based on age, citizenship and disability. The laws of most States also prohibit some or all of the above types of discrimination as well as some additional types such as discrimination based upon ancestry, marital status and sexual preference.

☐	Provide dates you attended school: Elementary From To; High School From To; College From To; Other (give name and dates)	☐	Number of dependents, including yourself
		☐	Are you a Vietnam veteran? ☐Yes ☐No
		☐	Sex ☐ Male ☐ Female
☐	Marital status ☐ Single ☐ Separated ☐ Engaged ☐ Divorced ☐ Married ☐ Widowed ☐ Date of marriage	☐	Are you a U.S. citizen? ☐Yes ☐No
☐	What was your previous address?	☐	How long at previous address? ______ years
☐	State names of relatives and friends working for us, other that your spouse.	☐	How long at present address? ______ years
☐	Have you ever been bonded? ☐Yes ☐No If "Yes," with what employers?	☐	Are you over 18 years of age? ☐Yes ☐No If not, employment is subject to verification of age.

READ THE FOLLOWING CAREFULLY, THEN SIGN AND DATE THE APPLICATION

The information provided in this Application for Employment is true, correct, and complete. If employed, any misstatement or omission of fact on this application may result in my dismissal. I understand that acceptance of an offer of employment does not create a contractual obligation upon the employer to continue to employ me in the future. If you decide to engage an investigative consumer reporting agency to report on my credit and personal history I authorize you to do so. If a report is obtained you must provide, at my request, the name of the agency so I may obtain from them the nature and substance of the information contained in the report.

If requested, I hereby agree to submit to binding arbitration all disputes and claims arising out of the submission of this application. I further agree, in the event that I am hired by the company, that all disputes that cannot be resolved by informal internal resolution which might arise out of my employment with the company, whether during or after that employment, will be submitted to binding arbitration. I agree that such arbitration shall be conducted under the rules of the American Arbitration Association. This application contains the entire agreement between the parties with regard to dispute resolution, and there are no other agreements as to dispute resolution, either oral or written.

Date: 7-2-20XX Signature: Jennifer M. Valasquez

Fig. 20.4, cont'd

10. Reread the entire form, word for word, to find any errors or omissions.

Letter of Introduction

Individuals spend days perfecting a résumé but throw together an e-mail message or cover letter in minutes. This is a mistake. The main goal of the cover letter is to get the employer to take notice of the potential employee and résumé. A cover letter may be in the form of an e-mail message, so make sure the subject line is clean and specific to the job you want (for example, "Bilingual health insurance specialist seeks billing position"). Messages or letters should be typed, addressed to a specific person, and customized to each potential employer. If you do not have the name of a person to send the letter to, address it as "Dear Sir or Madam," "To Whom It May Concern," or a less formal "Hello" or "Good Morning."

Do not repeat everything in the résumé in your letter of introduction. Begin with an attention grabber and get right to the point so that the employer knows what you want and why. The message or letter should explain how your qualifications and skills would benefit the employer. Use key words that appear in the "position wanted" advertisement. Employers use applicant tracking systems (ATSs) to find and screen candidates, so include skill-oriented key words to boost your chance of being discovered. End the message or letter by requesting an interview and be sure to attach or enclose a résumé. Always include telephone numbers (home and cell) and the time of day when you are available.

Reread the message or letter to check for typos and errors in grammar, punctuation, and spelling. Avoid the use of "I" in the sentence structure (Fig. 20.5).

Résumé

A traditional résumé is a data sheet designed to sell job qualifications to prospective employers. A résumé that highlights information related to the position the applicant is trying to obtain should be created and therefore résumés will differ for each job. There are several formats from which to choose:

- A chronologic résumé gives recent experiences first, with dates and descriptive data for each job.

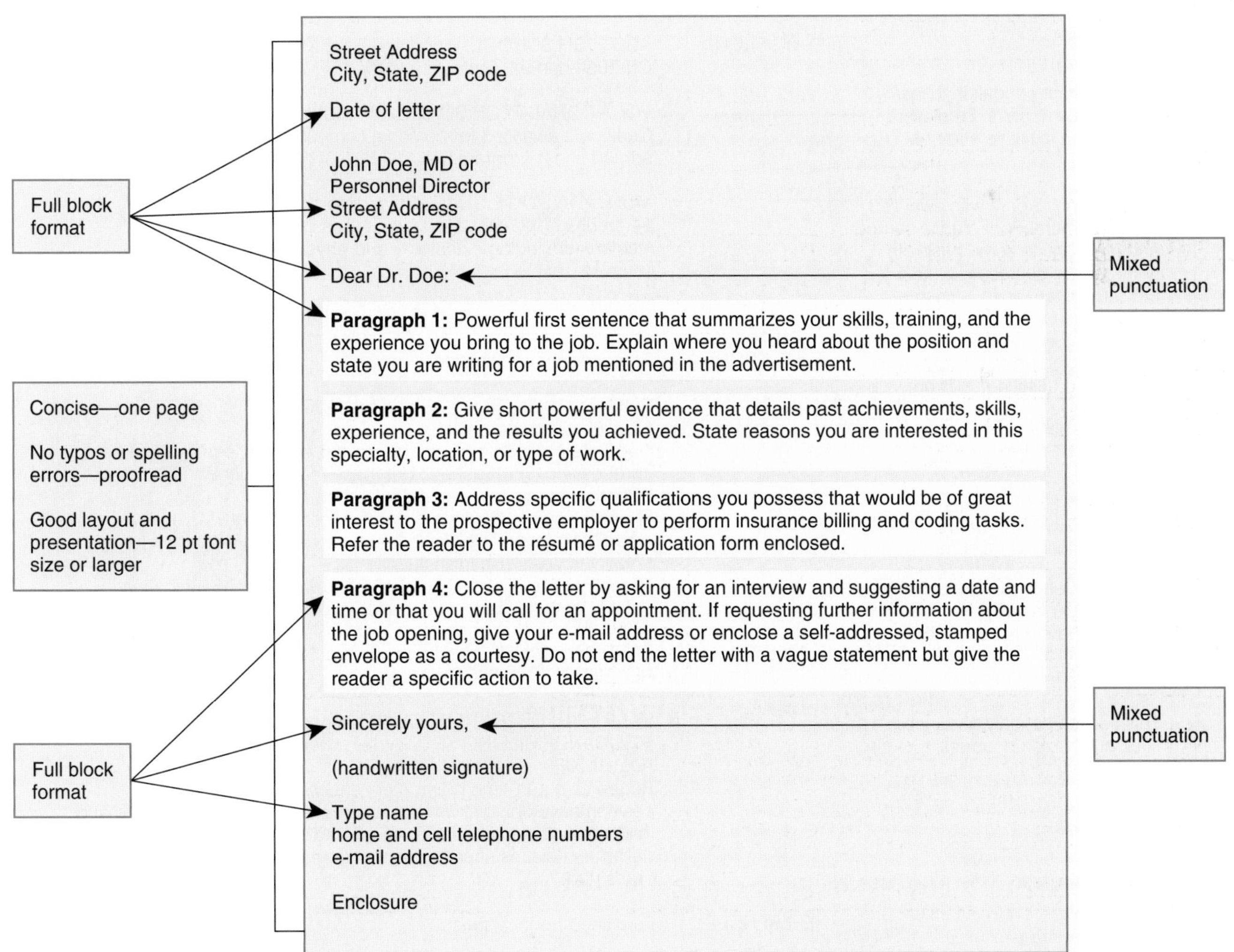

Fig. 20.5 Suggested content for a letter of introduction to accompany a résumé. Typed in full-block style with mixed punctuation.

- A **functional résumé** states the qualifications or skills that an individual can perform.
- A **combination résumé** summarizes the applicant's job skills as well as educational and employment history. The combination style is the best choice for an insurance billing specialist (Fig. 20.6).

The ideal length for a résumé is one page. It can be typed on an 8½- × 14-inch page and reduced to letter size. The résumé should be keyed or typed, not handwritten, on high-quality off-white or white paper. It should be single spaced internally with double spacing between main headings and balanced spacing for all four margins. Laser-printed résumés give a professional appearance. You might want to have a longer (two-page maximum) résumé on hand to offer during an interview.

Under the Civil Rights Act of 1964, enforced by the Equal Employment Opportunity Commission (**EEOC**), information about height, weight, birth date, marital status, Social Security number, and physical condition may be omitted. Additional items to omit are salary requirements, reason for leaving jobs, date of résumé preparation, date available to begin work, references, and vague references to time gaps. Questions about these items might be asked during an interview. If you were laid off and have a gap between jobs, get involved in volunteer projects or consulting opportunities, even if you work for free. This allows you to use your skills and can then be described on your résumé. Hobbies and outside interests that relate to the profession might be included. Membership or leadership positions held in professional organizations related to the medical

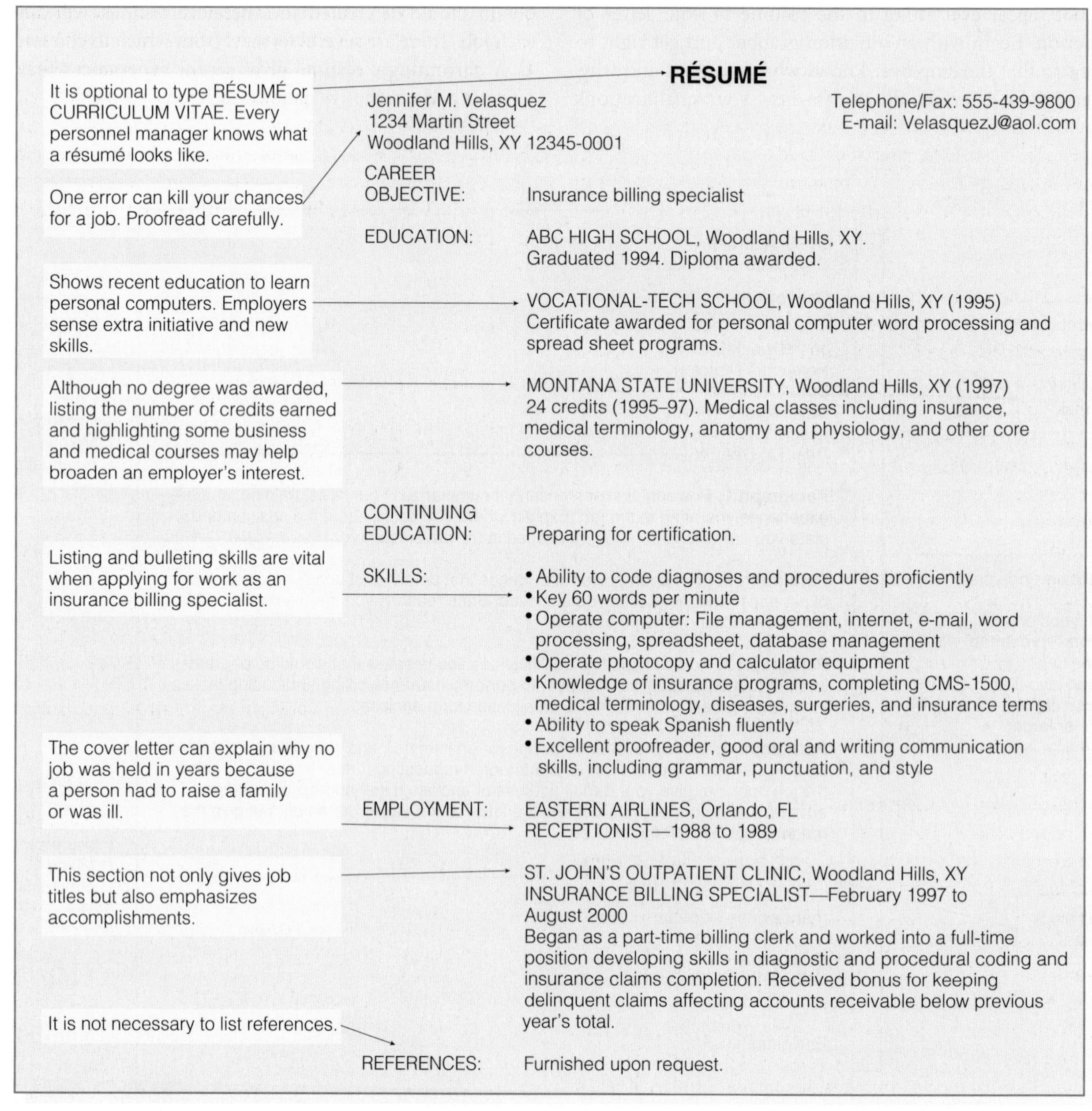

Fig. 20.6 Example of a combination résumé stressing education and skills. Personal data may be excluded as a result of the Civil Rights Act of 1964, enforced by the Equal Employment Opportunity Commission (EEOC).

field might be mentioned. A photograph is not necessary but might be included if it will be of value to the interviewer for recall purposes.

The format may include the following:

- *Title.* Résumé, Personal Data Sheet, Biographic Sketch, or Curriculum Vitae.
- *Heading.* At the beginning of the résumé, list your name, phone number, and e-mail address. Mailing addresses are being phased out, so simply noting your city and state is acceptable.
- *Summary.* This may be a statement as to why the employer should be interested in you. Use action words as shown in Fig. 20.6 and avoid the personal pronoun.
- *Education.* Name high school, college, any business school attended, and continuing education classes, city and state, degree, and date received. List in reverse chronologic order. Grade average and awards or scholastic honors may be included.
- *Professional experience.* Name all employers in reverse chronologic order with addresses, telephone numbers, and dates of employment. Include summer, full-time, part-time, and temporary jobs as well as externship and volunteer work. Detail achievements, not duties (for example, "possess strong communication, service to patients, and organizational skills" or "consistently surpassed collection goals by 10% or more each year").
- *Skills.* List keyboarding words per minute, computer equipment operated, experience with medical billing software programs, accurate procedure and diagnostic coding including knowledge of modifiers, expertise in insurance claims completion and submission, knowledge of medical terminology and insurance terminology, bookkeeping (posting charges, payments, and adjustments to accounts receivable journal), experience in preparing appeals for denied claims, resubmittal of delinquent claims, ability to explain insurance programs and plans (for example, benefits, requirements, and submission of claims), ability to abstract information from patients' medical and financial records, and ability to review insurance payments from explanation of benefits (EOB) documents. If you are fluent in another language, provide this information. Telephone and reception skills also might be mentioned. Skills might be placed near the top of the résumé where they will catch a résumé screener's eye.
- *References.* Type in the phrase "Furnished on request." Prepare approximately five references on a separate sheet and be sure to contact the persons referenced before an interview.
- *Final details.* It is acceptable to e-mail or fax a résumé to an employer who advertises a job opening but gives no guidelines on how to submit the résumé. It is wise to use every advantage possible in a competitive employment market in which time is of the essence (Fig. 20.7).

Proofread the résumé carefully for spelling, punctuation, grammar, and typographic errors. Ask a friend or professional individual with excellent English skills to read and critique it. Remember that the résumé is only a foot in the door and not what is going to land that job for you—you are!

Interview

After looking for a potential employer, preparing a résumé, and completing an application, the final step in landing a job is the face-to-face interview. An **interview** is a formal consultation with questions by an employer to evaluate the qualifications of a prospective job applicant (Fig. 20.8).

Make the best impression possible on the prospective employer as soon as you walk through the door. It is a well-known fact that the first 30 seconds makes either a positive or negative impression. Hiring depends on positive qualities. Display a warm, positive, and interested attitude. When speaking, employers want job candidates who are well spoken and articulate. Use proper grammar, avoid using slang, slow down your speaking, and always maintain eye contact.

Good grooming is essential and starts with cleanliness. Use a deodorant but avoid wearing any heavy fragrances. Applicants should dress conservatively in appropriate business attire and wear jewelry sparingly. Cosmetics should be minimal. It has been found that when applicants have similar skills and education, the decision to hire has been based on physical appearance at the interview.

Be poised and confident and focus on good posture. Eliminate nervous habits and do not smoke or chew gum. And above all turn off your cell phone before the interview begins. Do not be tempted to answer a call or send a text during the interview.

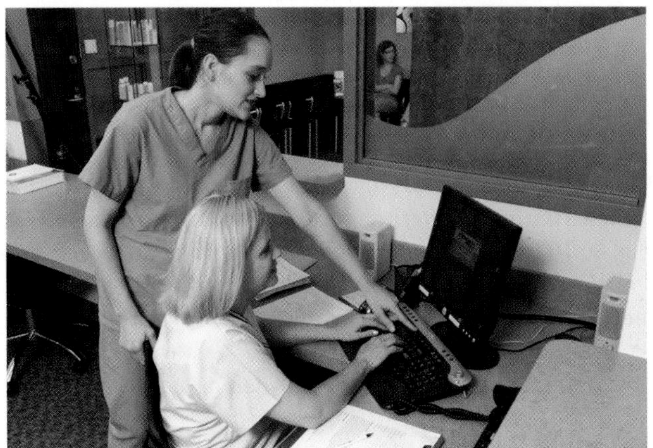

Fig. 20.7 Insurance billing student at an externship site.

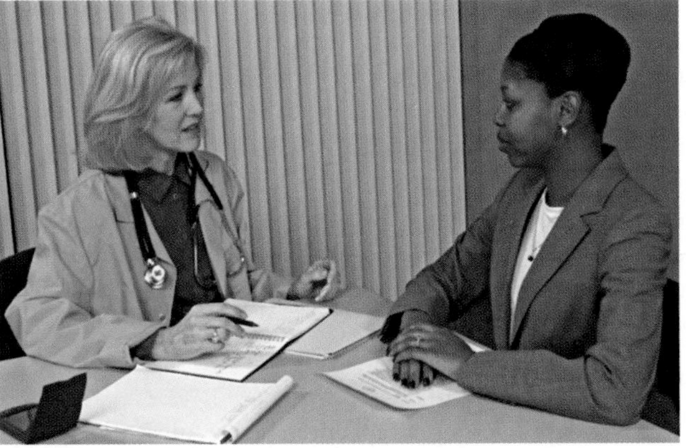

Fig. 20.8 Student being interviewed for an insurance billing position.

Fig. 20.9 is an example of an interview evaluation and reference investigation form. This form points out the areas an interviewer observes and how impressions are rated.

Research before the interview to know whether the salary (when offered) is acceptable. If you want to ask questions about benefits, do not appear to be overly interested in them.

If you are given a choice, avoid scheduling interviews for Mondays or Fridays. Mondays are usually catch-up, heavily scheduled days and Fridays are getaway days, so the interviewer may be rushed. Arrive promptly for the interview. Carry something in your hand (for example, portfolio with notepad, résumé, and other documents) so that you are not showing nervousness or anxiety.

Role-playing is a good method to use to prepare for an interview. Give a friend a list of questions to ask you and then try to answer the questions spontaneously without stumbling. Videotape or audiotape the session, if possible, to see or hear what the employer will experience.

Questions an interviewer might ask about personal life (marital status), family planning, pregnancy, provision for child care, religious preference, club memberships, height, weight, dependents, age (birth date), ethnic background, maiden name, native language, physical or psychiatric problems, spouse's employment and earnings, credit rating, and home and automobile ownership are illegal and do not have to be answered. (It is not considered discriminatory if an employer wants to know whether an applicant smokes.) Three suggestions for handling an illegal question follow:

1. Answer the question and ignore the fact that you know it is illegal.
2. Ask "Is this question relevant to the requirements of this position?"
3. Refuse to answer and contact the nearest EEOC office.

Shake the interviewer's hand at the conclusion of the meeting (Fig. 20.10). Ask how long it will be before a job offer or denial is forthcoming and then leave with a "thank you." If the job is offered at the interview and you are not sure about accepting, ask, "How soon do you need to know?" This will allow time to think and compare job offers before making a commitment.

Portfolio

Prepare in advance for the interview by organizing a **portfolio**. This may give you a leg up in the job market. Include letters of recommendation (from former employers, teachers, family physician, professional friends, or community leaders), school diplomas or degrees, transcripts, certificates, names and addresses of references, a résumé, timed keyboarding test certified by an instructor, insurance claim forms you may have completed with evidence of coding skills, and any other items related to prior education and work experience. You may also want to create a web-based portfolio by scanning the recommended documents and inserting a link to the portfolio for online job applications.

Proof of Citizenship

Within 3 days of being hired, an employee must provide their employer with proof of citizenship by completing an Employment Eligibility Verification Form I-9. The employee must also show proof of citizenship by providing appropriate documentation that may include a single document or combination of driver's license, Social Security card, birth certificate, US passport, naturalization certification, an alien registration receipt card, or an authorization card. The specific documentation requirements can be found on the US Citizenship and Immigration Services (**USCIS**) website (www.uscis.gov). Assemble your proof of citizenship documents and have them available in the event that it is requested by the prospective employer during the interview.

Follow-Up Letter

Write a follow-up letter or send an e-mail message within 24 hours of the interview. Thank the person for the interview and restate your interest in the position (Fig. 20.11). This keeps your name before the potential employer. Telephone to express continued interest in the position if no response is heard within the time frame given.

SELF-EMPLOYMENT

Setting Up an Office

When an individual wants to be his or her own boss (**self-employment**), it is usually wise to become educated and have some experience in the chosen career before undertaking this task. Having a positive and effective rapport with the public, as well as a strong background in insurance, is desirable for the individual who wants to work independently as an insurance billing specialist. Outpatient hospital and physician billing experience in several specialties is important if you choose to focus on professional billing and coding services. If you specialize in facility billing and coding services, experience is necessary, especially because it is not common for a hospital to outsource these services to a small billing company. If coding services are to be part of the billing company's offerings, the coding professional should be certified by a reputable professional organization, such as the AAPC or AHIMA.

! COMPLIANCE ALERT

Security Policies When Working from Home

The Health Insurance Portability and Accountability Act (HIPAA) security rules indicate that working from home requires the same security policies and practices as when working in the office. However, no specific policies are given. It is up to each covered entity to establish these documents based on its security risk assessment. Security measures should address the technical setup. For example, a typical security policy might stipulate that the telecommuter use a dedicated computer with a virtual private network solution, antivirus software, and firewall. Privacy compliance policies apply at home just as they do when working in an office. All oral, written and electronic information should be protected from family members and visitors.

One must have something to offer clients when marketing and selling one's services and skills. This knowledge and expertise can be gained only with years of experience and persistence. Full-time commitment, hard work, dedication, and many long hours to obtain clients are encountered when beginning a

INTERVIEW EVALUATION AND REFERENCE INVESTIGATION FORM

THIS IS	SUMMARY OF EVALUATION	
☐ 1ST INTERVIEW ☐ 2ND INTERVIEW ☐ 3RD INTERVIEW	POINTS FROM (21 CATEGORIES) APPLICATION AND INTERVIEW (FRONT)	
	POINTS FROM REFERENCES (1 TO 3 CATEGORIES FROM BACK)	
	TOTAL POINTS = (Front and Back)	
	OVERALL IMPRESSION: Divide total points by number of categories rated (24 maximum categories).	

NAME OF APPLICANT:	DATE
ADDRESS:	PHONE

RATING: EXCELLENT – 3 POINTS
GOOD – 2 POINTS
FAIR – 1 POINT
POOR – 0 POINTS

POSITION APPLIED FOR:

FROM APPLICATION FOR POSITION, GAUGE APPLICANT IN FOLLOWING AREAS		EXC	GOOD	FAIR	POOR
APPLICATION SECTION REFERENCE	1. NECESSARY SKILLS FOR THIS POSITION?				
	2. SUITABLE ADVANCEMENT HISTORY?				
	3. AN EMPLOYMENT HISTORY THAT POINTS TOWARD DEPENDABILITY?				
	4. STABILITY (REMAINED IN ONE PLACE OF RESIDENCE AND ONE JOB FOR A REASONABLE LENGTH OF TIME)?				
	5. THE PROPER EDUCATIONAL BACKGROUND TO FILL THE POSITION?				
	6. SALARY REQUIREMENT COMMENSURATE WITH POSITION?				
	7. LEGIBLE HANDWRITING?				
	8. LIMITATION ON WORKING HOURS?				
FROM THE PERSONAL INTERVIEW – (SHOULD BE SPECIFIC QUALITIES – OBJECTIVE)					
	9. SUFFICIENT CAPABILITY TO HANDLE ANY SITUATION THAT MAY ARISE WHEN ALONE IN OFFICE?				
	10. AN APPROPRIATE ATTITUDE TOWARD WORK?				
	11. APPROPRIATE DICTION, GRAMMAR, ARTICULATION?				
	12. POISE?				
	13. SELF CONFIDENCE (NOT OVER-CONFIDENCE)?				
	14. TACT?				
	15. SUFFICIENT MATURITY FOR JOB?				
	16. AN ABILITY TO EXPRESS ONESELF WELL?				
	17. AN INITIATIVE OR INTEREST IN LEARNING?				
	18. ABILITY TO WORK WITH OTHERS IN OFFICE?				
	19. APPROPRIATE APPEARANCE (NEAT, CLEAN; SUITABLE TO BUSINESS)				
	20. ENERGY, VITALITY, AND PERCEIVED ABILITY TO HANDLE PRESSURE OF POSITION?				
	21. EAGERNESS TO OBTAIN THE POSITION IN QUESTION?				
NOTES:	COLUMNAR TOTALS				
	TOTAL POINTS THIS PAGE				

DIRECTIONS FOR USE OF FORM:

1. Look over your ratings. A zero score on any one VITAL question should automatically eliminate applicant. Add up the total rating points and enter in the SUMMARY OF EVALUATION BLOCK in the upper right-hand corner of this page.
2. After finishing all interviews, choose the "best bets" and check their references using the reverse side of this form.
3. Enter, as above, the results of your reference check and then your overall impression (E – Excellent, G – Good, F – Fair, P – Poor).

ORDER # 72-120 • BIBBERO SYSTEMS, INC. • PETALUMA, CA. • (REV.07/03)
TO REORDER CALL TOLL FREE: (800) BIBBERO (800-242-2376) OR FAX (800) 242-9330 MFG IN U.S.A.

(PLEASE TURN OVER)

Fig. 20.9 Example of an interview evaluation and reference investigation form. (Courtesy Bibbero Systems, Inc., Petaluma, Calif. Telephone: [800] 242-2376; fax: [800] 242-9330; website: www.bibbero.com.)

NOTES:

RATING: 0 - POOR, 1 - FAIR, 2 - GOOD, 3 - EXCELLENT

REFERENCE INVESTIGATION

1.	OFFICE CONTACTED	PHONE: ( )	DATE
	PERSON CONTACTED	TITLE OR POSITION:	
	HOW LONG HAVE YOU KNOWN THIS PERSON?	TITLE/POSITION THIS PERSON HELD?	
	BETWEEN WHAT DATES WAS THIS PERSON EMPLOYED BY YOU?	FROM TO	
	RESPONSIBILITIES?	SATISFACTORILY COMPLETED?	
	WAS THIS PERSON CONSISTENTLY COOPERATIVE?	WHAT WERE SHORTCOMINGS?	
	DID THIS PERSON GET ALONG WELL WITH OTHERS?		
	WAS THIS PERSON TRUSTWORTHY/DEPENDABLE?		ATTENDANCE RECORD:
	REASON FOR LEAVING?		SALARY LEVEL:
	WOULD YOU REHIRE THIS PERSON?		
	NOTES:		
			RATING:
2.	OFFICE CONTACTED	PHONE: ( )	DATE
	PERSON CONTACTED	TITLE OR POSITION:	
	HOW LONG HAVE YOU KNOWN THIS PERSON?	TITLE/POSITION THIS PERSON HELD?	
	BETWEEN WHAT DATES WAS THIS PERSON EMPLOYED BY YOU?		
	RESPONSIBILITIES?		
	WAS THIS PERSON CONSISTENTLY COOPERATIVE?		
	DID THIS PERSON GET ALONG WELL WITH OTHERS?		
	WAS THIS PERSON TRUSTWORTHY/DEPENDABLE?		ATTENDANCE RECORD:
	REASON FOR LEAVING?		SALARY LEVEL:
	WOULD YOU REHIRE THIS PERSON?		
	NOTES:		
			RATING:
3.	OFFICE CONTACTED	PHONE: ( )	DATE
	PERSON CONTACTED	TITLE OR POSITION:	
	HOW LONG HAVE YOU KNOWN THIS PERSON?	TITLE/POSITION THIS PERSON HELD?	
	BETWEEN WHAT DATES WAS THIS PERSON EMPLOYED BY YOU?		
	RESPONSIBILITIES?		
	WAS THIS PERSON CONSISTENTLY COOPERATIVE?		
	DID THIS PERSON GET ALONG WELL WITH OTHERS?		
	WAS THIS PERSON TRUSTWORTHY/DEPENDABLE?		ATTENDANCE RECORD:
	REASON FOR LEAVING?		SALARY LEVEL:
	WOULD YOU REHIRE THIS PERSON?		
	NOTES:		
			RATING:

INTERVIEWER____________________ DATE:________ TOTAL POINTS THIS PAGE:

Fig. 20.9, cont'd

business. Be cautious when purchasing billing service software and obtain a complete picture of what hardware is necessary, how the program works, and the benefits it offers to your clients.

Networking is extremely important when starting and growing a successful business. Contacts that you have met in previous jobs may lead to future business partners. Many times, it is who the individual knows that may get a foot in the potential client's door.

An insurance billing specialist can work as an independent contractor to have flexible hours, work from home, and reduce a health care organization's overhead. Working at home requires self-discipline and one must develop a schedule and stick to it. Good time management is essential. It takes additional hours to advertise, obtain clients, bill, and perform bookkeeping tasks.

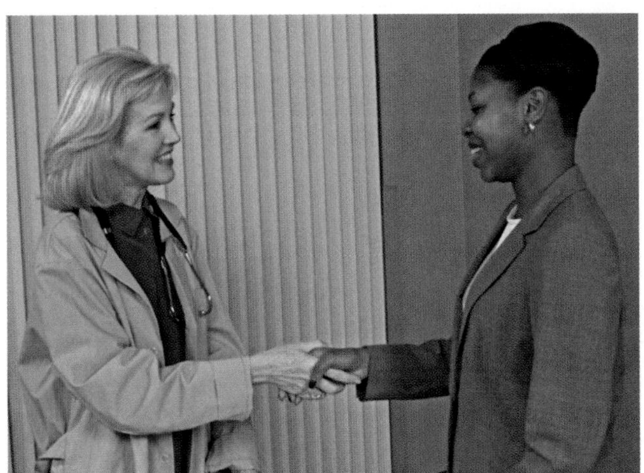

Fig. 20.10 Job applicant concluding an interview with an office manager.

Box 20.1 is a checklist of tasks that must be done to establish a new business.

Planning Your Business

Every successful business endeavor begins with a smart business plan. This is a road map that can guide your financial and business strategies from start-up to continuous success. A business plan addresses facts and figures pertinent to your business and financial abilities and assesses your objectives and goals. It would be wise to meet with an accountant, an attorney, or a business consultant to help get your company started in the right direction.

For more information about business planning, visit the US Small Business Association (SBA) website at www.sba.gov.

Professional Mailing Address

No doubt you will receive mail, so it is important to establish a professional address. Opting to rent a post office box creates a business-oriented mailing address, helps maintain confidentiality in mailings you receive about clients and patient accounts, and protects you from unwanted visitors to your home. Visit the website of the Internal Revenue Service (IRS) at www.irs.gov/Businesses/Small-Businesses-&-Self-Employed for self-employed and small business resources.

Finances to Consider

Taxes

You must decide on what form of business entity you will be (that is, sole proprietor, partnership, or corporation). It is advisable to seek the services of a lawyer, accountant, or both before legally establishing a business and making appropriate selection of the tax options involved. Set up detailed financial records

Street Address
City, State, ZIP code
Date of letter

John Doe, MD or
Personnel Director
Street Address
City, State, ZIP code

Dear Dr. Doe:

Thank you for spending your valuable time yesterday to interview me for the insurance billing specialist position in your clinic.

I hope that you will allow me the opportunity to prove my abilities as I feel that I am able to perform the work with expertise. Meeting your staff was most enjoyable, and it would certainly be pleasurable working with them as a team.

I am looking forward to hearing from you in the near future.

Sincerely yours,

(handwritten signature)

Type name

Fig. 20.11 Example of a thank-you letter sent after an interview.

BOX 20.1 New Business Checklist

The following is a checklist to help you in starting a new home business. This is not a complete list of items to consider nor the exact order to accomplish them in; however, important points are covered in this list.

- Define your services and construct a business plan. Make sure you forecast for success. Will this business be viable? Can you accomplish the services you will promise to carry out? Can you financially afford this endeavor?
- Research whether you need to obtain a business license from the business license section of your city hall. Regulations vary in each city licensing office. You might have to obtain a home occupation permit from the planning department and have it signed by your landlord if you are renting. The city may have guidelines on hours of business, pedestrian and vehicular activity, noise, and so on in residential areas. Determine whether your county has rules on operating a small business from home.
- Consider a name for your business. File a fictitious business name (doing business as [DBA]) at the county clerk's office by obtaining the proper form for completion. If you use your given name, you do not have to file a fictitious business name.
- Decide what address to use. You may want to obtain a post office box number instead of using your home address. This will help with a professional mailing address as well as protect you from unexpected visitors to your home.
- Consult with an accountant for advice on the tax structure of your company (for example, sole proprietor, corporation). Learn about what expenses are deductible. Depending on how you set up your business, some possible tax breaks are depreciation of office equipment; declaring a room of your home as an office; subscriptions to professional publications; dues to professional associations; expenses associated with your automobile; telephone, photocopying, and office supplies; promotion and advertising; and any expenses pertaining to meetings, conventions, workshops, or seminars.
- Obtain the insurance that you need: health insurance, disability insurance, life insurance, liability insurance, workers' compensation (if you have employees), and so on. Insurance called "release of information insurance" or "errors and omissions insurance" with a "hold harmless" clause is available to protect you against loss of material. Consider a retirement plan, such as an individual retirement account.
- Obtain a separate telephone number and possibly a fax number to separate "home" from "business." Having a business listing allows you to be listed in the Yellow Pages of your telephone directory.
- Create a website advertising your services, incorporating a video clip and web-based portfolio with other visuals as well as links to LinkedIn, Facebook, and Twitter.
- Open a bank account. Many banks offer small business accounts with nominal monthly fees.
- Create a professional image through business cards, stationery, and invoice billing forms. You can find resources on the internet or in software programs to print your own.
- Stay current in the industry with up-to-date reference books. Begin to assemble a library to include a good medical dictionary, procedural and diagnostic code books, compliance handbooks, trade journals, and so on.
- Start a contact database and begin to advertise your business using some of the following methods: visiting offices, mailing flyers, advertising in trade journals or your local newspaper, sending announcements, putting up signs (be sure to get permission), and sending personalized letters to prospects (hospitals, clinics, and physician's offices).
- If you have opened an office at a location outside of your home, make sure you have reviewed a proper lease before signing it and consider the finances needed for items such as utility deposits (that is, water, gas, and electricity). Rent, renovation, and janitorial or trash services must also be considered.
- Some contracts include a statement on confidentiality assuring the contracting facility that all patient data are handled in a confidential manner.

using the services of an accountant and simplified bookkeeping software for use on the computer. Expert advice is essential and helps develop a successful business.

Establishing a business in a home may result in some deductions, so obtain all the information you can from your accountant and the IRS regarding important laws concerning small business and self-employment taxes. Keep receipts and complete records of income and expenses. Retain records for the period stipulated by the IRS. The following is a sample record retention schedule for a small business:

- Bank statements and canceled checks: 7 years
- Expired contracts: 7 years
- Financial statements: permanently
- General correspondence: 1 to 5 years
- Payroll records and summaries: 7 years
- Income tax returns: permanently
- Worksheets and supporting documents: 7 years
- Business travel expenses and documentation of mileage: 7 years

Start-Up Expenses

Money is necessary for equipment, computer software, overhead, taxes, stationery, preprinted statements and forms, and myriad other expenses. It is vital that you accrue sufficient funds to run the business for a period of 1 year or more before vacating a full-time job. This will help to eliminate a lot of fear and anxiety associated with business start-up. A common reason for business failure is running out of the money necessary to keep the business going. It may take a year or more to begin seeing a profit, so one must be patient. This is where the business plan becomes a useful resource!

If an individual has had no business management experience, courses may be taken to gain knowledge and instill confidence in these areas before beginning a business. Attend workshops and lectures on starting a business that are offered by financial institutions, universities, community colleges, or private institutions.

Bank Account

Open a bank account that is separate from your own personal accounts. This smart approach saves a lot of time in the future when it comes to sorting out expenses and working on taxes. Also, think about the professional image that a business check will convey. Most banks have small business account services, including those for the self-employed.

Business Name and License

Some towns or counties require a license to operate a business. This may include working from your home office. Check with your local offices to determine whether an application or fee is required. This is the time to choose an appropriate business name and get applicable town and county licenses.

A business name should be easy to remember and explain what your company does. For example, ABC's #1 Medical Billing Service tells potential clients that the company works with health care related to billing and insurance claims.

Insurance

Business owners should protect income and property from unexpected loss. The following are types of insurance to investigate:

- Professional liability/errors and omissions protects you and your company from claims if your client holds you responsible for errors or the failure to perform as promised in your service contract. Coverage can include legal costs and may pay for resulting judgments against you.
- Business interruption insurance and property insurance in case of fire, theft, or disaster protects your assets and may help you in the recovery of data.
- Disability insurance if one becomes unable to work because of illness or injury can include yourself and/or an employee.
- Health and life insurance covers health care for you and/or employees as well as providing life insurance.

Business Associate Under the Health Insurance Portability and Accountability Act

HIPAA rules apply to most billing, coding, or consulting companies because they are considered to be business associates.

If your billing, coding, or consulting company gets personal health information from a covered entity to perform a function or activity on behalf of that covered entity, your relationship is likely that of a business associate and your responsibilities must be defined with a business associate agreement.

The Business Associate Agreement

The **business associate agreement** must give "satisfactory assurances" to the covered entity on whose behalf the business associate performs services and must include, according to HIPAA rules, the following terms as set forth in the regulation:

- Business Associate agrees to not use or disclose protected health information (PHI) other than as permitted or required by the Agreement or as required by law.
- Business Associate agrees to use appropriate safeguards to prevent use or disclosure of the PHI other than as provided for by this Agreement.
- Business Associate agrees to mitigate, to the extent practicable, any harmful effect that is known to Business Associate of a use or disclosure of PHI by Business Associate in violation of the requirements of this Agreement.
- Business Associate agrees to report to Covered Entity any use or disclosure of the PHI not provided for by this Agreement of which it becomes aware.
- Business Associate agrees to ensure that any agent including a subcontractor, to whom it provides PHI received from, or created or received by Business Associate on behalf of, Covered Entity agrees to the same restrictions and conditions that apply through this Agreement to Business Associate with respect to such information.
- Business Associate agrees to provide access, at the request of Covered Entity, and in the time and manner [insert negotiated terms], to PHI in a Designated Record Set, to Covered Entity or, as directed by Covered Entity, to an Individual to meet the requirements under 45 CFR § 164.524. (Not necessary if business associate does not have PHI in a designated record set.)
- Business Associate agrees to make any amendment(s) to PHI in a Designated Record Set that the Covered Entity directs or agrees to pursuant to 45 CFR § 164.526 at the request of Covered Entity or an Individual, and in the time and manner [insert negotiated terms]. (Not necessary if business associate does not have PHI in a designated record set.)
- Business Associate agrees to make internal practices, books, and records, including policies and procedures and PHI, relating to the use and disclosure of PHI received from, or created or received by Business Associate on behalf of, Covered Entity available [to the Covered Entity, or] to the Secretary, in a time and manner [insert negotiated terms] or designated by the Secretary, for purposes of the Secretary determining Covered Entity's compliance with the Privacy Rule.
- Business Associate agrees to document such disclosures of PHI and information related to such disclosures as would be required for Covered Entity to respond to a request by an Individual for an accounting of disclosures of PHI in accordance with 45 CFR § 164.528.
- Business Associate agrees to provide to Covered Entity or an Individual, in time and manner [insert negotiated terms], information collected in accordance with Section [insert section number in contract where provision (i) appears] of this Agreement, to permit Covered Entity to respond to a request by an Individual for an accounting of disclosures of PHI in accordance with 45 CFR § 164.528.[2]

Service Contract

The service contract is a separate document from the business associate agreement. The **service contract** is a necessary document that defines the duties and obligations of each party involved in the business relationship. Contracts or agreements should be made in writing, signed, and notarized. For example, a contract should define the following:

- Who is responsible for the coding (the health care organization or the billing service)?
- What will be the routine for claim submission?
- Is there a per-claim processing fee or is there a flat monthly fee?
- Who is responsible for follow-up on collection procedures (telephone calls or letters)?
- Who pays for rebilling, photocopying of records, mailing fees, and clearinghouse charges? Is this included in a flat monthly service fee?
- Under whose name will bills be sent to patients (the health care organization or the billing service)?
- Will the billing service telephone number appear on the statement or will a toll-free or local number be used?
- How will the telephone be answered?
- What are the charges for coding consultation services?
- What are the coverage arrangements for absence or illness?

- How will information be protected and handled between the client and billing company?

If there is any change in the terms of the agreements, write an addendum to the original agreement and have both parties sign to acknowledge the change. Be sure that all agreements and contracts have proper effective and termination dates. Remember that renegotiation is possible when the contract expires.

! COMPLIANCE ALERT

Confidentiality Statement

Some contracts may include a statement on confidentiality assuring the contracting facility that all patient data will be handled in a confidential manner.

Pricing Your Services

Define your services and work out a structured fee schedule. It is imperative that you get legal advice when creating contracts and agreements.

A variety of methods are used to price services, such as a percentage of reimbursement or an annual, hourly, or per-claim fee. Review state laws regarding percentage billing because it is illegal in some states. Deciding on which method depends on the type of client being served and the work to be done. For example, a coding specialist may bill a per-claim service, whereas a CAP may bill in 15-minute increments. Contact other billing and insurance services to learn what they are charging.

Security and Equipment

The most important consideration when starting your business is privacy and security of the health information and business documents that you will handle and be responsible for.

An initial equipment checklist may include the following:

- Computer
- Laser or ink jet printer
- Paper
- Current billing and coding manuals and books
- Desk supplies such as stapler, paper clips, and self-adhesive notes
- Locking file cabinets
- Fax machine

Also consider using separate computer backup protection (for example, a surge protector with battery power) to guard against faulty wiring or power failure. This gives you more than 10 minutes to back up your current project and then shut down. These are available at office stores for about $100.

Shop smart. Research upcoming sales and lease programs, rebates, upgrade trade-ins, and service plans.

Research the various medical billing software programs and ask for demonstration software before purchasing. Also look for a reputable clearinghouse. Compare functionality, customer service, technical support, and prices.

Marketing, Advertising, Promotion, and Public Relations

Marketing refers to how a business is presented or advertised to promote sales. Marketing strategies vary, depending on the section of the public that is targeted. When promoting a medical billing service, develop a well-organized marketing plan and follow basic guidelines to reach a specific target audience.

Ways to market a business and the reasons for marketing strategies are presented in Table 20.2.

At this point, you should be ready to start marketing your business. If you are creative, you can design your own business cards and have them printed. A classic white card with black

TABLE 20.2 Business Marketing and Strategies

Strategy	Reason
Obtain professionally printed stationery and business cards.	Enhances professional image.
Pass out business cards at professional meetings.	Advertises availability and services. Helps with networking.
Develop a business name and logo for the company.	Enables potential clients to identify that you are in business.
Ensure accuracy of all printed materials.	When items are not professionally assembled or proofread to eliminate typographical errors, a potential client receives a doubtful or negative image of the company.
Develop a professional flyer and distribute it to medical facilities and physicians' offices.	Introduces company name, advertises services, and describes benefits.
Follow up with a personal visit or telephone call.	A friendly voice and professional image offer personal services and let potential clients know that you are available and interested.
Advertise in the journal or newsletter of the county medical society and state medical association.	Potential clients read such publications and advertisements of this nature lend to your credibility.
Place an ad in the newspaper or on cable television.	Circulates business within the county.
Sign up for an ad on Google or put an ad in the local Yellow Pages.	Solicits a wider range of prospective clients.
Join a local chamber of commerce to network with members and network using social media, such as LinkedIn.	Networking and advertising can be the best public relations tool.
Promote your business with a professionally developed website.	Search engines will help find you. Websites deliver immediate, detailed information about your company.
Check with established businesses to determine whether they are overloaded with work, the owner needs a vacation, or they need help with a temporary situation because of illness.	Present your services as a help, not a threat to current office staff.

print conveys professionalism. When creating business brochures, obtain financial data to help convince clients that the service you are offering is better and can do more for their businesses than what they presently have. Save them time and money! Stress being honest, reliable, committed, efficient, and professional and offer them something they cannot do for themselves.

Put yourself in front of office managers and health care providers to advertise your services. Consider visiting the health care offices in your area, being cognizant of offices that have a sign stating, "No Soliciting." If you see this sign, respect it and jot down the address to mail them literature instead. Also, note that solicitation by fax is illegal according to the Federal Communications Commission.

Marketing can be tough and intimidating. Networking with other colleagues and professionals and persistence will pay off.

Business Incubator

Another way to develop a business and obtain management assistance is to seek the services of a business incubator. A *business incubator* is an environment that grows and nurtures small businesses through their early years of existence by offering an array of business assistance services, shared resources, and networking. An incubator facility can be an actual building that has several small business tenants. It is run by managers and staff who offer business advice and referral services to tenants and many additional services, such as high-speed internet; conference rooms; secretarial, mail, and courier service; fax; copier; printer; TV, DVD, and VCR; break room; and free parking.

Reassess and Continue With Success

Once your business is under way, you will find it necessary to routinely assess its overall health. Review your business plans and make sure you are following the guidelines. Make changes where applicable and revise your strategies and goals. Running your own successful business is challenging and highly rewarding both emotionally and financially.

ATTAINING PROFESSIONAL ADVANCEMENT

Whether you become the employee of a health care organization or you strike out as a self-employed contractor, advancing your skills and your career is essential to a successful and long-term career. As stated earlier in this chapter, it is important to join professional organizations and to seek certifications as part of your professional advancement. To be an expert in the ever-changing field of health care will require continuous learning and education on the part of the insurance billing specialist.

Networking

Networking is a core principal for success in developing any career. **Networking** is the exchange of information or services among individuals, groups, or institutions and making use of professional contacts. Networking has many benefits and can open the door to long-term friendships, business opportunities, advice, and positive influences.

As you develop your network, you are creating a community of people who provide information and emotional support to each other. You will learn of new developments in your field, new tools, and new processes, training programs, products, and services. You will identify the leaders in your network that you aspire to follow and mirror their image. And as you develop your career, you may have the satisfaction of providing support or a key piece of information that makes a difference in the life of one of those in your network.

Find A Mentor

A valuable vehicle for career development is to find a mentor in the business. A **mentor** is a guide or teacher who offers advice, criticism, wisdom, guidance, and perspective to an inexperienced but promising protégé to help reach a life goal. Decide what kind of help you want (for example, technical, general feedback, or managerial) and then look for a mentor whose background, values, and style are similar to yours. Be willing to face criticism with a positive attitude and express gratitude when excellence is praised.

PROCEDURE 20.1 Creating an Electronic Résumé

Once a medical position has been identified, a résumé may be e-mailed or a hard copy may be faxed. The basic steps for creating a résumé are as follows:

1. Compose a résumé using computer software with accurate spelling features and be sure to keep it simple. Each line should be no more than 65 characters in length.
2. Discard traditional résumé-writing techniques, such as focusing on action verbs. Instead, think of descriptive key words, such as *medical biller, education, work experience, skills, knowledge,* and *abilities.* To catch a résumé screener's eye, you might insert a section about skills at the top of the résumé.
3. Avoid the use of decorative graphics and complex typefaces, bulleted lists, complicated page formatting, symbols, underlining, and italics. These features may not appear the same on an employer's computer online.
4. When applying for an entry-level position, use only one page. However, if you are experienced, electronic résumés may be three to four pages. Save your résumé using a file name such as medical biller, medical coding specialist, or insurance biller because in some tracking systems this may help get you past the filters instead of using "myrésumé."
5. Proofread the résumé and save the electronic résumé in a job search file.
6. Study the potential employer's online guides presenting special procedures for sending e-mail and files.
7. Use the word processing software's "copy and paste" feature and enter the information in an e-mail, or, if you save it as an electronic file, it can be transmitted as an attachment to an e-mail message.
8. Do not post a letter of introduction when posting a résumé to a bulletin board. Upload the résumé to post online using the file transfer feature.
9. After you send a résumé electronically, mail a hard copy and call the hiring manager directly to follow up. Be assertive.

PROCEDURE 20.2 Compose, Format, Key, Proofread, and Print a Cover Letter

1. Assemble materials: computer, printer, letterhead paper, envelopes, attachments, thesaurus, English dictionary, medical dictionary, and pen or pencil.
2. Obtain recipient's name, address, and title and choose letterhead style (modified or full block format with mixed punctuation). Refer to Fig. 20.5.
3. Turn computer on and select the word processing software program (for example, Microsoft Word). Open a blank document.
4. Key the date line beginning three lines below letterhead and format in the location for the chosen style.
5. Double space down and insert the recipient's title, name, and address. If necessary, double space down for an attention line.
6. Double space down and key the salutation. Use open or mixed punctuation.
7. Double space down and key the reference line ("Re" or "Subject") in the location for chosen letter style.
8. Double space down and key the body (content) of the letter in single-spaced format. Paragraphs should match the chosen format. Always double space down between paragraphs. Save your file every 15 minutes.
9. Proofread the letter on screen for typos, spelling, grammar, and auto-correction errors.
10. If a second page is needed, key that page with a heading (name, page number, and date) in vertical or horizontal format.
11. Key a complimentary close, making sure it is in the location for the chosen style.
12. Drop four spaces down and key the sender's name and title with credentials as shown on the letterhead.
13. When keyboarding a letter for an individual, double space down and insert the sender's and typist's reference initials in lowercase letters, separating the two sets of initials with a colon or slash (for example, HWN:mtf). This step is eliminated when typing your own cover letter.
14. If enclosures or attachments accompany the letter, single or double space down to insert "CC" for copy or "Enc" for enclosures or attachments.
15. If necessary to insert a postscript, double space down to insert "P.S."
16. Save the file to the hard drive before printing a hard copy and proofread the letter, making final corrections.
17. Print two copies, one to be sent and one to be retained in the files.
18. Prepare an envelope. If the letter is to be sent registered or certified, insert mailing instructions on the envelope.
19. Sign the letter, fold it, and insert it with enclosures into the envelope for mailing.

PROCEDURE 20.3 Complete a Job Application Form

1. Assemble materials: job application form, notes of previous employment, pen or pencil.
2. Read the entire application before beginning.
3. If instructions say, "please print," "use pen only," or "put last name first," follow these directions precisely.
4. Complete the application in ink unless directed to use a pencil.
5. Block print if handwriting is illegible and abbreviate words only if there is a lack of space.
6. Insert data on the application form, stressing clarity and neatness.
7. Record dates of previous employment accurately because these data may be used for verification purposes. If there is a question asking you to state the reason you left a position, insert "To be discussed during the interview."
8. Specifically list all job skills that pertain to the position for which you are applying.
9. If salary expectation is requested, insert hourly wage or salary amount expected and then "negotiable" or "flexible" for further discussion during the interview.
10. Sign and date the completed application.

KEY POINTS

This is a brief chapter review, or summary, of the key issues presented. To further enhance your knowledge of the technical subject matter, review the key terms and key abbreviations for this chapter by locating the meaning for each in the Glossary at the end of this book, which appears in a section before the Index.

1. Use many ways to search for a job as an insurance billing specialist.
2. Access the internet to locate job offers by potential employers.
3. Prepare for and attend job fairs to make contact and network with potential employers.
4. Visit potential employers and complete job application forms.
5. Compose a letter of introduction and an updated résumé focused on the type of job you wish to obtain.
6. Prepare yourself for an interview so that you make a positive impression.
7. Organize a job portfolio by scanning in documents related to education, prior work experience, and skills.
8. Research thoroughly and begin the steps to establish a billing service.
9. Know all Health Insurance Portability and Accountability Act (HIPAA) security and confidentiality policy and practice requirements when working from a home-based business.
10. Pursue becoming certified or registered to convey a higher level of professionalism.
11. Become a member of a professional organization to network and keep current on technical data and federal regulations.

STUDENT ASSIGNMENT

- Study Chapter 20.
  - Answer the fill-in-the-blank, multiple-choice, and true/false review questions in the *Workbook* to reinforce the theory learned in this chapter and help you prepare for a future test.
- Complete the assignments in the *Workbook* to give you hands-on experience in completing an application for a position as an insurance billing specialist, preparing and typing a résumé, composing a cover letter to accompany the résumé, having someone evaluate you during an interview, and typing a follow-up thank-you letter after being interviewed.
- Turn to the Glossary at the end of this text for a further understanding of the key terms and key abbreviations used in this chapter.

REFERENCE

Federal Register; Department of Health and Human Services; Title 45, Section 164.528. https://www.usa.gov/federal-agencies/u-s-department-of-health-and-human-services.

Health Information Portability and Accountability Act of 1996, §160.103. https://www.hhs.gov/hipaa/index.html.

KEY ABBREVIATIONS

Chapter number(s) is (are) shown in parentheses after each term.

AAMA (American Association of Medical Assistants) (1)
AAPC (American Academy of Professional Coders) (20)
ABN (Advance Beneficiary Notice of Noncoverage) (6, 19)
ACA (Affordable Care Act) (4)
ADSM (active duty service member) (8)
AHA (American Hospital Association) (12)
AHIMA (American Health Information Management Association) (12, 20)
AIDS (acquired immunodeficiency syndrome) (10)
ALJ (administrative law judge) (16)
AMA (American Medical Association) (1, 19)
AME (agreed medical evaluator) (9)
ANSI (American National Standards Institute) (15, 19)
APC (ambulatory payment classification) (19)
APM (Advanced Alternative Payment Model) (6)
A/R (accounts receivable) (4, 17)
ARRA (American Recovery and Reinvestment Act) (2, 11)
ASC (ambulatory surgery category) (19)
ASC X12 (Accredited Standards Committee X12) (15)
ASCA (Administrative Simplification Compliance Act) (14)
ASET (Administrative Simplification Enforcement Tool) (15)
ASHD (arteriosclerotic heart disease) (1)
ASP (application service provider) (15)
ATM (automatic teller machine) (15, 17)
BCBSA (Blue Cross/Blue Shield Association) (5)
C (comprehensive [level of history or examination]) (11)
C and R (compromise and release) (9)
CAC (computer-assisted coding) (12)
CAP (claims assistance professional) (1, 20)
CC (chief complaint) (11, 12)
CC (complication/comorbidity) (19)
CCAP (Certified Claims Assistance Professional) (20)
CCI (Correct Coding Initiative) (6)
CCS (Certified Coding Specialist) (20)
CCS-P (Certified Coding Specialist–Physician) (20)
CCU (coronary care unit) (11)
CDHP (Consumer Directed Health Plan) (4)
CDI (clinical documentation improvement) (11)
CE (consultative examiner) (19)
CECP (Certified Electronic Claims Processor) (20)
CERT (Comprehensive Error Rate Testing) (3)
CF (conversion factor) (13)
CHAMPUS Civilian Health and Medical Program of the Uniformed Services (8)
CHAMPVA (Civilian Health and Medical Program of the Department of Veterans Affairs) (4, 8)
CHIP Children's Health Insurance Program (7)
CLIA (Clinical Laboratory Improvement Amendments) (3)
CM (Clinical Modification) (12)
CMA (Certified Medical Assistant) (20)
CMBS (Certified Medical Billing Specialist) (20)
CMG (case mix groups) (19)
CMP (Civil Monetary Penalty) (3)
CMP (competitive medical plan) (4)
CMRS (Certified Medical Reimbursement Specialist) (20)
CMS (Centers for Medicare and Medicaid Services) (2, 3, 6, 16, 19)
CMS-1500 (Centers for Medicare and Medicaid Services Health Insurance Claim Form) (14)
COB (coordination of benefits) (4)
COBRA (Consolidated Omnibus Budget Reconciliation Act) (4)
COLA Cost-of-living adjustment (10)
copay (copayment) (5)
CPC (Certified Professional Coder) (20)
CPC-A (Certified Professional Coder–Apprentice) (20)
CPC-H (Certified Professional Coder–Hospital) (20)
CPT (Current Procedural Terminology) (12, 13, 19)
CSRS (Civil Service Retirement System) (10)
D (detailed [level of history or examination]) (11)
DAB (departmental appeal board) (16)
DC (Doctor of Chiropractic) (6)
DDE (direct data entry) (15)
DDS (Disability Determination Services) (10)
DEERS (Defense Enrollment Eligibility Reporting System) (8)
DEFRA (Deficit Reduction Act) (7)
DHHS (Department of Health and Human Services) (2, 3, 6, 15)
DM (diabetes mellitus) (12)
DME (durable medical equipment) (6, 13, 14)
DNA (does not apply) (14)
DNFB (discharge not final billed) (19)
DOJ (Department of Justice) (3)
DOS (date of service) (4)
DRG (diagnosis-related group) (19)
DSL (digital subscriber line) (15)
dx or Dx (diagnosis) (11)
ECG (electrocardiogram) (13)
e-check (electronic check) (17)
ECP (electronic claims processor) (20)
ED or ER (emergency department or emergency room) (11, 13)
EDI (electronic data interchange) (15)
EEOC (Equal Employment Opportunity Commission) (20)
EFT (electronic funds transfer) (15)
EHR (electronic health record) (11, 15)
EIN (employer identification number) (2, 14)
E/M (evaluation and management) (11, 13)
e-mail (electronic mail) (1)
EMC (electronic medical claim) (15)
EMG (emergency) (14)
EMR (electronic medical record) (11)
EMTALA (Emergency Medical Treatment and Active Labor Act) (3, 19)
EOB (explanation of benefits) (13, 16)
EOMB (explanation of Medicare benefits) (15)
EPF (expanded problem focused [level of history or examination]) (11)
ePHI (electronic protected health information) (2)
EPO (exclusive provider organization) (4, 5)
EPSDT (Early and Periodic Screening, Diagnosis, and Treatment) (7, 14)
ERA (electronic remittance advice) (6, 15)
ERISA (Employee Retirement Income Security Act) (9, 16)
ESRD (end-stage renal disease) (6)
FACT (Fair and Accurate Credit Transactions) (17)
FBI (Federal Bureau of Investigation) (2)
FCA (False Claims Act) (3)
FCBA (Fair Credit Billing Act) (17)
FCRA (Fair Credit Reporting Act) (17)
FDCPA (Fair Debt Collection Practices Act) (17)
FDIC (Federal Deposit Insurance Corporation) (3)
FECA (Federal Employees' Compensation Act) (9)
FEHBA (Federal Employee Health Benefit Act) (17)
FERA (Federal Enforcement and Recovery Act of 2009) (3)
FERS (Federal Employees Retirement System) (10)
FH (family history) (11)
FMC (foundation for medical care) (4)
FPL (federal poverty level) (7)
FSA (flexible spending account) (4)
FTC (Federal Trade Commission) (13, 17)
FTP (file transfer protocol) (2)
GAF (geographic adjustment factor) (13)
GEMs (general equivalence mapping) (12)
GPCIs (geographic practice cost indices) (6, 13)
HAC (Health Administration Center) (19)
HBA (health benefits advisor) (8)
HC (high complexity [medical decision making]) (11)
HCERA (Health Care and Education Reconciliation Act) (4)
HCF (health care finder) (8)
HCFAC (Health Care Fraud and Abuse Control [program]) (3)
HCPCS (Healthcare Common Procedure Coding System) (13)
HDHP (high-deductible health plan) (4)
HEAT (Health Care Fraud Prevention and Enforcement Action Team) (3)
HIM (health information management) (11)
HIPAA (Health Insurance Portability and Accountability Act) (2, 16, 19)
HITECH (Health Information Technology for Economic and Clinical Health [Act]) (2)
HIV (human immunodeficiency virus) (10, 11, 12)
HMO (health maintenance organization) (4, 5)
HPI (history of present illness) (11)
HPID (health plan identifier) (15)
HRA (health reimbursement account) (4)
HRS (Health Care Reimbursement Specialist) (20)
HSA (health savings account) (4)
ICD-9-CM (*International Classification of Diseases,* Ninth Revision, Clinical Modifications) (12)
ICD-10-CM (*International Classification of Diseases,* Tenth Revision, Clinical Modifications) (12, 19)
ICD-10-PCS (*International Classification of Diseases,* Tenth Revision, Procedure Coding System) (12, 19)
ICD-11 (*International Classification of Diseases,* Eleventh Revision) (12)
ICR (intelligent character recognition or image copy recognition) (14)

ICU (intensive care unit) (6, 11)
IIHI (individually identifiable health information) (2)
IME (independent medical evaluator) (9)
IPA (independent [or individual] practice association) (4, 5)
IPF PPS Inpatient Psychiatric Facility Prospective Payment System (19)
IPO (inpatient only) [list] (19)
IPPS Inpatient Prospective Payment System (19)
IRF PAI Inpatient Rehabilitation Facility Patient Assessment Instrument (19)
IRF PPS Inpatient Rehabilitation Facility Prospective Payment System (19)
IRS (Internal Revenue Service) (15)
LC (low complexity [medical decision making]) (11)
LCD (local coverage determination) (6)
LGHP (large group health plan) (6)
LHWCA (Longshore and Harbor Workers' Compensation Act) (9)
listserv (list service) (1)
LLQ (left lower quadrant) (11)
LMP (last menstrual period) (14)
LTCH (long-term care hospital) (19)
LTCH PPS (long-term care hospital prospective payment system) (19)
LUQ (left upper quadrant) (11)
MA Plan Medicare Advantage Plan (6)
MAC (Medicare administrative contractor) (3, 6, 15, 19)
MACRA Medicare Access and CHIP Reauthorization Act of 2015 (6)
MBI Medicare Beneficiary Identifier (6)
MC (moderate complexity [medical decision making]) (11)
MCC (major complication/comorbidity) (19)
MCHP (Maternal and Child Health Program) (4)
MCO (managed care organization) (5)
MDC (major diagnostic category) (19)
MDM (medical decision making) (11)
Medi-Medi (Medicare/Medicaid) (4, 6)
MG (Medigap) (6)
MHS (Military Health System) (8)
MIP (Medicare Integrity Program) (3)
MIPAA (Medicare Improvements for Patients and Providers Act) (6)
MIPS (Merit-based Incentive Payment System) (6)
MMA (Medicare Prescription Drug, Improvement, and Modernization Act) (6)
MN (medically needy) (7)
MRI (magnetic resonance imaging) (12)
MSA (medical savings account) (4, 6)
MS-DRG (Medicare Severity Diagnosis-Related Group) (19)
MSN (Medicare Summary Notice) (6)
MSO (management services organization) (1)
MSP (Medicare secondary payer) (6, 7, 14)
MTF (Military Treatment Facility) (8)
NA or N/A (not applicable) (14, 17)
NAS (Nonavailability Statement) (8)
NC (no charge) (17)
NCCI (National Correct Coding Initiative) (13)
NCD (national coverage determination) (6)
NCHS (National Center for Health Statistics) (12)
NCICS (National Certified Insurance and Coding Specialist) (20)
NCQA (National Committee for Quality Assurance) (5)
NDC (National Drug Code) (15)
NEC (not elsewhere classifiable) (12)
NF (nursing facility) (6)
nonpar (nonparticipating [provider or physician]) (4, 6, 8)
NOS (not otherwise specified) (12)
NPI (National Provider Identifier) (2, 6, 14, 16)
NPP (non-physician practitioner) (1, 4, 11)
NPP (Notice of Privacy Practices) (2)
NSF (National Standard Format) (15)
NSF (nonsufficient funds or not sufficient funds) (17)
NUCC (National Uniform Claim Committee) (14)
OASDI (Old Age, Survivors, and Disability Insurance) (10)
OBRA (Omnibus Budget Reconciliation Act) (7)
OCR (Office of Civil Rights) (2, 14)
OHI (other health insurance) (8)
OIG (Office of the Inspector General) (2, 3)
OOY (over-one-year [claims]) (7)
OPPS (Outpatient Prospective Payment System) (19)
ORT (Operation Restore Trust) (3)
OSHA (Occupational Safety and Health Administration) (3, 9)
OWCP Office of Workers' Compensation Programs (9)
PA (physician advisor) (19)
P&P (policies and procedures) (2, 3)
P and S (permanent and stationary) (9)
PAHCOM (Professional Association of Health Care Office Management) (20)
par (participating [physician or provider]) (4, 6, 8)
PAT (preadmission testing) (19)
PC (professional component) (13)
PCM (primary care manager) (8)
PCP (primary care physician) (5, 11)
PD (permanent disability) (9)
PE or PX (physical examination) (11)
PF (problem focused [level of history or examination]) (11)
PFFS (private fee-for-service [plan]) (6)
PFSH (past, family, or social history) (11)
PH (past history) (11)
PHI (protected health information) (2)
PMS (practice management software or practice management system) (4, 15)
PO (privacy officer or privacy official) (2)
POA (present on admission) (19)
POMR system (problem-oriented medical record system) (11)
POS (place-of-service) (8)
POS machine (point of service machine) (7)
POS plan (point-of-service) (4, 5)
PPACA (Patient Protection and Affordable Care Act) (2, 4)
PPG (physician provider group) (5)
PPO (preferred provider organization) (4, 5)
PPS (prospective payment system) (6, 19)
PS (physical status) (13)
PSO (provider-sponsored organization) (6)
QC (qualifying circumstances) (13)
QI (Qualifying Individuals [program]) (7)
QIC (Qualified Independent Contractor) (16)
QIO (Quality Improvement Organization) (6, 19)
QISMC (Quality Improvement System for Managed Care) (5)
QMB (qualified Medicare beneficiary) (7)
QME (qualified medical evaluator) (9)
RA (remittance advice) (6, 7, 16)
RAC (Recovery Audit Contractor) (3)
RAC Initiative Recovery Audit Contractor Initiative (6)
RBRVS (resource-based relative value scale) (6, 13, 19)
RCM (revenue cycle management) (16)
RCU (respiratory care unit) (11)
RICs (Rehabilitation Impairment Category) (19)
RLQ (right lower quadrant) (11)
RMA (Registered Medical Assistant) (20)
RMC (Registered Medical Coder) (20)
R/O (rule out) (11)
ROA (received on account) (4)
ROM (range-of-motion) (9)
ROS (review of systems) (11)
RUQ (right upper quadrant) (11)
RVS (relative value studies or scale) (13)
RVU (relative value unit) (13)
SCHIP (State Children's Health Insurance Program) (4)
SDHP (Self-Directed Health Plan) (4)
SDI (State Disability Insurance) (4, 10)
SDP (Self-Disclosure Protocol) (3)
SF (straightforward [medical decision making]) (11)
SH (social history) (11)
SHCP (Supplemental Health Care Program) (8)
SHOP (Small Business Health Options Program) (4)
SIF (subsequent-injury fund) (9)
SLMB (Specified Low-Income Medicare Beneficiary) (6)
SOAP (subjective objective assessment plan) (11)
SOF (signature on file) (4, 14)
SOR (source-oriented record [system]) (11)
SSA (Social Security Administration) (10)
SSDI (Social Security Disability Insurance) (10)
SSI (Supplemental Security Income) (6, 7, 10)
SSN (Social Security number) (14)
TANF (Temporary Assistance to Needy Families) (7)
TC (technical component) (13)
TCS (Transaction and Code Set [rule]) (15)
TD (temporary disability) (9)
TDI (temporary disability insurance) (10)
TEFRA (Tax Equity and Fiscal Responsibility Act) (19)
TFL (TRICARE for Life) (8)
TILA (Truth in Lending Act) (17)
TMA (TRICARE Management Activity) (8)
TPO (treatment, payment, or health care operations) (2)
TPR (TRICARE Prime Remote) (8)
TSC (TRICARE service center) (8)
UB-04 (Uniform Bill–04) (19)
UCD (Unemployment Compensation Disability) (4, 10)
UCR (usual, customary, and reasonable) (13)
UM (utilization management (19)
UR (utilization review) (5)
USCIS (US Citizenship and Immigration Services) (20)
VA (Veterans Affairs) (4, 8, 10)
W2 (wage and tax statement) (17)
WC Workers' Compensation (4)
WCAB (Workers' Compensation Appeals Board) (9)
WHO (World Health Organization) (12)
WNL (within normal limits) (11)
WP (waiting period) (9)
ZPIC (Zone Program Integrity Contractor) (3)

GLOSSARY

Chapter number(s) is (are) shown in parentheses after each term.

72-hour rule (19) Medicare policy that states if a patient receives diagnostic tests and hospital outpatient services within 72 hours of admission to a hospital, all such tests and services are combined (bundled) with inpatient services only if services are related to the admission. Also called the 3-day payment window because it is 3 calendar days rather than 72 hours. Sometimes referred to as the 72/24-hour rule.

Abuse (3) Incidents or business practices, not usually considered fraudulent, that are inconsistent with accepted sound medical business or fiscal practices.

Accident (9) An unexpected happening, causing injury traceable to a definite time and place.

Accidental death and dismemberment (10) An insurance policy provision that protects the insured if he or she suffers loss of sight, loss of limb(s), or death by accident.

Accounts receivable (A/R) (17) The total amount of money owed for professional services rendered.

Accounts receivable management (4) The organization and administration of coding and billing in a health care organization or medical practice.

Accredited Standards Committee X12 (ASC X12) (15) The United States standards body formed by the American National Standards Institute (ANSI) for cross-industry development, maintenance, and publication of electronic data exchange standards.

Accredited Standards Committee X12 Version 5010 (15) System developed by the American National Standards Institute (ANSI) that meets Health Insurance Portability and Accountability Act (HIPAA) standards for the transmission of either ICD-9 or ICD-10 diagnostic code data.

Active duty service member (ADSM) (8) An active member of the United States government military services (for example, Army, Navy, Air Force, Marines, Coast Guard).

Acute (11) A medical condition that runs a short but relatively severe course.

Adjudication (6, 9) 1. The process of paying claims submitted or denying them after comparing the claim to benefit and coverage requirements; also known as a claim settlement. 2. In workers compensation cases, final determination of the issues involving settlement of a work-related accident and the rating of a case.

Adjustments (6) An adjustment refers to any change to the balance due of an account such as additional payment, partial payment, courtesy adjustment, write-off, discount, or change made to correct an error in billing or processing of a claim (overpayment or underpayment) or as a result of a retroactive rate change (late charges for a previously submitted bill).

Administrative Law Judge Hearing (ALJ) (16) The third level of Medicare appeals a health care provider may use if they disagree with a claims reconsideration decision. The hearing provides an opportunity to explain your position to an Administrative Law Judge.

Administrative Simplification Compliance Act (ASCA) (14) Legislation enacted by Congress to improve administration of the Medicare program by increasing efficiencies gained through electronic claim submission. The Act required all claims sent to the Medicare program to be submitted electronically.

Administrative Simplification Enforcement Tool (ASET) (15) A web-based tool implemented by the federal government to address issues of noncompliance with the HIPAA by enabling health care providers, payers, clearinghouses and others to submit complaints against a covered entity that fails to adopt and follow the HIPAA rules for transactions and code sets.

Admission (19) Formal acceptance of a patient into the hospital for care.

Admission review (19) A review for appropriateness and necessity of formal acceptance into the hospital for care.

Advance Beneficiary Notice of Noncoverage (ABN) (6) An agreement given to the patient to read and sign before rendering a service if the participating physician thinks it may be denied for payment because of medical necessity or limitation of liability by Medicare. The patient agrees to pay for the service; also known as a waiver of liability agreement or responsibility statement.

Advanced Alternative Payment Model (APM) (6) A system for medical reimbursement that provides additional compensation as an incentive for the delivery of high-quality and more cost-efficient health care by providers.

Adverse effect (12) An unfavorable, detrimental, or pathologic reaction to a drug that occurs when appropriate doses are given to humans for prophylaxis (prevention of disease), diagnosis, and therapy.

Affordable Care Act (ACA) (Obamacare) (4) Health insurance reform signed into law in 2010 to make health care available and affordable to Americans who did not have health insurance.

Against medical advice (AMA) (19) Situations when a patient insists upon leaving the hospital and the physician recommends that the patient needs continued hospitalization.

Age analysis (17) The procedure of systematically arranging the accounts receivable by age, from the date of service.

Aging report (16) Document that reports the status of insurance claims to the provider of the medical services and identifies individual transactions that need to be followed up (e.g., appeal or resubmit a corrected claim).

Allowable charge (8) An amount on which TRICARE figures the patient's cost share for covered care. This is based on 75% to 80% of the allowable charge.

Ambulatory payment classification (APC) (19) A system of outpatient hospital reimbursement based on procedures rather than diagnoses.

American Health Information Management Association (AHIMA) (20) A national professional organization that promotes the art and science of medical record management and improves the quality of comprehensive health information for the welfare of the public.

American Medical Association (AMA) (1) A national professional society of physicians.

American National Standards Institute (ANSI) (15) A private, nonprofit organizations that oversees development of voluntary consensus standards for products, services, processes, systems and personnel in the United States.

American Recovery and Reinvestment Act (ARRA) (2) A fiscal stimulus package that ended the Great Recession and signed into law by President Obama in 2009. Included in ARRA legislation is the Health Information Technology for Economic and Clinical Health (HITECH) Act which contained incentives for adopting health care information technology designed to speed up the adoption of electronic health record system in health care organizations.

Ancillary services (5) Supportive services other than routine hospital services provided by the facility, such as x-ray films and laboratory tests.

Appeal (16) A request for a review of an insurance claim that has been underpaid or denied by an insurance company in an effort to receive additional payment.

Application form (20) A request form to be completed with pertinent data when applying for employment.

Application service provider (ASP) (15) A practice management system available over the internet in which data are housed on the server of the ASP but the accounts are managed by the health care provider's staff.

Approved charges (6) A fee determined by an insurance carrier as to what a medical service is worth, which may or may not be the same as the amount billed. The patient may or may not be responsible for the difference.

Armed Services Disability (10) A disability occurring or aggravated while the patient is in military service.

Assignment (4, 6) In health care, this is an agreement signed by the patient to allow the insurance carrier to send payment directly to the service provider.

Assumption coding (3) Inappropriate assignment of diagnosis or procedure codes based on a review of clinical evidence in a patient's record rather than basing it on information specifically documented by the provider of services.

Attending physician (11) A medical staff member who is legally responsible for the care and treatment given to a patient.

Audit trail (15) Chronologic record of submitted data that can be traced to the source to determine the place or origin. Also referred to as audit log.

Auditing (3) A systemic and objective review of a transaction.

Auditor (20) An individual authorized to review and very the accuracy of business records; auditing titles vary according to what they are monitoring (coding auditor, revenue cycle auditor, compliance auditor).

Authorization (2) Under the Health Insurance Portability and Accountability Act (HIPAA) Privacy Rule, an individual's formal, written permission to use or disclose his or her personally identifiable health information for purposes other than treatment, payment, or health care operations.

Authorization form (2) A document signed by the patient that is needed for use and disclosure of protected health information that is not included in any existing consent form agreements.

Authorized provider (8) A physician or other individual authorized provider of care, or a hospital or supplier approved by TRICARE to provide medical care and supplies.

Automatic stay (17) A court order that goes into effect once a bankruptcy petition is filed; all other legal actions, such as attachments and foreclosures, are halted.

Balance (17) An amount owed on a credit transaction; also known as the outstanding or unpaid balance.

Bankruptcy (17) A condition under which a person or corporation is declared unable to pay debts.

Batch (15) A group of claims for different patients from one office submitted in one computer transmission.

Beneficiary (6, 8) An individual entitled to receive insurance policy or government program health care benefits. Also known as participant, subscriber, dependent, enrollee, or member.

Benefit period (6, 10) 1. A period of time during which payments for Medicare inpatient hospital benefits are available. A benefit period begins on the first day an enrollee is given inpatient hospital care (nursing care or rehabilitation services) by a qualified provider and ends when the enrollee has not been an inpatient for 60 consecutive days. 2. In workers' compensation cases, the maximum amount of time that benefits will be paid to the injured or ill person for the disability. 3. For disability insurance, the maximum amount of time that benefits will be paid to the injured or ill person for a disability.

Benign tumor (12) An abnormal growth that does not have the properties of invasion and metastasis and is usually surrounded by a fibrous capsule; also called a neoplasm.

Bilateral (13) When coding surgical procedures, this term refers to both sides of the body.

Birthday rule (4) An informal rule that the health insurance industry has adopted for the coordination of benefits when children are listed as dependents on two parents' health plans. Under the birthday rule, the health plan of the parent whose birthday comes first in the calendar year is designated as the primary plan.

Blanket contract (4) Comprehensive group insurance coverage through plans sponsored by professional associations for their members.

Blind mailing (20) To send a résumé with a cover letter to possible prospects whom the individual does not know personally and who have not advertised for a job opening.

Blue Cross/Blue Shield Association (5) A national association of approximately 36 independent, community-based and locally operated Blue/Cross/Blue Shield companies providing some form of health insurance in every state within the U.S. and a program for U.S. federal employees, retirees and their families.

Bonding (17) An insurance contract by which, in return for a stated fee, a bonding agency guarantees payment of a certain sum to an employer in the event of a financial loss to the employer by the act of a specified employee or by some contingency over which the employer has no control.

Breach of confidential communication (2) Breach means "breaking or violation of a law or agreement." In the context of the medical office, it means the unauthorized release of information about the patient.

Buffing (5) A physician's justifying the transference of sick, high-cost patients to other physicians in a managed care plan.

Bundled codes (13) To group more than one component (service or procedure) into one Current Procedural Terminology (CPT) code.

Business associate (2) A person who, on behalf of the covered entity, performs or assists in the performance of a function or activity involving the use or disclosure of individually identifiable health information, including claims processing or administration, data analysis, process or administration, utilization review, quality assurance, billing, benefit management, practice management, and repricing.

Business associate agreement (15, 20) Contract between the provider and a clearinghouse that submits the electronic claims on behalf of the provider.

Cable modem (15) A modem used to connect a computer to a cable television system that offers online services.

Cancelable (4) A renewal provision in an insurance agreement that grants the insurer the right to cancel the policy at any time and for any reason.

Capitation (4, 5, 19) A system of payment used by managed care plans in which physicians and hospitals are paid a fixed per capita amount for each patient enrolled over a stated period of time, regardless of the type and number of services provided; reimbursement to the hospital on a per-member/per-month basis to cover costs for the members of the plan. Capitation can also mean a set amount to be paid per claim.

Carcinoma in situ (12) Cancer confined to the site of origin without invasion of neighboring tissues.

Carve outs (5) Medical services not included within the capitation rate as benefits of a managed care contract and that may be contracted for separately.

Case mix groups (CMG) (19) A patient classification system to group together patients with similar characteristics (such as functional motor and cognitive scores and age) as a basis for describing the types of patients a hospital or other health care provider treats.

Cash flow (1, 17) In a health care organization or medical practice, the amount of actual cash generated and available for use within a given period of time.

Catastrophic cap (8) The maximum dollar amount that a member has to pay under TRICARE or CHAMPVA in any fiscal year or enrollment period for covered medical bills.

Catchment area (8) In the TRICARE program, an area, defined by zip codes, that is approximately 40 miles in radius surrounding each United States military treatment facility.

Categorically needy (7) Aged, blind, or disabled individuals or families and children who meet financial eligibility requirements for Aid to Families with Dependent Children (AFDC), Supplemental Security Income (SSI), or an optional state supplement.

Centers for Medicare and Medicaid Services (CMS) (6) A federal agency within the U.S. Department of Health and Human Services (DHHS), who administers the Medicare program. They are responsible for implementation of all rules, regulations and health related policies governing the Medicare program.

Certification (20) A statement issued by a board or association verifying that a person meets professional standards.

Certified Coding Specialist (CCS) (20) A title received by a person after appropriate training and by passing a certification examination administered by the American Health Information Management Association (AHIMA) for hospital-based coding.

Certified Coding Specialist–Physician (CCS-P) (20) A title received by a person after appropriate training and by passing a certification examination administered by the American Health Information Management Association (AHIMA) for physician-based coding.

Certified Medical Assistant (CMA) (20) A title received by a person after appropriate training and by passing a certification examination administered by the American Association of Medical Assistants (AAMA).

Certified Medical Billing Specialist (CMBS) (20) A title received by a person after appropriate training and by passing a certification examination administered by either the American Association of Medical Billers (AAMB) or the Medical Association of Billers (MAB).

Certified Professional Coder (CPC) (20) A title received by a person after appropriate training and the passing of a certification examination administered by the American Academy of Professional Coders (AAPC).

CHAMPVA (4, 8) See Veterans Health Administration.

Chargemaster (19) A list or database of all the services, supplies, equipment, and so forth provided by the hospital and the charge that is associated with it. Other data elements in the chargemaster include a unique identifier for each item, the department providing the service, a revenue code, and the procedure codes (discussed later in this section). Also called a charge description master.

Chargemaster Coordinator (20) An individual who oversees managing the contents of the chargemaster including tasks such as updating codes, adding new services, deleted services no longer provided, updating charges and working with the clinical services, billers, financial department and others to ensure the entries in the chargemaster meets their needs.

Chief complaint (CC) (11, 12) A patient's statement describing symptoms, problems, or conditions as the reason for seeking health care services from a physician.

Children's Health Insurance Program (CHIP) (7) A partnership between the federal and state governments that provides low-cost health coverage to children in families that earn too much money to qualify for Medicaid. In some states, CHIP also covers care for pregnant women.

Chronic (11) A medical condition persisting over a long period of time.

Chronologic résumé (20) A data sheet that outlines experience and education by dates.

Churning (5) When physicians see a high volume of patients—more than medically necessary—to increase revenue. May be seen in fee-for-service or managed care environments.

Civil False Claims Act (3) Legislation authorizing the United Stated federal government to recover monetary damages from people who file fraudulent claims for payment with the federal government.

Civil Monetary Penalty (CMP) (3) Federal statute that imposes fines and sanctions to combat health care fraud and abuse and is imposed on individuals or health care facilities that do not comply with the Centers for Medicare and Medicaid Services (CMS) regulations.

Civil Service Retirement System (CSRS) (10) A program for federal employees who work in civil service and become totally disabled.

Civilian Health and Medical Program of the Department of Veterans Affairs (CHAMPVA) (8) See Veterans Health Administration.

Claim (4) A bill sent to an insurance carrier requesting payment for services rendered; also known as encounter record.

Claim attachments (15) Documents that contain information, hard copy or electronic, related to a completed insurance claim that assists in validating the medical necessity or explains the medical service or procedure for payment (for example, operative report, discharge summary, invoice).

Claim denial management (16) The process of identifying and reviewing specific reasons for claim denials, followed by development of a process for appealing denied claims when appropriate.

Claims assistance professional (CAP) (1) A practitioner who works for the consumer and helps patients to organize, complete, file, and negotiate health insurance claims of all types to obtain maximum benefits as well as tells patients what checks to write to providers to eliminate overpayment.

Claims examiner (1, 9) A representative of the insurer who authorizes treatment and investigates, evaluates, and negotiates the patient's insurance claim and acts for the company in the settlement of claims; also known as claims adjuster, claims representative, and claims administrator.

Clean claim (14) A completed insurance claim form submitted within the program time limit that contains all necessary information without deficiencies so that it can be processed and paid promptly.

Clearinghouse (2, 15) An independent organization that receives insurance claims from a health care organization or a physician's office, performs software edits, and redistributes the claims electronically to various insurance carriers.

Clinical documentation improvement (11) The process of creating accurate and effective patient health records in an effort to improve patient outcomes, provide accurate data for quality measurement reporting, and to ensure proper reimbursement.

Clinical Documentation Improvement Specialist (20) An individual who works with physicians and other health care professionals to ensure that the documentation in the health record is complete and granular (at the appropriate level of detail).

Clinical Laboratory Improvement Amendments (CLIA) (3) Legislation which ensures quality lab testing through certification requirements for health care laboratories.

Cloned note (11) 1. Entry in a patient's medical record worded exactly like or similar to the previous entries. 2. Medical documentation that is worded exactly the same from patient to patient. Cloned notes are considered a misrepresentation of the medical necessity requirements for insurance coverage of medical services and can trigger audits.

Clustering (3) Reporting one level of service for all patient visits, regardless of the patient's presenting problem or the amount of work or time spent with the patient.

Code sets (15) Any set of codes with their descriptions used to encode data elements, such as tables of terms, medical concepts, medical diagnostic codes, or medical procedure codes.

Coding Specialist (20) An individual trained in assigning review health record documentation and extract the appropriate diagnosis and procedure codes that will be reported on the insurance claim.

Coinsurance (4, 5, 7) A cost-sharing requirement under a health insurance policy in which the insured will assume a percentage of the costs for covered services.

Collateral (17) Any possession, such as an automobile, furniture, stocks, or bonds, that secures or guarantees the discharge of an obligation.

Collection ratio (17) The relationship between the amount of money owed and the amount of money collected in reference to the doctor's accounts receivable.

Combination code (12) A code from one section of the procedural code book combined with a code from another section that is used to completely describe a procedure performed; in diagnostic coding, a single five-digit code used to identify etiology and secondary process (manifestation) or complication of a disease.

Combination résumé (20) A data sheet that combines specific dates or work experience with educational skills.

Comorbidity (11, 19) An ongoing condition that exists along with the condition for which the patient is receiving treatment; regarding diagnosis-related groups (DRGs), a preexisting condition that, because of its presence with a certain principal diagnosis, causes an increase in length of stay by at least 1 day in approximately 75% of cases. Also known as substantial comorbidity.

Competitive Medical Plan (CMP) (4) A type of managed care organization created by the 1982 Tax Equity and Fiscal Responsibility Act to facilitate the enrollment of Medicare beneficiaries into managed care plans. CMPs are organized and financed much like HMOs but are not bound by all the regulatory requirements HMOs must deal with.

Compliance (3) A process of meeting regulations, recommendations, and expectations of federal and state agencies that pay for health care services and regulate the industry.

Compliance plan (3) A management plan composed of policies and procedures to accomplish uniformity, consistency, and conformity in medical record keeping that fulfills official requirements.

Compliance Specialist (20) An individual who is responsible for the development and management of the health care organization's compliance with federal and state laws. Tasks include development of policies and procedures, auditing and monitoring, ensuring the programs are being followed, identifying risk areas and compliance issues, and developing corrective actions to be taken.

Complication/comorbidity (CC) (12, 19) A disease or condition arising during the course of or as a result of another disease modifying medical care requirements; for diagnosis-related groups (DRGs), a condition that arises during the hospital stay that prolongs the length of stay by at least 1 day in approximately 75% of cases. Also known as substantial complication. Also see Comorbidity.

Comprehensive (C) (11) A term used to describe a level of history or physical examination.

Comprehensive code (13) A single procedural code that describes or covers two or more CPT component codes that are bundled together as one unit.

Comprehensive Error Rate Testing (CERT (3) An audit program implemented by CMS to measure the accuracy of payments made by Medicare Administrative Contractors (MACs) and to identify OIG target issues.

Compromise and release (C and R) (8) An agreement arrived at, whether in or out of court, for settling a workers' compensation case after the patient has been declared permanent and stationary.

Computer-assisted coding (CAC) (12) Use of computer software that automatically generates a set of medical codes for review, validation, and use based on clinical documentation provided by health care practitioners. CAC uses two technology options: natural language processing (NLP) and structured input.

Concurrent care (11) The provision of similar services (for example, hospital visits) to the same patient by more than one physician on the same day. Usually a separate physical disorder is present.

Concurrent review (19) An evaluation of health care services to determine medical necessity and appropriateness of the care provided during the time services are being provided.

Conditionally renewable (4) An insurance policy renewal provision that grants the insurer a limited right to refuse to renew a health insurance policy at the end of a premium payment period.

Confidential communication (2) A privileged communication that may be disclosed only with the patient's permission.

Confidentiality (2) The state of treating privately or secretly, and not disclosing to other individuals or for public knowledge, the patient's conversations or medical records.

Consent (2) Verbal or written agreement that gives approval to some action, situation, or statement.

Consultation (11) Services rendered by a physician whose opinion or advice is requested by another physician or agency in the evaluation or treatment of a patient's illness or suspected problem.

Consultative examiner (CE) (10) A physician who is paid a fee to examine or test a person for disability under either the Social Security Disability Insurance (SSDI) or Supplemental Security Income (SSI) program.

Consulting physician (11) A provider whose opinion or advice about evaluation or management of a specific problem is requested by another physician.

Consumer Directed Health Plan (CDHP) (4) Type of health insurance that allows the consumer to design and customize the plan based on their specific needs and circumstances. Also referred to as Self-Directed Health Plan (SDHP).

Continued stay review (19) Examination of a patient's health records to determine whether or not the patient should stay in the hospital.

Continuing education (CE) (20) Formal education pursued by a working professional and intended to improve or maintain professional competence.

Continuity of care (11) When a physician sees a patient who has received treatment for a condition and is referred by the previous doctor for treatment of the same condition.

Contract (4) A legally enforceable agreement when relating to an insurance policy; for workers' compensation cases, an agreement involving two or more parties in which each is obligated to the other to fulfill promises made. (The contract exists between the physician and the insurance carrier.)

Conventions (12) Rules or principles for determining a diagnostic code when using diagnostic code books, such as each space, typefaces, indentations, punctuation marks, instructional notes, abbreviations, cross-reference notes, and specific usage of the words "and," "with," and "due to." These rules assist in the selection of correct codes for the diagnoses encountered.

Conversion factor (13) The dollars and cents amount that is established for one unit as applied to a procedure or service rendered. This unit is then used to convert various procedures into fee-schedule payment amounts by multiplying the relative value unit by the conversion factor.

Conversion privilege (4) An element of some group insurance policies which allow an insured to continue coverage under an individual policy if they are leaving the employer or organization or if the group contract is terminated.

Cooperative care (8) A term used when a patient is seen by a civilian physician or hospital for services cost-shared by TRICARE.

Coordination of benefits (COB) (4, 8) Two insurance carriers working together and coordinating the payment of their benefits so that there is no duplication of benefits paid between the primary and secondary insurance carriers.

Copayment (copay) (4, 5, 7) A type of cost-sharing that requires the patient to pay a predetermined fee to the health care provider at the time the service is rendered.

Correct Coding Initiative (CCI) (6) Federal legislation that attempts to eliminate unbundling or other inappropriate reporting of procedural codes for professional medical services rendered to patients.

Corrective action plan (3) A step by step plan of action that is developed to achieve resolution to errors or offenses that have been identified in a health care organization.

Cost-of-living adjustment (10) A disability insurance provision to increase monthly benefits.

Cost outlier (19) A typical case that has an extraordinarily high cost when compared with most discharges classified to the same diagnostic cost group (DCG).

Cost report (3) A summary of information CMS requires institutional health care providers to submit annually which identify operating costs.

Cost share (8) The portion of the allowable charges (20% or 25%) after the deductible has been met that the TRICARE patient is responsible for.

Counseling (11) A discussion between the physician and a patient, family, or both concerning the diagnosis, recommended studies or tests, prognosis, risks, and benefits of treatment, treatment options, patient and family education, and so on.

Cover letter (20) A letter of introduction prepared to accompany a résumé when seeking a job.

Covered entity (2, 15, 19) An entity that transmits health information in electronic form in connection with a transaction covered by the Health Insurance Portability and Accountability Act (HIPAA). The covered entity may be (1) a health care coverage carrier such as Blue Cross/Blue Shield, (2) a health care clearinghouse through which claims are submitted, or (3) a health care provider, such as a primary care physician (PCP), a hospital, or nursing home.

Covered services (7) Specific services and supplies for which Medicaid will provide reimbursement; these consist of a combination of mandatory and optional services as stated in the state's Medicaid plan.

Credit (17) 1. From the Latin *credere,* meaning "to believe" or "to trust"; trust regarding financial obligation. 2. Accounting entry reflecting payment by a debtor (patient) of a sum received on his or her account.

Credit card (17) A card issued by an organization and devised for the purpose of obtaining money, property, labor, or services on credit.

Creditor (17) A person to whom money is owed.

Criminal False Claims Act (3) Legislation enacted stating that anyone who knowingly makes or presents a false or fraudulent claim to any department or agency of the United States shall be imprisoned up to 5 years and shall be subject to a fine.

Critical care (11) In reference to coding professional services, this phrase relates to intensive care provided in a variety of acute life-threatening conditions requiring constant bedside attention by a physician.

Crossover claim (6) A bill for services rendered to a patient receiving benefits simultaneously from Medicare and Medicaid or from Medicare and a Medigap plan. Medicare pays first and then determines the amount of unmet Medicare deductible and coinsurance to be paid by the secondary insurance carrier. The claim is automatically transferred (electronically) to the secondary insurance carrier for additional payment. Also known as claims transfer.

Current Procedural Terminology (CPT) (13) A reference procedural code book using a five-digit numeric system to identify and code procedures established by the American Medical Association (AMA).

Customary fee (13) The amount a physician usually charges most of her or his patients.

Cycle (1) A complete set of events that are repeated on a regular basis.

Cycle billing (17) A system of billing accounts at spaced intervals during the month based on a breakdown of accounts by alphabet, account number, insurance type, or date of first service.

Data elements (15) Medical code sets used uniformly to document why patients are seen (diagnosis, ICD-10-CM) and what is done to them during their encounter (procedure, CPT-4, HCPCS).

Daysheet (4) A register for recording daily business transactions (charges, payments, or adjustments); also known as daybook, daily log, or daily record sheet.

Debit card (17) A card permitting bank customers to withdraw from any affiliated automated teller machine (ATM) and make cashless purchases from funds on deposit without incurring revolving finance charges for credit.

Debt (17) A legal obligation to pay money.

Debtor (17) A person owing money.

Deductible (4, 5) A type of cost-sharing that requires a specific dollar amount to be paid by the insured before a medical insurance plan or government program begins covering health care costs.

Defense Enrollment Eligibility Reporting System (DEERS) (8) An electronic database used to verify beneficiary eligibility for individuals in the TRICARE programs.

Degaussing (11) Method to dispose of confidential or sensitive information by use of electromagnetic fields to erase data.

Deleted claim (14) Insurance claim that has been canceled, deleted, or voided by a Medicare fiscal intermediary for the following reasons: CMS-1500 (08-05) or current CMS-1450 is not used, itemized charges are not provided, more than six line items are submitted on the CMS-1500 (08-05) claim form, patient's address is missing, internal clerical error was made, Certificate of Medical Necessity (CMN) was not with the Part B claim or was incomplete or invalid, and name of the store is not on the receipt that includes the price of the item.

Delinquent claim (16) An insurance claim submitted to an insurance company, for which payment is overdue.

Denied claim (16) An insurance claim submitted to an insurance company in which payment has been rejected owing to a technical error or because of medical coverage policy issues.

Department of Veterans Affairs (8) The federal agency that oversees health care services to military veterans and determines eligibility of beneficiaries.

Deposition (8) The process of taking sworn testimony from a witness out of court. This is usually done by an attorney.

Designated record sets (2) A specific set of information that is maintained by a health care organization on behalf of a patient which may include health records, billing and claim records, and health plan enrollment records. This information is used to make decisions about a patient.

Detailed (D) (11) A term used to describe a level of history or physical examination.

Diagnosis-related group (DRG) (19) A patient classification system that categorizes patients who are medically related with respect to diagnosis and treatment and statistically similar in length of hospital stay. Medicare hospital insurance payments are based on fixed dollar amounts for a principal diagnosis as listed in DRGs.

Diagnostic creep (DRG creep) (3, 19) Coding that is inappropriately altered to obtain a higher payment rate; also known as coding creep, DRG creep, or upcoding.

Digital subscriber line (DSL) (15) A high-speed connection through a telephone line jack; usually a means of accessing the internet.

Direct data entry (DDE) (15) Keying claim information directly into the payer system by accessing over modem dial-up or digital subscriber line (DSL). This is a technology to directly enter the information into the payer system via the access, whether it is dial-up or DSL.

Direct referral (5) Certain services in a managed care plan may not require preauthorization. The authorization request form is completed and signed by the physician and handed to the patient (for example, obstetric care or dermatology) to be done directly.

Dirty claim (14) A claim submitted with errors or one that requires manual processing to resolve problems or is rejected for payment.

Disability Determination Services (DDS) (10) A state Social Security division office that assesses a case for disability benefits.

Disability income insurance (4, 10) A form of health insurance that provides periodic payments to replace income when the insured is unable to work as a result of illness, injury, or disease and not as a result of a work-related accident or condition.

Disabled (6) An individual who is impaired or limited by a physical, mental, cognitive or developmental condition or incapacitated by illness or injury.

Discharge (19) Occurs when the physician writes an order releasing the patient from the hospital. This order should include where the patient should go. Possible locations include home, home with home health, another acute care hospital, rehabilitation, and more.

Discharge disposition (19) The location where the patient is being discharged to (home, nursing facility, etc.).

Discharge not final billed (DNCB) (19) A list of all hospital (inpatient and outpatient) claims that have not been submitted to the insurer due to a number of reasons such as: not coded, missing data, still in window of time waiting for late charges, missing discharge disposition, and more.

Disclosure (2) The release, transfer, provision of access to, or divulging in any other manner of information outside the entity holding the information.

Discount (17) A reduction of a normal charge based on a specific amount of money or a percentage of the charge.

Discounting (19) The reduction of APC reimbursement to the hospital occurring for a number of reasons such as, surgery is cancelled, or more than 1 surgery is performed at an operative session.

Disenrollment (5) A member's voluntary cancellation of membership in a managed care plan.

Documentation (11) 1. A chronologic detailed recording of pertinent facts and observations about a patient's health as seen in chart notes and medical reports; entries in the medical record, such as prescription refills, telephone calls, and other pertinent data. 2. For computer software, a user's guide to a program or piece of equipment.

Donut hole (6) A temporary limit on what a Medicare drug will pay. The coverage gap begins after the patient and the drug plan together have spent a certain amount for covered drugs.

Double indemnity (10) A feature in some life and disability insurance policies that provides for twice the face amount of the policy to be paid if death results to the insured from accidental causes.

Downcoding (13, 19) The practice of reporting a code for a lower level of care when the health record would support a higher level. This also occurs when the insurance carrier processing the claim converts the code submitted to a lower level of service, generating decreased payment.

DRG creep (3, 19) Slang expression for diagnostic creep. See Diagnostic creep.

Dun message (17) A message or phrase to inform or remind a patient about a delinquent account.

Durable medical equipment (DME) (6, 13, 14) Any equipment that provides therapeutic benefits to a patient in need because of certain medical conditions and/or illnesses.

Early and Periodic Screening, Diagnosis, and Treatment (EPSDT) (7) The EPSDT program covers screening and diagnostic services to determine physical or mental defects in recipients younger than 21 years of age and health care, treatment, and other measures to correct or ameliorate any defects and chronic conditions discovered. In New York, this is called the Child Health Assurance Program (CHAP).

Electronic claim (14) Digital files that are not printed on paper claim forms when submitted to the payer; instead, claims are submitted using a central processing unit (CPU), tape, diskette, direct data entry, direct wire, dial-in telephone, digital fax, or personal computer download or upload.

Electronic data interchange (EDI) (15) The process by which understandable data items are sent back and forth via computer linkages between two or more entities that function alternatively as sender and receiver.

Electronic funds transfer (EFT) (15) A paperless computerized system that enables funds to be debited, credited, or transferred, eliminating the need for personal handling of checks.

Electronic health record (EHR) (11) A patient record that is created using a computer with software. A template is brought up and by answering a series of questions, data are entered.

Electronic mail (1) Electronic message that is transmitted, received, stored, or forwarded text, voice messages, attachments, or images by computer from one person to another or from one person to a defined group or all users on a system.

Electronic media (2) The mode of electronic transmission (for example, internet, extranet, leased phone or dial-up phone lines, fax modems).

Electronic remittance advice (ERA) (15) An online transaction about the status of a claim.

Emancipated minor (4) A person younger than 18 years of age who lives independently, is totally self-supporting, and possesses decision-making rights.

Embezzlement (3, 17) A willful act by an employee of taking possession of an employer's money.

Emergency (8) A sudden and unexpected medical condition, or the worsening of a condition, that poses a threat to life, limb, or sight and requires immediate treatment to alleviate suffering (for example, shortness of breath, chest pain, drug overdose).

Emergency care (11) Health care services provided to prevent serious impairment of bodily functions or serious dysfunction to any body organ or part. Advanced life support may be necessary. Not all care provided in an emergency department of a hospital can be termed "emergency care."

Emergency department (13) Defined by CPT as an organized hospital-based facility, open 24 hours day, 7 days per week; for the provision of unscheduled episodic services to patients who present for immediate medical attention.

Emergency Medical Treatment and Labor Act (EMTALA) (3) Legislation requiring that anyone who comes to an emergency room, or is in active labor, be evaluated and stabilized regardless of their ability to pay.

Employer identification number (EIN) (14) An individual's federal tax identification number issued by the Internal Revenue Service (IRS) for income tax purposes.

Employment agency (20) A business organization that refers job applicants to potential employers.

Encoder (15) An add-on software program to practice management systems that can reduce the time it takes to build or review insurance claims before batch transmission to the carrier.

Encryption (15) To assign a code to represent data. This is done for security purposes.

End-stage renal disease (ESRD) (6) End-stage renal disease occurs when a patient who has chronic kidney disease has gradual loss of kidney function and reaches an advanced state; the kidneys are no longer able to work as they should to meet the body's needs.

Eponym (11, 12) The name of a disease, anatomic structure, operation, or procedure, usually derived from the name of a place where it first occurred or a person who discovered or first described it.

Errors and omissions insurance (1) A type of insurance that provides protection against loss of money caused by failure through error or unintentional omission on the part of the individual or service involved in any aspect of preparation or submission of an insurance claim.

Ergonomic (8) Science and technology that seek to fit the anatomic and physical needs of the worker to the workplace.

Essential modifiers (12) In ICD-10-CM, subterms that are indented two spaces to the right under main terms. They are referred to as essential modifiers because their presence changes the diagnostic code assignment.

Established patient (11) An individual who has received professional services within the past 3 years from the physician or another physician of the same specialty who belongs to the same group practice.

Estate administrator (17) One who takes possession of the assets of a decedent, pays the expenses of administration and the claims of creditors, and disposes of the balance of an estate in accordance with the statutes governing the distribution of decedent's estates.

Estate executor (17) One who takes possession of the assets of a decedent, pays the expenses of administration and the claims of creditors, and disposes of the balance of an estate in accordance with the decedent's will.

Ethics (1) Standards of conduct generally accepted as a moral guide for behavior by which an insurance billing or coding specialist may determine the appropriateness of his or her conduct in a relationship with patients, the physician, co-workers, the government, and insurance companies.

Etiology (12) The cause of disease; the study of the cause of a disease.

Etiquette (1) Customs, rules of conduct, courtesy, and manners of the medical profession.

Exchanges (4) Organized marketplace where uninsured individuals and small-business owners can find health insurance coverage and select from all of the qualified health plans available in their area. Also referred to as *Health Benefit Exchanges.*

Excludes 1 (12) Word with number that is one of the conventions used in the diagnostic code book titled *International Classification of Diseases,* Tenth Revision, Clinical Modification (ICD-10-CM). This indicates that the code excluded should never be used at the same time as the code above the Excludes 1 note. An Excludes 1 is when two conditions cannot occur together (for example, congenital form versus acquired form of a condition). A note instructs the reader to go to another code for the excluded condition.

Excludes 2 (12) Word with number that is one of the conventions used in the diagnostic code book titled *International Classification of Diseases,* Tenth Revision, Clinical Modification (ICD-10-CM). This note represents "Not included here" and indicates that the condition excluded is not part of the condition represented by the code but a patient may have both conditions at the same time. When an Excludes 2 note appears under a code, it is acceptable to use both the code and the excluded code together.

Exclusion(s) (4, 10) Provisions written into the insurance contract denying coverage or limiting the scope of coverage.

Exclusive provider organization (EPO) (4, 5) A type of managed health care plan that combines features of health maintenance organizations (HMOs) and preferred provider organizations (PPOs). It is referred to as "exclusive" because it is offered to large employers who agree not to contract with any other plan. EPOs are regulated under state health insurance laws.

Expanded problem focused (EPF) (11) A phrase used to describe a level of history or physical examination.

Explanation of benefits (EOB) (16) A document detailing services billed and describing payment determinations; also known in Medicare, Medicaid, and some other programs as a remittance advice (RA). In the TRICARE program, it is called a summary payment voucher.

Expressed contract (4) A verbal or written agreement.

External audit (11) A review done after claims have been submitted (retrospective review) of medical and financial records by an insurance company or Medicare representative to investigate suspected fraud or abusive billing practices.

External causes of morbidity (12) Classification of codes used for external causes of injury rather than disease. The code description refers to the circumstances that caused an injury rather than the nature of the injury. The codes are also used in coding adverse reactions to medications.

Extraterritorial (8) State laws effective outside the state by either specific provision or court decision. In workers' compensation cases, benefits under the state law that apply to a compensable injury of an employee hired in one state but injured outside that state.

Facility billing (1) Charging for services done in hospitals, acute care hospitals, skilled nursing or long-term care facilities, rehabilitation centers, or ambulatory surgical centers.

Facility provider number (14) A facility's (hospital, laboratory, radiology office, or nursing facility) provider number to be used by the facility to bill for services, or by the performing physician to report services done at that location.

Family history (FH) (11) A review of medical events in the patient's family, including diseases that may be hereditary or place the patient at risk.

Federal Deposit Insurance Corporation (FDIC) (3) Fraud and abuse laws associated with mailing and wiring of money or property.

Federal Employees' Compensation Act (FECA) (8) An Act instituted in 1908 providing benefits for on-the-job injuries to all federal employees.

Federal Employees Retirement System (FERS) (10) A retirement program for federal employees hired after 1984 or those hired before 1984 who switched from Civil Service Retirement System (CSRS) to FERS.

Federal poverty level (FPL) (7) A measure of income issued every year by the Department of Health and Human Services found in the *Federal Register;* used to determine eligibility for certain Medicaid programs.

Fee-for-service (FFS) (4, 5) A method of payment in which the patient pays the health care organization or provider for service performed from an established schedule of fees.

Fee schedule (13, 17) A list of charges or established allowances for specific medical services and procedures. See also Relative value studies (RVS).

Financial accounting record (17) An individual record indicating charges, payments, adjustments, and balances owed for services rendered; also known as a ledger.

Fiscal agent (7) An organization under contract to the state to process claims for a state Medicaid program.

Flexible Spending Account (4) An employee sponsored health plan which allows individuals to put aside a certain amount of wages for qualified medical expenses and dependent care. The amount is not subject to payroll taxes.

Formal referral (5) An authorization request (telephone, fax, or completed form) required by the managed care organization contract to determine medical necessity and grant permission before services are rendered or procedures performed.

Formulary (6) List of drugs that a health insurance plan covers as a benefit.

Fraud (3) An intentional misrepresentation of the facts to deceive or mislead another.

Fraud Enforcement and Recovery Act (FERA) (3) Legislation enacted in 2009 with a principal objective to increase enforcement and oversight of fraud and to provide the federal government with tools to investigate and prosecute violators.

Functional résumé (20) A data sheet that highlights qualifications and skills.

Future purchase option (10) See Cost-of-living adjustment.

Garnishment (17) A court order attaching a debtor's property or wages to pay off a debt.

Gatekeeper (5, 19) In the managed care system, this is the physician who controls patient access to specialists and diagnostic testing services.

Global surgery policy (13) A coding policy relating to surgical procedures in which preoperative and postoperative visits (24 hours before [major] and day of [minor]), usual intraoperative services, and complications not requiring additional trips to the operating room are included in one CPT code and reimbursed as one fee.

Group National Provider Identifier (group NPI) (14) A number assigned to a group of physicians submitting insurance claims under the group name and reporting income under one name.

Group practice model (5) Multispecialty physician group practices who contract with a managed care insurance company to provide all physician services to its' members. Physician are employed by the group practice.

Grouper (19) The computer software program that assigns diagnosis-related groups (DRGs) of discharged patients using the following information: patient's age, sex, principal diagnosis, complications/comorbid conditions, principal procedure, and discharge status.

Guaranteed renewable (4, 10) A clause in an insurance policy that means the insurance company must renew the policy as long as premium payments are made. However, the premium may be increased when it is renewed. These policies may have age limits of 60, 65, or 70 years or may be renewable for life.

Guarantor (4) An individual who promises to pay the medical bill by signing a form agreeing to pay or who accepts treatment, which constitutes an expressed promise.

Health benefits advisor (HBA) (8) An individual at military hospitals or clinics who is there to help TRICARE beneficiaries obtain medical care through the military and through TRICARE.

Healthcare and Education Reconciliation Act (HCERA) (4) Legislation enacted in 2010 and divided into two titles, one addressing health care reform and the other addressing student loan reform. The Act modified certain provisions of PPACA.

Health care finder (HCF) (8) Health care professionals, generally registered nurses, who are located at TRICARE service centers (TSCs) to act as a liaison between military and civilian providers, verify eligibility, determine availability of services, coordinate care, facilitate the transfer of records, and perform first level medical review. HCFs help TRICARE beneficiaries and providers with preauthorization of medical services.

Healthcare Common Procedure Coding System (HCPCs) (13) A coding system developed by the Medicare Program for reporting physician or supplier services and procedures; consists of 2 levels of coding: Level 1 (CPT codes) and Level II (National Codes).

Healthcare Fraud and Abuse Control (HCFAC) (3) A program under the joint direction of the Attorney General and the Secretary of the DHHS acting through the department's Inspector General (DHHS/OIG) to coordinate federal, state and local law enforcement activities to combat health care fraud and abuse.

Healthcare Fraud Prevention and Enforcement Action Team (HEAT) (3) Group created in 2009 by the Department of Justice and the Department of Health and Human Services to build and strengthen programs to combat Medicare and Medicaid fraud and to crack down on fraud perpetrators.

Healthcare organization (2) A group of healthcare professionals that provide medical or health services.

Health care provider (2) A provider of medical or health services.

Health Information Technology for Economic and Clinical Health Act (HITECH) (2) A provision of the ARRA which strengthened the patient privacy protections and security responsibilities of covered entities that were already established under HIPAA.

Health insurance (4) A contract between the policyholder or member and insurance carrier or government program to reimburse the policyholder or member for all or a portion of the cost of medical care rendered by health care professionals; generic term applying to lost income arising from illness or injury; also known as accident and health insurance or disability income insurance.

Health Insurance Claim Form (CMS-1500) (14) Known as CMS-1500. A universal insurance claim form developed and approved by the American Medical Association (AMA) Council on Medical Service and the Centers for Medicare and Medicaid Services (CMS). It is used by physicians and other professionals to bill outpatient services and supplies to TRICARE, Medicare, and some Medicaid programs as well as some private insurance carriers and managed care plans.

Health Insurance Portability and Accountability Act (HIPAA) (2, 19) A federal law that is made up of five titles and mandated a number of requirements including the privacy and security of protected health information. It also established standards for the sharing of data for administrative purposes.

Health maintenance organization (HMO) (4, 5) A medical insurance group that provides coverage of health services for a prepaid, fixed annual fee.

Health record (11) Written or graphic information documenting facts and events during the rendering of patient care.

Health Reimbursement Account (HRA) (4) A type of health plan which allows the employer to own the account and only the employer is eligible to make contributions. These plans are usually offered in tandem with high-deductible health plans.

Health Savings Account (HSA) (4) A type of savings account that lets you set aside money on a pre-tax basis to pay for qualified medical expenses such as deductibles, copayments and coinsurances.

Hearing (10) The second level of the appeal process for an individual applying for Social Security Disability Insurance (SSDI) or Supplemental Security Income (SSI). This is a hearing before an administrative law judge who had no part in the initial or reconsideration disability determination.

High complexity (HC) (11) A phrase used to describe a type of medical decision making when a patient is seen for an evaluation and management (E/M) service.

HIPAA Omnibus Rule Regulation that became effective in 2013 under the Health Insurance Portability and Accountability Act (HIPAA) that modified privacy and security rules for covered entities and their business associates.

HIPAA Transaction and Code Set (TCS) rule (15) This regulation under the Health Insurance Portability and Accountability Act (HIPAA) defines the standardized methods for transmitting electronic health information. The TCS process includes any set of HIPAA-approved codes with their descriptions used to encode data elements, such as tables of terms, medical concepts, medical diagnostic codes, or medical procedure codes. TCS regulations were implemented to streamline electronic data interchange.

History of present illness (HPI) (11) A chronologic description of the development of the patient's present illness from the first sign or symptom or from the previous encounter to the present.

Hospice (6) A public agency or private organization primarily engaged in providing pain relief, symptom management, and supportive services to terminally ill patients and their families in their own homes or in a homelike center.

Hospital acquired condition (HAC) (19) A number of conditions identified by CMS that indicate a quality of care issue if the patient developed these conditions while an inpatient at an acute care hospital. Some of these conditions include administration of wrong blood type, foreign body left in patient during surgery, trauma due to fall, and air embolism. If a patient developed one of the conditions while in the hospital, the hospital is not reimbursed by Medicare a higher weighted Medicare-Severity Diagnosis Related Group.

Hospital insurance (6) A program providing basic protection against the costs of hospital and related after-hospital services for individuals eligible under the Medicare program. Known as Medicare Part A.

Implied contract (4) A contract between physician and patient not manifested by direct words but implied or deduced from the circumstance, general language, or conduct of the patient.

Incidental use and disclosure (2) A limited use or disclosure of protected health information that occurs as a by-product of another permissible or required use or disclosure which could not have reasonably been prevented.

Incomplete claim (14) Any Medicare claim missing necessary information; such claims are identified to the provider so that they may be resubmitted.

Indemnity Health Insurance (4, 5) Traditional or fee-for-service health insurance plan that allows patients maximum flexibility and choice of provider for a fixed monthly premium. Medical services are paid at a percentage of covered benefits after an annual deductible is paid. Providers are paid each time a service is rendered on a fee-for-service basis. Also referred to as indemnity benefits plan.

Independent contractor (1) Individuals who have decided to establish their own self-operated business and provide services to health care organizations under contract.

Independent (or individual) practice association (IPA) (4, 5) A type of managed care organization in which a program administrator contracts with a number of physicians who agree to provide treatment to subscribers in their own offices. Physicians are not employees of the managed care organization (MCO) and are not paid salaries. They receive reimbursement on a capitation or fee-for-service basis.

Individually identifiable health information (IIHI) (2) Any part of an individual's health information, including demographic information (for example, address, date of birth) collected from the individual, that is created or received by a covered entity.

Injury (8) In a workers' compensation policy, this term signifies any trauma or damage to a body part or disease sustained, arising out of, and in the course of employment, including injury to artificial members and medical braces of all types.

Inpatient (19) A term used when a patient is admitted to the hospital for overnight stay.

Inpatient Prospective Payment System (IPPS) (19) The prospective reimbursement system used for Medicare inpatient claims. Reimbursement rates are predetermined and are made based on Medicare Severity – Diagnosis Related Groups (MS-DRGs); the hospital receives one MS-DRG payment for each admission.

Inpatient Psychiatric Facility Prospective Payment System (IPF PPS) (19) The reimbursement system used for psychiatric hospitals and acute care hospital's psychiatric units that are exempt from the MS-DRG system. The IPF PPS reimburses at a predetermined rate, per diem (a specific rate for each day that the patient is hospitalized; established each year by CMS).

Inpatient Rehabilitation Facility Patient Assessment Instrument (IRF PAI) (19) The discharge evaluation tool used to evaluate patient's functional motor and cognitive skills.

Inpatient Rehabilitation Facility Prospective Payment System (19) The reimbursement system used for rehabilitation hospitals. In order to qualify for this reimbursement system, 60% of the hospital's inpatients must be treated for one of 13 conditions.

Inpatient only (IPO) (19) Procedure lists created by insurers, including Medicare, that they consider to be too risky to be performed on an outpatient basis and will only reimburse hospitals if the procedure is performed on an inpatient basis. Examples include open heart procedures and amputations.

Inquiry (16) See Tracer.

Insurance adjuster (8) An individual at the workers' compensation insurance carrier overseeing an industrial case, authorizing diagnostic testing and medical treatment, and communicating with the provider of medical care.

Insurance billing specialist (1) A practitioner who carries out claims completion, coding, and billing responsibilities and may or may not perform managerial and supervisory functions; also known as an insurance claims processor, reimbursement specialist, medical billing representative, or senior billing representative.

Insurance payment poster (16) Individual working for a medical practice or hospital that inserts payments received, adjustments (credits or write-offs), and denials from insurance companies, patients, and governmental agencies into patient financial accounts. Also known as insurance payment poster, payment coordinator, payment representative, or reimbursement coordinator.

Insurance payment posting (16) Process of applying payments and adjustments (credits or write-offs) to patient financial accounts.

Intelligent character recognition (ICR) (14) Same as Optical character recognition.

Internal review (11) The process of going over financial documents before and after billing to insurance carriers to determine documentation deficiencies or errors.

International Classification of Diseases, Tenth Revision, Clinical Modification (ICD-10-CM) (12, 19) A diagnostic code book that uses a system for classifying diseases and operations to assist collection of uniform and comparable health information. It has been modified, was implemented on October 1, 2013, and replaces ICD-9-CM Volumes 1 and 2 when submitting insurance claims for billing hospital and physician office medical services.

International Classification of Diseases, Tenth Revision, Procedure Coding System (ICD-10-PCS) (12, 19) Procedural code system developed by 3M Health Information Systems (HIS) under contract with the Centers for Medicare and Medicaid Services (CMS). When implemented on October 1, 2014, it replaced ICD-9-CM Volume 3 for hospital inpatient procedure reporting in the United States.

Interview (20) Meeting an individual face to face for evaluating and questioning a job applicant.

Intoxication (12) A diagnostic coding term that relates to an adverse effect rather than a poisoning when drugs, such as digitalis, steroid agents, and so on, are involved.

Invalid claim (14) A claim that contains complete, necessary information but is illogical or incorrect (for example, listing an incorrect provider number for a referring physician). Invalid claims are identified to the provider and may be resubmitted.

Itemized statement (17) A detailed summary of all transactions of a patient's account: dates of service, detailed charges, payments (copayments and deductibles), date on which the insurance claim was submitted, adjustments, and account balance.

Jurisdiction (6) A defined geographical area over which a Medicare Administrative Contractor oversees processing of claims.

Late effect (12) An inactive residual effect or condition produced after the acute phase of an illness or injury has ended.

Laterality (12) defines the side of the body affected.

Legible (11) Pertaining to a health record, data that is easily recognizable by individuals outside of a medical practice who are unfamiliar with the particular handwriting.

Lien (8, 17) A claim on the property of another as security for a debt. In litigation cases, it is a legal promise to satisfy a debt owed by the patient to the physician out of any proceeds received on the case.

Life cycle of a claim (4) Also referred to as the revenue cycle of an insurance claim which includes the administrative and clinical functions that are required to capture and collect payment for services provided by a health care organization.

Limiting charge (6) A percentage limit on fees, specified by legislation, that nonparticipating physicians may bill Medicare beneficiaries above the fee schedule amount.

List service (listserv) (1) An online computer service run from a website where questions may be posted by subscribers.

Local coverage determination (LCD) (6) Decisions made by a Medicare contractor that are developed to decide whether to cover a particular service in accordance with CMS' definition of what is medically necessary and to provide coverage information for medical services. LCDs are only applicable to that Medicare contractor's jurisdiction.

Long term care hospital prospective payment system (LTCH PPS) (19) The prospective reimbursement system used by long-term care hospitals, who provide services to patients who no longer need acute care but their level of care is still significant. Long term care hospitals must provide an average length of stay of at least 25 days.

Long-term disability insurance (10) A provision to pay benefits to a covered disabled person to age 65.

Lost claim (16) An insurance claim that cannot be located after sending it to an insurer.

Low complexity (LC) (11) Phrase used to describe a type of medical decision making when a patient is seen for an evaluation and management (E/M) service.

Major complication/comorbidity (MCC) (19) Main underlying condition or other condition that arises or exists along with the condition for which the patient is receiving treatment. Used in diagnostic-related group (DRG) reimbursement.

Major diagnostic category (MDC) (19) A broad classification of diagnoses. There are 83 coding system–oriented MDCs in the original diagnosis-related groups (DRGs) and 23 body system–oriented MDCs in the revised set of DRGs.

Major medical (4) A health insurance policy designed to offset heavy medical expenses resulting from catastrophic or prolonged illness or injury.

Malignant tumor (12) An abnormal growth that has the properties of invasion and metastasis (for example, transfer of diseases from one organ to another). The word "carcinoma" refers to a cancerous or malignant tumor.

Managed care (5) Refers to a group of techniques intended to reduce the cost of providing healthcare while improving the access to care and the quality of care.

Mandated benefit (4) Health service (treatment or procedure) required by state and/or federal law that may be given to a patient for a specific health condition. This health service may be delivered by certain types of health care providers for some categories of dependents, such as children placed for adoption. Also referred to as mandated services.

Manifestation (12) An associated secondary process or disease.

Maternal and Child Health Program (MCHP) (4) A state service organization to assist children younger than 21 years of age who have conditions leading to health problems.

Medicaid (4, 6, 7) A federally aided, state-operated, and state-administered program that provides medical benefits for certain low-income persons in need of health and medical care.

Medi-Cal (7) California's version of the nationwide program known as Medicaid.

Medical billing representative (1) See Insurance billing specialist.

Medical decision making (MDM) (11) Health care management process done after performing a history and physical examination on a patient that results in a plan of treatment. It is based on establishing one or more diagnoses and/or selecting a management or treatment option, amount of data or complexity of data reviewed, and complications and/or morbidity or mortality.

Medical necessity (3, 4, 6, 11, 12, 16) The performance of services and procedures that are consistent with the diagnosis in accordance with standards of good medical practice, performed at the proper level, and provided in the most appropriate setting. Medical necessity must be established (via diagnostic or other information presented on the individual claim under consideration) before the carrier may make payment.

Medical Savings Account (MSA) (4) A type of tax-free savings account that allows individuals and their employers to set aside money to pay for health care expenses.

Medical service order (8) An authorization given to the physician, either written or verbal, to treat the injured or ill employee.

Medically necessary (4) See Medical necessity.

Medically needy (MN) (7) Persons in need of financial assistance or whose income and resources will not allow them to pay for the costs of medical care; also called medically indigent in some states.

Medically (or psychologically) necessary (8) Medical or psychological services considered appropriate care and generally accepted by qualified professionals to be reasonable and adequate for the diagnosis and treatment of illness, injury, pregnancy, and mental disorders or that are reasonable and adequate for well-baby care.

Medicare (4, 6) A nationwide health insurance program for people age 65 years of age and older and certain disabled or blind persons regardless of income, administered by Centers for Medicare and Medicaid Services (CMS).

Medicare administrative contractors (MAC) (3, 6, 19) A private insurance carrier that has been contracted by CMS to process Medicare Part A and Part B medical claims for Medicare fee-for-service (FFS) beneficiaries.

Medicare Advantage Plan (6) Private insurance companies who have been approved by Medicare to offer Medicare Part C coverage to patients eligible for Medicare benefits, as an alternative to traditional Medicare.

Medicare Access and CHIP Reauthorization Act of 2015 (MACRA) (6) Legislation enacted to establish quality payment programs as a new way to pay providers by giving incentives for high-quality and high-value care.

Medicare Beneficiary Identifier (MBI) (6) The 11 character beneficiary identifier used on Medicare insurance cards.

Medicare Claims Processing Manual – Internet Only Manual (6) The publication which provides Medicare's general billing requirements for various health care professionals and suppliers, as well as claims submission information.

Medicare Improvements for Patients and Providers Act (MIPPA) (6) A multi-faceted piece of legislation containing provisions and funding to states to help older adults, individuals with disabilities and their caregivers for special assistance. It also required CMS to implement quality incentives into the ESRD bundled payment system to promote high-quality services to outpatient dialysis facilities treating patients with ESRD.

Medicare Integrity Program (MIP) (3) A program designed to promote the integrity of the Medicare program through a series of audits and reviews of health care organization's claims and cost report data.

Medicare/Medicaid (Medi-Medi) (4, 6) Refers to an individual who receives medical or disability benefits from both Medicare and Medicaid programs; sometimes referred to as a Medi-Medi case or a crossover.

Medicare Part A (6) Hospital benefits of a nationwide health insurance program for persons age 65 years of age and older and certain disabled individuals regardless of income, administered by Centers for Medicare and Medicaid Services (CMS).

Medicare Part B (6) Medical insurance of a nationwide health insurance program for persons age 65 years of age and older and certain disabled individuals regardless of income, administered by Centers for Medicare and Medicaid Services (CMS). Local Social Security offices take applications and supply information about the program.

Medicare Part C (6) Medicare Plus (+) Choice plans offer a number of health care options in addition to those available under Medicare Part A and Part B. Plans may include health maintenance organizations (HMOs), fee-for-service plans, provider-sponsored organizations, religious fraternal benefit societies (RFBSs), and Medicare medical savings accounts.

Medicare Part D (6) Stand-alone prescription drug plan, presented by insurance and other private companies that offer drug coverage that meets the standards established by Medicare. Other names for these plans are Part D private prescription drug plans (PDPs) or Medicare Advantage prescription drug plans (MA-PDs).

Medicare Savings Programs (MSP) help low-income individuals with out-of-pocket costs for Medicare, including Medicare Part A and Part B premiums, deductibles, copayments and coinsurance. There are four types of Medicare Savings Programs:

- Qualified Medicare Beneficiary Program (QMB)
- Specified Low-Income Medicare Beneficiary Program (SLMB)
- Qualifying Individual Program (QI)
- Qualified Disabled and Working Individuals Program (QDWI)

All four types of MSP are run by state Medicaid programs. Each program addresses a different financial category and the monthly income figures are adjusted each year. Eligibility for the programs may differ from state to state.

Medicare savings program (MSP) (7) Programs developed by state Medicaid programs designed to help low-income individuals with out-of-pocket costs for Medicare, including Medicare Part A and B premiums, deductibles, copayments and coinsurance.

Medicare secondary payer (MSP) (6) The primary insurance plan of a Medicare beneficiary that must pay for any medical care or services first before Medicare is sent a claim.

Medicare Summary Notice (MSN) (6) A document received by the patient explaining amount charged, Medicare approved, deductible, and coinsurance for medical services rendered.

Medigap (MG) (6) A specialized supplemental insurance policy devised for the Medicare beneficiary that covers the deductible and copayment amounts typically not covered under the main Medicare policy written by a nongovernmental third-party payer.

Mentor (20) Guide or teacher who offers advice, criticism, wisdom, guidance, and perspective to an inexperienced but promising protégé to help reach a life goal.

Merit-Based Incentive Payment System (MIPS) (6) A quality payment program established under MACRA that will determine Medicare payment adjustments to providers.

Metastasis (12) Process in which tumor cells spread and transfer from one organ to another site.

Military Treatment Facility (MTF) (8) All uniformed service hospitals or health clinics; also known as military hospitals or uniformed service hospitals.

Minimum necessary rule (2) A requirement of the HIPAA privacy rule for covered entities to take reasonable steps to limit the use or disclosure of protected health information to only what is necessary to accomplish the intended purpose.

Mitigation (2) For a breach of privacy under the Health Insurance Portability and Accountability Act (HIPAA), this means to alleviate the severity, reduce, or make mild any harmful effects of such violation.

Moderate complexity (MC) (11) A phrase used to describe a type of medical decision making when a patient is seen for an evaluation and management (E/M) service.

Modifiers (13) In Current Procedural Terminology (CPT) coding, a two-digit add-on number placed after the usual procedure code number to indicate a procedure or service has been altered by specific circumstances. The two-digit modifier may be separated by a hyphen. In HCPCS Level II coding, one-digit or two-digit add-on alpha characters, placed after the usual procedure code number (Example G-1).

Example G-1 27372-51

Monitoring (3) A spot check for quality control; less structured than an audit.

Morbidity (11, 12) A diseased condition or state.

Mortality (11, 12) Death.

National Certified Insurance and Coding Specialist (NCICS) (20) An insurance and coding certification that is awarded by an independent testing agency, the National Center for Competency Testing (NCCT).

National Correct Coding Initiative (NCCI) (13) A code editing system implemented into the Medicare program in 1996, consistent with Medicare policies to eliminate unbundling or other inappropriate reporting of CPT codes.

National coverage determination (NCD) (6) Guidelines mandated by CMS at the federal level which all Medicare contractors must follow that are developed to decide whether to cover a particular service in accordance with CMS' definition of what is medically necessary and to provide coverage information for medical services.

National health insurance (6) A legally enforced system of health insurance that insures a countries' population against the costs of health care. It is usually established by national legislation, but may be administered by the public sector, the private sector, or a combination of both.

National Provider Identifier (NPI) (2, 6, 14) A lifetime number issued to health care organizations and providers and used to identify them on claim forms.

National Standard Format (NSF) (15) The name of the standardization of data to reduce paper and have more accurate information and efficient organization.

National Uniform Claim Committee (NUCC) (14, 19) A committee made up of health care industry stakeholders representing providers, payers, designated standards maintenance organizations, public health organizations, and vendors who are responsible for maintaining the integrity of the data sets and physical layout of the CMS-1500 claim form. It is further charged with the task of standardizing national instructions for completion of the claim form to be used by all payers.

Neoplasm (12) Benign or malignant tumor.

Netback (17) Evaluating a collection agency's performance by taking the amount of monies collected and subtracting the agency's fees.

Networking (20) Exchanging information or services among individuals, groups, or institutions and making use of professional contacts.

Never event (13) Incident related to a wrong surgical device, patient protection, care management, environment, or criminal occurrence that results in injury or death due to error in health care management or failure to follow standard care or institutional practices or policies. Also referred to as serious reportable event.

New patient (NP) (11) An individual who has not received any professional services from the physician or another physician of the same specialty who belongs to the same group practice within the past 3 years.

No charge (NC) (17) Waiving the entire fee owed for professional care.

Nonavailability statement (NAS) (8) A certification from a military hospital stating that it cannot provide the care needed by the beneficiary.

Noncancelable policy or clause (4, 10) An insurance policy clause that prevents the insurance company from increasing premium rates and requires them to renew the policy until the insured reaches the age stated in the contract. Some disability income policies have noncancelable terms.

Nondisability (ND) claim (8) A claim for an on-the-job injury that requires medical care but does not result in loss of working time or income.

Nonessential modifiers (12) In ICD-10-CM, modifiers that provide additional description and are enclosed in parentheses. They are referred to as nonessential modifiers because their presence or absence does not affect the diagnostic code assigned.

Nonexempt assets (17) One's total property (in bankruptcy cases) not falling in the exemption category, including money, automobile equity, and property, more than a specified amount, depending on the state in which the person lives.

Nonparticipating (nonpar) physician or provider (4, 6, 8) A health care organization, physician, or provider who has not entered into a contractual agreement with a specific insurance plan.

Non-physician practitioner (NPP) (11) Health care provider who meets state licensing requirements to provide specific medical services. Medicare allows payment for services furnished by NPPs, including but not limited to advance registered nurse practitioners (ARNPs), certified registered nurse practitioners, clinical nurse specialists (CNSs), licensed clinical social workers (LCSWs), physician assistants (PAs), nurse midwives, physical therapists, speech therapists, and audiologists. Also referred to as midlevel practitioner, midlevel provider, or physician extender.

Nonprivileged information (2) Information consisting of ordinary facts unrelated to the treatment of the patient. The patient's authorization is not required to disclose the data unless the record is in a specialty hospital or in a special service unit of a general hospital, such as the psychiatric unit.

Non-VA Medicare Care Program (10) A program which allows veterans to apply for and be granted medical care by a private physician rather than the nearest VA outpatient clinic if the VA facility is not within reasonable distance, when the veteran is too ill to travel to the nearest location, or when the condition needs prompt attention.

Not elsewhere classifiable (NEC) (12) This term is used in the ICD-9-CM diagnostic coding system when the code lacks the information necessary to code the term in a more specific category.

Not otherwise specified (NOS) (12) Unspecified. Used in ICD-9-CM numeric code system for coding diagnoses.

Notice of Privacy Practices (NPP) (2) Under the Health Insurance Portability and Accountability Act (HIPAA), a document given to the patient at the first visit or at enrollment explaining the individual's rights and the physician's legal duties in regard to protected health information (PHI).

Nursing facility (NF) (6) A specially qualified facility that has the staff and equipment to provide skilled nursing care and related services that are medically necessary to a patient's recovery; formerly known as a skilled nursing facility (SNF).

Observation (19) An outpatient place of service used to determine what is wrong with the patient and if inpatient services are needed. Observation patients may be admitted as an inpatient or sent home depending on what is found.

Occupational illness (or disease) (8) An abnormal condition or disorder caused by environmental factors associated with employment. It may be caused by inhalation, absorption, ingestion, or direct contact.

Occupational Safety and Health Administration (OSHA) (3, 8) A federal agency that regulates and investigates safety and health standards in work locations.

Office of Inspector General (OIG) (3) The largest inspector general's office in the Federal

Government, established to safeguard the Medicare and Medicaid programs by finding and eliminating fraud, abuse, and waste.

Office of Workers' Compensation Programs (OWCP) (8) The agency within the U.S. Department of Labor charged with administering four major disability compensation programs which provide wage replacement benefits, medical treatment, vocational rehabilitation, and other benefits to certain workers and their dependents who experience work-related injury or occupational disease.

Official Coding Guidelines for Coding and Reporting (12) Set of rules developed to accompany and complement the official conventions and instructions provided within the ICD-10-CM coding manual. The guidelines include definitions, standards, rules, general coding guidelines, and 21 chapter-specific guidelines. Adherence to the guidelines when assigning an ICD-10-CM diagnosis code is required under the Health Insurance Portability and Accountability Act (HIPAA) and has been adopted for all health care settings.

Operation Restore Trust (ORT) (3) A program launched in 1995 designed to combat fraud, waste, and abuse in the Medicare and Medicaid programs by allowing the public to report issues that might indicate fraud, abuse, or waste.

Optical character recognition (OCR) (14) A device that can read typed characters at very high speed and convert them to digitized files that can be saved on disk. Also known as intelligent character recognition (ICR).

Optionally renewable (4) An insurance policy renewal provision in which the insurer has the right to refuse to renew the policy on a date and may add coverage limitations or increase premium rates.

Ordering physician (11) The physician ordering non-physician services for a patient (for example, diagnostic laboratory tests, pharmaceutical services, or durable medical equipment [DME]) when an insurance claim is submitted by a non-physician supplier of services. The ordering physician also may be the treating or performing physician.

Ordinality of encounter (12) The determination as to whether a health care encounter is the patient's first for the condition being treated.

Other health insurance (OHI) (8) Health care coverage for TRICARE beneficiaries through an employer, an association, or a private insurer. A student in the family may have a health care plan through school.

Overpayment (16) Money paid over and above the amount due by the insurer or patient.

Paper claim (14) An insurance claim submitted on paper, including those optically scanned and converted to an electronic form by the insurance carrier.

Partial disability (10) A disability from an illness or injury that prevents an insured person from performing one or more of the functions of his or her regular job.

Participating (par) physician or provider (4, 5, 6, 8) A health care organization, physician, or provider who has entered into a contractual agreement with a specific insurance carrier.

Partnership program (8) A program that allows TRICARE-eligible individuals to receive inpatient or outpatient treatment from civilian providers of care in a military hospital or from uniformed services providers of care in civilian facilities.

Past history (PH) (11) A patient's past experiences with illnesses, operations, injuries, and treatments.

Patient dumping (3) The phrase coined through the occurrence of private hospitals refusing to examine or treat the poor or insured in the emergency department and transferring them to public hospitals.

Patient Protection and Affordable Care Act (PPACA) (ACA) (Obamacare) (2, 4) A comprehensive health care reform law enacted in March of 2010 which provides numerous rights and protections that make health coverage more fair and easy to understand, along with subsidies to make health care more affordable. The law also expanded the Medicaid program.

Payer of last resort (7) The insurance carrier to be billed when the patient is eligible for Medicaid and also has coverage under a group health insurance through an employer.

Peer review (16) The review of a patient's case by one or more physicians using federal guidelines to evaluate another physician regarding the quality and efficiency of medical care. This is done to discover overuse or misuse of a plan's benefits.

Pending claim (14) See Suspended claim.

Per capita (5) See Capitation.

Permanent and stationary (P and S) (8) A phrase used when a workers' compensation patient's condition has become stabilized and no improvement is expected. It is only after this declaration that a case can be rated for a compromise and release.

Permanent disability (PD) (8) An illness or injury (impairment of the normal use of a body part) expected to continue for the lifetime of the injured worker that prevents the person from performing the functions of his or her regular occupation, therefore impairing his or her earning capacity.

Petition (8) A formal written request commonly used to indicate an appeal; also means any request for relief other than an application.

Phantom bills (3) Bills for services not performed.

Physical examination (PE or PX) (11) Objective inspection or testing of organ systems or body areas of a patient by a physician.

Physical status modifier (13) A 2-character descriptor used in anesthesia coding to report the overall health of the patient by referencing patients who are healthy or those who have mild or severe systemic diseases.

Physically clean claim (14) Insurance claims with no staples or highlighted areas. The bar code area has not been deformed.

Physician provider group (PPG) (5) A physician-owned business that has the flexibility to deal with all forms of contract medicine and still offer its own packages to business groups, unions, and the general public.

Placeholder (12) Last or seventh character that composes an ICD-10-CM diagnostic code indicated by an "X" that is used to allow space for future code expansion or to meet the requirement of coding to the highest level of specificity.

Point-of-service (POS) option (8) Individuals under the TRICARE program can choose to get TRICARE-covered nonemergency services outside the prime network of providers without a referral from the primary care manager and without authorization from a health care finder.

Point-of-service (POS) plan (4, 5) A managed care plan in which members are given a choice as to how to receive services, whether through a health maintenance organization (HMO), preferred provider organization (PPO), or fee-for-service plan. The decision is made at the time the service is necessary (for example, "at the point of service"); sometimes referred to as open-ended HMOs, swing-out HMOs, self-referral options, or multiple option plans.

Poisoning (12) A condition resulting from an overdose of drugs or chemical substances or from the wrong drug or agent given or taken in error.

Portability (2) Under HIPAA, portability is defined as an employee's right to maintain health care benefits under a group health plan when leaving a job.

Portfolio (20) A compilation of items that represents a job applicant's skills.

Preadmission (19) The process of preparing for the patient's care by collecting demographic information and insurance information.

Preadmission testing (PAT) (19) Treatment, tests, and procedures done 48 to 72 hours before admission of a patient to the hospital.

Preauthorization (4, 8, 19) A requirement of some health insurance plans to obtain permission for a service or procedure before it is done and to see whether the insurance program agrees that it is medically necessary.

Precertification (4) A procedure done to determine whether treatment (surgery, tests, or hospitalization) is covered under a patient's health insurance policy.

Predetermination (4) A financial inquiry done before treatment to determine the maximum dollar amount the insurance company will pay for surgery, consultations, postoperative care, and so forth.

Preexisting conditions (2, 4) Illnesses or injuries acquired by the patient before enrollment in an insurance plan.

Preferred provider organization (PPO) (4, 5) A type of health benefit program in which enrollees receive the highest level of benefits when they obtain services from a physician, hospital, or other health care provider designated by their program as a "preferred provider." Enrollees may receive substantial, although reduced, benefits when they obtain care from a provider of their own choosing who is not designated as a "preferred provider" by their program.

Premium (4, 6) The cost of insurance coverage paid annually, semiannually, or monthly to keep the policy in force.

Prepaid group practice model (5) A plan under which specified health services are rendered by participating physicians to an enrolled group of persons, with fixed periodic payments made in advance, by or on behalf of each person or family. If a health insurance carrier is involved, it contracts to pay in advance for the full range of health services to which the insured is entitled under the terms of the health insurance contract.

Prepayment audit (11) Review of a submitted claim by an insurance carrier that is pended with a request to the physician to submit a copy of the patient's medical record to support the claim before payment is generated. The insurance carrier reviews the record to determine payment or nonpayment of the claim. Sometimes referred to as prospective audit.

Prepayment screen (6) Also referred to as prepayment edits which are put in place by insurance carriers to prevent payment for noncovered and incorrectly coded services. Also used to target claims for review prior to payment.

Present on admission (POA) (19) Determination as to whether the patient had a specific condition prior to admission into hospital care.

Primary care manager (PCM) (8) A physician who is responsible for coordinating and managing all of the TRICARE beneficiary's health care unless there is an emergency.

Primary care physician (PCP) (5, 11) A physician (for example, family practitioner, general practitioner, pediatrician, obstetrician/gynecologist, general internist) who oversees the care of patients in a managed health care plan and refers patients to specialists (for example, cardiologists, oncologists, surgeons) for services as needed. Also known as a gatekeeper.

Primary diagnosis (12) Initial identification of the condition or chief complaint for which the patient is treated for outpatient medical care.

Principal diagnosis (12, 19) A condition established after study that is chiefly responsible for the admission of the patient to the hospital.

Prior approval (PA) (7) The evaluation of a provider request for a specific service to determine the medical necessity and appropriateness of the care requested for a patient. Also called prior authorization in some states.

Privacy (2) The condition of being secluded from the presence or view of others.

Privacy officer, privacy official (PO) (2) An individual designated to help the provider remain in compliance by setting policies and procedures and by training and managing the staff regarding Health Insurance Portability and Accountability Act (HIPAA) and patient rights; usually the contact person for questions and complaints.

Private health insurance (5) An insurance plan marketed by the private health insurance industry rather than through government sponsored programs and generally offered through employers or other organizations.

Privileged information (2) Data related to the treatment and progress of the patient that can be released only when written authorization of the patient or guardian is obtained.

Problem focused (PF) (11) A phrase used to describe a type of medical decision making when a patient is seen for an evaluation and management (E/M) service.

Procedure code numbers (13) Five-digit numeric codes that describe each service the physician renders to a patient.

Professional billing (1) Charging for services performed by physicians or non-physician practitioners (NPPs).

Professional component (PC) (13) The portion of a test or procedure (containing both a professional and a technical component) that the physician performs (for example, interpreting an electrocardiogram [ECG], reading an x-ray, making an observation and determination using a microscope).

Professional courtesy (17) A discount or exemption from charges given to certain people at the discretion of the physician rendering the service. It is rarely used in current medicine.

Prophylaxis (12) Prevention of disease.

Prospective audit (11) See Prepayment audit.

Prospective payment system (PPS) (6, 19) A method of payment for Medicare hospital insurance based on diagnosis-related groups (DRGs) (a fixed dollar amount for a principal diagnosis).

Prospective review (11) The process of going over financial documents before billing is submitted to the insurance company to determine documentation deficiencies and errors.

Protected health information (PHI) (2) Any data that identify an individual and describe his or her health status, age, sex, ethnicity, or other demographic characteristics, whether or not that information is stored or transmitted electronically.

Psychotherapy notes (2) Notes recorded in any medium by a health care provider who is a mental health professional documenting or analyzing the contents of conversation during a private counseling session or a group, joint, or family counseling session and that are separate from the rest of the individual's medical record.

Qualified Independent Contractor (16) Independent contractors involved in Level 2 Medicare appeals who make reconsideration decisions and are expected to give weight to local and national coverage policies and conduct a panel review of denials when necessary.

Qualifying circumstance modifiers (QC) (13) Add-on codes for anesthesia services used when a patient's age or status has a significant effect on the service provided.

Quality Improvement Organization (QIO) (6, 19) A program that replaces the peer review organization program and is designed to monitor and improve the usage and quality of care for Medicare beneficiaries.

Query (11) A tool used by a clinical documentation improvement specialist to request additional clarification from the provider of services.

Qui tam (3) A provision under the FCA which offers financial incentives to private citizens who act as informants and report suspected fraud on behalf of the federal government.

Real time (15) Online interactive communication between two computer systems allowing instant transfer of information.

Reason for the encounter (19) First diagnosis stated or listed for an outpatient insurance claim.

Reasonable fee (13) A charge is considered reasonable if it is deemed acceptable after peer review even though it does not meet the customary or prevailing criteria. This includes unusual circumstances or complications requiring additional time, skill, or experience in connection with a particular service or procedure. In Medicare, the amount on which payment is based for participating physicians.

Rebill (resubmit) (16) To send another request for payment for an overdue bill to either the insurance company or the patient.

Recipient (7) A person certified by the local welfare department to receive the benefits of Medicaid under one of the specific aid categories; an individual certified to receive Medicare benefits.

Reconsideration (10) The first level of appeal process for an individual applying for Social Security Disability Insurance (SSDI) or Supplemental Security Income (SSI). It is a complete review of the claim by a medical or psychological consultant or disability examiner team who did not take part in the original disability determination.

Recovery Audit Contractor (RAC) (3) A company that contracts with Medicare to recoup money from inappropriately paid claims.

Recovery Audit Contractor (RAC) Initiative (6) Legislation enacted allowing CMS to contract with audit companies for identification of Medicare underpayments and overpayments and recover overpayments using automated review and complex review. An automated review is done electronically without human review and complex review is done using human review of the medical record.

Reexamination report (8) A detailed progress report sent to an insurance carrier to provide the status of a patient on temporary disability who has made significant changes following 2–4 weeks of treatment.

Referral (11) The transfer of the total or specific care of a patient from one physician to another. In managed care, a request for authorization for a specific service.

Referring physician (11) A physician who sends the patient for testing or treatment noted on the insurance claim when it is submitted by the physician performing the service.

Regional contractor (8) For TRICARE and CHAMPVA, the insurance company that handles the claims for care received within a particular state or country. Also known as claims processor and formerly known as fiscal agent, fiscal carrier, or fiscal intermediary. For Medicare, see Medicare administrative contractor (MAC).

Registered Medical Assistant (RMA) (20) A title earned by completing appropriate training and passing a registry examination administered by the American Medical Technologists (AMT).

Registered Medical Coder (RMC) (20) A registered title awarded after completion of coursework given by the Medical Management Institute (MMI) with recertification requirements.

Rehabilitation impairment category (RIC) (19) Categories used to group discharges based on patient's primary diagnosis/condition for which a patient is admitted to an IRF.

Assessment Instrument (IRF PAI). The CMGs is broken into four tiers based on

Reimbursement (16) Payment for services provided.

Reimbursement specialist (1) See Insurance billing specialist.

Rejected claim (14, 16) An insurance claim submitted to an insurance carrier that is discarded by the system because of a technical error (omission or erroneous information) or because it does not follow carrier instructions. It is returned to the provider for correction or change so that it may be processed properly for payment.

Relative value studies or scale (RVS) (13) A list of procedure codes for professional services and procedures that are assigned unit values that indicate the relative value of one procedure over another.

Relative value unit (RVU) (13) A monetary value assigned to each service on the basis of the amount of physician work, practice expenses, and cost of professional liability insurance. These three RVUs are then adjusted according to geographic area and used in a formula to determine Medicare fees.

Relative weight (19) The value assigned to MS-DRGs based on the average resources used to treat Medicare patients for that condition and used to determine the amount of reimbursement for the assigned MS-DRG. The MS-DRG relative weight is multiplied by the base rate.

Remittance advice (RA) (6, 16) A document sent by an insurance carrier to the provider of services, detailing services billed and describing payment determination issued; also known in some programs as an explanation of benefits (EOB).

Resident physician (11) A physician who has finished medical school and is performing one or more years of training in a specialty area on the job at a hospital (medical center).

Residual benefits (10) A term used in disability income insurance for disability that is not work related. It is the payment of partial benefits when the insured is not totally disabled.

Residual disability (10) A disability from an illness or injury that prevents an insured person from performing one or more of the functions of his or her regular job. This is sometimes referred to as partial disability. See also Partial disability.

Residual subcategories (12) Categories of codes in ICD-10-CM used to describe conditions that are specifically named in the health record but not specifically listed under a code description.

Resource-based relative value scale (RBRVS) (6, 13, 19) A prospective payment system that ranks physician services by units and provides a formula to determine a Medicare fee schedule.

Respite care (6) A short-term hospice inpatient stay for a terminally ill patient to give temporary relief to the person who regularly assists with home care of a patient.

Respondeat superior (1) "Let the master answer." Refers to a physician's liability in certain cases for the wrongful acts of his of her assistant(s) or employee(s).

Résumé (20) A summary of education, skills, and work experience, usually in outline form.

Retrospective review (11, 19) (1) The process of going over financial documents after billing an insurance carrier to determine documentation deficiencies and errors. (2) Review of services provided to a patient after the service is performed.

Revenue (1) The total income produced by a medical practice or health care organization for services provided to patients.

Revenue code (19) A four-digit code used to group similar charges together in the chargemaster, or database of all of the services, supplies, equipment, and so forth provided by the hospital and the charge that is associated with it.

Revenue cycle (4, 19) The administrative and clinical functions that are required to capture and collect payment for services provided by a health care organization.

Revenue cycle management (RCM) (16) The process that health care organizations use to track services provided and patient care episodes from registration and appointment scheduling to the final payment of the associated fees.

Revenue cycle manager (20) An individual responsible for overseeing the billing teams that manage accounts, communications with insurance, collections, contract analysis, cash posting, billing transactions with clients, report creation, and detecting problems in the billing system followed by implementation of process improvement initiatives.

Review (16) To look over a claim to assess how much payment should be made.

Review of systems (ROS) (11) An inventory of body systems obtained through a series of questions used to identify signs or symptoms that the patient might be experiencing or has experienced.

Rule-out (12) In reference to diagnosis coding, a rule-out diagnosis is one that has not been confirmed; however, the provider is keeping an open mind about the possibility of that diagnosis.

Secondary diagnosis (12) A reason subsequent to the primary diagnosis for an office or hospital encounter that may contribute to the condition or define the need for a higher level of care but is not the underlying cause. There may be more than one secondary diagnosis.

Second-injury fund (8) See Subsequent-injury fund (SIF).

Secured debt (17) A debt (an amount owed) in which a debtor pledges certain property (collateral), in a written security agreement, to the repayment of the debt.

Security officer (2) A person who protects the computer and networking systems within the practice and implements protocols, such as password assignment, backup procedures, firewalls, virus protection, and contingency planning for emergencies.

Security Rule (2) Health Insurance Portability and Accountability Act (HIPAA) regulations related to the security of electronic protected health information (ePHI) that, along with regulations related to electronic transactions and code sets, privacy, and enforcement, compose the Administrative Simplification provisions.

Self-Disclosure Protocol (SDP) (3) Established in 2006 as a vehicle for providers and health care organizations to voluntarily disclose self-discovered evidence of potential fraud and to work together with the OIG in resolving issues efficiently and fairly.

Self-employment (20) Working for oneself, with direct control over work, services, and fees.

Self-pay/Self-pay patient (1, 19) Individuals who do not have any medical insurance, who are liable for medical services received, and must pay out-of-pocket.

Self-referral (5) A patient in a managed care plan that refers himself or herself to a specialist. The patient may be required to inform the primary care physician (PCP).

Senior billing representative (1) See Insurance billing specialist.

Sequelae (8, 12) Diseased conditions after and usually resulting from a previous disease.

Sequencing (12) Listing diagnosis codes in the appropriate order as outlined in the ICD guidelines.

Service benefit program (8) A program (for example, TRICARE) that provides benefits without a contract guaranteeing the indemnification of an insured party against a specific loss; there are no premiums.

Service-connected injury (8) Injury incurred by a service member while on active duty or incurred during reserve duty with a military unit.

Service contract (20) A document that enumerates the obligations of a billing service and a medical practice stating the responsible party for each specific duty and task.

Service retiree (8) An individual who is retired from a career in the armed forces; also known as a military retiree.

Share of cost (7) The amount the patient must pay each month before he or she can be eligible for Medicaid; also known as liability or spend down.

Short-term disability insurance (10) A provision to pay benefits to a covered disabled person as long as he or she remains disabled, up to a specified period not exceeding 2 years.

Skip (17) A debtor who has moved and neglected to give a forwarding address (that is, skipped town).

Social history (SH) (11) An age-appropriate review of a patient's past and current activities (for example, smoking, diet intake, alcohol use).

Social Security Administration (SSA) (10) Administers Social Security Disability Insurance (SSDI) and Supplemental Security Income (SSI) programs for disabled persons.

Social Security Disability Insurance (SSDI) program (10) A federal entitlement program for long-term disability under Title II of the Social Security Act. It provides monthly benefits to workers and those self-employed who meet certain conditions.

Social Security number (SSN) (14) An individual's tax identification number issued by the federal government.

Sponsor (8) For the TRICARE program, the service person (active duty, retired, or deceased) whose relationship makes the patient (dependent) eligible for TRICARE.

Staff model (5) The type of health maintenance organization (HMO) in which the health plan hires physicians directly and pays them a salary.

Standard transactions (15) The electronic files in which medical data are compiled to produce a specific format.

State Children's Health Insurance Program (SCHIP) (4) A state-sponsored program that provides free or low-cost health coverage to low-income children.

State Disability Insurance (SDI) (4, 10) Insurance that covers off-the-job injury or sickness and is paid for by deductions from a person's paycheck. Also referred to as Unemployment Compensation Disability (UCD).

State license number (14) A number issued to a physician who has passed the state medical examination indicating his or her right to practice medicine in the state where issued.

State-run program (8) Workers' compensation programs which are administered by the state's department of labor, commerce, or industrial relations. Workers' compensation benefits are paid out by the state department responsible for administering the program; the state department acts like an insurance company.

Status indicator (19) In the OPPS, assignment of a measure to every CPT and HCPCs code which provides information about the procedure including whether or not it is covered, if it is subject to discounting, if it is an inpatient only procedure, and more.

Statute of limitations (17) A time limit established for filing lawsuits; may vary from state to state.

Stop loss (5) An agreement between a managed care company and a reinsurer in which absorption of prepaid patient expenses is limited; or limiting losses on an individual expensive hospital claim or professional services claim; form of reinsurance by which the managed care program limits the losses of an individual expensive hospital claim.

Straightforward (SF) (11) Phrase used to describe a type of medical decision making when a patient is seen for an evaluation and management (E/M) service.

Subacute (11) Refers to a condition that is both acute and chronic.

Subpoena (11) "Under penalty." A writ that commands a witness to appear at a trial or other proceeding and give testimony.

Subpoena duces tecum (11) "In his possession." A subpoena that requires the appearance of a witness with his or her records. Sometimes the judge permits the mailing of records and it is not necessary for the physician to appear in court.

Sub rosa films (8) Videotapes made without the knowledge of the subject; used to investigate suspicious claims in workers' compensation cases.

Subsequent-injury fund (SIF) (8) A special fund that assumes all or part of the liability for benefits provided to a worker because of the combined effect of a work-related impairment and a preexisting condition; also known as second-injury fund.

Summary payment voucher (8) The document that the fiscal agent sends to the provider or beneficiary, showing the service or supplies received, allowable charges, amount billed, amount TRICARE paid, how much deductible has been paid, and the patient's cost-share.

Supplemental benefits (10) Disability insurance provisions that allow benefits to the insured to increase the monthly indemnity or receive a percentage of the policy premiums if an individual keeps a policy in force for 5 or 10 years or does not file any claims.

Supplemental Security Income (SSI) (6, 7, 10) A program of income support for low-income aged, blind, and disabled persons established by Title XVI of the Social Security Act.

Surgical package (13) Surgical procedure code numbers include the operation; local infiltration, digital block, or topical anesthesia; and normal, uncomplicated postoperative care. This is referred to as a package and one fee covers the whole package.

Suspended claim (14, 16) An insurance claim that is processed by the insurance carrier but held in an indeterminate (pending) state about payment because of an error or the need for additional information.

Suspense (16) The pending indeterminate state of an insurance claim because of an error or the need for more information.

Swing bed (19) A bed in an acute care hospital that can be used for acute care or for skilled nursing facility.

Syndrome (12) Another name for a symptom complex (a set of complex signs, symptoms, or other manifestations resulting from a common cause or appearing in combination, presenting a distinct clinical picture of a disease or inherited abnormality).

T-1 (15) A T-carrier channel that can transmit voice or data channels quickly.

Tax Equity and Fiscal Responsibility Act of 1982 (TEFRA) (19) Legislation enacted which mandated the use of prospective payment systems for Medicare for acute care hospital's inpatient discharges.

Taxonomy codes (14, 15) Numeric and alpha provider specialty codes that are assigned and classify each health care provider when transmitting electronic insurance claims.

Teaching physician (11) A physician who is responsible for training and supervising medical students, interns, or residents and who takes them to the bedsides of patients in a teaching hospital to review course and treatment.

Technical component (13) Portion of a test or procedure (containing both a technical and a professional component) that pertains to the use of the equipment and the operator who performs it (for example, electrocardiogram [ECG] machine and technician, radiography machine and technician, microscope and technician).

Temporary disability (TD) (8, 10) The recovery period after a work-related injury during which the employee is unable to work and the condition has not stabilized; a schedule of benefits payable for the temporary disability.

Temporary disability insurance (TDI) (10) See Unemployment Compensation Disability (UCD).

Tertiary care (5) Services requested by a specialist from another specialist (for example, neurosurgeons, thoracic surgeons, intensive care units).

Third-party liability (8) Third-party liability exists if an entity is liable to pay the medical cost for injury, disease, or disability of a person hurt during the performance of his or her occupation and the injury is caused by an entity not connected with the employer.

Third-party subrogation (8) The legal process by which an insurance company seeks from a third party, who has caused a loss, recovery of the amount paid to the policyholder.

Total disability (10) A term that varies in meaning from one disability insurance policy to another. For example, a liberal definition might read: "The insured must be unable to perform the major duties of his or her specific occupation."

Total, permanent service-connected disability (8) A total, permanent disability incurred by a service member while on active duty.

Tracer (16) An inquiry made to an insurance company to locate the status of an insurance claim (for example, claim in review, claim never received).

Trading partner (15) See Business associate.

Trading partner agreement (15) See Business associate agreement.

Traditional insurance plan (5) Fee for service insurance plans offered by private health insurance companies. Insured individuals pay a fixed monthly premium and generally must meet an annual deducible and pay a coinsurance amount after the claim is processed.

Transaction (2) The transmission of information between two parties to carry out financial or administrative activities related to health care.

Transaction set (19) The collection of data that is exchanged in order to convey meaning between the parties engaged in an electronic data interchange.

Treating, or performing, physician (11) A provider who renders a service to a patient.

TRICARE (4, 8) A government-sponsored program that provides military and nonmilitary hospital and medical services. It covers spouses and dependents of active service personnel, retired service personnel and their dependents, and dependents of member who have died in active duty.

TRICARE Extra (8) A TRICARE coverage option offered to beneficiaries prior to January 1, 2018, and replaced with TRICARE Select.

TRICARE for Life (TFL) (8) A health care program that offers additional TRICARE benef as a supplementary payer to Medicare for formed service retirees, their spouses, a vivors age 65 years of age or older.

TRICARE Prime (8) A voluntary hea nance organization (HMO)–type o

TRICARE Select (8) A fee-for-service, self-managed, preferred provider network plan for TRICARE beneficiaries which became effective January 1, 2018, and replaced the TRICARE Standard, TRICARE Extra, and TRICARE Standard Overseas programs.

TRICARE service center (TSC) (8) An office staffed by TRICARE Health Care Finders and beneficiary service representatives.

TRICARE Standard (8) A TRICARE coverage option offered to beneficiaries prior to January 1, 2018, and replaced with TRICARE Select.

Turfing (5) Transferring the sickest high-cost patients to other physicians so that the provider appears as a "low-utilizer" in a managed care setting.

Unbundling (13) The practice of using numerous Current Procedural Terminology (CPT) codes to identify procedures normally covered by a single code; also known as itemizing, fragmented billing, exploding, or a la carte medicine; billing under Medicare Part B for non-physician services to hospital inpatients furnished to the hospital by an outside supplier or another provider.

Uncertain behavior (12) Phrase used to describe certain types of neoplasms or lesions when future cell response cannot be predicted.

Unemployment Compensation Disability (UCD) (4, 10) Insurance that covers off-the-job injury or sickness and is paid for by deductions from a person's paycheck. Also known as State Disability Insurance (SDI) or temporary disability insurance (TDI).

Uniform Bill 04 (UB-04) (19) Also known as the CMS 1450; the claims form used to submit paper claims for institutional health care facilities such as hospitals (acute care and specialty) and skilled nursing facilities.

Unsecured debt (17) Any debt (amount owed) that is not secured or backed by any form of collateral.

Upcoding (3, 13, 19) Deliberate manipulation of Current Procedural Terminology (CPT) codes for increased payment.

Urgent care (8) Medically necessary treatment that is required for illness or injury that would result in further disability or death if not treated immediately.

Use (2) The sharing, employment, application, utilization, examination, or analysis of individually identifiable health information (IIHI) within an organization that holds such information.

Usual, customary, and reasonable (UCR) (13) A method used by insurance companies to establish their fee schedules in which three fees are considered in calculating payment: (1) the usual fee is the fee typically submitted by the physician, (2) the customary fee falls within the range of usual fees charged by providers of similar training in a geographic area, and (3) the reasonable fee meets the aforementioned criteria or is considered justifiable because of special circumstances.

Utilization management (UM) (19) The evaluation of patient records to ensure that patient care needs are met, that care was medically necessary, appropriate and efficient use of the use of health care services, procedures, and facilities fall under the provisions of the applicable health benefits plan.

Utilization review (UR) (5) A process, based on established criteria, of reviewing and controlling the medical necessity for services and providers' use of medical care resources. Reviews are carried out by allied health personnel at predetermined times during the hospital stay to assess the need for the full facilities of an acute care hospital. In managed care systems, reviews are done to establish medical necessity, thus curbing costs. Also called utilization or management control.

Value based program (VBP) (6) Programs which reward health care organizations with incentive payments for the quality and efficiency of care they give with the shift away from paying providers based solely on their volumes of services. Also known as pay-for-performance programs.

Verbal referral (5) A primary care physician (PCP) informs the patient and telephones to the referring physician that the patient is being referred for an appointment.

Veteran (8) Any person who has served in the armed forces of the United States, especially in time of war; is no longer in the service; and has received an honorable discharge.

Veterans Affairs (VA) disability program (10) A program for honorably discharged veterans who file claim for a service-connected disability.

Veterans Affairs (VA) Outpatient Clinic (4) A facility where medical and dental services are rendered to a veteran who has a service-related disability.

Veterans Affairs (VA) outpatient clinic card (10) An identification card belonging to a retired member of the armed forces that is shown when receiving medical or dental services for service-related disabilities from a clinic.

Veterans Health Administration (CHAMPVA) (4, 8) Formerly known as Civilian Health and Medical Program of the Department of Veterans Affairs. A program for veterans with total, permanent, service-connected disabilities or surviving spouses and dependents of veterans who died of service-connected disabilities.

Voluntary disability insurance (10) A majority of employees of an employer voluntarily consent to be covered by an insured or self-insured disability insurance plan instead of a state plan.

Waiting period (WP) (8, 10) For disability insurance, the initial period of time when a disabled individual is not eligible to receive benefits even though unable to work; for workers' compensation, the days that must elapse before workers' compensation weekly benefits become payable. Also known as elimination period.

Waiver of premium (10) A disability insurance policy provision that an employee does not have to pay any premiums while disabled.

Withhold (5) A portion of the monthly capitation payment to physicians retained by the health maintenance organization (HMO) until the end of the year to create an incentive for efficient care. If the physician exceeds utilization norms, he or she will not receive it.

Work hardening (8) An individualized program of therapy using simulated or real job duties to build up strength and improve the worker's endurance so he or she can work up to 8 hours per day. Sometimes work site modifications are instituted to get the employee back to gainful employment.

Workers' Compensation Appeals Board (WCAB) (8) The board that handles workers' compensation liens and appeals.

Workers' compensation insurance (4, 8) A contract that insures a person against on-the-job injury or illness. The employer pays the premium for his or her employees.

Write-off (17) Assets or debts that have been determined to be uncollectable and are therefore adjusted off the accounting books as a loss.

Z codes (12) A classification of ICD-10-CM coding used to describe environmental events, circumstances, and conditions as the external cause of injury, poisoning, and other adverse effects. Z codes are also used in coding adverse reactions to medications.

zeroization (11) Method to dispose of confidential or sensitive information by writing repeated sequences of ones and zeros over the data.

Zone Program Integrity Contractor (ZPIC) (3) A fraud-investigating contractor hired by CMS to audit on their behalf and review claims that have suspicious billing patterns.

INDEX

Note: Page numbers followed by "f" indicate figures, "t" indicate tables, and "b" indicate boxes.

J

S